MUSCLE

Volume 2

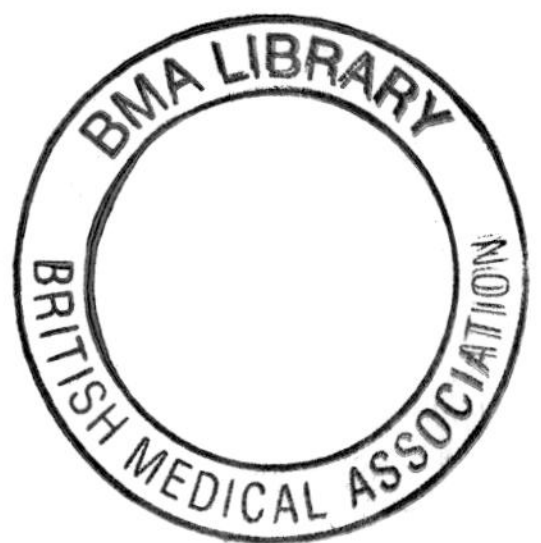

MUSCLE

Fundamental Biology and Mechanisms of Disease

Volume 2

Edited by

Joseph A. Hill and Eric N. Olson

Section Editors

**Kathy K. Griendling,
Richard N. Kitsis, James T. Stull,
and H. Lee Sweeney**

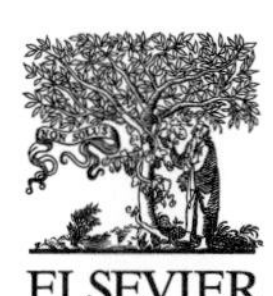

AMSTERDAM • BOSTON • HEIDELBERG • LONDON • NEW YORK • OXFORD
PARIS • SAN DIEGO • SAN FRANCISCO • SINGAPORE • SYDNEY • TOKYO
Academic Press is an imprint of Elsevier

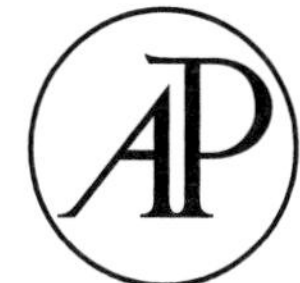

Academic Press is an imprint of Elsevier
32 Jamestown Road, London NW1 7BY, UK
225 Wyman Street, Waltham, MA 02451, USA
525 B Street, Suite 1800, San Diego, CA 92101-4495, USA

First edition 2012

British Library Cataloguing-in-Publication Data
A catalogue record for this book is available from the British Library

Library of Congress Cataloging-in-Publication Data
A catalog record for this book is available from the Library of Congress

ISBN: 978-0-12-381510-1 (Set)
ISBN: 978-0-12-415890-0 (Volume 1)
ISBN: 978-0-12-415889-4 (Volume 2)

For information on all Academic Press publications
visit our website at www.elsevierdirect.com

Typeset by MPS Limited, Chennai, India
www.adi-mps.com

Printed and bound in Canada

12 13 14 15 10 9 8 7 6 5 4 3 2 1

Contents

Section D: Therapeutics

PART IV
Smooth Muscle

Section A: Basic Physiology

Section B: Heterogeneities

Section C: Adaptations and Response

Section D: Smooth Muscle Disease

Volume 1

PART I
Introduction

PART II
Cardiac Muscle

Section A: Basic Physiology

Section B: Adaptations and Response

Section C: Myocardial Disease

List of Contributors

Numbers in parentheses indicate the chapter number of the author's contribution

Paul D. Allen, MD, PhD
(56), Department of Anesthesia, Perioperative and Pain Medicine, Brigham and Women's Hospital, Harvard Medical School, Boston, Massachusetts

Ovid C. Amadi, BS
(14), Harvard Stem Cell Institute and the Cardiovascular Division, Department of Medicine, Brigham and Women's Hospital and Harvard Medical School, Cambridge, Massachusetts

Mark Anderson, MD, PhD
(22), University of Iowa Carver College of Medicine, Iowa City, Iowa

Daniel C. Andersson, MD
(12), Department of Physiology and Cellular Biophysics, Clyde and Helen Wu Center for Molecular Cardiology, College of Physicians and Surgeons, Columbia University, New York, New York

Stephen L. Archer, MD, FRCP(C), FAHA, FACC
(38), Section of Cardiology, Department of Medicine, University of Chicago, Chicago, Illinois

Andrea L.H. Arnett, PhD
(76), Department of Neurology, Medical Scientist Training Program, and Program in Molecular and Cellular Biology, University of Washington, Seattle, Washington

Richard Arnoldi, MSc
(88), Department of Pathology and Immunology, Faculty of Medicine, University of Geneva, Geneva, Switzerland

Sarah Arrowsmith, PhD
(90), Department of Cellular and Molecular Physiology, University of Liverpool, Liverpool, UK

Elisabeth R. Barton, PhD
(80), School of Dental Medicine, Department of Anatomy and Cell Biology, University of Pennsylvania, Philadelphia, Pennsylvania

Rhonda Bassel-Duby, PhD
(61), Department of Molecular Biology, University of Texas Southwestern Medical Center, Dallas, Texas

Stephen L. Belmonte, PhD
(8), Aab Cardiovascular Research Institute, Department of Medicine, University of Rochester School of Medicine and Dentistry, Rochester, New York

Rabah Ben Yaou, MD
(72), Inserm, UMR S974; Université Pierre et Marie Curie-Paris 6, UM 76; CNRS, UMR7215; Institut de Myologie, IFR14; Association Institut de Myologie, Paris, France

Ivor J. Benjamin, MD
(43), Division of Cardiology, University of Utah School of Medicine, Salt Lake City, Utah

Bradford C. Berk, MD, PhD
(98), Aab Cardiovascular Research Institute, University of Rochester School of Medicine and Dentistry, Rochester, New York

Donald M. Bers, PhD
(11), Department of Pharmacology, University of California, Davis, Davis, California

Anne T. Bertrand, PhD
(72), Inserm, UMR S974; Université Pierre et Marie Curie-Paris 6, UM 76; CNRS, UMR7215; Institut de Myologie, IFR14, Paris, France

Matthew J. Betzenhauser, PhD
(12), Department of Physiology and Cellular Biophysics, Clyde and Helen Wu Center for Molecular Cardiology, College of Physicians and Surgeons, Columbia University, New York, New York

Morris J. Birnbaum, MD, PhD
(59), Institute for Diabetes, Obesity, and Metabolism, Perelman School of Medicine, University of Pennsylvania, Philadelphia, Pennsylvania

Brian L. Black, PhD
(3), Cardiovascular Research Institute, and Department of Biochemistry and Biophysics, University of California, San Francisco, California

Burns C. Blaxall, PhD
(8), Aab Cardiovascular Research Institute, Department of Medicine, University of Rochester School of Medicine and Dentistry, Rochester, New York

Roberto Bolli, MD
(28), Department of Medicine, Division of Cardiovascular Medicine, University of Louisville, Louisville, Kentucky

Elena Bonanno, MD
(105), Department of Biopathology and Diagnostic Imaging – Section of Anatomic Pathology, University of Rome "Tor Vergata", Rome, Italy

Gisèle Bonne, PhD
(72), Inserm, UMR S974; Université Pierre et Marie Curie-Paris 6, UM 76; CNRS, UMR7215; Institut de Myologie, IFR14; AP-HP, Groupe Hospitalier Pitié-Salpêtrière, UF Cardiogénétique et Myogénétique Moléculaire, Service de Biochimie Métabolique, Paris, France

Carsten G. Bönnemann, MD
(70), Neuromuscular and Neurogenetic Disorders of Childhood Section, National Institute of Neurological Disorders and Stroke/NIH, Porter Neuroscience Research Center, Bethesda, Maryland

Nina Bowens, MD
(82), Department of Surgery and University of Pennsylvania Cardiovascular Institute, Philadelphia, Pennsylvania

Hasse Brønnum, MSc PhD
(29), Division of Matrix Biology, Department of Medicine, Beth Israel Deaconess Medical Center and Harvard Medical School, Boston, Massachusetts

Benoit G. Bruneau, PhD
(3), Gladstone Institute of Cardiovascular Disease, San Francisco, California; Department of Pediatrics, University of California, and Cardiovascular Research Institute, University of California, San Francisco, California

Margaret Buckingham, DPhil
(52), CNRS URA 2578, Department of Developmental Biology, Institut Pasteur, Paris, France

Theodor Burdyga, PhD, DSc
(86), Department of Cellular and Molecular Physiology, Institute of Translational Medicine, University of Liverpool, Liverpool, UK

Gillian Butler-Browne, PhD
(77), Université Pierre et Marie Curie-Paris 6, UM76, INSERM U974, and CNRS UMR 7215, Institut de Myologie, Paris, France

Peter Buttrick, MD
(24), Division of Cardiology, University of Colorado, Denver, Denver, Colorado

P.A. Cahill, PhD
(92), School of Biotechnology, Faculty of Science and Health, Dublin City University, Dublin, Ireland

John W. Calvert, PhD
(6), Department of Surgery, Division of Cardiothoracic Surgery, Carlyle Fraser Heart Center, Emory University School of Medicine, Atlanta, Georgia

Kevin P. Campbell, PhD
(66), Howard Hughes Medical Institute, Department of Molecular Physiology and Biophysics, Department of Neurology, Department of Internal Medicine, Roy J. and Lucille A. Carver College of Medicine, The University of Iowa, Iowa City, Iowa

Stephen C. Cannon, MD, PhD
(73), University of Texas Southwestern Medical Center, Dallas, Texas

Paola Cattaneo, PhD
(25), Casa di Cura Multimedica, Istituto di Ricovero e Cura a Carattere Scientifico, Milan, Italy; Università di Bicocca, Dipartimento di Scienze Chirurgiche, Monza, Italy

Aravinda Chakravarti, PhD
(18), Center for Complex Disease Genomics, McKusick–Nathans Institute of Genetic Medicine, Johns Hopkins University School of Medicine, Baltimore, Maryland

Jeffrey S. Chamberlain, PhD
(76), Department of Neurology, Program in Molecular and Cellular Biology, Department of Biochemistry, and Department of Medicine, University of Washington, Seattle, Washington

Christine Chaponnier, PhD
(88), Department of Pathology and Immunology, Faculty of Medicine, University of Geneva, Geneva, Switzerland

Stephanie E. Chin, MD
(34), Department of Pediatrics, Division of Pediatric Cardiology, Mount Sinai School of Medicine, New York, New York

Ethan David Cohen, PhD
(32), Department of Medicine and Cardiovascular Institute, University of Pennsylvania, Philadelphia, Pennsylvania

Ronald D. Cohn, MD
(71), McKusick–Nathans Institute of Genetic Medicine and Johns Hopkins Center for Hypotonia, Johns Hopkins University School of Medicine, Baltimore, Maryland

Gianluigi Condorelli, MD, PhD
(25), Casa di Cura Multimedica, Istituto di Ricovero e Cura a Carattere Scientifico, and Consiglio Nazionale delle Ricerche (CNR), Istituto di Ricerca Genetica e Biomedica (IRGB), Milan, Italy; Department of Medicine, University of California, San Diego, La Jolla, CA

James H. Cummins, MS
(62), Stem Cell Research Center, Department of Orthopaedic Surgery, University of Pittsburgh, Pittsburgh, Pennsylvania

Kelvin P. Davies, PhD
(102), Albert Einstein College of Medicine, Bronx, New York

Bridget Deasy, PhD
(62), Stem Cell Research Center, Department of Orthopaedic Surgery, Department of Bioengineering, and McGowan Institute for Regenerative Medicine, University of Pittsburgh, Pittsburgh, Pennsylvania

Deeptankar DeMazumder, MD, PhD
(7, 41), Department of Internal Medicine (Cardiology), Johns Hopkins University School of Medicine, Baltimore, Maryland

Linda Demer, MD, PhD
(106), David Geffen School of Medicine at UCLA, Los Angeles, California

Cor de Wit, MD
(94), Department of Physiology, University of Lübeck, Lübeck, Germany

Harry C. Dietz III, MD
(71), Howard Hughes Medical Institute and Institute of Genetic Medicine, Departments of Pediatrics, Medicine, and Molecular Biology & Genetics, Johns Hopkins University School of Medicine, Baltimore, Maryland

Fabio Di Lisa, MD
(17), Department of Biomedical Sciences, University of Padua, Padua, Italy

Salvatore DiMauro, MD
(75), H. Houston Merritt Clinical Research Center for Muscular Dystrophy and Related Diseases, Columbia University Medical Center, New York, New York

Stephan Dobner, MD, PhD
(14), Harvard Stem Cell Institute and the Cardiovascular Division, Department of Medicine, Brigham and Women's Hospital and Harvard Medical School, Cambridge, Massachusetts

Gerald W. Dorn II, MD
(31), Center for Pharmacogenomics, Department of Internal Medicine, Washington University School of Medicine, St Louis, Missouri

Shirin Doroudgar, BS
(10), SDSU Heart Institute and Department of Biology, San Diego State University, San Diego, California

V. Reggie Edgerton, PhD
(55), Department of Integrative Biology and Physiology, University of California, Los Angeles, Los Angeles, California

Charles P. Emerson Jr, PhD
(69), Boston Biomedical Research Institute, Watertown, Massachusetts

Andrew G. Engel, MD
(53), Department of Neuroscience, Mayo Clinic, Rochester, Minnesota

Karyn A. Esser, PhD
(64), Center for Muscle Biology, Department of Physiology, College of Medicine, University of Kentucky, Lexington, Kentucky

Yong-Hu Fang, MD, PhD
(38), Section of Cardiology, Department of Medicine, University of Chicago, Chicago, Illinois

QiPing Feng, PhD
(67), Department of Medicine, Division of Clinical Pharmacology, Vanderbilt University Medical Center, Nashville, Tennessee

Glenn I. Fishman, MD
(40), New York University School of Medicine, Leon H. Charney Division of Cardiology, New York, New York

Thomas Force, MD
(47), Center for Translational Medicine, Thomas Jefferson University, Philadelphia, Pennsylvania

Nikolaos G. Frangogiannis, MD
(36), Department of Medicine, Albert Einstein College of Medicine, Bronx, New York

Clara Franzini-Armstrong, PhD
(53,58), Department of Cell and Developmental Biology, Perelman School of Medicine, University of Pennsylvania, Philadelphia, Pennsylvania

Norbert Frey, MD
(35), Department of Cardiology, University of Kiel, Kiel, Germany

Maria G. Frid, PhD
(103), University of Colorado Denver, Anschutz Medical Campus, Department of Pediatric Critical Care Medicine and Developmental Lung Biology Laboratory, Aurora, Colorado

Giulio Gabbiani, MD, PhD
(88), Department of Pathology and Immunology, Faculty of Medicine, University of Geneva, Geneva, Switzerland

Bruce D. Gelb, MD
(34), Child Health and Development Institute, Departments of Pediatrics and Genetics & Genetic Sciences, Mount Sinai School of Medicine, New York, New York

Eric M. George, PhD
(101), Department of Physiology and Biophysics and the Center for Excellence in Cardiovascular-Renal Research, University of Mississippi Medical Center, Jackson, Mississippi

A. Martin Gerdes, PhD
(5), New York College of Osteopathic Medicine at New York Institute of Technology, Old Westbury, New York

Burhan Gharaibeh, PhD
(62), Stem Cell Research Center, Department of Orthopaedic Surgery, Department of Bioengineering, and McGowan Institute for Regenerative Medicine, University of Pittsburgh, Pittsburgh, Pennsylvania

Hamilton S. Gillespie, MD
(43), Division of Cardiology, University of Utah School of Medicine, Salt Lake City, Utah

Christopher C. Glembotski, PhD
(10), SDSU Heart Institute and Department of Biology, San Diego State University, San Diego, California

Tommaso Gori, MD, PhD
(91), II Medical Clinic for Cardiology and Angiology, Mainz, Germany

Joey P. Granger, PhD
(101), Department of Physiology and Biophysics and the Center for Excellence in Cardiovascular-Renal Research, University of Mississippi Medical Center, Jackson, Mississippi

Kathy K. Griendling, PhD
(96), Department of Medicine, Division of Cardiology, Emory University, Atlanta, Georgia

Susan J. Gunst, PhD
(104), Department of Cellular and Integrative Physiology, Indiana University School of Medicine, Indianapolis, Indiana

Denis C. Guttridge, PhD
(65), Department of Molecular Virology, Immunology, and Medical Genetics, Human Cancer Genetics Program, The Ohio State University, Columbus, Ohio

Roger J. Hajjar, MD
(46), Cardiovascular Research Center, Mount Sinai School of Medicine, New York, New York

Ronald G. Haller, MD
(75), Department of Neurology, University of Texas Southwestern Medical Center and North Texas VA Medical Center, and Neuromuscular Center, Institute for Exercise and Environmental Medicine, Texas Health Presbyterian Hospital, Dallas, Texas

Erick O. Hernández-Ochoa, MD, PhD
(57), Department of Biochemistry and Molecular Biology, School of Medicine, University of Maryland, Baltimore, Maryland

Neil Herring, DPhil, MRCP
(20), Burdon Sanderson Cardiac Science Centre, Department of Physiology, Anatomy and Genetics, University of Oxford, Oxford, UK

Lula L. Hilenski, PhD
(96), Department of Medicine, Division of Cardiology, Emory University, Atlanta, Georgia

Joseph A. Hill, MD, PhD
(1, 7, 35), Departments of Internal Medicine (Cardiology) and Molecular Biology, University of Texas Southwestern Medical Center, Dallas, Texas

Michael A. Hill, PhD
(93), Dalton Cardiovascular Research Center and the Department of Medical Pharmacology and Physiology, University of Missouri, Columbia, Missouri

Charis L. Himeda, PhD
(69), Boston Biomedical Research Institute, Watertown, Massachusetts

Boris Hinz, PhD
(88), Laboratory of Tissue Repair and Regeneration, Matrix Dynamics Group, Faculty of Dentistry, University of Toronto, Toronto, Canada

Steven R. Houser, PhD
(11), Department of Physiology, Temple University School of Medicine, Philadelphia, Pennsylvania

Johnny Huard, PhD
(62), Cell Research Center, Department of Orthopaedic Surgery, Department of Bioengineering, McGowan Institute for Regenerative Medicine, Department of Pathology, and Departments of Molecular Genetics and Biochemistry, Physical Medicine and Rehabilitation, University of Pittsburgh, Pittsburgh, Pennsylvania

William F. Jackson, PhD
(89), Pharmacology and Toxicology, Michigan State University, East Lansing, Michigan

John Lynn Jefferies, MD, MPH
(33), The Heart Institute, Cincinnati Children's Hospital, Cincinnati, Ohio

Raghu Kalluri, MD, PhD
(29), Division of Matrix Biology, Department of Medicine, Beth Israel Deaconess Medical Center and Harvard Medical School, Boston, Massachusetts

Fadia A. Kamal, PhD
(8), Aab Cardiovascular Research Institute, Department of Medicine, University of Rochester School of Medicine and Dentistry, Rochester, New York

Ashish Kapoor, PhD
(18), Center for Complex Disease Genomics, McKusick–Nathans Institute of Genetic Medicine, Johns Hopkins University School of Medicine, Baltimore, Maryland

David A. Kass, MD
(21), Division of Cardiology, Department of Biomedical Engineering, Johns Hopkins University School of Medicine, Baltimore, Maryland

Arnold M. Katz, MD
(2), Professor of Medicine Emeritus, University of Connecticut School of Medicine, Farmington, Connecticut; Visiting Professor of Medicine and Physiology, Dartmouth Medical School, Hanover, New Hampshire; Visiting Professor of Medicine, Harvard Medical School, Boston, Massachusetts

Daniel P. Kelly, MD
(16), Sanford–Burnham Medical Research Institute, Orlando, Florida

Aarif Y. Khakoo, MD, MBA
(9, 47), Executive Director Research, Metabolic Disorders, Amgen, San Francisco, California

Sujay V. Kharade, PhD
(84), Department of Pharmacology and Toxicology, College of Medicine, University of Arkansas for Medical Sciences, Little Rock, Arkansas

Eugene Kim, MD
(40), New York University School of Medicine, Leon H. Charney Division of Cardiology, New York, New York

Jung A. Kim, PhD
(55), Department of Integrative Biology and Physiology, University of California, Los Angeles, Los Angeles, California

Richard N. Kitsis, MD
(31), Wilf Family Cardiovascular Research Institute, Departments of Medicine and Cell Biology, Albert Einstein College of Medicine, Bronx, New York

Yvonne M. Kobayashi, PhD
(66), Howard Hughes Medical Institute, Department of Molecular Physiology and Biophysics, Department of Neurology, Department of Internal Medicine, Roy J. and Lucille A. Carver College of Medicine, The University of Iowa, Iowa City, Iowa

Issei Komuro, MD, PhD
(51), Department of Cardiovascular Medicine, Osaka University Graduate School of Medicine, Osaka, Japan

Irina Kramerova, PhD
(78), Department of Neurology and Center for Duchenne Muscular Dystrophy at UCLA, Los Angeles, California

Callie S. Kwartler, BA
(97), Department of Internal Medicine, University of Texas Health Science Center at Houston, Houston, Texas

Edward G. Lakatta, MD
(44), Laboratory of Cardiovascular Science, Intramural Research Program, National Institute on Aging, National Institutes of Health, Baltimore, Maryland

Triona Lally, PhD
(92), School of Mechanical and Manufacturing Engineering, Dublin City University, Dublin, Ireland

Lars Larsson, MD, PhD
(74), Department of Neuroscience, Clinical Neurophysiology, Uppsala University Hospital, Uppsala, Sweden

Michael V.G. Latronico
(25), Casa di Cura Multimedica, Istituto di Ricovero e Cura a Carattere Scientifico, Milan, Italy

Sergio Lavandero, PhD
(30), Department of Internal Medicine (Cardiology), University of Texas Southwestern Medical Center at Dallas, Texas, and Center for Molecular Studies of the Cell, Faculty of Chemical and Pharmaceutical Sciences/Faculty of Medicine, University of Chile, Santiago, Chile

Mitra Lavasani, PhD
(62), Stem Cell Research Center, Department of Orthopaedic Surgery, School of Medicine, University of Pittsburgh, Pittsburgh, Pennsylvania

Richard T. Lee, MD
(14), Harvard Stem Cell Institute and the Cardiovascular Division, Department of Medicine, Brigham and Women's Hospital and Harvard Medical School, Cambridge, Massachusetts

Se-Jin Lee, MD, PhD
(79), Department of Molecular Biology and Genetics, Johns Hopkins University School of Medicine, Baltimore, Maryland

Young il Lee, PhD
(54), Section of Molecular Cell and Developmental Biology, School of Biological Sciences, University of Texas, Austin, Texas

David J. Lefer, PhD
(6, 28), Department of Surgery, Division of Cardiothoracic Surgery, Carlyle Fraser Heart Center, Emory University School of Medicine, Atlanta, Georgia

Leslie A. Leinwand, PhD
(13), University of Colorado at Boulder, Molecular, Cellular and Developmental Biology, Boulder, Colorado

Benjamin Levine, MD
(24), Institute for Exercise and Environmental Medicine, Texas Health Resources and University of Texas, Southwestern Medical Center, Dallas, Texas

Yong Li, PhD
(62), Stem Cell Research Center, Department of Orthopaedic Surgery, Department of Bioengineering, McGowan Institute for Regenerative Medicine, and Department of Pathology, University of Pittsburgh, Pittsburgh, Pennsylvania; Recently relocated to Department of Pediatric Surgery at The University of Texas, School of Medicine at Houston

Stephen B. Liggett, MD
(45), Departments of Medicine and Physiology, University of Maryland School of Medicine, Baltimore, Maryland

Zhiqiang Lin, PhD
(39), Department of Cardiology, Children's Hospital Boston, Boston, Massachusetts; Harvard Stem Cell Institute, Cambridge, Massachusetts

Ning Liu, PhD
(61), Department of Molecular Biology, University of Texas Southwestern Medical Center, Dallas, Texas

Jose R. Lopez, MD, PhD
(56), Department of Anesthesia, Perioperative and Pain Medicine, Brigham and Women's Hospital, Harvard Medical School, Boston, Massachusetts

Douglas W. Losordo, MD
(48), Feinberg Cardiovascular Research Institute, Northwestern University; and Program in Cardiovascular Regenerative Medicine, Northwestern Memorial Hospital, Chicago, Illinois

Calum A. MacRae, MD, PhD
(42), Cardiovascular Division, Department of Medicine, Brigham and Women's Hospital, and Harvard Medical School, Boston, Massachusetts

Yasuhiro Maejima, MD, PhD
(23), Department of Cell Biology and Molecular Medicine, University of Medicine and Dentistry of New Jersey, New Jersey Medical School, Newark, New Jersey

Mark W. Majesky, PhD
(108), Departments of Pediatrics and Pathology, Center for Cardiovascular Biology, Institute for Stem Cell and Regenerative Medicine, Seattle Children's Research Institute, University of Washington, Seattle, Washington

Andrew R. Marks, MD
(12), Department of Physiology and Cellular Biophysics, Clyde and Helen Wu Center for Molecular Cardiology, and Department of Medicine, College of Physicians and Surgeons, Columbia University, New York, New York

Melissa L. Martin, BS
(8), Aab Cardiovascular Research Institute, Department of Medicine, University of Rochester School of Medicine and Dentistry, Rochester, New York

Alessandro Mauriello, MD
(105), Department of Biopathology and Diagnostic Imaging – Section of Anatomic Pathology, University of Rome "Tor Vergata", Rome, Italy

Alicia Mayeuf, MSc
(52), CNRS URA 2578, Department of Developmental Biology, Institut Pasteur, Paris, France

John J. McCarthy, PhD
(64), Center for Muscle Biology, Department of Physiology, College of Medicine, University of Kentucky, Lexington, Kentucky

Elizabeth McNally, MD, PhD
(81), Department of Medicine, Section of Cardiology, Department of Human Genetics, University of Chicago, Chicago, Illinois

Gerald A. Meininger, PhD
(93), Dalton Cardiovascular Research Center and the Department of Medical Pharmacology and Physiology, University of Missouri, Columbia, Missouri

Mark Mercola, PhD
(49), Muscle Development and Regeneration Program, Sanford–Burnham Medical Research Institute, La Jolla, California

Joseph M. Miano, PhD
(95), Aab Cardiovascular Research Institute, University of Rochester School of Medicine and Dentistry, Rochester, New York

M. Carrie Miceli, PhD
(78), Departments of Microbiology, Immunology and Molecular Genetics, and Center for Duchenne Muscular Dystrophy, David Geffen School of Medicine at UCLA, Los Angeles, California

Dianna M. Milewicz, MD, PhD
(97), Department of Internal Medicine, University of Texas Health Science Center at Houston, Houston, Texas

Kathleen G. Morgan, PhD
(87), Health Sciences Department, Boston University, Boston, Massachusetts

Edward E. Morrisey, PhD
(32), Department of Medicine, Department of Cell and Developmental Biology, Cardiovascular Institute and Institute for Regenerative Medicine, University of Pennsylvania, Philadelphia, Pennsylvania

Vincent Mouly, PhD
(77), Université Pierre et Marie Curie-Paris 6, UM76, INSERM U974, and CNRS UMR 7215, Institut de Myologie, Paris, France

Thomas Münzel, MD
(91), II Medical Clinic for Cardiology and Angiology, Mainz, Germany

Anne Murphy, MD
(19), Department of Pediatrics, School of Medicine, Johns Hopkins University, Baltimore, Maryland

Anthony J. Muslin, MD
(37), Novartis Institutes for Biomedical Research, Inc., Cambridge, Massachusetts

R. Kannan Mutharasan, MD
(48), Department of Medicine, Northwestern University, Feinberg School of Medicine, Chicago, Illinois

Kanneboyina Nagaraju , DVM, PhD
(78), Research Center for Genetic Medicine, Children's National Medical Center, Washington, DC

Atsuhiko T. Naito, MD, PhD
(51), Department of Cardiovascular Medicine, Osaka University Graduate School of Medicine, Osaka, Japan

Carlo Napolitano, MD, PhD
(42), Molecular Cardiology Laboratories, IRCCS Salvatore Maugeri Foundation, Pavia, Italy; Cardiovascular Genetics, Leon Charney Division of Cardiology, Langone Medical Center, New York University School of Medicine, New York; Department of Cardiology, University of Pavia, Italy

Sandeep Nathan, MD, MSc
(38), Section of Cardiology, Department of Medicine, University of Chicago, Chicago, Illinois

Eva Nozik-Grayck, MD
(103), University of Colorado Denver, Anschutz Medical Campus, Department of Pediatric Critical Care Medicine and Developmental Lung Biology Laboratory, Aurora, Colorado

Julien Ochala, PhD
(74), Department of Neuroscience, Clinical Neurophysiology, Uppsala University Hospital, Uppsala, Sweden

Stefan Offermanns, MD
(85), Max-Planck-Institute for Heart and Lung Research, Department of Pharmacology, Bad Nauheim, Germany

Eric N. Olson, PhD
(35), Department of Molecular Biology, University of Texas Southwestern Medical Center, Dallas, Texas

Augusto Orlandi, MD
(105), Department of Biopathology and Diagnostic Imaging – Section of Anatomic Pathology, University of Rome "Tor Vergata", Rome, Italy

Roberto Papait, PhD
(25), Casa di Cura Multimedica, Istituto di Ricovero e Cura a Carattere Scientifico, and Consiglio Nazionale delle Ricerche (CNR), Istituto di Ricerca Genetica e Biomedica (IRGB), Milan, Italy

Michael S. Parmacek, MD
(82), Department of Medicine and University of Pennsylvania Cardiovascular Institute, Philadelphia, Pennsylvania

Amit R. Patel, MD
(38), Section of Cardiology, Department of Medicine, University of Chicago, Chicago, Illinois

David J. Paterson, DPhil, DSc
(20), Burdon Sanderson Cardiac Science Centre, Department of Physiology, Anatomy and Genetics, University of Oxford, Oxford, UK

Asif R. Pathan, MS
(84), Department of Pharmacology and Toxicology, College of Medicine, University of Arkansas for Medical Sciences, Little Rock, Arkansas

Cam Patterson, MD, MBA
(27), Departments of Medicine, Pharmacology, and Cell and Developmental Biology, University of North Carolina at Chapel Hill, Chapel Hill, North Carolina

Richard J. Paul, PhD
(86), Department of Molecular and Cellular Physiology, University of Cincinnati College of Medicine, Cincinnati, Ohio

Lin Piao, PhD
(38), Section of Cardiology, Department of Medicine, University of Chicago, Chicago, Illinois

Silvia G. Priori, MD, PhD
(42), Molecular Cardiology Laboratories, IRCCS Salvatore Maugeri Foundation, Pavia, Italy; Cardiovascular Genetics, Leon Charney Division of Cardiology, Langone Medical Center, New York University School of Medicine, New York; Department of Cardiology, University of Pavia, Italy

William T. Pu, MD
(39), Department of Cardiology, Children's Hospital Boston, Boston, Massachusetts; Harvard Stem Cell Institute, Cambridge, Massachusetts

Rashmi Ram, PhD
(8), Aab Cardiovascular Research Institute, Department of Medicine, University of Rochester School of Medicine and Dentistry, Rochester, New York

J. Eduardo Rame, MD, MPhil
(50), Mechanical Circulatory Support Program, Division of Cardiovascular Medicine, University of Pennsylvania, Philadelphia, Pennsylvania

Julian N. Ramos, BS
(76), Department of Neurology, and Program in Molecular and Cellular Biology, University of Washington, Seattle, Washington

E.M. Redmond, PhD
(92), Department of Surgery, University of Rochester Medical Center, Rochester, New York

Carlo Reggiani, MD
(60), Consiglio Nazionale delle Ricerche (CNR), Institute of Neurosciences, and Department of Human Anatomy and Physiology, University of Padua, Padua, Italy

Stuart Rich, MD
(38), Section of Cardiology, Department of Medicine, University of Chicago, Chicago, Illinois

Chiara Rinaldi, PhD
(63), Department of Integrative Biology and Physiology, University of California, Los Angeles, Los Angeles, California

Beverly A. Rothermel, PhD
(30), Departments of Internal Medicine (Cardiology) and Molecular Biology, University of Texas Southwestern Medical Center at Dallas, Texas

Roland R. Roy, PhD
(55), Brain Research Institute, University of California, Los Angeles, Los Angeles, California

Nancy J. Rusch, PhD
(84), Department of Pharmacology and Toxicology, College of Medicine, University of Arkansas for Medical Sciences, Little Rock, Arkansas

John J. Ryan, MB, BCh
(38), Section of Cardiology, Department of Medicine, University of Chicago, Chicago, Illinois

Junichi Sadoshima, MD, PhD
(23), Department of Cell Biology and Molecular Medicine, University of Medicine and Dentistry of New Jersey, New Jersey Medical School, Newark, New Jersey

Alejandra San Martín, PhD
(96), Department of Medicine, Division of Cardiology, Emory University, Atlanta, Georgia

Richard C. Scarpulla, PhD
(16), Department of Cell and Molecular Biology, Northwestern University Medical School, Chicago, Illinois

Stefano Schiaffino, MD
(60), Venetian Institute of Molecular Medicine (VIMM), and Consiglio Nazionale delle Ricerche (CNR), Institute of Neurosciences, Padua, Italy

Ernesto L. Schiffrin, MD, PhD
(99), Lady Davis Institute for Medical Research and Department of Medicine, Sir Mortimer B. Davis–Jewish General Hospital, McGill University, Montreal, QC, Canada

Jay W. Schneider, MD, PhD
(49), Department of Internal Medicine/Cardiology, University of Texas Southwestern Medical Center, Dallas, Texas

Martin F. Schneider, PhD
(57), Department of Biochemistry and Molecular Biology, School of Medicine, University of Maryland, Baltimore, Maryland

Andreas Schober, MD
(107), Institute for Molecular Cardiovascular Research, RWTH Aachen University, Aachen, Germany

Manuel Scimeca, MB
(105), Department of Biopathology and Diagnostic Imaging – Section of Anatomic Pathology, University of Rome "Tor Vergata", Rome, Italy

Luca Scorrano, MD, PhD
(17), Department of Cell Physiology and Medicine, Geneva, Switzerland

Tiffany L. Shih, BSE
(9), Medical Student, University of Texas MD Anderson Medical Cancer Center, Houston, Texas

Ichiro Shiojima, MD, PhD
(51), Department of Cardiovascular Medicine, Osaka University Graduate School of Medicine, Osaka, Japan

Marion J. Siegman, PhD
(83), Department of Molecular Physiology and Biophysics, Thomas Jefferson University, Philadelphia, Pennsylvania

Elaine Smolock, PhD
(98), Aab Cardiovascular Research Institute, University of Rochester School of Medicine and Dentistry, Rochester, New York

R. John Solaro, PhD
(13), Department of Physiology and Biophysics (M/C 901), University of Illinois at Chicago College of Medicine, Chicago, Illinois

Avril V. Somlyo, PhD
(83), Department of Molecular Physiology and Biological Physics, University of Virginia, Charlottesville, Virginia

James R. Sowers, MD
(100), MU Diabetes and Cardiovascular Center, Department of Medical Pharmacology & Physiology, University of Missouri-Columbia, Columbia, Missouri

Luigi Giusto Spagnoli, MD
(105), Department of Biopathology and Diagnostic Imaging – Section of Anatomic Pathology, University of Rome "Tor Vergata", Rome, Italy

Melissa J. Spencer, PhD
(78), Department of Neurology, and Center for Duchenne Muscular Dystrophy, David Geffen School of Medicine at UCLA, Los Angeles, California

David Spragg, MD
(50), Division of Cardiology, Johns Hopkins Hospital, Johns Hopkins Bayview Medical Center, Baltimore, Maryland

Miroslava Stastna, PhD
(19), Johns Hopkins Bayview Proteomics Center, Division of Cardiology, Department of Medicine, School of Medicine, Johns Hopkins University, Baltimore, Maryland; Institute of Analytical Chemistry of the ASCR, Brno, Czech Republic

Charles Steenbergen, MD, PhD
(36), Department of Pathology, Johns Hopkins Medical Institutions, Baltimore, Maryland

Kurt R. Stenmark, MD
(103), University of Colorado Denver, Anschutz Medical Campus, Department of Pediatric Critical Care Medicine and Developmental Lung Biology Laboratory, Aurora, Colorado

James B. Strait, MD, PhD
(44), Laboratory of Cardiovascular Science, Intramural Research Program, National Institute on Aging, National Institutes of Health, Baltimore, Maryland

H. Lee Sweeney, PhD
(58), Department of Physiology, Perelman School of Medicine, University of Pennsylvania, Philadelphia, Pennsylvania

Heinrich Taegtmeyer, MD, DPhil
(15), Department of Medicine/Cardiology, The University of Texas School of Medicine at Houston, Houston, Texas

Eiki Takimoto, MD
(21), Division of Cardiology, Department of Biomedical Engineering, Johns Hopkins University School of Medicine, Baltimore, Maryland

Keshari M. Thakali, PhD
(84), Department of Pharmacology and Toxicology, College of Medicine, University of Arkansas for Medical Sciences, Little Rock, Arkansas

Wesley J. Thompson, PhD
(54), Section of Molecular Cell and Developmental Biology, School of Biological Sciences, University of Texas, Austin, Texas

Charles Thornton, MD
(68), Department of Neurology, University of Rochester, Rochester, New York

James G. Tidball, PhD
(63), Molecular, Cellular & Integrative Physiology Program, Department of Integrative Biology and Physiology, and Department of Pathology and Laboratory Medicine, David Geffen School of Medicine at UCLA, University of California, Los Angeles, California

Yin Tintut, PhD
(106), David Geffen School of Medicine at UCLA, Los Angeles, California

Gordon F. Tomaselli, MD
(41), Division of Cardiology, Johns Hopkins University School of Medicine, Baltimore, Maryland

Rhian M. Touyz, MD, PhD
(99), Kidney Research Centre, Ottawa Hospital Research Institute, University of Ottawa, Ontario, Canada

Jeffrey A. Towbin, MD
(33), The Heart Institute, Cincinnati Children's Hospital, Cincinnati, Ohio

Kevin Tsai, MD
(38), Section of Cardiology, Department of Medicine, University of Chicago, Chicago, Illinois

Denis Vallese, MSc
(77), Université Pierre et Marie Curie-Paris 6, UM76, INSERM U974, and CNRS UMR 7215, Institut de Myologie, Paris, France

Jennifer E. Van Eyk, PhD
(19), Johns Hopkins Bayview Proteomics Center, Division of Cardiology, School of Medicine, Johns Hopkins University, Baltimore, Maryland

Eva Van Rooij, PhD
(26), miRagen Therapeutics, Inc., Boulder, Colorado

Susanne Vetterkind, PhD
(87), Health Sciences Department, Boston University, Boston, Massachusetts

Nicol C. Voermans, MD, PhD
(70), Department of Neurology, Radboud University Nijmegen Medical Center, Nijmegen, The Netherlands

Antonio Volpe, MB
(105), Department of Biopathology and Diagnostic Imaging – Section of Anatomic Pathology, University of Rome "Tor Vergata", Rome, Italy

Xuejun Wang, MD, PhD
(27), Division of Basic Biomedical Sciences, Sanford School of Medicine, The University of South Dakota, Vermillion, South Dakota

Yanggan Wang, MD, PhD
(7), Department of Pediatrics and Children's Healthcare of Atlanta, Emory University, Atlanta, Georgia

Yibin Wang, PhD
(22), David Geffen School of Medicine, University of California at Los Angeles, Los Angeles, California

Stephanie Ware, MD, PhD
(33), The Heart Institute, Cincinnati Children's Hospital, Cincinnati, Ohio

Christian Weber, MD
(107), Institute for Cardiovascular Prevention, Ludwig-Maximilians-University Munich, Munich, Germany

Adam Whaley-Connell, DO, MSPH
(100), Harry S. Truman VA Medical Center and the University of Missouri-Columbia School of Medicine, Department of Internal Medicine, Division of Nephrology and Hypertension, Columbia, Missouri

Russell A. Wilke, MD, PhD
(67), Department of Medicine, Division of Clinical Pharmacology, Vanderbilt University Medical Center, Nashville, Tennessee

Angela Wirth, PhD
(85), Max-Planck-Institute for Heart and Lung Research, Department of Pharmacology, Bad Nauheim, Germany; Institute of Pharmacology, University of Heidelberg, Heidelberg, Germany

Susan Wray, PhD
(90), Department of Cellular and Molecular Physiology, University of Liverpool, Liverpool, UK

Erica Yada, PhD
(77), Université Pierre et Marie Curie-Paris 6, UM76, INSERM U974, and CNRS UMR 7215, Institut de Myologie, Paris, France

Michael E. Yeager, PhD
(103), University of Colorado Denver, Anschutz Medical Campus, Department of Pediatric Critical Care Medicine and Developmental Lung Biology Laboratory, Aurora, Colorado

Katherine E. Yutzey, PhD
(4), Division of Molecular Cardiovascular Biology, Cincinnati Children's Hospital Medical Center, Cincinnati, Ohio

Daniela Zablocki, MS
(23), Department of Cell Biology and Molecular Medicine, University of Medicine and Dentistry of New Jersey, New Jersey Medical School, Newark, New Jersey

Cuihua Zhang, PhD, FAHA
(100), Division of Cardiovascular Medicine, Department of Internal Medicine, Department of Medical Pharmacology & Physiology, Dalton Cardiovascular Research Center, University of Missouri-Columbia, Columbia, Missouri

Hanrui Zhang, MS
(100), Dalton Cardiovascular Research Center, University of Missouri-Columbia, Columbia, Missouri

Pingbo Zhang, PhD
(19), Johns Hopkins Bayview Proteomics Center, Division of Cardiology, Department of Medicine, School of Medicine, Johns Hopkins University, Baltimore, Maryland

Zhou Zhe, PhD
(107), Institute for Molecular Cardiovascular Research, RWTH Aachen University, Aachen, German

Bin Zhou, PhD, MD
(39), Department of Cardiology, Children's Hospital Boston, Boston, Massachusetts; Institute for Nutritional Sciences, Shanghai Institutes for Biological Sciences, Chinese Academy of Sciences, Shanghai, China

Acknowledgments

Many people contributed directly and indirectly to this book, and without their input, *Muscle* would never have appeared in its present form. First, a host of thought leaders in muscle biology generously agreed to devote considerable time and energy to the book, recognizing that a work of this sort has never been attempted before. These authors, without exception, dedicated enormous energy and attention to providing a state-of-the-art snapshot of their area of expertise. Remarkably, some did this in the face of significant personal issues, which included an episode of appendicitis complicated by peritonitis, a co-author being detained in the Middle East during the Arab Spring, and a house fire!

Next, the Section Editors – Drs Kathy Griendling, Rick Kitsis, Jim Stull, Lee Sweeney – devoted near-countless hours to ensuring that the topics under their direction were covered in a comprehensive, rigorous, thoughtful, and unbiased manner, without overlooking – or over-treating – areas of importance. Their wide-ranging knowledge of their fields, combined with assiduous attention to detail, were critical to our success. This book is truly the result of their hard work.

Our colleagues at Elsevier, including Mara Conner, Janice Audet, and April Graham, deserve recognition and thanks for their support and patience throughout this journey.

A number of professional colleagues and personal friends have contributed importantly to the project. These include Drs Rhonda Bassel-Duby, Jay Schneider, Hesham Sadek, Beverly Rothermel, Thomas Gillette, and Anwarul Ferdous, our close scientific collaborators. Everything we do professionally relies critically on support from our administrative colleagues, including Cindy Lawson, Wanda Simpson, Christie Evans, and Jennifer Brown. We thank John Shelton for providing extraordinary images of cardiac, skeletal, and smooth myocytes for the cover.

Each of us is fortunate to work with an impressive cadre of scientific professionals and trainees, too numerous to mention, in our labs. These folks challenge us, enlighten us, occasionally frustrate us, but always strive to move the frontiers of science forward.

A long list of personal friends deserve recognition, including Joe Illick and Gina Browning, from whom we have learned much about life and art, and Mo Ghomi, from whom we have learned much about life and muscle.

Finally, we are grateful – indeed most grateful – to our families, who have listened to our frustrations, tolerated our whims, and shouldered an extra burden during this project. These include our wives, Beverly and Laurie, and our children, Christopher and Theodore (Teddy) [Hill] and Eric, Sarah, and Emily [Olson]. Without exception, they are the lights of our lives and – ultimately – the final motivators of our work.

Joseph A. Hill and Eric N. Olson

Part III

Skeletal Muscle

Section A

Basic Physiology

Chapter 52

Skeletal Muscle Development

Margaret Buckingham and Alicia Mayeuf

CNRS URA 2578, Department of Developmental Biology, Institut Pasteur, Paris, France

INTRODUCTION

Study of skeletal muscle formation began with classical morphological observations and experimental embryology which led to the first description of its somitic origin. The isolation of skeletal muscle cell lines, from the 1970s, made this a system of choice for trying to unravel molecular mechanisms that control tissue differentiation. This led to the identification of the MyoD family of myogenic regulatory factors, and indeed such *in vitro* studies still provide sophisticated insights into myogenic gene regulation. With the introduction of cloned probes, it became possible, at the beginning of the 1980s, to examine gene expression during myogenesis *in vivo*. The development of techniques for gene manipulation in the mouse and other organisms subsequently led to functional studies. In the past 10 years, upstream regulators of skeletal muscle formation, such as the *Pax3/7* genes in the trunk and limbs or *Pitx2* in the head, have been characterised and gene regulatory networks that underlie the behaviour of muscle stem cells are emerging.

In the following sections we discuss the current understanding of skeletal muscle development, with the aim of informing muscle biologists in general. We therefore present an overview, without entering into all the more detailed aspects of this fast-moving field. In general, we reference reviews where the primary literature can be found, except if the subject has not been reviewed or in the case of recent publications.

TRUNK AND LIMB MUSCLES

The Formation of Skeletal Muscles of the Trunk and Limbs

The Somitic Origin of Skeletal Muscle in the Body

Skeletal muscle of the trunk and limbs derives from somites (1). Somites are formed by progressive segmentation of paraxial mesoderm on either side of the axis, following an anterior to posterior gradient as the embryo develops (Figure 52.1A). Newly formed somites have an epithelial structure. This epithelium is subsequently maintained dorsally as the dermomyotome, while the ventral somite undergoes an epithelial to mesenchymal transition with formation of the sclerotome compartment. This gives rise to the cartilage and bone of the vertebral column and ribs. The dorsal-most part of the sclerotome constitutes another compartment, the syndetome, which is the source of connective tissue, including tendons associated with trunk muscles (2). Experiments in the chick embryo, together with clonal analysis in the mouse, have shown that cells in the dermomyotome are multipotent, giving rise to all skeletal muscles of the body and to the derm of the back, brown fat, as well as endothelial and smooth muscle cells of blood vessels (3,4).

The Onset of Myogenesis in the Trunk and Limbs

The first skeletal muscle to form is the myotome, in the central domain of the somite (1) (Figure 52.1A). This is a result of delamination of cells from the edges of the dermomyotome, mainly from the epaxial lip, adjacent to the neural tube, and then from the hypaxial lip, adjacent to the lateral mesoderm. As soon as they leave the dermomyotome, these cells differentiate into myocytes, which span the extent of the myotome, assuming an orientation parallel to the body axis. In the chick embryo, early myotome formation has been described in detail, with successive waves of delamination, firstly of pioneer cells from the epaxial domain which form a myocyte scaffold to organize the arrival of differentiating cells from the other edges of the dermomyotome (5).

As development proceeds, the central epithelial domain of the dermomyotome undergoes an epithelial to mesenchymal transition, releasing muscle progenitor cells into the underlying myotome (3). These cells provide a proliferating progenitor cell population that contributes to muscle growth throughout late embryonic and fetal development. By about 16 days in the mouse embryo, these cells begin to take up a satellite cell position under a

Muscle. DOI: http://dx.doi.org/10.1016/B978-0-12-381510-1.00052-1

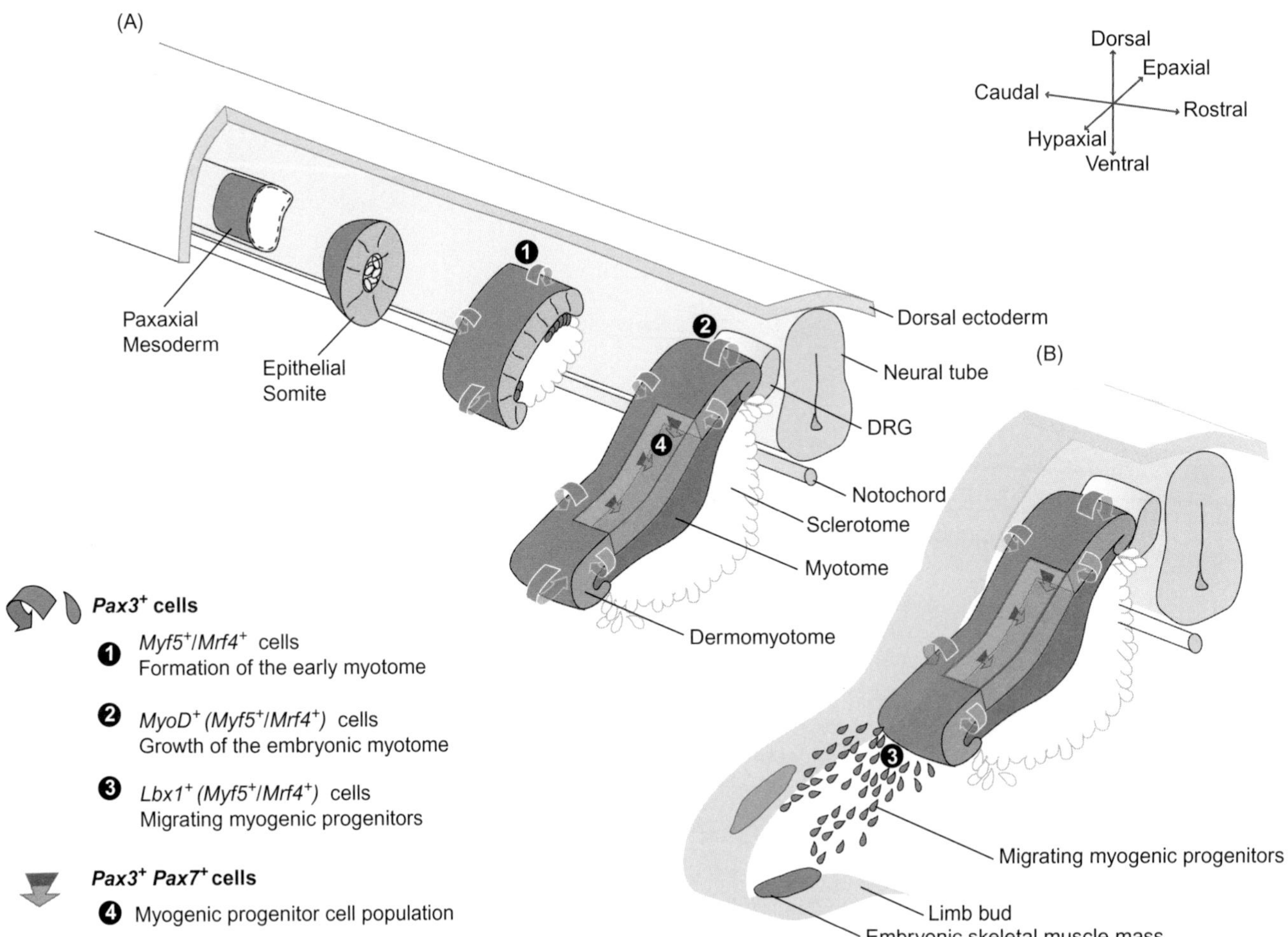

FIGURE 52.1 **Origin of skeletal muscles of the trunk and limbs.** (A) Somites are formed by the segmentation of paraxial mesoderm. Initially they have an epithelial structure and then their ventral part undergoes an epithelial-mesenchymal transition giving rise to the sclerotome. The epithelium is maintained in the dorsal part of the somite, as the dermomyotome, where all cells express *Pax3*. The first skeletal muscle, the myotome, is progressively established by delamination of progenitor cells (*Pax3* +), which have activated *Myf5/Mrf4* (blue arrows). The central part of the dermomyotome then breaks down and cells expressing both *Pax3* and *Pax7* enter the primary myotome (red arrows). The myotome subsequently grows to give rise to all trunk muscles. (B) At the level of the limb buds, *Pax3* + progenitors, present in the hypaxial lip of the dermomyotome, delaminate and migrate to the limbs where they form skeletal muscles. This process occurs from E9 to E11.5. (E, Embryonic day of mouse development; DRG, Dorsal root ganglion).

nascent basal lamina on muscle fibers. Somite grafting experiments in birds (3), together with genetic tracing and genetically engineered cell ablation experiments in mammals (6), indicate that the satellite cells of postnatal muscle derive from this progenitor cell population.

At the level of the fore- and hindlimbs, cells delaminate from the hypaxial dermomyotome and migrate into the early limb bud (1) where they subsequently differentiate into skeletal muscle or continue to proliferate as a progenitor cell population (Figure 52.1B). Delamination, followed by migration, also characterizes the behavior of cells that will form the muscle of the diaphragm. A variant on this theme has been described for progenitor cells for cloacal muscles, which first enter the hindlimb bud and then exit it to take up their final position in the ventral body cavity, where these muscles, which control urogenital function, will form (7). At the thoracic level, the transitory structure of the hypoglossal chord, which consists of a sheet of myogenic cells, extends anteriorly from the hypaxial dermomyotome of some occipital and cervical level somites, contributing somite-derived muscle cells to the throat, including some tongue muscles (1).

Skeletal Muscle Maturation

Most trunk muscles grow from the initial myotome, where the myocytes subsequently undergo cell fusion to form multinucleated muscle fibers (8), followed by cleavage and re-organization of the developing muscle masses (Figure 52.2). The epaxial myotome will give rise to the

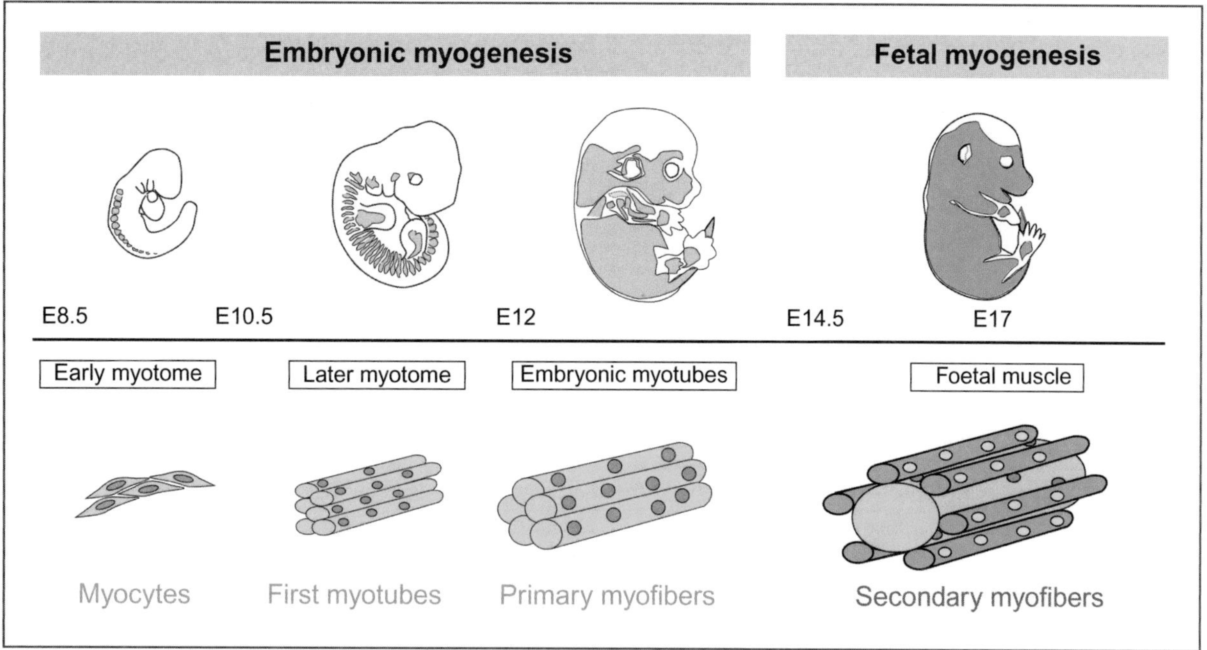

FIGURE 52.2 **Waves of skeletal muscle formation.** There is a first wave of skeletal muscle formation, termed embryonic or primary myogenesis. This is followed by a second wave of fetal or secondary myogenesis. The timing of this transition depends on the onset of innervation which varies at different sites in the embryo. E, Embryonic day of mouse development.

deep muscles of the back that are attached to the vertebrae. A recent study (9) of this process shows the close association of syndecan-derived connective tissue with the muscle fibers, potentially shaping the muscles as they grow. The hypaxial dermomyotome provides a major source of myotomal cells and the hypaxial myotome underlies most of the body wall musculature of the trunk, where, as for epaxial muscles, the developing muscle masses are fuelled by the myogenic progenitor cell pool. Limb musculature also follows a similar developmental progression towards the separation of individual muscle masses. In this case the role of connective tissue is more clearly defined. Classic experiments in the chick embryo have led to the notion of the naïve myogenic progenitor cell that is instructed where to locate and differentiate by the connective tissue of the limb (1). Subsequent cleavage of the initial dorsal and ventral muscle masses, to finally give the individual muscles of the limb, also depends on interactions with connective tissue (see section on signaling).

Secondary Myogenesis During Fetal Development

As development proceeds, neurons grow out towards the muscle fibers, which play an attractant role in axon guidance and the establishment of innervation. This includes both sensory innervation through the intrafusal fibers of muscle spindles, which retain a more embryonic contractile protein phenotype even in the adult (10) and motor innervation of muscle fibers which drives contraction (11). The establishment of definitive neuromuscular junctions and excitation–contraction coupling is associated with so-called secondary or fetal myogenesis, which gives rise to the bulk of fibers in post-natal muscle (12). This takes place from about two days after the first appearance of differentiated muscle, at about embryonic day (E) 14.5 in the mouse hindlimb, for example (13), and is characterized by the appearance of secondary muscle fibers which are initially much thinner (the nuclei have been described as "pearls on a string") than the previously formed primary fibers that they surround (Figure 52.2). These fibers can be distinguished by the contractile proteins that they express: for example, primary fibers contain slow as well as embryonic fast myosin whereas secondary fibers contain only fast myosin isoforms. Expression of muscle-specific isoforms of metabolic enzymes, such as β-enolase, is also a feature of secondary fibers. Previous work on secondary myogenesis had shown that it was preceded by a wave of progenitor cell proliferation to generate secondary myoblasts, which behave differently in culture and have a transcriptome that distinguishes them from primary or embryonic myoblasts (14). In postnatal muscle, when innervation by slow motor neurons leads to fibers with a classic slow phenotype, it is thought that many of these derive from the primary fibers of embryonic muscle, whereas the secondary fibers acquire mature fast phenotypes. In large mammals it has been proposed that a later third wave of myogenesis takes place to generate additional tertiary muscle fibers (15).

Transcription Factors that Control Skeletal Muscle Development

The Myogenic Regulatory Factors, which Determine Entry into the Myogenic Program

Entry into the myogenic programme depends on myogenic regulatory factors of the MyoD family of basic-helix-loop-helix (b-HLH) transcriptional regulators. Gene deletion experiments in the mouse have established that Myf5 and MyoD are essential for myogenic determination, with Mrf4 also playing this role at the outset of myogenesis in the somite (3). During muscle development, myogenic determination genes show different spatio-temporal expression patterns, with different functional roles (1,3) (Figure 52.3). Thus the formation of the early myotome depends on the activation of *Myf5* and *Mrf4*, at the edges of the dermomyotome (Figure 52.1A), in cells that will delaminate, although this process is not myogenic factor-dependent. *MyoD* is activated later in the hypaxial and then in the epaxial domain and this initially requires Myf5/Mrf4. Subsequently, in the absence of these factors, *MyoD* is expressed and myogenesis is initiated, without early myotome formation. In the absence of MyoD, *Myf5*, which is normally downregulated by late embryonic stages, continues to be expressed and skeletal muscle development proceeds. Based on Cre-mediated ablation experiments, it has been suggested that there are distinct MyoD- and Myf5-dependent myogenic lineages, however this interpretation depends on the level of *Myf5* regulated Cre expression (4). Although myogenic determination factors can substitute for each other, some sites of myogenesis are more affected by the absence of one member of this family. Thus, the diaphragm in *MyoD* mutants is functional, but is less robust so that on an *mdx* (dystrophic) mutant background it is partially compromised (16). During the onset of myogenesis in the limb, when both Myf5 and MyoD are normally present, *MyoD* mutant embryos show a delay in myogenesis, indicating that Myf5 alone cannot initiate the myogenic programme on time (1). In keeping with their function as myogenic determination factors, Myf5, MyoD, and also Mrf4, contain a protein domain that plays a role in chromatin remodeling, which is absent from the myogenic differentiation factor, Myogenin (17). Different targets of these myogenic determination factors, prior to activation of *Myogenin* and muscle differentiation, have not been characterized. However, it was shown recently that MyoD and Myf5 differ in their response to DNA damage, such that phosphorylation of MyoD results in a transient block of MyoD-activated gene expression, while DNA repair takes place, not seen for Myf5 which does not have the tyrosine residue targeted by the kinase (18).

Myogenic factors normally function as heterodimers with universally expressed members of the E12 family of b-HLH transcription factors. A number of proteins that interfere with myogenic factor function have been identified, including Id HLH proteins that sequester them as heterodimers. Id2/3 expression is high in somitic domains surrounding the myotome, thus preventing any premature transcriptional activity of the myogenic factor (1). Downregulation of Id2/3 is re-enforced by the presence of a transcriptional repressor, RP58 (Zfp238), in differentiating muscle (19). Micro RNAs represent another level of regulation and microRNA 31 has been shown to target the 3′UTR of *Myf5* messenger RNA and thus prevent Myf5 protein translation (20). This microRNA is not present in differentiating muscles like the myotome but it is present in the dermomyotome, particularly at the edges where *Myf5* is already transcribed. Absence of Myf5 protein would be consistent with the lack of Myf5 function, seen in the *Myf5* mutant, in the initial delamination of these cells (1). MicroRNA 31 is also expressed in regions of the central nervous system where unexpected transcription of *Myf5* had been detected, without detectable protein or evidence of a phenotype in the *Myf5*

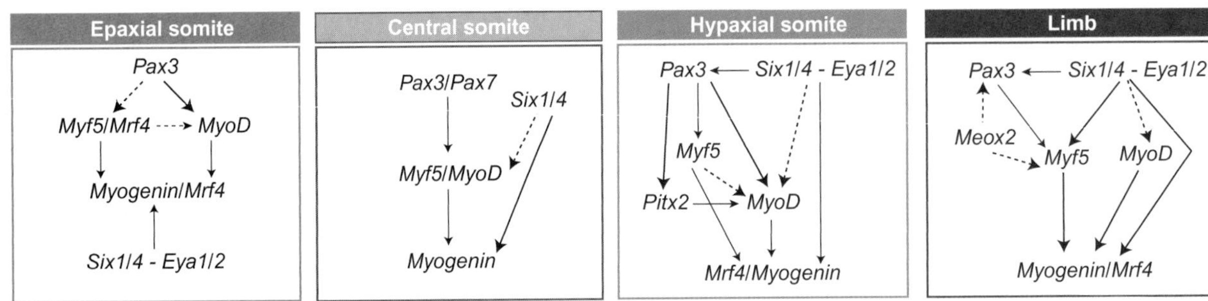

FIGURE 52.3 Genetic regulation of myogenesis in the trunk and limbs. Different genetic hierarchies regulate the onset of myogenesis in the epaxial, central or hypaxial domains of the somite or limb. Arrows indicate established genetic regulation, while dotted arrows indicate suggested interactions or regulation in a brief window of time.

mutant. This is an example where microRNA safeguards against inappropriate function of a tissue determination factor when the gene is inappropriately expressed. Thus both at the protein and the mRNA level there are mechanisms to reinforce the restriction of myogenic factor activity to sites of myogenesis.

The regulatory sequences of *Myf5,* which extend over more that 100 kb 5′, in a locus that also contains the closely linked *Mrf4* gene, have been extensively studied and illustrate the complexity of the upstream regulation of this early myogenic determination gene (21). Different enhancer elements control the activation of *Myf5* at different sites of myogenesis during development. This reflects the fact that skeletal muscle formation does not result from a single gene regulatory cascade, but from different regulatory inputs according to the timing and the site of skeletal muscle formation in the embryo. Indeed part of the differing responses of muscles to mutations that result in myopathies may be due to their different regulatory histories.

Pax3 and Pax7, as Upstream Regulators of Myogenic Stem Cells

Pax3 is a key upstream regulator of myogenic progenitor cells in the trunk and limbs (Figure 52.3). It is a member of the Pax family of transcriptional activators which play important roles in tissue specification and organogenesis during embryogenesis (22). Pax3, and its sister protein Pax7, have homeo-domains in addition to the characteristic paired domain. The expression of *Pax3* and *Pax7* is not confined to sites of myogenesis and indeed Pax3 is an important early regulator of neural crest cells. In the myogenic context, *Pax3* is activated in pre-somitic mesoderm and then is expressed throughout the newly formed epithelial somite before becoming restricted to the dermomyotome. At this stage *Pax7* is activated and expressed at a high level in the central domain of this epithelium (Figure 52.1A).

Pax3/Foxc2 Regulation of Cell Fate Choices

Foxc2 and *Pax3* are co-expressed in cells of the epithelial somite. Subsequently *Foxc2* expression remains high in the cells of the sclerotome, which will form cartilage and bone, and indeed the transcription factor, Foxc2, is required for this process. Low levels of *Foxc2* transcripts continue to be present in the dermomyotome and when Pax3 levels are reduced genetically, *Foxc2* transcription increases. Conversely, in *Foxc2* mutants, *Pax3* transcription increases. There is therefore reciprocal inhibition of these two genes in the multipotent cells of the dermomyotome. Non-myogenic cell fates, such as that of vascular endothelial and smooth muscle cells, depend on Foxc2. When *Foxc2* or *Pax3* are downregulated, more cells can be shown to acquire myogenic or vascular cell fates respectively. *Pax7* and *Foxc1* are also involved in this scenario. The model is that maintenance of multipotency depends on a balance of factors and that perturbation of the equilibrium, by external signals for example, will direct cells to a Pax-dependent myogenic fate or to a Foxc-dependent non-myogenic fate (23).

The Myogenic Progenitor Cell Population

Pax3-positive cells migrate from the dermomyotome and in the absence of Pax3 this process does not take place with a total absence of limb muscles, for example, in *Pax3* mutant embryos. Subsequently, hypaxial cell death is observed in these mutants. Both Pax3 and Pax7 mark the myogenic progenitor cells that derive from the central dermomyotome. In the absence of the two Pax factors, these cells fail to enter the myogenic programme and many of them die, leading to a major muscle deficit in the double mutants (3).

As development proceeds, *Pax3* is downregulated (from about E12 in the mouse) and Pax7 becomes the dominant factor. After birth, *Pax3* transcription is no longer detectable in the satellite cells of some muscles, such as those of the hindlimbs, whereas in many forelimb and trunk muscles, including the diaphragm, *Pax3* continues to be transcribed at a lower level. Genetic tracing and cell ablation experiments, using *Pax3-* and *Pax7-Cre* lines, show that Pax7-positive cells in the trunk and limbs are derived from Pax3-expressing cells (4). These experiments also demonstrated that satellite cells from adult muscle have a similar history and cell ablation directed by an inducible *Pax7Cre-ERT2* allele showed that the initial population of Pax3/7 cells that derive from the embryonic dermomyotome give rise to the satellite cells of adult muscle (6).

Pax3/7 Target Genes

Pax3, in the myogenic context, acts as a transcriptional activator (22) and repression of *Foxc2* is probably indirect, possibly through Hdac5 (23). Pax3 and Pax7 have overlapping functions during muscle development and are expected to share many of the same targets. Indeed when a Pax7 coding sequence is introduced into an allele of *Pax3*, embryos that express only Pax7 in place of Pax3 undergo normal myogenesis in the trunk, with minor perturbations observed only in certain limb muscles. (22). Delamination of cells that migrate away from the dermomyotome depends on *c-Met* and the gene encoding this tyrosine kinase receptor is a Pax3 target. Many other genes for components of signaling pathways involved in myogenesis, including *Fgfr4* which is a direct target (4), or for transcriptional regulators, were identified in a genetic screen for potential Pax3 targets in the embryo (24). Mutational analysis indicates that *Pax3* and *Pax7* lie genetically upstream of *Myf5* and *MyoD*. In the case of *Myf5*, a key regulatory element required for expression in the limbs and hypaxial somite has been shown to be a direct Pax3 target (22). *Dmrt2*, which encodes a transcriptional activator expressed in the dermomyotome, is a direct Pax3 target. Dmrt2, in turn, directly targets an enhancer responsible for early epaxial activation of *Myf5*, thus illustrating how Pax3 indirectly also modulates this aspect of *Myf5* expression (25). Direct activation of *MyoD* by Pax3/7 has not been demonstrated in the embryo, however a regulatory sequence upstream of *MyoD* has been shown to be a Pax7 target in satellite cells (4). Genetically, *MyoD* lies downstream of Pax3 as also shown by the absence of all trunk and limb muscles in *Pax3/Myf5* double mutants (1) (Figure 52.3).

Six1 and Six4, as Regulators of Myogenic Progenitor Cells

Another family of transcription factors that play an important upstream role in myogenesis is that of the Six homeodomain proteins (26) (Figure 52.3). Like the Pax family, Six proteins are implicated in the regulation of a number of tissue specific programmes. These functions are conserved during evolution and formation of the *Drosophila* eye provides an example of the cooperation between these factors (27). *Eyeless (Pax)* acts as a master regulator of eye formation controlling *sine oculis (Six)* which in turn, in conjunction with its co-factor *eyes absent (Eya)*, feeds back to regulate *eyeless,* as well as activating downstream genes leading to eye formation. In the mouse mammalian model, *Six1/4* are expressed in the dermomyotome and the double mutant embryos have major muscle defects. Notably, hypaxial trunk muscles and limb muscles are absent. *Pax3* is downregulated and myogenic factor activation is compromised in the surviving cells, notably Mrf4 is absent and *Myf5* activation is only retained epaxially and in the posterior lip of the dermomyotome, where *Pax3* also continues to be expressed. Mutation of the genes for Six co-activators Eya1/2 has a similar hypaxial phenotype, although myogenic cells derived from the central dermomyotome, where these genes are not expressed, are unaffected (4); other as yet unidentified Six co-activators may function in this domain. In *Six4* single mutants, limb myogenesis is abnormal, with effects on *Myf5* activation (4). The same limb regulatory element of the *Myf5* gene that is Pax3 dependent also has a Six binding site which, when mutated, does not abolish, but impairs transcriptional activity. Although, potentially, Six and Pax could interact through their homeodomains, there is no evidence of this and the factors appear to act independently through their adjacent DNA binding sites. An open question is why the myogenic determination genes are not activated in migrating Pax/Six-positive cells before they reach the limb. This may be due to other transcription factors, however the presence of the Six co-repressor, Dach, in these cells probably contributes to preventing premature entry into the myogenic programme (28).

Other Upstream Regulators of Somitic Cells that Migrate to the Limbs – Lbx1, Meox2

In addition to Pax3 and Six1/4, other transcription factors are implicated in the migration of myogenic cells from the somites (21). The homeobox gene, *Lbx1*, which is a potential Pax3 target (24), is activated in the hypaxial dermomyotome at the level of the limb buds and hypoglossal chord and is expressed in migrating cells. In *Lbx1* mutants, cells fail to migrate correctly and accumulate adjacent to the somites. Hindlimb and ventral forelimb muscles are absent (21). *Meox2,* which encodes another homeodomain protein, is expressed, together with *Meox*1, in paraxial mesoderm and later in the dermomyotome and in cells that migrate to the limbs. In *Meox2* mutants, muscle progenitors appear to migrate normally, but specific limb muscles are absent, notably in the forelimb, and *Pax3* and *Myf5* expression is reduced in myogenic cells in the limb (21). The interpretation of this phenotype is complicated by additional expression of *Meox2* in connective tissue which, in the mutant, may not signal correctly to myogenic progenitors.

Pitx2, as an Upstream Myogenic Regulator

At sites of myogenesis in the trunk and limbs, Pitx transcription factors (29) intervene downstream of Pax3 and indeed *Pitx2* is a potential Pax3 target (24) (Figure 52.3). *Pitx2* is expressed in both myogenic progenitor cells and in differentiating muscle cells. In the absence of Pitx2, *MyoD* is not activated in myogenic progenitor cells in the limb and this was shown to be a direct effect of Pitx2 acting through the *MyoD* embryonic enhancer. *Myf5* activation is not Pitx2-dependent and the early myotome forms normally, with correct initiation of *MyoD* expression (Figure 52.3). However, in the absence of Myf5 and Mrf4, Pitx2 contributes to the rescue of *MyoD* expression, indicating that it acts in this *Pax3* dependent genetic pathway (30).

Factors Implicated in Skeletal Muscle Differentiation

There is a very extensive literature on skeletal muscle differentiation, mainly based on experiments on myogenic cell lines, which includes data on interactions of the myogenic regulatory factors with the basic transcriptional machinery (31). During muscle development *in vivo*, Myogenin is the member of the MyoD family that is responsible for the activation of downstream muscle genes and *Myogenin* mutant mice have severe fetal muscle defects (21). At the onset of skeletal muscle differentiation in the embryo, Mrf4 performs this function and can replace Myogenin. Compound mutants show that Myf5 alone cannot activate differentiation, whereas MyoD, as well as Mrf4 and Myogenin, has this capacity (3). Other transcription factors are also important for muscle differentiation.

The Mef2 family (32) plays a role, with myogenic determination factors, in the activation of *Myogenin*. Subsequently Mef2 factors, that bind to A/T rich sites, are important for the activation of many downstream muscle genes; they can also interact with myogenic factors to increase transactivation efficiency. Several *Mef2* genes are co-expressed during skeletal muscle differentiation in the embryo and Mef2c is essential for early cardiac function making mutant analysis difficult. However, targeted deletion of *Mef2c* in skeletal muscle revealed its importance for sarcomeric gene regulation, particularly of M line proteins (33). Morpholino knock-down in zebrafish embryonic muscle indicates that Mef2d and Mef2c are essential for the transcription of genes encoding thick filament proteins (34). SRF, which like Mef2 is a widely expressed MADS box-containing factor, is also involved in the activation of many muscle genes, including those for sarcomeric actin of the thin filaments. Targeted deletion of SRF results in early skeletal muscle defects which become increasingly severe as the muscle matures (35). Other transcription factors such as the widely expressed Tead/Taf1 factors that target MCAT sites (36), and more muscle-specific Vestigial-like cofactors (37) are also implicated in skeletal muscle gene regulation, but mutant phenotypes have not yet been described in this context. MicroRNAs also intervene to regulate transcription factors associated with muscle differentiation, as in the case of miR133 or miR1-1 which directly, or indirectly, affect SRF or Mef2 activity respectively (3).

Pax factors do not play a role in muscle differentiation and they interfere with this process. Downregulation of Pax3 is assured by miR27 and manipulation of this microRNA in the embryo affects the balance between myogenic progenitor cells and differentiating muscle (38). In contrast to Pax3/7, Pitx2 and Six1/4, which are upstream regulators of myogenesis, also play a role in muscle differentiation. *Pitx2* is normally downregulated in differentiated muscle, where *Pitx3* is expressed, throughout the body and head. *Pitx3* expression depends on a muscle specific enhancer that is regulated by myogenic factors (39). In *Pitx3* mutants, Pitx2 levels remain high, suggesting negative feedback regulation of Pitx3 on *Pitx2* (40). The absence of a pronounced mutant phenotype points to overlapping functions between these Pitx factors. Activation of *Myogenin* depends on myogenic factors, like Myf5, acting via an E-box motif, and on Mef2, but also depends on a Mef3 site that binds Six factors. Downstream muscle genes also depend on Six1/4, as well as myogenic and other factors for transcriptional activation (3).

Fast versus Slow Muscle Gene Regulation

In adult muscle, Six1 and Eya1 are accumulated in fast muscle fibers, and ectopic overexpression of these factors in the slow-type soleus muscle results in a conversion of the slow oxidative phenotype to a fast glycolytic phenotype. Higher activity of Six1/Eya1in fast-type fibers is seen immediately postnatally, suggesting that it may have a precocious role in the activation of the fast-type programme, prior to slow/fast motor neuron activity.

A transcriptome analysis in the embryo shows that many genes encoding fast muscle isoforms are downregulated in the remaining myotome of *Six1/4* double mutants. The binding of Six1/4 to regulatory regions of fast muscle genes supports direct regulation by these factors in the embryo as well as the adult (3). In the mouse, both fast and slow isoforms are co-expressed in embryonic muscle cells. This is in contrast to the situation in the zebrafish, for example, where there is an early segregation of fast and slow muscle progenitors. In this case, Hedgehog signaling induces the transcriptional repressor, Prdm1/Blimp1, in adaxial cells, preventing the activation of fast muscle genes and of the gene for Sox6, a repressor of slow-type gene transcription, therefore conferring a slow phenotype on these cells. Prdm1 is expressed in the mouse myotome, but mutants do not have a fast phenotype, reflecting differences in regulation of slow muscle genes; in myotomal cells. *Sox6* null embryos only show upregulation of slow muscle gene expression at fetal stages (4).

Factors Implicated in Embryonic versus Fetal Myogenesis

At the fetal stage of muscle development when secondary myogenesis is initiated, a number of genes characteristic of secondary muscle fibers are activated and others expressed in primary fibers during embryonic myogenesis are downregulated (14). The molecular mechanisms underlying this transition have remained obscure, although regulatory sequences such as those of the *Myosin light chain (Mlc)1/3* gene that result in later expression of the Mlc3 isoform had been described (4). As a result of a transcriptome analysis on embryonic versus fetal myoblasts, a number of differentially expressed sequences encoding potential regulatory factors were identified. The homeodomain transcription factor, Arx, is present only in embryonic myoblasts where its interaction with Mef2c promotes muscle differentiation (4). On the other hand, the transcription factor, Nfix, is accumulated in fetal muscle where it forms a complex with PKCθ, which is also a marker of fetal myogenesis (41). This complex binds to, and phosphorylates, Mef2 in this case the Mef2a isoform, leading to transcriptional activation of later muscle genes such as *M-CPK*. Overexpression of Nfix in embryonic myoblasts leads to the downregulation of *slow myosin heavy chain* gene transcription and upregulation of fetal genes, whereas muscle specific mutation of *Nfix* results in the maintenance of the embryonic muscle program. Nfi factors have also been reported to bind to the *Myogenin* promoter and to enhance the binding of Myogenin to downstream muscle genes, so they may affect muscle differentiation at a number of levels. However the manipulation of the Nfix isoform in developing muscle points to its role in secondary myogenesis in the fetus. It has been suggested that Pax7, which predominates in myogenic progenitors at fetal stages, activates *Nfix*, however since Pax7 is present earlier in myogenic progenitors that arise from the central dermomyotome, other factors are also probably involved at fetal stages.

Signaling Pathways that Impact Myogenesis

The Onset of Myogenesis in the Somite

The somite is patterned by signals from surrounding tissues, which also regulate the onset of skeletal muscle formation (42). In general, Wnt signaling promotes and Tgfβ/BMP signaling inhibits myogenesis. Other signals also intervene, including those mediated by Sonic hedgehog (Shh), Notch, Integrins and Neuregulin (3,4) (Figure 52.4A).

The Epaxial Myotome

In the epaxial dermomyotome, canonical Wnt signaling (acting with β-catenin) from the dorsal neural tube directly activates *Myf5* expression through Tcf/Lef sites in the early epaxial enhancer of the *Myf5* gene (43) (Figure 52.4A). Wnt signaling also promotes proliferation of cells in the epaxial somite, thus helping to maintain the myogenic progenitor population (44). Canonical Wnt signaling, in the epaxial dermomyotome of the chick embryo, has been shown to activate non-canonical Wnt11 expression in myogenic progenitors, which subsequently plays a role, through the planar cell polarity pathway, in organizing the orientation of differentiating muscle cells in the myotome (4). The inhibitory effect of BMP signaling from the neural tube is counteracted by the expression of the BMP antagonists, Gremlin and Noggin, in the epaxial dermomyotome (24).

Sonic Hedgehog (Shh) signaling from the notochord and floor plate of the neural tube plays a major role as a survival factor. In the absence of Shh, there is somite cell death and most sclerotomal cells are lost. The dorsal somite is less affected, however effects on the survival of

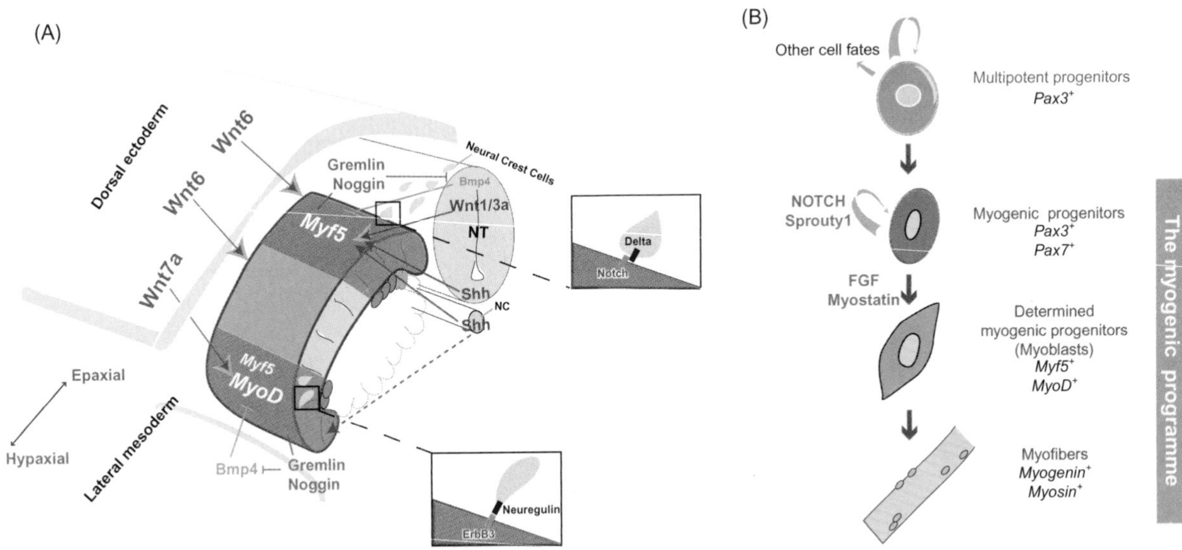

FIGURE 52.4 Control of myogenesis in the trunk and limbs. (A) Activation of the myogenic programme in the somite is under the control of signaling molecules from adjacent structures such as the dorsal ectoderm, the neural tube (NT), the notochord (Nc) and the lateral mesoderm. Wnts and Sonic hedgehog (Shh) have a positive effect on the activation of *Myf5* and *MyoD* in the epaxial (pink) or hypaxial (orange) dermomyotome respectively, while BMP4 inhibits the activation of myogenic determination genes. This effect is counteracted by the BMP inhibitors, Noggin and Gremlin, produced by the somite. Neural crest cells, migrating from the dorsal neural tube through the somite, promote myogenesis by activation of the Notch pathway in the epaxial dermomyotome, whereas they inhibit it in the hypaxial dermomyotome by activation of ErbB3 signaling. (B) The equilibrium between progenitor cell renewal and differentiation is under the control of the Notch, TGFβ (Myostatin) and FGF pathways. Notch and Sprouty1, which is an inhibitor of the FGF pathway, promote self-renewal of progenitors, whereas FGF and Myostatin promote entry into the myogenic programme.

myogenic progenitors in the dermomyotome, with consequences for myotomal patterning are also observed (3). Shh directly regulates the *Myf5* epaxial enhancer, through Gli binding sites, and early *Myf5* expression therefore also depends on this signaling pathway (43). Myogenic cells that delaminate from the dermomyotome and enter the myotome upregulate $\alpha6\beta1$ integrins, in response to Myf5/Mrf4 (45), while expression of *Lama1*, that encodes an integrin ligand, is regulated by Shh (46). The correct localization of myogenic cells prior to differentiation, myotome patterning, and formation of the basal lamina which separates this compartment from the sclerotome also depend on these laminin receptors.

Notch signaling has also now been implicated in the onset of myogensis in the epaxial somite (47). Neural crest cells, which delaminate from the dorsal neural tube, traverse this part of the somite where cells in the dermomyotome express the Notch receptor. Neural crest cells express the Notch ligand, Delta and, when they contact the dermomyotomal cells in a "kiss and run" type model, they activate this signaling pathway with promotion of *Myf5* expression in the epaxial dermomyotome (Figure 52.4A). Interference with neural crest and associated Notch signaling negatively affects the onset of myogenesis. These experiments were carried out in the chick embryo and it remains to be seen how Notch signaling directly or indirectly regulates the *Myf5* early epaxial enhancer, characterised in the mouse (43).

The Hypaxial Myotome

The hypaxial dermomyotome is influenced by signaling from lateral mesoderm, notably BMP signaling which is thought to retard the onset of myogensis in this domain of the somite (Figure 52.4A). Again, the presence of BMP antagonists subsequently dampens this negative effect. Manipulation of BMP signaling in the multipotent cells of the chick hypaxial dermomyotome has been shown to promote an endothelial cell fate of Pax3-positive progenitors. In this context, Notch signaling promotes a smooth muscle cell fate at the expense of skeletal muscle. The dorsal ectoderm, which overlies the dermomyotome, is also a source of signals, as seen for Wnt6 which is important for maintaining the epithelial structure of the dermomyotome, and the maintenance of *Pax3* expression. Activation of PCK activity, which depends on the presence of the ectoderm, also affects Pax3 phosphorylation and enhances its transcriptional activity, leading to downstream activation of *MyoD* (4). The effect of ectoderm on *MyoD* activation has also been proposed to depend on Wnt7a signaling (1). In the hypaxial dermomyotome, migrating neural crest cells delay the onset of myogenesis, promoting the maintenance of Pax3-positive progenitors. This is effected by Neuregulin signaling from neural crest to ErbB3 receptors on myogenic progenitor cells (48).

Breakdown of the Central Dermomyotome, with Release of Myogenic Progenitors

The epithelial to mesenchymal transition (EMT) which takes place in the central domain of the dermomyotome, as the somite matures, corresponds to the time when *Wnt6* transcription is down-regulated in the ectoderm. In addition to the consequences of loss of Wnt signaling on dermomyotome integrity, epithelial breakdown, with the release of Pax3/7 myogenic progenitors, is promoted by FGF signaling from the underlying myotome, as shown by experiments in the chick embryo. This triggers the MAPK/ERK pathway, leading to the activation of the transcription factor Snail in the dermomyotome, which is known to promote EMT (4).

Migration of Myogenic Progenitors from the Hypaxial Somite – Limb Myogenesis

Delamination and migration of cells from the hypaxial dermomyotome depends on signaling through the tyrosine kinase receptor, c-Met, via the signal transduction molecule Gab1, in response to HGF/Scatter factor. This is produced by the mesenchymal cells adjacent to the somite and along the route for myogenic progenitor cell migration, into the limb buds or towards the sites where the diaphragm or tongue muscles will form (21). The chemokine receptor, CXCR4, is also expressed in Pax3-positive cells in the hypaxial dermomyotome at the limb level. This gene is an Lbx1 target, whereas *c-met* is regulated by Pax3. CXCR4 responds to the chemokine SDF1, again produced by the mesenchyme. In the absence of c-Met, or its ligand, no myogenic cells delaminate and migrate away from the dermomyotome, whereas in the absence of CXCR4/SDF1 cells delaminate from the somite, but fail to migrate correctly, so that hindlimb muscles and dorsal muscles of the forelimb do not form (4). Cloacal muscles are also absent in the mutant (7).

Within the limb, the mesenchymal connective tissue, marked by Tcf4, a downstream target of Wnt signaling, is important for determining the location of myogenic progenitors and the patterning of developing muscle masses (49). The different signaling centers within the limb, such as Wnt from the dorsal ectoderm (3) or Shh from the zone of polarising activity are implicated in limb development and patterning (50).

Regulation of progenitor cell self-renewal versus differentiation

Pax3/7-positive progenitor cells in trunk or limb muscles play an essential role in muscle growth during development. It is therefore critical to maintain a balance between progression towards skeletal muscle differentiation and self-renewal of this population (4) (Figure 52.4B). Overactivation of Notch signaling had been shown to result in a reduction in MyoD-positive cells. From analysis of mutants in which RBP-J, the transcriptional effector of Notch signaling, or its ligand, Delta1, are mutated in *Pax3*-expressing cells, it is clear that this signaling pathway ensures self-renewal of myogenic progenitors (4). Manipulation of FGF signaling suggests that it is also implicated in the maintenance of this equilibrium, such that signaling through the Fgfr4 receptor, which promotes entry into the myogenic programme, is modulated by the intracellular inhibitors of this pathway, Sprouty1/2, mainly present in the progenitors (4).

Myostatin, a member of the TGFβ superfamily, is also expressed in skeletal muscle progenitors in the embryo where it has been shown to promote differentiation (51) (Figure 52.4B). It had also been reported to induce quiescence of embryonic cells. In keeping with a role in promoting differentiation, *Myostatin* mutant embryos have increased numbers of myogenic progenitors which results in increased secondary fiber formation at later stages (4). By postnatal stages the Myostatin receptor, Act RIIB, is downregulated on myogenic progenitor cells which are therefore less sensitive to Myostatin signaling. In contrast to the embryo, its major role postnatally is in skeletal muscle fibers, where the absence of Myostatin leads to muscle hypertrophy. Follistatin, present in embryonic muscle, binds to extracellular Myostatin, thus regulating its activity, and indeed *Follistatin* mutant mice have less skeletal muscle at birth, due to premature differentiation of progenitors which then do not contribute to muscle growth (51).

Later Stages of Muscle Development

Most studies on later muscle development have focussed on the limb. Comparison of myoblasts from embryonic and fetal limb muscles has shown that differentiation of the former is insensitive to TGFβ/BMP signaling, whereas secondary myoblast differentiation is blocked by these Smad-mediated pathways (14). In contrast to embryonic myogenesis, secondary myoblasts at fetal stages depend on Wnt/βcatenin signaling to promote proliferation (52).

Maturation of the muscle mass also involves signaling from adjacent cell types. This is illustrated by the later role of connective tissue. Genetic manipulation of *Tcf4* in this tissue reveals the importance of connective tissue fibroblasts in muscle fiber-type development and maturation (49). In *Tbx4/5* mutants, reduction in N-cadherin and β-catenin affect connective tissue behavior resulting in loss of some skeletal muscles and defects in others (53).

As muscles mature they become articulated with the developing skeleton. The establishment of myotendinous junctions in the developing limb, depends on interdependent FGF signaling in muscle fiber tips and adjacent mesenchyme, which will form tendon primordia (54). Separation of tendons from developing muscles also reveals interactions between these tissues, with retinoic acid signaling playing a role in tendon mediated muscle survival (55). Another example of crosstalk, between muscle and skeletal components, is provided by the requirement of muscle contraction for maintenance of joint progenitors, which depends on contraction-dependent regulation of the β-catenin signaling pathway required for joint formation (56).

HEAD MUSCLES

Origin of Head Muscles

In the anterior region of the embryo, somites do not form and the distinction between paraxial and lateral mesoderm is less clear-cut, partly reflecting an overall reduction in mesoderm. Skeletal muscles in the head derive from this cranial mesoderm (57–59) (Figure 52.5A). Whereas all muscles in the trunk and limbs, including some neck muscles, derive from somitic paraxial mesoderm, other muscles in the neck form from lateral mesoderm adjacent to the first three somites (60).

At the level of the pharynx, transitory structures, known as branchial or pharyngeal arches, form as protrusions on either side of the axis. They contain a core of cranial (pharyngeal) mesoderm surrounded by endoderm and ectoderm. The first arches will give rise to maxillary and mandibulary prominences and subsequently to the musculoskeletal structures of the upper and lower jaws (Figure 52.5A). Bone of the jaws forms from neural crest cells that invade the mesodermal core of the first arches, whereas the cranial mesoderm is the source of jaw muscles such as the masseter or temporalis. The mesodermal core of the second arches gives rise to facial expression muscles. Mesoderm of the more posterior arches contributes to laryngeal and pharyngeal muscles in the neck. Pharyngeal mesoderm also constitutes the anterior part of the second heart field which is a source of progenitor cells for outflow tract and right ventricular myocardium. The mesodermal core of the second arches contributes myocardium to the outflow tract of the heart and retrospective clonal analysis has shown that this shares a common progenitor with facial skeletal muscle. Jaw muscles derived from the first brachial arch show clonality with myocardial cells in the right ventricle. This close association between skeletal and cardiac muscle (58,61) is also indicated by overlapping gene expression patterns for major upstream regulators of cardiac versus skeletal myogenesis. Genetic tracing of the descendants of cells that had expressed cardiac regulatory genes, such as *Islet1*, in

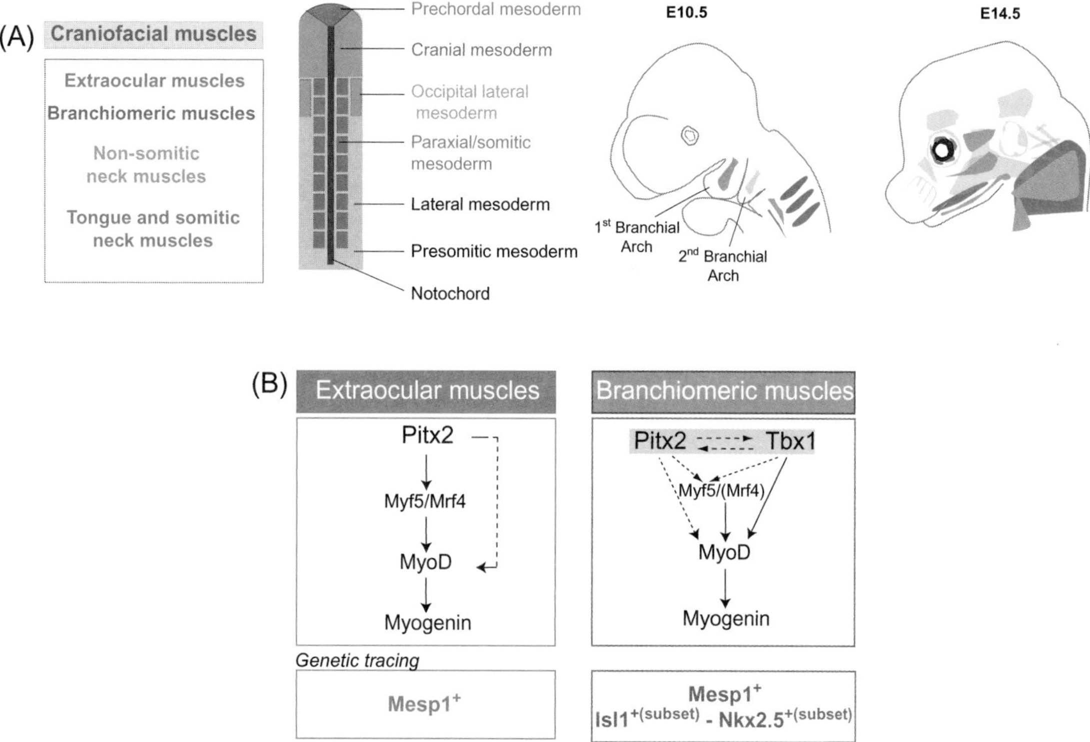

FIGURE 52.5 **Origin and genetic regulation of branchiomeric and extraocular muscles.** (A) Schematic representation of the anterior/posterior axis of a chordate embryo indicating the origin of anterior skeletal muscles. Extraocular muscles are derived mainly from prechordal mesoderm (red). Branchiomeric muscles derive from the mesodermal core of the first (dark blue) or second (light blue) branchial arches. Neck muscles derive from the occipital lateral mesoderm (purple) and somitic paraxial mesoderm (green), which also contributes to tongue muscles. (B) The genetic hierarchy regulating myogenesis is different between extraocular and branchiomeric muscles. Pitx2 is a key regulator for extraocular myogenesis and for the first branchial arches, whereas Tbx1 intervenes in branchiomeric myogenesis. Arrows indicate established genetic regulation, while dotted arrows indicate suggested interactions or regulation, which take place only in the first branchial arches. During development, progenitors of these different muscles have expressed different genes: genetic tracing experiments show that they are all derived from Mesp1-expressing cells, whereas only branchiomeric muscle progenitors have expressed the cardiac marker genes Isl1 and Nkx2.5.

the mouse demonstrate this overlap, with cardiac progenitors located in the more distal region of the arch mesodermal core, whereas skeletal progenitors extend more proximally (Figure 52.5B).

The most anterior muscles of the head, the extraocular muscles, derive from prechordal cranial mesoderm which is distinct from the cranial/pharyngeal mesoderm that lies on either side of the notochord (Figure 52.5A). Retrospective clonal analysis indicates that extraocular muscles also show clonality with first arch derivatives suggesting that they have two origins (61). Development of head muscles is intimately linked to neural crest which is involved in the positioning of muscle cells and the shaping of muscle masses, providing the connective tissue of the head (57).

Control of Head Muscle Myogenesis

In head muscles too, the myogenic factors are essential, but they are differentially expressed at sites of branchial arch or extraocular myogenesis and these muscles differ in their dependence on Myf5/Mrf4 or MyoD (59). Thus myogenic determination in extraocular muscles depends primarily on Myf5 and Mrf4 and cannot be rescued by MyoD, which plays a minor role, whereas brachial arch-derived muscles depend on Myf5/Mrf4 and MyoD (Figure 52.5B).

The upstream regulators of non-somitic myogenic progenitors in the head and neck are different from those in the body (58,59). *Pax3* is not expressed and *Pax7* is only activated later. Pitx2 plays a key role in the upstream regulation of these cells. Pitx2 is present in myogenic progenitor cells that will form extraocular muscles. In its absence these cells undergo apoptosis, without entering the myogenic programme. Conditional mutation of *Pitx2* at later stages impairs myogenic gene expression and it is proposed that there is a direct effect on *Myf5* and *MyoD* promoter activity. Pitx2 is also required for the differentiation and survival of myogenic progenitor cells in the mesodermal core of the first branchial arches. In addition to jaw muscle phenotypes *Pitx2*, mutants have malformations of the arterial pole of the heart, reflecting these arch defects, as well as other cardiac defects due to deficiencies in left/right patterning of the heart.

During the early stages of branchiometric muscle formation in the head, the T-box factor, Tbx1, expressed in the mesodermal core of the branchial arches, plays a role in ensuring robust activation of *Myf5* and *MyoD*; in its absence muscles are hypoplastic and often unilateral. Laryngeal muscles and part of the trapezius jaw muscle are particularly Tbx1-dependent. The *Tbx1* hypoplastic phenotype is much more severe when Myf5 is also absent. This indicates that Myf5 normally drives the Tbx1-independent aspects of myogenesis and that MyoD, which normally compensates for the lack of Myf5, is Tbx1 dependent (Figure 52.5B). Interestingly, the subset of head muscles affected in the *Tbx1* mutant are the same as those that derive from *Islet1*-expressing cells, as shown by genetic tracing. This cardiac link is also manifest in the severe arterial pole defects, particularly of the pulmonary trunk, seen in the hearts of *Tbx1* mutant embryos (58). TBX1 is implicated in DiGeorge syndrome where patients have cardiac and craniofacial muscle defects.

In branchial arch myogenesis, MyoR (Msc) and Capsulin (Tcf21), two b-HLH transcription factors, also play specific roles (58,59). They are both required for *Myf5* activation in the part of the first branchial arches (mandibular arches) that gives rise to jaw-closing muscles and in their absence cell death takes place in this mesodermal core. *Pitx2* lies genetically upstream of *Msc* in controlling proliferation and survival (Figure 52.5B).

Six1/4 are expressed during cranial myogenesis. In zebrafish, during branchial arch development, *Six1* is activated after *Myf5* and appears to be Tbx1-independent, also acting genetically upstream of *MyoD*. Downstream regulation of muscle differentiation appears to involve the same factors as in the trunk (62).

The striking difference in the upstream regulators of myogenesis in the head compared to the body is also seen for signaling pathways (58,59). Canonical Wnt signaling is known to activate *Pitx2*. However, in addition to this potential role, Wnt signaling delays the onset of myogenesis in pharyngeal arch mesoderm, promoting maintenance of the myogenic progenitor cells. This probably contributes to the late onset of myogenic differentiation in head muscles, which depend on the complex processes of jaw and head morphogenesis for their correct positioning. BMPs activate cardiogenesis, thus favoring the myocardial rather than the skeletal muscle cell fate. FGF signaling, which is regulated by Tbx1, is required to maintain the myogenic programme after specification by upstream regulators.

There are interesting evolutionary implications (59) in the distinct programme for activation of myogenesis in the head and the lineage relationship with heart progenitors. The development of the head, linked to the emergence of neural crest, is a characteristic of vertebrates and head muscles have therefore evolved more recently than those of the body, although the myogenic strategy may reflect older links between cardiac and skeletal myogenesis.

ACKNOWLEDGMENTS

Work on skeletal muscle in M.B.'s laboratory is supported by the Institut Pasteur and the CNRS (URA 2578), with grants from the AFM, and the EU programmes OPTISTEM (grant no. Health F4-2007, 200720) and EuroSyStem (grant no. FP7- Health 2007, 223098). A.M. benefits from a fellowship awarded by the University of Paris VI and additional support from the French Society of Myology.

REFERENCES

1. Tajbakhsh S, Buckingham M. The birth of muscle progenitor cells in the mouse: spatiotemporal considerations. *Curr Top Dev Biol* 2000;**48**:225–68.
2. Brent AE, Schweitzer R, Tabin CJ. A somitic compartment of tendon progenitors. *Cell* 2003;**113**:235–48.
3. Buckingham M. Myogenic progenitor cells and skeletal myogenesis in vertebrates. *Curr Opin Genet Dev* 2006;**16**:525–32.
4. Buckingham M, Vincent SD. Distinct and dynamic myogenic populations in the vertebrate embryo. *Curr Opin Genet Dev* 2009;**19**:444–53.
5. Kalcheim C, Ben-Yair R. Cell rearrangements during development of the somite and its derivatives. *Curr Opin Genet Dev* 2005;**15**:371–80.
6. Lepper C, Fan CM. Inducible lineage tracing of Pax7-descendant cells reveals embryonic origin of adult satellite cells. *Genesis* 2010;**48**:424–36.
7. Rehimi R, Khalida N, Yusuf F, Morosan-Puopolo G, Brand-Saberi B. A novel role of CXCR4 and SDF-1 during migration of cloacal muscle precursors. *Dev Dyn* 2010;**239**:1622–31.
8. Rochlin K, Yu S, Roy S, Baylies MK. Myoblast fusion: when it takes more to make one. *Dev Biol* 2010;**341**:66–83.
9. Deries M, Schweitzer R, Duxson MJ. Developmental fate of the mammalian myotome. *Dev Dyn* 2010;**239**:2898–910.
10. Maier A. Development and regeneration of muscle spindles in mammals and birds. *Int J Dev Biol* 1997;**41**:1–17.
11. Harris AJ. Embryonic growth and innervation of rat skeletal muscles. I. Neural regulation of muscle fiber numbers. *Philos Trans R Soc Lond B Biol Sci* 1981;**293**:257–77 II. Neural regulation of muscle cholinesterase. Philos Trans R Soc Lond B Biol Sci 293, 279–286.
12. Kelly AM, Zacks SI. The fine structure of motor endplate morphogenesis. *J Cell Biol* 1969;**42**:154–69.
13. Ontell M, Kozeka K. Organogenesis of the mouse extensor digitorum logus muscle: a quantitative study. *Am J Anat* 1984;**171**:149–61.
14. Biressi S, Molinaro M, Cossu G. Cellular heterogeneity during vertebrate skeletal muscle development. *Dev Biol* 2007;**308**:281–93.
15. Wilson SJ, McEwan JC, Sheard PW, Harris AJ. Early stages of myogenesis in a large mammal: formation of successive

generations of myotubes in sheep tibialis cranialis muscle. *J Muscle Res Cell Motil* 1992;**13**:534–50.
16. Inanlou MR, Dhillon GS, Belliveau AC, Reid GA, Ying C, Rudnicki MA, et al. A significant reduction of the diaphragm in mdx:MyoD-/- embryos suggests a role for MyoD in the diaphragm development. *Dev Biol* 2003;**261**:324–36.
17. Bergstrom DA, Tapscott SJ. Molecular distinction between specification and differentiation in the myogenic basic helix-loop-helix transcription factor family. *Mol Cell Biol* 2001;**21**:2404–12.
18. Innocenzi A, Latella L, Messina G, Simonatto M, Marullo F, Berghella L, et al. An evolutionarily acquired genotoxic response discriminates MyoD from Myf5, and differentially regulates hypaxial and epaxial myogenesis. *EMBO Rep* 2011;**12**:164–71.
19. Yokoyama S, Asahara H. The myogenic transcriptional network. *Cell Mol Life Sci* 2011;**68**:1843–9.
20. Daubas P, Crist CG, Bajard L, Relaix F, Pecnard E, Rocancourt D, et al. The regulatory mechanisms that underlie inappropriate transcription of the myogenic determination gene Myf5 in the central nervous system. *Dev Biol* 2009;**327**:71–82.
21. Buckingham M. Skeletal muscle formation in vertebrates. *Curr Opin Genet Dev* 2001;**11**:440–8.
22. Buckingham M, Relaix F. The role of Pax genes in the development of tissues and organs: Pax3 and Pax7 regulate muscle progenitor cell functions. *Annu Rev Cell Dev Biol* 2007;**23**:645–73.
23. Lagha M, Brunelli S, Messina G, Cumano A, Kume T, Relaix F, et al. Pax3:Foxc2 reciprocal repression in the somite modulates muscular versus vascular cell fate choice in multipotent progenitors. *Dev Cell* 2009;**17**:892–9.
24. Lagha M, Sato T, Regnault B, Cumano A, Zuniga A, Licht J, et al. Transcriptome analyses based on genetic screens for Pax3 myogenic targets in the mouse embryo. *BMC Genomics* 2010;**11**:696.
25. Sato T, Rocancourt D, Marques L, Thorsteinsdottir S, Buckingham M. A Pax3/Dmrt2/Myf5 regulatory cascade functions at the onset of myogenesis. *PLoS Genet* 2010;**6**:e1000897.
26. Kumar JP. The sine oculis homeobox (SIX) family of transcription factors as regulators of development and disease. *Cell Mol Life Sci* 2009;**66**:565–83.
27. Relaix F, Buckingham M. From insect eye to vertebrate muscle: redeployment of a regulatory network. *Genes Dev* 1999; **13**:3171–8.
28. Heanue TA, Reshef R, Davis RJ, Mardon G, Oliver G, Tomarev S, et al. Synergistic regulation of vertebrate muscle development by Dach2, Eya2, and Six1, homologs of genes required for Drosophila eye formation. *Genes Dev* 1999;**13**:3231–43.
29. Gage PJ, Suh H, Camper SA. Dosage requirement of Pitx2 for development of multiple organs. *Development* 1999;**126**:4643–51.
30. L'Honore A, Ouimette JF, Lavertu-Jolin M, Drouin J. Pitx2 defines alternate pathways acting through MyoD during limb and somitic myogenesis. *Development* 2010;**137**:3847–56.
31. Tapscott SJ. The circuitry of a master switch: Myod and the regulation of skeletal muscle gene transcription. *Development* 2005;**132**:2685–95.
32. Black BL, Olson EN. Transcriptional control of muscle development by myocyte enhancer factor-2 (MEF2) proteins. *Annu Rev Cell Dev Biol* 1998;**14**:167–96.
33. Potthoff MJ, Arnold MA, McAnally J, Richardson JA, Bassel-Duby R, Olson EN. Regulation of skeletal muscle sarcomere integrity and postnatal muscle function by Mef2c. *Mol Cell Biol* 2007;**27**:8143–51.
34. Hinits Y, Hughes SM. Mef2s are required for thick filament formation in nascent muscle fibers. *Development* 2007;**134**:2511–9.
35. Li S, Czubryt MP, McAnally J, Bassel-Duby R, Richardson JA, Wiebel FF, et al. Requirement for serum response factor for skeletal muscle growth and maturation revealed by tissue-specific gene deletion in mice. *Proc Natl Acad Sci USA* 2005;**102**:1082–7.
36. Yoshida T. MCAT elements and the TEF-1 family of transcription factors in muscle development and disease. *Arterioscler Thromb Vasc Biol* 2008;**28**:8–17.
37. Bonnet A, Dai F, Brand-Saberi B, Duprez D. Vestigial-like 2 acts downstream of MyoD activation and is associated with skeletal muscle differentiation in chick myogenesis. *Mech Dev* 2010;**127**:120–36.
38. Crist CG, Montarras D, Pallafacchina G, Rocancourt D, Cumano A, Conway SJ, et al. Muscle stem cell behavior is modified by microRNA-27 regulation of Pax3 expression. *Proc Natl Acad Sci USA* 2009;**106**:13383–7.
39. Coulon V, L'Honore A, Ouimette JF, Dumontier E, van den Munckhof P, Drouin J. A muscle-specific promoter directs Pitx3 gene expression in skeletal muscle cells. *J Biol Chem* 2007;**282**:33192–200.
40. L'Honore A, Coulon V, Marcil A, Lebel M, Lafrance-Vanasse J, Gage P, et al. Sequential expression and redundancy of Pitx2 and Pitx3 genes during muscle development. *Dev Biol* 2007; **307**:421–33.
41. Messina G, Biressi S, Monteverde S, Magli A, Cassano M, Perani L, et al. Nfix regulates fetal-specific transcription in developing skeletal muscle. *Cell* 2010;**140**:554–66.
42. Borycki AG, Emerson Jr. CP. Multiple tissue interactions and signal transduction pathways control somite myogenesis. *Curr Top Dev Biol* 2000;**48**:165–224.
43. Borello U, Berarducci B, Murphy P, Bajard L, Buffa V, Piccolo S, et al. The Wnt/beta-catenin pathway regulates Gli-mediated Myf5 expression during somitogenesis. *Development* 2006;**133**:3723–32.
44. Brauner I, Spicer DB, Krull CE, Venuti JM. Identification of responsive cells in the developing somite supports a role for beta-catenin-dependent Wnt signaling in maintaining the DML myogenic progenitor pool. *Dev Dyn* 2009;**239**:222–36.
45. Bajanca F, Luz M, Raymond K, Martins GG, Sonnenberg A, Tajbakhsh S, et al. Integrin alpha6beta1-laminin interactions regulate early myotome formation in the mouse embryo. *Development* 2006;**133**:1635–44.
46. Anderson C, Thorsteinsdottir S, Borycki AG. Sonic hedgehog-dependent synthesis of laminin alpha1 controls basement membrane assembly in the myotome. *Development* 2009; **136**:3495–504.
47. Rios AC, Serralbo O, Salgado D, Marcelle C. Neural crest regulates myogenesis through the transient activation of NOTCH. *Nature* 2011;**473**:532–5.
48. Van Ho AT, Hayashi S, Brohl D, Aurade F, Rattenbach R, Relaix F. Neural crest cell lineage restricts skeletal muscle progenitor cell differentiation through Neuregulin1-ErbB3 signaling. *Developmental Cell* 2011;**21**:273–87.
49. Mathew SJ, Hansen JM, Merrell AJ, Murphy MM, Lawson JA, Hutcheson DA, et al. Connective tissue fibroblasts and Tcf4 regulate myogenesis. *Development* 2011;**138**:371–84.

50. Duboc V, Logan MP. Building limb morphology through integration of signaling modules. *Curr Opin Genet Dev* 2009;**19**:497–503.
51. Otto A, Patel K. Signaling and the control of skeletal muscle size. *Exp Cell Res* 2010;**316**:3059–66.
52. Hutcheson DA, Zhao J, Merrell A, Haldar M, Kardon G. Embryonic and fetal limb myogenic cells are derived from developmentally distinct progenitors and have different requirements for beta-catenin. *Genes Dev* 2009;**23**:997–1013.
53. Hasson P, DeLaurier A, Bennett M, Grigorieva E, Naiche LA, Papaioannou VE, et al. Tbx4 and tbx5 acting in connective tissue are required for limb muscle and tendon patterning. *Dev Cell* 2010;**18**:148–56.
54. Eloy-Trinquet S, Wang H, Edom-Vovard F, Duprez D. Fgf signaling components are associated with muscles and tendons during limb development. *Dev Dyn* 2009;**238**:1195–206.
55. Rodriguez-Guzman M, Montero JA, Santesteban E, Ganan Y, Macias D, Hurle JM. Tendon-muscle crosstalk controls muscle bellies morphogenesis, which is mediated by cell death and retinoic acid signaling. *Dev Biol* 2007;**302**:267–80.
56. Kahn J, Shwartz Y, Blitz E, Krief S, Sharir A, Breitel DA, et al. Muscle contraction is necessary to maintain joint progenitor cell fate. *Dev Cell* 2009;**16**:734–43.
57. Noden DM, Francis-West P. The differentiation and morphogenesis of craniofacial muscles. *Dev Dyn* 2006;**235**:1194–218.
58. Kelly RG. Core issues in craniofacial myogenesis. *Exp Cell Res* 2010;**316**:3034–41.
59. Sambasivan R, Kuratani S, Tajbakhsh S. An eye on the head: the development and evolution of craniofacial muscles. *Development* 2011;**138**:2401–15.
60. Theis S, Patel K, Valasek P, Otto A, Pu Q, Harel I, et al. The occipital lateral plate mesoderm is a novel source for vertebrate neck musculature. *Development* 2010;**137**:2961–71.
61. Lescroart F, Kelly RG, Le Garrec JF, Nicolas JF, Meilhac SM, Buckingham M. Clonal analysis reveals common lineage relationships between head muscles and second heart field derivatives in the mouse embryo. *Development* 2010;**137**:3269–79.
62. Lin CY, Chen WT, Lee HC, Yang PH, Yang HJ, Tsai HJ. The transcription factor Six1a plays an essential role in the craniofacial myogenesis of zebrafish. *Dev Biol* 2009;**331**:152–66.

Chapter 53

Skeletal Muscle: Architecture of Membrane Systems

Clara Franzini-Armstrong[1] and Andrew G. Engel[2]

[1]Department of Cell and Developmental Biology, University of Pennsylvania, Philadelphia, PA, [2]Department of Neuroscience, Mayo Clinic, Rochester, MN

THE MEMBRANE SYSTEMS INVOLVED IN CALCIUM CYCLING

Calcium Cycling and the Control of Muscle Contraction: the EC Coupling Question

Normal contractile function in adult skeletal muscle requires large movements of calcium between cytoplasm and sarcoplasmic reticulum (SR). Exchanges with the extracellular spaces are considerably limited due to a variety of factors, namely the internal SR is a very efficient calcium sink; calcium entry through the plasmalemma's calcium channels is small; sodium/calcium exchange and calcium pumping at the plasmalemma are of small magnitude; and depletion of the SR rarely occurs, so that store operated calcium entry plays a restricted role. However, overall calcium homeostasis is affected by exchanges at the plasmalemma and even small imbalances have a deleterious effect (see Chapter 56).

Historical key findings led to the classical textbook list of the sequential steps involved in the activation of muscle fibers: depolarization of the plasmalemma; inward spread of the depolarization along the transverse (T) tubular system; release of calcium for the SR; binding of calcium to troponin C; release of the TN-TM block to cross-bridge action. The local stimulation experiments (1) initially identified transversely oriented elements that mediated the effect of a local depolarization. Correlation of the inward spread of activation sites with the positioning of specific elements of the membrane system, the triads (2), the identification of the central elements of the triad as direct invaginations of the plasmalemma (3) (Figure 53.1A), and evidence for their continuity all across the fiber – hence the name transverse, T, tubules (Figure 53.1B) – firmly established the first step in excitation–contraction (EC) coupling.

Working from the other end, calcium was shown to be the intracellular transmitter that removes the troponin–tropomyosin inhibition of actomyosin interaction (4), and the muscle homogenate containing SR-derived vesicles was shown to be capable of actively taking up calcium ions through an ATP-dependent calcium pump (5). The ability of SR to lower Ca concentration to very low levels (6) made this organelle the necessary and sufficient agent in promoting relaxation.

Thus two major EC coupling concepts – Ca cycling by the SR and the link provided by T-tubules – were in the literature in the very early 1960s. This focused attention on the connection between T-tubules and SR at the triads, but the specific transmission step that allowed transduction of T-tubule depolarization into SR Ca release turned out to be very hard to elucidate and was not fully unraveled until recent times.

T-tubules Are Surface Invaginations; the SR Is an Internal Membrane System

T-tubules have a random, mostly longitudinal, disposition between the myofibrils during their initial formation but even at this stage they immediately form junctions with SR elements. The mature position of T-tubules within planes perpendicular to the fiber long axis (Figure 53.1A, B) is acquired gradually during the coordinated differentiation of myofibrils and membrane system. This reorientation takes up to a month in chick and mouse muscles and the association of the whole triad assembly with the appropriate myofibril location drives it, perhaps via ankyrin and the giant protein obscurin. However, longitudinal remnants of the T network are still present in the adult. The T-tubules actually carry an action potential in some but perhaps not all fibers, but a depolarization of the tubules rather than the action potential is a triggering event in EC coupling (7).

The initial description of the SR (2) correctly identified this organelle as a differentiated form of the

Muscle. DOI: http://dx.doi.org/10.1016/B978-0-12-381510-1.00053-3

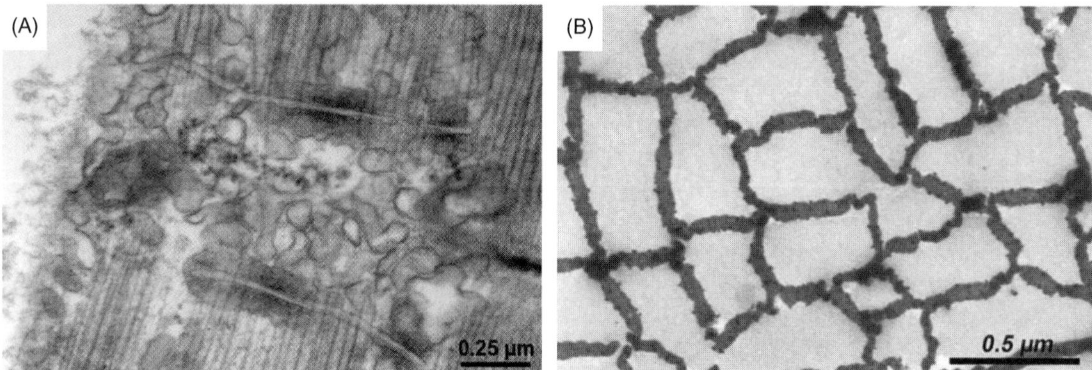

FIGURE 53.1 (A) The transverse (T) tubules (here overlaid in yellow) are invaginations of the surface membrane that penetrate transversely into the muscle fiber, carrying the electrical signal that initiates activation. The tubules establish close contacts with the sarcoplasmic reticulum (SR, in green), forming groups of three elements called triads. (B) T-tubules seen in a cross-section after the Golgi infiltration technique. This image establishes the continuity of the T-tubules network across the fiber and shows its sites of contact with the SR, where the tubules appear as flat ribbons.

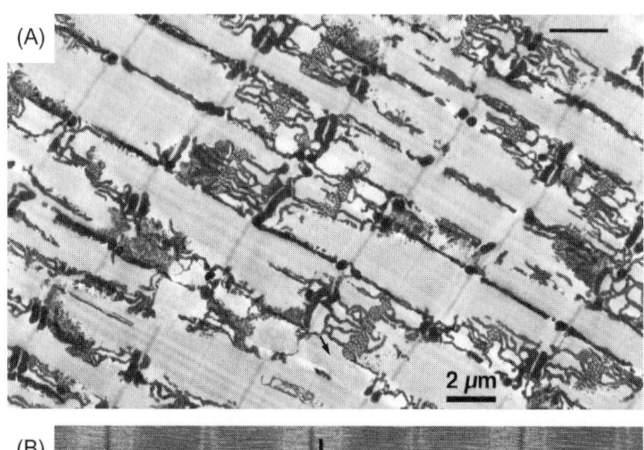

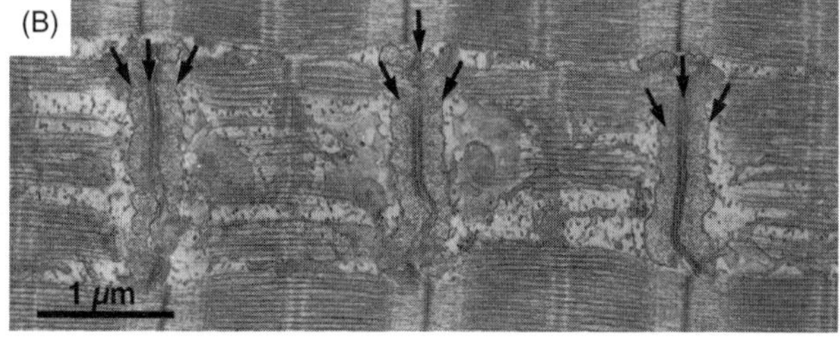

FIGURE 53.2 The SR, seen after Golgi "staining" (A) and in standard thin section (B), forms a complex, continuous network that surrounds the myofibrils. In these fibers from the frog the T-tubules (vertical arrows in B) are located at the Z-lines. The junctional domains of the SR (jSR, oblique arrows) are wide, contain calsequestrin and directly face the T-tubules. The triads are the sites of calcium release during muscle activation and thus they are also called calcium release units (CRUs).

ubiquitous endoplasmic reticulum (ER), characterized by its abundance and its precise positioning and relationship to the myofibrils (Figure 53.2). The SR is composed of elements that repeat longitudinally with a period equal to that of the sarcomere. In the case of frog muscle, shown in Figure 53.2, for example, the SR shows a network of longitudinal elements opposite the A band, connected to the two enlarged cisternae on either side of the Z-line. The T-tubules are located in the space between the two SR cisternae (Figure 53.2B) and the assembly of two SR and one T-tubule is called a triad. The SR, like the ER, is a totally internal membrane system that creates a segregated space: its lumen is not connected to either the cytoplasm or the extracellular space.

The SR appears to be divided into segments by the presence of T-tubules in triads. However, some longitudinal continuity, allowing equilibration of the luminal content through the length of the fiber, is provided by small connections that bypass the interruption introduced by the presence of the T network (arrow in Figure 53.2A). Thus the SR constitutes a reservoir of calcium whose content is equilibrated through the fiber.

Junctional SR and Junctional T-tubule Domains and Their Interaction at CRUs

By virtue of their architecture and molecular composition, both T-tubules and SR systems are divided into two domains that are functionally distinct, but in direct continuity with each other: the free and junctional domains. The junctional SR (jSR) domains, usually appearing as enlarged cisternae, face either the plasmalemma or the T-tubules and are linked to them within well-defined, apparently quite stable, junctions by virtue of "docking proteins", called junctophilins (type 1 and 2) (8–10). The free SR constitutes the rest of the SR and is dedicated to calcium reuptake. The T-tubules completely surround the myofibril and they in turn are composed of free T-tubules (fT) intercalated with short junctional (jT) segments. The latter face towards and are linked to the junctional SR domains. The SR–T-tubules and SR–plasmalemma junctions have different forms in different muscles and fibers. Triads, the most frequent configuration in adult skeletal

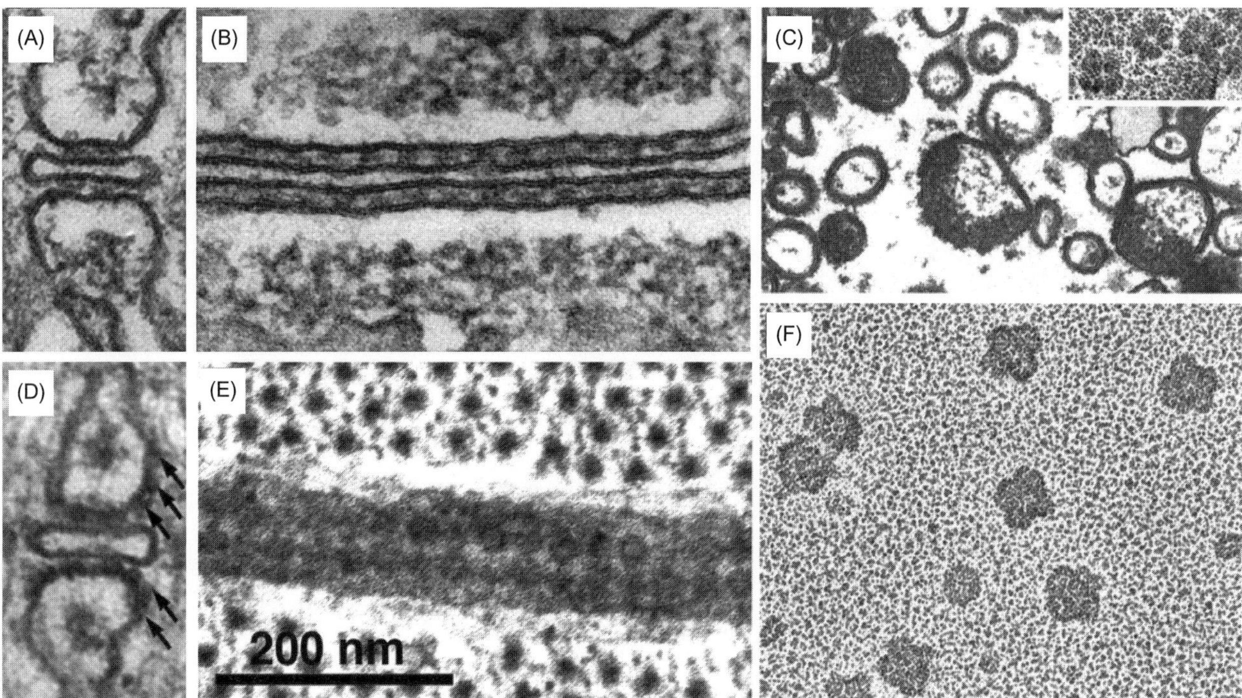

FIGURE 53.3 The jSR membrane of CRUs contains the SR calcium release channels or ryanodine receptors (RyR). The RyR's cytoplasmic domains appear as large projections (feet) that form two rows between the closely apposed jSR and T-tubule membranes (A and D). The rows are elongated (B) and they are clearly seen in a grazing view of the junction (E). Isolated jSR vesicles (C) show that RyRs belong to the SR membrane. The inset in (C) illustrates the four subunits of feet in situ that correspond to the structure of the purified RyR (F). In muscles that contain a high level of RyR type 3 in addition to the Type 1, the former is detected in a parajunctional position close to but not within the junctional gap between SR and T-tubules (arrows in D). All images are at the same magnification. (See references 11,12.)

muscle, are junctions between two jSR elements and a central T-tubule (Figures 53.2B, 53.3A and D). Dyads, formed by one SR and one T-tubule segment, are relatively infrequent in adult muscle, and are mostly found in slow fibers or in aging muscle. Peripheral couplings are junctions between a jSR domain and the plasmalemma that are initially formed during muscle differentiation and in most cases are lost in adult muscle. However, some muscle fibers retain peripheral couplings in parallel to triads in the differentiated state. All three types of SR junctions have the same molecular components and the same function: that of transducing the plasmalemma/T-tubule depolarization into a Ca release from the SR. On that basis these junctions are collectively named calcium release units or CRUs.

Molecular Composition of CRUs

The enlarged jSR cisternae (also called lateral sacs of the triads or terminal cisternae) have a very complex composition and novel proteins are currently still being discovered in them. Most of the jSR proteins are involved in calcium storage and calcium release.

Feet/ SR Calcium Release Channels/RyRs

The junctional gaps separating the two parallel membranes of SR and T-tubule/plasmalemma at CRUs are occupied by evenly spaced, large electron dense structures named "feet". In classical views of triads (Figure 53.3A and D) there are two feet on either side of the T-tubule. These are actually part of two parallel rows that are well seen in sections that cut along the length of the junctional gap (Figure 53.3B) or are the grazing to it (Figure 53.3E). The feet belong to the sarcoplasmic reticulum, as is readily demonstrated by examining a suspension of SR vesicles composing the "heavy microsomal" fraction from skeletal muscle (Figure 53.3C) (13). The vesicles have "feet" on their surface, and this is important, because vesicles from the same "heavy" fraction were shown to bind ryanodine with a high affinity (14) and to have, as important components, channels with a high permeability for calcium, the so-called SR calcium release channels (15). In shadow-cast images of the isolated heavy SR, the feet clearly display a tetrameric structure and their size can be quite well determined to be approximately 29 nm on the side (Figure 53.3C, inset). This structure and size allows an immediate identification

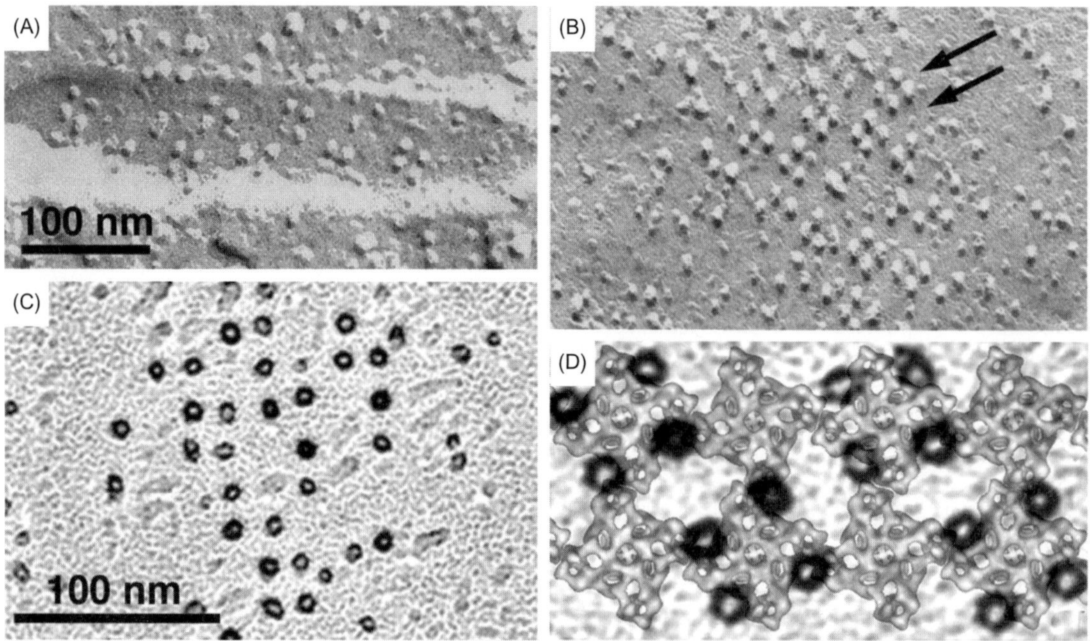

FIGURE 53.4 T-tubule (A) and plasmalemma (B) membranes facing arrays of junctional feet in CRUs contain arrays of DHPRs that are arranged into groups of four (tetrads). The positioning of tetrads is directly related to that of RyRs, so that when an array of rotary shadowed tetrads (C) is superimposed on an array of RyRs (D), the four components of the tetrads are precisely located relative to the four RyR subunits. This specific steric relationship supports a direct mechanical interaction between DHPR and RyR during excitation–contraction coupling (20,21).

of the heavy SR feet with the isolated and purified ryanodine receptor channels (RyR) that clearly have the same size and tetrameric structure (Figure 53.3F). RyRs are calcium channels with a large conductivity and they are the major sites of calcium release from the SR in skeletal muscle (16) The feet represent the large cytoplasmic domains of the ryanodine receptors, while the intramembrane, channel-forming domain is inserted in the jSR membrane. By virtue of their large cytoplasmic domains, ryanodine receptors completely bridge the gap between jSR and jT membranes, coming to very close proximity with the latter.

Skeletal muscles express two isoforms of RyRs: RyR1 and RyR3 in variable proportions, from 1:1 in frog and fish tail muscles, to 1:0.1 or 1:0 in some mammalian muscles. RyR1 is the channel directly involved in EC coupling by virtue of its interaction with DHPRs (see below), while RyR3 is likely to participate in EC coupling in a less direct manner. It is thus appropriate that RyR1 are located where they can directly interact with the components of T-tubules, while RyR3 are in an adjacent, but "parajunctional" position (Figure 53.3D) (17).

The content of RyR1s is fiber-type dependent. For example the number of "junctional feet" per μm^3 of fiber volume (excluding large areas of mitochondrial accumulation) is 230–300 in the superfast fibers of the toadfish swimbladder; 150–160 in fast twitch and 60 in slow twitch fibers of guinea pig (18,19).

L Type Calcium Channels and Voltage Sensing

The junctional segments of T-tubules in skeletal muscle are occupied by an identifiable set of intramembrane proteins with a highly specific disposition. Freeze-fractures of the jT membrane (Figure 53.4A) and of the plasmalemma at sites of peripheral couplings (Figure 53.4B) show clusters of large particles of homogenous size disposed in characteristic groupings of four particles occupying the corners of small squares. Each of these groupings (Figure 53.4A–B) is called a tetrad. Within jT profiles (Figure 53.4A), tetrads are arranged into two rows running parallel to the T-tubules' edges, but in alternate positions so that each tetrad in one row is opposite an empty space in the adjacent parallel row. The center-to-center distance between tetrads in each row is exactly double the center-to-center distance between the two rows of jSR feet (compare Figures 53.3E and 53.4A). Since the jT membrane overlies the two rows of feet, it appears that the tetrads overlay alternate feet. This is best apparent when the tetrad particles are rotary shadowed, bringing into evidence the precise orthogonal position of the particles in each tetrad (Figure 53.4C). After appropriate rotation, Figure 53.4C can be superimposed on an array of RyR profiles, to show that the four components of the tetrads assume a stereo-specific position relative to the four subunits of the feet/RyRs (Figure 53.4D), but that alternate RyRs are not associated with tetrads. At sites of peripheral couplings, the array of tetrads in the plasmalemma is large and comprises several repeated rows. However, here also it is possible to identify adjacent rows of tetrads that occupy alternate positioning, for example along the arrows in Figure 53.4B. So here also the tetrads are associated with alternate RyRs.

Immunolabeling for RyR and CaV1.1 (DHPR) confirms that both proteins are located at hot spots corresponding to the position of triads in the muscle fiber and of peripheral couplings in cultured myotubes.

The precise positioning of the four tetrad components relative to the four subunits of RyRs acquires a specific significance from the demonstration that the tetrad components are the L type calcium channels of T-tubules/plasmalemma. These channels are named CaV1.1, due to their function as voltage dependent channels, and also dihydropyridine receptors (DHPRs) due to the effect of these agents in their function. In dyspedic muscles lacking the main channel-forming α1 subunit of CaV1.1 the tetrads are absent, but they are reconstituted by expression of the appropriate cDNA (22). CaV1.1 have been identified as the voltage sensors of e-c coupling that is they are the components the T-tubules that respond to the change in membrane potential by affecting gating of the RyRs. RyRs in turn have a reciprocal interaction with CaV1.1, whose opening probability is dictated by an interaction with RyRs (21,23). This reciprocal interaction and the fact that skeletal muscle EC coupling does not require calcium permeation through CaV1.1 provide the best confirmation of the "mechanical hypothesis" of EC coupling (see Chapter 57). In cardiac muscle, the interaction between the equivalent components of CRUs (CaV1.2 and RyR2) is indirect, perhaps mediated by calcium ions, and the tetrad formation is absent.

T-tubule/SR interactions in a variety of fibers are matched to the requirements for EC coupling. The size of myofibrils affects the overall density of T-tubules: the difference is very obvious when one compares slow tonic to superfast fibers. In cases of smaller differences in contraction kinetics, such as in fast and slow twitch fibers of some mammals (cat, guinea pig), whose contraction times vary by a factor of 2, the overall density of T-tubules may be equal in the two types of fibers. However, jT segments occupy an approximately double percentage of the total lengths in fast than in slow fibers. Hence the double overall density of "feet" mentioned above is matched to a double overall content of CaV1.1 tetrads.

Co-localization of jSR Proteins: the SR as a Calcium Storage Compartment

Several proteins co-localize at the CRUs. RyRs, triadin, and junctin are in the jSR membrane calsequestrin of the jSR lumen. In electron micrographs, the lumen of the jSR is occupied by an extended gel of polymerized calsequestrin (CASQ, Figure 53.5), a high capacity, low affinity calcium binding protein that increases the SR capacitance for calcium storage while maintaining a relatively low free Ca concentration in the lumen. Fast twitch fibers express only type 1 CASQ, but slow twitch fibers also contain the cardiac type 2 isoform. Interestingly, mice carrying a null mutation for CASQ 1 are viable, despite a greatly decreased volume of the jSR cisternae in fast fibers and some evidence for impaired calcium handling (25). The male population has an additional extra sensitivity to heat and anesthetics resulting in sudden death (26). The effect of decreased luminal calcium buffering in the CASQ1 null mouse evidences the calcium dependence of CASQ's buffering power (27).

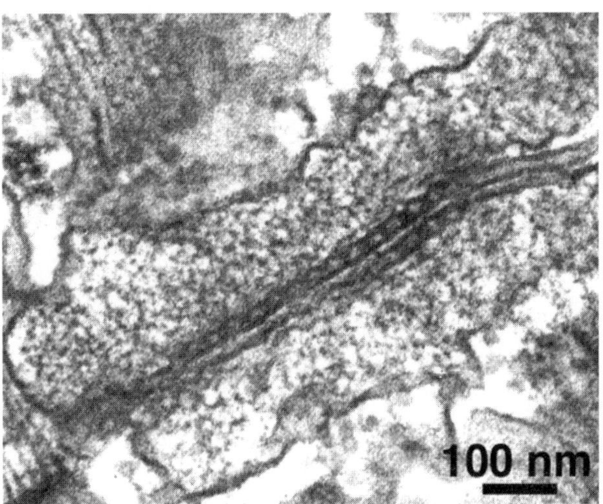

FIGURE 53.5 The jSR cisternae in CRUs are filled with a gel of long linear calsequestrin polymers randomly packed in the lumen, but showing evidence for grouping in proximity of the membrane occupied by RyRs (24).

Within the jSR lumen, the polymerized CASQ shows a complex structure that is consistent with a tight packing of long CASQ polymers that are randomly transected by the thin section (Figure 53.5). In proximity of the jSR membrane, particularly where feet are located, CASQ takes a fairly well-defined beaded appearance due to the presence of numerous small connections to the membrane. These have been traced to the presence of two other jSR proteins, triadin and junctin, that are known to be associated both with RyRs and with CASQ. Overexpression of triadin and junctin in cardiac muscle tightens the CASQ-membrane association (28), and lack of triadin in skeletal muscle reduces it (29). Lack of triadin affects the structure of triads in two ways. It induces a reorientation of the triads from transverse to longitudinal (29,30) an alteration that is also induced by lack of CASQ (25) and is frequent in pathological conditions (see below).

Muscle Relaxation: Free SR and the Calcium Pump

All SR surfaces that do not face directly towards T-tubules/plasmalemma are part of the free SR. This includes the lateral surface of triads as well as all the "longitudinal SR", a highly convoluted system of membranes with a large surface area that completely envelops the myofibrils. The free SR surface is at least 10-fold larger that the jSR surface facing T-tubules.

In skeletal muscle calcium is very effectively cycled within the muscle fiber, while exchanges between the cytoplasm and the extracellular spaces are functionally significant, but relatively small in magnitude (see Chapter 57). Essentially all the calcium that is released returns, in time, to the lumen of the SR through the function of the calcium ATPase or calcium pump, which constitutes 90% or more of the intrinsic membrane proteins in the free SR membrane.

The density of calcium ATPase in the SR is equal to that achieved in planar crystalline arrays. In freeze-fracture images of the SR cytoplasmic leaflet (Figure 53.6) the ATPase forms an uninterrupted carpet covering all visible SR membranes. Small protein-free lipid patches are only visible in the SR of slow twitch fibers. The freeze-fracture particles shown in Figure 53.6 actually represent small variable-size clusters of 2–6 molecules as shown by comparison of fractured SR membranes showing the intramembrane particles and freeze-dried SR tubules showing the ATPase tails on the cytoplasmic surface of the SR. On the basis of this type of image, it is estimated that the density of ATPase in the free SR membrane is $\sim 30{,}000/\mu m^2$. Combining this information with the morphometric measurements of SR surface area per fiber volume, the ATPase content in the myofibrillar areas of the fast toadfish swimbladder muscle is estimated to be $\sim 290{,}000/\mu m^3$, giving a ratio of ATPase to RyR of 1200–1800. Thus although calcium release at each twitch is not maximal in this sound-producing muscle, a large number of slow acting ATPase molecules are necessary to eventually mop up all the calcium that exits the SR via the highly conductive RyR channels.

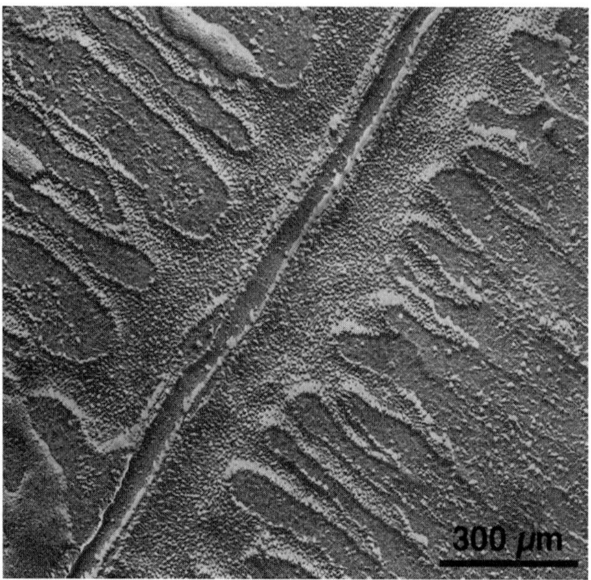

FIGURE 53.6 Freeze-fractures of free SR membranes. The numerous intramembrane particles covering the entire cytoplasmic leaflet of the fractured free SR represent small aggregates of 2–4 SERCA (CaATPase) molecules. The estimated density of molecules is ~30,000/μm2 of SR membrane (31).

A stunning series of crystal structures for the Ca-ATPase pump in nine different configurations of the pump cycle has been obtained (see 32,33 for reviews). From these images, a highly visual definition of the large molecular motions that transform the pumps' high calcium affinity cytoplasmic-facing site to a low affinity luminal through an occluded period has been derived, providing a compelling explanation of this complex pumping mechanism.

MITOCHONDRIA

Mitochondria occupy stereotyped positions relative to the myofibrils and to the membrane systems in skeletal muscle of mammals. However, it is also important to notice that the frequency, positioning and size of mitochondria differ quite significantly between muscle fibers of different functional types from the same organism and even more so between muscles from different organisms, particularly if one considers classes other than mammals.

In all mammalian muscle fibers there are two categories of mitochondria. One category is located within clusters at the fiber edge (not shown). The frequency of such clusters is highest in the slow twitch (type 1) fibers, lower in fast twitch oxidative (type IIA) fibers, and lowest in fast glycolytic fibers (type II B and IIX), particularly in larger mammals. Within the clusters the mitochondria profiles, when imaged in thin sections for electron microscopy, are mostly circular, indicating that the profiles belong to separate organelles. Mitochondria in the second category are located between the myofibrils and have two configurations. Some are fairly large cylindrical organelles that run longitudinally within small gaps separating myofibrils. The mitochondria adapt to the available space, being larger as they cross the I-Z-I level than where they run along the A band (Figure 53.7A). Elongated mitochondria of smaller diameter run transversely between the myofibrils closely surrounding them in a branching pattern at the level of the I band (Figure 53.7B). The longitudinal mitochondria can be

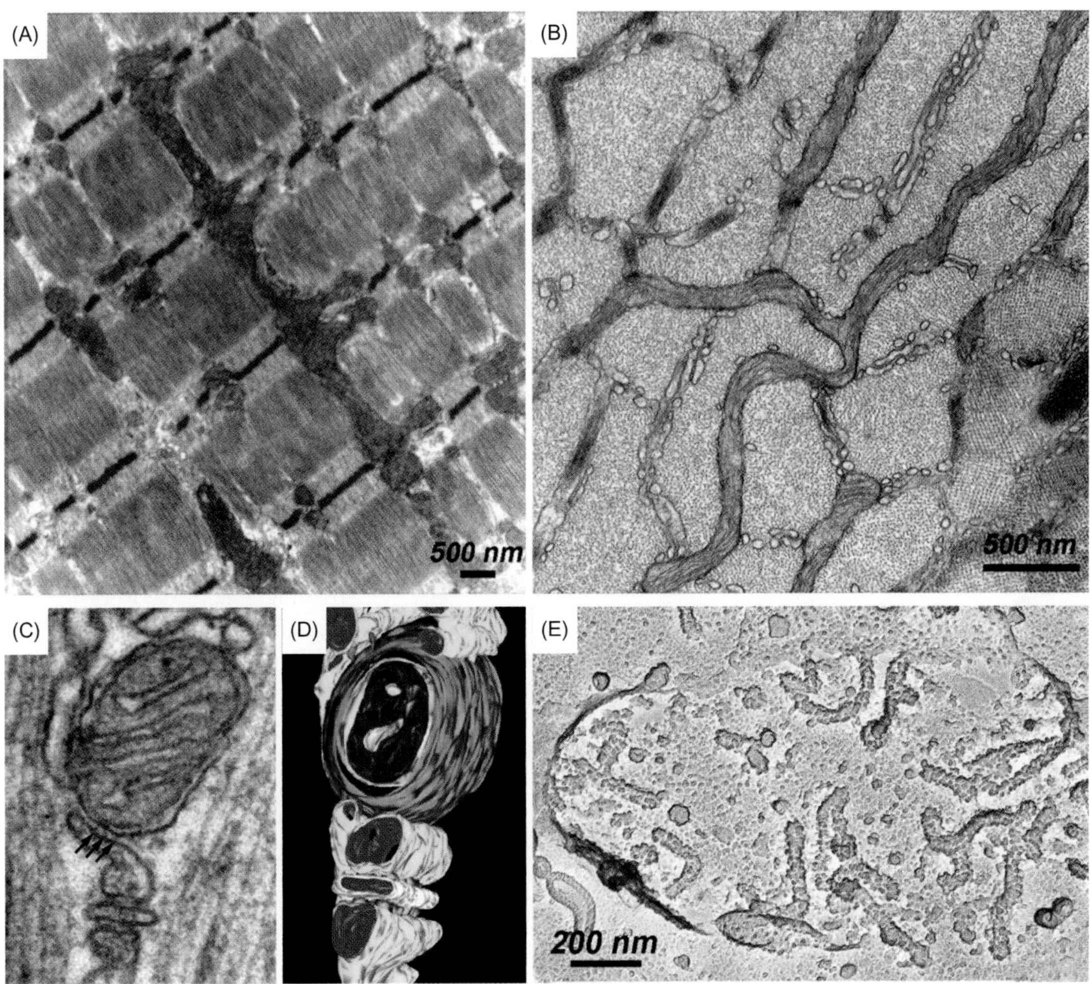

FIGURE 53.7 (A) Two dispositions of mitochondria in a mouse fiber. Two long mitochondria occupy a longitudinal slit between the myofibrils. Branches for the same mitochondria run transversely at the level of the I band. In a cross-section (B) the transverse mitochondrial branches run for long lengths. The transverse branches are closely apposed to triads, to which they are connected by numerous small tethers (C and D), the latter showing a 3D reconstruction of the SR-mitochondrion relationship from a tomogram (34). (E) Freeze-drying rotary shadowing image showing the cristae in an exploded mitochondrion.

occasionally followed without interruptions for the length of several sarcomeres. Additionally they are also seen to branch into transverse extensions at the I band level, thus continuing into the transversely located organelles. Combination of images such as shown in Figure 53.8(A, B), shows that skeletal muscle mitochondria are very extensive, although how far the continuity extends has not been determined.

In muscles from mammals, including human, the transverse branches of mitochondria have a very specific positioning: they closely follow the surface of the jSR sacs that are apposed to T-tubules in the triads. This apposition is more than casual: developmentally regulated specific tethering links between the jSR and mitochondria hold the two organelles together (Figure 53.7C,D) (36). The link is lost under pathological conditions and the mitochondria lose their specific positioning.

General principles regarding the functional significance of this disposition can be easily derived from a comparison of structural and functional observations. Mitochondria take up Ca^{2+}, but their contribution to skeletal muscle Ca^{2+} homeostasis under physiological conditions has been greatly debated given the fact that they have a low affinity for calcium. The concept of cellular microdomains (37) has come to the rescue in explaining how mitochondria can pick up calcium during skeletal (38) and cardiac (39,40) muscle contraction cycles. The idea is that if mitochondria are in close proximity to the calcium release sites, then for a brief period of time they will be exposed to a high calcium concentration and thus they will take up calcium. The mitochondria located in close proximity to the triads are in such position; those in peripheral clusters are not. Hence it can be shown that some mitochondria take up calcium during muscle

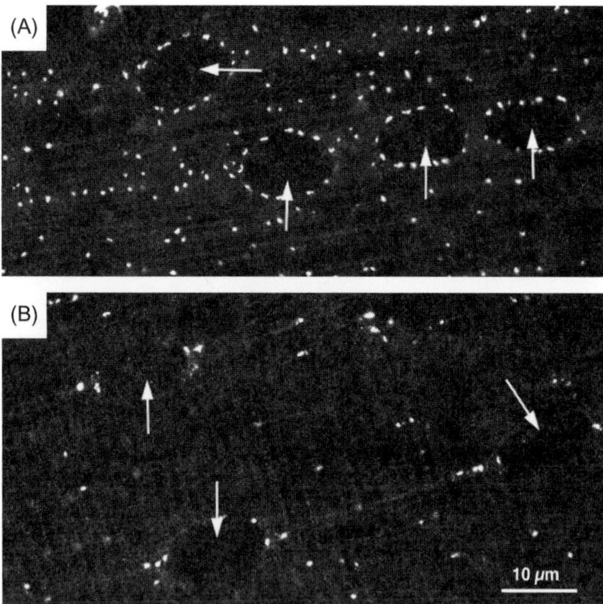

FIGURE 53.8 Distribution of Golgi complex elements detected by specific antibodies. In slow type I fibers of the soleus in rat (A) Golgi sites surround the nuclei (arrows) near the fiber surface. In fast and type IIB fibers of the tensor fasciae latae (B) Golgi sites are fewer and more scattered. (See reference 35). *(Courtesy of E. Ralston.)*

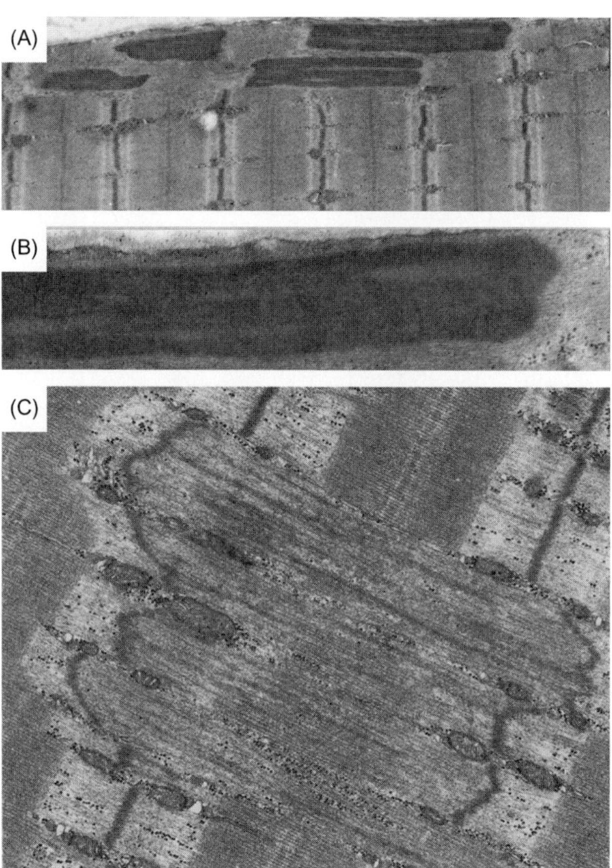

FIGURE 53.9 (A and B) Nemaline rods are elongated well-delimited regions of high electron density (from human congenital myopathy) (54). (C) Z-line streaming results in spread of Z-line components over the sarcomere and loss of structural organization (from human muscle with Kearns Sayre syndrome) (55,56).

activity, while others do not (41). It should be noted that while calcium uptake is of importance to the activation of the mitochondrial respiratory chains that are exposed to the internal matrix (Figure 53.7E), the total amount of calcium taken up by mitochondria is limited relative to that taken up by the SR. It is calculated that mitochondria take up approximately only 1% of the SR calcium uptake during a normal calcium transient even in cardiac muscle, with its high content of mitochondria and less efficient SR, although they integrate over time (42). Poisoning of mitochondria does slow down relaxation in skinned, mitochondria-rich skeletal muscle fibers stimulated by local application of calcium, presumably because in this case the mitochondria were allowed to take up a relatively high proportion of the applied calcium (43).

GOLGI AND ASSOCIATED ORGANELLES

Skeletal muscle cells maintain an extensive and highly differentiated membrane system and in addition they are actively secretory, being responsible for the production and secretion of numerous endocrine, autocrine, and bioactive factors (44). It is thus not surprising that muscle fibers have very extensive Golgi systems, the organelles responsible for "maturation" and trafficking of intrinsic membrane proteins and of secretary products. Golgi complexes of skeletal muscle are located in paranuclear areas and in other small portions of the cytoplasm that are not filled by myofibrils, Interestingly, immunolabeling for Golgi system protein markers reveals an unconventional distribution of multiple small organelles scattered in numerous sites rather than the more conventional single large complex (Figure 53.8). Additionally, the distribution of Golgi elements is strongly fiber-type-dependent (35,45,46). A very extensive microtubule network is related to Golgi distribution.

The SR of muscle fibers is a differentiated domain of the general ER and derives from it by proliferation and differentiation into specific domains dedicated to calcium handling, concurrent with the accumulation of a high density of SR-specific proteins, a decrease in housekeeping proteins and the association with the myofibrils and transverse tubules (47,48). The gradual differentiation starts in parallel with early myofibrillogenesis, with the early formation of CRUs at the fiber edge and later in the triads (49,50). Generic ER mostly remains located within small

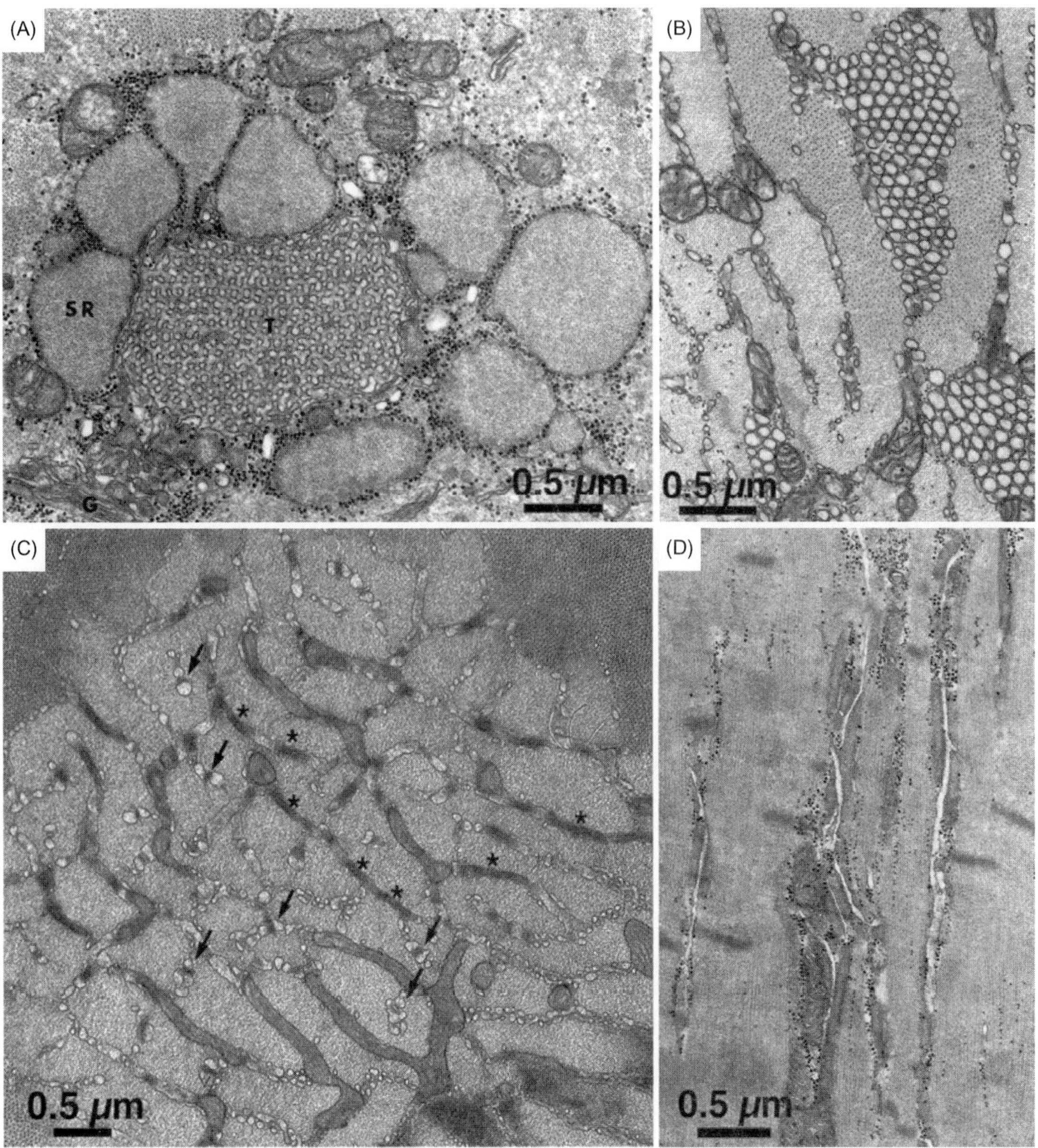

FIGURE 53.10 Alterations in T-tubules and SR dispositions. (A) A large 3D network of T-tubules (T) and enlarged of SR cisternae (SR) near a Golgi network in a muscle affected by polymyositis. (B) Aggregates of SR tubules in polymyositis. Similar aggregates are also seen in muscle fibers from the EDL of aging male mice (34). (C) Cross-section through a fiber of the mouse EDL in which many triads are oriented with their long axis in the longitudinal direction. Asterisks point to triads that have the standard transverse orientation and arrows to those that are longitudinally oriented. The triads maintain their positioning at the edges of the A band (34). (D) An unusual longitudinal position of T-tubules and triads in a case of botulism.

spaces in paranuclear positions, in association with the Golgi system, but general ER proteins are not excluded from the myofibrils-associated SR, demonstrating functional continuity within the entire endo-membrane system (51,52). Non-muscle cells also have some domains of the endoplasmic reticulum, the so-called calciosomes, that are basically equivalent to the SR in that they have calcium ATPase in the membrane and some calsequestrin (or calreticulin) in the lumen and thus are dedicated to calcium uptake (53). However, these domains are very small.

PATHOLOGY OF MYOFIBRILS AND MEMBRANE SYSTEMS

A number of structural alterations are common to aging, often resulting from accumulated effects of repeated low level attrition, and to a variety of pathological conditions.

Z Line Defects in Pathology

The Z-line is the most frequently affected component of the sarcomere under stress and pathological conditions but also in aging, probably because it is the element through which tension is transmitted along the myofibril and also because calcium-activated proteases specifically degrade Z-line proteins. Nemaline rods originate at Z disc and they basically represent an iteration of the Z-line architecture: they maintain the structural organization of Z-line, although extending it over large volumes (Figure 53.9A,B). When sectioned across, nemaline rods show a square lattice that is identical to that found in Z-lines under certain conditions and in longitudinal sections that have a periodicity of 14–20 nm also reminiscent of that found in wide Z-lines. A second very common reaction of Z-lines to a variety of myopathies, to excessive accumulation of cytoplasmic calcium, as well as to denervation, to eccentric contractions, and to aging is an initial streaming of Z-line material away from the standard Z-line location, followed by a gradual focal myofibrillar degeneration and disappearance of cell organelles (SR, T-tubules, mitochondria). Z-line streaming and its consequences may affect very small regions, a whole sarcomere (Figure 53.9C), or several sarcomeres and myofibrils. Alterations initiated by Z-line streaming probably lead to the development of featureless cores in central core diseases.

Defects of the Membrane Systems

Both T-tubules and SR respond to pathological stimuli (including those inherent with aging) by changing their frequency and configuration. Proliferating T-tubules often aggregate into complex honeycomb aggregates with a characteristic three-dimensional disposition during normal muscle differentiation. Normally, the honeycombs disappear in time, while a generic overall rearrangement of the T network from random to transverse occurs. This trend is reversed under certain pathological conditions, so that T aggregates become relatively frequent (Figure 53.10A) and the tubules acquire a disordered disposition. A second, frequent ultrastructural response is an enlargement of the longitudinal SR tubules, with an accumulation of an electron-dense content in the lumen that resembles, and most likely is, calsequestrin (Figure 53.10A). Excess SR also accumulates into "tubular aggregates" (Figure 53.10B), where SR tubules acquire an unusual straight configuration. Finally, the orientation of triads relative to the myofibrils may be altered from transverse to longitudinal, in two different configurations. In one case (Figure 53.10C) the T-tubules retain their appropriate position at the A–I junction level, but while the long axes of some triads have the appropriate transverse orientation, others are longitudinal. This has been detected during differentiation (50), as an early response to denervation (57,58) as a result of damage in eccentric contractions (59) as well as in the absence of calsequestrin (25). A second configuration occurs over a short period of time during differentiation and is also found in some pathological responses. In this case the overall T-tubule disposition is longitudinal and so are the triads' axes (Figure 53.10D).

ACKNOWLEDGMENTS

Supported by NIH RO1 HL48093 to C.F.A. and by NIH R01 NS6277 and a Research Grant from the Muscular Dystrophy Association to A.G.E.

REFERENCES

1. Huxley AF, Taylor RE. Local activation of striated muscle fibres. *J Physiol* 1958;**144**:426–41.
2. Porter KR, Palade GE. Studies on the endoplasmic reticulum. III. Its form and distribution in striated muscle cells. *J Biophys Biochem Cytol* 1957;**3**:269–300.
3. Franzini-Armstrong C, Porter KR. Sarcolemmal invaginations constituting the T system in fish muscle fibers. *J Cell Biol* 1964;**22**:675–96.
4. Weber A. On the role of calcium in the activity of adenosine 5'-triphosphate hydrolysis by actomyosin. *J Biol Chem* 1959; **234**:2764–9.
5. Ebashi S, Lipmann F. Adenosine triphosphate-linked concentration of calcium ions in a particulate fraction of rabbit muscle. *J Cell Biol* 1962;**14**:389–400.
6. Weber A, Herz R, Reiss I. On the mechanism of the relaxing effect of fragmented sarcoplasmic reticulum. *J Gen Physiol* 1963;**46**:679–702.
7. Costantin LL. Contractile activation in skeletal muscle. *Prog Biophys Mol Biol* 1975;**29**:197–224.
8. Ito K, Komazaki S, Sasamoto K, Yoshida M, Nishi M, Kitamura K. Deficiency of triad junction and contraction in mutant skeletal muscle lacking junctophilin type 1. *J Cell Biol* 2001;**154**:1059–67.
9. Komazaki S, Ito K, Takeshima H, Nakamura H. Deficiency of triad formation in developing skeletal muscle cells lacking junctophilin type 1. *FEBS Lett* 2002;**524**:225–9.
10. Takeshima H, Komazaki S, Nishi M, Iino M, Kangawa K. Junctophilins: a novel family of junctional membrane complex proteins. *Mol Cell* 2000;**6**:11–22.
11. Ferguson DG, Schwartz HW, Franzini-Armstrong C. Subunit structure of junctional feet in triads of skeletal muscle: a freeze-drying, rotary-shadowing study. *J Cell Biol* 1984;**99**:1735–42.
12. Franzini-Armstrong C, Ferguson DG. Density and disposition of Ca^{2+}-ATPase in sarcoplasmic reticulum membrane as determined by shadowing techniques. *Biophys J* 1985;**48**:607–15.
13. Campbell KP, Franzini-Armstrong C, Shamoo AE. Further characterization of light and heavy sarcoplasmic reticulum vesicles. Identification of the "sarcoplasmic reticulum feet" associated with heavy sarcoplasmic reticulum vesicles. *Biochim Biophys Acta* 1980;**602**:97–116.

14. Pessah IN, Waterhouse AL, Casida JE. The calcium-ryanodine receptor complex of skeletal and cardiac muscle. *Biochem Biophys Res Commun* 1985;**128**:449–56.
15. Smith JS, Coronado R, Meissner G. Single channel measurements of the calcium release channel from skeletal muscle sarcoplasmic reticulum. Activation by Ca^{2+} and ATP and modulation by Mg^{2+}. *J Gen Physiol* 1986;**88**:573–88.
16. Lai FA, Meissner G. The muscle ryanodine receptor and its intrinsic Ca^{2+} channel activity. *J Bioenergetics Biomembranes* 1989;**21**:227–46.
17. Felder E, Franzini-Armstrong C. Type 3 ryanodine receptors of skeletal muscle are segregated in a parajunctional position. *Proc Natl Acad Sci USA* 2002;**99**:1695–700.
18. Appelt D, Shen V, Franzini-Armstrong C. Quantitation of Ca ATPase, feet and mitochondria in superfast muscle fibres from the toadfish, *Opsanus tau*. *J Muscle Res Cell Motil* 1991;**12**: 543–52.
19. Franzini-Armstrong C, Ferguson DG, Champ C. Discrimination between fast- and slow-twitch fibres of guinea pig skeletal muscle using the relative surface density of junctional transverse tubule membrane. *J Muscle Res Cell Motil* 1988;**9**:403–14.
20. Block BA, Imagawa T, Campbell KP, Franzini-Armstrong C. Structural evidence for direct interaction between the molecular components of the transverse tubule/sarcoplasmic reticulum junction in skeletal muscle. *J Cell Biol* 1988;**107**:2587–600.
21. Paolini C, Fessenden JD, Pessah IN, Franzini-Armstrong C. Evidence for conformational coupling between two calcium channels. *Proc Natl Acad Sci USA* 2004;**101**:12748–52.
22. Takekura H, Bennett L, Tanabe T, Beam KG, Franzini-Armstrong C. Restoration of junctional tetrads in dysgenic myotubes by dihydropyridine receptor cDNA. *Biophys J* 1994;**67**:793–803.
23. Nakai J, Dirksen RT, Nguyen HT, Pessah IN, Beam KG, Allen PD. Enhanced dihydropyridine receptor channel activity in the presence of ryanodine receptor. *Nature* 1996;**380**:72–5.
24. Franzini-Armstrong C, Kenney LJ, Varriano-Marston E. The structure of calsequestrin in triads of vertebrate skeletal muscle: a deep-etch study. *J Cell Biol* 1987;**105**:49–56.
25. Paolini C, Quarta M, Nori A, Boncompagni S, Canato M, Volpe P, et al. Reorganized stores and impaired calcium handling in skeletal muscle of mice lacking calsequestrin-1. *J Physiol* 2007;**583**:767–84.
26. Dainese M, Quarta M, Lyfenko AD, Paolini C, Canato M, Reggiani C, et al. Anesthetic- and heat-induced sudden death in calsequestrin-1-knockout mice. *FASEB J* 2009;**23**:1710–20.
27. Royer L, Sztretye M, Manno C, Pouvreau S, Zhou J, Knollmann BC, et al. Paradoxical buffering of calcium by calsequestrin demonstrated for the calcium store of skeletal muscle. *J Gen Physiol* 2010;**136**:325–38.
28. Zhang L, Franzini-Armstrong C, Ramesh V, Jones LR. Structural alterations in cardiac calcium release units resulting from overexpression of junctin. *J Mol Cell Cardiol* 2001;**33**:233–47.
29. Oddoux S, Brocard J, Schweitzer A, Szentesi P, Giannesini B, Faure J, et al. Triadin deletion induces impaired skeletal muscle function. *J Biol Chem* 2009;**284**:34918–29.
30. Shen X, Franzini-Armstrong C, Lopez JR, Jones LR, Kobayashi YM, Wang Y, et al. Triadins modulate intracellular Ca(2+) homeostasis but are not essential for excitation-contraction coupling in skeletal muscle. *J Biol Chem* 2007;**282**:37864–74.
31. Ferguson DG, Franzini-Armstrong C, Castellani L, Hardwicke PM, Kenney LJ. Ordered arrays of Ca^{2+}-ATPase on the cytoplasmic surface of isolated sarcoplasmic reticulum. *Biophys J* 1985;**48**:597–605.
32. Toyoshima C. Structural aspects of ion pumping by Ca^{2+}-ATPase of sarcoplasmic reticulum. *Arch Biochem Biophys* 2008;**476**:3–11.
33. Toyoshima C. How Ca^{2+}-ATPase pumps ions across the sarcoplasmic reticulum membrane. *Biochim Biophys Acta* 2009;**1793**:941–6.
34. Boncompagni S, Protasi F, Franzini-Armstrong C. Sequential stages in the age-dependent gradual formation and accumulation of tubular aggregates in fast twitch muscle fibers: SERCA and calsequestrin involvement. Age (Dordr). ePub ahead of print, February 12, 2011, PMID: 21318331.
35. Ralston E, Lu Z, Ploug T. The organization of the Golgi complex and microtubules in skeletal muscle is fiber type-dependent. *J Neurosci* 1999;**19**:10694–705.
36. Boncompagni S, Rossi AE, Micaroni M, Beznoussenko GV, Polishchuk RS, Dirksen RT, et al. Mitochondria are linked to calcium stores in striated muscle by developmentally regulated tethering structures. *Mol Biol Cell* 2009;**20**:1058–67.
37. Rizzuto R, Pozzan T. Microdomains of intracellular Ca^{2+}: molecular determinants and functional consequences. *Physiol Rev* 2006;**86**:369–408.
38. Rudolf R, Mongillo M, Magalhaes PJ, Pozzan T. In vivo monitoring of Ca(2 +) uptake into mitochondria of mouse skeletal muscle during contraction. *J Cell Biol* 2004;**166**:527–36.
39. Andrienko TN, Picht E, Bers DM. Mitochondrial free calcium regulation during sarcoplasmic reticulum calcium release in rat cardiac myocytes. *J Mol Cell Cardiol* 2009;**46**:1027–36.
40. Robert V, Gurlini P, Tosello V, Nagai T, Miyawaki A, Di Lisa F, et al. Beat-to-beat oscillations of mitochondrial [Ca^{2+}] in cardiac cells. *EMBO J* 2001;**20**:4998–5007.
41. Shkryl VM, Shirokova N. Transfer and tunneling of Ca^{2+} from sarcoplasmic reticulum to mitochondria in skeletal muscle. *J Biol Chem* 2006;**281**:1547–54.
42. Trollinger DR, Cascio WE, Lemasters JJ. Mitochondrial calcium transients in adult rabbit cardiac myocytes: inhibition by ruthenium red and artifacts caused by lysosomal loading of Ca(2 +)-indicating fluorophores. *Biophys J* 2000;**79**:39–50.
43. Gillis JM. Inhibition of mitochondrial calcium uptake slows down relaxation in mitochondria-rich skeletal muscles. *J Muscle Res Cell Motil* 1997;**18**:473–83.
44. Vult von Steyern F, Kanje M, Tagerud S. Protein secretion from mouse skeletal muscle: coupling of increased exocytotic and endocytotic activities in denervated muscle. *Cell Tissue Res* 1993;**274**:49–56.
45. Ralston E. Changes in architecture of the Golgi complex and other subcellular organelles during myogenesis. *J Cell Biol* 1993; **120**:399–409.
46. Ralston E, Ploug T, Kalhovde J, Lomo T. Golgi complex, endoplasmic reticulum exit sites, and microtubules in skeletal muscle fibers are organized by patterned activity. *J Neurosci* 2001; **21**:875–83.
47. Villa A, Podini P, Nori A, Panzeri MC, Martini A, Meldolesi J, et al. The endoplasmic reticulum-sarcoplasmic reticulum connection. II. Postnatal differentiation of the sarcoplasmic reticulum in skeletal muscle fibers. *Exp Cell Res* 1993;**209**:140–8.

48. Volpe P, Villa A, Podini P, Martini A, Nori A, Panzeri MC, et al. The endoplasmic reticulum-sarcoplasmic reticulum connection: distribution of endoplasmic reticulum markers in the sarcoplasmic reticulum of skeletal muscle fibers. *Proc Natl Acad Sci USA* 1992;**89**:6142–6.
49. Flucher BE, Takekura H, Franzini-Armstrong C. Development of the excitation-contraction coupling apparatus in skeletal muscle: association of sarcoplasmic reticulum and transverse tubules with myofibrils. *Dev Biol* 1993;**160**:135–47.
50. Takekura H, Sun X, Franzini-Armstrong C. Development of the excitation–contraction coupling apparatus in skeletal muscle: peripheral and internal calcium release units are formed sequentially. *J Muscle Res Cell Motil* 1994;**15**:102–18.
51. Kaisto T, Metsikko K. Distribution of the endoplasmic reticulum and its relationship with the sarcoplasmic reticulum in skeletal myofibers. *Exp Cell Res* 2003;**289**:47–57.
52. Nori A, Bortoloso E, Frasson F, Valle G, Volpe P. Vesicle budding from endoplasmic reticulum is involved in calsequestrin routing to sarcoplasmic reticulum of skeletal muscles. *Biochem J* 2004;**379**:505–12.
53. Treves S, De Mattei M, Landfredi M, Villa A, Green NM, MacLennan DH, et al. Calreticulin is a candidate for a calsequestrin-like function in Ca2(+)-storage compartments (calciosomes) of liver and brain. *Biochem J* 1990;**271**:473–80.
54. Engel AG, Gomez MR. Nemaline (Z disk) myopathy: observations on the origin, structure, and solubility properties of the nemaline structures. *J Neuropathol Exp Neurol* 1967;**26**:601–19.
55. Banker BQ, Engel AG. Basic reactions of muscle. In: Engel AG, Franzini-Armstrong C, editors. *Myology*, vol. 1. 2nd ed. New York: McGraw Hill; 2004. p. 691–748.
56. Engel AG. Ultrastructural changes in diseased muscle. In: Engel AG, Franzini-Armstrong C, editors. *Myology*, vol 1. 2nd ed. New York: McGraw Hill; 2004. p. 889–1017.
57. Takekura H, Tamaki H, Nishizawa T, Kasuga N. Plasticity of the transverse tubules following denervation and subsequent reinnervation in rat slow and fast muscle fibres. *J Muscle Res Cell Motil* 2003;**24**:439–51.
58. Tomori K, Ohta Y, Nishizawa T, Tamaki H, Takekura H. Low-intensity electrical stimulation ameliorates disruption of transverse tubules and neuromuscular junctional architecture in denervated rat skeletal muscle fibers. *J Muscle Res Cell Motil* 2010;**31**: 195–205.
59. Takekura H, Fujinami N, Nishizawa T, Ogasawara H, Kasuga N. Eccentric exercise-induced morphological changes in the membrane systems involved in excitation–contraction coupling in rat skeletal muscle. *J Physiol* 2001;**533**:571–83.

Chapter 54

The Vertebrate Neuromuscular Junction

Young il Lee and Wesley J. Thompson
Section of Molecular Cell and Developmental Biology, School of Biological Sciences, University of Texas, Austin, TX

The common name given to the connection that muscle fibers receive from the central nervous system is "neuromuscular junction" (NMJ). This is the site where action potentials generated in motor neurons in the central nervous system result in the production of action potentials in the skeletal muscle fibers. The muscle fiber action potentials then trigger the calcium signals coordinated along the entire muscle fiber that result in fiber contraction. Because of its peripheral location (easy access), large size (it dwarfs CNS interneuronal synapses in size), ease of functional assay through the twitches that result from nerve stimulation and the early identification of the transmitter (acetylcholine or ACh) along with pharmacological agents that modulate transmission, the NMJ became an object for much early study. These studies have resulted in an astounding portion of our knowledge of synapses in general, and yielded information that is fundamental in neurobiology today. Some of these fundamental contributions are listed below. Some, but not all, of the topics in the list are treated briefly below. The reader is referred in each case to a review that treats each in greater detail.

Substantial contributions obtained by study of the NMJ:

1. the nature of chemical synaptic transmission across a synapse (1);
2. basic pharmacology of synaptic transmission (2);
3. the vesicular mechanisms of transmitter release (the quantal hypothesis) (3);
4. mechanisms of vesicle recycling (4);
5. the principle of numerical matching of projecting neuronal population to target population through the target-dependent cell death (5);
6. principle of overconnection during initial projections of axons in development and elimination of initial connections, i.e. "synapse elimination" (6);
7. principles of selective axon guidance that insure the motor neurons reach the correct target (7);
8. the clustering of postsynaptic receptors at synapses (8);
9. the importance of activity in shaping the properties of the synapses and the muscle (9).

This chapter will provide some fundamental background information and will attempt to illustrate some discoveries that continue to provide unexpected insights into this critical component of muscle biology.

THE STRUCTURE OF THE JUNCTION

The NMJ is commonly located near the center of each muscle fiber (see cartoon in Figure 54.1). With few exceptions (some fibers in the extraocular eye muscles being one), there is only one per fiber. The motor axons that enter the muscle usually run as a bundle through the center of the muscle. Branches emerge from this nerve and approach the contact area on each fiber. As a result there is a "band" of junctions that commonly lies across the center of the muscle (Figure 54.1). The motor axons in each such band come from a discrete subset of neurons in the spinal cord, a so-called "motor pool" whose cell bodies are located in a crude topographic map relative to the muscles. The crudeness of the map is shown by the intermixture of motor neurons innervating different muscles. Each motor neuron in a given motor pool branches several times in the muscle and there captures the exclusive innervation of a set of fibers (Figure 54.1). These fibers and their innervating motor neuron constitute a "motor unit". Given that each NMJ is designed to transmit faithfully across the synapse (see below), this means that each action potential in the motor neuron evokes a contraction in the fibers in its motor unit. Since these fibers are in parallel, their tensions sum. Gradation in force production by a muscle can be achieved by the number of simultaneously active motor neurons, as will be discussed again below.

The NMJ can be easily visualized these days by light microscopy, especially in mice where transgenic expression of the different spectral variants of fluorescent proteins can be used to pre-label components of the junction (10). Such labeling with cytoplasmic fluorescent proteins is illustrated in Figure 54.2. A promoter active in motor neurons has been used to express a blue fluorescent

Muscle. DOI: http://dx.doi.org/10.1016/B978-0-12-381510-1.00054-5

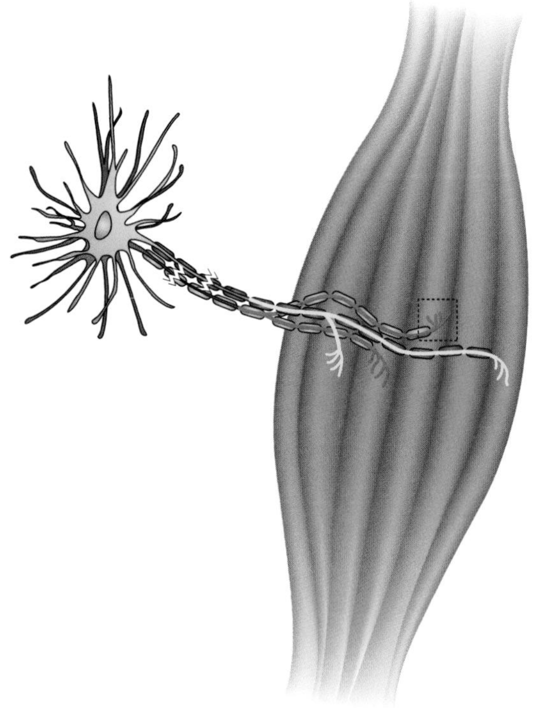

FIGURE 54.1 Cartoon illustration of muscle innervation. Shown for simplification are two motor neurons in the spinal cord, their peripheral axons, and only two nerve terminals for each. The terminals lie in a band across the center of the muscle. There is only one terminal per fiber. Each motor neuron and the fibers it innervates is a motor unit. The boxed area indicates the NMJ. Light micrographs of such a NMJ are shown in Figure 54.2.

protein that is present even in the distal axons and portrays the terminal arbor. On the surface of this one muscle fiber within its NMJ, this axon divides into a number of branches that are apposed to the muscle surface. These processes actually occupy a slight depression in the muscle surface known as the "synaptic gutter". A promoter active in Schwann cells that drives expression of a green fluorescent protein was used in the case in Figure 54.2 to label Schwann cells. These cells, a non-myelinating variety of the same cells that myelinate the axon as it exits the spinal cord and approaches the muscle and the muscle fiber, have cell bodies above the junction itself and extend processes that cover the nerve terminal (11). The processes of these Schwann cells are always associated with the nerve terminal except for processes that connect to the cell body and occasional processes that run without a terminal branch between synaptic gutters. In electron micrographs (see below), these Schwann cells are seen to cover the nerve terminal almost completely and to be more closely associated with the terminal than the terminal is with the muscle fiber. We will have more to say about the Schwann cells and their role at the junction below.

The labeling of the junction in Figure 54.2 also illustrates the location of the acetylcholine receptors (AChR). These ligand-gated ion channels are transmembrane proteins in the muscle fiber membrane. They bind the acetylcholine (ACh) released from the nerve terminal. They can be labeled with a snake venom component named alpha-bungarotoxin (Btx) conjugated to a fluorochrome (12). Btx competes with ACh for sites on AChR and binds to these receptors in an essentially irreversible manner, blocking transmission. This toxin has been of enormous benefit to the community of scientists studying the NMJ, enabling study of the molecular and cell biology of this receptor. In Figure 54.2, rhodamine-conjugated Btx is used to label AChR. AChR are distributed so that they lie right beneath the nerve terminal. This concentration of receptors (more than 1,000-fold greater than outside the synapse) has intrigued neuroscientists for some time. It clearly is due to the presence of the nerve, as the receptors appear in muscle membrane outside the junction following denervation (13) (creating so-called "denervation hypersensitivity", see below). A careful examination of the pattern of labeling with the rhodamine-bungarotoxin reveals that the labeling is in stripes. These stripes are a consequence of the folding of the muscle membrane beneath the nerve terminal within the synaptic gutter (14). These folds of membrane, called "postsynaptic folds" or "secondary folds" reach into the muscle cytoplasm (the primary fold being the synaptic gutter itself).

Still another snake toxin, fasciculin-2, binds to and inhibits an enzyme located at the synaptic site called acetylcholine esterase (AChE) (15). Like bungarotoxin, fasciculin-2 can be conjugated to a fluorochrome and made into a fluorescent probe for this component of the junction (Figure 54.2). AChE breaks down the ACh released from the nerve terminal into acetate and choline, terminating the ability of this ACh to bind to and activate AChR. The AChE ensures that the released ACh has a short lifetime at the synapse and provides only a brief activation of the AChR. The AChE is located in the synaptic gutter between the nerve terminal and the muscle fiber. It is synthesized largely by the muscle fiber and becomes concentrated at the synapse bound to collagen components of the "synaptic basal lamina", a specialized protein matrix that exists between the nerve terminal and the muscle fiber and extends down into the depths of the secondary folds (16).

Still another fluorescent label, DAPI was applied to the preparation in Figure 54.2. This shows the location of nuclei present at the synapse. Some of these are those present in the cell bodies of the SCs. Some are fibroblasts that are known to be present at the junction (17). But many of these nuclei are myonuclei. These synaptic nuclei or "sole plate nuclei" are specialized in their transcriptional program (18). Many genes transcribed here are

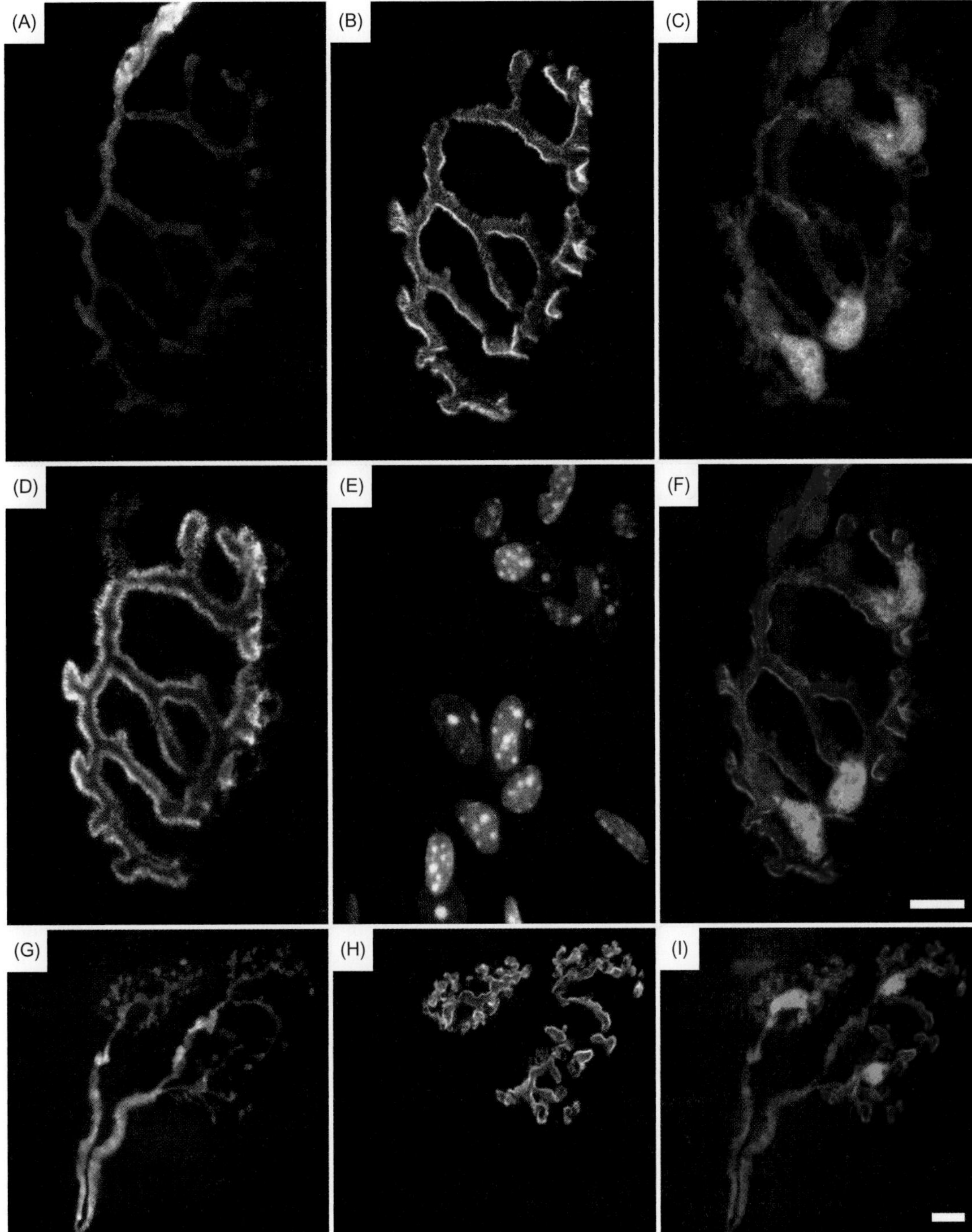

FIGURE 54.2 Light micrographs of a normal young adult NMJ (A–F) and an aged (22-month-old) NMJ, both from the mouse sternomastoid muscle. (A) shows fluorescent protein (CFP) expression in the motor neuron; (B) labeling of AChR with rhodamine-bungarotoxin; (C) fluorescent protein (GFP) expression in Schwann cells; (D) labeling of AChE with Alexa647-fasciculin-2; (E) label of nuclei with DAPI; (F) colored superposition of terminal (blue), Schwann cells (green), and AChR (red); G shows fluorescent protein (CFP) in the motor neuron, (H) labeling of AChR with rhodamine-bungarotoxin, (I) colored superposition with the colors as in (F). The junction in the aged animal is fragmented and the nerve terminal varicose. Scale bars = 10 μm in each case.

transcribed poorly (if at all) in other nuclei in the muscle. For example, the genes for the AChR are transcribed here. This so-called "synapse-specific gene expression" and how it is encoded is critical to understanding the specializations at the synapse. This transcription is a partial explanation for the concentration of certain components at the synapse. It will be a subject for some of the discourse below.

There are, of course, other crucial molecular components that are known to be present at the NMJ but are not shown in Figure 54.2. Some of these will come up in the discussion below, but one is important for a discussion of synaptic transmission. Use of iodinated Btx and autoradiography in electron microscopy shows that AChR are concentrated at the top of the folds where the membrane is nearest the site of the release of ACh (19). Another component, voltage-activated Na channels, are concentrated at the bottom of these folds along with anchoring proteins, giving this membrane a high sensitivity to depolarization (20). Thus, the depolarization of the muscle fiber membrane evoked by the ACh-mediated opening of the AChR can act on concentrated Na channels to bring the muscle fiber membrane to threshold. This arrangement of ion channels at the NMJ is designed for efficient transfer of activity in the nerve terminal to action potential activity in the muscle fiber. In fact, the "safety factor", i.e. the amount the depolarization exceeds threshold for a muscle fiber action potential, is such that about 70% of AChR can be blocked and the junction will still transmit (21).

THE ULTRASTRUCTURE OF THE JUNCTION

The NMJ was one of the earliest synapses to fall under the scrutiny of the electron microscope (22). Synaptic vesicles were first encountered at this site. An ultrathin section through the junction stained with osmium and lead citrate is shown in Figure 54.3. This micrograph shows a slice through one of the terminal branches and its apposition to the muscle surface. The nerve terminal, filled with mitochondria and synaptic vesicles lies within the synaptic gutter. Some of the synaptic vesicles in the terminal occur in clumps docked on the membrane facing the muscle fiber. These so-called "active zones" are the sites of fusion of vesicles with this terminal membrane resulting in the dumping of the vesicular contents into the extracellular space between the terminal and muscle known as the synaptic cleft. Within the synaptic cleft is the basal lamina. Atop the nerve terminal and closely apposed to it sits the processes of the Schwann cells, very tightly apposed to the nerve terminal itself.

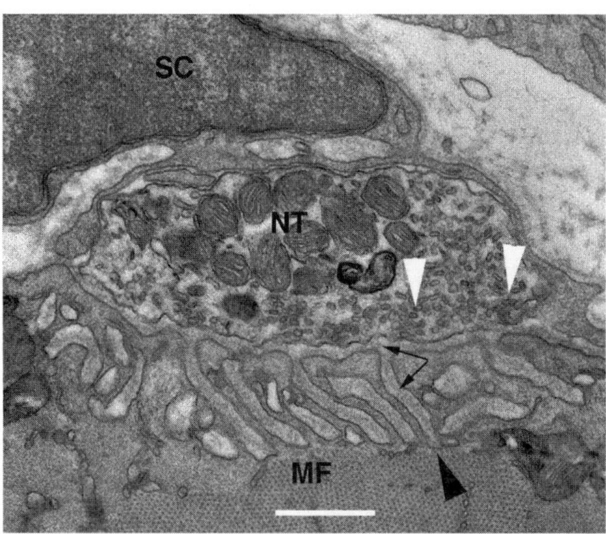

FIGURE 54.3 Transmission electron micrograph of a section through one of the terminal branches at a mouse NMJ. The nerve terminal (NT) lies in a "synaptic gutter" in the surface of the muscle fiber (MF). The NT is covered by a Schwann cell. White arrowheads indicate active zones. Black arrowhead indicates a secondary fold. Smaller black arrows indicate the basal lamina. Scale bar = 500 nm.

CLUSTERING OF AChR AT THE SYNAPSE

The high density of receptors underneath the junction (and their sparseness elsewhere on the muscle fiber membrane) has fascinated scientists investigating the NMJ for a number of years. How is this accumulation achieved? A beautiful set of simple, compelling experiments led to the discovery that molecules deposited in the basal lamina at the synapse (the "synaptic basal lamina") specify the accumulation of high densities of receptors. These studies led ultimately to the identification of the protein agrin (23). A specific splice form produced by motor neurons and deposited into the synaptic basal lamina is capable of causing this aggregation. Knockouts of this agrin gene in mice are lethal at birth as the mice have no NMJs that are capable of activating the muscle fibers (24).

If agrin is capable of aggregating receptors like this, then there had to be a receptor for agrin located in the muscle fibers. About 15 years ago a transmembrane "muscle specific kinase" (MuSK) was identified as a crucial part of the agrin signaling pathway (25). MuSK activation initiates a complex, still incompletely understood cascade of signaling that leads to synaptic accumulation of AChR, likely through other proteins known to associate with receptors. The crucial role of MuSK was demonstrated by the lack of NMJs in knockout mice and their perinatal death. However, no direct association between MuSK and agrin could be demonstrated, suggesting the existence of a co-receptor.

In the past two years, good evidence has accumulated that Lrp4, a member of the low density lipoprotein receptor family of proteins, is the agrin receptor (26,27). Lrp4 binds agrin and stimulates its interaction with and activation of MuSK. Muscle cells without Lrp4 expression, like those from MuSK knockouts, lack the ability to aggregate AChR in response to agrin.

Certainly there are many pieces of the puzzle still to be worked out, but a major outline of how an accumulation of receptors develops at the junction is now apparent, from the release of a specific factor from the motor neuron to an activation of a signaling cascade in the muscle. A beautiful demonstration of the primacy of agrin in dictating the differentiation of neuromuscular synapses comes from investigation of formation of synapses at ectopic locations on muscle fibers (28,29). It has been known since 1917 that one can transplant a nerve containing motor axons onto the surface of a muscle, but the motor neurons, while they grow across the muscle, are incapable of synaptogenesis, at least while the fibers are still innervated at the original NMJs and are activated by this innervation (30). Denervation of the muscle can induce formation of ectopic NMJs by these implanted motor axons, showing that new synapses can form even in adult muscle under certain circumstances. It was logical then to ask if agrin by itself without the nerve could effect this same sort of synaptic differentiation. Transfection of muscle fibers with constructs encoding the active (i.e. neural) isoform of agrin, caused these muscle fibers to express and release the protein. This expression induced (in the absence of any nerve), fully differentiated sites on the adjoining fibers exposed to the agrin (28,29). These sites contained all the postsynaptic specializations: synaptic gutters filled with AChR aggregates, AChE, secondary folds, and the accumulation of nuclei. Synapse specific gene expression was even induced. Clearly agrin does more than just direct the accumulation of receptors – it appears to be a master switch capable of initiating a program for synaptic differentiation.

A MODIFICATION TO THE AGRIN HYPOTHESIS: MUSCLE PRE-PATTERNING OF RECEPTORS

The discovery of agrin made the initial establishment of the neuromuscular contact during development seem straightforward: the axons of the motor neurons were proposed to enter the developing muscle at the time the muscle fibers were quite short. These axon terminals would induce, through their release of agrin, the differentiation of a synaptic site on the surface of each muscle fiber. The muscle would then grow by addition of myoblasts to each end of these fibers and the result would be long muscle fibers with NMJs near their centers. Initial examination of agrin null mice at the late embryonic stage supported this scheme, as AChR clusters were missing (24).

A challenge to this neurocentric view of NMJ formation came from examination of mice in which motor neurons were ablated during early development (31). These muscles that had never seen a motor neuron had clusters of AChR in the center of their fibers. There was synapse-specific gene expression in this region of the fibers as well. These features constitute the "pre-pattern". Re-examination of the agrin null mice at an earlier stage of development showed that clusters of AChR had formed; however, these clusters subsequently disappeared. Agrin expression by the motor neurons appears to be necessary to maintain the AChR clustered underneath the initial synaptic contacts. Indeed, it appears that ACh released by the nerve terminal acts as a negative modulator of AChR clustering, and motor neuron-derived agrin opposes this effect at the site of synaptic contact (32,33). The discovery of the pre-pattern gives the muscle fiber a role in determining the site of synaptogenesis, a role that is much more like postsynaptic neurons in the CNS. Recent experiments also show us that the agrin-signaling components within the muscle are responsible for the formation of the pre-pattern and that this pre-pattern may guide growth of motor axons across the muscle (34).

RETROGRADE SIGNALING

Another issue that has fascinated neuroscientists is the possibility that factors produced by the target, possibly in reaction to an initial synaptic contact, might influence the differentiation of the nerve terminal and/or the neurons that form the synapses. This process has been referred to as retrograde signaling. Numerous experiments, most prominently those of Mu-ming Poo and collaborators (35), have provided evidence for such influences on the formation and strength of the synapse. The pre-patterning of AChR in the muscle prior to the arrival of the nerve is a clear example of a retrograde influence. Our discussion below will include just two of the many additional examples that could be discussed here: target-mediated cell death and the alignment of pre- and postsynaptic specializations.

Embryologists studying the early development of the spinal cord noted that there was an overproduction of neurons, most of which subsequently died. This is particularly obvious in the motor neuron pools in the spinal cord. The excess in motor neuron production is as high as three-fold, and the cell death is mostly complete before the time of birth in the rodent (36). Hamburger and colleagues showed that ablation of the target leads to death of most motor neurons and augmentation of the peripheral targets (for example implantation of an extra limb bud in the chick) allowed the survival of many more motor neurons (37). These results were explained by proposing a competition among the motor neurons for targets: those that succeeded in establishing contact with a target muscle survived whereas those that failed, died. These findings led directly to the discovery of factors produced in the targets and support cells that were named trophic factors that allowed the survival of the neurons (38). With the advent of mouse knockout technology, it has been possible to show that defects in certain trophic factor signaling lead to neuromuscular pathologies (39).

One particularly perplexing issue with the above schema of competition for targets is how, if the motor neurons are predetermined as to their muscle target and perhaps the fibers within these targets they are to innervate, how an appropriate set of differentiated motor neurons is selected from the initially projecting population for each muscle. The problem is this selection occurs when the muscle itself has not yet reached its adult size or fiber composition, as cell death is completed even before the muscle has finished the last wave of myogenesis. It will be interesting to know exactly when the differentiation of motor neurons and the fibers in their units are determined and exactly how much of this is determined by factors within the developing limb itself (see also below).

A second powerful example of a retrograde influence concerns the alignment of specializations in the postsynaptic muscle fiber and the presynaptic nerve terminal. The active zones in the presynaptic nerve terminal, the sites for docking and release of synaptic vesicles, align with the opening of the synaptic folds, placing the site of release of transmitter optimally across from the site where it is to act (40). Transmitter release occurs via the depolarization of the nerve terminal by the action potential arriving over the axon, the activation of voltage-gated calcium channels (VGCC), and the influx of calcium. This calcium triggers the fusion of synaptic vesicles at the active zone and the release of the neurotransmitter. Calcium channels in turn are tightly associated with the material that constitutes the active zone, thus ensuring that the maximum change in calcium concentration occurs in the region of the nerve terminal where vesicle fusion occurs. Laminin molecules containing a beta-2 chain are produced by the muscle fiber and enriched in those areas of the basal lamina apposed to clusters of AChR; therefore the laminin also appears to be organized by agrin signaling. This isoform binds directly to the extracellular domain of VGCC in the membrane of the nerve terminal (40). This interaction, seemingly reinforced by other components of the basal lamina, ensures the clustering of VGCC across the synaptic cleft from the laminin-beta-2. Indeed, laminin-beta-2 is shown not only to cluster calcium channels but intracellular components of the transmitter release machinery (40). Clearly the postsynaptic cell coordinates the organization of machinery in the presynaptic nerve terminal.

STRUCTURAL BIOLOGY OF THE NERVE TERMINAL VIA ELECTRON MICROSCOPY

Standard thin section electron micrographs have provided us with many details of the structure of the synapse. However, these micrographs do not provide any information about the dimension that occurs through the thickness of the thin slice, typically something like 50 nm. This is the size of a typical synaptic vesicle. In essence, structures within this thickness, even though they are resolved by the microscope, are projected into a single flat image. Thus, much of the structural information present is missed. This problem can be solved by taking electron micrographs as the specimen is tilted through a series of angles and tomography used to prepare images representing virtual slices of the volume, which can then be viewed from any vantage point. U. J. McMahan and his colleagues (41) have developed and exploited this technique to reveal previously unrecognized structures within the release machinery in the active zone of the frog NMJ. The ridges of material right next to the presynaptic membrane are not amorphous blobs. Rather, there are regular, repeating structural units. So far three units have been identified and called beams, ribs, and pegs. Beams are rods arranged end-to-end along the length of the ridge. Ribs extend laterally from beams at regular intervals and attach to docked synaptic vesicles that in the frog are generally present as two parallel rows, one on each side of the active zone ridge. Pegs attach to the ribs and to proteins in the nerve terminal membrane believed to be calcium channels. Thus, there appears to be machinery to anchor synaptic vesicles in the anticipated places and moreover there are attachments of this machinery to the proteins that trigger the release process. This tomographic analysis has been extended to mouse junctions (42): the same components are present; they have the same connections to each other and to synaptic vesicles and calcium channels. However, the mouse active zones are not arrayed into repeated arrays, contain only a pair of docked vesicles per zone, and the beams and ribs occupy a different position than that in the frog. This preparation is rich with possibilities for examining the detailed structural biology of transmitter release and the processes by which synaptic vesicles are brought to the active zone.

THE LIFE HISTORY OF THE NEUROMUSCULAR JUNCTION

So how does the elaborate structure that constitutes the NMJ come about during development? How does this synapse mature and grow as the muscle grows? What happens as animals age?

Muscle fibers become innervated very quickly after they begin to be generated (43). The synapse forms in the pre-patterned area described above. The receptors present are concentrated in an oval area called a "plaque". Unlike in the adult, the processes of several motor neurons contact the muscle fiber within this plaque. The plaque gradually transforms into a "pretzel", i.e. the branched shape shown in Figure 54.2 (43). This transformation involves the elimination of AChR from portions of the original plaque and holes in the plaque appear. The mechanism of this elimination has always been presumed to be a consequence of the elimination of nerve terminals (see next), but this is now less certain: myotubes grown in culture with certain substrates develop pretzels of AChR that look very much like those present on fibers in the living animal in the absence of any innervation (44).

As described above, several axons contact the NMJs at nascent muscle fibers. Surprisingly, this "multiple innervation" or "polyneuronal innervation" persists for some time – in rodents, out into the second week of postnatal life (45). There is a gradual elimination of all but one of these inputs from each fiber. This elimination does not involve death of motor neurons – the massive die-off of motor neurons precedes the elimination. Rather, analysis of motor units, both physiologically and anatomically, shows that synapse elimination is a rearrangement of the distribution of terminal branches by the same population of motor neurons that is present in the muscle in the adult (45,46). Each motor neuron initially just makes many more terminal branches and contacts more muscle fibers. The process has always been viewed as a competition between the innervating axons for contact with each fiber, largely on the basis of the end result: inputs are eliminated so only one remains and there appears to be no period of time in which all inputs are lost (45,46). A major advance in our understanding of the process has come from vital imaging pioneered in the Lichtman lab (46). It is possible to label a small complement of the AChR at a living synapse with a low concentration of fluorochrome-conjugated Btx. Because of the large safety factor of transmission of this synapse, it is possible to vitally label a portion of the receptors without altering transmission at the synapse. With expression of a fluorescent protein (FP) in motor axons, it is possible to vitally image the motor axon terminals as well. The sternomastoid muscle in the neck is a convenient muscle that can be imaged in the anesthetized mouse; individual junctions can be viewed with a wide-field fluorescence microscope by inserting a dipping objective through a small opening in the skin (47). Moreover, owing to the unique pretzel morphology of each NMJ (and the surrounding NMJs), it is possible to image an individual junction, allow the animal to recover, and then come back at a later time and re-image the very same junction, observing what happens pre- and postsynaptically during the process. Even more powerful observations are made possible by variegation in the expression of FPs and different spectral variants of the colors of these proteins (10). Apparently because of random integration of the transgenes during the preparation of mouse transgenics and other poorly understood mechanisms, transgene expression can vary widely in amount and in which particular cells it is expressed. Some lines of mice express the FP in only a small subset of motor (10). If this "subset mouse" is crossed with another transgenic line that expresses another color of FP in all motor axons, then one can visualize the extent of a single axon at a NMJ as well as the axons of all its competitor axons. This allows one to determine the behavior of individual axon terminals at the NMJ. These experiments show that competition is quite dynamic, with axons withdrawing and extending over the plaque on each fiber. At least a major portion of the competition is between the different terminals for contact within the synaptic site and its AChR (46). It appears that the territory within the site occupied by one terminal expands as the others retract, although reversals in the apparent "winner" occur. The competition ends when one axon remains and all the others have been withdrawn from the synaptic site.

Because of fascination with the effects of experience on the nervous system in general and the development of the visual system in particular as well as the impact of the ideas of Donald Hebb as to how the strength of synapses in the nervous system could be changed by a particular pattern of use (48), there have been a number of experimental efforts made to examine the role of the activity among the motor neurons in the competition occurring during this synapse elimination. Clearly activity plays a major role and three sets of experiments are particularly compelling. One set of experiments examined the role of activity in a similar episode of synapse elimination that occurs in adult muscles during reinnervation (49). Regenerating axons commonly establish polyneuronal innervation of fibers and this polyneuronal innervation is lost with time following reinnervation. The Na channel blocker tetrodotoxin was applied to the nerve far from the muscle; this blocks conduction of action potentials past the application site. Since the activity in these nerves emanates from the spinal cord, these motor neurons fell silent. Such a block delays the removal of polyneuronal innervation from the muscle. A stimulating electrode was placed around the nerve distal to the block site. In this manner, it was possible to precisely control the activity of the motor neurons (the only activity present was that imposed by the stimulation). The synchronous activity evoked in the nerve by the stimulation significantly delayed synapse elimination even beyond that by the block alone. This shows that the relative timing of the activity in the set of axons is important in the elimination process. Synchronous activity promotes retention of inputs. Asynchronous activity promotes removal.

A second set of experiments used a sophisticated transgenic approach, employing a tamoxifen-inducible activation of cre-mediated excision of a floxed choline acetyltransferase (ChAT) in motor neurons (50). ChAT is the enzyme responsible for the synthesis of ACh, so motor neurons in which ChAT is inactivated fall silent and cannot activate muscle fibers at their NMJs. The tamoxifen administration allows the timing of the inactivation to be controlled and the amount of tamoxifen administered controls the fraction of the motor neurons in which excision effectively takes place. Motor axon terminals with and without ChAT can be identified by immunostaining for this molecule. It was shown that the motor neurons expressing ChAT "win" in the competition with axons that do not have ChAT and therefore do not release ACh. This shows active motor neurons win out over inactive ones.

A third set of experiments tested changes in the firing patterns of early motor neurons. Experiments discussed above suggested that synchronous activity among the innervating motor neurons favors retention of polyneuronal innervation where as asynchronous activity favored its removal. These experiments sought to determine how much synchrony was present in motor neurons during the period of polyneuronal innervation. Single unit electromyograms were recorded from early postnatal mouse muscles (51). These electromyograms record the muscle fiber action potentials occurring as a result of the activity of single motor units in the muscle. The waveform and amplitude of these recordings allow the identification of single motor units. Motor units in early postnatal life have a tendency to be active together; this tendency disappears with postnatal development during the period of synapse elimination. So why does the synchronous activity diminish as the motor neurons mature? It was shown that at least a partial explanation for the synchrony was the presence of gap junctions among the motor neurons. Gap junction coupling decreased during development as the synchrony disappeared (52). The gap junctions, since they spread excitation among the linked motor neurons, would be expected to help synchronize their action potential activity. Thus, one factor driving the development of asynchrony and the elimination of polyneuronal innervation is the reduction in gap junctional coupling. Indeed a precocious loss of polyneuronal innervation occurs in mice that lack expression of the predominant gap junctional protein in motor neurons (52).

As a result of synapse elimination, almost all NMJs in rodents are singly innervated by the second week of postnatal life and the NMJ has achieved its mature pretzel morphology by the end of this period. However, the muscle has not attained its adult size – it grows considerably in the subsequent weeks by an increase in the diameter of its fibers. How does the junction accommodate the growth of the muscle fiber and how stable is the synapse? A definitive answer to this question was achieved by vital imaging (53). The take-home message is that the NMJ retains its pattern of branching by expanding (or contracting in the cases of atrophy) in synchronization with the muscle fiber. It does this through intercalary growth (or shrinkage) so the pretzel just becomes a larger (or smaller) version of itself. The junction itself is very stable over many months of adult life.

However, aging does impact the junction. As mice approach 2 years of life, this stability disappears and their junctions begin to change dramatically (see Figure 54.2) (54,55). The nerve terminal changes from the predominantly smooth tubes apposed to the muscle surface to one that has varicose swellings dangling from it. There are corresponding changes in the AChR in the muscle membrane which change from the pretzel to islands located at the sites of the varicosities. The cause of such change in this normally stable synapse is unknown but has been presumed to be a gradual, aging-induced decline in the mechanisms maintaining the synapse. However, recent experiments suggest that the age-related changes are sudden and are explained by injury occurring to the muscle fibers in the region of the NMJ (56).

SPECIFICITY OF MUSCLE INNERVATION

During development, individual motor neurons achieve a specification so they have an identity, i.e. they come to receive an appropriate set of connections within the central nervous system as well as project to the correct muscles in the periphery (57). That axons grow into the periphery to reach their muscle targets in a selective manner during early development was made apparent by the elegant experiments of Landmesser and colleagues in which they mapped motor neurons according to the peripheral nerves they entered and the muscles to which they projected (7). They showed that these neurons would reroute themselves to achieve their intended targets if the spinal cord was rotated, as long as the rotation was not so large as to make this impossible. This was a demonstration not only of motor neuron specification but of axonal pathfinding. Investigations by Jessell and colleagues (57) have shown us mechanisms by which motor neurons themselves are specified by gradients of morphogens that initiate expression of specific transcription factors as well as how a series of gradients can specify motor neuron identity. Since the pathways of motor neurons in the peripheral nerves and the muscles and fiber types within the muscles they innervate are highly stereotyped, these properties are likely specified by gradients of peripheral morphogens, some of which are already known (57).

MUSCLE PLASTICITY MEDIATED BY THE NMJ

Activity is not only involved in synapse elimination. Muscle itself is exquisitely sensitive to the activity imposed on it by its motor neurons (9).

An immediate example is denervation hypersensitivity. When a muscle is denervated by damaging the axons that innervate it, that muscle becomes sensitive to ACh in the membrane all along the fiber (13,58). One does not have to denervate the muscle. Paralyzing the muscle produces the same result. The hypersensitivity is produced by synthesis of AChR outside the NMJ, i.e. the myonuclei that normally do not transcribe AChR come to do so as the muscle becomes inactive. These receptors then appear on the surface membrane (13). The activity normally imposed on the muscle fiber by its innervation suppresses the synthesis of AChR by these "extrajunctional" nuclei. Not only does this activity suppress AChR, it also determines the ability of the muscle to accept innervation by a nerve implanted outside the junction (see above). It is not necessary to denervate a muscle to obtain the ability of these nerves to form synapses, only to paralyze it. On the other hand stimulation of a denervated muscle, i.e. evoking action potentials by depolarization of the fibers themselves with implanted electrodes, can suppress the ability of an implanted nerve to engage in synaptogenesis (30).

Muscles and the fibers within them are specialized in their contractile properties; these specializations are often described as different "fiber types" because they involve a whole array of expression of different protein isoforms that enable different types of contractile performance (9). These differences have long fascinated neurobiologists, in large part because each motor unit is composed of fibers of one type (59). Moreover, the fiber types in each motor unit are matched in their contractile abilities to the activity patterns of their motor neuron. For example, motor neurons that fire long trains of action potentials that occur at low frequency are said to be "slow" and they form motor units whose muscle fibers contract more slowly but are capable of sustained contractions. Motor neurons that fire shorter duration trains of action potentials at higher frequency form motor units whose fibers contract more rapidly but can fatigue more quickly (60).

So how is the fiber type selective innervation by individual motor neurons set up in development? Many issues here seem to be poorly resolved. It is clear that the type of any particular fiber is not immutable as innervation or even activity can transform types (9). However, some compelling experiments suggest that the adaptation might be incomplete or only work within an "adaptive range" (61). Fiber types begin to emerge quite early in development and the patterns that emerge are clearly muscle-specific and even region-specific within individual muscles (62). Experiments with cultured myoblasts suggest that lineage can play a role in the differentiation of certain types (63), but innervation and even environment within the limb also plays a major role (64). In any case, it is clear that the early patterns can form even in the absence of innervation (65). Some experiments suggest that innervation of a set of fibers might emerge by selective elimination of innervation of inappropriate fiber types (66,67). Other experiments suggest that the innervation of single motor units is quite biased as to type at a time when all fibers remain polyneuronally innervated (68). It seems likely that this important issue is going to be determined by many factors: axon guidance, positional gradients within the limb, timing of development and lineage of myoblasts, axon preference, the adaptability of muscles to different activity patterns imposed by the nerve, and the emergence of these different activity patterns during development.

SOME ISSUES IN THE DEVELOPMENT OF MOTOR UNITS

One of the basic principles of motor control is the so-called "size principle" (69). As mentioned above contractions in muscle are produced through the activation of individual motor units and the amount of tension generated can be varied through the number of simultaneously active motor units. The fineness with which muscle force can be controlled depends on the number of these motor units and their individual size (i.e. how many muscle fibers they contain). Moreover, in each muscle there is an order to the recruitment of motor units. The small motor units are recruited first and the larger units last.

Since the organization of motor programs is so dependent on this orderly recruitment of motor units according to their size, it is crucial that the appropriate sizes of units be created within muscles during development. It is yet unclear how this is achieved, but the process of synapse elimination seems obviously suited to such a purpose. For example, if a motor neuron retained contact with most of the fibers it initially polyneuronally innervated, a large motor unit would be generated. That such a mechanism might be in play is suggested by experiments examining the status of polyneuronally innervated NMJs in mice in which two sets of motor neurons were transgenically labeled with two different fluorescent proteins (70). In this way, the investigators could examine axon terminals of these two different motor neurons and determine, on the basis of their morphology, which one was likely winning in the competition for the NMJ and which one was losing. They found that, in cases where the two neurons co-innervated the same muscle fibers, one of the axons appeared to be winning at most of these NMJs and displacing the other axon. However, both axons could be winning or losing at other NMJs where they were competing with different axons. These results suggest there is a hierarchy of different competitive vigor among the motor axons and that this could ultimately drive differences in motor unit size.

THE ROLE OF SYNAPTIC GLIA

The NMJ has glial investments. There are a set of "terminal" Schwann cells that associate with the terminal nerve branches. The function of these cells has been an object of several studies. Some of the prominent studies are outlined here.

Are the terminal glia really important? Do they provide support crucial for the maintenance of the synapse? The obvious way to address this question is to delete the cells. The cells can be removed by preventing their formation by genetic deletion of a trophic signaling important for their early survival. When such deletion is achieved prenatally, the motor axons, after initially contacting their muscles, withdraw from innervation and the mice are born dead (71–73). This suggests these glia (or the glia along the nerves) play a crucial role in maintaining NMJs after they form. Ko and colleagues have performed deletion experiments on the "perisynaptic" Schwann cells at the frog NMJ (74), using an antibody that binds selectively to the surface of these cells, followed by a complement-mediated lysis. Killing the Schwann cells in the adult animal does not immediately impact the nerve terminal but leads to gradual withdrawal of the nerve and a decrease in the efficacy of the synapse. In the developing tadpole, such ablation leads to failure of the nerve terminal to grow. Such responses are supported by more recent experiments suggesting Schwann cells express factors important for the nerve terminal (75–77).

Experiments in frog and mouse have also shown that the glial cells eavesdrop on the conversation occurring between the nerve and the muscle (78). The Schwann cells have purinergic and muscarinic receptors whose activation by release of ACh and ATP as a cotransmitter can lead to calcium elevations in the cells. These calcium elevations can result in feedback to the nerve terminal that can change the nature of transmitter release during repeated stimulation.

Schwann cells appear to play an important role in the removal of the losing motor axons during postnatal synapse elimination. Axons that lose in the competition at nms "withdraw" back into their parent axon (46). The process of withdrawal can be followed by imaging FP-expressing axons in living mice and in short-term explants during the period of synapse elimination. The Schwann cell wrapping the losing axon plays a major role in this withdrawal. It sends out short processes that subdivide the axon into small fragments and then consumes these fragments, creating so-called "axosomes" (79). Schwann cells thus participate in the destruction of eliminated axons at developing NMJs.

SCHWANN CELLS PLAY A ROLE IN REPAIR OF MUSCLE INNERVATION AFTER NERVE DAMAGE

Peripheral axons, in contrast to those in the central nervous system, regenerate following disconnection from their targets. One of the major factors in this regeneration is the presence of Schwann cells. These glia support regrowth of axons in the periphery and will do in the central nervous system if transplanted there (80). The Schwann cells extend processes across gaps placed in peripheral nerves by injury and form a pathway that supports axon regeneration into the distal end of the nerve (81). Generally, the Schwann cells are confined within the nerve sheaths in the distal stump of the nerve and here appear to play a similar role in growth support. The guidance offered by the nerve sheaths that persist following the degeneration of the axon explains why motor axons generally grow back to synaptic sites within the muscle (82). Indeed, it is not surprising, since these guides confine the growth of the axon, that the precision with which an old site is reinnervated by the same axon depends heavily on the navigation of axons across a crush or cut in the nerve (82). A simple crush leaves this guidance intact and the axons generally return to their original targets. A gap placed in the nerve means the axon entering the nerve sheath is likely not to be the axon that previously did so.

There are additional mechanisms that the Schwann cells use in the attempt to restore innervation to denervated muscle fibers. The phenomenon is called "sprouting" and refers here to growth of axons induced within the muscle. For example, in the case of damage to a portion of the innervation to the muscle, the remaining motor units begin to sprout processes that grow to innervate at least some of the denervated muscle fibers. This growth occurs along Schwann cell processes (11,83). These processes emerge from the Schwann cells at denervated synaptic sites in the muscle, grow to adjacent NMJs and guide the growth of the axons back to the denervated sites. This same mechanism appears to play a role in reinnervation, allowing axons innervating one site to grow to adjacent sites. The role of the Schwann cells here appears to be to maximize the chances for the reinnervation of as many fibers as possible by whatever axons manage to return to the muscle.

Taken all together, these experiments suggest that glial cells have substantial roles to play in maintaining and repairing neuromuscular connections. Just as the NMJ has taught us much about the nature of synapses, their construction, operation, and maintenance, so too will the NMJ have much more to teach us about the roles of glia.

ACKNOWLEDGMENTS

Some of the work described here was supported by NIH grant NS20480. We thank Gwen Gage for artwork and Michelle Mikesh for the electron micrograph.

REFERENCES

1. Hubbard JI, Quastel DM. Micropharmacology of vertebrate neuromuscular transmission. *Annu Rev Pharmacol* 1973;**13**:199–216.
2. Colquhoun D. Mechanisms of drug action at the voluntary muscle endplate. *Annu Rev Pharmacol* 1975;**15**:307–25.
3. Katz B. Neural transmitter release: from quantal secretion to exocytosis and beyond. The Fenn Lecture. *J Neurocytol* 1996;**25**:677–86.
4. Rizzoli SO, Betz WJ. Synaptic vesicle pools. *Nat Rev Neurosci* 2005;**6**:57–69.
5. Buss RR, Sun W, Oppenheim RW. Adaptive roles of programmed cell death during nervous system development. *Annu Rev Neurosci* 2006;**29**:1–35.
6. Lichtman JW, Colman H. Synapse elimination and indelible memory. *Neuron* 2000;**25**:269–78.
7. Lance-Jones C, Landmesser L. Pathway selection by chick lumbosacral motoneurons during normal development. *Proc R Soc Lond B Biol Sci* 1981;**214**:1–18.
8. Wu H, Xiong WC, Mei L. To build a synapse: signaling pathways in neuromuscular junction assembly. *Development* 2010;**137**:1017–33.
9. Schiaffino S, Sandri M, Murgia M. Activity-dependent signaling pathways controlling muscle diversity and plasticity. *Physiology (Bethesda)* 2007;**22**:269–78.
10. Feng G, Mellor RH, Bernstein M, Keller-Peck C, Nguyen QT, Wallace M, et al. Imaging neuronal subsets in transgenic mice expressing multiple spectral variants of GFP. *Neuron* 2000;**28**:41–51.
11. Kang H, Tian L, Thompson. W. Terminal Schwann cells guide the reinnervation of muscle after nerve injury. *J Neurocytol* 2003;**32**:975–85.
12. Ravdin P, Axelrod D. Fluorescent tetramethyl rhodamine derivatives of alpha-bungarotoxin: preparation, separation, and characterization. *Anal Biochem* 1977;**80**:585–92.
13. Berg DK, Kelly RB, Sargent PB, Williamson P, Hall ZW. Binding of bungarotoxin to acetylcholine receptors in mammalian muscle (snake venom-denervated muscle-neonatal muscle-rat diaphragm-SDS-polyacrylamide gel electrophoresis). *Proc Natl Acad Sci USA* 1972;**69**:147–51.
14. Marques MJ, Conchello JA, Lichtman JW. From plaque to pretzel: fold formation and acetylcholine receptor loss at the developing neuromuscular junction. *J. Neurosci.* 2000;**20**:3663–75.
15. Peng HB, Xie H, Rossi SG, Rotundo RL. Acetylcholinesterase clustering at the neuromuscular junction involves perlecan and dystroglycan. *J Cell Biol* 1999;**145**:911–21.
16. Patton BL. Basal lamina and the organization of neuromuscular synapses. *J Neurocytol* 2003;**32**:883–903.
17. Court FA, Gillingwater TH, Melrose S, Sherman DL, Greenshields KN, Morton AJ, et al. Identity, developmental restriction and reactivity of extralaminar cells capping mammalian neuromuscular junctions. *J Cell Sci* 2008;**121**(Pt 23):3901–11.
18. Merlie JP, Sanes JR. Concentration of acetylcholine receptor mRNA in synaptic regions of adult muscle fibres. *Nature* 1985;**317**:66–8.
19. Fertuck HC, Salpeter MM. Localization of acetylcholine receptor by 125I-labeled alpha-bungarotoxin binding at mouse motor endplates. *Proc Natl Acad Sci USA* 1974;**71**:1376–8.
20. Flucher BE, Daniels MP. Distribution of Na^+ channels and ankyrin in neuromuscular junctions is complementary to that of acetylcholine receptors and the 43 kD protein. *Neuron* 1989;**3**:163–75.
21. Lingle CJ, Steinbach JH. Neuromuscular blocking agents. *Int Anesthesiol Clin* 1988;**26**:288–301.
22. Robertson JD. Electron microscopy of the motor end-plate and the neuromuscular spindle. In: Bowman HD, Woolf AL, editors. *Utrecht Symposium on the Innervation of Muscle*. Baltimore, MD: Williams and Wilkins;1960. p. 181–223.
23. McMahan UJ. The agrin hypothesis. *Cold Spring Harb Symp Quant Biol* 1990;**55**:407–18.
24. Gautam M, Noakes PG, Moscoso L, Rupp F, Scheller RH, Merlie JP, et al. Defective neuromuscular synaptogenesis in agrin-deficient mutant mice. *Cell* 1996;**85**:525–35.
25. DeChiara TM, Bowen DC, Valenzuela DM, Simmons MV, Poueymirou WT, Thomas S, et al. The receptor tyrosine kinase MuSK is required for neuromuscular junction formation in vivo. *Cell* 1996;**85**:501–12.
26. Kim N, Stiegler AL, Cameron TO, Hallock PT, Gomez AM, Huang JH, et al. Lrp4 is a receptor for Agrin and forms a complex with MuSK. *Cell* 2008;**135**:334–42.
27. Zhang B, Luo S, Wang Q, Suzuki T, Xiong WC, Mei L. LRP4 serves as a coreceptor of agrin. *Neuron* 2008;**60**:285–97.
28. Cohen I, Rimer M, Lomo T, McMahan UJ. Agrin-induced postsynaptic-like apparatus in skeletal muscle fibers in vivo. *Mol Cell Neurosci* 1997;**9**:237–53.
29. Jones G, Meier T, Lichtsteiner M, Witzemann V, Sakmann B, Brenner HR. Induction by agrin of ectopic and functional postsynaptic-like membrane in innervated muscle. *Proc Natl Acad Sci USA* 1997;**94**:2654–9.
30. Jansen JK, Lomo T, Nicolaysen K, Westgaard RH. Hyperinnervation of skeletal muscle fibers: dependence on muscle activity. *Science* 1973;**181**:559–61.
31. Arber S, Burden SJ, Harris AJ. Patterning of skeletal muscle. *Curr Opin Neurobiol* 2002;**12**:100–3.
32. Brandon EP, Lin W, D'Amour KA, Pizzo DP, Dominguez B, Sugiura Y, et al. Aberrant patterning of neuromuscular synapses in choline acetyltransferase-deficient mice. *J Neurosci* 2003;**23**:539–49.
33. Misgeld T, Burgess RW, Lewis RM, Cunningham JM, Lichtman JW, Sanes JR. Roles of neurotransmitter in synapse

formation: development of neuromuscular junctions lacking choline acetyltransferase. *Neuron* 2002;**36**:635–48.
34. Kim N, Burden SJ. MuSK controls where motor axons grow and form synapses. *Nat Neurosci* 2008;**11**:19–27.
35. Fitzsimonds RM, Poo MM. Retrograde signaling in the development and modification of synapses. *Physiol Rev* 1998;**78**:143–70.
36. Lance-Jones C. Motoneuron cell death in the developing lumbar spinal cord of the mouse. *Dev Brain Res* 1982;**4**:473–9.
37. Hamburger V. Trophic interactions in neurogenesis: a personal historical account. *Annu Rev Neurosci* 1980;**3**:269–78.
38. Hamburger V. The history of the discovery of the nerve growth factor. *J Neurobiol* 1993;**24**:893–7.
39. Pitts EV, Potluri S, Hess DM, Balice-Gordon. RJ. Neurotrophin and Trk-mediated signaling in the neuromuscular system. *Int Anesthesiol Clin* 2006;**44**:21–76.
40. Nishimune H, Sanes JR, Carlson SS. A synaptic laminin-calcium channel interaction organizes active zones in motor nerve terminals. *Nature* 2004;**432**:580–7.
41. Harlow ML, Ress D, Stoschek A, Marshall RM, McMahan UJ. The architecture of active zone material at the frog's neuromuscular junction. *Nature* 2001;**409**:479–84.
42. Nagwaney S, Harlow ML, Jung JH, Szule JA, Ress D, Xu J, et al. Macromolecular connections of active zone material to docked synaptic vesicles and presynaptic membrane at neuromuscular junctions of mouse. *J Comp Neurol* 2009;**513**:457–68.
43. Bennett MR, Pettigrew AG. The formation of synapses in striated muscle during development. *J Physiol* 1974;**241**:515–45.
44. Kummer TT, Misgeld T, Lichtman JW, Sanes JR. Nerve-independent formation of a topologically complex postsynaptic apparatus. *J Cell Biol* 2004;**164**:1077–87.
45. Brown MC, Jansen JKS, Van Essen. D. Polyneuronal innervation of skeletal muscle in new-born rats and its elimination during maturation. *J Physiol* 1976;**261**:387–422.
46. Walsh MK, Lichtman JW. In vivo time-lapse imaging of synaptic takeover associated with naturally occurring synapse elimination. *Neuron* 2003;**37**:67–73.
47. Van Mier P, Balice-Gordon R, Lichtman J. Synaptic plasticity studied in vivo using vital dyes, lasers, and computer-assisted fluorescence microscopy. *Neuroprotocols* 1994;**5**:91–101.
48. Stent GS. A physiological mechanism for Hebb's postulate of learning. *Proc Natl Acad Sci USA* 1973;**70**:997–1001.
49. Favero M, Buffelli M, Cangiano A, Busetto G. The timing of impulse activity shapes the process of synaptic competition at the neuromuscular junction. *Neuroscience* 2010;**167**:343–53.
50. Buffelli M, Burgess RW, Feng G, Lobe CG, Lichtman JW, Sanes JR. Genetic evidence that relative synaptic efficacy biases the outcome of synaptic competition. *Nature* 2003;**424**:430–4.
51. Personius KE, Balice-Gordon RJ. Loss of correlated motor neuron activity during synaptic competition at developing neuromuscular synapses. *Neuron* 2001;**31**:395–408.
52. Personius KE, Chang Q, Mentis GZ, O'Donovan MJ, Balice-Gordon RJ. Reduced gap junctional coupling leads to uncorrelated motor neuron firing and precocious neuromuscular synapse elimination. *Proc Natl Acad Sci USA* 2007;**104**:11808–13.
53. Balice-Gordon RJ, Lichtman JW. In vivo visualization of the growth of pre- and postsynaptic elements of neuromuscular junctions in the mouse. *J Neurosci* 1990;**10**:894–908.
54. Balice-Gordon RJ. Age-related changes in neuromuscular innervation. *Muscle Nerve* 1997;**Suppl. 5**:S83–7.
55. Valdez G, Tapia JC, Kang H, Clemenson Jr GD, Gage FH, Lichtman JW, et al. Attenuation of age-related changes in mouse neuromuscular synapses by caloric restriction and exercise. *Proc Natl Acad Sci USA* 2010;**107**:14863–8.
56. Li Y, Lee Y, Thompson WJ. Changes in aging mouse neuromuscular junctions are explained by degeneration and regeneration of muscle fiber segments at the synapse. *J Neurosci* 2011; [submitted]
57. Dasen JS, Jessell TM. Hox networks and the origins of motor neuron diversity. *Curr Top Dev Biol* 2009;**88**:169–200.
58. Lømo T, Rosenthal J. Control of ACh sensitivity by muscle activity in the rat. *J Physiol* 1972;**221**:493–513.
59. Burke RE, Levine DN, Salcman M, Tsairis P. Motor units in cat soleus muscle: physiological, histochemical and morphological characteristics. *J Physiol* 1974;**238**:503–14.
60. Hennig R, Lømo T. Firing patterns of motor units in normal rats. *Nature* 1985;**314**:164–6.
61. Ausoni S, Gorza L, Schiaffino S, Gundersen K, Lømo T. Expression of myosin heavy chain isoforms in stimulated fast and slow rat muscles. *J Neurosci* 1990;**10**:153–60.
62. Condon K, Silberstein L, Blau HM, Thompson WJ. Development of muscle fiber types in the prenatal rat hindlimb. *Dev Biol* 1990;**138**:256–74.
63. Stockdale FE. Myogenic cell lineages. *Dev Biol* 1992;**154**:284–98.
64. Cho M, Webster SG, Blau HM. Evidence for myoblast-extrinsic regulation of slow myosin heavy chain expression during muscle fiber formation in embryonic development. *J Cell Biol* 1993;**121**:795–810.
65. Condon K, Silberstein L, Blau HM, Thompson WJ. Differentiation of fiber types in aneural musculature of the prenatal rat hindlimb. *Dev Biol* 1990;**138**:275–95.
66. Fladby T, Jansen JKS. Development of homogeneous fast and slow motor units in the neonatal mouse soleus muscle. *Development* 1990;**109**:723–32.
67. Jones SP, Ridge RMAP, Rowlerson A. The non-selective innervation of muscle fibres and mixed composition of motor units in a muscle of neonatal rat. *J Physiol* 1987;**386**:377–94.
68. Thompson WJ, Sutton LA, Riley DA. Fibre type composition of single motor units during synapse elimination in neonatal rat soleus muscle. *Nature* 1984;**309**:709–11.
69. Henneman E. The size-principle: a deterministic output emerges from a set of probabilistic connections. *J Exp Biol* 1985;**115**:105–12.
70. Kasthuri N, Lichtman. JW. The role of neuronal identity in synaptic competition. *Nature* 2003;**424**:426–30.
71. Jaworski A, Burden SJ. Neuromuscular synapse formation in mice lacking motor neuron- and skeletal muscle-derived Neuregulin-1. *J Neurosci* 2006;**26**:655–61.
72. Woldeyesus MT, Britsch S, Riethmacher D, Xu L, Sonnenberg-Riethmacher E, Abou-Rebyeh F, et al. Peripheral nervous system defects in erbB2 mutants following genetic rescue of heart development. *Genes Dev* 1999;**13**:2538–48.
73. Wolpowitz D, Mason TB, Dietrich P, Mendelsohn M, Talmage DA, Role. LW. Cysteine-rich domain isoforms of the neuregulin-1 gene are required for maintenance of peripheral synapses. *Neuron* 2000;**25**:79–91.
74. Reddy LV, Koirala S, Sugiura Y, Herrera AA, Ko CP. Glial cells maintain synaptic structure and function and promote

development of the neuromuscular junction in vivo. *Neuron* 2003;**40**:563–80.
75. Feng Z, Ko CP. Schwann cells promote synaptogenesis at the neuromuscular junction via transforming growth factor-beta1. *J Neurosci* 2008;**28**:9599–609.
76. Peng HB, Yang JF, Dai Z, Lee CW, Hung HW, Feng ZH, et al. Differential effects of neurotrophins and schwann cell-derived signals on neuronal survival/growth and synaptogenesis. *J Neurosci* 2003;**23**:5050–60.
77. Ullian EM, Harris BT, Wu A, Chan JR, Barres BA. Schwann cells and astrocytes induce synapse formation by spinal motor neurons in culture. *Mol Cell Neurosci* 2004;**25**:241–51.
78. Rousse I, Robitaille R. Calcium signaling in Schwann cells at synaptic and extra-synaptic sites: active glial modulation of neuronal activity. *Glia* 2006;**54**:691–9.
79. Bishop DL, Misgeld T, Walsh MK, Gan WB, Lichtman JW. Axon branch removal at developing synapses by axosome shedding. *Neuron* 2004;**44**:651–61.
80. David S, Aguayo AJ. Axonal elongation into peripheral nervous system "bridges" after central nervous system injury in adult rats. *Science* 1981;**214**:931–3.
81. Son YJ, Thompson WJ. Schwann cell processes guide regeneration of peripheral axons. *Neuron* 1995;**14**:125–32.
82. Nguyen QT, Sanes JR, Lichtman JW. Pre-existing pathways promote precise projection patterns. *Nat. Neurosci.* 2002;**5**: 861–7.
83. Son YJ, Thompson WJ. Nerve sprouting in muscle is induced and guided by processes extended by Schwann cells. *Neuron* 1995;**14**:133–41.

Chapter 55

Neuromechanical Interactions that Control Muscle Function and Adaptation

Jung A. Kim[1], Roland R. Roy[1,4] and V. Reggie Edgerton[1,2,3,4]

[1]Departments of Integrative Biology and Physiology, [2]Neurobiology, [3]Neurosurgery, [4]Brain Research Institute, University of California, Los Angeles, Los Angeles, CA

IMPACT OF MOTOR UNIT ORGANIZATION ON MUSCLE FUNCTION

In the evolution of the neuromuscular system of virtually every species, and perhaps all species, a remarkable level of synergism between the neural and musculoskeletal systems has resulted in highly predictable kinematics, kinetics, and metabolic responses to any given neural motor demand and the consequential movement. Recognition of the details of the properties that have been conserved in this evolutionary process provides a basis for a unifying perspective and understanding of the limitations of our movement capability and the metabolic consequences that are largely attributable to skeletal muscle tissue, and oftentimes define the nature of a given movement. For example, once a decision has been made regarding the nature of a movement, i.e., which motor pools and consequently muscles will be activated by the nervous system, the intensity (power) of activation of each of the motor pools, the patterns of activation and inactivation (work–rest duty cycles), and the relative metabolic consequences are largely already determined, assuming that all other supportive systems are functioning appropriately. This is not to say that the absolute magnitude of the metabolic consequences in response to a movement with a given intensity will be identical in every individual or among different species, for that will depend on the unique relative characteristics of the motor unit phenotypes, combined with the physiological state of the cardiovascular, pulmonary, and other supportive systems of the individual or species. For example, the relative magnitude of a metabolic response will differ in an individual that is well-trained compared to non-trained and among the species that have adapted toward endurance type activities, such as the hunting dog compared to those that have been genetically adapted to speed-power, such as the Greyhound. On the other hand, within any given animal the relative changes in the metabolic responses to a specific motor task will be qualitatively similar over different recruitment intensities and the work-to-rest ratio of the recruitment.

The predictability of these responses to the nature of the exercise is clearly illustrated in numerous examples of maximal performances as defined by world records in athletes. The relationship between the world record time and the average speed of movement for a wide range of athletic events is highly predictable for each track event, ranging from the 100-meter dash to the 20,000-meter run. A similar relationship is noted between the 100-meter and the 5000-meter swim. The difference is essentially in the particular motor pools and muscles that are recruited and the number of motor units activated within each of those motor pools. The pattern of the relationship between time and speed will be similar because of the relatively fixed relationship between motor unit and muscle fiber phenotypes. These relationships are entirely predictable based on the physiological–biochemical properties of the motor units within a given motor pool.

What is the basis for this stereotypical and predictable metabolic and subsequent performance response? There are two fundamental properties of the evolved neuromusculoskeletal systems that underlie this constancy. First, the neural strategies for defining the level of recruitment of motoneurons within a motor pool is to define how many and which motoneurons will be activated. How many motoneurons will be activated is a function of an individual's "effort" in performing a specific movement, thus rendering the specific movement and the metabolic consequences a voluntary "choice". This can be explained by the fact that which motoneurons within a given motor pool will be recruited for any given movement is decided automatically by the spinal neural circuitry. This relatively fixed order of recruitment from the lowest to the highest effort translates into recruitment of the smallest to the largest motoneurons. Because of the constancy of recruitment from smallest to largest motor

Muscle. DOI: http://dx.doi.org/10.1016/B978-0-12-381510-1.00055-7

units and the constancy of the widely ranging metabolic phenotypes among motor units within a motor pool among muscles and species, the metabolic consequences of an effort is determined by what is largely known as the "size principle" of recruitment within each motor pool (1,2).

But how does this order of recruitment define the metabolic consequences of the muscular effort? This highly predictable response is the consequence of a highly synchronized gene expression between the components of a motor unit, i.e., a motoneuron and all of the muscle fibers that it innervates. For example, the motoneuron largely defines the specific kind and number of proteins expressed in the muscle fibers it innervates (3–6). It also is known that this neural control of gene expression occurs through both activity-dependent and activity-independent mechanisms (4). This neural control of gene expression is manifested as motor unit phenotypes: there is a highly synergistic relationship between the metabolic and contractile properties of the muscle fibers and the metabolic and electrophysiological properties of the motoneuron within a motor unit (3,4,7).

The smallest motoneurons innervate the smallest number of muscle fibers that are, in general, relatively small, resulting in motor units that produce relatively low forces (8). In addition, the muscle fibers and motoneurons have genes that support a high capacity for oxidative phosphorylation, a high mitochondrial density, and a more modest capability for metabolizing glucose through glycogenolysis and glycolysis (9,10). In addition, the maximum capacity for utilizing ATP at the actomyosin cross-bridges of the slow, oxidative fibers is modest relative to the faster muscle phenotypes. These, among other properties, define the slow motor unit phenotype that is highly resistant to fatigue, but generates relatively low forces and power. Based on the size principle these are the motor units that are recruited first in almost all types of movements (Figure 55.1).

At the other end of the spectrum, the largest motoneurons innervate the largest number of muscle fibers that are, in general, relatively large, resulting in motor units that produce relatively high forces. In addition, the muscle fibers and motoneurons have genes that support a very high capacity for providing glycolytic substrates through glycolysis, while its potential for restoring high-energy phosphates via oxidative phosphorylation is rather limited and the relative expression of mitochondrial proteins is modest (11,12). These motor units are recruited only in the most intense efforts when speed and power, not endurance, becomes a priority. The metabolic consequences are highly predictable because this muscle fiber phenotype has a very high capability for utilizing ATP at a relatively fast rate due to the high actomyosin ATPase activity and fast myosin isoform (11). Thus this fast-fatigable motor unit phenotype is recruited only for short bursts of high power activity and is highly fatigable (Figures 55.1, 55.2).

The net effect of this motor unit phenotype is that the motor units that are recruited the most often and for the more prolonged periods have muscle fibers that are well defined for this pattern of activity. This striking level of synergism of gene expression between the motoneuron and muscle fibers and among muscle fibers within the motor unit must be present for there to be motor unit phenotypes. This level of coordinated gene expression within a motor unit reflects the fact that the genes within the single nucleus of a motoneuron basically controls, or at least strongly modulates, the gene expression in hundreds of thousands of myonuclei among all of the muscle fibers of each motor unit (13–16). This degree of amplification of gene control of the motoneuron nucleus is a striking example of how the nervous system not only determines when and how a movement will occur, but it has already predetermined how long this movement can persist and the metabolic consequences of that movement. The combination of the highly synergistic properties of the motoneurons and muscle fibers resulting from highly programmed and coordinated gene expression provide the underlying basis for the highly predictable relationship of the speed and duration that characterizes practically all world records in athletic events.

Given this generalization throughout the evolution of the neuromuscular system among species, as in all of biology there are exceptions and considerable focus has been placed on these exceptions. For example, there are molecular differences among the "slow" and "fast" myosins and there are even multiple myosins expressed within the same muscle fiber, but the frequency of this occurrence differs substantially from species to species and from muscle to muscle and within different physiological or adaptive states of the muscle (17–19). Much of this variability can be attributed to ongoing activity-dependent mechanisms that can induce changes in gene expression. In spite of this intrinsic variability, however, the physiological consequences do not seem to be substantial. To some extent this heterogeneity within the muscle fibers and even among muscle fibers of the same motor unit must be present if there is some capability for varying levels of activation of gene expression within and among nuclei of the same fiber and across fibers of the same motor unit. Otherwise there would have to be an instantaneous and complete reformation of the proteins within the sarcomeric structure whenever there is some adaptive event. At the same time there has been some argument regarding the level of homogeneity among muscle fibers of the motor unit (20,21). In spite of initial claims of perfect homogeneity within the motor unit, it is now clear that there is a significant level of heterogeneity of

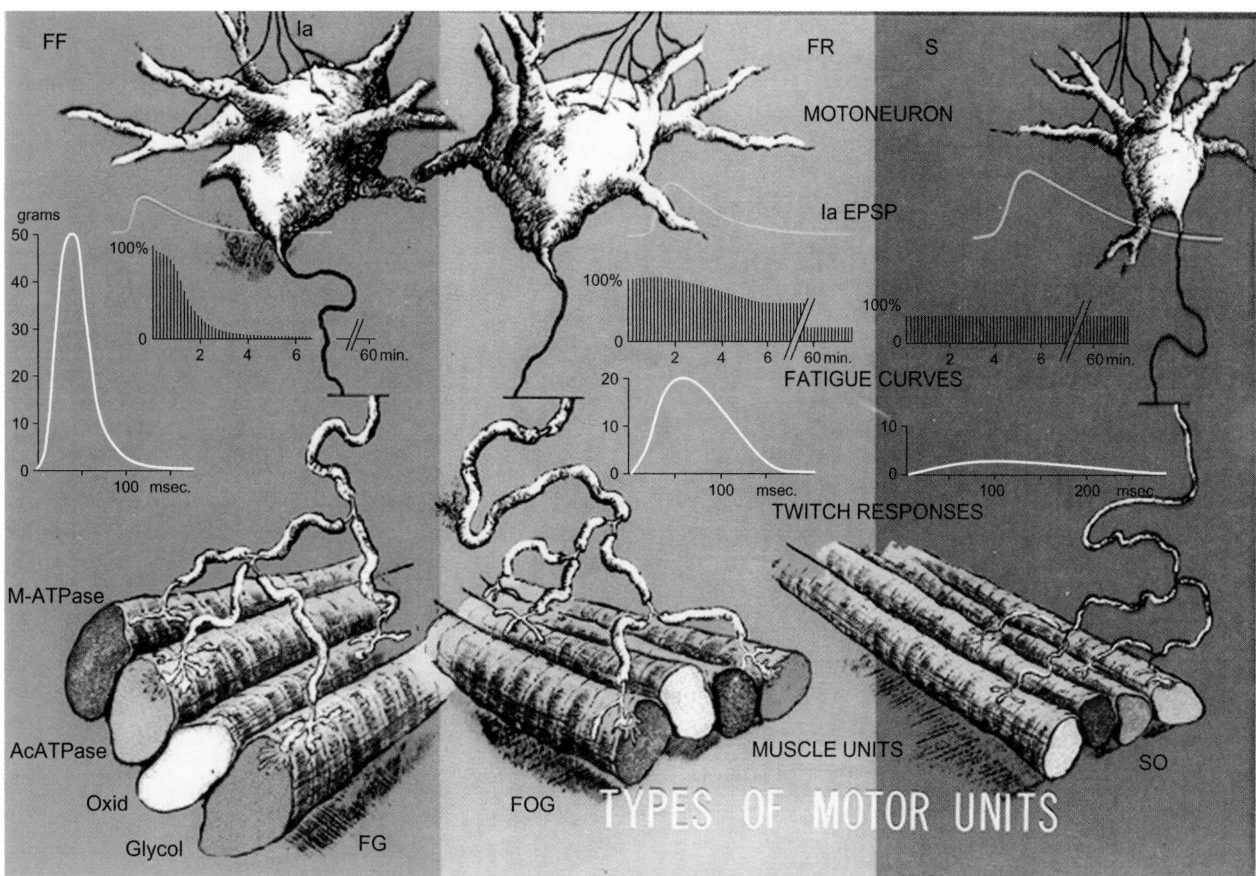

FIGURE 55.1 Schematic summarizing the most important features of the organization of the three major motor unit types identified in a typical predominantly fast mammalian muscle: FF, fast fatigable; FR, fast fatigue resistant; and S, slow fatigue resistant. The size of the motoneurons, axons, and muscle fibers are scaled appropriately for each motor unit type based on observations from a population of motoneurons. The density of Ia terminals and size of Ia excitatory post-synaptic potentials (EPSPs) are S > FR > FF, whereas the number of Ia terminals per motoneuron are approximately the same for each motor unit type. The shading of the muscle fibers denotes the relative staining intensity for each of the histochemical reactions identified in the fibers of the FF motor unit: M-ATPase, myofibrillar adenosinetriphosphatase, alkaline preincubation; AcATPase, myofibrillar ATPase, acid preincubation; Oxidative, a representative marker of oxidative metabolic capacity; and Glycolytic, a representative marker of glycolytic metabolic capacity. The M-ATPase staining is closely linked to the expression of specific myosin isoforms identified immunohistochemically. The fatigue resistance to repetitive stimulation and the isometric twitch contraction time are S > FR > FF. The neurons with the largest cell bodies also have the largest dendritic trees and axons. The largest axons have the fastest conduction velocities. The larger axons also branch intramuscularly more times and innervate more muscle fibers than the smaller axons. FG, fast glycolytic fiber; FOG, fast oxidative glycolytic fiber; S slow oxidative fiber. *(From Edington D and Edgerton VR, The biology of physical activity. Boston: Houghton Mifflin; 1976. Reproduced courtesy of Dr VR. Edgerton; all rights reserved.)*

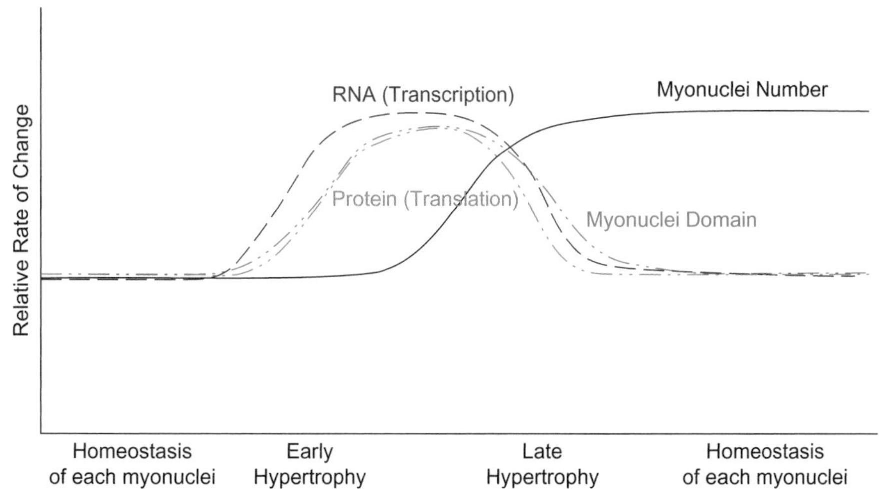

FIGURE 55.2 A hypothetical schematic illustrating the relative rate of change in the cellular events associated with homeostasis, and at the early and late phases of muscle hypertrophy. Note that transcription (blue) and translation (red) increase first prior to addition of more myonuclei (black) and that the changes in myonuclear domain (green) are in parallel to that observed with protein synthesis. More importantly note that the number of myonuclei increases and the myonuclear domain decreases proportionally, thus permitting the homeostatic state of each myonuclei to return to the pre-adaptative state.

multiple phenotypic characteristics, including activities of different mitochondrial proteins, among muscle fibers of the same motor unit (13–15).

Probably the most striking level of heterogeneity within the motor unit is in the fiber diameter. There is extensive overlap in cross-sectional area (CSA) of the fibers among different motor units (8,13,14). Similarly, there can be several-fold differences in the CSA of muscle fibers within the same motor unit (8). There is no underlying mechanism known for this phenomenon and it raises an intriguing question, given the commonly presumed concept that the activity of the muscle fiber is a dominating factor in determining its size. Ironically, in fact, the generalization of the size principle as described above leaves us with the observation that the largest fibers are the least active fibers. What are these activity-independent factors that control fiber CSA and therefore its force generating potential?

CONTROL OF MUSCLE FIBER DIAMETER AND LENGTH

The mechanisms that control the size, shape, and number of cells in a given organ largely define the qualitative and quantitative features of their functional capacities. Skeletal muscle fibers are unique in that they are relatively long and multinucleated cells that show a tremendous propensity for plasticity (16). Multiple factors influence the size, length, and shape of muscle fibers, including neural, mechanical, and hormonal influences. Here we focus on the CSA and length of skeletal muscle fibers and how the acute and chronic modification of these anatomical features affects the functional properties of the muscle. This is not to imply that the dynamics of gene expression does not play a role in defining their function, for these aspects of the plasticity of muscle are intricately linked to those molecular decisions that determine how a protein is placed within the organizational structure of a muscle fiber. For example, contractile proteins arranged *in parallel* contribute to the magnitude of force production of a fiber, whereas contractile proteins added *in series* enhance the displacement and indirectly the velocity potential of the fiber (22–24).

While we know little about the mechanisms associated with the architectural assembly of proteins *in parallel* or *in series*, there are numerous clues as to the role of myogenesis (increase in the number of myonuclei) and apoptosis (loss of myonuclei) in determining a sustainable CSA, and thus force potential, of a muscle fiber (25). In the earliest stage in the formation of a muscle fiber from a myotube during development, the CSA of a fiber is approximately the diameter of a single myonucleus (26,27). As the fiber develops there is a close relationship between the number of myonuclei and the CSA, although an adult-like ratio is not established until about 21 days in rats (28). This relatively constant relationship in homeostatic conditions has led to the concept of a myonuclear domain, i.e., the amount of cytoplasm per myonucleus (25,29). In spite of this myonuclear domain concept, a consistent anatomical feature during fiber growth is that the myonuclei are uniformly displaced to the periphery of the fiber and are rarely found embedded within the myofibrillar structure, i.e., in the center of the fiber. Another feature of the non-random placement of myonuclei is that there is some clustering of myonuclei in specialized regions of the muscle fiber, e.g., near the neuromuscular junction where these myonuclei have a unique RNA profile that probably reflects specialized functions associated with neuromuscular transmission (30,31), and to some degree at the region of the myotendinous junction where the myonuclei most likely are associated with longitudinal growth of the fibers (32). The focus here, however, is on the myonuclei distributed throughout the length of each muscle fiber, for these myonuclei seem to be responsive to and play a role in the adaptive processes associated with muscle hypertrophy and atrophy (25,33).

Over the past 15 years much has been written about the role of the modulation of myonuclei number in the atrophic and hypertrophic processes in skeletal muscles. Considerable differences remain, however, in the interpretation of data supporting or not supporting a role of myonuclei number modulation as a component of the mechanisms underlying atrophy and hypertrophy. We suggest that the experimental data present a rather clear picture of the role of modulation of the number of myonuclei as a fundamental process of fiber adaptation and the maintenance of homeostatic processes among muscle fibers. A primary reason for the controversy that surrounds this issue is the absence of recognizing that all adaptation processes consists of multiple adjustments occurring over different time frames. The initial and immediate cellular responses are those that can be engaged rapidly but not necessarily designed as the ultimate solution to the new demands. These initial responses rarely provide the long-term solution to a lesser or greater demand on the cellular processes and their control features. Multiple and sequential processes among any multiphase adaptive syndrome are widely recognized as the General Adaptation Syndrome (34). In fact, the data related to muscle hypertrophy (and atrophy) are uniformly consistent with this interpretation (35,36).

What are the observations suggesting this interpretation? When the rat plantaris muscle is induced to hypertrophy by removing synergistic muscles, the muscle fibers can hypertrophy significantly with little or no increase in total myonuclei for the first 2–4 weeks (37,38). By 10 weeks, however, the mean CSA of all fiber types is significantly larger than control (36–90%) and the average number of myonuclei across fiber types increases (61–109%) in proportion to the increase in CSA, thus maintaining a near normal myonuclear domain size (39). Furthermore, some fast fibers are estimated to have increased the number of myonuclei after training by as much as four-fold above normal. Similarly, after atrophy was induced in the soleus muscle of mice by hindlimb unloading, the muscle recovered substantial mass within one week of terminating the unloading without any increase in myonuclear number (40,41). During the second week of recovery, however, the increase in muscle mass was dependent on the presence of satellite cells and proliferation of myonuclei. The role of satellite cells and myonuclei addition in the growth of the fibers also has been clearly demonstrated in studies using low levels of irradiation to eliminate active satellite cells after chronic functional overload of a muscle: in these studies fiber hypertrophy was less in irradiated than non-irradiated functionally overloaded muscles (42–44). In effect, these studies demonstrate that overloaded muscles do not sustain substantial hypertrophy without eventually adding myonuclei.

We hypothesize that the "logic" (biological strategy) underlying this phasic response is that there is a normal range within which genes in each myonucleus can sustain their regulatory processes that enable continuous and relative immediate adaptation. The multiphasic adaptive feature allows the cell to respond acutely and then in a more chronic mode. When marked muscle hypertrophy is induced there are immediate increases in the rates of transcriptional and translational events, perhaps demanding the maximum of those processes (Figure 55.3). This immediate solution, however, is not likely the most effective adaptive response for the long term. It has been suggested that the disadvantage of increasing the number of myonuclei eventually could be that the supply of satellite cells will decline earlier as one ages (45,46). No evidence to date has shown this to be the case. An alternative logic would be that the myonuclei could be over-stressed and consequently die earlier as a result of the necessity to sustain a high rate of transcription and translation. We suggest that the end result of increasing myonuclei in the chronic hypertrophic state is that this provides a strategy that enables the gene function of all myonuclei to function within its normal/usual range, i.e., rather than fewer myonuclei being consistently overloaded, a larger number of myonuclei can work within their optimal range. If the myonuclear domain is re-established to a near-normal range, then the gene regulatory processes of all myonuclei can function as they did when the fiber was smaller and in its original homeostatic state.

Although this regulatory and adaptive hypothesis has not been demonstrated with certainty, there are some obvious experiments that can be performed to test it definitively. For example, can a hypertrophied fiber without an increase in myonuclei sustain that hypertrophied state as long as a hypertrophied fiber that has maintained a more normal myonuclei domain by the addition of myonuclei? Also, with respect to muscle atrophy and apoptosis, there remains some controversy about the importance of maintaining myonuclear domain (25,47), but again the apparent differences in interpretation given the limitations in the data of any given paper, seem to contribute to this issue. Studying one component of a highly multi-phasic and multi-dimensional process severely limits the generalizations that can be made for a complex *in vivo* phenomenon.

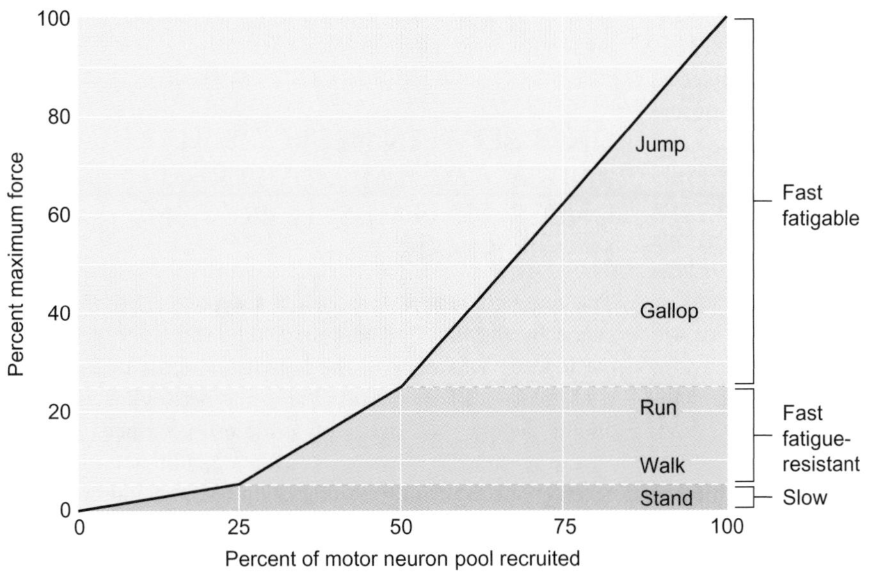

FIGURE 55.3 The recruitment of motoneurons in the cat medial gastrocnemius muscle under different behavioral conditions. Slow motor units provide the tension required for standing. Fast fatigue-resistant units provide the additional force needed for walking and running. Fast fatigable units are recruited for the most strenuous activities. *(Reprinted with permission from Sinauer Associates, Inc.)*

A final issue is "how is the number of myonuclei being modulated under atrophic and hypertrophic conditions"? The major source of new myonuclei most likely is the satellite cell (48–50). Satellite cells divide and one daughter cell enters the myofiber, but it is not known what triggers the fusion event. It appears, for example, multiple divisions of satellite cells and the daughter cells can occur without there being a fusion after each satellite cell division. This delayed fusion, theoretically, would provide a greater potential for providing more new myonuclei, more rapidly. The rate and frequency that satellite cells can divide and a daughter cell fuses with the muscle fiber *in vivo* is unknown, but in culture these cells can divide as many as 35–45 times (51) and can double the number of myonuclei in an individual fiber in 4 days (52). One hypothesis has been that there are a limited number of divisions of a satellite cell and therefore continued demands would eventually exhaust the satellite cell and limit the adaptability of a muscle fiber (53).

INTEGRATION OF ACTIVE AND PASSIVE ELEMENTS OF NEUROMUSCULAR COMPONENTS, *IN VIVO*

Extensive examination and progress in understanding the contractile process of myofibrillar proteins has been made using a variety of experimental techniques to isolate the contractile protein function from the passive elements to which it is attached, both *in series* and *in parallel*. A. V. Hill and his peers (54,55) went to great extremes to isolate the output of contractile protein without the complexities of its integration with the associated connective tissues and the variety of other proteins that directly or indirectly bind to the contractile protein. Because of his success in this isolation he was able to describe a virtually universal property of skeletal muscle with rather impressive precision that defines the output properties of activated contractile protein of skeletal muscle. His objective was not to describe the underlying mechanism of muscle actions *in vivo* with the contractile protein fully integrated in its passive matrices. It is ironic that in spite of Hill's objective to understand the mechanism of the contractile proteins without interference of the passive elements, his model remains the one used most to understand *in vivo* neuromuscular function.

There also has been an extensive examination of the non-contractile elements of skeletal muscle, but again, these efforts, have largely been to understand the mechanical properties of the non-contractile elements in isolation, not as it is integrated with the contractile elements *in vivo*. Largely for these reasons, our understanding of the underlying mechanics of the different contractile and non-contractile elements as they are fully integrated *in vivo* is superficial at best. The best information is based on *in vivo* functions of the whole muscle in different types of movements (56–58). Almost no information has been available on the intricacies of the interactions of different levels of recruitment of motor units and the importance of their differing phenotypes (59–62).

We do have some understanding, however, of the forces and velocities of length changes of skeletal muscle–tendon complexes, largely at moderate speeds of locomotion (56,63,64). These data are consistent in demonstrating the ability of this complex to store mechanical energy and recapture some of this energy in the relaxing phases of a contraction. Given the structural heterogeneity within any muscle–tendon complex and what we know about recruitment of segments of a muscle complex, however, it cannot be assumed that the mechanics observed in an isolated muscle–tendon complex or even under *in vivo* conditions that all of the muscle fibers are stimulated maximally and simultaneously and to its maximum (65,66). These are not events that occur in normally functioning muscle–tendon units *in vivo*. This has been shown clearly in recent work illustrating routine and extensive temporal and spatial heterogeneity in the length changes among and along the length of the fascicles and muscle fibers (67), even in the more mechanically simple *in vivo* isometric contractions in human subjects (65,66,68,69) (Figure 55.4). For example, during isometric contractions the degree of shortening of fibers along their length can differ substantially (66). Similarly, during a voluntary isometric contraction at one phase there can be a strain of the associated connected elements while simultaneously nearby connective tissue elements can even shorten during a muscle contraction, suggesting that the contractile elements of one part of a muscle can unload other subunits of muscle-tendon units. These observations as well as recent modeling results question the validity of most current models of the musculoskeletal system which assume strict homogeneity throughout a muscle–tendon complex (70).

LINKS BETWEEN NEUROMECHANICAL AND MOLECULAR MECHANISMS UNDERLYING MUSCLE PROTEIN HOMEOSTASIS

The mature skeletal muscle phenotype is strongly influenced by the level of neuromuscular activation and muscle loading. Changes in the activity patterns of a muscle can induce either an atrophic or hypertrophic response and/or adapt the kinds of proteins sustained without changing muscle fiber size. Many conditions including disease, age, and injury disrupt this balance and there is a marked change in protein degradation and synthesis, modifying the functional capacity of the affected muscles

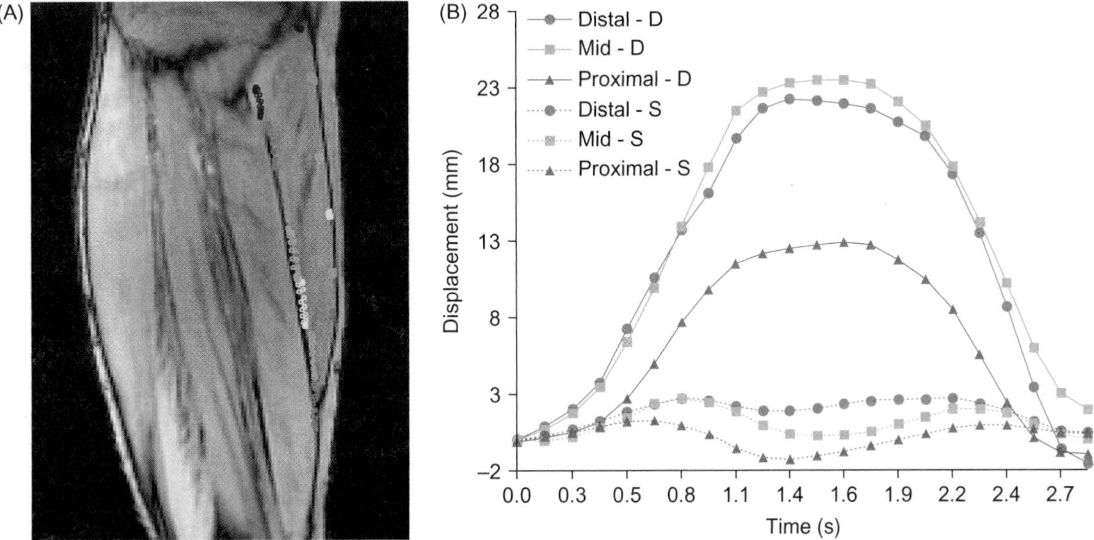

FIGURE 55.4 Displacement of regions of interest (ROIs) during a passive ankle dorsiflexion–plantarflexion cycle. (A) Seven pairs of ROIs corresponding to the ends of muscle fascicles on deep (D) and superficial (S) aponeuroses. The deep aponeurosis is the proximal extension of the Achilles tendon and therefore moves substantially with ankle rotation. The superficial aponeurosis is the tendon of origin for the medial gastrocnemius muscle and moves minimally during the contraction. (B) Graph showing the vertical displacement of the origin and insertion points of muscle fascicles on the aponeuroses. Downward (distal) movements of the ROIs are plotted as positive displacement. The colors correspond to the ROIs in (A). Note that the origins of the fascicles are almost stationary relative to movement of the insertions of the fascicles. *(From Shin et al., 2009 (69), reprinted with permission from the American Physiological Society.)*

(16,42,71–73). Given the magnitude of the motoneuron effect on protein expression in skeletal muscle, the question arises as to the importance of neuromechanical-mediated signals in exerting an influence on a coordinated expression of genes among the hundreds of thousands of myonuclei within a motor unit. Furthermore, given the multiple protein systems that are controlled in a highly coordinated fashion in muscle fibers resulting in different phenotypes, how responsive are the genes that modulate synthesis and degradation of those proteins associated with fiber phenotype to the absence and presence of varying patterns of neuromuscular activity? For example, significant modulation of the metabolic pathways that enhance endurance can be achieved by upregulating specific genes pharmacologically or genetically (74,75). It is well established that many cell types respond to mechanical signals, but there are still large gaps in our knowledge about how these signals are transduced into chemical signals that, in turn, regulate gene expression.

Recent evidence shows the presence of a well-regulated series of events in skeletal muscle concerning the control of net protein balance that are mediated by the relative rates controlling protein synthesis vs. protein degradation (76). For example, IGF-1 stimulates muscle protein synthesis and hypertrophy via the Akt/mammalian target of rapamycin (mTOR) pathway that leads to the concomitant activation of initiation and elongation factors resulting in the elevation of protein translation and the downregulation of ubiquitin proteasome components through Forkhead-box O (FoxO) transcription factors, e.g., atrogin-1 and muscle-specific ring finger 1 (MuRF-1) (35,77,78). In contrast, downregulation of Akt signaling leads to net protein degradation and subsequent atrophy due to the upregulation of atrogin-1 and MuRF-1 (79,80) (Figure 55.5). Together, these data demonstrate a well-coordinated balance between catabolic and anabolic pathways of multiple protein systems that are regulated and maintained to sustain homeostatic and adaptive events in skeletal muscle.

Stretch has been shown to be a powerful stimulation of muscle protein synthesis and growth (81). Numerous studies show that a critical variable in the maintenance of muscle mass, particularly for the muscle to be able to generate force, is that it must generate strain that, in turn, triggers a series of tissue adaptive events. For example, chronically stretching the muscle can increase protein synthesis by adding sarcomeres *in parallel* and *in series* so that the sarcomere length is adjusted back to the optimum for force generation, velocity, and hence power output (23,82,83). Furthermore, when chronic muscle stretch is combined with electrical stimulation, there is a pronounced additive effect on the enhancement of protein synthesis (84). Even in this case, however, the controlling variable could be attributable to the mechanical strain imposed or to biochemical events that could be directly attributable to energy-associated events triggered by action potentials of the motoneurons and subsequently the muscle fibers.

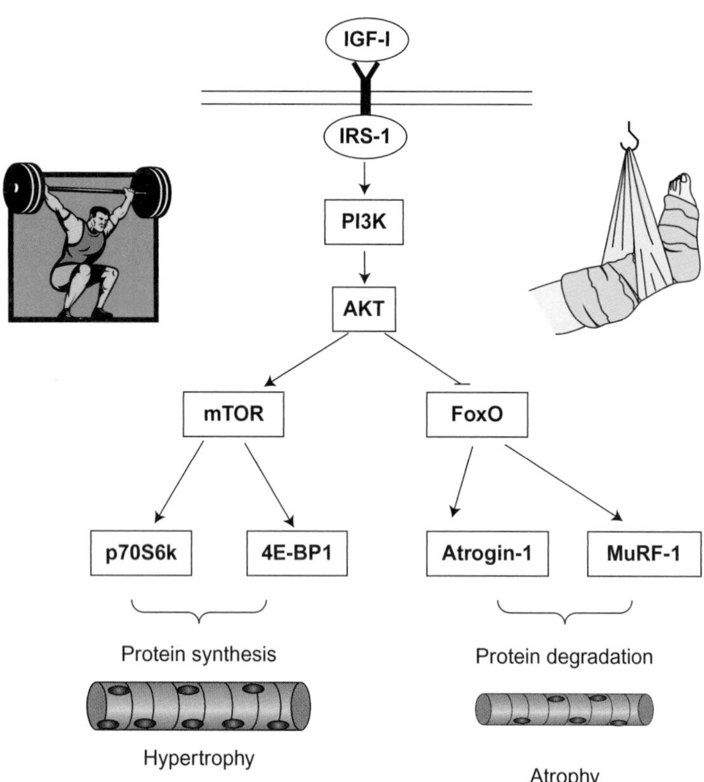

FIGURE 55.5 Schematic and simplified diagram illustrating the IGF-1-mediated pathway involved in protein synthesis and degradation that subsequently leads to muscle hypertrophy or atrophy. Detailed description of the modulation of this pathway has been reviewed by Favier et al. (46). *(Modified from Kim et al., 2010 (93).)*

The increase in mass in response to functional overload of a muscle by removing its synergists is directly proportional to the increases in amino acid incorporation (85). Similarly, in animals and humans, there is a marked increase in protein synthesis within a few hours after an acute bout of resistance exercise or after 2 weeks of resistance training (86). Myofibrillar protein synthesis also is increased with eccentric, concentric, and isometric contraction paradigms in both fast and slow muscles (79,87–89). Although the rate of protein degradation is elevated after a single bout of resistance exercise, there is a greater net increase in protein synthesis, shifting the balance toward greater protein synthesis (89).

Similar adaptive phenomena in protein synthesis and degradation occur with models of decreased use, disuse, and injury, i.e., protein synthesis is decreased and protein degradation is increased, leading to net protein loss as observed with denervation (90), hindlimb unloading (91), spinal cord injury (SCI) (92–94), bedrest (95), limb immobilization (96), microgravity (26,97), and in elderly human subjects (86). Considerable progress has been made in blunting the deleterious effects observed in skeletal muscle after decreased use, disuse, or injury using a variety of pharmacological, electromechanical, and rehabilitative interventions (98,99). For example, weight-supported treadmill training for as little as 30 min per day can lessen the high degree of muscle atrophy and functional deficits associated with a complete spinal cord transection at a mid-thoracic level in adult cats (100,101). Similarly in humans, functional electrical stimulation (FES) has been used commonly to counteract the marked atrophy that occurs after a SCI. The effects of FES on improving muscle mass is largely dependent on the time between the injury and beginning of training, with fewer deficits observed when FES is applied during the acute phase of the injury, i.e., $<$3 months (102,103), but is still effective after more prolonged periods (104,105). In addition, when FES is combined with some form of resistance training, i.e., cycle ergometry, muscle atrophy is further attenuated and there is a marked decrease in muscle protein degradation (102,106) and increase in power output (103).

The potential of electrical stimulation to ameliorate atrophy also has been studied in other models of decreased neuromuscular activity such as hindlimb unloading (107) and in models of inactivity such as denervation (108,109) and spinal cord isolation (92–94,110,111). Stimulating denervated muscles directly with patterns of activity that resemble the normal motor unit activity can restore some muscle properties to near normal, i.e., fiber size, metabolic enzymes, and myosin heavy chain composition (112–115). In addition, when the hindlimb muscles that were otherwise nearly completely electrically silent (via spinal cord isolation) were stimulated for a few min per day (4–9 min over a 24-hr period), the relative muscle mass was maintained near control in both rats and cats (110,111). Combined, these studies demonstrate the importance of motoneuron input, as well as activity, for maintaining muscle mass.

REFERENCES

1. Henneman E. Relation between size of neurons and their susceptibility to discharge. *Science* 1957;**126**:1345–7.
2. Henneman E, Olson CB. Relations between structure and function in the design of skeletal muscles. *J Neurophysiol* 1965;**28**:581–98.
3. Burke RE, Edgerton VR. Motor unit properties and selective involvement in movement. *Exerc Sport Sci Rev* 1975;**3**:31–81.
4. Edgerton VR, Bodine-Fowler S, Roy RR, Ishihara A, Hodgson JA. Neuromuscular adaptation. In: Rowell LB, Shepherd JT, editors. *Handbook of physiology. Section 12. Exercise: regulation and integration of multiple systems*. New York: Oxford University Press; 1996. p. 54–88.
5. Salmons S, Sreter FA. Significance of impulse activity in the transformation of skeletal muscle type. *Nature* 1976;**263**:30–4.
6. Pette D, Vrbova G. What does chronic electrical stimulation teach us about muscle plasticity? *Muscle Nerve* 1999;**22**:666–77.
7. Stuart DG, Enoka RM. *Motoneurons, motor units, and the size principle*. New York: Churchill Livingstone;1983.
8. Bodine SC, Roy RR, Eldred E, Edgerton VR. Maximal force as a function of anatomical features of motor units in the cat tibialis anterior. *J Neurophysiol* 1987;**57**:1730–45.
9. Barnard RJ, Edgerton VR, Furukawa T, Peter JB. Histochemical, biochemical, and contractile properties of red, white, and intermediate fibers. *Am J Physiol* 1971;**220**:410–4.
10. Pette D, Ramirez BU, Muller W, Simon R, Exner GU, Hildebrand R. Influence of intermittent long-term stimulation on contractile, histochemical and metabolic properties of fibre populations in fast and slow rabbit muscles. *Pflugers Arch* 1975;**361**:1–7.
11. Peter JB, Barnard RJ, Edgerton VR, Gillespie CA, Stempel KE. Metabolic profiles of three fiber types of skeletal muscle in guinea pigs and rabbits. *Biochem J* 1972;**11**:2627–33.
12. Pette D, Staron RS. Cellular and molecular diversities of mammalian skeletal muscle fibers. *Rev Physiol Biochem Pharmacol* 1990;**116**:1–76.
13. Pierotti DJ, Roy RR, Bodine-Fowler SC, Hodgson JA, Edgerton VR. Mechanical and morphological properties of chronically inactive cat tibialis anterior motor units. *J Physiol* 1991;**444**:175–92.
14. Roy RR, Garfinkel A, Ounjian M, Payne J, Hirahara A, Hsu E, et al. Three dimensional structure of cat tibialis anterior motor units. *Muscle Nerve* 1995;**18**:1187–95.
15. Unguez GA, Bodine-Fowler S, Roy RR, Pierotti DJ, Edgerton VR. Evidence of incomplete neural control of motor unit properties in cat tibialis anterior after self-reinnervation. *J Physiol* 1993; **472**:103–25.
16. Edgerton VR, Roy RR. Regulation of skeletal muscle fiber size, shape and function. *J Biomech* 1991;**24** (Suppl. 1):123–33.
17. Caiozzo VJ, Baker MJ, Baldwin KM. Novel transitions in MHC isoforms: separate and combined effects of thyroid hormone and mechanical unloading. *J Appl Physiol* 1998;**85**:2237–48.
18. Pette D. The adaptive potential of skeletal muscle fibers. *Can J Appl Physiol* 2002;**27**:423–48.
19. Talmadge RJ. Myosin heavy chain isoform expression following reduced neuromuscular activity: potential regulatory mechanisms. *Muscle Nerve* 2000;**23**:661–79.
20. Edgerton VR, Martin TP, Bodine SC, Roy RR. How flexible is the neural control of muscle properties? *J Exp Biol* 1985;**115**:393–402.
21. Nemeth PM, Solanki L, Gordon DA, Hamm TM, Reinking RM, Stuart DG. Uniformity of metabolic enzymes within individual motor units. *J Neurosci* 1986;**6**:892–8.
22. Lieber RL. *Skeletal muscle structure, function and plasticity. The physiological basis of rehabilitation*. 2nd ed. Baltimore, MD: Lippincott Williams & Wilkins; 2002.
23. Spector SA, Gardiner PF, Zernicke RF, Roy RR, Edgerton VR. Muscle architecture and force-velocity characteristics of cat soleus and medial gastrocnemius: implications for motor control. *J Neurophysiol* 1980;**44**:951–60.
24. Sacks RD, Roy RR. Architecture of the hind limb muscles of cats: functional significance. *J Morphol* 1982;**173**:185–95.
25. Allen DL, Roy RR, Edgerton VR. Myonuclear domains in muscle adaptation and disease. *Muscle Nerve* 1999;**22**:1350–60.
26. Ohira Y, Jiang B, Roy RR, Oganov V, Ilyina-Kakueva E, Marini JF, et al. Rat soleus muscle fiber responses to 14 days of spaceflight and hindlimb suspension. *J Appl Physiol* 1992;**73**:51S–7S.
27. Kawano F, Takeno Y, Nakai N, Higo Y, Terada M, Ohira T, et al. Essential role of satellite cells in the growth of rat soleus muscle fibers. *Am J Physiol Cell Physiol* 2008;**295**:C458–67.
28. Mantilla CB, Sill RV, Aravamudan B, Zhan WZ, Sieck GC. Developmental effects on myonuclear domain size of rat diaphragm fibers. *J Appl Physiol* 2008;**104**:787–94.
29. Hall ZW, Ralston E. Nuclear domains in muscle cells. *Cell* 1989;**59**:771–2.
30. Ketterer C, Zeiger U, Budak MT, Rubinstein NA, Khurana TS. Identification of the neuromuscular junction transcriptome of extraocular muscle by laser capture microdissection. *Invest Ophthalmol Vis Sci* 2010;**51**:4589–99.
31. Milanic T, Kunstelj A, Mar T, Grubi Z. Morphometric characteristics of myonuclear distribution in the normal and denervated fast rat muscle fiber. *Chem Biol Interact* 1999;**119**:321–6.
32. Allouh MZ, Yablonka-Reuveni Z, Rosser BWC. Pax7 reveals a greater frequency and concentration of satellite cells at the ends of growing skeletal muscle fibers. *J Histochem Cytochem* 2008;**56**:77–87.
33. Teixeira CE, Duarte JA. Myonuclear domain in skeletal muscle fibers. A critical review. *Arch Exerc Health Dis* 2011;**2**:92–101.
34. Selye H. *The stress of life*. New York: McGraw-Hill; 1956.
35. Sacheck JM, Hyatt JPK, Raffaello A, Jagoe RT, Roy RR, Edgerton VR, et al. Rapid disuse and denervation atrophy involve transcriptional changes similar to those of muscle wasting during systemic diseases. *FASEB J* 2007;**21**:140–55.
36. Thomason DB, Booth FW. Atrophy of the soleus muscle by hindlimb unweighting. *J Appl Physiol* 1990;**68**:1–12.
37. Blaauw B, Canato M, Agatea L, Toniolo L, Mammucari C, Masiero E, et al. Inducible activation of Akt increases skeletal muscle mass and force without satellite cell activation. *FASEB J* 2009;**23**:3896–905.
38. van der Meer SF, Jaspers RT, Jones DA, Degens H. The time course of myonuclear accretion during hypertrophy in young adult and older rat plantaris muscle. *Ann Anat* 2011;**193**:56–63.

39. Roy RR, Monke SR, Allen DL, Edgerton VR. Modulation of myonuclear number in functionally overloaded and exercised rat plantaris fibers. *J Appl Physiol* 1999;**87**:634–42.
40. Mitchell PO, Pavlath GK. A muscle precursor cell-dependent pathway contributes to muscle growth after atrophy. *Am J Physiol Cell Physiol* 2001;**281**:C1706–15.
41. Zhang BT, Yeung SS, Liu Y, Wang HH, Wan YM, Ling SK, et al. The effects of low frequency electrical stimulation on satellite cell activity in rat skeletal muscle during hindlimb suspension. *BMC Cell Biol* 2010;**11**:87.
42. Adams GR, Caiozzo VJ, Haddad F, Baldwin KM. Cellular and molecular responses to increased skeletal muscle loading after irradiation. *Am J Physiol Cell Physiol* 2002;**283**:C1182–95.
43. Li P, Akimoto T, Zhang M, Williams RS, Yan Z. Resident stem cells are not required for exercise-induced fiber-type switching and angiogenesis but are necessary for activity-dependent muscle growth. *Am J Physiol Cell Physiol* 2006;**290**:C1461–8.
44. Rosenblatt JD, Yong D, Parry DJ. Satellite cell activity is required for hypertrophy of overloaded adult rat muscle. *Muscle Nerve* 1994;**17**:608–13.
45. Brack AS, Bildsoe H, Hughes SM. Evidence that satellite cell decrement contributes to preferential decline in nuclear number from large fibres during murine age-related muscle atrophy. *J Cell Sci* 2005;**118**:4813–21.
46. Favier FB, Benoit H, Freyssenet D. Cellular and molecular events controlling skeletal muscle mass in response to altered use. *Pflugers Arch* 2008;**456**:587–600.
47. Gundersen K, Bruusgaard JC. Nuclear domains during muscle atrophy: nuclei lost or paradigm lost? *J Physiol* 2008;**586**:2675–81.
48. Adams GR. Satellite cell proliferation and skeletal muscle hypertrophy. *Appl Physiol Nutr Metab* 2006;**31**:782–90.
49. Hawke TJ, Garry DJ. Myogenic satellite cells: physiology to molecular biology. *J Appl Physiol* 2001;**91**:534–51.
50. Schiaffino S, Pierobon Bormioli S, Aloisi M. The fate of newly formed satellite cells during compensatory muscle hypertrophy. *Virchows Arch B Cell Pathol* 1976;**21**:113–8.
51. Blau HM, Webster C, Pavlath GK. Defective myoblasts identified in Duchenne muscular dystrophy. *Proc Natl Acad Sci USA* 1983;**80**:4856–60.
52. Bischoff R. Analysis of muscle regeneration using single myofibers in culture. *Med Sci Sports Exerc* 1989;**21**:S164–72.
53. Scimè A, Rudnicki MA. Anabolic potential and regulation of the skeletal muscle satellite cell populations. *Curr Opin Clin Nutr Metab Care* 2006;**9**:214–9.
54. Hill AV. The heat of shortening and the dynamic constant. *Proc R Soc Lond B Biol Sci* 1938;**126**:136–95.
55. Hill AV. *First and last experiments in muscle mechanics*. New York: Cambridge University Press; 1970.
56. Gregor RJ, Roy RR, Whiting WC, Lovely RG, Hodgson JA, Edgerton VR. Mechanical output of the cat soleus during treadmill locomotion: in vivo vs in situ characteristics. *J Biomech* 1988;**21**:721–32.
57. Maas H, Gregor RJ, Hodson-Tole EF, Farrell BJ, Prilutsky BI. Distinct muscle fascicle length changes in feline medial gastrocnemius and soleus muscles during slope walking. *J Appl Physiol* 2009;**106**:1169–80.
58. Prilutsky BI, Herzog W, Allinger TL. Mechanical power and work of cat soleus, gastrocnemius and plantaris muscles during locomotion: possible functional significance of muscle design and force patterns. *J Exp Biol* 1996;**199**:801–14.
59. Clamann HP, Schelhorn TB. Nonlinear force addition of newly recruited motor units in the cat hindlimb. *Muscle Nerve* 1988;**11**:1079–89.
60. Emonet-Denand F, Laporte Y, Proske U. Summation of tension in motor units of the soleus muscle of the cat. *Neurosci Lett* 1990;**116**:112–7.
61. Horcholle-Bossavit G, Jami L, Petit J, Vejsada R, Zytnicki D. Ensemble discharge from Golgi tendon organs of cat peroneus tertius muscle. *J Neurophysiol* 1990;**64**:813–21.
62. Perreault EJ, Day SJ, Hulliger M, Heckman CJ, Sandercock TG. Summation of forces from multiple motor units in the cat soleus muscle. *J Neurophysiol* 2003;**89**:738–44.
63. Walmsley B, Hodgson JA, Burke RE. Forces produced by medial gastrocnemius and soleus muscles during locomotion in freely moving cats. *J Neurophysiol* 1978;**41**:1203–16.
64. Whiting WC, Gregor RJ, Roy RR, Edgerton VR. A technique for estimating mechanical work of individual muscles in the cat during treadmill locomotion. *J Biomech* 1984;**17**:685–94.
65. Kinugasa R, Kawakami Y, Sinha S, Fukunaga T. Unique spatial distribution of in vivo human muscle activation. *Exp Physiol* 2011;**96**:938–48.
66. Kinugasa R, Shin D, Yamauchi J, Mishra C, Hodgson JA, Edgerton VR, et al. Phase-contrast MRI reveals mechanical behavior of superficial and deep aponeuroses in human medial gastrocnemius during isometric contraction. *J Appl Physiol* 2008;**105**:1312–20.
67. Monti RJ, Roy RR, Zhong H, Edgerton VR. Mechanical properties of rat soleus aponeurosis and tendon during variable recruitment in situ. *J Exp Biol* 2003;**206**:3437–45.
68. Finni T, Hodgson JA, Lai AM, Edgerton VR, Sinha S. Nonuniform strain of human soleus aponeurosis-tendon complex during submaximal voluntary contractions in vivo. *J Appl Physiol* 2003;**95**:829–37.
69. Shin DD, Hodgson JA, Edgerton VR, Sinha S. In vivo intramuscular fascicle-aponeuroses dynamics of the human medial gastrocnemius during plantarflexion and dorsiflexion of the foot. *J Appl Physiol* 2009;**107**:1276–84.
70. Chi SW, Hodgson J, Chen JS, Reggie Edgerton V, Shin DD, Roiz RA, et al. Finite element modeling reveals complex strain mechanics in the aponeuroses of contracting skeletal muscle. *J Biomech* 2011;**43**:1243–50.
71. Booth FW, Tseng BS, Fluck M, Carson JA. Molecular and cellular adaptation of muscle in response to physical training. *Acta Physiol Scand* 1998;**162**:343–50.
72. Caiozzo VJ, Richmond H, Kaska S, Valeroso D. The mechanical behavior of activated skeletal muscle during stretch: effects of muscle unloading and MyHC isoform shifts. *J Appl Physiol* 2007;**103**:1150–60.
73. Roy RR, Baldwin KM, Edgerton VR. The plasticity of skeletal muscle: effects of neuromuscular activity. *Exerc Sport Sci Rev* 1991;**19**:269–312.
74. Narkar VA, Downes M, Yu RT, Embler E, Wang YX, Banayo E, et al. AMPK and PPARdelta agonists are exercise mimetics. *Cell* 2008;**134**:405–15.
75. Wang YX, Zhang CL, Yu RT, Cho HK, Nelson MC, Bayuga-Ocampo CR, et al. Regulation of muscle fiber type and running endurance by PPARdelta. *PLoS Biol* 2004;**2**:e294.

76. Goll DE, Neti G, Mares SW, Thompson VF. Myofibrillar protein turnover: the proteasome and the calpains. *J Anim Sci* 2008;**86**: E19–35.
77. Bodine SC, Stitt TN, Gonzalez M, Kline WO, Stover GL, Bauerlein R, et al. Akt/mTOR pathway is a crucial regulator of skeletal muscle hypertrophy and can prevent muscle atrophy in vivo. *Nat Cell Biol* 2001;**3**:1014–9.
78. Leger B, Cartoni R, Praz M, Lamon S, Deriaz O, Crettenand A, et al. Akt signalling through GSK-3beta, mTOR and Foxo1 is involved in human skeletal muscle hypertrophy and atrophy. *J Physiol* 2006;**576**:923–33.
79. Latres E, Amini AR, Amini AA, Griffiths J, Martin FJ, Wei Y, et al. Insulin-like growth factor-1 (IGF-1) inversely regulates atrophy-induced genes via the phosphatidylinositol 3-kinase/Akt/mammalian target of rapamycin (PI3K/Akt/mTOR) pathway. *J Biol Chem* 2005;**280**:2737–44.
80. Sandri M, Sandri C, Gilbert A, Skurk C, Calabria E, Picard A, et al. Foxo transcription factors induce the atrophy-related ubiquitin ligase atrogin-1 and cause skeletal muscle atrophy. *Cell* 2004;**117**:399–412.
81. Goldspink G. Changes in muscle mass and phenotype and the expression of autocrine and systemic growth factors by muscle in response to stretch and overload. *J Anat* 1999;**194**:323–34.
82. Tabary JC, Tabary C, Tardieu C, Tardieu G, Goldspink G. Physiological and structural changes in the cat's soleus muscle due to immobilization at different lengths by plaster casts. *J Physiol* 1972;**224**:231–44.
83. Loughna P, Goldspink G, Goldspink DF. Effect of inactivity and passive stretch on protein turnover in phasic and postural rat muscles. *J Appl Physiol* 1986;**61**:173–9.
84. Goldspink G, Scutt A, Loughna PT, Wells DJ, Jaenicke T, Gerlach GF. Gene expression in skeletal muscle in response to stretch and force generation. *Am J Physiol* 1992;**262**:R356–63.
85. Goldberg AL. Protein synthesis during work-induced growth of skeletal muscle. *J Cell Biol* 1968;**36**:653–8.
86. Yarasheski KE, Zachwieja JJ, Bier DM. Acute effects of resistance exercise on muscle protein synthesis rate in young and elderly men and women. *Am J Physiol* 1993;**265**:E210–4.
87. MacDougall JD, Tarnopolsky MA, Chesley A, Atkinson SA. Changes in muscle protein synthesis following heavy resistance exercise in humans: a pilot study. *Acta Physiol Scand* 1992;**146**:403–4.
88. Moore DR, Phillips SM, Babraj JA, Smith K, Rennie MJ. Myofibrillar and collagen protein synthesis in human skeletal muscle in young men after maximal shortening and lengthening contractions. *Am J Physiol Endocrinol Metab* 2005;**288**:E1153–9.
89. Phillips SM, Tipton KD, Aarsland A, Wolf SE, Wolfe RR. Mixed muscle protein synthesis and breakdown after resistance exercise in humans. *Am J Physiol Endocrinol Metab* 1997;**273**:E99–107.
90. Goldspink DF. The effects of denervation on protein turnover of rat skeletal muscle. *Biochem J* 1976;**156**:71–80.
91. Goldspink DF, Morton AJ, Loughna P, Goldspink G. The effect of hypokinesia and hypodynamia on protein turnover and the growth of four skeletal muscles of the rat. *Pflugers Arch* 1986;**407**:333–40.
92. Haddad F, Roy RR, Zhong H, Edgerton VR, Baldwin KM. Atrophy responses to muscle inactivity. II. Molecular markers of protein deficits. *J Appl Physiol* 2003;**95**:791–802.
93. Kim JA, Roy RR, Kim SJ, Zhong H, Haddad F, Baldwin KM, et al. Electromechanical modulation of catabolic and anabolic pathways in chronically inactive, but neurally intact, muscles. *Muscle Nerve* 2010;**42**:410–21.
94. Kim SJ, Roy RR, Zhong H, Suzuki H, Ambartsumyan L, Haddad F, et al. Electromechanical stimulation ameliorates inactivity-induced adaptations in the medial gastrocnemius of adult rats. *J Appl Physiol* 2007;**103**:195–205.
95. Ferrando AA, Lane HW, Stuart CA, Davis-Street J, Wolfe RR. Prolonged bed rest decreases skeletal muscle and whole body protein synthesis. *Am J Physiol Endocrinol Metab* 1996;**270**: E627–33.
96. Booth FW, Seider MJ. Early change in skeletal muscle protein synthesis after limb immobilization of rats. *J Appl Physiol* 1979;**47**:974–7.
97. Baldwin KM, Herrick RE, Ilyina-Kakueva E, Oganov VS. Effects of zero gravity on myofibril content and isomyosin distribution in rodent skeletal muscle. *FASEB J* 1990;**4**:79–83.
98. Edgerton VR, Roy RR, Allen DL, Monti RJ. Adaptations in skeletal muscle disuse or decreased-use atrophy. *Am J Phys Med Rehabil* 2002;**81**:S127–47.
99. Fong AJ, Roy RR, Ichiyama RM, Lavrov I, Courtine G, Gerasimenko Y, et al. Recovery of control of posture and locomotion after a spinal cord injury: solutions staring us in the face. *Prog Brain Res* 2009;**175**:393–418.
100. Roy RR, Acosta Jr L. Fiber type and fiber size changes in selected thigh muscles six months after low thoracic spinal cord transection in adult cats: exercise effects. *Exp Neurol* 1986;**92**:675–85.
101. Roy RR, Talmadge RJ, Hodgson JA, Oishi Y, Baldwin KM, Edgerton VR. Differential response of fast hindlimb extensor and flexor muscles to exercise in adult spinalized cats. *Muscle Nerve* 1999;**22**:230–41.
102. Baldi JC, Jackson RD, Moraille R, Mysiw WJ. Muscle atrophy is prevented in patients with acute spinal cord injury using functional electrical stimulation. *Spinal Cord* 1998;**36**:463–9.
103. Demchak TJ, Linderman JK, Mysiw WJ, Jackson R, Suun J, Devor ST. Effects of functional electrical stimulation cycle ergometry training on lower limb musculature in acute SCI individuals. *J Sports Sci Med* 2005;**4**:263–71.
104. Chilibeck PD, Jeon J, Weiss C, Bell G, Burnham R. Histochemical changes in muscle of individuals with spinal cord injury following functional electrical stimulated exercise training. *Spinal Cord* 1999;**37**:264–8.
105. Mohr T, Andersen JL, Biering-Sorensen F, Galbo H, Bangsbo J, Wagner A, et al. Long-term adaptation to electrically induced cycle training in severe spinal cord injured individuals. *Spinal Cord* 1997;**35**:1–16.
106. Crameri RM, Weston A, Climstein M, Davis GM, Sutton JR. Effects of electrical stimulation-induced leg training on skeletal muscle adaptability in spinal cord injury. *Scand J Med Sci Sports* 2002;**12**:316–22.
107. Diffee GM, Caiozzo VJ, McCue SA, Herrick RE, Baldwin KM. Activity-induced regulation of myosin isoform distribution: comparison of two contractile activity programs. *J Appl Physiol* 1993;**74**:2509–16.
108. Dow DE, Cederna PS, Hassett CA, Kostrominova TY, Faulkner JA, Dennis RG. Number of contractions to maintain mass and force of a denervated rat muscle. *Muscle Nerve* 2004;**30**:77–86.

109. Hennig R, Lomo T. Effects of chronic stimulation on the size and speed of long-term denervated and innervated rat fast and slow skeletal muscles. *Acta Physiol Scand* 1987;**130**:115–31.

110. Kim SJ, Roy RR, Kim JA, Zhong H, Haddad F, Baldwin KM, et al. Gene expression during inactivity-induced muscle atrophy: effects of brief bouts of a forceful contraction countermeasure. *J Appl Physiol* 2008;**105**:1246–54.

111. Roy RR, Zhong H, Hodgson JA, Grossman EJ, Siengthai B, Talmadge RJ, et al. Influences of electromechanical events in defining skeletal muscle properties. *Muscle Nerve* 2002; **26**:238–51.

112. Hennig R, Lomo T. Firing patterns of motor units in normal rats. *Nature* 1985;**314**:164–6.

113. Lomo T, Westgaard RH, Dahl HA. Contractile properties of muscle: control by pattern of muscle activity in the rat. *Proc R Soc Lond B Biol Sci* 1974;**187**:99–103.

114. Melichna J, Gutmann E. Stimulation and immobilization effects on contractile and histochemical properties of denervated muscle. *Pflugers Arch* 1974;**352**:165–78.

115. Riley DA, Allin EF. The effects of inactivity, programmed stimulation, and denervation on the histochemistry of skeletal muscle fiber types. *Exp Neurol* 1973;**40**:391–413.

Chapter 56

Control of Resting Ca^{2+} Concentration in Skeletal Muscle

Jose R. Lopez and Paul D. Allen

Department of Anesthesia, Perioperative and Pain Medicine, Brigham and Women's Hospital, Harvard Medical School, Boston, MA

INTRODUCTION

Ca^{2+} is a critical signaling molecule within cells (1). Many cellular functions are directly or indirectly regulated by intracellular calcium concentration ($[Ca^{2+}]_i$), and because cells extract specific information from changes in $[Ca^{2+}]_i$ over time, in space and in amplitude all three parameters must be very tightly regulated.

Under resting conditions, skeletal muscle cells maintain $[Ca^{2+}]_i$ in a narrow range near 100 nM. This low cytosolic concentration has been described in both frog (2) and mammalian skeletal muscle (3–5). Because the gradient between resting myoplasmic free calcium and the extracellular space and internal stores is about 10,000-fold, to constantly keep $[Ca^{2+}]_i$ in the nM concentration range muscle cells use a complex dynamic equilibrium of Ca^{2+} fluxes among pumps (plasma membrane Ca^{2+} ATPase, and sarcoplasmic reticulum Ca^{2+} ATPase) and an exchanger (Na^+/Ca^{2+}exchanger) opposed by sarcoplasmic reticulum (SR) leak channels (ryanodine-insensitive "Ca^{2+} leak") as well as basal sarcolemmal Ca^{2+} influx (6) which tunes myoplasmic Ca^{2+} homeostasis at rest (see Figure 56.1).

MECHANISMS FOR Ca^{2+} REMOVAL FROM THE MYOPLASM OF MUSCLE CELLS

Sarcolemmal Outward Ca^{2+} Transport Mechanisms

It is generally accepted that the control of resting $[Ca^{2+}]_i$ in mammalian muscle cells is via plasmalemmal Ca^{2+} extrusion via the sodium calcium exchanger (NCX) and the calmodulin-regulated plasma membrane Ca-ATPase (PMCA).

Sodium Calcium Exchanger (NCX)

The NCX is an electrogenic ($3Na^+/1Ca^{2+}$) and reversible counter transport system with a well-established role in Ca^{2+} homeostasis in a variety of cells (7), including amphibian and mammalian skeletal muscle and mammalian myotubes (8–10). Three mammalian isoforms of the NCX protein that are products of three different genes have been cloned (11–13) and appear to have very similar properties (14). In its forward mode, NCX can operate as a high capacity and low affinity system for Ca^{2+} transport, extruding Ca^{2+} against its transmembrane electrochemical gradient, making use of the Na^+ electrochemical gradient (7). Given the right balance between the respective electrochemical gradients, the NCX can also operate in the reverse mode, transporting Ca^{2+} into cells and Na^+ out (7).

Although both NCX1 and NCX3 isoforms have been found in the transverse tubule (T-tubule) and the sarcolemma (10,15) in mammalian skeletal muscle, the physiological role for NCX in muscle has not yet been defined. Muscle fibers from amphibian skeletal muscle (8,16) and human myotubes (10) have been shown to exhibit Na^+-dependent Ca^{2+} efflux (forward and reverse mode). Recently we have found that NCX in its reverse mode may play an important role in the regulation of resting $[Ca^{2+}]_i$ in muscle fibers which express RyR1s with mutations associated with malignant hyperthermia. A possible explanation for this is the high resting $[Na^+]$i (15 mM) that we have found in these cells. In practical terms the elevation of $[Ca^{2+}]_i$ during contraction activates the NXC forward mode, and an elevation of $[Na^+]_i$ above normal resting values will result in enhanced Ca^{2+} influx via the NCX-reverse mode (Lopez et al., unpublished results).

Plasma Membrane Ca^{2+}-ATPase (PMCA)

Plasma membrane calcium pumps, also known as the plasma membrane Ca^{2+}-ATPase or PMCA, are responsible for the expulsion of Ca^{2+} from the cytosol of all eukaryotic cells. Together with NCX, they are the major plasma membrane transport system responsible for the long-term regulation of the resting $[Ca^{2+}]_i$. Like the

Muscle. DOI: http://dx.doi.org/10.1016/B978-0-12-381510-1.00056-9

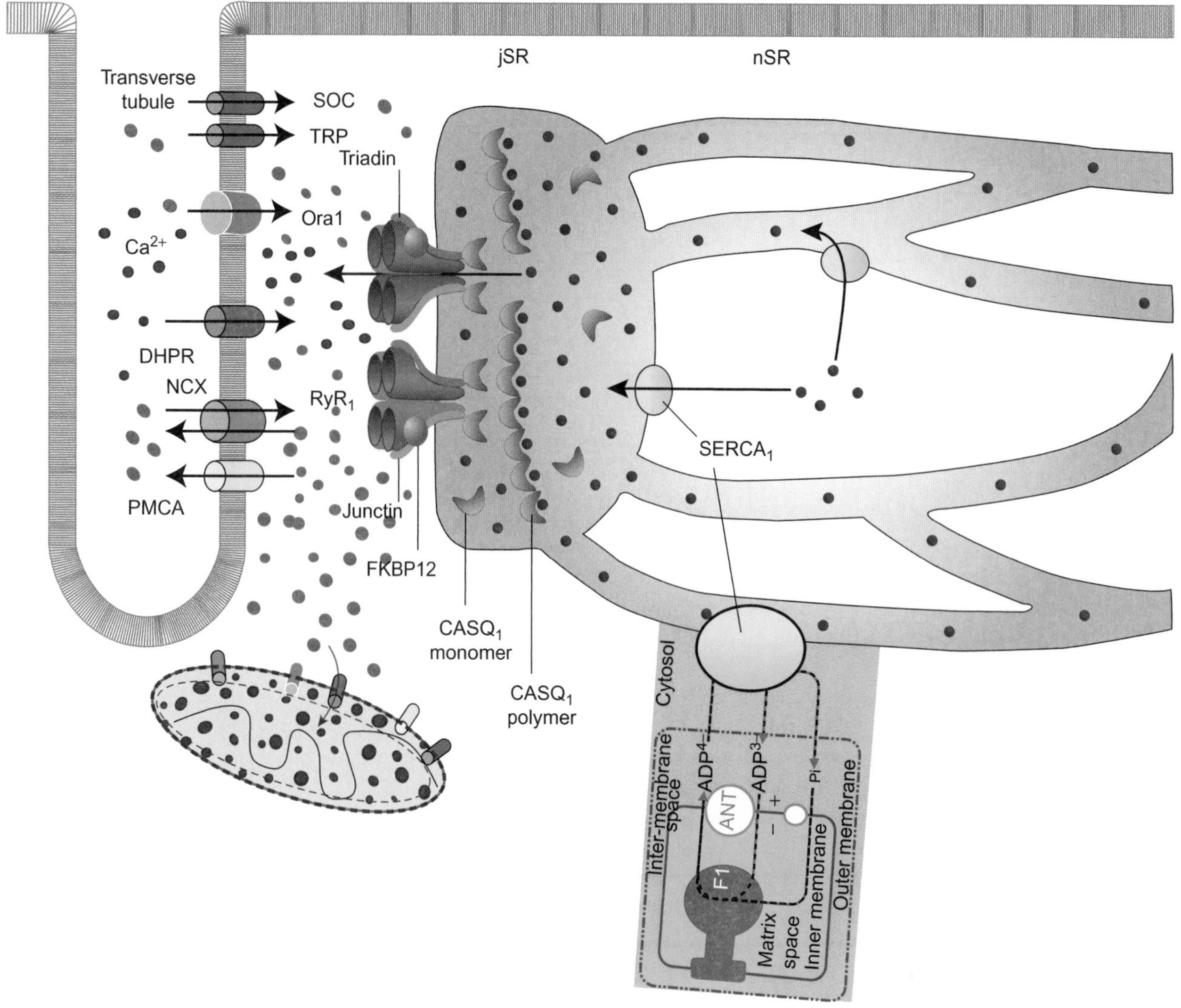

FIGURE 56.1 Cartoon model of skeletal muscle showing all of the proposed involved proteins in the macromolecular CRU complex that play a significant role in controlling Ca^{2+} homeostasis at rest.

Ca^{2+} pump of the sarcoplasmic/endoplasmic reticulum (SERCA), which pumps Ca^{2+} from the cytosol into the SR, PMCA belong to the family of P-type, named so because these calcium-transport proteins undergo autophosphorylation in which the γ-phosphate of ATP is transferred to a highly conserved aspartyl residue in the cytoplasmic portion of the protein (17). Mammalian PMCA are encoded by four separate genes and additional isoform variants are generated via alternative RNA splicing of the primary gene transcripts (18,19). The expression of different PMCA isoforms and splice variants is regulated in a developmental, tissue- and cell type-specific manner, suggesting that these pumps are functionally adapted to the physiological needs of particular cells and tissues. Different PMCA isoforms have different basal activities, affinities for calmodulin and rates of activation and inactivation (20), suggesting they may have different physiological roles.

The PMCA has low capacity but high affinity for Ca^{2+} transport with a 1:1 Ca^{2+}/ATP stoichiometry. Work on purified protein reconstituted in liposomes had suggested electroneutrality (21) while other experiments have suggested that it is a partially electrogenic 1:1 Ca^{2+}:H^+ transport process (22). The activity of the pump in native membranes has been found to be insensitive to the variation of the membrane potential, strongly supporting an electroneutral H^+/Ca^{2+} reaction (23). Under conditions found in the cell, the K_d of the pump for Ca^{2+} is in the 200–500 nM range. Although the Ca^{2+} affinity of the PMCA pump is lower than that of SERCA, it is high enough to enable it to operate with reasonable efficiency at Ca^{2+} concentrations such as those prevailing in the myoplasm at rest. Accordingly, the PMCA has been conventionally defined as the fine tuner of cytosolic [Ca^{2+}]. However the physiological contribution of PMCA to the intracellular Ca^{2+} homeostasis in skeletal muscle still is not fully defined. One significant reason for this is that there are no specific pharmacological inhibitors for any of the PMCA isoforms or splice variants and until muscle-specific genetic manipulation, i.e., selective "knock out or knock down" or overexpression of specific PMCA isoforms is done in skeletal muscle its regulation of contraction/relaxation in adult animals will be unknown.

SR Ca^{2+} Reuptake: the SERCA Pump

It is well established that active transport is required to import Ca^{2+} into the lumen of SR after muscle activation (for review see 24). The SR of skeletal muscle is an extensively developed network of tubules and cisternae that is arranged in a precise geometric relationship to the contractile elements (25) and represents the primary calcium-storage organelle in striated muscle.

The 100 kDa ATP-dependent Ca^{2+} pump (SERCA) is an intrinsic component of the SR membrane in muscle cells, which makes up 50–80% of the total protein of endoplasmic reticulum (26). SERCA-mediated SR calcium reuptake controls the rate of muscle relaxation in skeletal muscle and is responsible for maintaining a 10,000-fold calcium gradient across the SR membrane. Like the PMCA, SERCA is a member of the family of P-type Ca^{2+}-ATPases (17). The ATP-dependent Ca^{2+} pump is evenly distributed throughout the free SR and catalyzes the electrogenic transport of 2 Ca^{2+} coupled to the hydrolysis of 1 mol of ATP, against a large electrochemical gradient of Ca^{2+}. Unlike the PMCA, SERCA is relatively insensitive to calmodulin (27,28).

Brody's disease is a rare recessive genetic disease associated with mutation in SERCA characterized by impaired relaxation, painless cramps, and stiffness following exercise (29). Three mutations in the SERCA1 gene have been identified in two affected families (30). These patients can still relax their muscles, although at a significantly reduced rate. This suggests that some compensation by ectopic expression of other SERCA isoforms (SERCA2 or SERCA3), and/or that Ca^{2+} removal from the cytosol by the PMCA pump and/or the Na^+/Ca^{2+} exchanger could limit the defect in the Ca^{2+}-clearing activity of the SR.

Although it has been generally thought that the only function of SERCA1 is the reuptake of Ca^{2+} after muscle contraction and that the overall control of resting cytosolic [Ca^{2+}] is via the pumps and exchangers at the sarcolemma, recent studies suggest that this is not the case. Goonasakera et al. have shown that by overexpressing SERCA1 in skeletal muscle of mice with three severe myopathic conditions that the pathologic changes associated with these myopathies could be abrogated (31). Because some, and it is likely all, of these conditions are associated with increased resting $[Ca^{2+}]_i$ these data suggest that the control of resting $[Ca^{2+}]_i$ is not limited to the sarcolemma but may also be mediated by SR Ca^{2+} uptake.

MECHANISMS FOR Ca^{2+} ENTRY INTO THE MYOPLASM IN SKELETAL MUSCLE

Sarcolemmal Ca^{2+} Entry Mechanisms

It was established decades ago that excitation–contraction (EC) coupling relies on the depolarization-dependent release of stored calcium in the SR for skeletal muscle contraction (32,33). More recently, growing evidence suggests that alternative calcium signaling pathways rely on sarcolemmal calcium entry (34–36). Two forms of Ca^{2+} entry have been characterized in skeletal muscle fibers: excitation-coupled calcium entry (ECCE), which is activated in muscle cells during prolonged membrane depolarization and is independent of the filling state, and store-operated calcium entry (SOCE) (37), which occurs in response to depletion of the internal stores (for reviews see 38, 39).

Excitation-Coupled Ca^{2+} Entry (ECCE)

It has been reported that the interaction between the DHPR and RYR1 during activation promotes entry of extracellular Ca^{2+} into the myoplasm in skeletal myotubes (5,37) and adult muscle fibers (40). This form of Ca^{2+} entry is termed excitation-coupled Ca^{2+} entry (ECCE). Although the molecular identity of the ECCE pore remains undefined, some authors have suggested it is the L-type calcium channel (41–43). ECCE requires the expression of both the DHPR and RYR1, as it is absent in both dysgenic ($Ca_V1.1$-null) and dyspedic (RYR1-null) myotubes (37). Interestingly, ECCE is enhanced by conformational changes in RYR1 such as those caused by ryanodine, certain cysteine mutations and mutations that are associated with malignant hyperthermia (5,40,44). Pharmacologically, ECCE can be blocked by 2-aminoethyl diphenylborate (2-APB), SKF 96356, La^{3+}, Gd^{3+}, and dantrolene (37,43,45). ECCE is independent of stores and can occur both without any store depletion (36,37,40,45) and in cells in which stores are fully depleted (37,46). Thus, it appears that ECCE may be important in normal skeletal muscle in helping to maintain force generation during tetanic stimulation, and accentuated ECCE may contribute to the pathophysiological increase in myoplasmic Ca^{2+} in malignant hyperthermia.

Store-Operated Ca^{2+} Entry (SOCE)

Capacitative Ca^{2+} entry, or store-operated Ca^{2+} entry (SOCE), was first described and characterized in non-excitable cells, where it constitutes a major pathway for Ca^{2+} influx (38). The electrical manifestation of this Ca^{2+} entry in the continuous presence of extracellular Ca^{2+} is a Ca^{2+} current, Icrac, whose mechanism has recently been described as an interaction between Orai1 in the plasmalemma and STIM1 in the ER (47). Activation of SOCE is not restricted to non-excitable cells, but is also observed in excitable cells including neurons, cardiac myocytes, and smooth muscle cells (48). This mode of Ca^{2+} entry has also been described in myotubes and in adult skeletal muscle fibers, where release from SR Ca^{2+} stores is operated by RyRs (6,35,49–51).

The physiological role of SOCE in skeletal muscle is not well understood, but it is likely to be important for sustaining calcium stores to prevent muscle weakness and contribute calcium needed to modulate muscle-specific gene expression (52). Although other mechanisms have been proposed as the basis of SOCE in skeletal muscle, such as activation of SOCE channels by IP_3 receptors (50) or RyR1 as the SR Ca^{2+} sensor (53,54) and via TRPC proteins as the SOCE channel (53,55,56), it has recently been shown that SOCE in muscle is the result of highly Ca^{2+}-selective CRAC channel activation (57,58), resulting from store depletion causing STIM1 aggregation and reorganization in diverse regions of the SR that interact and activate Ca^{2+} entry via Orai1 channels sarcolemma (57).

Transient Receptor Potential Channels (TRPs)

TRP channels show a great diversity in activation and ion selectivity. Transcripts for TRPC subfamily members 1, 2, 3, 4, and 6 have been found in skeletal muscle and confirmed by Western blot. Immunohistochemical staining shows the presence of TRPC1, 3, 4, and 6 in the sarcolemma (55,59–61), however in other studies TRPC1, 4, and 6 showed a sarcolemmal localization while TRPC3 was preferentially found in the intracellular compartment, both in isolated fibers (61) and muscle cross-sections (59) but comparisons of TRPC channel expression between different skeletal muscles revealed significant variations (60). TRPC1, 2, 3, 4, and 6 mediate the transmembrane flux of cations down their electrochemical gradients, and because they are not selective for Ca^{2+} their activation can increase both the intracellular Ca^{2+} and Na^+ concentrations. The mechanism by which TRPC channels are activated is unknown but possible mechanisms include (i) hydrolysis of phosphatidylinositol bis-phosphate (PIP2); (ii) diacylglycerol (DAG); (iii) by inositol (1,4,5) tris-phosphate (IP3); (iv) direct activation by changes in temperature, mechanical stimuli or inorganic ions (Ca^{2+} and Mg^{2+}) (62). Co-immunoprecipitation and co-localization experiments suggested an association of TRPC1, TRPC4, and α-syntrophin in cultured myotubes (61,63). These data suggest that TRPC1 is associated via syntrophin to the complex of dystrophin-associated glycoproteins (DAG) and that TRPC1 may form a Ca^{2+} channel or at least contributes to as a subunit of a Ca^{2+} influx channel. In addition, connecting to the DAG complex, TRPC1 co-localizes with the scaffolding protein Homer 1 in skeletal muscle fibers (63). Knockdown of TRPC3 by small interference RNAs did not impair muscle differentiation and neither SOCE nor ECCE were impaired; however the association of TRPC3 with the calcineurin-NFAT (nuclear factor of activated T cells) signal transduction pathway is thought to couple extracellular Ca^{2+} influx with regulation of gene expression (64).

Resting Ca^{2+} Entry and Resting $[Ca^{2+}]_i$

In quiescent muscle cells resting $[Ca^{2+}]_i$ is maintained, in part, by a continuous Ca^{2+} influx that is not mediated by ECCE or SOCE. This resting Ca^{2+} entry (R_{CaE}) appears to play an important role in preserving the resting $[Ca^{2+}]_i$ in skeletal muscle (6). The cation channels responsible for R_{CaE}, most probably TRPCs, show a variable Ca^{2+}/Na^+ ratio (65). Recent work demonstrated that R_{CaE} could be blocked either by the I_{crac} blocker BTP2 or overexpression of a dominant negative form of Orai1 (E190Q) with a result being a reduction in resting $[Ca^{2+}]_i$ (6). In addition, we have recently found that Gd^{3+} and GsMTx-4 (Chilean Rose Tarantula) can also block R_{CaE} in muscle cells, and lower resting $[Ca^{2+}]_i$ and $[Na^+]_i$ (Eltit et al., unpublished results). Together these data suggest a possible participation of both TRPCs and Orai in this novel Ca^{2+} entry pathway. Additional investigation is required to completely identify the mechanisms that may be involved in the regulation of resting Ca^{2+} entry in skeletal muscle.

SR Ca^{2+} Leak

A significant part of the Ca^{2+} leak pathway from the SR into the cytoplasm arises from a ryanodine-insensitive constitutively open ($P_O \sim 1$) low conductance conformation of RyR1 (6,66). Bastadin 5, a brominated macrocyclic derivative of dityrosine isolated from the marine sponge *Iathella basta* (67), modulates RyR1 gating behavior and can be used as a pharmacological tool to convert RyR1 from its leak conformation into a gating conformation (67). It is well known that the DHPR and the RyR1 engage in bidirectional signaling (68) and that physical coupling between them is essential for skeletal excitation–contraction coupling. Freeze-fracture images have shown that DHPRs are clustered in groups of four particles (tetrads), which due to steric hindrance are associated with alternate RyR1s in each Ca^{2+} release unit (CRU). Thus alternate RyR1 channels are not physically coupled with DHPRs and the function of the uncoupled RyR1 population is unknown (69–71).

Recently, Eltit and colleagues have identified a previously undiscovered orthograde signal from the DHPR to RyR1 that appears to dictate the ratio of actively gating RyR1 channels vs. those in the leak conformation (72). They speculate that since the RyR1 population not coupled to DHPRs in muscle should have a higher propensity to be in the leak conformation, this may be determinant in maintaining normal intracellular Ca^{2+} homeostasis and is needed to keep myoplasmic $[Ca^{2+}]$ and the SR Ca^{2+} content in the physiological range (Figure 56.2).

METHODS FOR MEASUREMENTS RESTING $[Ca^{2+}]_I$ IN MUSCLE CELLS

Measuring resting $[Ca^{2+}]_i$ in skeletal muscle has become an important issue for muscle physiologists. Two main approaches have been used for the determination of resting $[Ca^{2+}]_i$ in muscle: the introduction of indicators into muscle cells, by various means, which give luminescence, absorbance, or fluorescence signals that are proportional to the $[Ca^{2+}]_i$ and electrophysiologically using Ca^{2+}-selective microelectrodes.

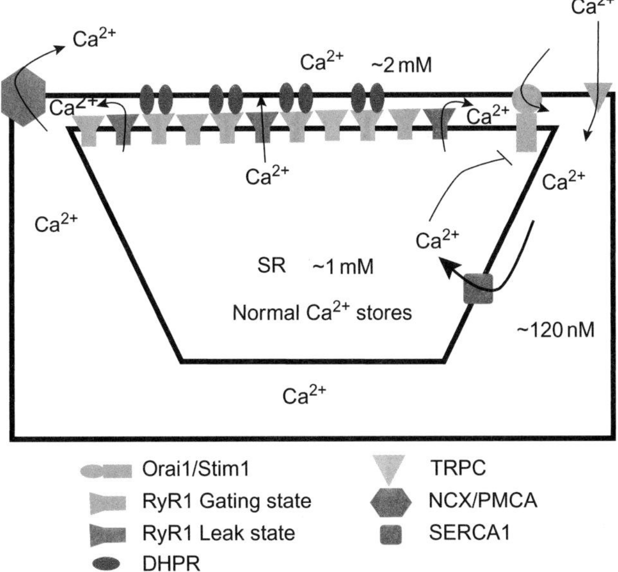

FIGURE 56.2 Cartoon showing DHPR control of RyR1 "leaks" and mechanisms for Ca^{2+} entry into and extrusion from the cytoplasm.

Optical Indicators

Three major classes of indicators have been used: (i) bioluminescent calcium-activated photoproteins; (ii) metalochromic indicators; and (iii) tetracarboxylate Ca^{2+} chelator dyes. The first two are mentioned largely for historical interest.

Photoproteins

Aequorin (73) is the best known of the two photoproteins that have been used as intracellular Ca^{2+} indicators and has to be either microinjected into the cell or loaded when the cell membrane is partially permeabilized and then allowed to reseal. Measurements of resting $[Ca^{2+}]_i$ with aequorin are problematic both because its signal is very small at calcium concentrations that resemble the normal myoplasmic resting free calcium in muscle fibers determined by other methods, calibration of the signal into absolute $[Ca^{2+}]$ is not easy, because the signal is influenced by a variety of experimental variable (ionic strength, temperature, $[Mg^{2+}]$ and its emission proportional roughly to the $[Ca^{2+}]$ to the power 2.5 (74), and because it has a luminescence signal that is independent of $[Ca^{2+}]$ which has been reported at very low $[Ca^{2+}]$ (74). Resting $[Ca^{2+}]_i$ values in the range of 39–80 nM have been reported in skeletal muscle microinjected with aequorin (75,76).

Metalochromic Dyes

Metallochromic dyes change color on binding Ca^{2+} and several different metallochromic dyes have been used in living muscle cells (77–81) as intracellular Ca^{2+} indicators, however it was found that the properties of these dyes made them unsuitable and no one has used them to determine resting $[Ca^{2+}]_i$ in muscle cells. Three important limitations of metallochromic Ca^{2+} indicators are: (1); that a major fraction of the dye molecules are bound to both soluble and fixed proteins in the muscle cell, making them inaccessible to sense Ca^{2+} ionic activity in the resting state (79,81); (2) it has been estimated that two-thirds of the dye is not freely available in the cytoplasm (79); and (3) sulfhydryl groups reduce metallochromic Ca^{2+} indicators to form azo anion radicals that inhibit SERCA function (82).

Tetracarboxylate Fluorescent Ca^{2+} Chelator Dyes

Most currently used fluorescent Ca^{2+} indicators (high-affinity or low-affinity) are members of a family of tetracarboxylate derivatives of BAPTA (Fura-2, Indo-1, Fluo-3, Fluo-4, Rhod-2, Calcium Green, etc.), which for the most part have a high selectivity for calcium over

Mg^{2+} and monovalent ions (83–85). One of the most attractive features of these Ca^{2+} indicators is the ease with which they can be introduced into the muscle cells. Although as salts they are highly charged and alone cannot diffuse across the plasma membrane, in their acetomethyl ester (AM) salt form they become lipid-soluble and can penetrate the plasma membrane where the ester group is hydrolyzed by cytoplasmic esterases and the charged form of the tetracarboxylate derivative is trapped in the cytoplasm. Several studies have been conducted in diverse non-diseased muscle cells using these indicators to measure resting $[Ca^{2+}]_i$ (86–91). Unfortunately, a number of problems must be considered when tetracarboxylate indicators are used for the determination of resting $[Ca^{2+}]_i$ in muscle cells. (i) As BAPTA derivatives all have a chelator effect on Ca^{2+} they reduce $[Ca^{2+}]_i$. Thus in most cases the $[Ca^{2+}]_i$ that have been reported in muscle cells using this method have been significantly lower (range 20–80 nM) compared with those reported using Ca^{2+} selective microelectrodes. (ii) The esterases capable of hydrolyzing the AM esters of these indicators are not located exclusively in the cytoplasm. They have been found in some cellular organelles such as SR and mitochondria, which can allow the indicator to be accumulated internally (92–94). (iii) Incomplete hydrolysis of the ester may occur in the interior of the muscle cell and different hydrolysis sub-products are generated whose properties are unknown (93). (iv) These indicators can leak out the cell in their unesterified or free acid form using an undefined active transport system, which is highly temperature-dependent (84,95,96). The leakage can be slowed by reducing the temperature or by treatment with probenecid. Unfortunately these interventions can also modify $[Ca^{2+}]_i$. (v) All BAPTA-derivative fluorescent Ca^{2+} indicators are subject to photobleaching and the product of the photobleaching is both fluorescent and relatively insensitive to Ca^{2+}(97). (vi) The fluorescence spectra or the calcium binding properties of these fluorescent Ca^{2+} indicators are sufficiently altered in an intracellular environment to make the calibration curves done in aqueous buffers inappropriate (86,87,98,99). As an example, one indicator's calculated Kd was smaller in aqueous solution alone than when it was measured with a myoplasmic protein, like aldolase, added to the buffer solution (100).

Ca^{2+}-Selective Microelectrodes

The basis for this technique is the use of a Ca^{2+} selective membrane (ligand) that separates two aqueous solutions containing Ca^{2+} and the readout is the electrical potential difference established between the solutions. In practice, the membrane in the Ca^{2+}-selective microelectrodes is a short column of Ca^{2+}-selective neutral carrier ligand, which separates two different solutions, a microelectrode filling solution (usually pCa7) and the solution outside the microelectrode tip. Neutral carriers are uncharged organic molecules that bind specific ions, generating an electrical potential (100,101). Current available neutral ligand sensors, ETH-1001 (102) and ETH-129 (103), have an adequate selectivity against Na^+, K^+, and H^+ and have negligible interference from Mg^2. Ca^{2+}-selective microelectrodes made with these ligands can give a well-calibrated measurement of $[Ca^{2+}]_i$, over the full range of $[Ca^{2+}]_i$ of biological interest from pCa3 to below pCa8 in single muscle cells. Typically their response is Nernstian (29.5 mV/pCa unit at room temperature) from pCa3–7 and the signal down to pCa8 is useable. When Ca^{2+}-selective microelectrodes made with either ETH-1001 (103) or ETH-127 (104) have been used to measure $[Ca^{2+}]_i$ in skeletal muscle, the majority of values reported in normal muscle have been in the vicinity of 100 nM (2,4,5,6,85,105,106).

However, Ca^{2+}-selective microelectrodes have some drawbacks. The most important is that they respond very slowly to changes in $[Ca^{2+}]_i$ due to the high electrical resistance of the neutral ligand. For measurements of resting $[Ca^{2+}]_i$ in quiescent muscle cells (steady-state), this slow response is not a limiting factor but it does make their use inappropriate to track rapid changes $[Ca^{2+}]_i$, such as those observed during muscle activation. Another potential disadvantage of Ca^{2+}-selective microelectrodes lies in that they sample $[Ca^{2+}]_i$ from just one point which could under certain circumstances not represent the $[Ca^{2+}]_i$ in all parts of the cell. However, in skeletal muscle there is no evidence of intracellular Ca^{2+} gradients at rest (107), so this problem is moot. Lastly this method is very demanding technically and requires special skills, and because with repeated use their sensitivity to Ca^{2+} may change in the course of the experiments, a calibration curve must be carried out both before and after intracellular measurements.

It has been suggested by some investigators that Ca^{2+} measurements carried out using Ca^{2+} selective microelectrodes do not represent the true intracellular Ca^{2+} concentration due to membrane damage caused by electrode impalement (90,91). In general any muscle cell damage due to microelectrode impalements appears to be associated with either the use of microelectrodes with a tip size greater than 1 μm or inadequate care during cell impalement. In this regard we have monitored microelectrode impalements in muscle cells previously loaded with Indo-1 AM or Fluo-4 AM and we have not observed any detectable increase in the fluorescence signal during or after the impalement was carried out, ruling out any potential membrane damage and leakage of Ca^{2+} around the microelectrode (Yang et al., unpublished observations). In addition, measurements of $[Ca^{2+}]_i$ in muscle cells done after impalement in high extracellular $[Ca^{2+}]$ solutions (12.5 mM) (105), are not different than those obtained when the impalement is done in normal Ringer solution (2 mM).

SUMMARY

In summary, maintenance of the gradient between resting $[Ca^{2+}]_i$ inside muscle cells and the extracellular space and internal stores requires a complex dynamic equilibrium of Ca^{2+} fluxes among pumps (PMCA, and SERCA) and an exchanger (NCX) which is opposed by sarcoplasmic reticulum (SR) leak channels (ryanodine insensitive "Ca^{2+} leak") as well as basal sarcolemmal Ca^{2+} influx. Against what has been commonly thought and has been stated as the boundary theorem (108) which supposes that $[Ca^{2+}]_i$ is controlled solely by the sarcolemmal Ca^{2+} fluxes, it is clear from recent data that this is not the case. Although sarcolemmal Ca^{2+} fluxes do play an important role, the contribution of Ca^{2+} fluxes in and out of the internal store must be considered in the overall equation.

ACKNOWLEDGMENTS

The authors wish to express their thanks to Dr Jose M. Eltit for reading the manuscript and Francisco Altamirano for his help in preparation. Funding for the unpublished data was supported by grants to P.D.A. from NIH/NIAMS (AR43140, AR052354, and AR055104).

REFERENCES

1. Brini M, Manni S, Carafoli E. A study of the activity of the plasma membrane Na/Ca exchanger in the cellular environment. *Ann NY Acad Sci* 2002;**976**:376–81.
2. Lopez JR, Alamo L, Caputo C, DiPolo R, Vergara S. Determination of ionic calcium in frog skeletal muscle fibers. *Biophys J* 1983;**43**:1–4.
3. Lopez JR, Briceno LE, Sanchez V, Horvart D. Myoplasmic (Ca^{2+}) in Duchenne muscular dystrophy patients. *Acta Cient Venez* 1987;**38**:503–4.
4. Lopez JR, Allen PD, Alamo L, Jones D, Sreter FA. Myoplasmic free $[Ca^{2+}]$ during a malignant hyperthermia episode in swine. *Muscle Nerve* 1988;**11**:82–8.
5. Yang T, Esteve E, Pessah IN, Molinski TF, Allen PD, Lopez JR. Elevated resting $[Ca(^{2+})](i)$ in myotubes expressing malignant hyperthermia RyR1 cDNAs is partially restored by modulation of passive calcium leak from the SR. *Am J Physiol Cell Physiol* 2007;**292**:C1591–8.
6. Eltit JM, Yang T, Li H, Molinski TF, Pessah IN, Allen PD, et al. RyR1-mediated Ca^{2+} leak and Ca^{2+} entry determine resting intracellular Ca^{2+} in skeletal myotubes. *J Biol Chem* 2010;**285**:13781–7.
7. Blaustein MP, Lederer WJ. Sodium/calcium exchange: its physiological implications. *Physiol Rev* 1999;**79**:763–854.
8. Cifuentes F, Vergara J, Hidalgo C. Sodium/calcium exchange in amphibian skeletal muscle fibers and isolated transverse tubules. *Am J Physiol Cell Physiol* 2000;**279**:C89–97.
9. Deval E, Levitsky DO, Constantin B, Raymond G, Cognard C. Expression of the sodium/calcium exchanger in mammalian skeletal muscle cells in primary culture. *Exp Cell Res* 2000;**255**:291–302.
10. Deval E, Levitsky DO, Marchand E, Cantereau A, Raymond G, Cognard C. $Na(^{+})/Ca(^{2+})$ exchange in human myotubes: intracellular calcium rises in response to external sodium depletion are enhanced in DMD. *Neuromuscul Disord* 2002;**12**:665–73.
11. Li Z, Matsuoka S, Hryshko LV, Nicoll DA, Bersohn MM, Burke EP, et al. Cloning of the NCX2 isoform of the plasma membrane $Na(^{+})$-Ca^{2+} exchanger. *J Biol Chem* 1994;**269**:17434–9.
12. Nicoll DA, Longoni S, Philipson KD. Molecular cloning and functional expression of the cardiac sarcolemmal $Na(^{+})$-Ca^{2+} exchanger. *Science* 1990;**250**:562–5.
13. Nicoll DA, Quednau BD, Qui Z, Xia YR, Lusis AJ, Philipson KD. Cloning of a third mammalian Na^{+}-Ca^{2+} exchanger, NCX3. *J Biol Chem* 1996;**271**:24914–21.
14. Linck B, Qiu Z, He Z, Tong Q, Hilgemann DW, Philipson KD. Functional comparison of the three isoforms of the Na^{+}/Ca^{2+} exchanger (NCX1, NCX2, NCX3). *Am J Physiol* 1998;**274**: C415–23.
15. Sacchetto R, Margreth A, Pelosi M, Carafoli E. Colocalization of the dihydropyridine receptor, the plasma-membrane calcium ATPase isoform 1 and the sodium/calcium exchanger to the junctional-membrane domain of transverse tubules of rabbit skeletal muscle. *Eur J Biochem* 1996;**237**:483–8.
16. Caputo C, Bolanos P. Effect of external sodium and calcium on calcium efflux in frog striated muscle. *J Membr Biol* 1978;**41**:1–14.
17. Apell HJ. Structure-function relationship in P-type ATPases – a biophysical approach. *Rev Physiol Biochem Pharmacol* 2003;**150**:1–35.
18. Carafoli E. The Ca^{2+} pump of the plasma membrane. *J Biol Chem* 1992;**267**:2115–8.
19. Strehler EE, Zacharias DA. Role of alternative splicing in generating isoform diversity among plasma membrane calcium pumps. *Physiol Rev* 2001;**81**:21–50.
20. Bilmen JG, Khan SZ, Javed MH, Michelangeli F. Inhibition of the SERCA Ca^{2+} pumps by curcumin. Curcumin putatively stabilizes the interaction between the nucleotide-binding and phosphorylation domains in the absence of ATP. *Eur J Biochem* 2001;**268**:6318–27.
21. Niggli V, Sigel E, Carafoli E. The purified Ca^{2+} pump of human erythrocyte membranes catalyzes an electroneutral Ca^{2+}-H^{+} exchange in reconstituted liposomal systems. *J Biol Chem* 1982;**257**:2350–6.
22. Hao L, Rigaud JL, Inesi G. Ca^{2+}/H^{+} countertransport and electrogenicity in proteoliposomes containing erythrocyte plasma membrane Ca-ATPase and exogenous lipids. *J Biol Chem* 1994;**269**:14268–75.
23. Thomas RC. The plasma membrane calcium ATPase (PMCA) of neurones is electroneutral and exchanges 2 H^{+} for each Ca^{2+} or Ba^{2+} ion extruded. *J Physiol* 2009;**587**:315–27.
24. Inesi G, Prasad AM, Pilankatta R. The Ca^{2+} ATPase of cardiac sarcoplasmic reticulum: physiological role and relevance to diseases. *Biochem Biophys Res Commun* 2008;**369**:182–7.

25. Franzini-Armstrong C. Structure of sarcoplasmic reticulum. *Fed Proc* 1980;**39**:2403–9.
26. Martonosi AN, Dux L, Terjung RL, Roufa D. Regulation of membrane assembly during development of sarcoplasmic reticulum: the possible role of calcium. *Ann NY Acad Sci* 1982;**402**:485–514.
27. MacLennan DH, Reithmeier RAF. In: Martonosi A, editor. *Membranes and transport*, vol. 1. New York: Plenum Press;1982. p. 567–71.
28. Martonosi A, Beeler TJ. In: Peachey LD, Adrian RH, editors. *Handbook of physiology: skeletal muscle*, vol. 1. Bethesda, MD: American Physiological Society;1983. p. 417–85.
29. Brody IA. Muscle contracture induced by exercise. A syndrome attributable to decreased relaxing factor. *N Engl J Med* 1969;**281**:187–92.
30. Odermatt A, Taschner PE, Khanna VK, Busch HF, Karpati G, Jablecki CK, et al. Mutations in the gene-encoding SERCA1, the fast-twitch skeletal muscle sarcoplasmic reticulum Ca^{2+} ATPase, are associated with Brody disease. *Nat Genet* 1996;**14**:191–4.
31. Goonasekera SA, Lam CK, Millay DP, Sargent MA, Hajjar RJ, Kranias EG, et al. Mitigation of muscular dystrophy in mice by SERCA overexpression in skeletal muscle. *J Clin Invest.* 2011;**121**:1044–52.
32. Caputo C, Gimenez M. Effects of external calcium deprivation on single muscle fibers. *J Gen Physiol* 1967;**50**:2177–95.
33. Luttgau HC, Oetliker H. The action of caffeine on the activation of the contractile mechanism in straited muscle fibres. *J Physiol* 1968;**194**:51–74.
34. Dirksen RT. Checking your SOCCs and feet: the molecular mechanisms of Ca^{2+} entry in skeletal muscle. *J Physiol* 2009;**587**:3139–47.
35. Kurebayashi N, Ogawa Y. Depletion of Ca^{2+} in the sarcoplasmic reticulum stimulates Ca^{2+} entry into mouse skeletal muscle fibres. *J Physiol* 2001;**533**:185–99.
36. Lyfenko AD, Dirksen RT. Differential dependence of store-operated and excitation-coupled Ca^{2+} entry in skeletal muscle on STIM1 and Orai1. *J Physiol* 2008;**586**:4815–24.
37. Cherednichenko G, Hurne AM, Fessenden JD, Lee EH, Allen PD, Beam KG, et al. Conformational activation of Ca^{2+} entry by depolarization of skeletal myotubes. *Proc Natl Acad Sci USA* 2004;**101**:15793–8.
38. Putney Jr JW. A model for receptor-regulated calcium entry. *Cell Calcium* 1986;**7**:1–12.
39. Putney Jr JW. New molecular players in capacitative Ca^{2+} entry. *J Cell Sci* 2007;**120**:1959–65.
40. Cherednichenko G, Ward CW, Feng W, Cabrales E, Michaelson L, Samso M, et al. Enhanced excitation-coupled calcium entry in myotubes expressing malignant hyperthermia mutation R163C is attenuated by dantrolene. *Mol Pharmacol* 2008;**73**:1203–12.
41. Bannister RA, Grabner M, Beam KG. The alpha(1S) III-IV loop influences 1,4-dihydropyridine receptor gating but is not directly involved in excitation-contraction coupling interactions with the type 1 ryanodine receptor. *J Biol Chem* 2008;**283**:23217–23.
42. Bannister RA, Pessah IN, Beam KG. The skeletal L-type $Ca(^{2+})$ current is a major contributor to excitation-coupled $Ca(^{2+})$ entry. *J Gen Physiol* 2009;**133**:79–91.
43. Hurne AM, O'Brien JJ, Wingrove D, Cherednichenko G, Allen PD, Beam KG, et al. Ryanodine receptor type 1 (RyR1) mutations C4958S and C4961S reveal excitation-coupled calcium entry (ECCE) is independent of sarcoplasmic reticulum store depletion. *J Biol Chem* 2005;**280**:36994–7004.
44. Treves S, Vukcevic M, Jeannet PY, Levano S, Girard T, Urwyler A, et al. Enhanced excitation-coupled $Ca(^{2+})$ entry induces nuclear translocation of NFAT and contributes to IL-6 release from myotubes from patients with central core disease. *Hum Mol Genet* 2011;**20**:589–600.
45. Yang T, Riehl J, Esteve E, Matthaei KI, Goth S, Allen PD, et al. Pharmacologic and functional characterization of malignant hyperthermia in the R163C RyR1 knock-in mouse. *Anesthesiology* 2006;**105**:1164–75.
46. Gach MP, Cherednichenko G, Haarmann C, Lopez JR, Beam KG, Pessah IN, et al. Alpha2delta1 dihydropyridine receptor subunit is a critical element for excitation-coupled calcium entry but not for formation of tetrads in skeletal myotubes. *Biophys J* 2008; **94**:3023–34.
47. Smyth JT, Hwang SY, Tomita T, DeHaven WI, Mercer JC, Putney JW. Activation and regulation of store-operated calcium entry. *J Cell Mol Med* 2010;**14**:2337–49.
48. Parekh AB, Putney Jr JW. Store-operated calcium channels. *Physiol Rev* 2005;**85**:757–810.
49. Gonzalez Narvaez AA, Castillo A. Ca^{2+} store determines gating of store operated calcium entry in mammalian skeletal muscle. *J Muscle Res Cell Motil* 2007;**28**:105–13.
50. Launikonis BS, Barnes M, Stephenson DG. Identification of the coupling between skeletal muscle store-operated Ca^{2+} entry and the inositol trisphosphate receptor. *Proc Natl Acad Sci USA* 2003;**100**:2941–4.
51. Launikonis BS, Rios E. Store-operated Ca^{2+} entry during intracellular Ca^{2+} release in mammalian skeletal muscle. *J Physiol* 2007;**583**:81–97.
52. Launikonis BS, Murphy RM, Edwards JN. Toward the roles of store-operated Ca^{2+} entry in skeletal muscle. *Pflugers Arch* 2010;**460**:813–23.
53. Kiselyov KI, Shin DM, Wang Y, Pessah IN, Allen PD, Muallem S. Gating of store-operated channels by conformational coupling to ryanodine receptors. *Mol Cell* 2000;**6**:421–31.
54. Pan Z, Yang D, Nagaraj RY, Nosek TA, Nishi M, Takeshima H, et al. Dysfunction of store-operated calcium channel in muscle cells lacking mg29. *Nat Cell Biol* 2002;**4**:379–83.
55. Lee EH, Cherednichenko G, Pessah IN, Allen PD. Functional coupling between TRPC3 and RyR1 regulates the expressions of key triadic proteins. *J Biol Chem* 2006;**281**:10042–8.
56. Sampieri A, Diaz-Munoz M, Antaramian A, Vaca L. The foot structure from the type 1 ryanodine receptor is required for functional coupling to store-operated channels. *J Biol Chem* 2005;**280**:24804–15.
57. Feske S, Gwack Y, Prakriya M, Srikanth S, Puppel SH, Tanasa B, et al. A mutation in Orai1 causes immune deficiency by abrogating CRAC channel function. *Nature* 2006;**441**:179–85.
58. Vig M, Peinelt C, Beck A, Koomoa DL, Rabah D, Koblan-Huberson M, et al. CRACM1 is a plasma membrane protein essential for store-operated Ca^{2+} entry. *Science* 2006; **312**:1220–3.
59. Kruger J, Kunert-Keil C, Bisping F, Brinkmeier H. Transient receptor potential cation channels in normal and dystrophic mdx muscle. *Neuromuscul Disord* 2008;**18**:501–13.

60. Kunert-Keil C, Bisping F, Kruger J, Brinkmeier H. Tissue-specific expression of TRP channel genes in the mouse and its variation in three different mouse strains. *BMC Genomics* 2006;**7**:159.
61. Vandebrouck C, Martin D, Colson-Van Schoor M, Debaix H, Gailly P. Involvement of TRPC in the abnormal calcium influx observed in dystrophic (mdx) mouse skeletal muscle fibers. *J Cell Biol* 2002;**158**:1089–96.
62. Ramsey IS, Delling M, Clapham DE. An introduction to TRP channels. *Annu Rev Physiol* 2006;**68**:619–47.
63. Sabourin J, Lamiche C, Vandebrouck A, Magaud C, Rivet J, Cognard C, et al. Regulation of TRPC1 and TRPC4 cation channels requires an alpha1-syntrophin-dependent complex in skeletal mouse myotubes. *J Biol Chem* 2009;**284**:36248–61.
64. Rosenberg P, Hawkins A, Stiber J, Shelton JM, Hutcheson K, Bassel-Duby R, et al. TRPC3 channels confer cellular memory of recent neuromuscular activity. *Proc Natl Acad Sci USA* 2004;**101**:9387–92.
65. Venkatachalam K, Montell C. TRP channels. *Annu Rev Biochem* 2007;**76**:387–417.
66. Pessah IN, Molinski TF, Meloy TD, Wong P, Buck ED, Allen PD, et al. Bastadins relate ryanodine-sensitive and -insensitive Ca^{2+} efflux pathways in skeletal SR and BC3H1 cells. *Am J Physiol* 1997;**272**:C601–14.
67. Mack MM, Molinski TF, Buck ED, Pessah IN. Novel modulators of skeletal muscle FKBP12/calcium channel complex from Ianthella basta. Role of FKBP12 in channel gating. *J Biol Chem* 1994;**269**:23236–49.
68. Nakai J, Dirksen RT, Nguyen HT, Pessah IN, Beam KG, Allen PD. Enhanced dihydropyridine receptor channel activity in the presence of ryanodine receptor. *Nature* 1996;**380**:72–5.
69. Franzini-Armstrong C, Kish JW. Alternate disposition of tetrads in peripheral couplings of skeletal muscle. *J Muscle Res Cell Motil* 1995;**16**:319–24.
70. Takekura H, Bennett L, Tanabe T, Beam KG, Franzini-Armstrong C. Restoration of junctional tetrads in dysgenic myotubes by dihydropyridine receptor cDNA. *Biophys J* 1994;**67**:793–803.
71. Protasi F, Franzini-Armstrong C, Allen PD. Role of ryanodine receptors in the assembly of calcium release units in skeletal muscle. *J Cell Biol* 1998;**140**:831–42.
72. Eltit JM, Li H, Ward CW, Molinski TF, Pessah IN, Allen PD, et al. An orthograde DHPR signal regulates RyR1 passive leak. *Proc Natl Acad Sci USA* 2011;**108**:7046–51.
73. Allen DG, Blinks JR, Prendergast FG. Aequorin luminescence: relation of light emission to calcium concentration – a calcium-independent component. *Science* 1977;**195**:996–8.
74. Blinks JR, Wier WG, Hess P, Prendergast FG. Measurement of Ca^{2+} concentrations in living cells. *Prog Biophys Mol Biol* 1982;**40**:1–114.
75. Blatter LA, Blinks JR. Simultaneous measurement of Ca^{2+} in muscle with Ca electrodes and aequorin. Diffusible cytoplasmic constituent reduces $Ca(^{2+})$-independent luminescence of aequorin. *J Gen Physiol* 1991;**98**:1141–60.
76. Blinks JR, Moore ED. Practical aspects of the use of photoproteins as biological calcium indicators. *Soc Gen Physiol Ser* 1986;**40**:229–38.
77. Baylor SM, Chandler WK, Marshall MW. Dichroic components of Arsenazo III and dichlorophosphonazo III signals in skeletal muscle fibres. *J Physiol* 1982;**331**:179–210.
78. Baylor SM, Chandler WK, Marshall MW. Use of metallochromic dyes to measure changes in myoplasmic calcium during activity in frog skeletal muscle fibres. *J Physiol* 1982;**331**:139–77.
79. Baylor SM, Hollingworth S, Hui CS, Quinta-Ferreira ME. Properties of the metallochromic dyes Arsenazo III, Antipyrylazo III and Azo1 in frog skeletal muscle fibres at rest. *J Physiol* 1986;**377**:89–141.
80. Baylor SM, Quinta-Ferreira ME, Hui CS. Comparison of isotropic calcium signals from intact frog muscle fibers injected with Arsenazo III or Antipyrylazo III. *Biophys J* 1983;**44**:107–12.
81. Beeler TJ, Schibeci A, Martonosi A. The binding of arsenazo III to cell components. *Biochim Biophys Acta* 1980;**629**:317–27.
82. Beeler T. Oxidation of sulfhydryl groups and inhibition of the $(Ca^{2+} + Mg^{2+})$-ATPase by arsenazo III. *Biochim Biophys Acta* 1990;**1027**:264–7.
83. Grynkiewicz G, Poenie M, Tsien RY. A new generation of Ca^{2+} indicators with greatly improved fluorescence properties. *J Biol Chem* 1985;**260**:3440–50.
84. Rink TJ, Pozzan T. Using quin2 in cell suspensions. *Cell Calcium* 1985;**6**:133–44.
85. Tsien RY, Rink TJ. Neutral carrier ion-selective microelectrodes for measurement of intracellular free calcium. *Biochim Biophys Acta* 1980;**599**:623–38.
86. Avila G, Dirksen RT. Functional effects of central core disease mutations in the cytoplasmic region of the skeletal muscle ryanodine receptor. *J Gen Physiol* 2001;**118**:277–90.
87. Avila G, O'Brien JJ, Dirksen RT. Excitation–contraction uncoupling by a human central core disease mutation in the ryanodine receptor. *Proc Natl Acad Sci USA* 2001;**98**:4215–20.
88. Dainese M, Quarta M, Lyfenko AD, Paolini C, Canato M, Reggiani C, et al. Anesthetic- and heat-induced sudden death in calsequestrin-1-knockout mice. *FASEB J* 2009;**23**:1710–20.
89. Ducreux S, Zorzato F, Ferreiro A, Jungbluth H, Muntoni F, Monnier N, et al. Functional properties of ryanodine receptors carrying three amino acid substitutions identified in patients affected by multi-minicore disease and central core disease, expressed in immortalized lymphocytes. *Biochem J* 2006;**395**:259–66.
90. Iaizzo PA, Klein W, Lehmann-Horn F. Fura-2 detected myoplasmic calcium and its correlation with contracture force in skeletal muscle from normal and malignant hyperthermia susceptible pigs. *Pflugers Arch* 1988;**411**:648–53.
91. Iaizzo PA, Seewald M, Oakes SG, Lehmann-Horn F. The use of Fura-2 to estimate myoplasmic $[Ca^{2+}]$ in human skeletal muscle. *Cell Calcium* 1989;**10**:151–8.
92. DeFeo TT, Morgan KG. A comparison of two different indicators: quin 2 and aequorin in isolated single cells and intact strips of ferret portal vein. *Pflugers Arch* 1986;**406**:427–9.
93. Spurgeon HA, Stern MD, Baartz G, Raffaeli S, Hansford RG, Talo A, et al. Simultaneous measurement of Ca^{2+}, contraction, and potential in cardiac myocytes. *Am J Physiol* 1990;**258**:H574–86.
94. Williams DA, Fogarty KE, Tsien RY, Fay FS. Calcium gradients in single smooth muscle cells revealed by the digital imaging microscope using Fura-2. *Nature* 1985;**318**:558–61.
95. Murphy E, Jacob R, Lieberman M. Cytosolic free calcium in chick heart cells. Its role in cell injury. *J Mol Cell Cardiol* 1985;**17**:221–31.

96. Tsien R, Pozzan T. Measurement of cytosolic free Ca^{2+} with quin2. *Methods Enzymol* 1989;**172**:230–62.
97. Becker PL, Fay FS. Photobleaching of fura-2 and its effect on determination of calcium concentrations. *Am J Physiol* 1987;**253**: C613–8.
98. David-Dufilho M, Montenay-Garestier T, Devynck MA. Fluorescence measurements of free Ca^{2+} concentration in human erythrocytes using the Ca^{2+}-indicator fura-2. *Cell Calcium* 1988;**9**:167–79.
99. Malgaroli A, Milani D, Meldolesi J, Pozzan T. Fura-2 measurement of cytosolic free Ca^{2+} in monolayers and suspensions of various types of animal cells. *J Cell Biol* 1987;**105**: 2145–55.
100. Kurebayashi N, Harkins AB, Baylor SM. Use of fura red as an intracellular calcium indicator in frog skeletal muscle fibers. *Biophys J* 1993;**64**:1934–60.
101. Alvarez-Leefmans FJ, Gamino SM, Giraldez F, Gonzalez-Serratos H. Intracellular free magnesium in frog skeletal muscle fibres measured with ion-selective micro-electrodes. *J Physiol* 1986;**378**:461–83.
102. Tsien RY, Rink TJ. Ca^{2+}-selective electrodes: a novel PVC-gelled neutral carrier mixture compared with other currently available sensors. *J Neurosci Methods* 1981;**4**:73–86.
103. Oehme M, Kessler M, Simon W. Neutral carrier Ca^{2+} microelectrodes. *Chimia* 1976;**30**:204–6.
104. Schefer U, Ammann D. Neutral carrier based Ca^{2+} selective electrode with detection limit in the subnanomolar range. *Anal Chem* 1986;**58**:2282.
105. Lopez JR, Linares N, Pessah IN, Allen PD. Enhanced response to caffeine and 4-chloro-m-cresol in malignant hyperthermia-susceptible muscle is related in part to chronically elevated resting $[Ca^{2+}]i$. *Am J Physiol Cell Physiol* 2005;**288**:C606–12.
106. Lopez JR, Rojas B, Gonzalez MA, Terzic A. Myoplasmic Ca^{2+} concentration during exertional rhabdomyolysis. *Lancet* 1995;**345**:424–5.
107. Westerblad H, Lee JA, Lamb AG, Bolsover SR, Allen DG. Spatial gradients of intracellular calcium in skeletal muscle during fatigue. *Pflugers Arch* 1990;**415**:734–40.
108. Rios E. RyR1 expression and the cell boundary theorem. *J Biol Chem* 2010;**285**:le13 [author reply le14].

Chapter 57

Skeletal Muscle Excitation–Contraction Coupling

Martin F. Schneider and Erick O. Hernández-Ochoa
Department of Biochemistry and Molecular Biology, School of Medicine, University of Maryland, Baltimore, MD

OVERVIEW OF STEPS IN SKELETAL MUSCLE EXCITATION–CONTRACTION COUPLING

The process of physiological activation of a skeletal muscle fiber involves an action potential propagating along the muscle fiber in both directions away from the neuromuscular junction, where a single muscle fiber action potential is initiated in response to each action potential in the motor neuron. In addition to propagating longitudinally along the fiber, the action potential also propagates radially into the fiber via the transverse tubular (TT) network, a mesh of interconnected tubular invaginations of the fiber surface membrane extending radially into the fiber. The resulting TT depolarization causes the activation of Ca^{2+} release from the sarcoplasmic reticulum (SR), a separate membrane system that forms an intracellular storage depot for Ca^{2+} in relaxed muscle, and for Ca^{2+} release in response to TT depolarization. The released Ca^{2+} binds to thin filament troponin C molecules, resulting in a conformational change in thin filament tropomyosin which allows force-generating cross-bridges from the thick myosin-containing contractile filaments to bind to the regulated actin filaments and produce force or shortening. When Ca^{2+} release terminates, Ca^{2+} is returned to the SR via the ATP-dependent Ca^{2+} pump in the SR membrane, restoring the initial resting state of the fiber. Excitation–contraction (EC) coupling, a phrase coined by Alexander Sandow in his classic review in 1952 (1), encompasses the steps from membrane depolarization to thin filament activation.

The classical physiological studies of EC coupling compared the initial and final steps, muscle fiber depolarization and force production, in the EC coupling process. Subsequent studies examined the intervening steps of TT voltage sensor charge movement and the myoplasmic $[Ca^{2+}]$ signal and its underlying SR Ca^{2+} release flux. These phenomenological studies will be considered first here. Later work delved into the molecular components and mechanisms that constitute and link TT depolarization to SR Ca^{2+} release during muscle activation, as well as the reversal of these steps during muscle relaxation. These molecular mechanisms will be considered in the latter part of this chapter.

THE MUSCLE FIBER ACTION POTENTIAL ACTIVATES FORCE PRODUCTION

A single action potential in a vertebrate twitch skeletal muscle fiber consists of a change in fiber membrane potential from the inside negative resting potential of about −80 to −90 mV to a positive membrane potential and then rapid and slower phases of return to the resting potential, with the full duration at half maximum depolarization lasting just a few milliseconds (Figure 57.1A,B, red trace, normalized to peak amplitude and shown at lower and higher time resolution in (A) and (B), respectively). These and all other records in Figures 57.1 and 57.2 represent a synthesis of various results in mammalian (mouse) fast twitch muscle fibers at room temperature, with slow twitch fibers being roughly twice as slow as fast twitch fibers. In frog fibers at or below room temperature speed would be even slower than mammalian slow twitch fibers. The muscle fiber action potential is initiated physiologically by the local muscle fiber depolarization produced by the neurotransmitter acetylcholine released at the motor neuron nerve endings as a result of the neuron action potential, and propagates along the muscle fiber in both directions away from the muscle end plate. Alternatively, the muscle action potential can be initiated experimentally by direct electric field stimulation of the muscle or of an isolated muscle fiber.

The action potential triggers a "twitch contraction" (Figure 57.1, blue), which begins a few milliseconds after the action potential and has rising and falling phases lasting some tens of milliseconds, with exact time course depending on the fiber type under examination. Again, and as also the case for the Ca^{2+} transients described

Muscle. DOI: http://dx.doi.org/10.1016/B978-0-12-381510-1.00057-0

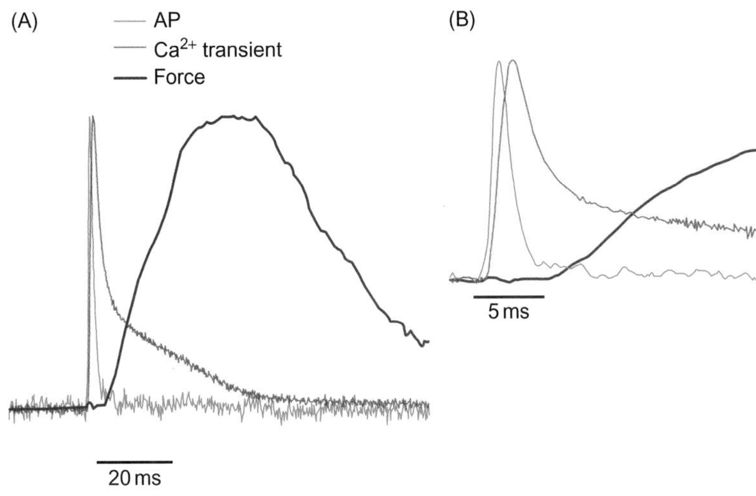

FIGURE 57.1 Action potential (red), myoplasmic Ca^{2+} transient (green), and force (blue) records normalized and superimposed on two time scales. Unpublished records from our lab of action potentials recorded with the membrane potential sensitive dye di-8-ANEPPS and of Ca^{2+} transients recorded using Magfluo-4 in intact fibers dissociated from mouse flexor digitorum brevis (FDB) muscle or unpublished records of muscle force from tibialis anterior muscle in anesthetized mice. *(Muscle force courtesy of Drs R. Lovering and B. Prosser.)*

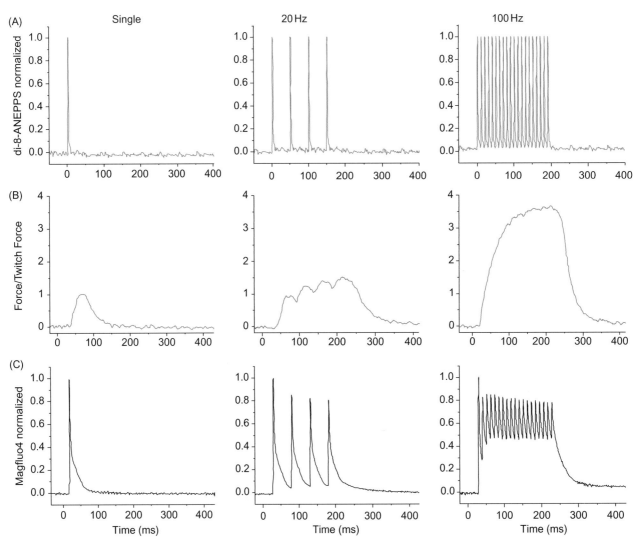

FIGURE 57.2 Action potentials (A), muscle force (B), and Ca^{2+} transients (C) for a single action potential (left; same records as Figure 57.1, but now on compressed time scale) and for 200 ms trains of action potentials at 20 Hz (center) and 100 Hz (right). Note that the action potential trains for the 20 and 100 Hz train were simulated by repositioning the single action potential record following published results (2). *(Muscle force courtesy of Drs R. Lovering and B. Prosser.)*

below, contraction speed is in decreasing order for mammalian fast twitch > mammalian slow twitch > frog fiber, and with all parameters decreased in speed with decreasing temperature for each type of fiber. A single brief stimulus gives a single action potential, which is followed by a single twitch contraction (Figure 57.2A and B, left). When the muscle fiber is repetitively stimulated at a relatively low frequency (e.g., less than 10 Hz) each muscle fiber action potential results in a distinct twitch contraction (not shown). However, when stimuli are applied more rapidly (e.g., 20 Hz), a single muscle fiber action potential is still triggered by each stimulus (Figure 57.2A, center), but the individual contractions initiated by each action potential begin to partially fuse in time (Figure 57.2B, center). As the stimulation frequency is further increased, the contractions with each action potential eventually fuse into a smooth "tetanic" contraction (Figure 57.2B, right), even though the action potentials remain distinct (Figure 57.2A, right). The tetanic force is the maximum force that the muscle fiber can generate during high frequency repetitive stimulation, and is similar to the force that the fiber contractile apparatus can generate under experimental conditions of full contractile filament activation (see below). Thus, high frequency repetitive action potentials result in full activation of the muscle contractile apparatus during fused tetanic contractions.

A RISE IN MYOPLASMIC [CA^{2+}] LINKS FIBER DEPOLARIZATION TO FORCE ACTIVATION

Myoplasmic Ca^{2+} ions serve a key second messenger function in skeletal muscle activation, coupling the muscle fiber action potential with force production (3). In response to a single muscle fiber action potential, a transient rise and fall of cytosolic free Ca^{2+} concentration $[Ca^{2+}]$, the "Ca^{2+} transient" (Figure 57.1, green), occurs between the action potential (Figure 57.1, red) and fiber force generation (Figure 57.1, blue), closely following the action potential in time. For trains of action potentials at a moderate frequency that give partial force summation (e.g., 20 Hz; Figure 57.2B, center), the Ca^{2+} transients remain almost distinct, with Ca^{2+} decaying almost to resting levels between action potentials (Figure 57.2C, center), whereas at frequencies giving a smooth fused tetanus (e.g., 100 Hz; Figure 57.2B, right) the Ca^{2+} signals only partial decay between action potentials (Figure 57.2C, right). Note that even though the second and later Ca^{2+} transients in the 100 Hz train start from an elevated Ca^{2+} level, the peaks reached are actually smaller than for the first action potential. This foreshadows the fact that the Ca^{2+} released from the SR during rapid trains of action potentials decreases drastically after the first action potential in the train due to release inactivation (see below).

DURING STEADY EXPERIMENTAL DEPOLARIZATION, MAXIMUM FORCE INCREASES OVER A NARROW VOLTAGE RANGE

In order to quantitatively characterize any membrane potential- and time-dependent processes, such as muscle activation, it is convenient to experimentally impose controlled voltage steps and monitor the resulting response with time at a variety of set voltages, as done in the classic studies of Hodgkin and Huxley on ionic channels in nerve axons (4). Since the $[K^+]$ ratio across the fiber membrane sets the membrane potential (V_m) for K^+-permeable membranes as in muscle fibers, Hodgkin and Horowicz (5) used application of solutions with various elevated $[K^+]$ concentrations to produce a range of step depolarizations in manually dissected frog single muscle fibers. These studies established that in single frog skeletal muscle fibers the maximum force generated during a several second depolarization increased steeply with voltage from the threshold voltage of about −50 mV to about −20 mV, and then remained constant for further depolarization.

During any suprathreshold $[K^+]$ contracture depolarization, the force first increased with time, then remained relatively constant at the maximum level for that depolarization, and finally declined with time and decayed to zero after several seconds despite the continued depolarization, indicating the development of a "mechanically refractory state" during maintained fiber depolarization (5). It was found that the fiber must be repolarized (= "repriming") to allow reactivation of the fiber by a subsequent depolarization, and that the repriming process was also membrane potential-dependent (5). The mechanically refractory state is not due to depletion of Ca^{2+} since application of caffeine, a pharmacological activator of Ca^{2+} release from the SR, is able to cause force development in fully depolarized and mechanically refractory fibers. Later studies indicated that the refractory state and the recovery from the refractory state are instead related to inactivation and restoration of the TT voltage sensors for SR Ca^{2+} release (see below).

LARGE DEPOLARIZATIONS ACTIVATE FORCE WITHIN MILLISECONDS

The preceding studies utilized depolarizations that were orders of magnitude longer than the few millisecond duration of a muscle action potential. To be more comparable to the physiological time scale, subsequent studies used controlled electrical depolarization of muscle fibers by passing electrical current across the membrane using internal or external electrodes together with a "voltage clamp" feedback circuit that controlled fiber membrane potential at any specified "command" time course, now allowing characterization of muscle fiber activation on a ms time scale. Using depolarizations of set amplitude but variable duration it was possible to determine the pulse duration for just detectable contraction at any given depolarization above the threshold voltage, and by using a range of depolarizations the "strength duration curve" for detectable contraction was determined. As in the case of long depolarizations (above), no detectable contraction was produced unless the fiber was depolarized to about −50 mV. With further depolarization shorter pulses could elicit contraction, indicating faster activation kinetics at larger depolarizations comparable to the duration of an action potential. Interestingly, these voltage clamp studies of muscle fiber activation also showed that fiber depolarization with the known plasma membrane and TT membrane channel currents blocked using a range of channel inhibitors still causes muscle fiber contractile activation, supporting the notion that movement of ions into (or out of) the fiber, including Ca^{2+} ions, is *not* needed for skeletal muscle fiber activation.

BIOPHYSICAL CHARACTERIZATION OF THE TT VOLTAGE SENSORS

The classic studies of A. F. Huxley and collaborators (6,7) established that the transverse tubular system, which forms two TT networks per sarcomere in mammalian (or lizard) muscle fibers and one per sarcomere in frog fibers, carries the electrical depolarization of the action potential into the fiber interior. Even though the TT and SR membranes are closely apposed at the triad junction, where each TT is flanked by junctional SR membrane through which the Ca^{2+} release flux occurs (below), the SR is *not* electrically connected to the adjacent TT system. Thus the membrane potential sensitive mechanism activating SR Ca^{2+} release must be physically located in the TT membrane, which is the membrane depolarized during an action potential or during experimental depolarization of the muscle fiber. In their classic work characterizing the voltage-sensitive membrane currents in squid axons, Hodgkin and Huxley (4) predicted that any membrane potential sensitive process would be regulated by charged or dipolar molecules that could alter their distribution in the membrane in response to changes in membrane potential, and that such rearrangements of charged intramembrane "voltage sensors" would generate small membrane currents. Such "gating current" was first detected in skeletal muscle, and was suggested to be the voltage sensor for EC coupling (8). Under voltage clamp depolarizations the relatively small amplitude intramembrane voltage sensor charge movement currents I_Q can be monitored (Figure 57.3, left) by blocking ionic currents and subtracting linear capacitive currents. Studies showing that pulses along the strength duration curve for just detectable contraction (above) caused the same amount of charge movement, that the shortening of the test pulse duration for just detectable contraction that was produced by a subthreshold prepulse could be predicted by the time required to move the prepulse charge at the test pulse voltage (10) and that the restoration of contractile ability after prolonged depolarization agreed with the kinetics of restoration of charge movement during the repriming protocol (11) all strongly supported the hypothesis that the measured charge movement was the voltage sensor for EC coupling. The activation of detectable SR Ca^{2+} release flux, calculated as described in the next section, requires larger depolarizations than needed for activating detectable charge movement, and increases relatively more steeply with depolarization than the charge moved (Figure 57.3, right). This is consistent with release being controlled by the movement of several charged intramembrane molecules which must move to turn on the SR Ca^{2+} release channel. For frog skeletal muscle fibers the amounts and time courses of charge moved and of Ca^{2+} release activation are consistent with a model in which 4 voltage sensors activate each Ca^{2+} release channel, since the release amplitude and time course was proportional to the 4th power of the charge moved (12).

CA^{2+} RELEASE FLUX FROM THE SR EXHIBITS AN EARLY PEAK AND RAPID INACTIVATION DURING DEPOLARIZATION

Skeletal muscle cytosolic calcium transients are detected in muscle fibers by introducing Ca^{2+} indicator dyes into the myoplasm (13–16). These Ca^{2+} indicators change their optical properties (absorbance and/or fluorescence) when Ca^{2+} ion binds to a dye molecule forming a Ca^{2+}–dye complex. If the speed of equilibration of the free Ca^{2+} with the dye is rapid compared to the free Ca^{2+} time course, the indicator provides an accurate estimate of the free Ca^{2+} time course in the fiber. In contrast, if the dye does not rapidly equilibrate with the change in free Ca^{2+}, then the optical signal lags the Ca^{2+} transient, and must be corrected for the delay in the Ca^{2+}/dye reaction. Using rapid dyes, which also have low Ca^{2+} affinity due to their relatively high rate constants for the dissociation of the Ca^{2+}/dye complex, the free Ca^{2+} transient in response to a single action potential lasts a few

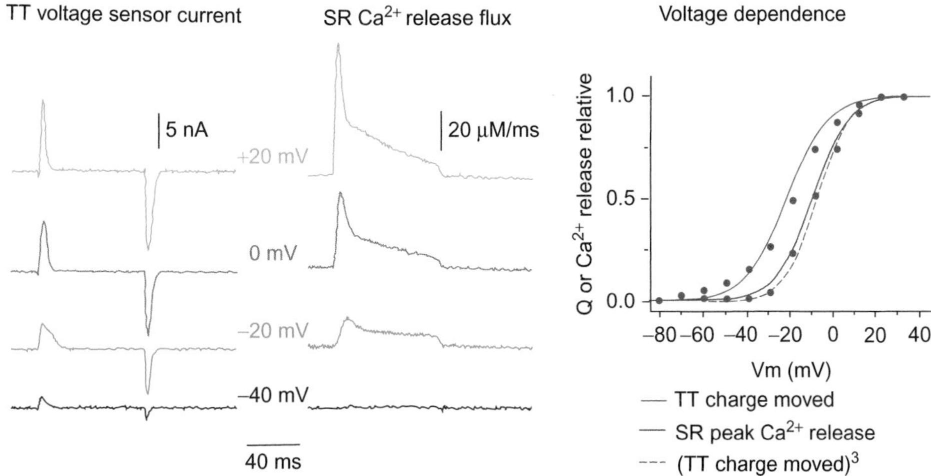

FIGURE 57.3 TT voltage sensor charge movement currents (left) and SR Ca^{2+} release flux (center) and their voltage dependence (right) in whole cell voltage-clamped mouse fast skeletal muscle fibers. (Left) Charge movement recorded with the "P/4" pulse protocol (9) to eliminate linear currents in fibers exposed to solutions to block all ionic conductances. (Center) Ca^{2+} release flux calculated from the same fiber under the same conditions. (Right) Voltage dependence of charge moved by the TT voltage sensor (left points and fit, blue colored) and peak Ca^{2+} release flux (right data set and solid curve, brown colored). The dashed blue curve is the voltage dependence of charge movement (solid blue curve) to the third power, which would be consistent with the observed peak release flux if activation of each release flux channel required the simultaneous movement of all three of a group of three voltage sensor charged groups. Unpublished results from whole cell voltage clamped FDB fiber with 20 mM total EGTA in the fiber interior to eliminate fiber contraction.

milliseconds and reaches a peak of about 10–20 μM (17), with little or no further summation of peak free Ca^{2+} during tetanic stimulation (Figure 57.2C, right). In comparison to the 10–20 μM peak free [Ca^{2+}], the concentration of regulatory Ca^{2+} binding sites on the thin filament troponin C molecules, which are occupied for full fiber contractile activation, is of the order of 200 μM. Thus, in a fiber fully activated for contraction, the Ca^{2+} bound to troponin C would be an order of magnitude higher than the free myoplasmic [Ca^{2+}]. Consequently, in order to determine the rate of Ca^{2+} movement out of the SR during fiber activation, it is crucial to examine not only the free myoplasmic Ca^{2+} monitored directly by the dye, but also the Ca^{2+} bound to all other myoplasmic binding sites, including the relatively rapidly equilibrating sites on troponin C and the more slowly equilibrating sites on the soluble relaxing protein parvalbumin present in fast twitch fibers, as well as Ca^{2+} that is bound to and transported by the SR Ca^{2+} pump (below) and the Ca^{2+} bound to the indicator dye (17,18). Such calculations give the total Ca^{2+} released from the SR, and the time derivative of the total Ca^{2+} released is equal to the rate of release of Ca^{2+} from the SR or the "Ca^{2+} release flux". The resulting calculated Ca^{2+} release flux is brief for a single action potential, reaching its peak prior to the peak free Ca^{2+}, and then rapidly decaying. For a train of repetitive action potentials at relatively rapid rate, the Ca^{2+} release flux is much reduced for the second and following action potentials in the train, even though the voltage wave forms of the successive action potentials are essentially the same. Similarly, during relatively large voltage clamp step depolarizations, the Ca^{2+} release flux (Figure 57.3, center) reaches an early peak, and then exhibits an initial rapid decay (attributed to Ca^{2+} dependent inactivation of the SR Ca^{2+} release channel) and then a slower decay with time that is attributed to depletion of Ca^{2+} from the SR lumen during continued depolarization (19,20). Since charge movement does not seem to be altered during these events, the decay in release does not seem to be due to any change at the level of the TT voltage sensor.

MOLECULAR COMPONENTS FOR T-TUBULE MEMBRANE POTENTIAL CONTROL OF SR CA^{2+} RELEASE

As considered above, two separate but closely apposed membranes, the TT and junctional SR membranes, mediate the TT voltage-dependent regulation of the SR Ca^{2+} release flux. The molecular entities mediating these functional properties were later found to be the dihydropyridine receptor (DHPR) as the TT voltage sensor for activating SR Ca^{2+} release (21–23), and the ryanodine receptor (RyR) as the SR Ca^{2+} release channel (24,25). In addition to considering the functions and properties of each of these molecules individually, it is also essential to address their inter-molecular interactions in the generation of TT membrane-dependent SR Ca^{2+} release. As described above, the functional properties of these molecules were well defined prior to their molecular identification. We now consider the molecular basis for those functional properties.

THE DIHYDROPYRIDINE RECEPTOR IS THE SKELETAL MUSCLE TT VOLTAGE SENSOR FOR EC COUPLING

The alpha 1 subunit of the skeletal muscle dihydropyridine receptor (DHPR, a member of the family of voltage-operated Ca^{2+} channels, also known as Cav1.1), hereafter, for chronological reasons, simply referred to as "the DHPR" or sometimes as the "skeletal DHPR" to distinguish it from the cardiac DHPR isoform unless otherwise identified, was first cloned and sequenced as the receptor for Ca^{2+} channel blockers (i.e., 1,4-dihydropyridine derivatives) isolated from the TTs of skeletal muscle (23), the membrane that exhibits the highest concentration of DHPR. However, in skeletal muscle the Ca^{2+} current through the DHPR is small, activates more slowly than Ca^{2+} release, and is not needed for muscle activation (26–28).

In contrast, the presence of the DHPR is essential for EC coupling. The DHPR is well established as the EC coupling voltage sensor based on the findings that skeletal muscle myotubes cultured from embryonic muscle from the homozygous mutant dysgenic mice, which die at birth due to respiratory failure resulting from failure of skeletal muscle activation, express no DHPR and lack the EC coupling components of charge movement and depolarization activated Ca^{2+} transients, as well as lacking L-type calcium current (29,30). Expression of skeletal muscle DHPR restores EC coupling, charge movement, calcium current, and Ca^{2+} transients (22). Interestingly, skeletal muscle EC coupling does not require Ca^{2+} influx, and the restored EC coupling due to expression of skeletal DHPR in dysgenic myotubes also does not require Ca^{2+} influx. However, if instead the cardiac DHPR was expressed in the dysgenic skeletal myotubes, then the restored EC coupling was of the cardiac variety in that it required Ca^{2+} entry for activation (31). Thus, the nature of the DHPR isoform, skeletal or cardiac, dictated whether the restored EC coupling was of the skeletal or cardiac phenotype. The DHPR has four transmembrane domains, each containing six transmembrane alpha helical segments, with the domains linked by cytosolic loops. When skeletal/cardiac chimeras were expressed in dysgenic myotubes, a chimera that was fully cardiac except for the cytoplasmic loop between the 2nd and 3rd transmembrane domain which had the skeletal sequence, exhibited "skeletal" EC coupling (i.e., independent of Ca^{2+} entry), indicating that this segment could be sufficient for skeletal EC coupling in the context of an otherwise cardiac DHPR (31,32). Subsequent studies identified other important interacting components for skeletal EC coupling, including the beta subunit of the TT Ca^{2+} channel. The molecular details of the coupling mechanism are still under investigation (below). The fourth transmembrane alpha helical segment in each DHPR transmembrane domain possesses several positively charged residues which are believed to be the charges that move in the TT membrane in response to TT depolarization, and to thus generate the voltage sensor charge movement current (8,21,33). The resulting molecular conformational change in the DHPR is thought to be the switch for activating the adjacent SR Ca^{2+} release channel, as well as for the opening of the TT Ca^{2+} channel in the DHPR itself, which results in TT Ca^{2+} current. However, Ca^{2+} release activation occurs more rapidly than the activation of the TT Ca^{2+} current.

THE RYANODINE RECEPTOR IS THE SR CALCIUM RELEASE CHANNEL

Isolation of junctional ("heavy") SR membrane vesicles, purification, and electronmicroscopic visualization of junctional SR proteins and their incorporation into lipid planar bilayer membranes, led to identification of a >2 MD protein homotetramer as the Ca^{2+} release channel of the SR (24,34,35). This channel binds and is activated by the plant alkaloid ryanodine, and thus is called the ryanodine receptor (RyR). Ultrastructural studies of purified RyR revealed a quadrafoil-like particle when viewed face-on from the TT membrane, and subsequent image analysis and structure reconstruction algorithms based on thousands of particle images have led to a sub-nanometer resolution image of the RyR (36–39). The RyR has a large cytosolic domain, that spans the gap between the TT and SR membranes, which can be visualized in electronmicroscopic thin sections of skeletal muscle fibers as the "junctional feet", periodic densities positioned touching each other in a line in the cytosolic space (i.e., gap) between the TT and SR membranes (40). RyR isolation, purification, and reconstitution into planar lipid bilayers gives calcium channel activity similar to that obtained from incorporation of native SR vesicles.

SR CALCIUM RELEASE CHANNELS CAN BE STUDIED DIRECTLY IN FRAGMENTED SYSTEMS, BUT GENERALLY LACK THE TT VOLTAGE SENSOR

Membrane vesicles formed from SR membrane take up calcium from the bathing medium and, if formed from junctional SR, exhibit calcium release properties when the RyR channels are activated. "Triad" vesicle preps, which contain TT membrane vesicle still attached to junctional SR vesicle, exhibit TT depolarization-induced calcium release that can be initiated by ionic composition changes that depolarize the TT component. In contrast, SR vesicles that are *not* attached to TT vesicles, as well as SR vesicles or purified RyR incorporated into lipid bilayer membranes, lack a key element of EC coupling, namely the TT voltage sensor or DHPR, which controls the physiological activation and deactivation of the RyR Ca^{2+} channel. Thus, although the ligand-dependent gating of RyR Ca^{2+} channels in these preparations lacking TTs may reveal ligands that promote or inhibit RyR Ca^{2+} channel opening, the actions of these agents are probably modulatory rather than causative for physiological activation of RyR channels in response to the TT voltage sensor during TT depolarization. In such uncoupled channel preparations, $[Ca^{2+}]$ (1–10 μM) and ATP (~300 μM) serve as physiologically present ligands that have activating effects, Mg^{2+} (~1 mM) competes with Ca^{2+} for binding to the activating site but does not have the activating effect and thus inhibits Ca^{2+} activation and caffeine (1–10 mM) and ryanodine (Ry, ~10 nM) are experimental (i.e., non-physiological) activating ligand molecules (32,39,40). Ligand inhibitors of activity of isolated SR Ca^{2+} release channels include high concentrations of Ca^{2+} and Mg^{2+} (1–10 mM (both binding to an inhibitory site) and higher concentrations of Ry (~100 μM), as well as the muscle relaxant dantrolene (41–43). Interestingly, certain peptides derived from the RyR itself also promote channel opening. This has led to the concept of stabilization of the RyR channel closed configuration by interdomain interactions between neighboring domains within the RyR, termed channel "zipping" (44–46). When these interdomain interactions are disrupted, as when added "domain peptide" binds to its cognate site and thereby competes for and disrupts the normal interdomain interaction, then the RyR is destabilized ("unzipped") and the channel is more likely to open both with and without voltage sensor activation.

PHYSIOLOGICAL MECHANISM FOR ACTIVATION OF THE SR CALCIUM RELEASE CHANNELS IN MUSCLE FIBERS

A complete understanding of the molecular mechanism that couples voltage-dependent, charge moving conformational changes in the DHPR to the transition of the RyR to its open state are not yet fully defined, and probably will only be known at the molecular and submolecular levels of detail when the structure of the entire multimolecular complex of all the interacting components is established. As mentioned above, the interaction of the DHPR TT voltage sensor with the RyR appears to require the skeletal (but not the cardiac) II-III loop of the DHPR alpha 1 subunit (32,47). TT depolarization causes the reorientation of intramembrane positively charged helices in the DHPR toward the TT lumen, i.e., away from the RyR (Figure 57.4), which would occur during the action potential depolarization of the TT (Figure 57.4B). A straightforward hypothesis is that movement of the DHPR charged helices away from the RyR removes an inhibitory influence on Ca^{2+} release, and thereby activates release (48), and it has been proposed that the conformational change of the DHPR may result in decreased Mg^{2+}

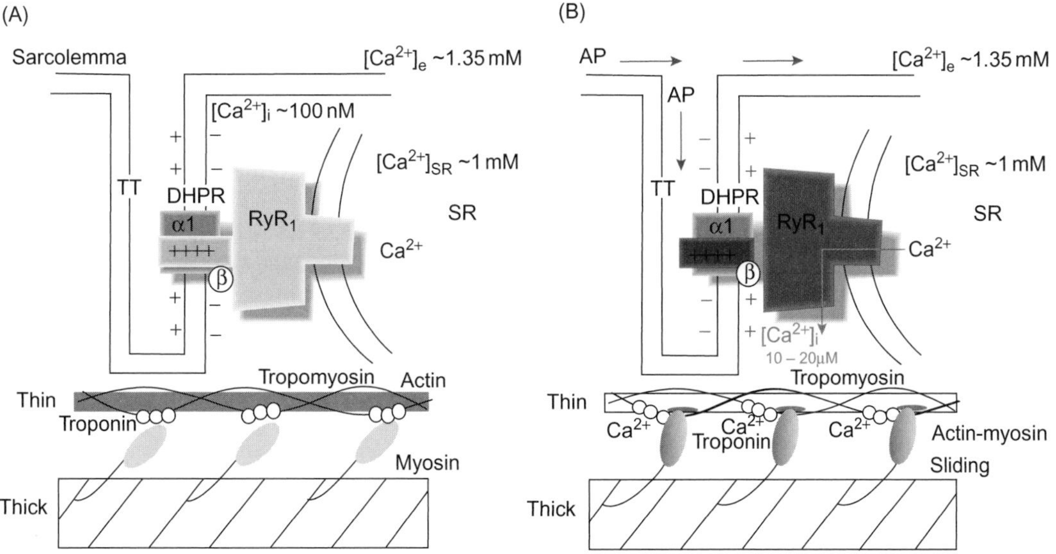

FIGURE 57.4 Cartoon representation of the EC coupling apparatus (A) in the resting state with TT polarized and (B) in the activated state due to TT depolarization during an action potential (AP). Membrane elements are depicted at the top and contractile filaments at the bottom, although both are interspersed throughout an actual fiber. Communication between membranes and filaments is mediated by myoplasmic Ca^{2+} released from the SR during fiber depolarization. Major changes during ECC activation are illustrated in red on panel (B).

affinity of the RyR, and thereby remove the Mg^{2+} suppression of RyR channel opening (49). In addition, the DHPR's beta subunit also seems to participate in the interaction (50), together with other accessory cytoplasmic (e.g., calmodulin, FKBP, S100A1) and junctional membrane and SR luminal proteins (e.g., triadin, junctin, calsequestrin) (51–56) that may modulate DHPR-RyR activation (not shown in Figure 57.4). In addition to the "orthograde" coupling from DHPR to RyR (21,32,57) described above, there is also a "retrograde" coupling whereby activation of the RyR feeds back to promote and modify the calcium current via the DHPR Ca^{2+} channel (58–61).

It is also noteworthy that only half of the RyR Ca^{2+} release channels in the mammalian TT-SR junction are believed to be structurally coupled to TT voltage sensors (62). One possibility for activation of such "uncoupled" RyR channels is secondary activation by calcium-induced calcium release mediated by calcium released via immediately adjacent RyR channels that are coupled to TT voltage sensors. Another possibility is lateral "coupled gating" between neighboring RyRs (63).

UNITARY CA^{2+} RELEASE EVENTS: CA^{2+} SPARKS

Brief, highly localized "spontaneous" stochastic elevations of myoplasmic Ca^{2+}, termed Ca^{2+} "sparks", are readily detectable in mammalian cardiac myocytes as well as in frog skeletal muscle fibers, and reflect underlying unitary calcium release events (64–66). In both cardiac myocytes and frog skeletal muscle fibers such unitary events are observed to occur at much higher frequency during relatively small cell depolarization. Under conditions of low likelihood of release activation, Ca^{2+} sparks have been shown to summate during larger depolarizations to constitute the global Ca^{2+} transient, with the timing of occurrence of sparks during a relatively large step depolarization giving rise to the time course of the macroscopic Ca^{2+} transient. Although in principal unitary Ca^{2+} release events are also anticipated to occur in mammalian skeletal muscle fibers, they have not been clearly resolved under physiological conditions, possibly because of being too small and/or too brief for resolution with current techniques. However, cardiac/frog skeletal muscle-like Ca^{2+} sparks are detected in mammalian embryonic or neonatal skeletal muscle, disappear during the postnatal period and reappear in adult fibers undergoing dedifferentiation in culture, changes that parallel the radial organization and disorganization of the TT system, with corresponding formation and dissociation of TT-SR junctions in development and dedifferentiation respectively (67–71). In addition, cardiac/frog skeletal muscle-like Ca^{2+} sparks are detected in mammalian skeletal muscle fibers under conditions of osmotic or mechanical stress (72), which may disrupt the TT–SR coupling. These diverse observations have led to the concept that the occurrence of cardiac/frog skeletal-like Ca^{2+} sparks requires local groups of RyRs that are uncoupled from DHPRs, which is the case for all cardiac RyRs and for the "parajunctional" RyRs in frog skeletal muscle (73,74). In contrast, when alternate RyRs are coupled to DHPRs and larger groups of uncoupled RyRs are *not* present, as is the case in adult mammalian skeletal muscle fibers under physiological conditions, the Ca^{2+} sparks may be smaller and/or briefer, and thus less readily detected. The type of Ca^{2+} sparks that appear in mammalian fibers when RyRs are decoupled from DHPRs may also appear in muscle disease or degenerative states due to disruption of DHPR–RyR coupling (72).

CALCIUM DEPENDENT CONTRACTILE FILAMENT ACTIVATION

As described above, a major fraction of the Ca^{2+} released in response to an action potential binds to the "Ca^{2+} specific" regulatory Ca^{2+} binding sites on troponin C molecules in the thin filament (Figure 57.4B) (75). Such Ca^{2+} binding to troponin C causes changes in thin filament structure, including rearrangement of tropomyosin molecules in the thin filament, resulting in the availability of previously unavailable binding sites for myosin on the thin filament actin molecules. This allows the myosin heads (cross-bridges) from the thick filaments to bind to thin filament actin molecules and produce force and/or shortening. This is the basic "ON/OFF switch" for mechanical activation of skeletal muscle, which simply requires Ca^{2+} binding and a resulting macromolecular conformational change, and is thus relatively rapid. In parallel, and by a slower enzymatic reaction, the speed and efficiency of the myosin ATPase, and thus the cross-bridge mechanochemical cycle kinetics, is modulated by the Ca^{2+}-calmodulin dependent activation of myosin light chain kinase and the resulting phosphorylation of myosin light chains (76,77).

RELAXATION

In addition to the RyR Ca^{2+} release channels in the junctional SR, the entire SR membrane contains a high concentration of Ca^{2+} ATPase molecules, the SR/ER (SERCA) Ca^{2+} pump (78,79). This transport system translocates Ca^{2+} ions up their concentration gradient and establishes the resting 4-order of magnitude concentration gradient of roughly 0.1 μM cytosolic $[Ca^{2+}]$ and 1 mM or higher SR luminal $[Ca^{2+}]$. In the resting fiber the cytosolic $[Ca^{2+}]$ is low and the SERCA pump cycles correspondingly slowly. When cytosolic Ca^{2+} rises, Ca^{2+} ions bind to and are transported by the pump. Considering that the concentration of pump sites in the myoplasmic volume is similar to the concentration of troponin C Ca^{2+} regulatory sites (also referred to the myoplasmic volume), the simple binding of previously released Ca^{2+} ions to the pump could relax the muscle after a twitch, but cycling is required for successive activation and relaxation. In fast twitch fibers, the soluble Ca^{2+} binding protein parvalbumin provides a way station for binding Ca^{2+} during relaxation prior to its ultimate return to the SR (80,81). The final uptake of released Ca^{2+} back into the SR, mediated by the ATP dependent Ca^{2+} pump in the SR membrane, restores the initial state of the resting fiber, with essentially all of the released Ca^{2+} returned to the SR Ca^{2+} pool, and terminates the excitation–contraction coupling process.

REFERENCES

1. Sandow A. Excitation–contraction coupling in muscular response. *Yale J Biol Med* 1952;**25**:176–201.
2. Capote J, DiFranco M, Vergara JL. Excitation–contraction coupling alterations in mdx and utrophin/dystrophin double knockout mice: a comparative study. *Am J Physiol Cell Physiol* 2010;**298**: C1077–86.
3. Berchtold MW, Brinkmeier H, Muntener M. Calcium ion in skeletal muscle: its crucial role for muscle function, plasticity, and disease. *Physiol Rev* 2000;**80**:1215–65.
4. Hodgkin AL, Huxley AF. A quantitative description of membrane current and its application to conduction and excitation in nerve. *J Physiol* 1952;**117**:500–44.
5. Hodgkin AL, Horowicz P. Potassium contractures in single muscle fibres. *J Physiol* 1960;**153**:386–403.
6. Huxley AF, Niedergerke R. Structural changes in muscle during contraction; interference microscopy of living muscle fibres. *Nature* 1954;**173**:971–3.
7. Huxley AF, Taylor RE. Local activation of striated muscle fibres. *J Physiol* 1958;**144**:426–41.
8. Schneider MF, Chandler WK. Voltage dependent charge movement of skeletal muscle: a possible step in excitation–contraction coupling. *Nature* 1973;**242**:244–6.
9. Armstrong CM, Bezanilla F. Charge movement associated with the opening and closing of the activation gates of the Na channels. *J Gen Physiol* 1974;**63**:533–52.
10. Horowicz P, Schneider MF. Membrane charge moved at contraction thresholds in skeletal muscle fibres. *J Physiol* 1981; **314**:595–633.
11. Adrian RH, Chandler WK, Rakowski RF. Charge movement and mechanical repriming in skeletal muscle. *J Physiol* 1976; **254**:361–88.
12. Simon BJ, Hill DA. Charge movement and SR calcium release in frog skeletal muscle can be related by a Hodgkin–Huxley model with four gating particles. *Biophys J* 1992;**61**:1109–16.
13. Ridgway EB, Ashley CC. Calcium transients in single muscle fibers. *Biochem Biophys Res Commun* 1967;**29**:229–34.
14. Kovacs L, Rios E, Schneider MF. Calcium transients and intramembrane charge movement in skeletal muscle fibres. *Nature* 1979;**279**:391–6.
15. Baylor SM, Chandler WK, Marshall MW. Sarcoplasmic reticulum calcium release in frog skeletal muscle fibres estimated from Arsenazo III calcium transients. *J Physiol* 1983;**344**:625–66.
16. Melzer W, Rios E, Schneider MF. Time course of calcium release and removal in skeletal muscle fibers. *Biophys J* 1984;**45**:637–41.
17. Baylor SM, Hollingworth S. Sarcoplasmic reticulum calcium release compared in slow-twitch and fast-twitch fibres of mouse muscle. *J Physiol* 2003;**551**:125–38.
18. Melzer W, Rios E, Schneider MF. A general procedure for determining the rate of calcium release from the sarcoplasmic reticulum in skeletal muscle fibers. *Biophys J* 1987;**51**:849–63.
19. Schneider MF, Simon BJ, Szucs G. Depletion of calcium from the sarcoplasmic reticulum during calcium release in frog skeletal muscle. *J Physiol* 1987;**392**:167–92.
20. Schneider MF, Simon BJ. Inactivation of calcium release from the sarcoplasmic reticulum in frog skeletal muscle. *J Physiol* 1988;**405**:727–45.
21. Rios E, Brum G. Involvement of dihydropyridine receptors in excitation–contraction coupling in skeletal muscle. *Nature* 1987;**325**:717–20.
22. Tanabe T, Beam KG, Powell JA, Numa S. Restoration of excitation–contraction coupling and slow calcium current in dysgenic muscle by dihydropyridine receptor complementary DNA. *Nature* 1988;**336**:134–9.
23. Tanabe T, Takeshima H, Mikami A, Flockerzi V, Takahashi H, Kangawa K, et al. Primary structure of the receptor for calcium channel blockers from skeletal muscle. *Nature* 1987;**328**:313–8.
24. Imagawa T, Smith JS, Coronado R, Campbell KP. Purified ryanodine receptor from skeletal muscle sarcoplasmic reticulum is the Ca^{2+}-permeable pore of the calcium release channel. *J Biol Chem* 1987;**262**:16636–43.
25. Takeshima H, Nishimura S, Matsumoto T, Ishida H, Kangawa K, Minamino N, et al. Primary structure and expression from complementary DNA of skeletal muscle ryanodine receptor. *Nature* 1989;**339**:439–45.
26. Armstrong CM, Bezanilla FM, Horowicz P. Twitches in the presence of ethylene glycol bis(-aminoethyl ether)-N,N'-tetracetic acid. *Biochim Biophys Acta* 1972;**267**:605–8.
27. Stanfield PR. A calcium dependent inward current in frog skeletal muscle fibres. *Pflugers Arch* 1977;**368**:267–70.
28. Sanchez JA, Stefani E. Inward calcium current in twitch muscle fibres of the frog. *J Physiol* 1978;**283**:197–209.
29. Beam KG, Knudson CM, Powell JA. A lethal mutation in mice eliminates the slow calcium current in skeletal muscle cells. *Nature* 1986;**320**:168–70.
30. Knudson CM, Chaudhari N, Sharp AH, Powell JA, Beam KG, Campbell P. Specific absence of the alpha 1 subunit of the dihydropyridine receptor in mice with muscular dysgenesis. *J Biol Chem* 1989;**264**:1345–8.
31. Tanabe T, Mikami A, Numa S, Beam KG. Cardiac-type excitation–contraction coupling in dysgenic skeletal muscle injected with cardiac dihydropyridine receptor cDNA. *Nature* 1990;**344**:451–3.
32. Tanabe T, Beam KG, Adams BA, Niidome T, Numa S. Regions of the skeletal muscle dihydropyridine receptor critical for excitation–contraction coupling. *Nature* 1990;**346**:567–9.

33. Catterall WA. Structure and regulation of voltage-gated Ca^{2+} channels. *Annu Rev Cell Dev Biol* 2000;**16**:521–55.
34. Smith JS, Coronado R, Meissner G. Single channel measurements of the calcium release channel from skeletal muscle sarcoplasmic reticulum. Activation by Ca^{2+} and ATP and modulation by Mg^{2+}. *J Gen Physiol* 1986;**88**:573–88.
35. Inui M, Saito A, Fleischer S. Purification of the ryanodine receptor and identity with feet structures of junctional terminal cisternae of sarcoplasmic reticulum from fast skeletal muscle. *J Biol Chem* 1987;**262**:1740–7.
36. Radermacher M, Wagenknecht T, Grassucci R, Frank J, Inui M, Chadwick C, et al. Cryo-EM of the native structure of the calcium release channel/ryanodine receptor from sarcoplasmic reticulum. *Biophys J* 1992;**61**:936–40.
37. Serysheva II, Hamilton SL, Chiu W, Ludtke SJ. Structure of Ca^{2+} release channel at 14 A resolution. *J Mol Biol* 2005;**345**:427–31.
38. Serysheva II, Ludtke SJ, Baker ML, Cong Y, Topf M, Eramian D, et al. Subnanometer-resolution electron cryomicroscopy-based domain models for the cytoplasmic region of skeletal muscle RyR channel. *Proc Natl Acad Sci USA* 2008;**105**:9610–5.
39. Samso M, Feng W, Pessah IN, Allen PD. Coordinated movement of cytoplasmic and transmembrane domains of RyR1 upon gating. *PLoS Biol* 2009;**7**:e85.
40. Franzini-Armstrong C, Nunzi G. Junctional feet and particles in the triads of a fast-twitch muscle fibre. *J Muscle Res Cell Motil* 1983;**4**:233–52.
41. Meissner G, Darling E, Eveleth J. Kinetics of rapid Ca^{2+} release by sarcoplasmic reticulum. Effects of Ca^{2+}, Mg^{2+}, and adenine nucleotides. *Biochemistry* 1986;**25**:236–44.
42. Fill M, Copello JA. Ryanodine receptor calcium release channels. *Physiol Rev* 2002;**82**:893–922.
43. Suarez-Isla BA, Orozco C, Heller PF, Froehlich JP. Single calcium channels in native sarcoplasmic reticulum membranes from skeletal muscle. *Proc Natl Acad Sci USA* 1986;**83**:7741–5.
44. Yamamoto T, El-Hayek R, Ikemoto N. Postulated role of interdomain interaction within the ryanodine receptor in Ca(2+) channel regulation. *J Biol Chem* 2000;**275**:11618–25.
45. Ikemoto N, Yamamoto T. Regulation of calcium release by interdomain interaction within ryanodine receptors. *Front Biosci* 2002;**7**:d671–83.
46. Yamamoto T, Ikemoto N. Spectroscopic monitoring of local conformational changes during the intramolecular domain–domain interaction of the ryanodine receptor. *Biochemistry* 2002;**41**:1492–501.
47. Nakai J, Adams BA, Imoto K, Beam KG. Critical roles of the S3 segment and S3-S4 linker of repeat I in activation of L-type calcium channels. *Proc Natl Acad Sci USA* 1994;**91**:1014–8.
48. Chandler WK, Rakowski RF, Schneider MF. A non-linear voltage dependent charge movement in frog skeletal muscle. *J Physiol* 1976;**254**:245–83.
49. Lamb GD, Stephenson DG. Effect of Mg^{2+} on the control of Ca^{2+} release in skeletal muscle fibres of the toad. *J Physiol* 1991;**434**:507–28.
50. Gregg RG, Messing A, Strube C, Beurg M, Moss R, Behan M, et al. Absence of the beta subunit (cchb1) of the skeletal muscle dihydropyridine receptor alters expression of the alpha 1 subunit and eliminates excitation–contraction coupling. *Proc Natl Acad Sci USA* 1996;**93**:13961–6.
51. Brillantes AB, Ondrias K, Scott A, Kobrinsky E, Ondriasova E, Moschella MC, et al. Stabilization of calcium release channel (ryanodine receptor) function by FK506-binding protein. *Cell* 1994;**77**:513–23.
52. Chen SR, MacLennan DH. Identification of calmodulin-, Ca(2+)-, and ruthenium red-binding domains in the Ca^{2+} release channel (ryanodine receptor) of rabbit skeletal muscle sarcoplasmic reticulum. *J Biol Chem* 1994;**269**:22698–704.
53. Tripathy A, Xu L, Mann G, Meissner G. Calmodulin activation and inhibition of skeletal muscle Ca^{2+} release channel (ryanodine receptor). *Biophys J* 1995;**69**:106–19.
54. Prosser BL, Wright NT, Hernandez-Ochoa EO, Varney KM, Liu Y, Olojo RO, et al. S100A1 binds to the calmodulin-binding site of ryanodine receptor and modulates skeletal muscle excitation–contraction coupling. *J Biol Chem* 2008;**283**:5046–57.
55. Treves S, Vukcevic M, Maj M, Thurnheer R, Mosca B, Zorzato F. Minor sarcoplasmic reticulum membrane components that modulate excitation–contraction coupling in striated muscles. *J Physiol* 2009;**587**:3071–9.
56. Beard NA, Wei L, Dulhunty AF. Ca(2+) signaling in striated muscle: the elusive roles of triadin, junctin, and calsequestrin. *Eur Biophys J* 2009;**39**:27–36.
57. Nakai J, Tanabe T, Konno T, Adams B, Beam KG. Localization in the II-III loop of the dihydropyridine receptor of a sequence critical for excitation–contraction coupling. *J Biol Chem* 1998; **273**:24983–6.
58. Nakai J, Dirksen RT, Nguyen HT, Pessah IN, Beam KG, Allen PD. Enhanced dihydropyridine receptor channel activity in the presence of ryanodine receptor. *Nature* 1996;**380**:72–5.
59. Sheridan DC, Takekura H, Franzini-Armstrong C, Beam KG, Allen PD, Perez CF. Bidirectional signaling between calcium channels of skeletal muscle requires multiple direct and indirect interactions. *Proc Natl Acad Sci USA* 2006;**103**:19760–5.
60. Nakai J, Sekiguchi N, Rando TA, Allen PD, Beam KG. Two regions of the ryanodine receptor involved in coupling with L-type Ca^{2+} channels. *J Biol Chem* 1998;**273**:13403–6.
61. Protasi F, Paolini C, Nakai J, Beam KG, Franzini-Armstrong C, Allen PD. Multiple regions of RyR1 mediate functional and structural interactions with alpha(1S)-dihydropyridine receptors in skeletal muscle. *Biophys J* 2002;**83**:3230–44.
62. Block BA, Imagawa T, Campbell KP, Franzini-Armstrong C. Structural evidence for direct interaction between the molecular components of the transverse tubule/sarcoplasmic reticulum junction in skeletal muscle. *J Cell Biol* 1988;**107**:2587–600.
63. Marx SO, Ondrias K, Marks AR. Coupled gating between individual skeletal muscle Ca^{2+} release channels (ryanodine receptors). *Science* 1998;**281**:818–21.
64. Cheng H, Lederer WJ, Cannell MB. Calcium sparks: elementary events underlying excitation–contraction coupling in heart muscle. *Science* 1993;**262**:740–4.
65. Tsugorka A, Rios E, Blatter LA. Imaging elementary events of calcium release in skeletal muscle cells. *Science* 1995;**269**:1723–6.
66. Klein MG, Cheng H, Santana LF, Jiang YH, Lederer WJ, Schneider MF. Two mechanisms of quantized calcium release in skeletal muscle. *Nature* 1996;**379**:455–8.
67. Conklin MW, Barone V, Sorrentino V, Coronado R. Contribution of ryanodine receptor type 3 to Ca(2+) sparks in embryonic mouse skeletal muscle. *Biophys J* 1999;**77**:1394–403.

68. Shirokova N, Shirokov R, Rossi D, Gonzalez A, Kirsch WG, Garcia J, et al. Spatially segregated control of Ca^{2+} release in developing skeletal muscle of mice. *J Physiol* 1999;**521**(Pt 2): 483–95.
69. Chun LG, Ward CW, Schneider MF. Ca^{2+} sparks are initiated by Ca^{2+} entry in embryonic mouse skeletal muscle and decrease in frequency postnatally. *Am J Physiol Cell Physiol* 2003;**285**:C686–97.
70. Zhou J, Yi J, Royer L, Launikonis BS, Gonzalez A, Garcia J, et al. A probable role of dihydropyridine receptors in repression of Ca^{2+} sparks demonstrated in cultured mammalian muscle. *Am J Physiol Cell Physiol* 2006;**290**:C539–53.
71. Brown LD, Rodney GG, Hernandez-Ochoa E, Ward CW, Schneider MF. Ca^{2+} sparks and T tubule reorganization in dedifferentiating adult mouse skeletal muscle fibers. *Am J Physiol Cell Physiol* 2007;**292**:C1156–66.
72. Wang X, Weisleder N, Collet C, Zhou J, Chu Y, Hirata Y, et al. Uncontrolled calcium sparks act as a dystrophic signal for mammalian skeletal muscle. *Nat Cell Biol* 2005;**7**:525–30.
73. Felder E, Franzini-Armstrong C. Type 3 ryanodine receptors of skeletal muscle are segregated in a parajunctional position. *Proc Natl Acad Sci USA* 2002;**99**:1695–700.
74. Pouvreau S, Royer L, Yi J, Brum G, Meissner G, Rios E, et al. Ca(2+) sparks operated by membrane depolarization require isoform 3 ryanodine receptor channels in skeletal muscle. *Proc Natl Acad Sci U S A* 2007;**104**:5235–40.
75. Ebashi S. Regulatory mechanism of muscle contraction with special reference to the Ca-troponin-tropomyosin system. *Essays Biochem* 1974;**10**:1–36.
76. Manning DR, Stull JT. Myosin light chain phosphorylation and phosphorylase A activity in rat extensor digitorum longus muscle. *Biochem Biophys Res Commun* 1979;**90**:164–70.
77. Sweeney HL, Bowman BF, Stul JTl. Myosin light chain phosphorylation in vertebrate striated muscle: regulation and function. *Am J Physiol* 1993;**264**:C1085–1095.
78. Hasselbach W. ATP-driven active transport of calcium in the membranes of the sarcoplasmic reticulum. *Proc R Soc Lond B Biol Sci* 1964;**160**:501–4.
79. Hasselbach W. The Ca(2+)-ATPase of the sarcoplasmic reticulum in skeletal and cardiac muscle. An overview from the very beginning to more recent prospects. *Ann NY Acad Sci* 1998;**853**: 1–8.
80. Gerday C, Gillis JM. J Physiol. *Proceedings: The possible role of parvalbumins in the control of contraction* 1976;**258**:96P–7P.
81. Pechere JF, Derancourt J, Haiech J. The participation of parvalbumins in the activation-relaxation cycle of vertebrate fast skeletal-muscle. *FEBS Lett* 1977;**75**:111–4.

Chapter 58

The Contractile Machinery of Skeletal Muscle

Clara Franzini-Armstrong[1] and H. Lee Sweeney[2]
[1]Department of Cell and Developmental Biology, [2]Department of Physiology, Perelman School of Medicine, University of Pennsylvania, Philadelphia, PA

SARCOMERES ARE REPEATING UNITS OF THE MYOFIBRILS

The contractile material within a skeletal muscle fiber (or cardiomyocyte) is bundled into small cylinders, the myofibrils, which in turn are composed of contractile myofilaments. In adult muscle fibers, the myofibrils fill the entire fiber, leaving small spaces for nuclei and associated Golgi system, for mitochondria and SR, glycogen granules, etc.

The myofibrils are composed of repeating units, or segments a few microns in length, called sarcomeres (Figure 58.1). By convention, the sarcomere starts and ends at the Z-lines or Z-bands: thin bands containing a high density of protein, with a high refractive index and a high electron density in the electron microscope. Between Z-lines are a series of bands with variable light optical and electron optical properties that are determined by their structural components.

BANDS AND FILAMENTS

The center of the sarcomere is occupied by the A-band, which is optically anisotropic (hence the name) or birefringent, that it has different refractive indices in two different directions relative to the incident light beam. The A-band is also electron dense (Figure 58.1). Both properties are due to the presence and parallel alignment of "thick" filaments composed mostly of myosin. A-band length is the same (1.6 μm) in all vertebrate skeletal muscles, and the edges of the A-band are sharp because the thick filaments have uniform length. A complete list of the many proteins associated with myosin in the A-band is given by Craig (1; also see reference 2).

The I-band, on either side of the A-band and bisected by the Z-line, is not totally isotropic as its name (I) would imply, but it is only weakly birefringent, since it is constituted of thin filaments composed of actin and associated proteins. Thin actin filaments are thinner, more flexible, and mostly less well aligned than the thick myosin filaments (1). Thin filaments run from the Z-line across the I-band into the A-band, where they overlap with the thick filaments and reach up to the edges of the H-zone. Thus the two outer regions of the A-band are denser than the central segments, because they contain overlapping thin and thick filaments (Figures 58.1, 58.2A), while the H-zone is lighter (Figures 58.1, 58.2B).

Thin and thick filaments are disposed in a double hexagonal array: in cross-sections of the overlap region the thick filaments are at the corners of perfect hexagons and six thin filaments surround each thick filament, forming a second hexagonal array (Figure 58.2A). Within the A-band each thin filament is equidistant from three adjacent thick filaments with which it interacts (trigonal position).

Within the H-band (or H-zone), thick filaments are the only longitudinally running elements (Figure 58.2B), yet three different segments are well defined within this region. The very central region of the H-zone, the M-band, is quite dense due to the presence of cross-links connecting thick filaments into a network (Figures 58.1, 58.2B), see also below. Immediately adjacent to the M-band, on either side of it, is a narrow lighter band, the L (for light) or bridge-free zone. In the L-zone, and also through the M-band, no myosin cross-bridges project from the surface of the thick filament. In cross-sections the thick filament profiles immediately adjacent to the M-band have a triangular shape and are smaller than the profiles in the rest of the A-band (compare Figures 58.2A and B). The rest of the H-zone is denser than the L line because cross-bridges (the heads of the myosin molecules) cover the surface of the thick filaments and/or project out from it (Figure 58.1).

Sarcomere shortening results in the sliding of thin filaments past the thick filaments into the A-band, so that the I-band and H-zone shorten, while the widths of Z-line, A-band M-line and the bridge-free region do not change.

Muscle. DOI: http://dx.doi.org/10.1016/B978-0-12-381510-1.00058-2

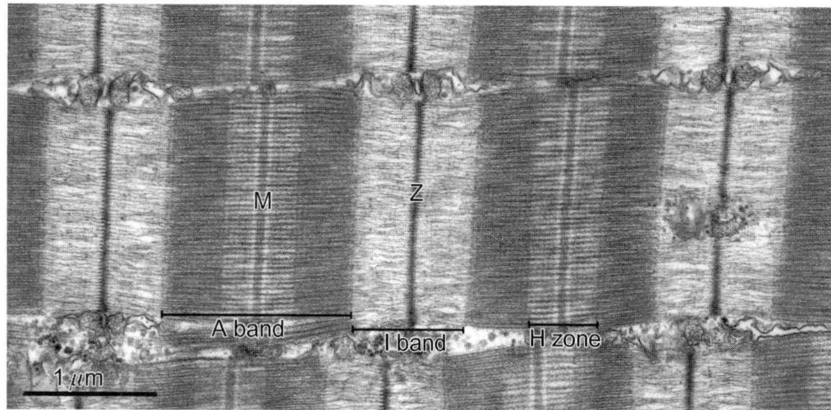

FIGURE 58.1 Longitudinal section through a muscle fiber from the frog, the fiber long axis is horizontal. Two complete sarcomeres are shown, elements of the sarcoplasmic reticulum separate myofibrils in the longitudinal direction. The major bands and lines are indicated. The relative densities of the bands in this electron micrograph are related to their content of protein. The light band on either side of the M-line shows the extent of the bridge-free region of the thick filaments. The fine transverse periodicity across the A-band, at approximately 43 nm, is due to the periodic structure of the thick filament backbone, which in turn determines the position of relaxed cross-bridges on the surface of the filaments and is enhanced by the presence of accessory proteins.

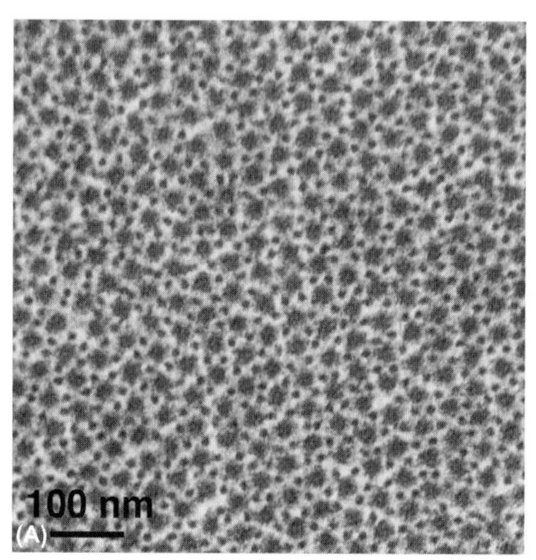

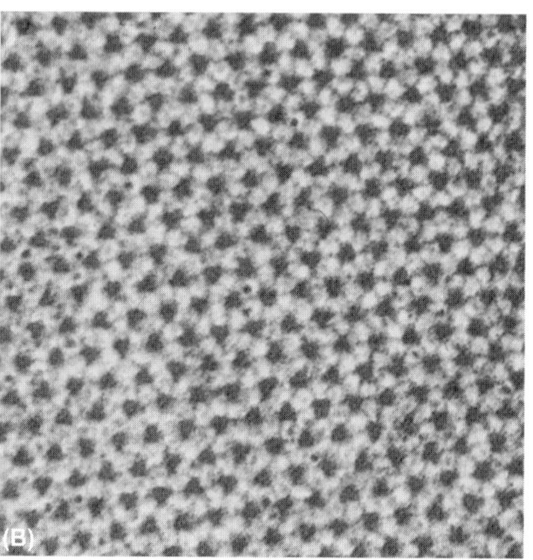

FIGURE 58.2 Cross-sections through the overlap region of the A-band (A) and the bridge-free region and the M-line (B). The double hexagonal array of thick and thin filaments (A) shows six thin filaments surrounding each thick filament. The thin filaments are in the trigonal position, so that one thin filament interacts with three thick filaments. The overall ratio is 2:1. The lower left corner of (B) shows cross-sections of the thick filaments' central region, which is bridge-free and has a triangular shape. In the upper right corner, M-line cross-links connect thick filaments and hold them in a precise hexagonal array.

This was first described in detail by Huxley and Hanson, and Huxley and Niedergerke in 1954 (3,4) and formed the basis of the Sliding Filament Theory of muscle contraction.

Actin Molecules Polymerize into Long Thin Filaments with a Helical Structure

At physiological ionic strength, and in the presence of Mg^{++} and K^{+}, actin monomers (G-actin) polymerize into long thin filaments (F-actin), in which the molecules form a tightly wound "genetic" helix, with a pitch of 5.9 nm. A further twist of the helix gives the filament the appearance of two twisted strands of beads, with crossover points at ~37 nm.

ATP is hydrolyzed to ADP during polymerization. This is not essential for polymerization itself, but it is important in giving different properties to the two ends of the filament and thus allowing thread milling (polymerization at one end and depolymerization at the other), a property that is very important for non-sarcomeric actin filaments. The length of actin filaments is not stable and thus not uniquely determined, particularly for "cytoplasmic" actin, but it can be stabilized by capping proteins that block loss and/or addition of monomers at the ends of the filaments. In skeletal muscle, the length of actin filaments depends on the species and muscles in question. For example, actin filaments in the tail myotomes of fish are considerably shorter than those in rabbit muscle.

Due to the uniform orientation of actin monomers within the filament, and to the fact that the four major domains of the monomers are not identical, the filament has an intrinsic structural and functional polarity, which is evidenced in the high-resolution images and in the different properties of the two ends. Direct evidence for the polarity of actin filaments was provided by fully

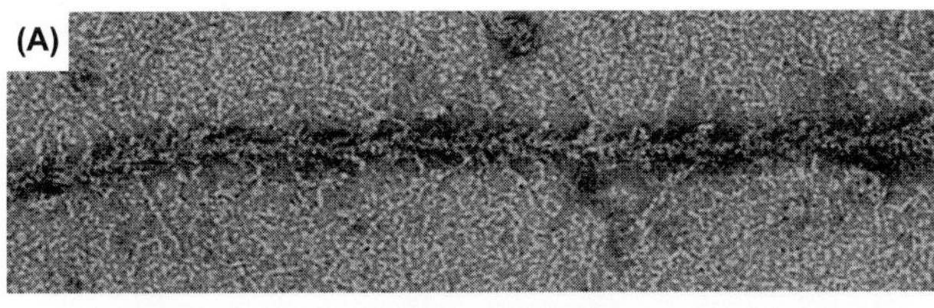

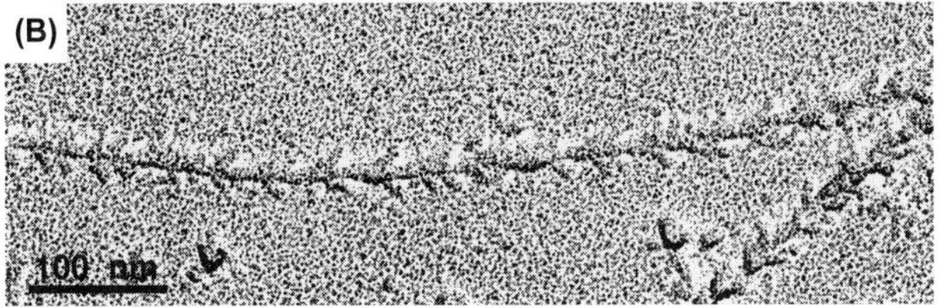

FIGURE 58.3 Negatively stained (A) and rotary shadowed (B) images of "natively decorated" thin filaments. These were obtained by dissociating the myosin filament backbone of myofibrils from a crustacean muscle after establishing rigor conditions, in the absence of ATP. The cross-bridges remain attached to the thin filaments in the original periodic positioning. Compare with Figure 58.7B.

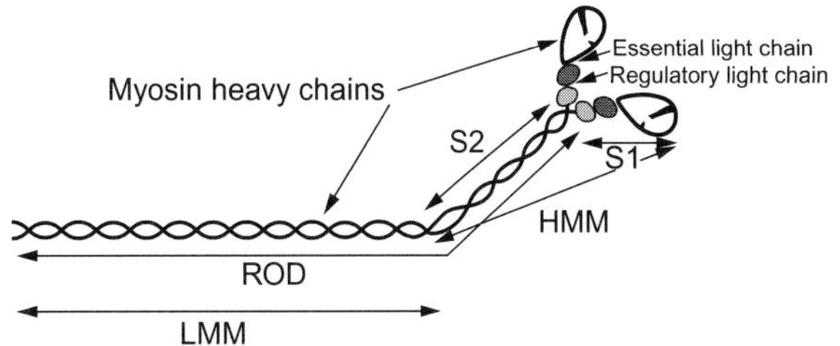

FIGURE 58.4 Myosin molecule and its proteolytic fragments. Illustrated is the myosin molecule of muscle, myosin II, and the fragments that have been generated by limited proteolysis and widely studied. The catalytic portion of the molecule is in the two S1 fragments, each of which contains a nucleotide binding site and an actin binding site. The S1 fragment is commonly referred to as the myosin head. The rest of the myosin molecule, comprised of the S2 and LMM fragments, forms an alpha-helical coiled coil. The C-terminal portion of the LMM is necessary for myosin filament formation. A two-headed, catalytically active fragment of myosin known as HMM can also be generated. The HMM fragments do not form filaments and thus have been used extensively for solution biochemistry.

decorating the filaments with myosin heads. Due to the twist of the long actin helix and to the angle of the myosin head attachment, the decorated actin filament seems to be covered by arrowheads. The arrowheads point away from the Z-lines and thus the direction of the myosin–actin interaction reverses at the Z-line, in a manner that is appropriate for the sliding of filaments during muscle shortening.

Figure 58.3 shows a negatively stained (A) and a shadowed (B) image of "natively decorated" actin filaments, These were isolated from a crayfish muscle in rigor by dissociating the backbone of the thick filament and the Z-lines in a high molarity solution (3 M KCl). The images show not only the clear polarity of the filaments, but also the fact that the attachment sites of myosin heads, which retain the position they had in the intact "rigor" sarcomere, are periodically spaced. At every ~36 nm (corresponding to the pitch of the actin helix) either a singe or two closely spaced cross-bridges, most composed of the two heads from a myosin molecule, are attached. See below for further details.

Actin filaments polymerize from the edges of the Z-line, with the "barbed" end at the Z-line end. Anchoring of thin filaments to the Z-line and/or nucleation, a necessary step in the initiation of actin polymerization are mediated by Cap Z, also called beta actinin (5,6). A second set of proteins, part of the formin family, also regulates actin assembly and/or maintenance in striated muscle, perhaps acting as elongating factors (7). In some muscles such as the frog muscle shown in Figure 58.1, the edges of the H-zone are quite sharp, indicating that the majority of the thin filaments have the same maximum length. Capping of the pointed (slow growing) end of the filaments (away from the Z-lines) is important in maintaining the thin filaments' lengths (8,9). However, the thin filament lengths are well specified in different muscles and thus in addition to capping a yardstick is necessary, and nebulin is thought to play this role.

While the factors defined above determine the overall length of the majority of the thin filaments, live muscle fibers, particularly those that support prolonged periods of contractile activity, have a population of shorter filaments. This is thought to be due to attrition in which a small proportion of the relatively weak thin filaments break and need to be continuously regenerated.

The Myosin Motor of Muscle

Myosin is the force generator of skeletal, cardiac, and smooth muscle. The myosin found in muscle was the first protein discovered in what is now a large superfamily of motor proteins (10). The form isolated from muscle is now referred to as myosin II, or conventional myosin. The nonmuscle form of this same type of myosin is found in nearly all eukaryotic cells and is the motor that powers cytokinesis and plays a role in cellular locomotion (11).

Muscle myosin is a hexameric protein consisting of four light chains and two heavy chains (Figure 58.4). The heavy chains contain the two distinct regions: the head and the rod. The rod is an alpha-helical coiled coil structure approximately 1500 Å long and 20 Å in diameter (12). Via a flexible linkage (13), the rod connects to the two globular regions, or heads. The rod is necessary for assembly of myosin molecules into filaments. The head is the enzymatic region, containing the site of ATP hydrolysis and actin binding. Biochemical studies (14–16) and the first high resolution crystal structure (17) identified regions in the myosin heavy chain head that are involved in nucleotide binding, actin binding, and light chain binding.

Each of the two heavy chains is approximately 200 kDa (18). Associated with each of the two heads are two light chains (thus a total of four light chains per myosin molecule). One of the light chains associated with each head is about 18.5 kDa; the other ranges from 16.5 kDa to 24 kDa (19,20).

The myosin light chains have been referred to by a variety of names through the years. The 18.5 kDa light chain can be dissociated from myosin using DTNB (21), and thus has been called the DTNB light chain. Since it is generally the second largest of the light chains of fast twitch muscle, it is also known as light chain 2 (LC2). To denote the fact that it is LC2 from fast twitch muscle, it is referred to as $LC2_f$. This light chain can be phosphorylated (22), and thus has been referred to as the P-light chain (23). In fact, this phosphorylation event forms the on/off switch for smooth and non-muscle myosin activity, hence it is known as the regulatory light chain (11). Regulatory light chain (RLC) is the term in current use for this light chain and is used throughout this chapter.

The other class of light chains have been referred to as the alkali light chains, since treatment of myosin at pH 11 removes them (24). Using this nomenclature, the two light chains of fast skeletal myosin have been referred to as Al (21 kDa) and A2 (16.5 kDa) (20). These specific light chains from mammalian fast twitch muscle have more often been denoted LCl_f and $LC3_f$, respectively. This class of light chains is most commonly referred to as the essential light chains, based on an early observation that they could not be removed without loss of myosin activity. The term essential light chain (ELC) is the most general and currently used and is the term used below.

The myosin molecule is divided into two pieces by limited tryptic or chymotryptic digestion: heavy meromyosin and light meromyosin. The heavy meromyosin (HMM) fragment of MHC (~150 kDa) contains the enzymatically functional head (S1) and N-terminal portion (S2) of the rod (Figure 58.4). The HMM and S1 proteolytic fragments of all types of muscle myosin have been used extensively for the delineation of actin-myosin kinetics in solution, since they do not aggregate at the low ionic strengths used in such assays.

With further tryptic digestion the myosin head, or S1 region, can be divided into three subfragments (14). Moving from the N-terminus, these subfragments are: Mr 25,000, Mr 50,000, and Mr 20,000. These tryptic subfragments are created by cleavage of flexible loops that are generally not resolvable in the high resolution X-ray structures of myosin. This nomenclature derived from myosin proteolysis was adapted by Rayment et al. (17) to describe the subdomains that the high-resolution crystal structure revealed for the skeletal muscle myosin head. This initial description of the subdomains has been modified as depicted in Figure 58.5B.

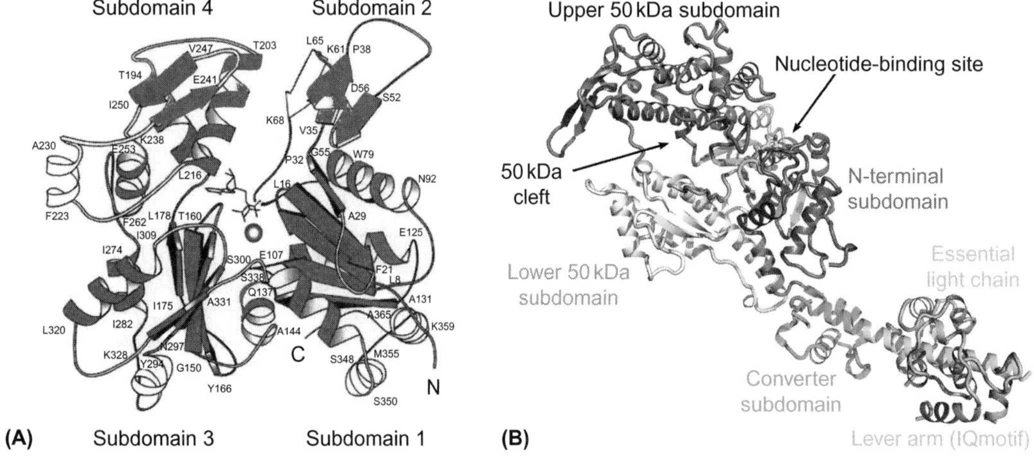

FIGURE 58.5 Structures of actin and the myosin head. (A) High-resolution structure of G-actin. In this ribbon diagram of the G-actin structure, the first and last amino acid residues in the helices and sheet strands are specified. The first actin structure was in a complex with DNAse I (25), and a number of subsequent structures have validated it. The four actin subdomains are thought to rearrange when G-actin forms filaments (F-actin), and subdomains 1 and 2 may further rearrange when myosin binds to actin. Subdomain 1 is thought to contribute most of the myosin-binding site, with contributions from subdomain 2 from a second actin monomer in the filament. The need for a contribution to the interface from two separate actin monomers explains why F-actin, but not G-actin, can activate the myosin ATPase activity. Based on the structures of thin filaments of muscle fibers, models of F-actin have been proposed (26). (B) High-resolution crystal structure of the myosin head. A ribbon diagram of a myosin head structure in the post-rigor (MgATP-bound) state is shown. Note that only the first light chain (ELC) is included, and that the RLC is bound next to the ELC on the extended lever arm helix. In the case of myosin II, his helix contains two "IQ motifs". The subdomains of the myosin head are labeled and move relative to each other as myosin goes through the force-generating ATPase cycle depicted in Figure 58.6B. Connectors between the subdomains are shown in various colors, including Switch II in orange, the relay in yellow, and the SH1 helix in red.

The Myosin Lever Arm Hypothesis

The first high resolution X-ray structure of myosin was published in 1993 (27). The structure was of the entire S1 fragment (head) of chicken fast skeletal myosin. While two and a half decades of biochemistry had given a general picture of what to expect, many of the details were unanticipated. Two key features of the structure generated immediate predictions as to the myosin mechanism. First was the presence of a large cleft (see Figure 58.5B) in the middle of the head that ran from the nucleotide binding site to the actin interface (identified as such on the basis of earlier cross-linking studies). Rayment et al. (17) suggested that this cleft likely closes when myosin loses its hydrolysis products upon strong binding to actin. A high-resolution structure of a myosin (chicken myosin V) motor without nucleotide revealed that this cleft can indeed close (28).

The second striking feature and prediction focused on the myosin light chains. The light chains (members of the calmodulin superfamily) were bound to the C-terminal portion of the heavy chain, which formed an extended alpha-helix. It appeared that the light chains bound to the heavy chain in calmodulin-like conformations, and in essence formed a lever arm that could likely amplify small movements within the rest of the head, which Rayment et al. (17) referred to as the motor domain. This has come to be known as the lever arm hypothesis (29), depicted diagrammatically in Figure 58.6A.

The structure of the unconventional myosin, myosin V, reveals many details of the rigor structure of myosin (28), albeit not bound to actin. It shows major rearrangements of the subdomains and cleft closure in this final rigor state, as compared to the so-called post-rigor state, but the lever arm position does appear to be similar in both instances (30). Thus there is no reversal of the lever arm swing when ATP binds to myosin attached to actin to induce dissociation. There is good evidence that myosin II and likely most other members of the myosin superfamily generate movement and force by this mechanism.

Comparison of these structures shows that the myosin motor domain is functionally made up of four major subdomains (Figure 58.5B) that are linked by four flexible structural connectors (so-called "joints") that are highly conserved in sequence (28,31). The connectors are found at the periphery of the subdomains and can readily change conformation, in coordination with the movement of the subdomains relative to one another. Among these subdomains, the converter (that leads directly to the lever arm) has by far the greatest potential for movement since it is connected to the lower 50 kDa and N-terminal subdomains by only two deformable joints (the relay and the SH1 helix, shown in yellow and red in Figure 58.5B, respectively). Rotation of the converter and lever arm can thus amplify relatively small conformational changes of the motor domain. Internal coupled rearrangements of the subdomains allow direct communication between the nucleotide-binding site, the actin binding interface and the lever arm. Coupling between the actin and nucleotide-binding sites is mediated via the large cleft between the upper and lower 50 kDa subdomains, that separates the actin-binding site in two distinct subdomains and communicates with the nucleotide-binding site via a third connector, called Switch II (shown in orange in Figure 58.5B).

Kinetic measurements (see below) had led to the proposal that force generation by myosin involves a structural change on actin after initially binding and sequentially releasing the hydrolysis products, inorganic phosphate, and MgADP. Experimental support for the swinging lever arm hypothesis (Figure 58.6A) for myosin force generation comes primarily from two types of studies. First, electron density maps from cryo-electron microscopy that compare actomyosin either in rigor or with ADP bound to the myosin reveals that, for some myosins, the lever arm moves upon dissociation of ADP (32). Further support comes from *in vitro* motility and single molecule mechanical studies that show that the velocity and/or unitary displacement of the myosin are related to lever arm length (33–35).

The displacement of the lever arm that was deduced by comparing the pre-powerstroke state and post-rigor structures (36,37) formed the initial structural evidence in support of the lever arm hypothesis (29). However, since neither of those structural states constitutes a force-bearing state when bound to actin (they both have weak affinities for actin), they cannot truly represent extremes of the powerstroke. The rigor state of myosin V directly supports the lever arm hypothesis, by revealing that the lever arm position in a nucleotide free, strong actin binding state has indeed moved in the appropriate direction away from the lever arm position in the pre-powerstroke-state and is in a position nearly identical to that of the post-rigor state (30). By this same reasoning, one anticipates that in the yet unseen phosphate-release state (see Figure 58.6B), the lever arm position will be similar to that of the pre-powerstroke state.

Many years of kinetic studies of the actin–myosin interaction have defined an ATP consuming cycle that is catalyzed by actin association (Figure 58.6B). This cycle contains many more states than have been seen in structural studies (38). The ATPase activity of myosin resides in its conserved motor domain, which interacts with actin, hydrolyses ATP, and produces the force necessary for movement along actin filaments. During the actomyosin ATPase cycle, weak ($K_d > \mu M$) actin-binding states (ATP and ADP-P_i states) alternate with strong ($K_d << \mu M$) actin-binding states (ADP states and nucleotide-free or

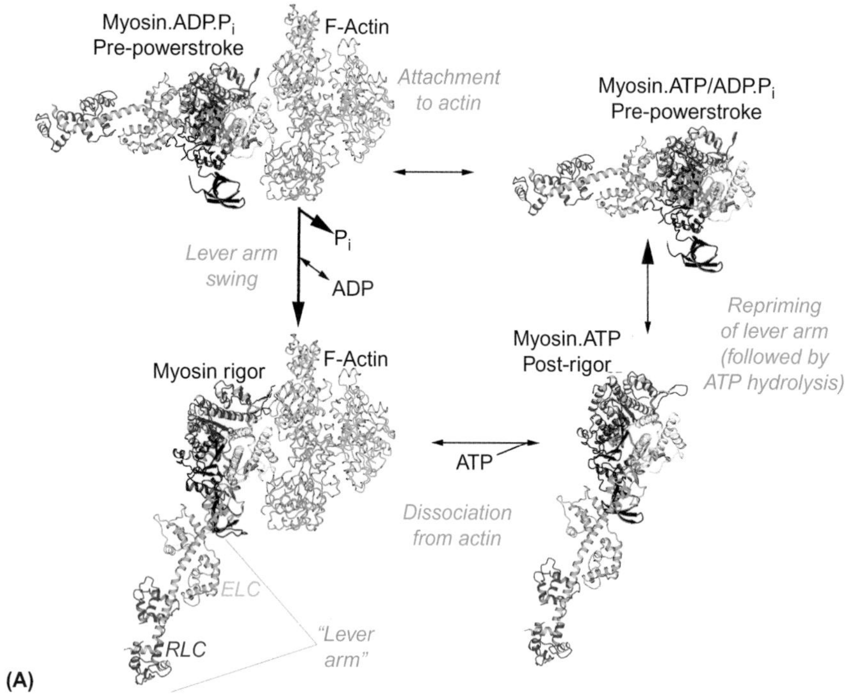

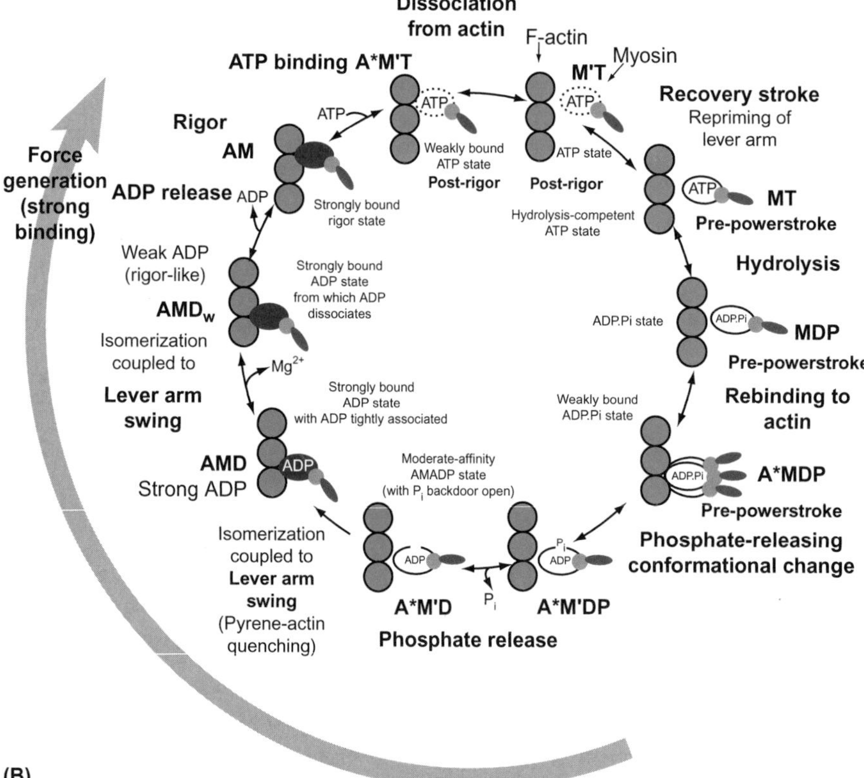

FIGURE 58.6 The lever arm hypothesis and the actin-myosin cross-bridge cycle. (A) Lever arm hypothesis. The myosin structural states for which we have high-resolution structures are positioned within the force-generating cycle. The lever arm hypothesis is in fact not based on structures of force-generating states, but is based on the structure transition that occurs in the absence of actin, in going from the MgATP bound post-rigor state to the hydrolysis competent pre-powerstroke state (29), in order to re-prime the lever arm (the recovery stroke). The myosin II S1 fragment (or head) is depicted in three structural states: rigor (nucleotide-free, docked to F-actin), post-rigor (detached from F-actin, bound to MgATP), and

(Continued)

pre-powerstroke (bound to MgADP. P_i), representing post-hydrolysis of MgATP with MgADP and P_i trapped at the active site. The lever arm is composed of a heavy-chain helix (cyan) surrounded by the light chains (magenta and purple) of myosin II, the essential light chain (ELC) in magenta, and the regulatory light chain (RLC) in purple. The lever arm position is controlled by the position of the converter (green), which swings relative to the rest of the motor domain. The distance measured at the distal end of the lever arm in pre-powerstroke versus the rigor-like state is ~12 nm for this S1 fragment. Three actin monomers are indicated as ribbon diagrams to represent the F-actin filament. Note that the actin–myosin interface is thought to be composed of subdomain 1 of one actin monomer (the upper monomer in the figure) and subdomain 2 of a second actin monomer (the lower monomer in the figure). (B) Actin–myosin ATPase cycle. Shown is a general kinetic scheme for all myosin family members. In the case of the myosin II isoforms expressed in muscle, the rate of phosphate (P_i) is slow and ADP release is fast, which leads to the low duty ratio characteristic of sarcomeric myosins. Note that the strong ADP state is not populated in the absence of strain for some myosin isoforms, including vertebrate fast skeletal myosin II. The affinity for actin of the phosphate release state is labeled as moderate, but no direct measurement of its affinity exists. This is mainly done to indicate that the actin affinity of each strongly bound, force-generating state is greater than that for the state that precedes it. The transition that immediately follows phosphate release (the pyrene-actin quenching step) appears to be virtually irreversible in the absence of strain. Whether it takes place as single or multiple distinct structural transitions is unknown, but it represents the primary powerstroke. The final lever arm rotation that follows is necessary to release MgADP and creates strain-dependent ADP release.

rigor state). Biochemical, kinetic, and mechanical studies on conventional myosins have established that ATP binding dissociates the actomyosin complex, and that ATP hydrolysis is rapid when myosin is not associated with actin. Phosphate release precedes ADP release and both product release steps are accelerated considerably upon actin binding. Force development occurs when myosin binds strongly to actin and is associated with actin-induced acceleration of phosphate release.

Several additional pieces of kinetic evidence are worth noting. First, it is clear that hydrolysis requires a structural transition (39) commonly denoted as from M' to M". It is now clear that M' is the post-rigor state of myosin, while M" is the pre-powerstroke state (Figure 58.6). It is also now clear that phosphate cannot be released from the pre-powerstroke state, so another state (a phosphate release state) must form to allow phosphate release (38). It is likely, but unproven, that this state can bind strongly enough to actin to bear force, or alternatively, rapidly leads to formation of a strongly bound state. Such a scheme would be consistent with skeletal muscle fiber data (40). Following release of phosphate, a strong actin-binding, strong ADP-binding state ($A.M.D^S$) is formed. This state is populated for slow skeletal/cardiac myosin and smooth muscle myosin (32), but it is not populated for fast skeletal myosin II, at least in the absence of strain. This state is then followed by a strain-dependent isomerization to a strong actin-binding, weak ADP-binding state ($A.M.D^W$) (30). ADP is released from this state, forming the rigor complex. These modifications are depicted in Figure 58.6B. Note that in Figure 58.6B, only the predominate steady state pathway is shown, and not all known possible kinetic states. Since strain can slow the isomerization that allows rapid ADP release, increasing load leads to progressive slowing of cross-bridge turnover in all types of muscle.

Understanding the chemo-mechanical coupling in the myosin motor requires assigning structural states to the distinct steps of the actomyosin cycle characterized by kinetic studies. We have little insight into the structural intermediates between the initial weak interaction of the pre-powerstroke state with actin, and the release of inorganic phosphate and formation of strong actin binding. However, studies on muscle fibers suggest that force generation, and thus strong actin binding, occurs prior to phosphate release (40).

Skeletal Muscle Myosin Isoforms

The expression of different myosin isoforms in different skeletal muscle fiber types, as well as co-expression of different myosin isoforms within a given fiber, allows for the creation of skeletal muscle fibers and muscles that have a range of contractile properties. This is coordinated with differential expression of other contractile protein isoforms, such as the thin filament regulatory protein isoforms, and metabolic changes to create the mammalian fiber types (see Chapter 57). Mammalian skeletal muscle fibers express members of three gene families of myosin II heavy chains (fast skeletal, slow skeletal/cardiac, and nonmuscle) and potentially three additional sarcomeric myosin heavy chain genes (superfast, slow A, and slow B) (41). The fast skeletal muscle locus is comprised of six distinct heavy chain genes. These are embryonic, perinatal (or neonatal), fast type IIa, fast type IIx (or IId), fast type IIb, and extraocular. These myosin heavy chain forms are expressed only in skeletal muscle. Interestingly, there is no evidence that human muscles ever express the IIb isoform, which is abundant in the muscles of smaller mammals, and rodents in particular. [Note that the original use of the type I, IIa, and IIb nomenclature was for histochemical fiber typing by Brooke and Kaiser (42).] It is unfortunate that when three adult fast twitch myosin heavy chains were found in rodents, it was not known that only two of them were expressed in the corresponding human muscles. Thus the IIb human fibers of Brooke and Kaiser contain the myosin heavy chain isoform that Schiaffino and colleagues named IIx (43). Embryonic and perinatal are expressed during muscle development, and re-expressed in the adult during muscle regeneration (44). The other heavy chains are expressed in adult muscles, with the order listed above reflecting increasing speed (velocity of shortening and actin-activated ATPase activity) of the myosins that they form. All of the fast skeletal myosin heavy chain genes are found as part of a multigene locus (on chromosome 17p13 in humans) (44,45). In mammals, there is an additional myosin heavy chain, which is called superfast, and is highly expressed in jaw muscles of most mammals, but not in humans. This myosin gene is on chromosome 7 in humans, but does not code for functional protein in humans due to a two base deletion resulting in a frameshift in the coding sequence (46). The loss of this myosin expression in humans has been suggested to be a major event in human evolution (46). Two additional sarcomeric myosin heavy chains of unknown distribution of tissue expression and function have been found on human chromosomes 3 and 20 (41).

The two cardiac heavy chain genes (alpha and beta) are found in tandem on human chromosome 14q12 (47). The cardiac beta heavy chain is expressed in slow skeletal muscle fibers, and thus the slow skeletal myosin is also the predominate myosin found in the human heart. The cardiac alpha heavy chain is infrequently expressed in some skeletal muscles, but is apparently confined to muscles within the head and neck.

Just as there are multiple heavy chain isoforms expressed in mammalian muscles, there is also a range of myosin light chain isoforms (48). There are likely functional differences associated with this light chain diversity. This can come about in one of two ways. Since the essential light chain (ELC) has direct associations with the converter subdomain, it can potentially affect transitions between structural states. Secondly, alterations in the interactions of both the ELC and regulatory light chain (RLC) with the heavy chain helix can alter the compliance of the lever arm, which will affect all strain-dependent state transitions (49).

The cyclic interaction of myosin and actin must be regulated in all muscle and non-muscle cells that utilize actomyosin-based motility. In all cases the signal to initiate contraction is an increase in the cytoplasmic calcium concentration. In striated muscle (skeletal and cardiac muscle) regulation is via calcium binding to the thin filament protein, troponin (see below).

The regulatory light chains of skeletal muscle are highly homologous. They contain a high affinity divalent cation-binding site near the N-terminus, that mutational analysis has demonstrated is necessary for proper binding of the light chain to the myosin II heavy chain (50). For nonmuscle and smooth muscle myosins, the increase in $[Ca^{2+}]$ leads to activation of myosin II cross-bridges via phosphorylation of the myosin regulatory light chains (11,51). The regulatory light chain of non-muscle and smooth muscle myosin IIs prevents the myosin cross-bridge from binding to actin (hence the term "regulatory"), unless it is phosphorylated at a specific site near its amino-terminus. While phosphorylation of the RLC is not an on/off switch in striated muscle myosins, it does modulate the actin–myosin activity. The phosphorylation alters the force–calcium relationship (increased calcium sensitivity) and increases the rate of force redevelopment (52). The striated muscles of a number of invertebrates may be dually regulated, requiring both phosphorylation of the myosin light chain and calcium binding to troponin C to be activated (53).

Myosin Filaments and Myosin Cross-Bridges

The myosin II of skeletal, cardiac, and smooth muscle thick filaments polymerizes at physiological ionic strength by an interaction of the LMM portions of the molecules that aggregate to form the filament backbone. The S1 (head) region of the HMM molecule domain remains on the filament surface, to form the cross-bridges that interact with actin. Each myosin molecule contributes two cross-bridges that may either remain closely apposed to each other or assume partly independent positions. The S2 region forms a movable link between the two heads. In vertebrate skeletal muscles, the length of the myosin filament is constant (1.6 μm) regardless of muscle type and/or species of origin, and in sarcomeres with a well-structured M-line (see below) the edges of the A-band are well delineated in electron micrographs (see Figure 58.1).

The position of the cross-bridges, and therefore the fine structure of thick filaments and of the entire A-band, is determined by the functional state of the muscle. In the relaxed condition (in the presence of MgATP and at very low calcium levels), the cross-bridges lie in close proximity to the surface of the thick filament, basically wrapping fairly tightly around the surface of the shaft (Figure 58.7). The two heads of each molecule have slightly different positions within this order and at least on some filaments have specific interactions with each other (54). The highly ordered disposition of cross-bridges on the surface of the relaxed thick filament depends on the position of the sites of junction between the cross-bridge and the surface of the thick filaments, which describe a helical path (Figure 58.7). In skeletal muscle, there are three parallel helices winding around the filament and thus the filament is said to be three-stranded. The distance between adjacent levels containing cross-bridges ("crowns", as defined by M.K. Reedy) is 14.3 nm and the repeat of the helix (that is the distance at which one subunit is at the same azymuthal position as one below or above it) is 3×14.3, or ~ 43 nm. In some arthropods, the thick filament is four-stranded and the helix has different parameters (such

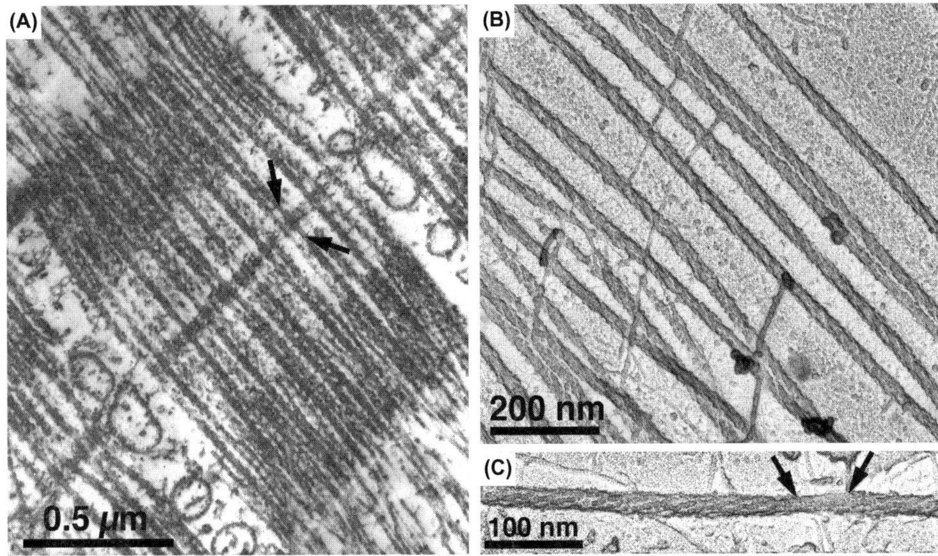

FIGURE 58.7 Myosin heads in the relaxed configuration are closely apposed to the surface of the thick filament and form a helical arrangement with spacings dictated by the configuration of the filament core. (A) A-band from a rabbit myofibril that was prepared by rapid freezing (see reference 55). (B) Thick filaments isolated from an arthropod muscle, freeze-dried, and rotary shadowed. The overall diameter of the thick filaments is narrower in the bridge free region where myosin heads (cross-bridges) are not present (between arrows in A and C).

as repeat), but the distance between crowns, which is dictated by parameters of the myosin molecules, remains 14.3 nm. The helical periodicity is prominent on the surface of thick filaments from sarcomeres fixed by rapid freezing which preserves the cross-bridge disposition (Figure 58.7). It is also clear in isolated thick filaments with contrast enhanced either by negative staining or by platinum shadow (see Figure 58.4). In thicker sections of relaxed sarcomeres, 11 transverse lines at a 43 nm repeat are visible in electron micrographs in the A-band. The bands are due to the superimposition of the cross-bridge profiles and of accessory C and H proteins (1).

There are two deviations from a perfect helical arrangement of relaxed cross-bridges. One is the fact that myosin's second layer line at 22 nm is less visible than the first and third order (43 and 14.3 nm), indicating a perturbation from a perfect helix. The second is the lack of one set of cross-bridges near the ends of the filaments, which results in a thin lighter cross line near the edges of the A-band (Figure 58.8). The center of the thick filaments is devoid of cross-bridges and this is visible both in the isolated filament and in the A-band, where the alignment of the bridge-free regions results in two thin pale lines (the L for light lines) on either side of the M-line (Figures 58.1, 58.7A, 58.8). The bridge-free central region is due to the fact that it is composed of the LMM segments from the myosin molecules of the two sides that abut tail to tail against each other (12). The myosin heads project out of the thick filament shaft in two different orientations on the two sides of the A-band, so that the thick filament reverses polarity on the middle of the sarcomere, as required for appropriate sliding action (12).

In the absence of ATP, regardless of the calcium concentration, the cross-bridges are attached to "target zones" of actin filaments with high affinity, in a configuration equivalent to the end of the powerstroke, creating a strongly cross-linked A-band in the rigor state. This is evidenced by a strong ~36 nm periodicity in the overlap region of the A-band (Figure 58.8). Even in the non-overlap zone of the A-band, where thin filaments are missing, the myosin heads become detached from the thick filament surface and project outwards in a slightly disorganized manner so that a slightly fuzzy particulate material fills the space between the filaments (Figure 58.8 and see reference 56).

The shift of myosin mass from myosin- to actin-centered resulting from the attachment of the myosin heads to actin can be detected both by X-rays and by optical diffraction of electron micrographs. Practically all myosin heads (cross-bridges) are attached to actin in the rigor state, and in most cases both heads of a single myosin molecule are attached to adjacent actin monomers, making double-headed cross-bridges (57,58).

Studies of the steady state rigor configuration have played a major role in determining the parameters of actin–myosin interactions within the constraints of the sarcomere, particularly in defining the range of longitudinal and azymuthal motions of which the myosin head is capable. The attachment of myosin cross-bridges is centered on actin filaments' target zones that are spaced at distances of ~36 nm (one-half of the double-stranded actin helical repeat) creating a strong cross periodicity that can be easily seen in thin sections for electron microscopy (Figure 58.8). This pattern is due to the fact at each twist of the actin helix one actin monomer presents itself at the best azymuthal angle for an interaction with the cross-bridges of the adjacent myosin filament. One to two actin monomers on either side of this central one are also appropriately if not optimally oriented, so that they can receive cross-bridges from the myosin

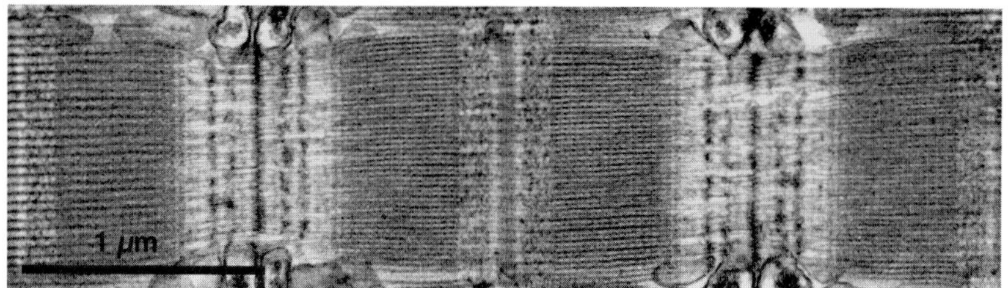

FIGURE 58.8 Sarcomeres from a fish muscle fiber that was fixed under rigor conditions. In comparison with the relaxed sarcomere (Figure 58.1) this shows an enhanced cross-periodicity in the overlap region of the A-band, which is dictated by the association of the rigor cross-bridges with the "active zones" of actin filaments at a spacing of approximately 36 nm. In the central area of no overlap with thin filaments, the cross-bridges are also detached from the thick filament backbone but are disordered. The two N-lines on either side of the Z-line are visible in this image.

filament. As a result, the actin target zone extends for up to four actin monomers and also it can receive cross-bridges from two adjacent myosin crowns.

Occupancy of actin target zones by rigor cross-bridges depends on three factors: the extent by which cross-bridges can flex and reach out in both the azymuthal and longitudinal directions to find an appropriate interaction site; the relative positioning of thin and thick filaments in the double hexagonal array of the A-band, and the relationship between helical parameters of actin and myosin filaments. Vertebrate skeletal muscle is a worst case. The thin filaments are located in the trigonal position at the center of a triangle delimited by three myosin filaments. Since the actin filament has a bilateral symmetry, this means that the positioning of its monomers cannot be equally optimized for the three adjacent filaments. Additionally, actin and myosin helices never achieve a matching period within each half sarcomere. As a result, tagging of active zones is highly variable: many receive only one (single- or double-headed) cross-bridge, some have no attached cross-bridges and only a portion of the zones have two cross-bridges attached (Figure 58.9A). In muscles of arthropods on the other hand, the thin filament is in a dyadic position, thus looking equally to the two adjacent thick filaments and the actin and myosin helical, repeat match periodically (at least for the Lethocerus muscle). As a result, most target zones are fully occupied by two double-headed cross-bridges, so that each actin monomer in the zone interacts with myosin (Figure 58.9B).

The orderly disposition of filaments and cross-bridges has permitted use of X-ray diffraction to study their behavior. The first major contribution was the early evidence from the high angle diffraction pattern that myosin did not fold or coil during contraction. The most revealing information, however, came from the low angle patterns dealing with larger structures of the same order of dimensions as filaments and cross-bridges. The first evidence for two separate sets of filaments and for cross-bridges linking them preceded by a few years the stunning 1957 electron microscope images illustrating for the first time the structure of skeletal muscle sarcomeres (59). The contracting sarcomere (in the presence of calcium and ATP) contains an asynchronous mixture of cross-bridges in all configurations of the active cross-bridge cycle. This provides a very interesting challenge to methodologies (such as X-ray diffraction) that rely on averaging the behavior of a large population of cross-bridges. Thanks to the use of powerful beams obtained from synchrotron radiation and subsequent improvements in synchrotron and X-ray detector technology, initially time resolved X-ray diffraction patterns could be detected and ultimately, with the appropriate selection of a muscle with an extremely highly ordered structure, the triumphant recording of real-time X-ray diffraction movies of actively contracting muscle has been possible (60). The combination of these and other approaches (including a novel second-harmonic generation polarization anisotropy and a close examination of specific equatorial and meridional X-ray reflections (61,62) have allowed detection of specific cross-bridge movements associated with activation and contraction in live muscle fibers. For example, the movement of mass from myosin- to an actin-centered and tropomyosin–troponin (see below) movements were shown to be early events, followed by other modifications related to changes in cross-bridges disposition. The fraction of cross-bridges that are attached at a point in time has been determined. A very interesting, novel finding is that rapid stretch of an actively contracting muscle brings into rapid action the second myosin head which is mostly not involved in the active cross-bridge cycle (63).

Overall, X-ray diffraction of live tissue and optical diffraction of actively contracting sarcomeres preserved in action by rapid freezing show that both myosin-based and actin-based periodicities change in a manner similar to the changes between relaxed and rigor, although with different time courses, indicating that the general rules derived from studies of rigor muscle are applicable to normal muscle contraction. Actin-based periodicities, due to marking of the actin helix by the myosin heads, appear shortly after calcium is released to the myofibrils and get stronger in time. The evidence indicates that attachment

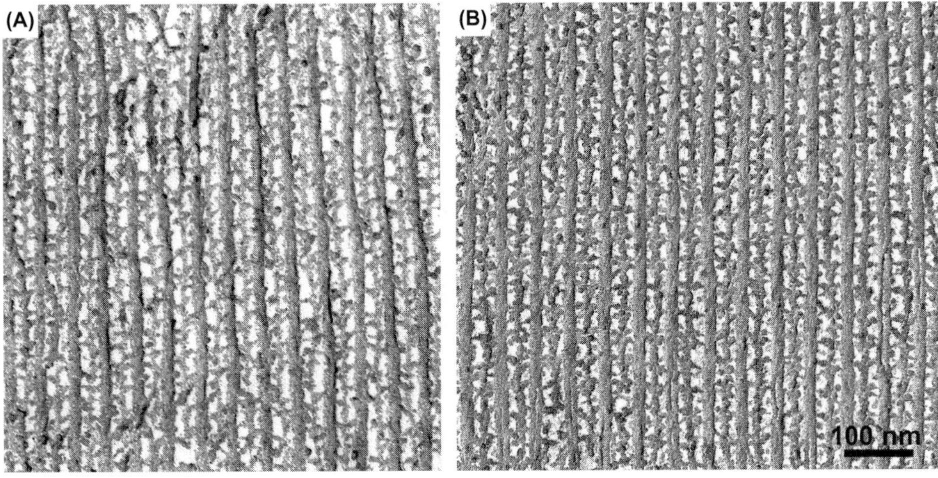

FIGURE 58.9 Deep-etch, rotary shadowed images of rigor A-bands from a vertebrate (fish, A) and an arthropod (crayfish, B). In both cases the cross-bridges fully decorate actin filaments target zones, but the arrangement is clearly more ordered in the invertebrate muscles (compare also with Figure 58.3). This is due to a better match of the actin and myosin periodicities and to the dyadic rather than trigonal position of thin filaments in muscles of arthropods. (See references 57,58.)

of the cross-bridges is followed by other minor structural changes. Myosin periodicities become initially weaker, indicating loss of helical order, but then recover.

Detailed information on the conformational changes in the myosin head during the cross-bridge active cycle required the imaging of individual molecules and this could be best obtained by tomographic 3D reconstruction of thin sections from a highly ordered muscle (Lethocerus) preserved by rapid freezing during active tension maintenance (64). Fitting of the active cross-bridge profiles in the filtered electron micrographs with the crystal structure of the myosin head determined by crystallography revealed two movements. One smaller movement involves a small tilt and slew of the motor domain relative to the actin filament axis, presumably corresponding to the change from weak to strong binding. A second larger movement involves a swing of the head's lever arm through an axial angle of $\sim 35^{\circ}$ and represent the active working stroke of 4–6 nm.

Axial tilt of the myosin head related to the active powerstroke is confirmed by X-ray diffraction of live muscle. A very useful interference between the diffraction patterns generated by the actin-associated myosin heads from the two halves of the same sarcomere is evident in the optical diffraction pattern of actively contracting muscle shown in Figure 58.5. This interference pattern, which is also clearly present in the X-ray diffraction pattern, is very sensitive to axial motions of the myosin head and clever advantage has been taken of this phenomenon in order to detect changes in myosin tilt under conditions that synchronize the working stroke following a rapid decrease in length or load during active contraction (65).

Cross-Linking Elements: the Z- and M-Lines

The Z-lines delimit the ends of the sarcomere and their components act both as cross linkers of the actin filaments and in the transmission of tension along the myofibrils. In proximity of the Z-line of skeletal muscle, actin filaments are held in a precise orthogonal disposition, obviously quite different from the hexagonal array within the overlap region of the A-band. The transition between the two dispositions is gradual at resting or longer sarcomere lengths in those muscles that have fairly long thin filaments and thus a wide I-band. However, the transition becomes abrupt and it generates a considerable problem when the sarcomere is shortened and the edges of the A-band are very close to the Z-lines.

In images of thin cross-sections, the orthogonal thin filaments pattern from each sarcomere is visible on either side of the Z-line (for example, in the upper left and bottom right corners of Figure 58.10B and E). Within the Z-line itself, the two patterns overlap because they are both present within the thickness of the section. The Z-line is constituted of cross-links (composed of alpha-actinin) that connect the ends of each thin filament from one sarcomere with the four nearest thin filaments from the adjacent sarcomere. In the simplest Z-lines (Figure 58.10A–D) the thin filaments terminate at the edges of the Z-line and are connected across it by the alpha-actinin cross links, generating a well visible zigzag pattern (Figure 58.10A–B). Even the "simple" Z-lines vary considerably in structure because the length and disposition of the connecting links and thus the width of the Z-lines vary in a species-dependent manner. The Z-line from fish, for example (Figure 58.10A) is very narrow and the links form a simple woven pattern in cross-sections (Figure 58.10F). The wider Z-line of frog (Figure 58.10C–D) has longer connecting links, which take two different configurations in cross-sections (Figure 58.10E,H), apparently depending on the state of the sarcomere. Further complexity is introduced in wider Z-lines, mostly in mammalian muscles in which the thin filaments from the two adjacent sarcomeres overlap with

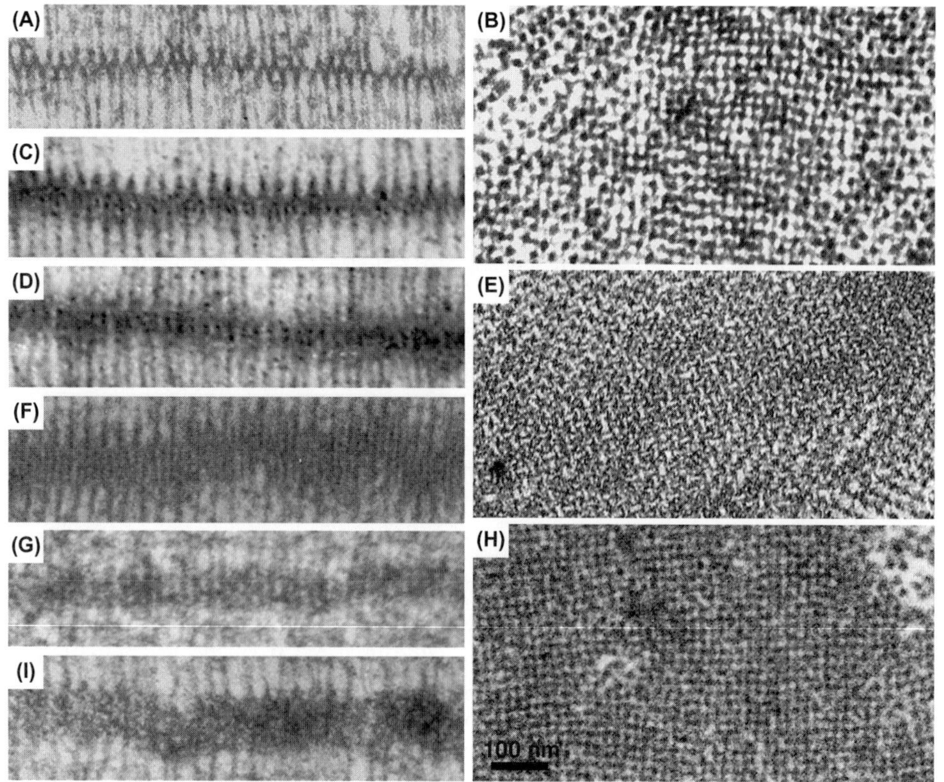

FIGURE 58.10 Z-lines cross-link the thin filaments of adjacent sarcomeres, thus allowing transmission of tension along the myofibril. The simplest Z-lines (A, from a fish) are narrow and the alpha-actinin links directly connect the thin filaments from the two adjacent sarcomeres (B). In slightly wider Z-lines (B, D, from the frog), the links are less direct and form two types of patterns on cross-sections (E, H). Finally, a variety of Z-line widths are obtained by staking up multiple copies of Z-lines. Thin filaments and the C terminus of nebulin overlap within the wider Z-lines. In cross-sections the more complex Z-lines take two different configurations (E and H). The latter is found in normal Z-lines as well as in nemaline rods, from which the image derives. (See reference 66.)

each other and several (two or more) tiers of periodically disposed cross-links connect them (Figure 58.10F–I). In general, Z-lines are wider and have a larger number of connecting tiers in fibers that sustain more prolonged activity (including cardiac muscle).

The Z-line is a complex of a number of proteins. In addition to the main structural components mentioned above: alpha-actinin and actin filaments (the latter within the wide Z-lines) and the actin nucleating/capping proteins, other components, with less clear roles, have been identified (67). The C terminal of nebulin, a component of thin filaments, is thought to continue into the wider Z-lines.

In the center of the A-band the thick filaments are linked to each other by a complex of proteins constituting the M-band, that stabilize the hexagonal array of thick filaments across the bridge-free region (Figure 58.11A–B). In its most complete pattern, found in fast twitch fibers, the M-line shows three levels of struts that connect directly thick filaments to each other (Figure 58.11D). The shaft of the thick filament within the M-band region is thicker than in the adjacent L-line, indicating that some components of the M-line wrap tightly around the surface of the thick filaments. Like the Z-line, the M-line has a complex composition (M protein, myomesin, and creatine kinase). Myomesin is particularly important as it provides structural linkage between the thick filaments as it is the major cross-linking protein of the M-line (69).

The extent of thick filaments cross-linking at the level of the M-band is fiber type-dependent. It is most extensive in fast twitch fibers (Figures 58.1, 59.8), somewhat incomplete in slow twitch fibers, and completely missing in slow tonic fibers (Figure 58.11C). This is true for all vertebrates. In mammals complete lack of M-line is found only in some extraocular muscles.

Both M- and Z-lines of myofibrils are peripherally associated with obscurin and ankyrin, proteins that mediate the interaction between myofibrils and the cytoskeleton.

THIN FILAMENT REGULATION OF MUSCLE CONTRACTION

In addition to the actin backbone, native thin filaments from skeletal and cardiac muscle contain the two major proteins tropomyosin and troponin that together confer calcium regulation to the contractile system. Tropomyosin (Tm) is a thin, elongated, two-stranded alpha-helical coiled coil molecule, with a molecular weight of $\sim$70,000 and a length of $\sim$41 nm. Two continuous strands of tropomyosins occupy the two grooves of the actin helix in the native thin filament. The

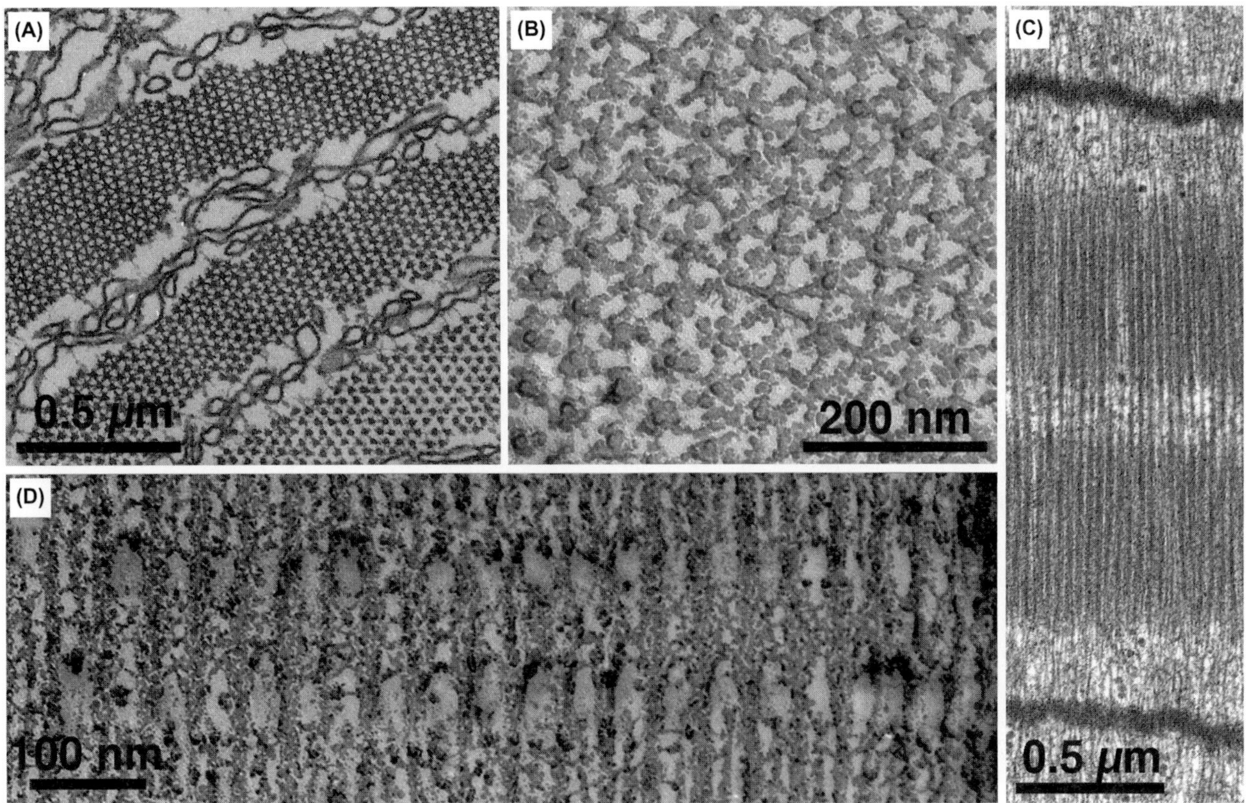

FIGURE 58.11 The M-lines directly connect adjacent thick filaments in the middle of the sarcomeres, here shown in thin section (A) and in deep etching, rotary shadowing (B). The connections form a complex pattern (D) with 2–5 tiers depending on the muscle fiber. Slower muscle fibers have either weaker (some slow twitch fibers) or totally missing M-lines (C). (See reference 68.)

specific structure of tropomyosin, with repeated actin binding sites, makes it most appropriate for its position and role in strengthening and stabilizing the actin filament (70,71).

Troponin (Tn) is a complex of three subunits (TnT, TnI, and TnC). TnT is an elongated molecule that allows attachment of the troponin complex to actin. The other two molecules are globular and they attach to TnT and actin. TnT is attached near one end of the tropomyosin molecule and TnC and TnI are located about one-third of the way along the molecule (Figure 58.12A). The specific location of the Tn complex on Tm, determines the ~40 nm intervals for the location of two complete Tn molecules along the actin filaments, producing a fine cross-periodicity that is sometimes visible in thin sections of the I-band (for example in Figure 59.8). The Tm/Tn repeat is longer than the pitch of the actin helix, so that the position of Tn bears no relationship to the azymuthal orientation of actin monomers relative to the thick filaments.

The two long strings of tropomyosin molecules are located in the grooves of the actin filament, essentially creating steric blocking of the actin–myosin interaction (Figure 58.12B) in the resting (i.e. low free calcium) muscle fiber (72). The ability of calcium to activate contraction (i.e. actin–myosin interaction) when released from the sarcoplasmic reticulum (see Chapter 57) is mediated by binding to the low affinity N-terminal calcium binding site(s) of TnC of the Tn complex. (There are two isoforms of TnC in skeletal muscle; fast TnC, which has two functional N-terminal calcium binding sites and slow/cardiac TnC, which has one functional site.) The consequence of calcium binding to the low affinity binding site(s) of TnC is that Tm is released from its steric blocking position, allowing myosin to interact with actin and generate force. This is mediated via conformational changes in the TnI component, transmitted to Tm via the Tm-linked TnT. Strong binding associations of myosin cross-bridges to actin have a synergistic effect, helping to further reduce Tm's steric hindrance and thus reveal a cooperativity in the thin filament activation (73). To recapitulate, in skeletal and cardiac muscle, Ca^{2+} binds to the low-affinity, N-terminal site(s) on TnC, which removes the inhibition of myosin binding to actin by causing (through interactions mediated by TnI and TnT) steric alterations in

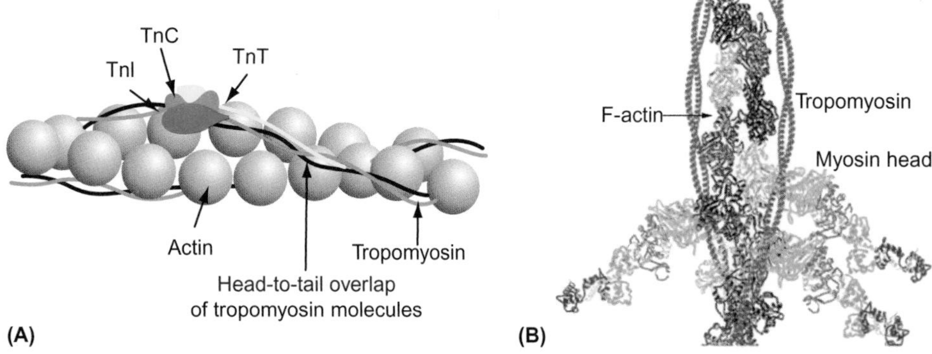

FIGURE 58.12 Thin filament regulation. (A) Regulatory subunits of the thin filament. Regulation in striated muscle is derived from the actions of the thin filament proteins, tropomyosin, and troponin. Tropomyosin is an elongated, coiled molecule that binds to the surface of the actin filament. Troponin is made up of three subunits, troponin T (TnT), which binds to tropomyosin, troponin I (TnI), which binds to both actin and tropomyosin, and troponin C (TnC), which confers calcium-sensitivity to the system. The relative position of these proteins on the actin filament is schematized. (B) Steric blocking model of thin filament regulation. Depicted is the position of tropomyosin at resting cytoplasmic calcium levels. The tropomyosin covers the actin-binding site of myosin so that the myosin cross-bridges cannot undergo phosphate release and enter the force-generating cycle (Figure 58.6B). If cytoplasmic calcium levels increase sufficiently for calcium to bind to the low-affinity calcium-binding sites of troponin C, then tropomyosin moves from this blocking position allow force generation via the actin-myosin interaction to occur.

tropomyosin, revealing potential actin binding sites for myosin. This is known as thin filament regulation. (For review see 74.)

For the special case of stretch activation of the asynchronous insect muscles, the steric hindrance hypothesis of tropomyosin–troponin action has also been shown to hold. In stretch-activated muscles, calcium alone is not sufficient to activate contraction, but stretch is additionally necessary. Evidence for the periodic movement of tropomyosin during stretch-activated contraction/relaxation cycles, presumably due to the action of direct myosin–tropomyosin cross-bridges, has been directly obtained by X-ray diffraction in live insect muscle (60).

THE SCAFFOLDING PROTEINS GIVE STABILITY AND ELASTICITY TO THE SARCOMERE

Titin (also called connectin) is a giant molecule ($\sim 3 \times 10^6$ mw) associated with the thick filaments. The C terminus of titin is at the M-line. Between the M-line and the edges of the A-band titin lies over the surface of the thick filament. Titin continues free along the I-band and attaches to the Z-band, probably interacting both with actin and with alpha-actinin at its N terminus. At least six titin molecules are associated with the thick filament, three on either side of the M-line. Along the thick filament, titin may act as a molecular ruler. Within the A-band the molecule has 11 identical copies of repeats containing immunoglobulin and fibronectin sequences. These presumably align with the 11 bands along which C and H proteins are located.

The I-band region of titin is stretchable and is responsible for elasticity of the resting muscle, that is for the increase in resting tension with stretches above a certain length. It is debated whether the PEVK region of the molecule, a stretch containing prevalently Pro (P), Glu (E), Val (V), and Lys (K) residues, is responsible for the elasticity. In favor of this hypothesis, the PEVK region of titin in cardiac muscle (which is quite stiff) is shorter than that in skeletal muscle (which is more easily stretchable).

A result of titin's elasticity within the I-band is that titin keeps the A-band centered in the sarcomere during contraction and/or stretching of the muscle (75). Nebulin is a second scaffolding protein. It is located along the filament and since its length varies in parallel to that of the thin filaments in different fibers, it is thought that nebulin may act as a ruler to determine thin filament length.

THE Z-LINE IS INVOLVED IN SIGNALING

Given that it transmits the force generated by the actin–myosin interaction, the Z-line is an ideal place to locate force sensors that can signal adaptation in muscle in response to load. The Z-line proteins that are thought to have potential signaling as well as structural roles include three families of proteins: myotilin, FATZ, and enigma (76). The myotilin family includes myotilin, paladin, and myopalladin. These proteins have immunoglobulin domains and bind α-actinin, filamin, and FATZ. The FATZ family includes FATZ (also called casarcin and myozenin) and their binding partners include myotilin, filamin, telethonin, α-actinin, and ZASP. FATZ-1 and FATZ-3 occur in fast-twitch muscles and FATZ-2 occurs in slow-twitch and cardiac muscles. Proteins of the enigma family have an amino-terminal PDZ domain and 0-3 LIM domains at the COOH terminal. Cypher/ZASP/ Oracle is the most studied enigma member (77–79). Cypher/ZASP may serve as a linker-strut by binding to α-actinin via its PDZ domain and may be involved in signaling as it binds protein kinase C via its LIM domains. Cypher is essential for maintaining Z-band structure and muscle integrity (79). Mutations in Cypher lead to dilated cardiomyopathy and skeletal muscle myopathies that are termed zaspopathies.

FAULTS IN THE CROSS-STRIATION ALIGNMENT

The bands of adjacent myofibrils are (for the most part) aligned across the fiber, creating alternating bands, or cross striations, traversing the entire muscle fiber. However, within each muscle fiber and particularly in the slow twitch fibers, Vernier displacements of the striation are often observed. At a Vernier site, *n* sarcomeres in the myofibrils on one side of the fault line face *n* + *1* sarcomeres in the myofibrils on the other side. At the top and bottom of the fault the Z-lines are aligned, but within the Verniers they are mismatched, so that the planes containing Z-lines (and T-tubules in frog fibers) define a helicoid (Figure 58.13) (80). Interestingly, a disarrangement of the sarcomere that initiates at the Z-lines and so is called "Z-line streaming" (see below), is often related to the position of Vernier striation mismatches, perhaps as a result of mechanical stress as nearby sarcomeres with slightly different thin/thick filaments overlaps are simultaneously activated.

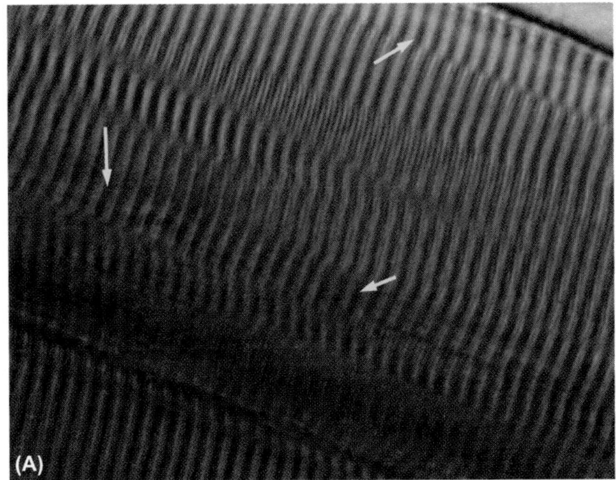

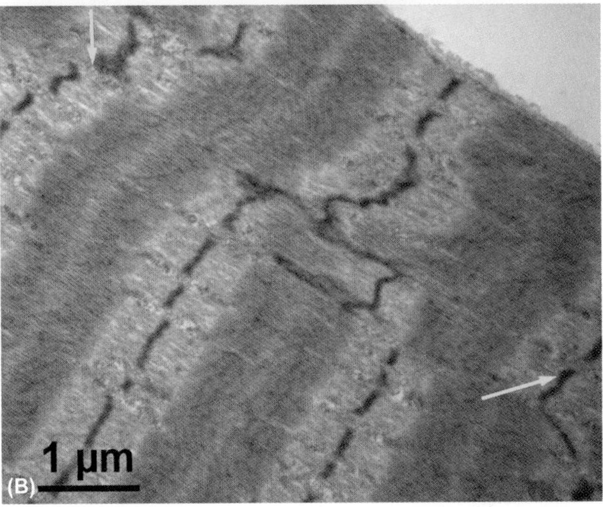

FIGURE 58.13 Images of cross-striation in phase contrast light microscopy (A) and in thin section electron microscopy (B) showing the presence of Verniers mismatch (between arrows) of the cross-striation arising from the presence of one extra sarcomere on one side. Where the mismatch involves just a few sarcomeres (B) distortions often arise and Z-line streaming occurs.

Z-LINE DEFECTS IN PATHOLOGY

The Z-line is the most frequently affected component of the sarcomere under stress and pathological conditions, but also in aging, probably because it is the elements through which force is transmitted along the myofibril and also because calcium-activated proteases specifically degrade Z-line proteins. Nemaline rods originate at the Z-disc and they basically represent an iteration of the Z-line architecture: they maintain the structural organization of Z-line, although extending it over large volumes (Figure 58.14A,B). When sectioned across, nemaline rods show a square lattice that is identical to that found in Z-lines under certain conditions (see Figure 58.10H) and in longitudinal sections that have a periodicity of 14–20 nm also reminiscent of that found in wide Z-lines. A second very common reaction of Z-lines to a variety of myopathies, to excessive accumulation of cytoplasmic calcium, as well as to denervation, to eccentric contractions, and to aging is an initial streaming of Z-line material away from the standard Z-line location, followed by a gradual focal myofibrillar degeneration and disappearance of cell organelles (SR, T-tubules, mitochondria). Z-line streaming and its consequences may affect very small regions (Figure 58.13B), a whole sarcomere (Figure 58.14C), or several sarcomeres and myofibrils. Alterations initiated by Z-line streaming probably lead to the development of featureless cores in central core diseases.

Myofibrillar myopathy (MFM) is a muscle disorder of the Z-line. MFM is a distinct group of pathologies of skeletal and cardiac muscle characterized by disintegration of the Z-line and abnormal protein accumulation (84). MFM is caused by mutations in the genes for proteins involved in maintaining the structural integrity of the Z-line, including desmin, αB-crystallin, myotilin, and ZASP.

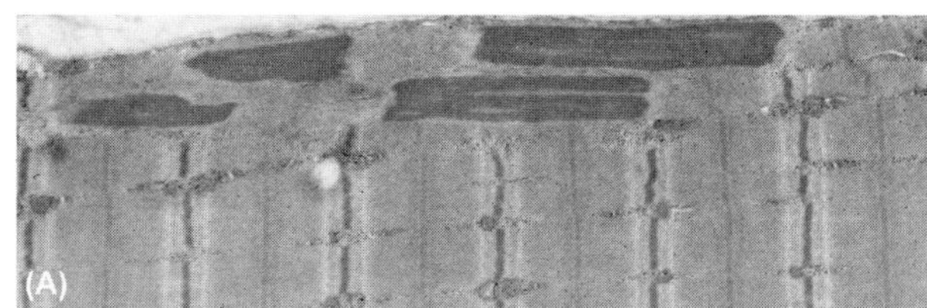

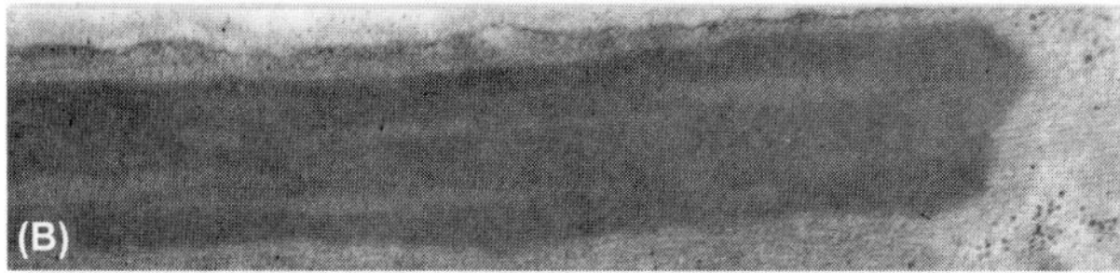

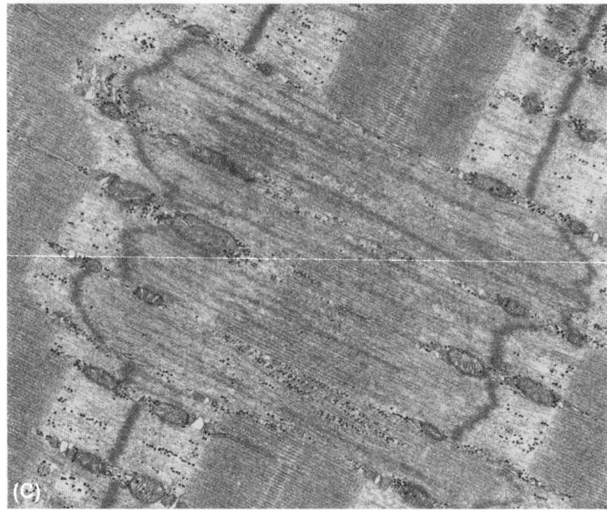

FIGURE 58.14 (A and B) Nemaline rods are elongated well-delimited regions of high electron density. They display the same structure as Z-lines in thin sections (see Figure 58.10H). From human congenital myopathy (see reference 81). (C) Z-line streaming, probably started as in Figure 58.10B, results in spread of Z-line components over the sarcomere and loss of structural organization. From human muscle with Kearns Sayre syndrome (see references 82,83).

ACKNOWLEDGMENTS

Supported by NIH grants HL48093 to C.F.A. and by AR35661 and DC009100 to H.L.S.

REFERENCES

1. Craig RW. *Molecular structure of the sarcomere*. 2nd ed. New York: McGraw-Hill; 2004.
2. Hidalgo C, Padron R, Horowitz R, Zhao FQ, Craig R. Purification of native myosin filaments from muscle. *Biophys J* 2001;**81**:2817–26.
3. Huxley HE, Hanson J. Changes in the cross-striations of muscle during contraction and stretch and their structural interpretation. *Nature* 1954;**173**:973.
4. Huxley AF, Niedergerke R. Structural changes in muscle during contraction. Interference microscopy of living muscle fibres. *Nature* 1954;**173**:971.
5. Casella JF, Casella SJ, Hollands JA, Caldwell JE, Cooper JA. Isolation and characterization of cDNA encoding the alpha subunit of Cap Z(36/32), an actin-capping protein from the Z-line of skeletal muscle. *Proc Natl Acad Sci USA* 1989;**86**:5800–4.
6. Maruyama K. beta-Actinin, Cap Z, connectin and titin: what's in a name? *Trends Biochem Sci* 2002;**27**:264–6.
7. Taniguchi K, Takeya R, Suetsugu S, Kan OM, Narusawa M, Shiose A, et al. Mammalian formin fhod3 regulates actin assembly and sarcomere organization in striated muscles. *J Biol Chem* 2009;**284**:29873–81.
8. Gregorio CC, Weber A, Bondad M, Pennise CR, Fowler VM. Requirement of pointed-end capping by tropomodulin to maintain actin filament length in embryonic chick cardiac myocytes. *Nature* 1995;**377**:83–6.
9. Almenar-Queralt A, Lee A, Conley CA, Ribas de Pouplana L, Fowler VM. Identification of a novel tropomodulin isoform, skeletal tropomodulin, that caps actin filament pointed ends in fast skeletal muscle. *J Biol Chem* 1999;**274**:28466–75.
10. Odronitz F, Kollmar M. Drawing the tree of eukaryotic life based on the analysis of 2,269 manually annotated myosins from 328 species. *Genome Biol* 2007;**8**:R196.
11. Bresnick AR. Molecular mechanisms of nonmuscle myosin-II regulation. *Curr Opin Cell Biol* 1999;**11**:26–33.
12. Huxley HE. Electron microscope studies on the structure of natural and synthetic protein filaments from striated muscle. *J Mol Biol* 1963;**7**:281.
13. Slayter HS, Lowey S. Substructure of the myosin molecule as visualized by electron microscopy. *Proc Natl Acad Sci USA* 1967;**58**:1611.
14. Mornet D, Bertrand R, Pantel P, Audemand E, Kassab R. Proteolytic approach to structure and function of actin recognition site in myosin heads. *Biochemistry* 1981;**20**:2110–20.
15. Sutoh K. An actin-binding site on the 20 K fragment of myosin subfragment 1. *Biochemistry* 1982;4800–4.
16. Sutoh K. Mapping of actin-binding sites on the heavy chain of myosin subfragment 1. *Biochemistry* 1983;**22**:1579–85.
17. Rayment I, Holden HM, Whitaker M, Yohn CB, Lorenz M, Holmes KC, et al. Structure of the actin-myosin complex and its implications for muscle contraction. *Science* 1993;**261**:58–61.
18. Biró NA, Szilágy L, Bálint M. Studies on the helical segment of the myosin molecule. *Cold Spring Harbor Symp Quant Biol* 1972;**37**:55.
19. Lowey S, Risby D. Light chains from fast and slow muscle myosins. *Nature* 1971;**234**:81–5.
20. Frank G, Weeds AG. The amino-acid sequence of the alkali light chains of rabbit skeletal-muscle myosin. *Eur J Biochem* 1974;**44**:317.
21. Weeds AG. Light chains of myosin. *Nature* 1969;**223**:1362.
22. Perrie WT, Smillie LB, Perry. SV. A phosphorylated light chain component of myosin from skeletal muscle. *Biochem J* 1973;**135**:151.
23. Morgan M, Perry SV, Ottaway J. Myosin light-chain phosphatase. *Biochem J* 1976;**157**:687.
24. Kominz DR, Carroll WR, Smith EN, Mitchell ER. A subunit of myosin. *Arch Biochem Biophys* 1959;**79**:191.
25. Kabsch W, Mannherz HG, Suck D, Pai EF, Holmes KC. Atomic structure of the actin:DNase I complex. *Nature* 1990;**347**:37–44.
26. Oda T, Iwasa M, Aihara T, Maéda Y, Narita A. The nature of the globular- to fibrous-actin transition. *Nature* 2009;**457**:441–5.
27. Rayment I, Rypniewski WR, Schmidt-Bäde K, Smith R, Tomchick DR, Benning MM, et al. Three-dimensional structure of myosin subfragment-1: a molecular motor. *Science* 1993;**261**:50–8.

28. Coureux PD, Wells AL, Ménétrey J, Yengo CM, Morris CA, Sweeney HL, et al. A structural state of the myosin V motor without bound nucleotide. *Nature* 2003;**425**:419–23.
29. Holmes KC, Geeves MA. Structural mechanism of muscle contraction. *Annu Rev Biochem* 1999;**68**:687–728.
30. Coureux PD, Sweeney HL, Houdusse A. Three myosin V structures delineate essential features of chemo-mechanical transduction. *EMBO J* 2004;**23**:4527–37.
31. Houdusse A, Szent-Györgyi AG, Cohen C. Three conformational states of scallop myosin S1. *Proc Natl Acad Sci USA* 2000;**97**:11238–43.
32. Whitaker M, Wilson-Kubalek EM, Smith JE, Faust L, Milligan RA, Sweeney HL. A 35-Å movement of smooth muscle myosin on ADP release. *Nature* 1995;**378**:748–51.
33. Uyeda TQ, Abramson PD, Spudich JA. The neck region of the myosin motor domain acts as a lever arm to generate movement. *Proc Natl Acad Sci USA* 1996;**93**:4459–64.
34. Warshaw DM, Guilford WH, Freyzon Y, Krementsova E, Palmiter KA, Tyska MJ, et al. The light chain binding domain of expressed smooth muscle heavy meromyosin acts as a mechanical lever. *J Biol Chem* 2000;**275**:37167–72.
35. Purcell TJ, Morris C, Spudich JA, Sweeney HL. Role of the lever arm in the processive stepping of myosin V. *Proc Natl Acad Sci USA* 2002;**99**:14159–64.
36. Fisher AJ, Smith CA, Thoden JB, Smith R, Sutoh K, Holden HM, et al. X-ray structures of the myosin motor domain of *Dictyostelium discoideum* complexed with MgADP.BeFx and MgADP.AlF4-. *Biochemistry* 1995;**34**:8960–72.
37. Dominguez R, Freyzon Y, Trybus KM, Cohen C. Crystal structure of a vertebrate smooth muscle myosin motor domain and its complex with the essential light chain: visualization of the pre-power stroke state. *Cell* 1998;**94**:559–71.
38. Sweeney HL, Houdusse A. Structural and functional insights into the Myosin motor mechanism. *Annu Rev Biophys* 2010;**39**:539–57.
39. Málnási-Csizmadia A, Pearson DS, Kovács M, Woolley RJ, Geeves MA, Bagshaw CR. Kinetic resolution of a conformational transition and the ATP hydrolysis step using relaxation methods with a Dictyostelium myosin II mutant containing a single tryptophan residue. *Biochemistry* 2001;**40**:12727–37.
40. Dantzig JA, Goldman YE, Millar NC, Lacktis J, Homsher E. Reversal of the cross-bridge force-generating transition by photogeneration of phosphate in rabbit psoas muscle fibres. *J Physiol* 1992;**451**:247–78.
41. Desjardins PR, Burkman JM, Shrager JB, Allmond LA, Stedman HH. Evolutionary implications of three novel members of the human sarcomeric myosin heavy chain gene family. *Mol Biol Evol* 2002;**19**:375–93.
42. Brooke MH, Kaiser KK. Muscle fiber types: how many and what kind? *Arch Neurol* 1970;**23**:369.
43. DiNardi C, Ausoni S, Moretti P, Gorza L, Velleca M, Buckingham M, et al. Type 2X myosin heacy hain is coded by a muscle fiber type-specific and developmentally regulated gene. *J Cell Biol* 1993;**123**:823–35.
44. Mahdavi V, Strehler EE, Periasamy M, Wieczorek D, Izumo S, Grund S, et al. Sarcomeric myosin heavy chain gene family: organization and pattern of expression. In: Emerson FD, Nadal-Ginard B, Siddique MA, editors. *Molecular biology of muscle development*. New York: Alan R. Liss.; p. 345–61.
45. Weiss A, McDonough D, Wertman B, Acakpo-Satchivil L, Montgomery K, Kucherlapati R, et al. Organization of human and mouse skeletal myosin heavy chain gene clusters is highly conserved. *Proc Natl Acad Sci USA* 1999;**96**:2958–63.
46. Stedman HH, Kozyak BW, Nelson A, Thesier DM, Su LT, Low DW, et al. Myosin gene mutation correlates with anatomical changes in the human lineage. *Nature* 2004;**428**:415–8.
47. Mahdavi V, Chambers AP, Nadal-Ginard B. Cardiac alpha and beta myosin heavy chain genes are organized in tandem. *Proc Natl Acad Sci USA* 1984;**81**:2626–30.
48. Collins JH. Myosin light chains and troponin C: structural and evolutionary relationships revealed by amino acid sequence comparisons. *J Muscle Res Cell Motil* 1991;**12**:3–25.
49. Lowey S, Waller GS, Trybus KM. Skeletal muscle myosin light chains are essential for physiological speeds of shortening. *Nature* 1993;**365**:454–6.
50. Reinach FC, Nagai K, Kendrick-Jones J. Site directed mutagenesis of the regulatory light-chain Ca^{+2}/Mg^{+2} binding sites and its role in hybrid myosins. *Nature* 1986;**322**:80–3.
51. Trybus KM. Regulation of smooth muscle myosin. *Cell Motil Cytoskel* 1991;**18**:81–5.
52. Sweeney HL, Bowman BF, Stull JT. Myosin light chain phosphorylation in striated muscle. *Am J Physiol* 1993;**264**:C1085–95.
53. Wang F, Martin BM, Sellers JR. Regulation of actomyosin interactions in Limulus muscle proteins. *J Biol Chem* 1993;**268**:3776–80.
54. Woodhead JL, Zhao FQ, Craig R, Egelman EH, Alamo L, Padron R. Atomic model of a myosin filament in the relaxed state. *Nature* 2005;**436**:1195–9.
55. Lenart TD, Murray JM, Franzini-Armstrong C, Goldman YE. Structure and periodicities of cross-bridges in relaxation, in rigor, and during contractions initiated by photolysis of caged Ca^{2+}. *Biophys J* 1996;**71**:2289–306.
56. Padron R, Craig R. Disorder induced in nonoverlap myosin cross-bridges by loss of adenosine triphosphate. *Biophys J* 1989;**56**:927–33.
57. Varriano-Marston E, Franzini-Armstrong C, Haselgrove JC. The structure and disposition of crossbridges in deep-etched fish muscle. *J Muscle Res Cell Motil* 1984;**5**:363–86.
58. Bard F, Franzini-Armstrong C, Ip W. Rigor crossbridges are double-headed in fast muscle from crayfish. *J Cell Biol* 1987;**105**:2225–34.
59. Huxley HE. The double array of filaments in cross-striated muscle. *J Biophys Biochem Cytol* 1957;**3**:631–48.
60. Perz-Edwards RJ, Irving TC, Baumann BA, Gore D, Hutchinson DC, Krzic U, et al. X-ray diffraction evidence for myosin-troponin connections and tropomyosin movement during stretch activation of insect flight muscle. *Proc Natl Acad Sci USA* 2011;**108**:120–5.
61. Nucciotti V, Stringari C, Sacconi L, Vanzi F, Fusi L, Linari M, et al. Probing myosin structural conformation in vivo by second-harmonic generation microscopy. *Proc Natl Acad Sci USA* 2010;**107**:7763–8.
62. Brunello E, Fusi L, Reconditi M, Linari M, Bianco P, Panine P, et al. Structural changes in myosin motors and filaments during relaxation of skeletal muscle. *J Physiol* 2009;**587**:4509–21.
63. Brunello E, Reconditi M, Elangovan R, Linari M, Sun YB, Narayanan T, et al. Skeletal muscle resists stretch by rapid binding of the second motor domain of myosin to actin. *Proc Natl Acad Sci USA* 2007;**104**:20114–9.

64. Taylor KA, Schmitz H, Reedy MC, Goldman YE, Franzini-Armstrong C, Sasaki H, et al. Tomographic 3D reconstruction of quick-frozen, Ca^{2+}-activated contracting insect flight muscle. *Cell* 1999;**99**:421–31.
65. Reconditi M, Linari M, Lucii L, Stewart A, Sun YB, Narayanan T, et al. Structure-function relation of the myosin motor in striated muscle. *Ann NY Acad Sci* 2005;**1047**:232–47.
66. Macdonald RD, Engel AG. The cytoplasmic body: another structural anomaly of the Z disk. *Acta Neuropathol* 1969;**14**:99–107.
67. Faulkner G, Lanfranchi G, Valle G. Telethonin and other new proteins of the Z-disc of skeletal muscle. *IUBMB Life* 2001; **51**:275–82.
68. Varriano-Marston E, Franzini-Armstrong C, Haselgrove JC. Structure of the M-band. *J Electron Microsc Tech* 1987;**6**:131–41.
69. Lange S, Himmel M, Auerbach D, Agarkova I, Hayess K, Furst DO, et al. Dimerisation of myomesin: implications for the structure of the sarcomeric M-band. *J Mol Biol* 2005;**345**:289–98.
70. Hitchcock-DeGregori SE, Singh A. What makes tropomyosin an actin binding protein? A perspective. *J Struct Biol* 2010; **170**:319–24.
71. Hitchcock-DeGregori SE, Varnell TA. Tropomyosin has discrete actin-binding sites with sevenfold and fourteenfold periodicities. *J Mol Biol* 1990;**214**:885–96.
72. Xu C, Craig R, Tobacman L, Horowitz R, Lehman W. Tropomyosin positions in regulated thin filaments revealed by cryoelectron microscopy. *Biophys J* 1999;**77**:985–92.
73. Weber A, Murray JM. Molecular control mechanisms in muscle contraction. *Physiol Rev* 1973;**53**:612–73.
74. Lehman W, Craig R. Tropomyosin and the steric mechanism of muscle regulation. *Adv Exp Med Biol* 2008;**644**:95–109.
75. Horowits R, Podolsky RJ. The positional stability of thick filaments in activated skeletal muscle depends on sarcomere length: evidence for the role of titin filaments. *J Cell Biol* 1987; **105**:2217–23.
76. von Nandelstadh P, Ismail M, Gardin C, Suila H, Zara I, Belgrano A, et al. A class III PDZ binding motif in the myotilin and FATZ families binds enigma family proteins: a common link for Z-disc myopathies. *Mol Cell Biol* 2009;**29**:822–34.
77. Faulkner G, Pallavicini A, Formentin E, Comelli A, Ievolella C, Trevisan S, et al. ZASP: a new Z-band alternatively spliced PDZ-motif protein. *J Cell Biol* 1999;**146**:465–75.
78. Passier R, Richardson JA, Olson EN. Oracle, a novel PDZ-LIM domain protein expressed in heart and skeletal muscle. *Mech Dev* 2000;**92**:277–84.
79. Zhou Q, Chu PH, Huang C, Cheng CF, Martone ME, Knoll G, et al. Ablation of Cypher, a PDZLIM domain Z-line protein, causes a severe form of congenital myopathy. *J Cell Biol* 2001; **155**:605–12.
80. Peachey LD, Eisenberg BR. Helicoids in the T system and striations of frog skeletal muscle fibers seen by high voltage electron microscopy. *Biophys J* 1978;**22**:145–54.
81. Engel AG, Gomez MR. Nemaline (Z disk) myopathy: observations on the origin, structure, and solubility properties of the nemaline structures. *J Neuropathol Exp Neurol* 1967;**26**:601–19.
82. Banker BQ, Engel AG. *Basic reactions of muscle*. 2nd ed. *Myology*, vol. 1. New York: McGraw-Hill; 2004.
83. Engel AG. *Ultrastructural changes in diseased muscle*. 3rd ed. *Myology*, vol. 1. New York: McGraw-Hill; 2004.
84. Selcen D, Engel AG. Mutations in myotilin cause myofibrillar myopathy. *Neurology* 2004;**62**:1363–71.

Chapter 59

Skeletal Muscle Metabolism

Morris J. Birnbaum
Institute for Diabetes, Obesity, and Metabolism, Perelman School of Medicine, University of Pennsylvania, Philadelphia, PA

In order to carry out its primary purpose of generating power, skeletal muscle has evolved a complicated set of regulatory networks to provide the requisite metabolic energy for different work loads during times of variable nutritional content and quality. Perhaps the most taxing metabolic challenge is accommodating the extraordinary range of energetic requirements in the mammalian muscle. ATP consumption in muscle can vary well over 100-fold, achieving rates of greater than 1.5 kg ATP/minute during strenuous exercise in an average-size human. Yet, ATP concentrations change remarkably little, decreasing less than 20–50% even under maximal exercise. Muscle achieves this through a number of specialized adaptions including (i) heterogeneity in the metabolic capacities of muscle fibers; (ii) the ability to utilize stored and exogenous substrates; (iii) profound "metabolic flexibility", i.e. the capacity to consume fuels of different composition; and (iv) utilization of phosphagen as an energy storage pool. Critical to provision of adequate energy throughout periods of muscle work is the efficient storage of nutrients during the absorptive period.

MUSCLE METABOLISM DURING THE ABSORPTIVE STATE

Skeletal muscle demonstrates remarkable flexibility in its ability to consume and store energy derived from either carbohydrate or lipid, depending in the nutritional state. The "default" state, designed for conditions of fasting when it is advantageous to spare glucose for tissues requiring this substrate, involves little consumption of exogenous sugars but rather the oxidation of the more efficient energetic storage form, lipid. After a meal, the muscle switches to the utilization of carbohydrate by two important signals: the hormone insulin, itself secreted by the pancreas in response to an increase in nutrients, and the rise in circulating blood glucose levels. Abnormalities in the process caused by an absolute or relative deficiency in insulin define the prevalent human diseases Type 1 and Type 2 diabetes mellitus, respectively. Thus, the mechanism by which insulin elicits accelerated glucose metabolism has been studied in some detail and, though there are a number of open questions, a generalized understanding of both the physiology and biochemistry has emerged in recent years.

The first critical insights into the regulation of muscle glucose metabolism date back to the middle of the previous century. At that time, it was generally recognized that both glucose concentration and insulin could increase the rate at which muscle utilizes glucose (1). However, there was little understanding of the precise site of insulin action within the muscle. In a seminal series of experiments, Rachmiel Levine administered the non-metabolized sugar galactose to eviscerated dogs in the absence and presence of insulin (2). Insulin reduced the concentration of galactose at equilibrium, indicating that the hormone increased the sugar's volume of distribution from about 40% to 70% of body weight (3). From these data, Levine had the insight that insulin must be working by affecting the permeability of the muscle membrane selectively towards glucose, such that the fundamental step being controlled was transport into the cell (4). This hypothesis represented a fundamental change in thinking about insulin action, in which regulated compartmentalization rather than enzyme catalysis represents the primary site of metabolic control. With appreciation of the role of membrane-spanning proteins in accelerating the selective uptake of hydrophilic substrates across the lipid bilayer, the question became whether insulin enhanced transport by increasing the activity of resident sarcolemmal carriers or by enhancing their number. Two groups resolved this question independently, each developing a method for measuring the number of glucose transport proteins in adipocytes independent of their activity in the intact cell (5,6). When cells were treated with insulin, disrupted, and the subcellular compartments fractionated, the quantity of transporter protein co-sedimenting with plasma membrane markers increased while those in a still poorly-defined intracellular compartment decreased. Thus, the model that emerged is one in which glucose transporter proteins are stored within the cell interior and the major stimulus for increased uptake is the insulin-dependent translocation to the cell surface

Muscle. DOI: http://dx.doi.org/10.1016/B978-0-12-381510-1.00059-4

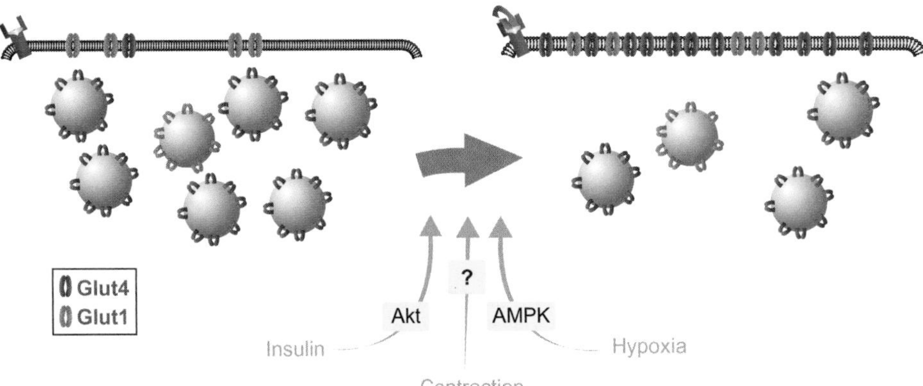

FIGURE 59.1 Translocation of glucose transport proteins to the cell surface in response to insulin, contraction or hypoxia. Glut4 is largely sequestered in a compartment in the cell interior till one of the indicated stimuli induce its translocation to the cell surface.

(Figure 59.1). Though originally determined for rat adipocytes, the "translocation hypothesis" was soon shown to be also applicable to skeletal muscle (7).

In spite of the attractiveness of the translocation model, there persisted doubt about its validity based on a lack of correlation between the extent of transporter redistribution as ascertained by the change of glucose uptake versus its abundance as assayed by Western immunoblot (8). The resolution to this problem was provided by the discovery of a novel glucose transporter protein expressed exclusively in insulin target tissues such as adipocytes and muscle, to which the then current antisera did not react (9). Cloning of the cDNA encoding the "insulin-responsive" glucose transporter, now known as Glut4, demonstrated it to be the product of a distinct gene and to have the unique characteristic of being retained within the interior of the cell until the latter is exposed to insulin (Figure 59.1) (10,11). Skeletal muscle also expresses considerably lower levels of other glucose transporter isoforms, including Glut1, a more ubiquitously expressed protein with great relative basal presence on the cell surface (8).

The nature of the intracellular compartment in which Glut4 resides in the basal state remains imperfectly understood. Some have likened it to a secretory compartment, while others a subdomain of the endosomal system. Morphologically, Glut4 storage vesicles (GSV) are tubulovesicular structures located adjacent to the trans Golgi network and, to a lesser extent, endosomes (12). Following treatment with insulin, Glut4 moves to sarcolemma and transverse tubules and increases in abundance in endosomes, consistent with dynamic recycling of transporters in the stimulated state (12,13). It is well established that following removal of hormone, cell surface transporters return to their resident intracellular compartment by endocytosis (14). Some data suggest that this process is itself regulated by insulin, though the major effect is on externalization (15–19). Internalizing Glut4 transits through clathrin coated vesicles as well as a route dependent on cholesterol. A novel clathrin heavy chain isoform has been implicated in trafficking of Glut4 from endosomes to the trans Golgi network in human skeletal muscle (20,21). The general consensus is that internalized Glut4 passes through an endosomal compartment to be sorted into GSV, which fuse with the sarcolemma and T-tubules in the absence and presence of insulin, but with a greatly enhanced rate in the presence of hormone (22–24).

The signaling pathway by which insulin transmits the stimulus for Glut4 stimulation has been studied in some depth and many though not all of the biochemical steps have been elucidated (Figure 59.2) (24,25). As is true in all tissues, insulin initiates its actions in skeletal muscle by binding to a prototypical protein tyrosine kinase receptor, a heterotetramer spanning the cell membrane (26–28). Binding induces a "transphosphorylation" event in which one subunit phosphorylates a tyrosine in the activation loop of the other catalytic domain (29–31). This yields a constitutively active receptor, which then phosphorylates itself and other proteins on defined tyrosine residues. The substrate of greatest physiological importance is represented by a family of related proteins termed insulin receptor substrates (IRS), of which IRS1 and IRS2 are most critical to metabolic regulation (32–34). IRS serves as a scaffold to dock signaling proteins that bind to phosphorylated tyrosines via cognate src homology 2 (SH2) domains (35). Again, most critical to the pathway that controls muscle glucose uptake is a Class 1 phosphoinositide 3′-kinase, which consists of an inhibitory p85 subunit containing 2 SH2 domains and a catalytic subunit. PI3K catalyzes the conversion of phosphoinositide 3,4 tris phosphate (PIP_2) to phosphoinositide 3,4,5 tris phosphate (PIP_3), a potent signaling lipid that binds to pleckstrin homology (PH) domains on target proteins (35–40). Two such PH domain-containing molecules are the kinases phosphoinositide-dependent kinase 1 (PDK1) and Akt (also known as protein kinase B, PKB), which are brought together at the cytoplasmic surface of membranes, recruited by the accumulation in PIP_3 in response to insulin (41–44). For maximal activation, Akt

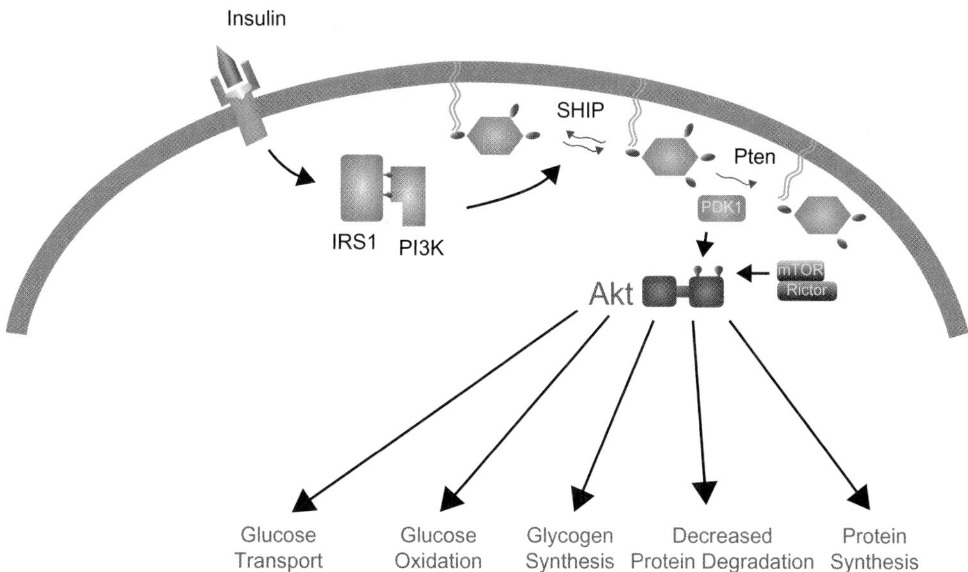

FIGURE 59.2 Insulin signaling pathway. Insulin interacts with its receptor tyrosine kinase, which phosphorylates the scaffold protein IRS. This docks a number of signaling complexes, including PI-3′-kinase. The latter generates PIP_3 that, through binding to PH domains, results in phosphorylation and activation of Akt/PKB.

has to be also phosphorylated at a conserved serine in a hydrophobic motif at its carboxyl terminus by mammalian target of rapamycin complex 2 (mTORC2) (45). There are three Akt isoforms, each the product of a distinct gene; Akt2 (PKBβ) appears to be most important to the regulation of muscle glucose transport by insulin (46,47). Akt is both necessary and sufficient for maximal activation of glucose uptake and translocation of Glut4, though the latter has yet to be tested in skeletal muscle *in vivo* (47–53).

In a search in cultured adipocytes for substrates of Akt that might be important to the regulation of Glut4 translocation, Lienhard and his colleagues identified the putative small G protein Rab GTPase activator protein (GAP) AS160, also known as TBC1D4 (54–56). Though Rab10 is a leading candidate for physiological substrate of AS160, other possible small G proteins include Rab8a, Rab13 and Rab14 (57–63). The consensus model is that AS160 exerts a constitutive inhibitory action on its target Rab protein, which is relieved by Akt phosphorylation. This allows the Rab to act as a positive regulator of Glut4 translocation. Though most of the experiments investigating this pathway have been performed in adipocytes, there are substantial data supporting a role for AS160 in transmitting the signaling from insulin and Akt to enhanced glucose uptake and Glut4 translocation in muscle (56,64–67). In particular, mice in which the major Akt phosphorylation site in AS160/TBC1D4 has been ablated using knockin technology displays glucose intolerance and impaired glucose uptake in to muscle (68).

One persistent controversy has been whether glucose transport is the exclusive determinate of the rate of glucose uptake in skeletal muscle under all conditions. The uptake of circulating glucose into muscle can be viewed as a three-step process: (1) delivery of glucose to muscle, (2) transport of glucose into the muscle by Glut4, and (3) phosphorylation of glucose within the muscle by a hexokinase (HK) (69). Once phosphorylated, the glucose is trapped in the muscle cell by its hydrophilicity. The principal fate of glucose transported into non-contracting skeletal muscle is glycogen, which accounts for about 80% of the sugar that is taken up (70). In the normal individual with circulating glucose levels in the physiological range, it is likely that glucose transport catalyzed by Glut4 is the primary if not sole determinant of the rate at which glucose is taken up and metabolized by the muscle cell. Support for this assertion derives from several lines of investigation. The first and perhaps most important biochemical evidence in this regard was reported in 1939 by Lundsgaard who found that even at near saturating concentrations of extracellular glucose, in the presence of insulin the intracellular concentration of glucose remained close to zero (quoted in 71). A sophisticated analysis based on infusion of three different radioactive tracers into the forearms of human subjects led to much the same conclusion, i.e. that transport is rate-limiting for glucose uptake under physiological insulin concentrations (72). The more modern approach has been genetic, using transgenic mice to overexpress glucose transporter proteins and assess the impact on glucose uptake. In such experiments, either Glut1 or Glut4 increases hexose uptake, supporting a major contribution of transport in the determination of rates of glucose utilization (73,74). In contrast, in at least some studies, overexpression of hexokinase does not affect glucose uptake or blood glucose levels (75). Nonetheless, it is likely that under conditions of high glucose transport and utilization such as exercise, hexokinase also contributes to the determination of flux rates (69,76,77). Once phosphorylated, the two predominant fates of glucose are conversion to glycogen or glycolysis. Under typical postprandial conditions, the majority of glucose follows the non-oxidative route, that is, storage as glycogen. Mice lacking the muscle form of glycogen synthase have relatively normal glucose metabolism under non-stressed conditions but lack muscle and cardiac glycogen (78,79). Thus, the actual amount of newly synthesized glycogen is determined both by the rate of glucose transport as well as the activity of glycogen synthase.

The mechanism by which glycogen synthesis is regulated has been well studied. Glycogen synthesis is initiated by glycogenin, a glycosyltransferase that catalyzes the formation of an approximately 10 residue glucose polymer from uridine diphosphate glucose (UDP-glucose) in an auto-glucosylation reaction. Glycogenin deficiency leads to an absence of glycogen in skeletal muscle and heart and causes a cardiomyopathy (80). Further storage of glucose is performed by glycogen synthase, which catalyzes the elongation of glycogen with α-1,4-glycosidic linkages of glycogen using UDP-glucose as the donor (81). The enzyme is one of the first recognized to be controlled by reversible protein phosphorylation (82,83). Phosphorylation of a cluster of seven sites in the carboxyl terminus of muscle glycogen synthase inhibits its catalytic activity. Two sites in particular, termed 3a and 3b, are phosphorylated by glycogen synthase kinase 3 (GSK3) in an hierarchical manner and have the greatest influence on enzyme activity (81). Since GSK3 is phosphorylated and inhibited by Akt, a pathway by which insulin increases glycogen accumulation through Akt → GSK3 → glycogen synthase has been favored (84). There is also some evidence that glycogen synthase is activated by a pathway in which insulin increases the activity of a glycogen synthase phosphatase (85). Given the abundance of data showing control of glycogen synthase by covalent modification, a recent report revealing that the primary mode of regulation *in vivo* is allosteric was quite surprising (86). Glycogen synthase is activated directly by the binding of glucose-6-phosphate such that maximal activity can be achieved even when the enzyme is fully phosphorylated. Bouskila et al. utilized mouse knockin technology to ablate the glucose-6-phosphate binding site in muscle glycogen synthase, thereby demonstrating the predominant reliance on allostery for increased activity in response to insulin (86). Enhanced glucose transport and phosphorylation elevates the level of glucose-6-phosphate within the muscle cell, which then activates glycogen synthase.

MUSCLE METABOLISM DURING FASTING

As noted above, in the postadsorptive period skeletal muscle shifts from the utilization of glucose to the oxidation of fatty acids for the production of energy (87). Though much of this is dictated by the reduction in blood glucose and insulin concentrations, the latter leading to the return of Glut4 to its intracellular storage site, there are also refined regulatory mechanisms for the control of substrate utilization. Increases in circulating fatty acids, such as those that occur during fasting, decrease glucose transport and glycogen synthesis in skeletal muscle (88). Randle proposed that this was due to an accumulation of metabolites that inhibit hexokinase; however, it is now clear that the regulation by fatty acids is at the level of Glut4 translocation (89).

One of the most important sites for the control of fatty acid oxidation is the allosteric regulation of carnitine palmitoyl transferase 1 (CPT1) by malonyl-CoA (Figure 59.3) (90). The first step in fatty acid metabolism is the "charging" of fatty acids by their ligation to Coenzyme A (CoA) by the enzyme acyl-CoA synthase. By coupling this initial reaction to the hydrolysis of ATP to AMP, the early steps in fat oxidation become energetically favorable at physiological concentrations of substrate. The acyl group must then be transferred across the mitochondrial membrane, as the enzymes of fatty acid oxidation are located within the mitochondrial matrix (91). This transport step is accomplished by transfer of the acyl group to carnitine by CPT1, movement of acyl carnitine across the mitochondrial membrane and regeneration of fatty acyl-CoA by CPT2 (92). The latter is then metabolized by repetitive rounds of oxidation and generation of acetyl CoA in the process of beta oxidation, at each round generating an acetyl CoA and NADH. Acetyl CoA enters the citric acid (or tricarboxylic acid, TCA) cycle by condensation with oxaloacetate in a reaction catalyzed by citrate synthase. One turn of the cycle generates three NADH and one FADN molecules, whose complete oxidation leads to the production of 11 molecules of ATP, and one ATP from GTP.

As noted above, malonyl-CoA generated by acetyl CoA carboxylase (ACC) and degraded by malonyl-CoA carboxylase (MCD) serves as the primary allosteric regulator of beta oxidation, inhibiting CPT1 and thus blocking the first step of fatty acid transport into the mitochondrion (Figure 59.3) (90). ACC is expressed as two isoforms, ACC-1 (ACC-α) and ACC-2 (ACC-β), corresponding to the roles of the enzyme as the rate-determining step in de novo lipogenesis in liver and adipose tissue and as a

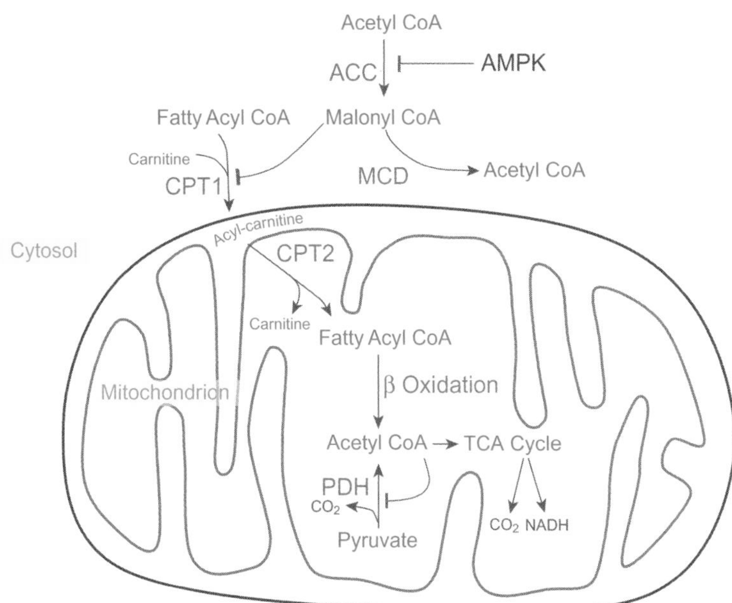

FIGURE 59.3 Selected metabolic pathways responsible for the generation of energy using carbohydrate or lipid oxidation. Acyl groups are transported into the mitochondrion using an acyl-carnitine shuttle and catalyzed by CPT1 and CPT2. The acyl groups are oxidized to acetyl-CoA, which enters the TCA cycle. ACC catalyzes the production of malonyl-CoA, which is an inhibitor of CPT1 and fatty acid oxidation. Carbohydrate enters the TCA through PDH, which catalyzed the decarboxylation of pyruvate to acetyl-CoA.

major control point for fatty acid oxidation in muscle, respectively. Deletion of ACC-2 in mice by targeted mutagenesis leads to increased fatty acid oxidation without a major change in organism bioenergetics (93). ACC-2 is regulated both by covalent and allosteric mechanisms. It is activated directly by citrate, and inhibited by long chain fatty acyl-CoA and malonyl-CoA (94). AMP-activated protein kinase (AMPK, see below) phosphorylates ACC-2 on a single residue resulting in inhibition of the enzyme by decreasing its V_{max} and increasing the K_a for citrate. Compared to ACC-1, ACC-2 has a 140 amino acid extension that targets the protein to the outer mitochondrial membrane (95). This has been interpreted as consistent with ACC-2 role as a regulator of beta oxidation in muscle. MCD is widely distributed among rodent and humans tissues and its level of expression correlates with the oxidative capacity of muscle fibers (95). Though the mechanism of regulation of MCD has not been studied in detail, its activity is increased in muscle by contraction or the AMPK activator, 5-aminoimidazole-4-carboxamide-1-beta-D-ribofuranoside (AICAR) (96). Thus, the complex control of cytoplasmic malonyl-CoA serves as an indirect way of regulating fatty acid metabolism.

Another site of regulation is at the level of substrate selection for entry into the TCA cycle. Pyruvate dehydrogenase (PDH) is a complex of multiple copies of three catalytic components, two regulatory components and one noncatalytic protein. It catalyzes the oxidative decarboxylation of pyruvate to acetyl-CoA, NADH and CO_2. PDH is required for complete aerobic metabolism glucose and thus serves as a major control point for the determination of substrate utilization. When PDH activity is low, acetyl CoA produced by fatty acids metabolism serves as the major source for generation of energy through the TCA cycle and oxidative phosphorylation. Acetyl-CoA inhibits PDH allosterically, thus reducing glucose oxidation when rates of fatty acid turnover are high. PDH is also negatively regulated by phosphorylation by a family of kinases, the pyruvate dehydrogenase kinases (PDK1-4), which themselves are controlled transcriptionally (97). Expression of the major isoform in muscle, PDK4, is induced during starvation in both slow and fast twitch muscle fibers (98). The net effect is that PDH is inhibited, thus shifting the substrate entering the TCA cycle from carbohydrate to fat. Mice lacking PDK4 demonstrate decreased blood glucose and increased fatty acids during starvation, consistent with increased glucose and pyruvate and decreased fatty acid oxidation compared to wild-type mice (97). PDH is also regulated by dephosphorylation and activation catalyzed by PDH phosphate phosphatase, whose activity in muscle is decreased during starvation (99).

MUSCLE METABOLISM DURING EXERCISE

Exercise, i.e. muscle contraction, represents a need for increased generation of energy, thus putting extra demands on the metabolic state of the cell. This is often accompanied by hypoxia, which necessitates the muscle relying on anaerobic metabolism for part or all of its ATP production. The selection of the stored or circulating fuel used to generate ATP is generally well matched to the nature and duration of the work being performed. The energy density of fat is much higher than that of protein or carbohydrate, largely because the former can be stored without associated water but also because it is more reduced. However, the poor solubility of lipid limits its availability and necessitates binding proteins for both extra- and intracellular transport. In addition to being more soluble, carbohydrate also has the advantage of being able to generate energy under anaerobic conditions. Nonetheless, at least under conditions of limited oxygen availability at high altitude, exercising muscle derives the same fraction of energy from carbohydrate as it does at sea level (100). Even under conditions of extreme exercise, ATP levels are maintained remarkably well, in part due to the reliance on the phosphagen, creatine phosphate, for the regeneration of ATP. Creatine kinase catalyzes the reversible reaction phosphocreatine + ADP$\leftrightharpoons$creatine + ATP, which is close to equilibrium at physiological concentration of substrate. The reaction is sensitive to small changes in ADP/ATP ratio and thus has the effect of buffering ATP concentrations (101). Moreover, when ATP decreases, the creatine kinase reaction generates ADP, a substrate and limiting factor in oxidative phosphorylation. Creatine phosphate functions not only as an energy store, but also as a means of shuttling ATP out of the mitochondrion to the cytoplasm, where it can support contraction.

The major fuels utilized during exercise are carbohydrate and lipids, as even though protein turnover increases during exercise, it accounts for only a small percentage of the ATP generated (102,103). Exercise does suppress protein synthesis in muscle (104). The most significant sources of fuels for skeletal muscle are (1) muscle glycogen, (2) muscle triacylglycerol, (3) glucose released from the liver from glycogen breakdown or gluconeogenesis, a process primarily under the control of the hormone glucagon, and (4) circulating free fatty acids (FFA) derived from adipocytes (69,105). As a rule, muscles with the greatest oxidative capacity tend to rely more on intracellular stores of substrate (105). Early work on muscle substrate selection showed that exercise is associated with increased utilization of carbohydrate, which is positively correlated with exercise intensity (106). The switch in fuels is thought due at least in part to limited flux of lipids and decreased activity of CPT1. There is a close relationship between metabolism of glucose and fatty acids, such that increases in one fuel suppress oxidation of the other, a phenomenon known as the Randle Cycle (107). Pyruvate dehydrogenase (PDH) is critical enzyme in fuel source selection, as was described above in reference to starvation. The high ratios of NADH/NAD$^+$ and acetyl-CoA/CoA that occur during fat metabolism suppress PDH, thus limiting the utilization of carbohydrate (107). PDH is also negatively regulated by phosphorylation by PDH phosphorylation kinase (PDK), which is itself inhibited by pyruvate and stimulated by acetyl-CoA and NADH. On the other hand, enhanced glucose metabolism and flux through PDH leads to an increase in cytosolic malonyl-CoA and inhibition of CPT1 and long chain fatty acid oxidation (91,94). Another mechanism by which carbohydrate may inhibit fatty acid oxidation is via depletion of carnitine by acetylation (108).

During contraction and/or hypoxia, a major site of regulation of glucose uptake is mediated by translocation of Glut4 glucose transporter from the cell interior to the sarcolemma and T-tubules (Figure 59.1) (109). Since under most conditions (see below) transport is rate-limiting for exogenous glucose metabolism, the total cellular content of Glut4 determines the maximal rate of glycolysis and glucose oxidation. Though, like insulin, exercise enhances glucose transport by means of Glut4 translocation, the signaling pathways by which the two responses are mediated are distinct (40,110,111). Contraction does not activate PI3K or Akt as part of the pathway by which it stimulates hexose transport, as inhibition of these signaling molecules blocks the response to insulin but not exercise or electrical stimulation (112,113). Moreover, maximal concentrations of insulin and electrically-stimulated contraction are additive in terms of stimulation of glucose transport, whereas hypoxia and contraction are not additive.

Several years ago, there developed the attractive hypothesis that AMP-activated protein kinase (AMPK) was the major signal connecting contraction to increased glucose uptake. AMPK is a phylogenetically conserved protein kinase, whose expression spans all eukaryotes from budding yeast to man. It is a heterotrimer consisting of a catalytic alpha subunit, a beta scaffold and a regulatory gamma subunit. In mammals there are three alpha isoforms, two beta and two gamma, creating the ability to generate 12 different oligomeric proteins (114,115). As its name suggests, AMPK can be activated allosterically by AMP about two-fold but considerably more by phosphorylation of the alpha subunit at a conserved residue, threonine 172. The major kinases capable of phosphorylating AMPK are Lkb1, a tumor suppressor deleted in Peutz–Jeghers syndrome, and calmodulin-dependent kinase kinase beta, though there might be others (116–119). The activity of Lkb1 appears not to be regulated but is either constitutively active towards AMPK or phosphorylates AMPK more efficiently when the latter binds AMPK. The major mode of regulation is probably the regulation of dephosphorylation of AMPK, which is largely abrogated by binding of nucleotide (120,121). Because only AMP can allosterically activate AMPK, until recently it was not recognized that ADP is as efficient in preventing AMPK dephosphorylation as AMP. Given the considerably higher intracellular concentrations of ADP, it is likely that this nucleotide represents the physiological regulator of AMPK (122–124).

A number of observations supported the idea that AMPK might mediate the effects of contraction and hypoxia on glucose transport (115). First, since AMPK is regulated by energy charge, increased muscle activity activates it in the absence of decreases in ATP, as occurs due to replenishment by creatine kinase. In fact, considerable data showed that contraction *ex vivo*, hypoxia or exercise increase AMPK phosphorylation and activity in a manner correlating well with glucose uptake. Thus, it was quite surprising when it was found that suppression of AMPK activity by expression of a dominant-inhibitory mutant in skeletal muscle of mice prevented the increase in glucose transport and Glut4 translocation in response to hypoxia, but not contraction (125,126). One explanation for this might be the presence in muscle of AMPK-like kinases also phosphorylated and activated by Lkb1 (127). However, there still exists no plausible mechanism to explain how contraction could activate these other kinases. In addition to the postulated role of AMPK in glucose transport, the same kinase appears to be an important determinant of utilization of other substrates. AMPK was initially identified in the context of its anti-anabolic functions, i.e. its suppression of cholesterol and fatty acid synthesis. However, it also has a positive effect on oxidative metabolism, which has been invoked as important to ATP generation during exercise. As alluded to above, AMPK phosphorylates and inhibits ACC, thus reducing the concentration of malonyl-CoA, itself an inhibitor of CPT1 (94). Thus, the net effect of acute AMPK activation is to increase fatty acid oxidation as well as glucose uptake. Chronic activation of AMPK leads to an increase in mitochondrial biogenesis and oxidative capacity, mimicking the metabolic effects of exercise training (128). Under conditions of expanded mitochondrial mass, the muscle maintains unchanged basal metabolic activity by developing mild uncoupling of oxidative phosphorylation (129). AMPK exerts its effects at least in part by stimulating the transcriptional co-activator peroxisome proliferator-activated receptor gamma coactivator-1α (PGC-1α) (128,130–132). Ablation of PGC-1α in muscle leads to a reduction in oxidative capacity (133–135). A number of genes that are co-activated by PGC-1α contribute to the increased expression of nuclear-encoded mitochondrial genes; these include PPARs, estrogen-related receptor, thyroid receptor, nuclear respiratory factor 1 (NRF1), NRF2, and MEF2 (136). Another downstream target of long-term AMPK activation is the NAD^+-dependent Type III deacetylase SIRT1, a direct activator of PGC-1α and forkhead box O (FOXO) transcription factors (137).

The interest in AMPK as a mediator of signals that increase Glut4 translocation spurred an effort to uncover relevant downstream targets. While initial attention focused on AS160/TBC1D4, which contains consensus putative phosphorylation sites for AMPK as well as Akt, interest soon shifted to a closely related Rab GAP family member TBC1D1, which is expressed as high levels in muscle. TBC1DI phosphorylation is increased in response to insulin, the AMPK activator AICAR, or contraction and expression of an inhibitor blocks TBC1D1 phosphorylation following at least some activators (138–139). A mutation of TBC1D1 (R125W) has been identified in human families and found to be associated with increased risk of familial obesity (140,141). Moreover, forced expression in skeletal muscle of a form of TBC1D1 containing the R125W mutation inhibits insulin-dependent glucose transport (142). One attractive model has been that insulin works predominantly through AS160/ TBC1D4, whereas contraction and hypoxia utilize TBC1D1 as an intermediary signaling molecular, though more likely both proteins integrate multiple independent signals (143,144). Interestingly, TBC1D1 contains a putative calmodulin-binding domain, raising the possibility that it is regulated by calcium, either alone or in synergy with phosphorylation.

During exercise, in addition to blood glucose, another more limited but readily accessible source of carbohydrate is muscle glycogen. The rate determining step in glycogenolysis catalyzed by glycogen phosphorylase is the phosphorolysis of the a-1,4-glycosidic linkages of glycogen yielding glucose-1-P and shorter chain length glycogen (81). The enzyme is phosphorylated at a single serine residue, which induces structural changes resulting in activation. Glycogen phosphorylase is also activated allosterically by AMP, which is competed by ATP and glucose-6-phosphate, which by virtue of adenylate kinase reaction makes glycogen breakdown exquisitely sensitive to ATP utilization. A single enzyme, phosphorylase kinase, which is composed of four copies of four subunits, phosphorylates and activates glycogen phosphorylase (145). A rise in calcium stimulates the enzyme by binding to calmodulin protein directly associated with phosphorylase kinase. Adrenergic agents such as epinephrine increase the intracellular levels of cyclic AMP; this activates protein kinase A, which then phosphorylates and stimulates phosphorylase kinase. Thus, glycogen breakdown is triggered by hormones of stress, the increase in calcium associated with contraction, and reduction in energy charge.

In addition to carbohydrate, lipid is an important source of energy during exercise. Though fatty acids from the circulation are the major source of lipid during exercise, triglyceride is also stored in the muscle cell as droplets surrounded by a phospholipid monolayer (146,147). During moderate exercise by fasted, endurance-trained athletes, about 40–60% of the lipids oxidized are provided by circulating free fatty acids (FFA), the rest consisting largely of fatty acids derived from intramuscular triglyceride and extracted from lipoprotein particles (106,148,149). Van Loon et al. performed a detailed study using isotope tracer techniques in human subjects to quantitate fat metabolism during moderate exercise (150). At rest after an overnight fast, FFA contributes about 48% of the energy utilized, while other sources of lipid supply about 17%. During exercise, the absolute amount of fat oxidized increases about six-fold, but as a percentage of all substrate utilized FFA acid consumption declines to 43% while other sources remain constant at 15% (150). These data indicate that intracellular triglyceride is likely to be an important source of energy during exercise. Nonetheless, utilization of intramuscular triglyceride during exercise has been a source of much controversy over the years, most likely due to the confounding effect of adipose tissue contaminating muscle biopsies. Studies that have used magnetic resonance spectroscopy or confocal microscopy, techniques more specific for intramuscular lipids, have revealed more consistent decreased in triglyceride, at least in normal lean individuals (151). Endurance athletes demonstrate an increased capacity for lipid storage, oxidation, and triglyceride hydrolysis in skeletal muscle (152).

In addition to the AMPK-dependent inhibition of malonyl-CoA formation described above, there are a number of others sites at which fatty acid utilization is controlled. For example, triglyceride lipolysis is increased in response to catecholamines or muscle contraction (153). For many years it was thought that hormone sensitive lipase (HSL) represents the rate limiting triglyceride lipase in muscle, as its activity is regulated by the same stimuli that modulate lipolysis (154). However, more recently it has been appreciated that the major lipase and the true rate determinant is adipose triglyceride lipase (ATGL) and that HSL is most likely a diacylglycerol lipase (DAG) lipase *in vivo* (155–157). As might be expected, ATGL is expressed at higher levels in Type 1 oxidative than type 2 glycolytic muscle fibers (158). Maximal activation of ATGL requires association with another lipid droplet protein, comparative gene identification-58 (CGI-85), whose absence causes neutral lipid storage disease in humans, as does mutation in ATGL (159–161). ATGL is critical to the maintenance of normal exercise capacity, though the relative contributions of defects in muscle triglyceride hydrolysis versus FFA release by adipose tissue have not been quantitated (162). The mechanism which lipolysis is regulated in muscle is not understood.

MUSCLE INSULIN RESISTANCE

Some of the most common diseases associated with modern societies, including obesity, the metabolic syndrome and Type 2 diabetes mellitus, are associated with muscle insulin resistance (163,164). This is generally defined in terms of insulin's action on glucose metabolism, such that resistance in muscle refers to an inability of the hormone to activate glucose transport and Glut4 translocation appropriately. Often the response to contraction is preserved, one of several factors contributing to the efficaciousness of exercise as a therapy. One consequence of muscle insulin resistance is "metabolic inflexibility" in that the ratio of carbohydrate to fat oxidized does not undergo the normal nutritional variation (165). The causes of muscle insulin resistance have been elusive, though a number of candidates have received experimental support. Perhaps the leading idea is that accumulation of intracellular neutral lipid in the form of diacylglycerol inhibits insulin signaling (89,164). The elucidation of the sequence of events leading to insulin resistance is critical to the rational design of therapeutics to treat this epidemic syndrome.

REFERENCES

1. Bouckaert JP, de Duve C. The action of insulin. *Physiol Rev* 1947;**27**:39–71.
2. Levine R, Goldstein M. The action of insulin on the distribution of galactose in eviscerated nephrectomized dogs. *J Biol Chem* 1949;**179**:985.
3. Goldstein MS, Henry WL, Huddlestun B, Levine R. Action of insulin on transfer of sugars across cell barriers; common chemical configuration of substances responsive to action of the hormone. *Am J Physiol* 1953;**173**:207–11.
4. Levine R, Haft DE. Carbohydrate homeostasis. *N Engl J Med* 1970;**283**:237–46.
5. Cushman SW, Wardzala LJ. Potential mechanism of insulin action on glucose transport in the isolated rat adipose cell. Apparent translocation of intracellular transport systems to the plasma membrane. *J Biol Chem* 1980;**255**:4758–62.
6. Suzuki K, Kono T. Evidence that insulin causes translocation of glucose transport activity to the plasma membrane from an intracellular storage site. *Proc Natl Acad Sci USA* 1980;**77**:2542–5.
7. Wardzala LJ, Jeanrenaud B. Potential mechanism of insulin action on glucose transport in the isolated rat diaphragm. Apparent translocation of intracellular transport units to the plasma membrane. *J Biol Chem* 1981;**256**:7090–3.
8. Bimbaum MJ. The insulin-sensitive glucose transporter. *Int Rev Cytol* 1992;**137**(Pt 1):239–97.
9. James DE, Brown R, Navarro J, Pilch PF. Insulin-regulatable tissues express a unique insulin-sensitive glucose transport protein. *Nature* 1988;**333**:183–5.
10. Birnbaum MJ. Identification of a novel gene encoding an insulin-responsive glucose transporter protein. *Cell* 1989;**57**:305–15.
11. James DE, Strube M, Mueckler M. Molecular cloning and characterization of an insulin-regulatable glucose transporter. *Nature* 1989;**338**:83–7.
12. Ploug T, van Deurs B, Ai H, Cushman SW, Ralston E. Analysis of glut4 distribution in whole skeletal muscle fibers: identification of distinct storage compartments that are recruited by insulin and muscle contractions. *J Cell Biol* 1998;**142**:1429–46.
13. Wang W, Hansen PA, Marshall BA, Holloszy JO, Mueckler M. Insulin unmasks a COOH-terminal Glut4 epitope and increases glucose transport across T-tubules in skeletal muscle. *J Cell Biol* 1996;**135**:415–30.

14. Bogan JS, Kandror KV. Biogenesis and regulation of insulin-responsive vesicles containing Glut4. *Curr Opin Cell Biol* 2010;**22**:506–12.
15. Robinson L, Pang S, Harris D, Heuser J, James D. Translocation of the glucose transporter (Glut4) to the cell surface in permeabilized 3T3-L1 adipocytes: effects of ATP insulin, and GTP gamma S and localization of Glut4 to clathrin lattices. *J Cell Biol* 1992;**117**:1181–96.
16. Blot V, McGraw TE. Glut4 is internalized by a cholesterol-dependent nystatin-sensitive mechanism inhibited by insulin. *EMBO J* 2006;**25**:5648–58.
17. Antonescu CN, Díaz M, Femia G, Planas JV, Klip A. Clathrin-dependent and independent endocytosis of glucose transporter 4 (Glut4) in myoblasts: regulation by mitochondrial uncoupling. *Traffic* 2008;**9**:1173–90.
18. Parton RG, Molero JC, Floetenmeyer M, Green KM, James DE. Characterization of a distinct plasma membrane macrodomain in differentiated adipocytes. *J Biol Chem* 2002;**277**:46769–78.
19. Nishimura H, Zarnowski MJ, Simpson IA. Glucose transporter recycling in rat adipose cells. Effects of potassium depletion. *J Biol Chem* 1993;**268**:19246–53.
20. Vassilopoulos SP, Esk C, Hoshino S, Funke BH, Chen C-Y, Plocik AM, et al. A role for the CHC22 clathrin heavy-chain isoform in human glucose metabolism. *Science* 2009;**324**:1192–6.
21. Esk C, Chen C-Y, Johannes L, Brodsky FM. The clathrin heavy chain isoform CHC22 functions in a novel endosomal sorting step. *J Cell Biol* 2010;**188**:131–44.
22. Pilch PF. The mass action hypothesis: Formation of glut4 storage vesicles, a tissue-specific, regulated exocytic compartment. *Acta Physiologica* 2008;**192**:89–101.
23. Hou JC, Pessin JE. Ins (endocytosis) and outs (exocytosis) of Glut4 trafficking. *Curr Opin Cell Biol* 2007;**19**:466–73.
24. Rowland AF, Fazakerley DJ, James DE. Mapping insulin/Glut4 circuitry. *Traffic* 2011;**12**:672–81.
25. Gross DN, Wan M, Birnbaum MJ. The role of FoxO in the regulation of metabolism. *Curr Diab Rep* 2009;**9**:208–14.
26. Taniguchi CM, Emanuelli B, Kahn CR. Critical nodes in signalling pathways: insights into insulin action. *Nat Rev Mol Cell Biol* 2006;**7**:85–96.
27. Ullrich A, Schlessinger J. Signal transduction by receptors with tyrosine kinase activity. *Cell* 1990;**61**:203–12.
28. Avruch J. Insulin signal transduction through protein kinase cascades. *Mol Cell Biochem* 1998;**182**:31–48.
29. Hubbard SR. Crystal structure of the activated insulin receptor tyrosine kinase in complex with peptide substrate and atp analog. *EMBO J* 1997;**16**:5572–81.
30. Hubbard SR, Wei L, Hendrickson WA. Crystal structure of the tyrosine kinase domain of the human insulin receptor. *Nature* 1994;**372**:746–54.
31. Rosen OM, Herrera R, Olowe Y, Petruzzelli LM, Cobb MH. Phosphorylation activates the insulin receptor tyrosine protein kinase. *Proc Natl Acad Sci USA* 1983;**80**:3237–40.
32. White MF. Irs proteins and the common path to diabetes. *Am J Physiol Endocrinol Metabol* 2002;**283**:E413–22.
33. Sun XJ, Rothenberg P, Kahn CR, Backer JM, Araki E, Wilden PA, et al. Structure of the insulin receptor substrate irs-1 defines a unique signal transduction protein. *Nature* 1991;**352**: 73–7.
34. Sun XJ, Wang L-M, Zhang Y, Yenush L, Myers Jr MG, Glasheen E, et al. Role of IRS-2 in insulin and cytokine signalling. *Nature* 1995;**377**:173–7.
35. Myers Jr MG, White MF. The new elements of insulin signaling. Insulin receptor substrate-1 and proteins with SH2 domains. *Diabetes* 1993;**42**:643–50.
36. Shepherd PR, Withers DJ, Siddle K. Phosphoinositide 3-kinase: The key switch mechanism in insulin signalling. *Biochem J* 1998;**333**:471–90.
37. Shoelson SE, Chatterjee S, Chaudhuri M, White MF. YMXM motifs of IRS-1 define substrate specificity of the insulin receptor kinase. *Proc Natl Acad Sci USA* 1992;**89**:2027–31.
38. Folli F, Saad MJ, Backer JM, Kahn CR. Insulin stimulation of phosphatidylinositol 3-kinase activity and association with insulin receptor substrate 1 in liver and muscle of the intact rat. *J Biol Chem* 1992;**267**:22171–7.
39. Myers MG, Backer JM, Sun XJ, Shoelson S, Hu P, Schlessinger J, et al. IRS-1 activates phosphatidylinositol 3′-kinase by associating with SRC homology 2 domains of p85. *Proc Natl Acad Sci USA* 1992;**89**:10350–4.
40. Yeh JI, Gulve EA, Rameh L, Birnbaum MJ. The effects of Wortmannin on rat skeletal muscle. Dissociation of signaling pathways for insulin- and contraction-activated hexose transport. *J Biol Chem* 1995;**270**:2107–11.
41. Mora A, Komander D, van Aalten DM, Alessi DR. Pdk1, the master regulator of AGC kinase signal transduction. *Semin Cell Dev Biol* 2004;**15**:161–70.
42. Gonzalez E, McGraw TE. The akt kinases: Isoform specificity in metabolism and cancer. *Cell Cycle* 2009;**8**:2502–8.
43. Whiteman EL, Cho H, Birnbaum MJ. Role of Akt/protein kinase B in metabolism. *Trends Endocrinol Metab* 2002;**13**:444–51.
44. Brozinick Jr JT, Birnbaum MJ. Insulin, but not contraction, activates Akt/PKB in isolated rat skeletal muscle. *J Biol Chem* 1998;**273**:14679–82.
45. Zoncu R, Efeyan A, Sabatini DM. Mtor: From growth signal integration to cancer, diabetes and ageing. *Nat Rev Mol Cell Biol* 2011;**12**:21–35.
46. Hill MM, Clark SF, Tucker DF, Birnbaum MJ, James DE, Macaulay SL. A role for protein kinase B-beta/AKT2 in insulin-stimulated Glut4 translocation in adipocytes. *Mol Cell Biol* 1999;**19**:7771–81.
47. Kohn AD, Summers SA, Birnbaum MJ, Roth RA. Expression of a constitutively active Akt Ser/Thr kinase in 3T3-L1 adipocytes stimulates glucose uptake and glucose transporter 4 translocation. *J Biol Chem* 1996;**271**:31372–8.
48. Hajduch E, Alessi DR, Hemmings BA, Hundal HS. Constitutive activation of protein kinase B alpha by membrane targeting promotes glucose and system a amino acid transport, protein synthesis, and inactivation of glycogen synthase kinase 3 in 16 muscle cells. *Diabetes* 1998;**47**:1006–13.
49. Ng Y, Ramm G, Lopez JA, James DE. Rapid activation of Akt2 is sufficient to stimulate Glut4 translocation in 3T3-L1 adipocytes. *Cell Metab* 2008;**7**:348–56.
50. Hausdorff SF, Fingar DC, Morioka K, Garza LA, Whiteman EL, Summers SA, et al. Identification of wortmannin-sensitive targets in 3T3-L1 adipocytes. *J Biol Chem* 1999;**274**:24677–84.
51. Kohn AD, Barthel A, Kovacina KS, Boge A, Wallach B, Summers SA, et al. Construction and characterization of a

conditionally active version of the serine/threonine kinase Akt. *J Biol Chem* 1998;**273**:11937–43.

52. Cho H, Mu J, Kim JK, Thorvaldsen JL, Chu Q, Crenshaw 3rd EB, et al. Insulin resistance and a diabetes mellitus-like syndrome in mice lacking the protein kinase Akt2 (PKB beta). *Science* 2001;**292**:1728–31.
53. Cleasby ME, Reinten TA, Cooney GJ, James DE, Kraegen EW. Functional studies of Akt isoform specificity in skeletal muscle in vivo; maintained insulin sensitivity despite reduced insulin receptor substrate-1 expression. *Mol Endocrinol* 2007;**21**:215–28.
54. Sano H, Kane S, Sano E, Miinea CP, Asara JM, Lane WS, et al. Insulin-stimulated phosphorylation of a Rab GTPase-activating protein regulates glut4 translocation. *J Biol Chem* 2003; **278**:14599–602.
55. Kane S, Sano H, Liu SCH, Asara JM, Lane WS, Garner CC, et al. A method to identify serine kinase substrates. *J Biol Chem* 2002;**277**:22115–8.
56. Sakamoto K, Holman GD. Emerging role for as160/TBC1D4 and TBC1D1 in the regulation of Glut4 traffic. *Am J Physiol Endocrinol Metab* 2008;**295**:E29–37.
57. Sun Y, Bilan PJ, Liu Z, Klip A. Rab8a and Rab13 are activated by insulin and regulate Glut4 translocation in muscle cells. *Proc Natl Acad Sci USA* 2010;**107**:19909–14.
58. Larance M, Ramm G, Stöckli J, van Dam EM, Winata S, Wasinger V, et al. Characterization of the role of the Rab GTPase-activating protein as160 in insulin-regulated Glut4 trafficking. *J Biol Chem* 2005;**280**:37803–13.
59. Sano H, Roach WG, Peck GR, Fukuda M, Lienhard GE. Rab10 in insulin-stimulated Glut4 translocation. *Biochem J* 2008; **411**:89–95.
60. Sano H, Eguez L, Teruel MN, Fukuda M, Chuang TD, Chavez JA, et al. Rab10, a target of the as160 Rab gap, is required for insulin-stimulated translocation of Glut4 to the adipocyte plasma membrane. *Cell Metab* 2007;**5**:293–303.
61. Roach WG, Chavez JA, Miinea CP, Lienhard GE. Substrate specificity and effect on glut4 translocation of the rab gtpase-activating protein tbc1d1. *Biochem J* 2007;**403**:353–8.
62. Eguez L, Lee A, Chavez JA, Miinea CP, Kane S, Lienhard GE, et al. Full intracellular retention of glut4 requires as160 Rab GTPase activating protein. *Cell Metab* 2005;**2**:263–72.
63. Ishikura S, Bilan PJ, Klip A. Rabs 8a and 14 are targets of the insulin-regulated Rab-Gap as160 regulating Glut4 traffic in muscle cells. *Biochem Biophys Res Commun* 2007;**353**:1074–9.
64. Kramer HF, Witczak CA, Taylor EB, Fujii N, Hirshman MF, Goodyear LJ. As160 regulates insulin- and contraction-stimulated glucose uptake in mouse skeletal muscle. *J Biol Chem* 2006; **281**:31478–85.
65. Thong FS, Bilan PJ, Klip A. The Rab GTPase-activating protein as160 integrates Akt, protein kinase C, and AMP-activated protein kinase signals regulating Glut4 traffic. *Diabetes* 2007;**56**:414–23.
66. Karlsson HK, Zierath JR, Kane S, Krook A, Lienhard GE, Wallberg-Henriksson H. Insulin-stimulated phosphorylation of the akt substrate as160 is impaired in skeletal muscle of type 2 diabetic subjects. *Diabetes* 2005;**54**:1692–7.
67. Bruss MD, Arias EB, Lienhard GE, Cartee GD. Increased phosphorylation of Akt substrate of 160 kDa (AS160) in rat skeletal muscle in response to insulin or contractile activity. *Diabetes* 2005;**54**:41–50.
68. Chen S, Wasserman DH, MacKintosh C, Sakamoto K. Mice with as160/TBC1D4-Thr649Ala knockin mutation are glucose intolerant with reduced insulin sensitivity and altered Glut4 trafficking. *Cell Metab* 2011;**13**:68–79.
69. Wasserman DH, Kang L, Ayala JE, Fueger PT, Lee-Young RS. The physiological regulation of glucose flux into muscle in vivo. *J Exp Biol* 2011;**214**:254–62.
70. Shulman GI, Rothman DL, Jue T, Stein P, DeFronzo RA, Shulman RG. Quantitation of muscle glycogen synthesis in normal subjects and subjects with non-insulin-dependent diabetes by 13C nuclear magnetic resonance spectroscopy. *New Engl J Med* 1990;**322**:223–8.
71. Ploug T, Vinten JR. Counterpoint: glucose phosphorylation is not a significant barrier to glucose uptake by the working muscle. *J Appl Physiol* 2006;**101**:1805–6.
72. Saccomani MP, Bonadonna RC, Bier DM, DeFronzo RA, Cobelli C. A model to measure insulin effects on glucose transport and phosphorylation in muscle: a three-tracer study. *Am J Physiol Endocrinol Metabol* 1996;**270**:E170–85.
73. Ren JM, Marshall BA, Mueckler MM, McCaleb M, Amatruda JM, Shulman GI. Overexpression of glut4 protein in muscle increases basal and insulin-stimulated whole body glucose disposal in conscious mice. *J Clin Invest* 1995;**95**:429–32.
74. Ren JM, Marshall BA, Gulve EA, Gao J, Johnson DW, Holloszy JO, et al. Evidence from transgenic mice that glucose transport is rate-limiting for glycogen deposition and glycolysis in skeletal muscle. *J Biol Chem* 1993;**268**:16113–5.
75. Hansen PA, Marshall BA, Chen M, Holloszy JO, Mueckler M. Transgenic overexpression of hexokinase II in skeletal muscle does not increase glucose disposal in wild-type or Glut1-overexpressing mice. *J Biol Chem* 2000;**275**:22381–6.
76. Halseth AE, Bracy DP, Wasserman DH. Limitations to exercise- and maximal insulin-stimulated muscle glucose uptake. *J Appl Physiol* 1998;**85**:2305–13.
77. Halseth AE, Bracy DP, Wasserman DH. Overexpression of hexokinase II increases insulinand exercise-stimulated muscle glucose uptake in vivo. *Am J Physiol* 1999;**276**:E70–7.
78. Pederson BA, Chen H, Schroeder JM, Shou W, DePaoli-Roach AA, Roach PJ. Abnormal cardiac development in the absence of heart glycogen. *Mol Cell Biol* 2004;**24**:7179–87.
79. Pederson BA, Schroeder JM, Parker GE, Smith MW, Depaoli-Roach AA, Roach PJ. Glucose metabolism in mice lacking muscle glycogen synthase. *Diabetes* 2005;**54**:3466–73.
80. Moslemi A-R, Lindberg C, Nilsson J, Tajsharghi H, Andersson B, Oldfors A. Glycogenin-1 deficiency and inactivated priming of glycogen synthesis. *N Engl J Med* 2010;**362**:1203–10.
81. Roach PJ. Glycogen and its metabolism. *Curr Mol Med* 2002;**2**:101–20.
82. Soderling TR. Regulation of glycogen synthetase. Specificity and stoichiometry of phosphorylation of the skeletal muscle enzyme by cyclic 3′:5′-amp-dependent protein kinase. *J Biol Chem* 1975; **250**:5407–12.
83. Roach PJ, Takeda Y, Larner J. Rabbit skeletal muscle glycogen synthase. I. Relationship between phosphorylation state and kinetic properties. *J Biol Chem* 1976;**251**:1913–9.
84. Lawrence Jr JC, Roach PJ. New insights into the role and mechanism of glycogen synthase activation by insulin. *Diabetes* 1997;**46**:541–7.

85. Dent P, Lavoinne A, Nakielny S, Caudwell FB, Watt P, Cohen P. The molecular mechanism by which insulin stimulates glycogen synthesis in mammalian skeletal muscle. *Nature* 1990; **348**:302–8.
86. Bouskila M, Hunter RW, Ibrahim AFM, Delattre L, Peggie M, van Diepen JA, et al. Allosteric regulation of glycogen synthase controls glycogen synthesis in muscle. *Cell Metab* 2010; **12**:456–66.
87. Andres R, Cader G, Zierler KL. The quantitatively minor role of carbohydrate in oxidative metabolism by skeletal muscle in intact man in the basal state; measurements of oxygen and glucose uptake and carbon dioxide and lactate production in the forearm. *J Clin Invest* 1956;**35**:671–82.
88. Kelley DE, Mokan M, Simoneau JA, Mandarino LJ. Interaction between glucose and free fatty acid metabolism in human skeletal muscle. *J Clin Invest* 1993;**92**:91–8.
89. Samuel VT, Petersen KF, Shulman GI. Lipid-induced insulin resistance: Unravelling the mechanism. *Lancet* 2010; **375**:2267–77.
90. Ruderman NB, Saha AK, Vavvas D, Witters LA. Malonyl-Coa, fuel sensing, and insulin resistance. *Am J Physiol* 1999;**276**: E1–18.
91. Rasmussen BB, Wolfe RR. Regulation of fatty acid oxidation in skeletal muscle. *Annu Rev Nutr* 1999;**19**:463–84.
92. Eaton S, Bartlett K, Pourfarzam M. Mammalian mitochondrial beta-oxidation. *Biochem J* 1996;**320**(Pt 2):345–57.
93. Hoehn KL, Turner N, Swarbrick MM, Wilks D, Preston E, Phua Y, et al. Acute or chronic upregulation of mitochondrial fatty acid oxidation has no net effect on whole-body energy expenditure or adiposity. *Cell Metab* 2010;**11**:70–6.
94. Saggerson D. Malonyl-Coa, a key signaling molecule in mammalian cells. *Annu Rev Nutr* 2008;**28**:253–72.
95. Voilley N, Roduit R, Vicaretti R, Bonny C, Waeber G, Dyck JR, et al. Cloning and expression of rat pancreatic beta-cell malonyl-Coa decarboxylase. *Biochem J* 1999;**340**(Pt 1):213–7.
96. Saha AK, Schwarsin AJ, Roduit R, Masse F, Kaushik V, Tornheim K, et al. Activation of malonyl-Coa decarboxylase in rat skeletal muscle by contraction and the AMP-activated protein kinase activator 5-aminoimidazole-4-carboxamide-1-beta-d-ribofuranoside. *J Biol Chem* 2000;**275**:24279–83.
97. Jeoung NH, Wu P, Joshi MA, Jaskiewicz J, Bock CB, Depaoli-Roach AA, et al. Role of pyruvate dehydrogenase kinase isoenzyme 4 (pdhk4) in glucose homoeostasis during starvation. *Biochem J* 2006;**397**:417–25.
98. Sugden MC, Kraus A, Harris RA, Holness MJ. Fibre-type specific modification of the activity and regulation of skeletal muscle pyruvate dehydrogenase kinase (PDK) by prolonged starvation and refeeding is associated with targeted regulation of PDK isoenzyme 4 expression. *Biochem J* 2000;**346**:651–7.
99. Hagg SA, Taylor SI, Ruberman NB. Glucose metabolism in perfused skeletal muscle. Pyruvate dehydrogenase activity in starvation, diabetes and exercise. *Biochem J* 1976;**158**:203–10.
100. McClelland GB, Hochachka PW, Weber J-M. Carbohydrate utilization during exercise after high-altitude acclimation: a new perspective. *Proc Natl Acad Sci USA* 1998;**95**:10288–93.
101. Kushmerick MJ, Conley KE. Energetics of muscle contraction: the whole is less than the sum of its parts. *Biochem Soc Trans* 2002;**30**:227–31.
102. Rennie MJ, Edwards RH, Krywawych S, Davies CT, Halliday D, Waterlow JC, et al. Effect of exercise on protein turnover in man. *Clin Sci* 1981;**61**:627–39.
103. Carraro F, Naldini A, Weber JM, Wolfe RR. Alanine kinetics in humans during low-intensity exercise. *Med Sci Sports Exerc* 1994;**26**:348–53.
104. Rose AJ, Richter EA. Regulatory mechanisms of skeletal muscle protein turnover during exercise. *J Appl Physiol* 2009; **106**:1702–11.
105. Weber J-M. Metabolic fuels: regulating fluxes to select mix. *J Exp Biol* 2011;**214**:286–94.
106. van Loon LJC, Greenhaff PL, Constantin-Teodosiu D, Saris WHM, Wagenmakers AJM. The effects of increasing exercise intensity on muscle fuel utilisation in humans. *J Physiol* 2001;**536**:295–304.
107. Hue L, Taegtmeyer H. The randle cycle revisited: a new head for an old hat. *Am J Physiol Endocrinol Metab* 2009;**297**:E578–591.
108. Kiens B. Skeletal muscle lipid metabolism in exercise and insulin resistance. *Physiol Rev* 2006;**86**:205–43.
109. Ploug T, Galbo H, Ohkuwa T, Tranum-Jensen J, Vinten J. Kinetics of glucose transport in rat skeletal muscle membrane vesicles: effects of insulin and contractions. *Am J Physiol* 1992;**262**:E700–11.
110. Lund S, Holman GD, Schmitz O, Pedersen O. Contraction stimulates translocation of glucose transporter glut4 in skeletal muscle through a mechanism distinct from that of insulin. *Proc Natl Acad Sci USA* 1995;**92**:5817–21.
111. Fazakerley DJ, Holman GD, Marley A, James DE, Stockli J, Coster AC. Kinetic evidence for unique regulation of glut4 trafficking by insulin and amp-activated protein kinase activators in l6 myotubes. *J Biol Chem* 2010;**285**:1653–60.
112. Whitehead JP, Soos MA, Aslesen R, O'Rahilly S, Jensen J. Contraction inhibits insulin-stimulated insulin receptor substrate-1/2-associated phosphoinositide 3-kinase activity, but not protein kinase B activation or glucose uptake, in rat muscle. *Biochem J* 2000;**349**:775–81.
113. Sakamoto K, Arnolds DE, Fujii N, Kramer HF, Hirshman MF, Goodyear LJ. Role of Akt2 in contraction-stimulated cell signaling and glucose uptake in skeletal muscle. *Am J Physiol Endocrinol Metab* 2006;**291**:E1031–7.
114. Richter EA, Ruderman NB. AMPK and the biochemistry of exercise: implications for human health and disease. *Biochem J* 2009;**418**:261–75.
115. Steinberg GR, Kemp BE. AMPK in health and disease. *Physiol Rev* 2009;**89**:1025–78.
116. Hawley SA, Boudeau J, Reid JL, Mustard KJ, Udd L, Makela TP, et al. Complexes between the LKB1 tumor suppressor, STRAD alpha/beta and MO5 alpha/beta are upstream kinases in the AMP-activated protein kinase cascade. *J Biol* 2003;**2**:28.
117. Woods A, Johnstone SR, Dickerson K, Leiper FC, Fryer LG, Neumann D, et al. LKB1 is the upstream kinase in the AMP-activated protein kinase cascade. *Curr Biol* 2003;**13**:2004–8.
118. Hawley SA, Pan DA, Mustard KJ, Ross L, Bain J, Edelman AM, et al. Calmodulin-dependent protein kinase kinase-beta is an alternative upstream kinase for AMP-activated protein kinase. *Cell Metab* 2005;**2**:9–19.
119. Woods A, Dickerson K, Heath R, Hong SP, Momcilovic M, Johnstone SR, et al. Ca^{2+}/calmodulin-dependent protein kinase

kinase-beta acts upstream of AMP-activated protein kinase in mammalian cells. *Cell Metab* 2005;**2**:21–33.

120. Suter M, Riek U, Tuerk R, Schlattner U, Wallimann T, Neumann D. Dissecting the role of 5′-AMP for allosteric stimulation, activation, and deactivation of AMP-activated protein kinase. *J Biol Chem* 2006;**281**:32207–16.
121. Sanders MJ, Grondin PO, Hegarty BD, Snowden MA, Carling D. Investigating the mechanism for amp activation of the amp-activated protein kinase cascade. *Biochem J* 2007;**403**:139–48.
122. Bland ML, Birnbaum MJ. Adapting to energetic stress. *Science* 2011;**332**:1387–8.
123. Oakhill JS, Steel R, Chen Z-P, Scott JW, Ling N, Tam S, Kemp BE. AMPK is a direct adenylate charge-regulated protein kinase. *Science* 2011;**332**:1433–5.
124. Xiao B, Sanders MJ, Underwood E, Heath R, Mayer FV, Carmena D, et al. Structure of mammalian ampk and its regulation by ADP. *Nature* 2011;**472**:230–3.
125. Holmes BF, Lang DB, Birnbaum MJ, Mu J, Dohm GL. AMP kinase is not required for the Glut4 response to exercise and denervation in skeletal muscle. *Am J Physiol Endocrinol Metab* 2004;**287**:E739–43.
126. Mu J, Brozinick Jr JT, Valladares O, Bucan M, Birnbaum MJ. A role for AMP-activated protein kinase in contraction- and hypoxia-regulated glucose transport in skeletal muscle. *Mol. Cell* 2001;**7**:1085–94.
127. Koh H-J, Toyoda T, Fujii N, Jung MM, Rathod A, Middelbeek RJ-W, et al. Sucrose nonfermenting AMPK-related kinase (SNARK) mediates contraction-stimulated glucose transport in mouse skeletal muscle. *Proc Natl Acad Sci USA* 2010;**107**:15541–6.
128. Zong H, Ren JM, Young LH, Pypaert M, Mu J, Birnbaum MJ, et al. AMP kinase is required for mitochondrial biogenesis in skeletal muscle in response to chronic energy deprivation. *Proc Natl Acad Sci USA* 2002;**99**:15983–7.
129. Befroy DE, Petersen KF, Dufour S, Mason GF, Rothman DL, Shulman GI. Increased substrate oxidation and mitochondrial uncoupling in skeletal muscle of endurance-trained individuals. *Proc Natl Acad Sci USA* 2008;**105**:16701–6.
130. Garcia-Roves PM, Osler ME, Holmstrom MH, Zierath JR. Gain-of-function r225q mutation in AMP-activated protein kinase gamma3 subunit increases mitochondrial biogenesis in glycolytic skeletal muscle. *J Biol Chem* 2008;**283**:35724–34.
131. Rockl KS, Hirshman MF, Brandauer J, Fujii N, Witters LA, Goodyear LJ. Skeletal muscle adaptation to exercise training: AMP-activated protein kinase mediates muscle fiber type shift. *Diabetes* 2007;**56**:2062–9.
132. Irrcher I, Ljubicic V, Kirwan AF, Hood DA. AMP-activated protein kinase-regulated activation of the PGC-1alpha promoter in skeletal muscle cells. *PLoS One* 2008;**3**:e3614.
133. Handschin C, Chin S, Li P, Liu F, Maratos-Flier E, Lebrasseur NK, et al. Skeletal muscle fiber-type switching, exercise intolerance, and myopathy in PGC-1alpha muscle-specific knock-out animals. *J Biol Chem* 2007;**282**:30014–21.
134. Leone TC, Lehman JJ, Finck BN, Schaeffer PJ, Wende AR, Boudina S, et al. PGC-1alpha deficiency causes multi-system energy metabolic derangements: muscle dysfunction, abnormal weight control and hepatic steatosis. *PLoS Biol* 2005;**3**:e101.
135. Lin J, Wu PH, Tarr PT, Lindenberg KS, St-Pierre J, Zhang CY, et al. Defects in adaptive energy metabolism with CNS-linked hyperactivity in PGC-1alpha null mice. *Cell* 2004;**119**:121–35.
136. Yan Z, Okutsu M, Akhtar YN, Lira VA. Regulation of exercise-induced fiber type transformation, mitochondrial biogenesis, and angiogenesis in skeletal muscle. *J Appl Physiol* 2011;**110**:264–74.
137. Canto C, Gerhart-Hines Z, Feige JN, Lagouge M, Noriega L, Milne JC, et al. AMPK regulates energy expenditure by modulating Nad+ metabolism and SIRT1 activity. *Nature* 2009;**458**:1056–60.
138. Pehmøller C, Treebak JT, Birk JB, Chen S, MacKintosh C, Hardie DG, et al. Genetic disruption of AMPK signaling abolishes both contraction- and insulin-stimulated TBC1D1 phosphorylation and 14-3-3 binding in mouse skeletal muscle. *Am J Physiol Endocrinol Metabol* 2009;**297**:E665–75.
139. Taylor EB, An D, Kramer HF, Yu H, Fujii NL, Roeckl KSC, et al. Discovery of TBC1D1 as an insulin-, aicar-, and contraction-stimulated signaling nexus in mouse skeletal muscle. *J Biol Chem* 2008;**283**:9787–96.
140. Meyre D, Farge M, Lecoeur C, Proenca C, Durand E, Allegaert F, et al. R125w coding variant in TBC1D1 confers risk for familial obesity and contributes to linkage on chromosome 4p14 in the French population. *Hum Mol Genet* 2008;**17**:1798–802.
141. Stone S, Abkevich V, Russell DL, Riley R, Timms K, Tran T, et al. TBC1D1 is a candidate for a severe obesity gene and evidence for a gene/gene interaction in obesity predisposition. *Hum Mol Genet* 2006;**15**:2709–20.
142. An D, Toyoda T, Taylor EB, Yu H, Fujii N, Hirshman MF, et al. TBC1D1 regulates insulin- and contraction-induced glucose transport in mouse skeletal muscle. *Diabetes* 2010;**59**:1358–65.
143. Geraghty KM, Chen S, Harthill JE, Ibrahim AF, Toth R, Morrice NA, et al. Regulation of multisite phosphorylation and 14-3-3 binding of as160 in response to IGF-1, EGF, PMA and AICAR. *Biochem J* 2007;**407**:231–41.
144. Chen S, Murphy J, Toth R, Campbell DG, Morrice NA, Mackintosh C. Complementary regulation of TBC1D1 and AS160 by growth factors, insulin and AMPK activators. *Biochem J* 2008;**409**:449–59.
145. Brushia RJ, Walsh DA. Phosphorylase kinase: the complexity of its regulation is reflected in the complexity of its structure. *Front Biosci* 1999;**4**:D618–41.
146. Havel RJ, Naimark A, Borchgrevink CF. Turnover rate and oxidation of free fatty acids of blood plasma in man during exercise: studies during continuous infusion of palmitate-1-C14. *J Clin Invest* 1963;**42**:1054–63.
147. Ahlborg G, Felig P, Hagenfeldt L, Hendler R, Wahren J. Substrate turnover during prolonged exercise in man. Splanchnic and leg metabolism of glucose, free fatty acids, and amino acids. *J Clin Invest* 1974;**53**:1080–90.
148. Sidossis LS, Wolfe RR, Coggan AR. Regulation of fatty acid oxidation in untrained vs. trained men during exercise. *Am J Physiol* 1998;**274**:E510–5.
149. Romijn JA, Coyle EF, Sidossis LS, Gastaldelli A, Horowitz JF, Endert E, et al. Regulation of endogenous fat and carbohydrate metabolism in relation to exercise intensity and duration. *Am J Physiol* 1993;**265**:E380–91.

150. van Loon LJC, Koopman R, Stegen JHCH, Wagenmakers AJM, Keizer HA, Saris WHM. Intramyocellular lipids form an important substrate source during moderate intensity exercise in endurance-trained males in a fasted state. *J Physiol* 2003;**553**:611–25.
151. Shaw CS, Clark J, Wagenmakers AJM. The effect of exercise and nutrition on intramuscular fat metabolism and insulin sensitivity. *Annu Rev Nutr* 2010;**30**:13–34.
152. Moro C, Bajpeyi S, Smith SR. Determinants of intramyocellular triglyceride turnover: implications for insulin sensitivity. *Am J Physiol Endocrinol Metab* 2008;**294**:E203–13.
153. Jocken JWE, Blaak EE. Catecholamine-induced lipolysis in adipose tissue and skeletal muscle in obesity. *Physiol Behav* 2008;**94**:219–30.
154. Roepstorff C, Vistisen B, Donsmark M, Nielsen JN, Galbo H, Green KA, et al. Regulation of hormone-sensitive lipase activity and Ser563 and Ser565 phosphorylation in human skeletal muscle during exercise. *J Physiol* 2004;**560**:551–62.
155. Haemmerle G, Lass A, Zimmermann R, Gorkiewicz G, Meyer C, Rozman J, et al. Defective lipolysis and altered energy metabolism in mice lacking adipose triglyceride lipase. *Science* 2006;**312**:734–7.
156. Zimmermann R, Strauss JG, Haemmerle G, Schoiswohl G, Birner-Gruenberger R, Riederer M, et al. Fat mobilization in adipose tissue is promoted by adipose triglyceride lipase. *Science* 2004;**306**:1383–6.
157. Haemmerle G, Zimmermann R, Hayn M, Theussl C, Waeg G, Wagner E, et al. Hormone-sensitive lipase deficiency in mice causes diglyceride accumulation in adipose tissue, muscle, and testis. *J Biol Chem* 2002;**277**:4806–15.
158. Jocken JW, Smit E, Goossens GH, Essers YP, van Baak MA, Mensink M, et al. Adipose triglyceride lipase (atgl) expression in human skeletal muscle is type i (oxidative) fiber specific. *Histochem Cell Biol* 2008;**129**:535–8.
159. Chanarin I, Patel A, Slavin G, Wills EJ, Andrews TM, Stewart G. Neutral-lipid storage disease: A new disorder of lipid metabolism. *Br Med J* 1975;**1**:553–5.
160. Lefevre C, Jobard F, Caux F, Bouadjar B, Karaduman A, Heilig R, et al. Mutations in CGI-58, the gene encoding a new protein of the esterase/lipase/thioesterase subfamily, in Chanarin–Dorfman syndrome. *Am J Hum Genet* 2001;**69**:1002–12.
161. Fischer J, Lefevre C, Morava E, Mussini JM, Laforet P, Negre-Salvayre A, et al. The gene encoding adipose triglyceride lipase (PNPLA2) is mutated in neutral lipid storage disease with myopathy. *Nat Genet* 2007;**39**:28–30.
162. Schoiswohl G, Schweiger M, Schreiber R, Gorkiewicz G, Preiss-Landl K, Taschler U, et al. Adipose triglyceride lipase plays a key role in the supply of the working muscle with fatty acids. *J Lipid Res* 2010;**51**:490–9.
163. Abdul-Ghani MA, Defronzo RA. Pathogenesis of insulin resistance in skeletal muscle. *J Biomed Biotechnol* 2010;**2010**:1–20.
164. Petersen KF, Shulman GI. Pathogenesis of skeletal muscle insulin resistance in type 2 diabetes mellitus. *Am J Cardiol* 2002;**90**:11–8.
165. Storlien L, Oakes ND, Kelley DE. Metabolic flexibility. *Proc Nutr Soc* 2004;**63**:363–8.

Chapter 60

Skeletal Muscle Fiber Types

Stefano Schiaffino[1,2] and Carlo Reggiani[2,3]
[1]*Venetian Institute of Molecular Medicine (VIMM),* [2]*Consiglio Nazionale delle Ricerche (CNR) Institute of Neurosciences,* [3]*Department of Biomedical Sciences, University of Padua, Padua, Italy*

The existence of muscle heterogeneity has been recognized since the 17th century, when Lorenzini first described white and red muscles in the elasmobranch *Torpedo*, and functional differences between skeletal muscles were described in the 19th century, when Ranvier first reported that rabbit red muscles contracted more slowly than white muscles. More recent studies have revealed the existence of a variety of muscle fiber types with distinct morphological, biochemical, and physiological properties. In this chapter we will mostly focus on fiber types in mammalian skeletal muscle (see reference 1 for a more comprehensive recent review).

DIVERSITY OF MUSCLES, MOTOR UNITS, AND MUSCLE FIBER TYPES

The human body, like the body of all vertebrates, contains a variety of skeletal muscles which differ in anatomical features (location, shape, size, color, tendon and bone insertions, innervation), embryological origin (somitic vs. non somitic origin), and physiological properties (type of movement, force, speed of shortening, power, resistance to fatigue). Muscle heterogeneity reflects the presence of distinct muscle functional units, the motor units, and distinct fiber types.

Major Muscle Fiber Types

Mammalian muscle fibers have been traditionally classified, using enzyme histochemical reactions for myosin ATPase, as type 1 or slow and type 2 or fast fibers, the latter comprising two subsets, type 2A and 2B (see reference 2 for the evolution of the notion of muscle fiber types). The current nomenclature, based on myosin heavy chain (MyHC) isoform composition, includes an additional fast fiber type, called type 2X. These four fiber populations can be identified by immunofluorescence staining using specific anti-MyHC antibodies (3) (Figure 60.1) or by in situ hybridization using probes specific for the corresponding mRNAs (4). An alternative method is the electrophoretic separation of the MyHCs as distinct bands in SDS-PAGE gels of single muscle fibers (5). Both approaches show that, in addition to pure fiber types, skeletal muscles contain hybrid fibers with mixed MyHC composition, supporting the existence of a spectrum of fiber types: 1 ↔ 1/2A ↔ 2A ↔ 2A/2X ↔ 2X ↔ 2X/2B ↔ 2B. Physiological studies of single fibers have shown that MyHC distribution correlates with speed of shortening, which is progressively higher from type 1 to type 2A, 2X, and 2B fibers. Muscle fibers also differ in metabolic properties, specifically in the relative prevalence of oxidative vs. glycolytic metabolism: type 1 fibers have abundant oxidative enzyme and myoglobin complement and lower levels of glycolytic enzymes, whereas at the other extreme, type 2B fibers have an opposite metabolic profile. Thus muscles with prevalent type 1 fiber type profile appear as red muscles to the naked eye, whereas muscles with prevalent type 2B fiber composition appears as white muscles. Type 2A and 2X fibers are also highly oxidative in mouse and rat, but less so in human muscle (see below). The oxidative enzyme level in the various fibers reflects the relative abundance of mitochondria, as determined by electron microscopy; other discriminating ultrastructural features are the volume and surface area of the sarcoplasmic reticulum, which is greater in type 2 compared to type 1 fibers, and the structure of the Z-disc of the sarcomeres, which is thicker in type 1 and 2A compared to type 2B fibers (6,7).

Motor Unit Diversity

Muscle fibers are organized in motor units, each composed of a group of fibers with similar MyHC profile innervated by a single α-motor neuron. The classic work of Kugelberg (8) and Burke (9) has led to the demonstration of the homogeneous fiber type composition of each motor unit and the identification of three major types of units: slow (S), fast-fatigue resistant (FR), and fast-fatigable (FF), composed of type 1, 2A, and 2B fibers, respectively. An additional motor unit type with intermediate

Muscle. DOI: http://dx.doi.org/10.1016/B978-0-12-381510-1.00060-0

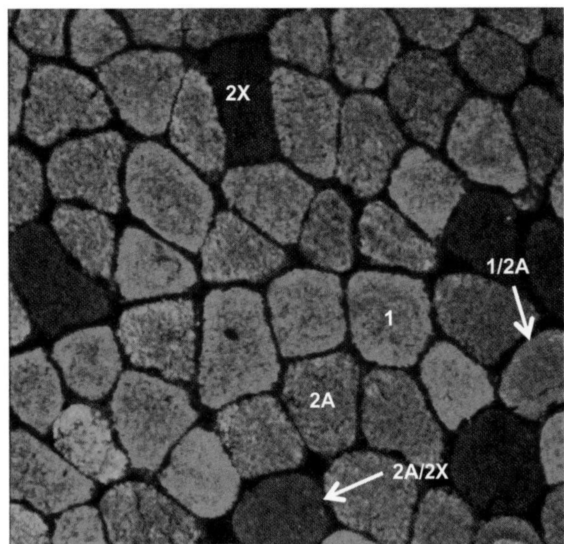

FIGURE 60.1 **Distribution of different MyHCs detected by immunofluorescence in the mouse slow soleus muscle.** This muscle is composed predominantly of type 1 fibers, expressing MyHC-β/slow, and type 2A fibers, expressing MyHC-2A. Rare unstained type 2X fibers are also present, whereas type 2B fibers are absent in this muscle. Hybrid type1/2A and type 2A/2X fibers are indicated by arrows. *(From Schiaffino, 2010 (2); courtesy of S. Ciciliot.)*

properties, composed of type 2X fibers, was subsequently identified (10). The motor unit resistance to fatigue is closely correlated with the oxidative enzyme activity in the component muscle fibers: FF units composed of glycolytic type 2B fibers cannot maintain force production for more than a few minutes following repetitive stimulation, whereas units composed of mitochondria-rich type 2A fibers are much more resistant to fatigue, though less so than slow units (8). Slow motor neurons are smaller in size and more easily recruited, as determined by intracellular recording of individual motor neurons. Unfortunately, no specific molecular marker for fast and slow α-motor neurons is presently available. A distinctive feature is the motor neuron firing pattern, which has been characterized using continuous electromyography recording of single motor units in freely moving animals. Rat slow motor units are continuously active for many hours (5–8 hours over 24 hours) with long-lasting trains (300–500 s) and relatively low frequency of firing (~20 Hz). In contrast, fast motor units show sporadic bursts of higher frequency of firing (~50–90 Hz) and comprise two types of units: motor units with very low amount of activity per day (0.5–3 min over 24 hr) and short duration of the trains (<3 s), probably corresponding to units composed of 2B fibers, and motor units with greater activity per day (23–72 min over 24 hr) and longer train duration (60–140 s), presumably corresponding to units composed of 2A or 2X fibers (11). The properties of the various muscle fiber types, including membrane properties, Ca^{2+} homeostasis, contractile mechanism and energy metabolism, are adapted to these different patterns of activity (see below).

Species and Individual Variability in Muscle Fiber Type Profile

The fiber type profile of skeletal muscles shows major variations among species (see reference 1). In small mammals, like the mouse, most muscles are composed of type 2B and 2X fibers with abundant mitochondrial complement, and type 1 fibers are confined to rare muscles, such as the soleus. The muscles of the common shrew, the smallest mammalian species, contain exclusively type 2X and 2B fibers, and mitochondrial volume represent more than 35% of the fiber volume. In contrast, human skeletal muscles, like the muscle of many large mammals, consist predominantly of type 1 and 2A fibers, and mitochondrial volume density is about 2–5% of the fiber volume. In addition, MyHC-2B is not detectable in most human muscles, although the corresponding *MYH4* gene is present in the genome, and fibers previously classified as type 2B based on ATPase histochemistry are in fact type 2X based on MyHC composition (12). The relative proportion of fiber types also varies between individuals: in the human vastus lateralis muscle, type 1 fibers may vary from 15% to 85% of the whole fiber population (13). These variations, which are largely due to genetic factors (14), are of interest in sport physiology, as they are often, but not always, associated with better performance in specific sports – for example type 2 fibers tend to predominate in sprint runners and type 1 fibers in endurance runners.

Minor Fiber Populations in Head Muscles and in Muscle Spindles

In addition to the four major fiber type populations, widely distributed in all body muscles, there are several minor fiber types with restricted distribution to specialized head and neck muscles, including extraocular, jaw and pharyngeal muscles, and in the proprioceptive sensory organs of skeletal muscles, the muscle spindles. With the recent demonstration that *MYH7b* and *MYH15* genes code for MyHCs selectively expressed in extraocular muscles and muscle spindles at the protein level (15), a complete picture of sarcomeric MyHC protein distribution in mammalian skeletal muscles is now available (Figure 60.2). Other MyHCs with restricted distribution to head muscles and muscle spindles include MyHC-EO, present in extraocular muscles, MyHC-M, present in jaw muscles in some mammalian species (carnivores and primates, except man), MyHC-α, which is normally expressed only in cardiac muscle but is present in jaw

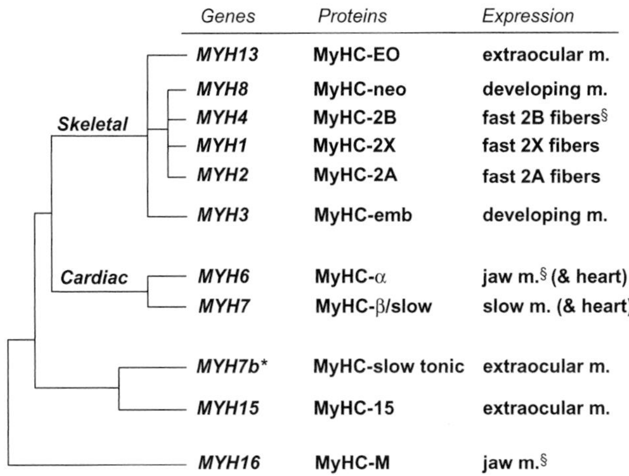

Genes
Proteins
Expression
Skeletal
Cardiac
MYH13 MyHC-EO extraocular m.
MYH8 MyHC-neo developing m.
MYH4 MyHC-2B fast 2B fibers§
MYH1 MyHC-2X fast 2X fibers
MYH2 MyHC-2A fast 2A fibers
MYH3 MyHC-emb developing m.
MYH6 MyHC-α jaw m.§ (& heart)
MYH7 MyHC-β/slow slow m. (& heart)
MYH7b* MyHC-slow tonic extraocular m.
MYH15 MyHC-15 extraocular m.
MYH16 MyHC-M jaw m.§

FIGURE 60.2 **Sarcomeric *MYH* genes with the corresponding protein products and their expression pattern in mammalian striated muscles.** The evolutionary relationship between *MYH* genes is indicated in the phylogenetic tree on the left (spacing and length of the branches not in scale). §Expression detected only in some mammalian species. **MYH7b* is expressed in both slow muscles and heart at the transcript level, but only in extraocular muscles at the protein level (15). *(Scheme modified from Schiaffino and Reggiani, 2011 (1) and Rossi et al., 2010 (15).)*

muscles in some mammalian species, as well as MyHCs typical of developing muscle, MyHC-emb, and MyHC-neo, which are also expressed in adult extraocular muscles.

MUSCLE FIBER TYPES DURING DEVELOPMENT AND AGING

Heterogeneity of Myoblast Lineages and Emergence of Fiber Types in Developing Muscle

The notion that muscle fiber diversification in embryonic skeletal muscle is independent of innervation, first proposed by Stockdale for avian muscle (16), has been confirmed in mammals with the demonstration that fiber types with different MyHC composition, in particular with differential distribution of MyHC-neo and MyHC-β/slow, are detectable in aneural muscles of E20 rat fetuses following β-bungarotoxin-mediated elimination of motor neurons prior to hindlimb muscle innervation (17). Muscle is formed in successive waves during embryonic development: primary and secondary generation fibers differ in myosin composition, and the latter show a greater dependence on innervation for their formation and survival (18). The existence of an intrinsic heterogeneity of myoblast lineages in developing skeletal muscle is further supported by the finding that head muscles, which have unique MyHC composition, derive from presomitic cranial mesoderm rather than from the somites like most body muscles, and during embryonic development show a distinct requirement for transcription factors involved in myogenesis, for example are dependent on *Pitx2* and *Tbx1* rather than *Pax3* and *Pax7* like trunk and limb muscles. The homeodomain transcription factor of the Six family and their coactivator, such as the protein phosphatase Eya1, are implicated in fiber type specification during embryonic development. Six factors appear to control the fast gene program, as *Six1*-*Six4* double knockout mice show specific downregulation of many fast-type genes already in E10.5 somites (19). On the other hand the slow program in embryonic muscle is controlled by the transcription factor Sox6, as a fast-to-slow switch is induced by Sox6 knockout (see below). Unique regulatory mechanisms are involved in the differentiation of intrafusal fibers, whose formation is dependent on sensory innervation (see reference 1).

Heterogeneity of Satellite Cells in Regenerating Muscles

Myogenic cell heterogeneity is apparently maintained in adult muscle satellite cells, the myogenic stem cells responsible for muscle regeneration. Satellite cells isolated from cat jaw muscles were found to express in culture the unique myofibrillar proteins of jaw muscles, which are not detected in cultures of satellite cells from leg muscles (20). However, MyHCs specific to extraocular muscles were not detected in cultures of satellite cells from adult extraocular muscles (21). Even satellite cells from leg fast twitch and slow twitch muscles are not apparently identical, as suggested by stimulation experiments in regenerating muscles. In this model, the regenerating rat slow soleus muscle acquires the typical slow phenotype only in the presence of innervation, whereas a default fast-like gene program is activated in the absence of innervation (22–24). The effect of the nerve can be reproduced by electrical stimulation with an impulse pattern typical of slow motor neurons. However, the same stimulation pattern is unable to induce significant upregulation of the slow program in a regenerating denervated fast muscle, suggesting the existence of intrinsic differences between satellite cell populations from fast and slow muscles (25).

Changes in Fiber Types during Postnatal Development, Adulthood, and Aging

A number of changes take place in rat and mouse skeletal muscles during the first weeks of postnatal development. The most important is the upregulation of fast 2A, 2X, and 2B MyHC transcripts and proteins with the emergence of the corresponding fiber types (4). This occurs concomitantly with the progressive disappearance of the developmental myosins, MyHC-emb and -neo, which tend to persist for longer periods in type 2A fibers (26). Neonatal denervation experiments show that the switch from developmental to adult fast myosins takes place independently of innervation (27), but is likely dependent on thyroid hormone, which rises at birth (28). In contrast, the maintenance of fiber type profile in slow muscles is dependent on innervation, as slow myosin progressively decreases in the rat soleus after neonatal denervation and is no longer detectable by one month (29). Further remodeling of the fiber type profile occurs throughout postnatal development in mouse and rat skeletal muscles: in the rat, type 2A fibers are transformed into type 1 fibers in the developing slow soleus muscle, whereas in the mouse, type 1 fibers present in neonatal fast muscles disappear during later stages. The reported slight increase in type 1 fibers described in some transgenic models might thus simply reflect the persistence of a neonatal profile rather than a real switch in fiber type composition.

Skeletal muscle fibers can change their phenotype during adulthood under the influence of hormones and in relation to motor neuron firing pattern. Among hormones, glucocorticoids can induce a fast-to-slow transition (30), while thyroid hormones and, to a lesser extent, catecholamines trigger a shift towards a fast phenotype (31,32). As initially demonstrated by cross-innervation experiments (33), neural influence is a major determinant of fiber type specification. Denervation of a slow muscle is followed by a shift towards fast phenotype (34). Chronic electrical stimulation with an impulse pattern characterized by high amounts of daily activity with low frequency of discharge leads to development of a slow fiber phenotype, while low amounts of activity with short high frequency bursts are associated with a fast fiber phenotype (35,36). The study of the effects of thyroid state (hypothyroidism and hyperthyroidism) and of electrical stimulation has supported the development of a model of sequential transition of fiber types (Figure 60.3A). The changes in the fiber phenotype are generally incomplete, suggesting the existence of intrinsic differences between muscles and of "adaptive ranges" of fiber transformations (Figure 60.3B,C).

During aging, skeletal muscles undergo progressive decrease in size and force, with muscle fiber atrophy, loss of muscle fibers and motor neurons, and remodeling of motor units due to denervation–reinnervation processes (38). In humans, type 2 fibers undergo greater atrophy than type 1 fibers, leading to a global reduction of fast MyHCs but without significant changes in the fiber type profile (39). In aging rat skeletal muscles, the contraction and half-relaxation time of the isometric twitch tend to increase, due to (i) changes in sarcoplasmic reticulum volume and function (40) and (ii) age-related type 2B to 2X fiber type switching (41).

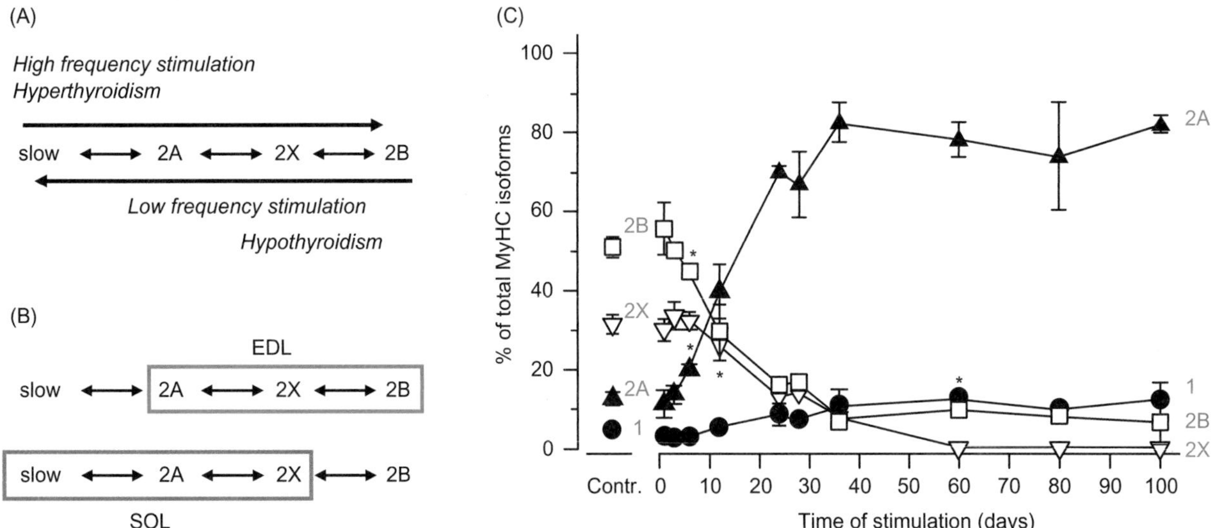

FIGURE 60.3 **Modulation of the fiber type profile and its limits.** (A) High frequency stimulation, typical of the firing pattern of fast motor neurons, as well as hyperthyroidism, tend to induce fiber type shifts in the direction slow → 2A → 2X → 2B, whereas low frequency stimulation, mimicking the firing pattern of slow motor neurons, as well as hypothyroidism, induce fiber type shifts in the opposite direction 2B → 2X → 2A → slow. (B) Adaptive ranges of fiber type plasticity. In fast rodent muscles, such as the extensor digitorum longus (EDL), it is possible to induce changes in the range 2A ↔ 2X ↔ 2B, but it is difficult to induce a shift from fast to slow fiber type. In contrast, in the slow soleus (SOL), it is possible to induce changes in the range slow ↔ 2A ↔ 2X, but it is difficult to induce a shift to the 2B fiber type. (C) Time course of changes in relative concentrations of MyHC protein isoforms in rat EDL in response to chronic low-frequency stimulation. *, First time points at which changes of the individual MyHC isoforms showed significant difference from control. *(Modified from Jaschinski et al., 1998 (37).)*

MOLECULAR AND FUNCTIONAL DIFFERENCES AMONG MUSCLE FIBER TYPES

When muscle fine structure is examined by electron microscopy, the similarity between muscle fibers in all animal species is remarkable. For example, the structure of the sarcomere is highly conserved in all muscle fibers of all vertebrates. The same holds true for the molecular architecture, as all muscle fibers are virtually composed of the same proteins. However, in spite of the apparent similarity, muscle fibers show high diversity in their functional properties, such as mechanical power output, speed of shortening, and resistance to fatigue. Although most studies usually focus on contractile response and metabolism as the two major areas of muscle fiber heterogeneity, fiber type diversity extends to any subcellular system, including sarcolemma and sarcoplasmic reticulum (SR).

Muscle Fiber Excitability: Neuromuscular Junctions and Sarcolemma

As discussed above, motor neuron discharge pattern is highly different in slow and fast motor units, and the structure of the neuromuscular junctions (NMJs) is adapted to these patterns (11). NMJs are specialized to achieve a greater safety of transmission in short and high-frequency bursts of fast motor units and to resist synaptic depression during prolonged repetitive stimulation in slow motor units (42). In NMJs of fast fibers, the greater transmission safety is achieved with a higher number of acetylcholine quanta released after each action potential from the nerve terminal, a greater density of acetylcholine receptors, a greater density of voltage-dependent sodium channels in the postsynaptic folds and in the surrounding region. In NMJs of slow fibers, a lower synaptic depression allows a sustained response to motor neurons during repetitive discharge.

The ionic conductances of the sarcolemma in the different fiber types are dictated by the motor neuron discharge patterns. Fast fibers are required to respond with an action potential following high-frequency discharge, while slow fibers must be able to keep their electrical response during prolonged period of activity. When compared to slow fibers, fast fibers shows a more negative resting membrane potential, possibly in relation to higher ionic conductances at rest (Cl and K) (43), and show higher Na conductance during action potential and specific inactivation kinetics (44). The T-tubules, invaginations of the sarcolemma, are more extensively developed in fast fibers (45). In addition, voltage sensor calcium channels, i.e. the skeletal muscle isoforms of dihydropyridine receptor (DHPR), are more abundant in the T-tubules of fast fibers: this is likely instrumental to a more efficient coupling between membrane depolarization and calcium release (46). Ca entry, however, is greater in slow compared to fast fibers both at rest and during depolarization (47,48). Na/K pump plays an essential role in keeping ionic gradients, not only at rest but also during contractile activity. The activity of Na/K pump is higher in fast than in slow fibers at rest, but such ratio is inverted during prolonged activity due to more efficient activation of the pump in slow fibers (49).

Mechanical Properties during Contraction and at Rest: Sarcomeric Motors and Cytoskeleton

The scarce daily amount of activity of the fast muscle fibers is closely related to their contractile specialization, as such fibers are able to develop high tension and high mechanical power and are, therefore, employed for rapid and strong movements. In contrast, slow fibers are employed in tasks requiring less power and tension, but are specialized to minimize energy expenditure and to avoid fatigue. The molecular basis of the specialized contractile performance can be found in the specific isoforms of sarcomeric proteins expressed by fast and slow fibers (Figure 60.4). Actually, the conversion of the chemical energy of ATP into mechanical energy (work) and heat occurs at different rates depending mainly on the specific myosin isoforms. Fast fibers, with their subtypes 2A, 2X, and 2B, develop more tension than slow fibers during maximal contraction (50,51) and, if allowed to shorten, reach a higher speed of shortening against any given load, thus producing different force velocity curves (50) (Figure 60.5A). Also, mechanical power, which is the rate of generation of work and is the most relevant parameter for limb or body movement, reaches different values in relation to the myosin isoform expressed by the fibers (Figure 60.5B). The values of both shortening velocity and peak power progressively increase from slow to fast 2A, fast 2X, and fast 2B. The ATP hydrolysis rate also differs between slow and fast fibers. The cost of tension development in ATP is much lower in slow than in fast fibers (53,54), while the ATP hydrolysis rate during shortening is approximately in proportion to power output and this implies a similar efficiency of chemo-mechanical energy conversion regardless of myosin isoform expression (55). On the whole, the mechanical and energetic parameters of the contractile response make slow fibers more suitable for low intensity and long-lasting activity and fast fibers for short and strong contractile performance.

The myofibrils, where myosin and actin interaction produce force and movement, are part of the cytoskeleton, i.e. the cellular scaffolding responsible not only for determining

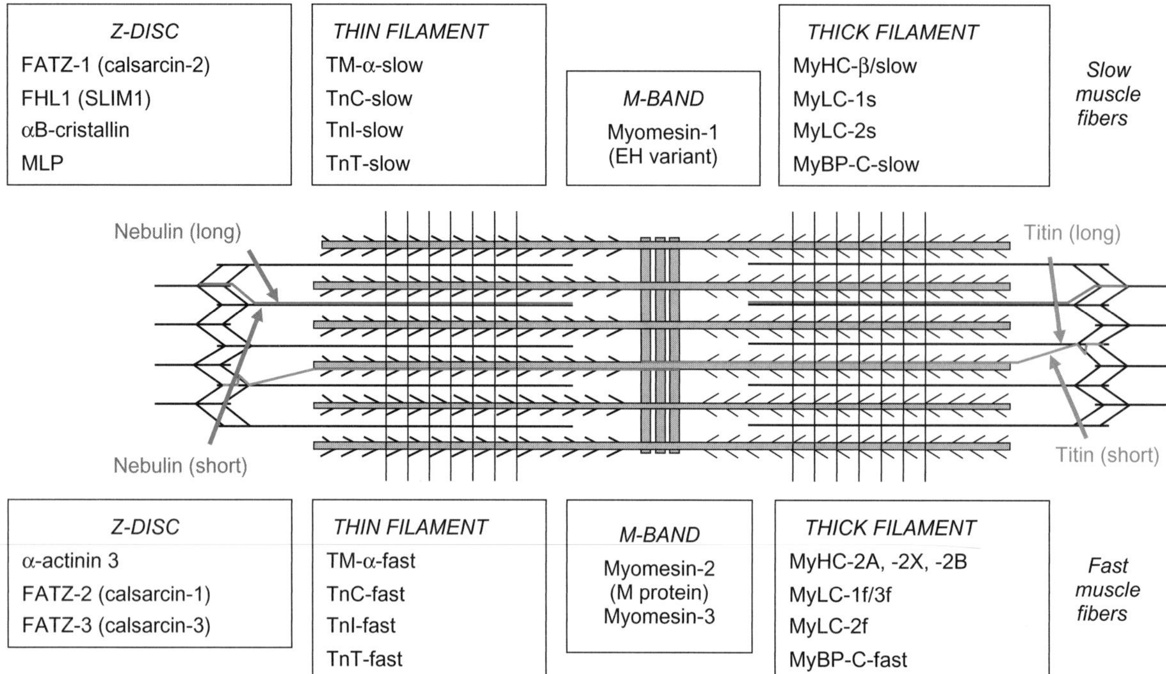

FIGURE 60.4 **Main contractile and cytoskeletal proteins of the sarcomere which show differential distribution between fast and slow muscles.** Isoforms prevalent in slow muscles are indicated in the upper part of the figure, fast isoforms in the lower part. Slow muscles are also characterized by longer nebulin and titin isoforms compared to fast muscles. FHL1, four and a half LIM domains 1; MLP, muscle LIM protein; TM, tropomyosin; Tn, troponin; MyHC, myosin heavy chain; MyLC, myosin light chain; MyBP-C, myosin binding protein C.

the shape and size (length) of muscle fibers, but also for transmitting the force and movement to the extracellular fibrous skeleton. Diversity among fibers is also detectable in the cytoskeleton, in particular in transversal protein aggregates forming the Z-discs, M-bands, and in longitudinally oriented sarcomeric giant proteins (titin and nebulin) (Figure 60.4). Slow fibers have thicker Z-discs and M-band, a feature that is probably related to the ability to withstand active force (56). Titin, the major determinant of resting tension, is present in slow fibers with longer and more extensible isoforms, thus allowing passive elongation with less mechanical resistance compared to fast fibers (different resting tension-length curve and viscoelasticity) (57). Slow fibers are also characterized by longer nebulin and actin filaments, which might imply that active tension-length curve and optimal length are shifted towards longer sarcomere length (57,58). It is worth recalling that, although fast fibers develop higher tension during isometric contractions, the difference disappears in eccentric contractions where the highest forces are generated (59). In such conditions, the ability to withstand tension without damage is greater in slow than in fast fibers (60).

Intracellular Ca^{2+} Kinetics

According to the classical nomenclature, fast twitch and slow twitch muscles are classified (61) with direct reference to time parameters, such as time to peak tension and half relaxation time, which characterize the isometric twitch, i.e. the contractile response to a single electrical stimulus. Such time parameters reflect the diversity in intracellular calcium kinetics and myofibrillar contractile response between fast twitch and slow twitch muscle fibers. In particular:

1. Fast fibers show lower cytosolic-free calcium concentration at rest than slow fibers, likely due to more powerful cytosolic buffering (parvalbumin, troponin C) and less calcium entry from extracellular space (47).
2. In fast fibers, the calcium transient following an action potential shows a greater amplitude and faster decay kinetics (Figure 60.5C) and this is due to a more developed SR (7,45) and a greater abundance of calcium release channels (ryanodine receptor, RyR), calcium pumps (sarcoplasmic endoplasmic reticulum Ca ATPase, SERCA), intraluminal calcium binding protein (calsequestrin, CASQ), and cytosolic buffers (parvalbumin) (62). It is not clear whether the different SERCA and CASQ isoforms (SERCA1a and CASQ1 in fast fibers, SERCA2a and both CASQ1 and CASQ2 in slow fibers) contribute to these differences.
3. Finally, while the myofibrils of slow fibers respond to lower calcium concentration (lower threshold), fast fibers are characterized by a higher calcium affinity

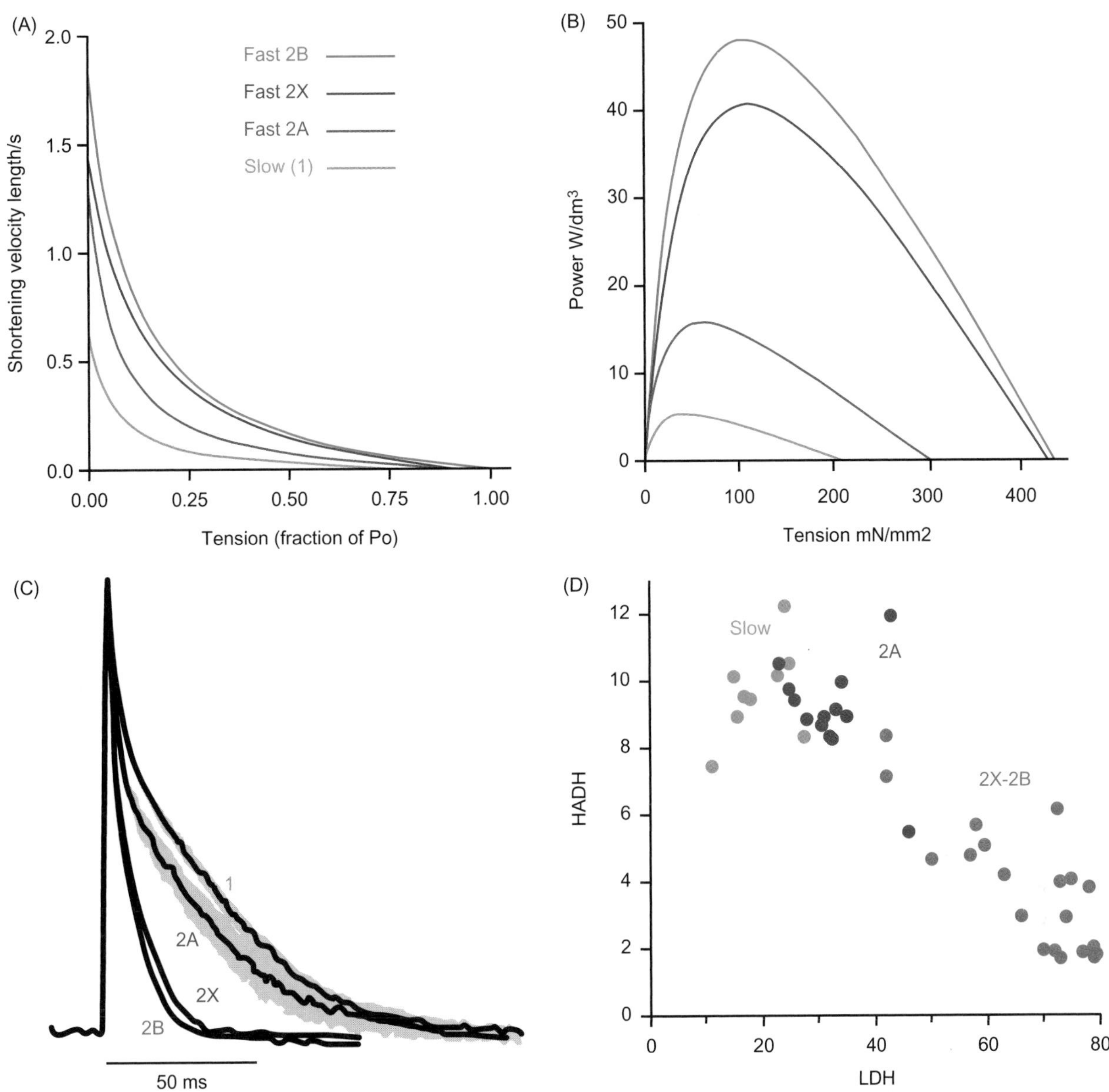

FIGURE 60.5 Diversity of functional parameters among muscle fiber types. (A) Force velocity curves of rat single fibers, maximally calcium activated at 12 °C, classified according to their myosin isoform content (redrawn from the data reported in Bottinelli et al. (50), table 3, according to the equation V = Vo.b.(1 − P/Po)/(Po.(P/Po + a). (B) Power force curves of the same four types of rat muscle fibers (same data as in panel A, equation W′ = P.V.Po). (C) Average cytosolic calcium transients following a single electrical stimulus detected with MagFluo-4AM in the four fiber types of mouse skeletal muscle, identified on the basis of their myosin isoform content. Peak amplitude has been equalized in all transients to better show the diversity in decay kinetics. (D) Lactate dehydrogenase (LDH) and hydroxyacyl CoA dehydrogenase (HADH) activities in rat plantaris single fibers assigned to their types on the basis of ATPase staining after alkali and acid preincubation. *(Panels (C) and (D) from Hintz et al., 1984 (52).)*

(or sensitivity, pCa50%) and a higher cooperativity in the response to calcium (63). This allows fast fibers to respond more quickly with tension to the rise of cytosolic calcium level. Such diversity in calcium sensitivity finds its molecular basis in the presence of specific isoforms of the regulatory proteins, troponin, and tropomyosin (64) (Figure 60.4).

Energy Supply: Glycolytic and Oxidative Metabolism

In contrast to the modest metabolic activity of muscle fibers at rest (65,66), during contraction large amounts of ATP are hydrolysed by the myosin motors (approximately 70% of the total) and by the ionic pumps, such as SERCA and Na/K ATPase (67). The available stores of ATP can provide energy to support contractile activity for only a few seconds, a time shorter in fast than in slow fibers. The earliest ATP regeneration is supported by creatine kinase (CK) and partly (up to 15%) by adenylate kinase (AK). AK is more active in fast than in slow fibers, thus causing greater AMP accumulation in fast than in slow fibers. AMP accumulation has two main effects: (i) activation of AMP kinase (AMPK) which is more effective in slow than in fast fibers and stimulates glucose intake and β-oxidation (68), and (ii) activation of AMP deaminase which produces IMP more effectively in fast than in slow fibers. IMP and AMP activate glycogenolysis more rapidly in fast than in slow fibers (69). ADP and creatine accumulation also follows the contractile activity and are important for triggering mitochondrial activation.

The second source of ATP regeneration is the glycolytic pathway which is about two times more effective in fast than in slow fibers (70). The end product of glycolysis is pyruvate, which can be either converted to lactate through lactate dehydrogenase (LDH) and exported or decarboxylated to acetyl-CoA through pyruvate dehydrogenase (PDH). PDH regulation via kinase (PDK) and phosphatase (PDP) is the switch between the two alternative pathways, the balance being inclined towards acetyl-CoA generation in slow fibers and towards conversion to lactate in fast fibers. Acetyl-CoA is the supply to the ATP regeneration based on tricarboxylic acid (TCA) cycle in the mitochondria and is more effective in slow than in fast fibers in relation to (i) greater mitochondrial density (71) and (ii) greater TCA cycle fuelling via β-oxidation which is about three times higher in slow oxidative than in fast glycolytic fibers (52). Thus, as shown in Figure 60.5D, in individual fibers the activity of LDH, typical of fast glycolytic fibers, and the activity of hydroxyacyl CoA dehydrogenase (HADH), typical of slow oxidative fibers, are inversely related (52). It is important to underline that in slow fibers, due to the lower ATP consumption, ATP regeneration based on mitochondrial respiration is sufficient to achieve a complete metabolic balance, which is a prerequisite to optimize resistance to fatigue. Such balance is never achieved in fast fibers.

SIGNALING PATHWAYS INVOLVED IN FIBER TYPE SPECIFICATION AND REMODELING

Different signaling pathways have been implicated in the specification of fast and slow fibers in embryonic muscle and in remodeling of the fiber type profile in adult skeletal muscles. However, a definitive picture is still missing and published diagrams depicting complex networks of transduction pathways and transcription factors potentially implicated in the fast/slow fiber type specification are often based on tenuous evidence. The differential distribution of a given factor in different fiber types is by no means evidence for a specific role, and the physiological significance of the effect of overexpression experiments in transgenic mice is doubtful. Only loss-of-function approaches are functionally relevant. Let us consider the postulated role of the myogenic regulatory factor myogenin. A role for myogenin was suggested by the higher level in slow muscle fibers (72) and by glycolytic-to-oxidative switch induced by myogenin overexpression in transgenic mice (73). However, myogenin gene inactivation induced after birth (myogenin knockout is lethal) is also accompanied by an increase in the proportion of oxidative fibers and type 1 fibers, and by increased endurance in treadmill running and voluntary wheel running (74). We will therefore consider here only those signaling pathways whose role is supported by loss-of-function experiments.

Calcineurin

The calcineurin-NFAT pathway is probably the best characterized signaling pathway with respect to muscle fiber type diversification. Calcineurin is a phosphatase activated by Ca^{2+} and calmodulin, whose major targets are the nuclear factor of activated T cells (NFAT) transcription factors. When dephosphorylated, NFATs translocate to the nucleus and modulate the expression of target genes. A slow-to-fast fiber type switch is induced by inactivation of the catalytic CnAα and CnAβ subunits of calcineurin in double null mice (75). A similar effect can be induced in adult slow muscles by treatment with the calcineurin inhibitor cyclosporin A (76), and by transfection with the calcineurin inhibitory protein domain from cain/cabin-1 (77). Accordingly, upregulation of the slow gene program in regenerating rat slow muscle, which is dependent on slow motor neuron activity, is completely prevented by transfection *in vivo* with the calcineurin inhibitory protein domain from cain/cabin-1 or by treatment with the calcineurin inhibitors, cyclosporin A, and FK506 (77). The effect of two other inhibitors of calcineurin, Rcan1 and calsarcin (FATZ, myozenin), is consistent with this role of calcineurin. Transgenic mice overexpressing Rcan1 have a normal fiber type profile at birth but then undergo a complete slow-to-fast switch with complete disappearance of slow fibers, suggesting that calcineurin signaling is not required for muscle fiber type specification in embryonic muscle but is essential for the slow motor neuron activity-dependent maintenance of the slow gene program (78). Inactivation of the calsarcin-1 gene leads to an increase in the number of slow fibers (79), while knockout of calsarcin-2 causes an increase of type 2A fast oxidative fibers and improved fatigue-resistance in fast muscle (80).

NFAT

NFAT transcription factors exist as four isoforms (NFATc1, c2, c3, and c4). They act as activity sensors in skeletal muscle, as shown by the finding that an NFATc1-GFP fusion protein has predominantly cytoplasmic localization in fast muscle but can be induced to translocate to the nucleus by low frequency stimulation, whereas it has a predominantly nuclear localization in slow muscle but translocates to the cytoplasm after denervation (81,82). An NFAT-luciferase reporter is likewise more active in slow than fast muscles, but is upregulated by stimulation in fast and downregulated by denervation in slow muscle (83). Selective inactivation of NFATc1 is embryonic lethal, while knockout of NFATc2 or NFATc3 has no apparent effect on fiber type profile, possibly due to redundant role of the various isoforms. However, the peptide inhibitor VIVIT, which blocks the interaction of all NFATs with calcineurin, blocks the upregulation of slow myosin in regenerating rat soleus and causes a rapid downregulation of MyHC-slow and upregulation of MyHC-2X and -2B transcripts in adult rat soleus (83). Selective silencing of NFAT isoform gene expression by RNAi suggests that NFATs may also be involved in the regulation of type 2 fiber subsets, as MyHC-2X and -2A promoter activity is inhibited by NFATc2, -c3 or -c4 RNAi, but not by NFATc1 knockdown, whereas MyHC-2B promoter activity is inhibited by NFATc4 RNAi, but not by NFATc1, -c2 or -c4 knockdown (84).

Other Signaling Pathways

The effect of NFAT in regulating the muscle fiber type can be potentiated by the transcription factors of the MEF2 gene family (MEF2a, -2b, -2c, -2d), as suggested by the finding that MEF2 activity is activated by calcineurin. Type 1 fibers in the mouse soleus are decreased by knockout of *Mef2c* or *Mef2d*, and increased by overexpression of an activated *Mef2c* (85). MEF2 activity is repressed by class II histone deacetylases (HDACs), such as HDAC-4, -5, -7, and -9. *Hdac5* and *Hdac9* double knockout mice showed increased proportion of slow fibers in soleus and increased levels of MyHC-β/slow and MyHC-2A transcripts in both soleus and plantaris (85). MEF2 activity is controlled by various HDAC kinases, such as calcium- and calmodulin-dependent protein kinase (CaMK) and protein kinase D1 (PKD1), that cause phosphorylation and nuclear export of HDAC. However, a role of these kinases on muscle fiber type is not demonstrated: indeed, PKD1 knockout mice have normal fiber type profile.

Peroxisome proliferator-activated receptor β/δ (PPAR-β/δ) and peroxisome proliferator-activated receptor gamma coactivator-1α (PGC-1α) have also been implicated in fiber type regulation. PPARs are members of the nuclear receptor superfamily that bind DNA as heterodimers with retinoid X receptors (RXRs). There are three isoforms in mammals, α (NR1C1), β/δ (NR1C2), and γ (NR1C3), which are activated by lipids and affect lipid metabolism. PGC-1α physically associates with PPAR-β/δ in muscle tissue and can powerfully activate it even in the absence of ligands (86). Both PPAR-β/δ and PGC-1α are expressed at higher levels in slow-oxidative than fast-glycolytic muscles and are induced by exercise in both rodents and humans. Muscle-specific PPAR-β/δ knockout causes a slow-to-fast switch in mouse soleus muscle and downregulation of some slow contractile protein genes and of PGC-1α (87). Selective inactivation of PGC-1α in skeletal muscle causes reduction in mitochondrial gene expression, partial fiber type shift from type 2A to type 2X and 2B and reduced exercise tolerance (88). PPAR-β/δ or PGC-1α overexpression in skeletal muscle induce a glycolytic-to-oxidative and a partial fast-to-slow switch (89). PGC-1α stimulates oxidative enzyme gene expression and mitochondrial biogenesis by inducing nuclear respiratory factors (NRF)-1 and -2, which control the transcription of many mitochondrial genes, and co-activating their transcriptional activity; NRFs in turn induce mitochondrial transcription factor A (mtTFA), which is essential for the replication and transcription of mitochondrial DNA.

AMP-activated protein kinase (AMPK) is a major energy sensor in all cells, including muscle cells (90). Various isoforms of AMPK catalytic and regulatory subunits are differentially distributed in different fiber types. AMPK activity is induced by exercise via two upstream kinases: LKB1 activated by the increase in AMP concentration secondary to ATP consumption, and CaMKK activated by the increase in Ca^{2+} concentration. Exercise intolerance is induced by a dominant negative form of AMPK (91) and by muscle-specific LKB1 knockout, that causes lower levels of cytochrome c and PGC-1α protein expression in the red region of the quadriceps (92). The shift from MyHC-2B to -2A and -2X induced by running exercise was reduced in mice expressing a muscle-specific AMPKα2 inactive subunit. AMPK activation induced by the AMP mimetic drug AICAR leads to increased levels of mitochondrial oxidative enzymes (93) and enhanced running endurance (94): this effect is probably mediated by PGC-1α, as the effect of AMPK on mitochondrial gene expression is drastically reduced in mice deficient in PGC-1α and AMPK can directly phosphorylate PGC-1α (95).

Coordinated Regulation of Fast and Slow Gene Programs

When a slow-to-fast switch in fiber type profile takes place, the activation of the fast muscle-specific genes

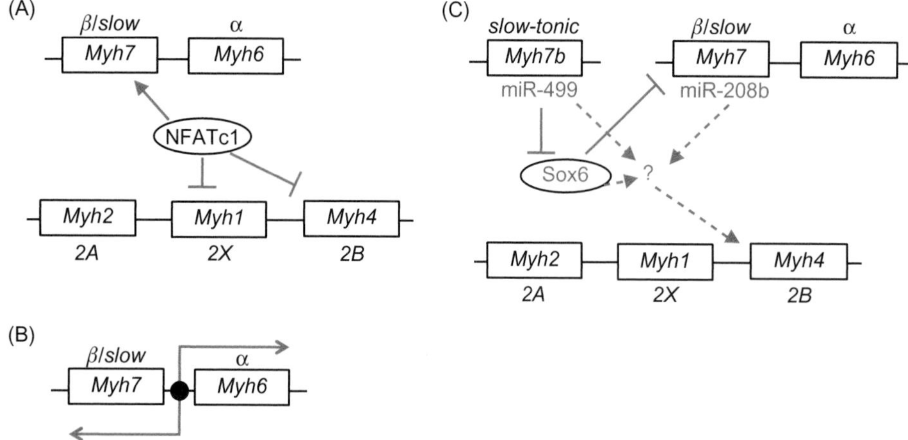

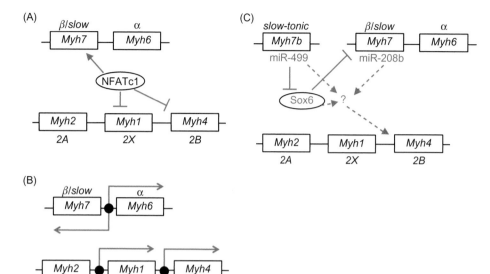

FIGURE 60.6 Different mechanisms may account for the coordinated antithetic regulation of MyHC genes during muscle fiber type switching. (A) Transcription factors, such as NFAT, may act as both activators (green) and repressors (red) of different *Myh* genes. (B) Bidirectional promoters may generate both sense (green) and antisense (red) transcripts of clustered genes. (C) microRNAs contained in *Myh* genes, like miR-499, embedded in *Myh7b*, and mir-208b, embedded in *Myh7*, may inhibit transcriptional repressors, like the transcription factor Sox6. Dotted lines indicate that the mechanism of repression of fast *Myh* genes is indirect and as yet undefined. *(Modified from Schiaffino and Reggiani, 2011 (1).)*

must be accompanied by the repression of the slow genes and vice versa, which implies the existence of mechanisms able to coordinate the antithetic regulation of the discordant gene programs. The switch between different subpopulations of type 2 fibers, for example a 2B-to-2X fiber type switch, likewise requires the simultaneous upregulation of one gene set and downregulation of another gene set. Three mechanisms are potentially implicated in this process (Figure 60.6). The first possibility, that the same transcription factor acts as both activator and repressor, is illustrated by the effect of calcineurin-dependent NFAT transcription factors on different MyHC gene promoters. Thus a constitutively active NFATc1 mutant was found to activate MyHC-β/slow but repress MyHC-2B promoter activity in adult rat skeletal muscle (83). A second possibility is that intergenic bidirectional promoters control in an opposite manner the expression of neighboring MyHC genes within the same gene cluster. For example, a bidirectional promoter located in the intergenic region between *Myh1* (coding for MyHC-2X) and *Myh4* (coding for MyHC-2B) controls the generation of a sense MyHC-2B transcript and an antisense of the upstream MyHC-2X transcript (96). The rapid shift from MyHC-2B to MyHC-2X expression induced by exercise was found to be accompanied by downregulation of this promoter, suggesting that *Myh1* and *Myh4* genes are functionally linked via the bidirectional promoter.

Another mechanism for coordinated regulation of fast and slow gene programs is mediated by microRNAs (miRNAs) located within MyHC genes and thus co-expressed with these genes (97). Two microRNAs, miR-499 located in an intron of *Myh7b*, and miR-208b located in an intron of *Myh7*, appear to be involved in muscle fiber type specification. Overexpression of miR-499 causes a fast-to-slow switch in the mouse soleus and a 2B-to-2X switch in fast muscles, while double knockout of miR-208b and miR-499 leads to slow-to-fast switch (97). The transcriptional repressor Sox6 is a target of mir-499 and Sox6 mRNA levels are reduced in skeletal muscles of miR-499 transgenic mice. Sox6 acts as a repressor of the slow gene program, as shown by the fast-to-slow switch in *Sox6*-deficient muscles, with upregulation of MyHC-slow and other slow genes and down-regulation of MyHC-2B and other fast genes (98–101). While the effect on MyHC-slow appears to be mediated by direct binding of Sox6 to a Sox consensus sequence present in the promoter of MyHC-slow, it remains to be established how the effect on fast genes is mediated. It is also possible that other targets of miR-208b and miR-499 mediate the upregulation of fast MyHC-2X and -2B genes in the double knockout of miR-208b and miR-499.

REFERENCES

1. Schiaffino S, Reggiani C. Fiber types in mammalian skeletal muscle. *Physiol Rev* 2011;**91**:1447–531.
2. Schiaffino S. Fibre types in skeletal muscle: a personal account. *Acta Physiol (Oxf)* 2010;**199**:451–63.
3. Schiaffino S, Gorza L, Sartore S, Saggin L, Ausoni S, Vianello M, et al. Three myosin heavy chain isoforms in type 2 skeletal muscle fibres. *J Muscle Res Cell Motil* 1989;**10**:197–205.
4. DeNardi C, Ausoni S, Moretti P, Gorza L, Velleca M, Buckingham M, et al. Type 2X-myosin heavy chain is coded by a muscle fiber type-specific and developmentally regulated gene. *J Cell Biol* 1993;**123**:823–35.
5. Termin A, Staron RS, Pette D. Myosin heavy chain isoforms in histochemically defined fiber types of rat muscle. *Histochemistry* 1989;**92**:453–7.
6. Eisenberg BR, Kuda AM. Discrimination between fiber populations in mammalian skeletal muscle by using ultrastructural parameters. *J Ultrastruct Res* 1976;**54**:76–88.

7. Schiaffino S, Hanzlikova V, Pierobon S. Relations between structure and function in rat skeletal muscle fibers. *J Cell Biol* 1970;**47**:107–19.
8. Edstrom L, Kugelberg E. Histochemical composition, distribution of fibres and fatiguability of single motor units. Anterior tibial muscle of the rat. *J Neurol Neurosurg Psychiatry* 1968;**31**:424–33.
9. Burke RE, Levine DN, Zajac 3rd FE. Mammalian motor units: physiological-histochemical correlation in three types in cat gastrocnemius. *Science* 1971;**174**:709–12.
10. Larsson L, Edstrom L, Lindegren B, Gorza L, Schiaffino S. MHC composition and enzyme-histochemical and physiological properties of a novel fast-twitch motor unit type. *Am J Physiol* 1991;**261**:C93–101.
11. Hennig R, Lomo T. Firing patterns of motor units in normal rats. *Nature* 1985;**314**:164–6.
12. Smerdu V, Karsch-Mizrachi I, Campione M, Leinwand L, Schiaffino S. Type IIx myosin heavy chain transcripts are expressed in type IIb fibers of human skeletal muscle. *Am J Physiol* 1994;**267**:C1723–8.
13. Simoneau JA, Bouchard C. Human variation in skeletal muscle fiber-type proportion and enzyme activities. *Am J Physiol* 1989;**257**:E567–72.
14. Simoneau JA, Bouchard C. Genetic determinism of fiber type proportion in human skeletal muscle. *FASEB J* 1995;**9**: 1091–5.
15. Rossi AC, Mammucari C, Argentini C, Reggiani C, Schiaffino S. Two novel/ancient myosins in mammalian skeletal muscles: MYH14/7b and MYH15 are expressed in extraocular muscles and muscle spindles. *J Physiol* 2010;**588**:353–64.
16. Stockdale FE, Miller JB. The cellular basis of myosin heavy chain isoform expression during development of avian skeletal muscles. *Dev Biol* 1987;**123**:1–9.
17. Condon K, Silberstein L, Blau HM, Thompson WJ. Differentiation of fiber types in aneural musculature of the prenatal rat hindlimb. *Dev Biol* 1990;**138**:275–95.
18. Harris AJ, Fitzsimons RB, McEwan JC. Neural control of the sequence of expression of myosin heavy chain isoforms in foetal mammalian muscles. *Development* 1989;**107**:751–69.
19. Niro C, Demignon J, Vincent S, Liu Y, Giordani J, Sgarioto N, et al. Six1 and Six4 gene expression is necessary to activate the fast-type muscle gene program in the mouse primary myotome. *Dev Biol* 2010;**338**:168–82.
20. Kang LH, Rughani A, Walker ML, Bestak R, Hoh JF. Expression of masticatory-specific isoforms of myosin heavy-chain, myosin-binding protein-C and tropomyosin in muscle fibers and satellite cell cultures of cat masticatory muscle. *J Histochem Cytochem* 2010;**58**:623–34.
21. Sambasivan R, Gayraud-Morel B, Dumas G, Cimper C, Paisant S, Kelly R, et al. Distinct regulatory cascades govern extraocular and pharyngeal arch muscle progenitor cell fates. *Dev Cell* 2009;**16**:810–21.
22. Esser K, Gunning P, Hardeman E. Nerve-dependent and -independent patterns of mRNA expression in regenerating skeletal muscle. *Dev Biol* 1993;**159**:173–83.
23. Whalen RG, Harris JB, Butler-Browne GS, Sesodia S. Expression of myosin isoforms during notexin-induced regeneration of rat soleus muscles. *Dev Biol* 1990;**141**:24–40.
24. Jerkovic R, Argentini C, Serrano-Sanchez A, Cordonnier C, Schiaffino S. Early myosin switching induced by nerve activity in regenerating slow skeletal muscle. *Cell Struct Funct* 1997;**22**:147–53.
25. Kalhovde JM, Jerkovic R, Sefland I, Cordonnier C, Calabria E, Schiaffino S, et al. 'Fast' and 'slow' muscle fibres in hindlimb muscles of adult rats regenerate from intrinsically different satellite cells. *J Physiol* 2005;**562**:847–57.
26. Schiaffino S, Gorza L, Pitton G, Saggin L, Ausoni S, Sartore S, et al. Embryonic and neonatal myosin heavy chain in denervated and paralyzed rat skeletal muscle. *Dev Biol* 1988;**127**:1–11.
27. Butler-Browne GS, Bugaisky LB, Cuenoud S, Schwartz K, Whalen RG. Denervation of newborn rat muscle does not block the appearance of adult fast myosin heavy chain. *Nature* 1982;**299**:
830–3.
28. Russell SD, Cambon N, Nadal-Ginard B, Whalen RG. Thyroid hormone induces a nerve-independent precocious expression of fast myosin heavy chain mRNA in rat hindlimb skeletal muscle. *J Biol Chem* 1988;**263**:6370–4.
29. Gambke B, Lyons GE, Haselgrove J, Kelly AM, Rubinstein NA. Thyroidal and neural control of myosin transitions during development of rat fast and slow muscles. *FEBS Lett* 1983;**156**:335–9.
30. Dekhuijzen P, Gayan-Ramirez G, Bisschop A, de Bock V, Dom R, Decramer M. Corticosteroid treatment and nutritional deprivation cause a different pattern of atrophy in rat diaphragm. *J Appl Physiol* 1995;**78**:629–37.
31. Simonides WS, van Hardeveld C. Thyroid hormone as a determinant of metabolic and contractile phenotype of skeletal muscle. *Thyroid* 2008;**18**:205–16.
32. Zeman RJ, Ludemann R, Easton TG, Etlinger JD. Slow to fast alterations in skeletal muscle fibers caused by clenbuterol, a beta 2-receptor agonist. *Am J Physiol* 1988;**254**:E726–32.
33. Buller AJ, Eccles JC, Eccles RM. Differentiation of fast and slow muscles in the cat hind limb. *J Physiol* 1960;**150**:399–416.
34. Huey K, Bodine S. Changes in myosin mRNA and protein expression in denervated rat soleus and tibialis anterior. *Eur J Biochem* 1998;**256**:45–50.
35. Ausoni S, Gorza L, Schiaffino S, Gundersen K, Lomo T. Expression of myosin heavy chain isoforms in stimulated fast and slow rat muscles. *J Neurosci* 1990;**10**:153–60.
36. Pette D, Vrobva G. Adaptation of mammalian skeletal muscle fibers to chronic electrical stimulation. *Rev Physiol Biochem Pharmacol* 1992;**120**:115–202.
37. Jaschinski F, Schuler M, Peuker H, Pette D. Changes in myosin heavy chain mRNA and protein isoforms of rat muscle during forced contractile activity. *Am J Physiol* 1998;**274**:C365–70.
38. Larsson L, Ansved T, Edstrom L, Gorza L, Schiaffino S. Effects of age on physiological, immunohistochemical and biochemical properties of fast-twitch single motor units in the rat. *J Physiol* 1991;**443**:257–75.
39. Lexell J, Taylor CC, Sjostrom M. What is the cause of the ageing atrophy? Total number, size and proportion of different fiber types studied in whole vastus lateralis muscle from 15- to 83-year-old men. *J Neurol Sci* 1988;**84**:275–94.
40. Larsson L, Salviati G. Effects of age on calcium transport activity of sarcoplasmic reticulum in fast- and slow-twitch rat muscle fibres. *J Physiol (Lond)* 1989;**419**:253–64.

41. Larsson L, Biral D, Campione M, Schiaffino S. An age-related type IIB to IIX myosin heavy chain switching in rat skeletal muscle. *Acta Physiol Scand* 1993;**147**:227–34.
42. Wood SJ, Slater CR. Safety factor at the neuromuscular junction. *Prog Neurobiol Dis* 2001;**64**:393–429.
43. Pierno S, Desaphy JF, Liantonio A, De Bellis M, Bianco G, De Luca A, et al. Change of chloride ion channel conductance is an early event of slow-to-fast fibre type transition during unloading-induced muscle disuse. *Brain* 2002;**125**:1510–21.
44. Ruff RL, Whittlesey D. Na^{+} current densities and voltage dependence in human intercostal muscle fibres. *J Physiol* 1992;**458**:85–97.
45. Luff AR, Atwood HL. Changes in the sarcoplasmic reticulum and transverse tubular system of fast and slow skeletal muscles of the mouse during postnatal development. *J Cell Biol* 1971; **51**:369–83.
46. Delbono O, Meissner G. Sarcoplasmic reticulum Ca^{2+} release in rat slow- and fast-twitch muscles. *J Membr Biol* 1996;**151**: 123–30.
47. Fraysse B, Desaphy JF, Pierno S, De Luca A, Liantonio A, Mitolo CI, et al. Decrease in resting calcium and calcium entry associated with slow-to-fast transition in unloaded rat soleus muscle. *FASEB J* 2003;**17**:1916–8.
48. Payne AM, Zheng Z, González E, Wang ZM, Messi ML, Delbono O. External $Ca(^{2+})$-dependent excitation–contraction coupling in a population of ageing mouse skeletal muscle fibres. *J Physiol* 2004;**560**:137–55.
49. Everts ME, Clausen T. Activation of the Na-K pump by intracellular Na in rat slow- and fast-twitch muscles. *Acta Physiol Scand* 1992;**145**:353–62.
50. Bottinelli R, Schiaffino S, Reggiani C. Force-velocity relations and myosin heavy chain isoform compositions of skinned fibres from rat skeletal muscle. *J Physiol (Lond)* 1991;**437**:655–72.
51. Bottinelli R, Canepari M, Pellegrino MA, Reggiani C. Force-velocity properties of human skeletal muscle fibres: myosin heavy chain isoform and temperature dependence. *J.Physiol* 1996;**495**:573–86.
52. Hintz CS, Coyle EF, Kaiser KK, Chi MM, Lowry OH. Comparison of muscle fiber typing by quantitative enzyme assays and by myosin ATPase staining. *J Histochem Cytochem* 1984;**32**:655–60.
53. Bottinelli R, Canepari M, Reggiani C, Stienen GJ. Myofibrillar ATPase activity during isometric contraction and isomyosin composition in rat single skinned muscle fibres. *J Physiol (Lond)* 1994;**481**:663–75.
54. Stienen GJM, Kiers J, Bottinelli R, Reggiani C. Myofibrillar ATPase activity in skinned human skeletal muscle fibres:fibre type and temperature dependence. *J.Physiol* 1996;**493**:299–307.
55. He Z-H, Bottinelli R, Pellegrino MA, Ferenczi MA, Reggiani C. ATP consumption and efficiency of human single muscle fibers with different myosin isoform composition. *Biophys J* 2000;**79**:945–61.
56. Luther P. The vertebrate muscle Z-disc: sarcomere anchor for structure and signalling. *J Muscle Res Cell Motil* 2009;**30**:171–85.
57. Prado LG, Makarenko I, Andresen C, Kruger M, Opitz CA, Linke WA. Isoform diversity of giant proteins in relation to passive and active properties of rabbit skeletal muscles. *J Gen Physiol* 2005;**126**:461–80.
58. Castillo A, Nowak R, Littlefield KP, Fowler VM, Littlefield RS. A nebulin ruler does not dictate thin filament lengths. *Biophys J* 2009;**96**:1856–65.
59. Linari M, Bottinelli R, Pellegrino M, Reconditi M, Reggiani C, Lombardi V. The mechanism of the force response to stretch in human skinned muscle fibres with different myosin isoforms. *J Physiol* 2004;**554**:335–52.
60. Macpherson PC, Schork MA, Faulkner JA. Contraction-induced injury to single fiber segments from fast and slow muscles of rats by single stretches. *Am J Physiol* 1996;**271**:C1438–46.
61. Close R. Dynamic properties of mammalian skeletal muscles. *Physiol Rev* 1972;**52**:129–97.
62. Calderon JC, Bolanos P, Caputo C. Myosin heavy chain isoform composition and $Ca(^{2+})$ transients in fibres from enzymatically dissociated murine soleus and extensor digitorum longus muscles. *J Physiol* 2010;**588**:267–79.
63. Ruff RL. Calcium sensitivity of fast- and slow-twitch human muscle fibers. *Muscle Nerve* 1989;**12**:32–7.
64. Gordon AM, Homsher E, Regnier M. Regulation of contraction in striated muscle. *Physiol Rev* 2000;**80**:853–924.
65. Blei ML, Conley KE, Kushmerick MJ. Separate measures of ATP utilization and recovery in human skeletal muscle. *J Physiol* 1993;**465**:203–22.
66. Barclay CG, Constable JK, Gibbs CL. Energetics of fast- and slow-twitch muscles of the mouse. *J Physiol* 1993;**472**:61–80.
67. Homsher E. Muscle enthalpy production and its relationship to actomyosin ATPase. *Annu Rev Physiol* 1987;**49**:673–90.
68. Winder WW, Thomson DM. Cellular energy sensing and signaling by AMP-activated protein kinase. *Cell Biochem Biophys* 2007;**47**:332–47.
69. Aragon JJ, Tornheim K, Lowenstein JM. On a possible role of IMP in the regulation of phosphorylase activity in skeletal muscles. *FEBS Lett* 1980;**117**:K56–64.
70. Spamer C, Pette D. Activity patterns of phosphofructokinase, glyceraldehydephosphate dehydrogenase, lactate dehydrogenase and malate dehydrogenase in microdissected fast and slow fibres from rabbit psoas and soleus muscle. *Histochemistry* 1977;**52**:201–16.
71. Eisenberg BR. Quantitative ultrastructure of mammalian skeletal muscle. In: Peachey L, Adrian R, Geiger S, editors. *Handbook of physiology*. Bethesda, MD: Williams & Wilkins;1983. p. 73–112.
72. Hughes SM, Taylor JM, Tapscott SJ, Gurley CM, Carter WJ, Peterson CA. Selective accumulation of MyoD and myogenin mRNAs in fast and slow adult skeletal muscle is controlled by innervation and hormones. *Development* 1993;**118**:1137–47.
73. Hughes SM, Chi MM, Lowry OH, Gundersen K. Myogenin induces a shift of enzyme activity from glycolytic to oxidative metabolism in muscles of transgenic mice. *J Cell Biol* 1999;**145**:633–42.
74. Flynn J, Meadows E, Fiorotto M, Klein W. Myogenin regulates exercise capacity and skeletal muscle metabolism in the adult mouse. *PLoS One* 2010;**5**:e13535.
75. Parsons SA, Wilkins BJ, Bueno OF, Molkentin JD. Altered skeletal muscle phenotypes in calcineurin Aalpha and Abeta gene-targeted mice. *Mol Cell Biol* 2003;**23**:4331–43.
76. Chin ER, Olson EN, Richardson JA, Yang Q, Humphries C, Shelton JM, et al. A calcineurin-dependent transcriptional pathway controls skeletal muscle fiber type. *Genes Dev* 1998;**12**: 2499–509.

77. Serrano AL, Murgia M, Pallafacchina G, Calabria E, Coniglio P, et al. Calcineurin controls nerve activity-dependent specification of slow skeletal muscle fibers but not muscle growth. *Proc Natl Acad Sci USA* 2001;**98**:13108–13.
78. Oh M, Rybkin II, Copeland V, Czubryt MP, Shelton JM, van Rooij E, et al. Calcineurin is necessary for the maintenance but not embryonic development of slow muscle fibers. *Mol Cell Biol* 2005;**25**:6629–38.
79. Frey N, Barrientos T, Shelton JM, Frank D, Rutten H, Gehring D, et al. Mice lacking calsarcin-1 are sensitized to calcineurin signaling and show accelerated cardiomyopathy in response to pathological biomechanical stress. *Nat Med* 2004;**10**:1336–43.
80. Frey N, Frank D, Lippl S, Kuhn C, Kogler H, Barrientos T, et al. Calsarcin-2 deficiency increases exercise capacity in mice through calcineurin/NFAT activation. *J Clin Invest* 2008; **118**:3598–608.
81. Liu Y, Cseresnyes Z, Randall WR, Schneider MF. Activity-dependent nuclear translocation and intranuclear distribution of NFATc in adult skeletal muscle fibers. *J Cell Biol* 2001;**155**:27–39.
82. Tothova J, Blaauw B, Pallafacchina G, Rudolf R, Argentini C, Reggiani C, et al. NFATc1 nucleocytoplasmic shuttling is controlled by nerve activity in skeletal muscle. *J Cell Sci* 2006;**119**:1604–11.
83. McCullagh KJ, Calabria E, Pallafacchina G, Ciciliot S, Serrano AL, Argentini C, et al. NFAT is a nerve activity sensor in skeletal muscle and controls activity-dependent myosin switching. *Proc Natl Acad Sci USA* 2004;**101**:10590–5.
84. Calabria E, Ciciliot S, Moretti I, Garcia M, Picard A, Dyar KA, et al. NFAT isoforms control activity-dependent muscle fiber type specification. *Proc Natl Acad Sci USA* 2009;**106**:13335–40.
85. Potthoff MJ, Wu H, Arnold MA, Shelton JM, Backs J, McAnally J, et al. Histone deacetylase degradation and MEF2 activation promote the formation of slow-twitch myofibers. *J Clin Invest* 2007;**117**:2459–67.
86. Wang YX, Lee CH, Tiep S, Yu RT, Ham J, Kang H, et al. Peroxisome-proliferator-activated receptor delta activates fat metabolism to prevent obesity. *Cell* 2003;**113**:159–70.
87. Schuler M, Ali F, Chambon C, Duteil D, Bornert JM, Tardivel A, et al. PGC1alpha expression is controlled in skeletal muscles by PPARbeta, whose ablation results in fiber-type switching, obesity, and type 2 diabetes. *Cell Metab* 2006;**4**:407–14.
88. Handschin C, Chin S, Li P, Liu F, Maratos-Flier E, Lebrasseur NK, et al. Skeletal muscle fiber-type switching, exercise intolerance, and myopathy in PGC-1alpha muscle-specific knock-out animals. *J Biol Chem* 2007;**282**:30014–21.
89. Lin J, Wu H, Tarr PT, Zhang CY, Wu Z, Boss O, et al. Transcriptional co-activator PGC-1 alpha drives the formation of slow-twitch muscle fibres. *Nature* 2002;**418**:797–801.
90. Hardie DG, Sakamoto K. AMPK: a key sensor of fuel and energy status in skeletal muscle. *Physiology* 2006;**21**:48–60.
91. Mu J, Brozinick Jr. JT, Valladares O, Bucan M, Birnbaum MJ. A role for AMP-activated protein kinase in contraction- and hypoxia-regulated glucose transport in skeletal muscle. *Mol Cell* 2001;**7**:1085–94.
92. Thomson DM, Porter BB, Tall JH, Kim HJ, Barrow JR, Winder WW. Skeletal muscle and heart LKB1 deficiency causes decreased voluntary running and reduced muscle mitochondrial marker enzyme expression in mice. *Am J Physiol Endocrinol Metab* 2007;**292**: E196–202.
93. Winder WW, Holmes BF, Rubink DS, Jensen EB, Chen M, Holloszy JO. Activation of AMP-activated protein kinase increases mitochondrial enzymes in skeletal muscle. *J Appl Physiol* 2000;**88**:2219–26.
94. Narkar VA, Downes M, Yu RT, Embler E, Wang YX, Banayo E, et al. AMPK and PPARdelta agonists are exercise mimetics. *Cell* 2008;**134**:405–15.
95. Jager S, Handschin C, St-Pierre J, Spiegelman BM. AMP-activated protein kinase (AMPK) action in skeletal muscle via direct phosphorylation of PGC-1α. *Proc Natl Acad Sci USA* 2007;**104**:12017–22.
96. Rinaldi C, Haddad F, Bodell PW, Qin AX, Jiang W, Baldwin KM. Intergenic bidirectional promoter and cooperative regulation of the IIx and IIb MHC genes in fast skeletal muscle. *Am J Physiol Regul Integr Comp Physiol* 2008;**295**:R208–18.
97. van Rooij E, Quiat D, Johnson BA, Sutherland LB, Qi X, Richardson JA, et al. A family of microRNAs encoded by myosin genes governs myosin expression and muscle performance. *Dev Cell* 2009;**17**:662–73.
98. Hagiwara N, Ma B, Ly A. Slow and fast fiber isoform gene expression is systematically altered in skeletal muscle of the Sox6 mutant, p100H. *Dev Dyn* 2005;**234**:301–11.
99. Hagiwara N, Yeh M, Liu A. Sox6 is required for normal fiber type differentiation of fetal skeletal muscle in mice. *Dev Dyn* 2007;**236**:2062–76.
100. Quiat D, Voelker KA, Pei J, Grishin NV, Grange RW, Bassel-Duby R, et al. Concerted regulation of myofiber-specific gene expression and muscle performance by the transcriptional repressor Sox6. *Proc Natl Acad Sci USA* 2011;**108**:10196–201.
101. An CI, Dong Y, Hagiwara N. Genome-wide mapping of Sox6 binding sites in skeletal muscle reveals both direct and indirect regulation of muscle terminal differentiation by Sox6. *BMC Dev Biol* 2011;**11**:59.

Section B

Adaptations and Response

Chapter 61

Regulation of Skeletal Muscle Development and Function by microRNAs

Ning Liu and Rhonda Bassel-Duby
Department of Molecular Biology, University of Texas Southwestern Medical Center, Dallas, TX

microRNA BIOGENESIS AND FUNCTION

microRNAs (miRNAs) are a class of ~22 nucleotide, non-coding RNAs that are evolutionarily conserved from plants to mammals and negatively regulate gene targets by inhibiting protein translation or enhancing mRNA degradation (1). The human genome is estimated to encode as many as 1000 miRNAs, which are either transcribed from their own transcriptional units or embedded in the introns of protein-coding genes and co-transcribed with the host genes (1). Approximately half of all miRNAs are encoded by polycistronic transcription units that generate multiple miRNAs (1).

The biogenesis pathway of miRNAs is outlined in Figure 61.1. Similar to protein-coding mRNAs, miRNAs are transcribed by RNA polymerase II as pri-miRNAs encoding one or multiple miRNAs (2,3). Pri-miRNAs fold into imperfectly base-paired stem–loop structures and are processed in the nucleus by the endonuclease Drosha and its cofactor DGCR8 into ~70 nucleotide hairpins, known as pre-miRNAs (3–5). The pre-miRNAs are exported to the nuclease where they are processed by the endonuclease Dicer to yield imperfect RNA duplexes containing miRNAs (6). The mature miRNA is released from Dicer and incorporated into the RNA-induced silencing complex (RISC) where it binds to the 3′ untranslated region (UTR) of target mRNAs via imperfect Watson–Crick base pairing and represses its expression by translational inhibition, mRNA degradation, or sequestering target mRNA into cytoplasmic P bodies (7). Nucleotides 2–8 at the 5′ end of the miRNA, termed "seed sequences", are essential for target recognition and binding (8). miRNAs can be detected in circulating plasma microvesicles (exosomes), indicating that they may mediate intercellular communication (9,10).

miRNA-dependent gene regulation is a complex and highly orchestrated process. In contrast to transcription factors, which generally act as "on-and-off" switches on their target genes, most miRNAs exert their inhibitory effects through subtle modulations of their targets, also referred to as "fine-tuning" (8). Strikingly, miRNAs have numerous targets, averaging about 300 conserved targets per miRNA family, and many of the targets regulate the same biological process (8). Thus, although the effects of an individual miRNA on a specific mRNA target may be relatively modest, the combined effects of a miRNA on multiple targets functioning within a common biological pathway can be synergetic (11,12). Each mRNA can be regulated by multiple miRNAs, allowing redundancy and cooperation between miRNAs. The multiplicity of miRNA and target regulation adds complexity and robustness to gene-regulatory networks.

The majority of miRNAs are evolutionarily conserved, indicative of their important function in gene regulation. However, many miRNAs can be deleted in mice or other animals without apparent defects in development. Intriguingly, there are numerous examples of miRNAs whose expression and actions are sensitized under pathological and physiological stress, implicating a more pronounced role of miRNAs in exacerbating or protecting the organism during stress or disease (12).

SKELETAL MUSCLE WITHOUT miRNAs

An essential role for miRNAs in skeletal muscle development was shown by the loss-of-function studies of Dicer, the RNase essential for miRNA biogenesis. Deletion of a conditional Dicer allele in embryonic skeletal muscle using a MyoD-Cre recombinase transgene results in skeletal muscle hypoplasia (fewer myofiber numbers), increased apoptosis and lethality within minutes after birth (13). In this study, expression of many muscle-specific miRNAs is downregulated in skeletal muscle (13). The severe phenotype in mice lacking Dicer in skeletal muscle is likely

Muscle. DOI: http://dx.doi.org/10.1016/B978-0-12-381510-1.00061-2

due to the absence of the collective functions of numerous miRNAs rather than the action of a single miRNA in skeletal muscle development.

SKELETAL MUSCLE-SPECIFIC miRNAs

The most widely studied muscle-specific miRNAs are the miR-1/206 family comprised of miR-1-1, miR-1-2, and miR-206, and the miR-133 family comprised of miR-133a-1, miR-133a-2, and miR-133b. These miRNAs are co-transcribed from bicistronic transcripts on three separate chromosomes (Figure 61.2). miR-1-1 and miR-1-2 are identical and differ from miR-206 by four nucleotides, while miR-133a-1 and miR-133a-2 are identical and differ from miR-133b by two nucleotides (11). The miR-1-1/133a-2 and miR-1-2/133a-1 genes are expressed in both cardiac and skeletal muscle, whereas the miR-206/133b locus is expressed only in skeletal muscle (11).

Cardiac and skeletal muscle expression of miR-1-1/133a-2 and miR-1-2/133a-1 are regulated by two separate enhancers (upstream and intragenic enhancer) controlled by combinations of transcription factors, serum response factor (SRF), MyoD, and myocyte enhancer factor-2 (MEF2) (14–16). MyoD also directly activates transcription of miR-206/133b in skeletal muscle by binding to the E-box in the upstream regulatory region (17). Thus, the same transcription factors that activate protein-coding genes involved in muscle function, such as the sarcomeric genes, also regulate muscle specific miRNAs, demonstrating an interconnected relationship between muscle-specific miRNAs and muscle-specific mRNAs.

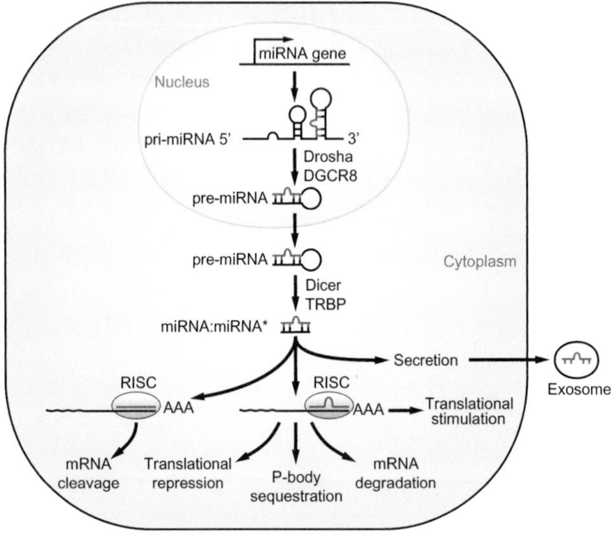

FIGURE 61.1 **microRNAs biogenesis and function.** miRNAs are transcribed as long precursors (pri-miRNAs), which are processed by Drosha and DGCR8 into hairpins called pre-miRs, which are processed by Dicer and TRBP to form mature miRNAs as a heteroduplex with miRNA*. miRNAs regulate numerous processes as shown. *(Redrawn from Figure 1 of Liu and Olson, 2010 (11).)*

miR-206 IN SKELETAL MUSCLE FUNCTION AND DISEASE

The miR-206/133b gene cluster is exclusively expressed in skeletal muscle. miR-206 regulates many aspects of skeletal muscle biology, including reinnervation of neuromuscular junctions and skeletal muscle regeneration. It is also involved in the pathogenesis of various muscle diseases, including amyotrophic lateral sclerosis (ALS), muscular dystrophies, and rhabdomyosarcoma.

Neuromuscular Synapse Reinnervation

Denervation of motor neurons in skeletal muscle causes axon degeneration and muscle atrophy. Subsequently, the motor axons regenerate through the nerve stump to the skeletal muscle and form new neuromuscular junctions (NMJs). Reinnervation in skeletal muscle after injury is a complex process and is regulated by factors secreted from both motor neurons and muscle fibers (18). Interestingly, miR-206 expression is enriched in synaptic regions of the

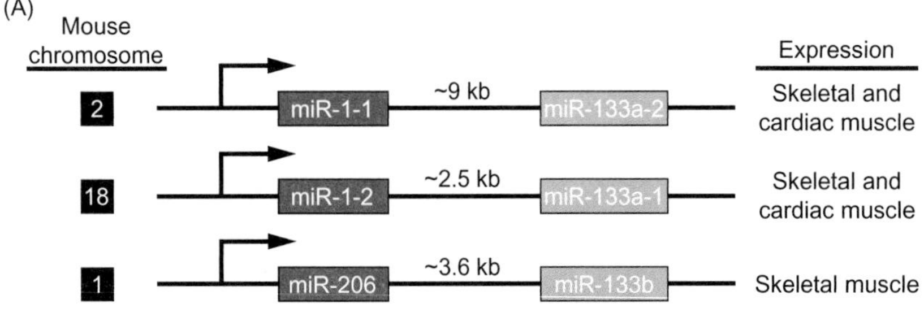

FIGURE 61.2 **Genomic organization of the miR-1/133 cluster.** (A) Three bicistronic miRNA genes encoding miR-1–1/miR-133a-2, miR-1–2/miR-133a-1, and miR-206/miR-133b are shown. Each pair of miRNAs is transcribed from left to right. Chromosomal locations of each miRNA gene and the muscle tissues in which they are expressed in mice are shown. (B) Sequences homologies among muscle-specific miRNAs are shown. Black letters indicate non-homology. *(Modified from Figure 1 of Liu et al., 2008 (53).)*

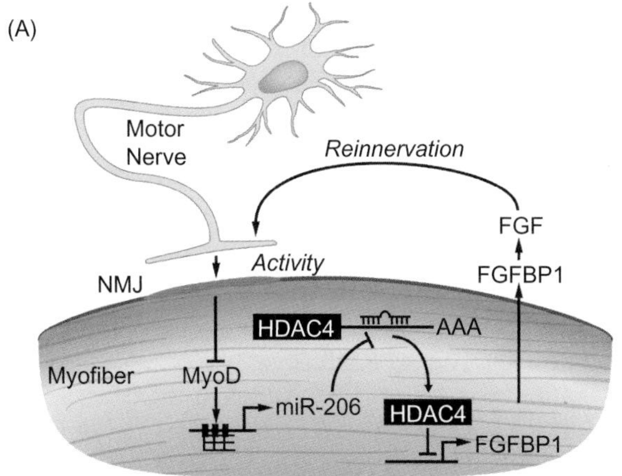

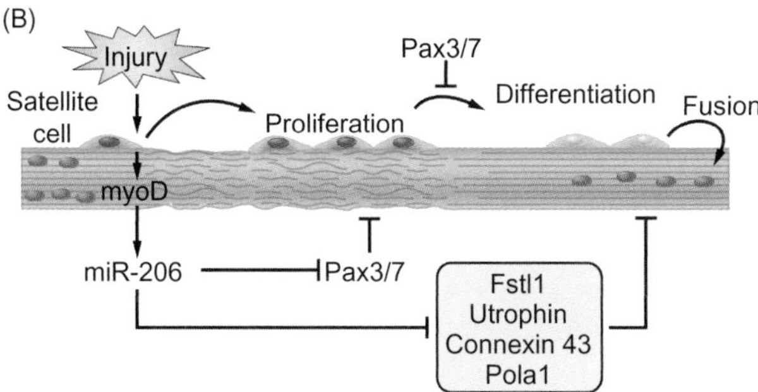

FIGURE 61.3 Functions of miR-206 in skeletal muscle. (A) Model of miR-206-dependent reinnervation of neuromuscular junctions (NMJs). (B) Model of miR-206 function in satellite cell activation and differentiation upon injury. *(Panel (A) modified from Figure 4K of Williams et al., 2009 (19).)*

muscle fibers (19). Upon denervation of the sciatic nerve, miR-206 is dramatically upregulated (Figure 61.3A). Denervation-responsive upregulation of miR-206 is activated by myogenic proteins, MyoD, and myogenin via the three E-boxes in the upstream enhancer region of the miR-206/133b gene (19). Consistent with the denervation-responsive upregulation of miR-206, mice deficient of miR-206 showed significant delay in reinnervation of NMJs in response to denervation. In mice lacking miR-206, axon regrowth towards the denervated NMJs was normal, but innervation of the junctional endplates (the muscle fiber membrane at the junction between muscles and nerves) was delayed (19). Moreover, the newly formed NMJs were morphologically defective (19). Loss of miR-206 did not affect normal formation or maturation of NMJs (19). Therefore, although miR-206 is not necessary for normal development, it promotes the regeneration of neuromuscular synapses upon denervation.

How does miR-206, a muscle-specific miRNA, affect innervation of NMJs? Studies by Williams et al. elegantly showed that miR-206 represses histone deacetylase 4 (HDAC4), which inhibits nerve reinnervation by inhibiting expression of fibroblast growth factor binding protein 1 (FGFBP1) (Figure 61.3A) (19). FGFBP1 is secreted from muscle and it can promote innervation by activating FGF proteins on distal motor neuron (19). Therefore, miR-206 serves as a sensor of motor innervation and regulates a retrograde signaling pathway required for the nerve–muscle interactions.

ALS Pathogenesis

ALS, also known as Lou Gehrig's disease, is the most common adult motor neuron disease. It causes the deterioration of the upper and lower motor neurons (20). The hallmark of this disease is the dysfunction and eventual death of motor neurons, leading to muscle atrophy, paralysis of lower limb and respiratory muscles, and death (21). miR-206 is highly upregulated in the muscle of the ALS mouse model (G93A-SOD1 transgenic mice) that expresses a mutant form of superoxide dismutase protein (SOD1) that triggers adult-onset motor neuron death (19,22,23). Upregulation of miR-206 coincides with the progression of the disease (19). More importantly, using mutant mouse models it was shown that the absence of miR-206 in the ALS (G93A-SOD1) mouse results in an acceleration of the initiation of symptoms and a decrease in survival of the ALS mice (19). These findings indicate that miR-206 protects against ALS and the upregulation of miR-206 expression is required to delay the onset of ALS. Therefore, the discovery of miR-206 as a modifier of ALS reveals an unappreciated role of muscle-derived factors in the pathogenesis of ALS and suggests the applicability of miRNA-mediated therapy for ALS.

Skeletal Muscle Regeneration

Skeletal muscle can regenerate after injury, exercise or disease. The regenerative potential of skeletal muscle relies on skeletal muscle stem cells (called satellite cells), which reside underneath the basal lamina of myofibers (24,25). Adult satellite cells, which are usually quiescent, are activated in response to injury and start to proliferate into myogenic precursor cells (myoblasts), which terminally differentiate and fuse into multi-nucleated myotubes (24,25). Activated satellite cells also divide to generate progeny that restore the pool of quiescent satellite cells (26). Paired-box protein Pax7 is expressed in both quiescent and activated satellite cells and is required for maintenance and self-renewal of quiescent satellite cells (27).

Activation of satellite cells promotes MyoD expression, which then activates the myogenic pathways leading to formation of myotubes. When satellite cells differentiate into myotubes, Pax7 expression is decreased (28). In addition to activating the skeletal muscle myogenic pathways, MyoD upregulates expression of microRNAs. In particular, miR-206 is significantly upregulated in activated satellite cells (29,30). Consistently, miR-206 targets Pax7 3′ UTR and directly represses Pax7 expression to restrict the proliferation of satellite cells and facilitate differentiation. Anti-miRs (antagomiRs) that knockdown miR-206 expression result in enhanced satellite cell proliferation and increased Pax7 expression, which inhibits differentiation (29,30). Of note, miR-206 also targets and represses Pax3, which is essential for survival of satellite cells (31). Therefore, following activation of satellite cells, MyoD not only activates myogenic genes that promote differentiation of satellite cells into myotubes, but also represses satellite cell survival and self-renewal via direct upregulation of miR-206 expression, thus further pushing them towards the differentiation pathway.

Three days after muscle injury by administration of cardiotoxin, miR-206 is downregulated in skeletal muscle (29). However, miR-206 expression is strongly upregulated beginning at day 4 post-injury and continues to remain upregulated (32). Remarkably, miR-206 expression is enriched in regenerating fibers, implying its involvement in the regeneration process (32). In this regard, miR-206 is also upregulated during myoblast differentiation. It is believed to induce differentiation by repressing a subunit of DNA polymerase alpha (Pola1), connexin43, as well as, follistatin-like 1 (Fstl1) and utrophin (Figure 61.3b) (31,33–35). However, the *in vivo* significance of miR-206 in regulating myoblast differentiation remains a conundrum given that mice lacking miR-206 have normal skeletal muscle development.

Muscular Dystrophies

Muscular dystrophy comprises a large group of over 30 different inherited disorders, characterized by progressive muscle wasting and degeneration of skeletal muscle (36). Mutations in the X-linked dystrophin gene cause both Duchenne muscular dystrophy (DMD), the most common and severe type of muscular dystrophies, and the milder phenotypes of Becker muscular dystrophy (BMD) (37). Loss of the sarcolemma protein dystrophin in DMD patients causes fragility of myofibers to mechanical damage, leading to muscle degeneration, chronic inflammation, and increased fibrosis (38).

miR-206 is highly upregulated in both diaphragm and tibialis anterior (TA) muscles of *mdx* mice, a mouse model of DMD (32,39). Satellite cells in *mdx* mice are continuously activated to generate new myofibers to repair damaged and degenerated myofibers caused by loss of expression of the dystrophin gene (38). In *mdx* mice, miR-206 is enriched in newly formed myofibers (32). Given the increased expression of miR-206 in *mdx* mice, it would be extremely interesting to explore whether miR-206 plays a protective role in the disease progression of *mdx* mice, as well as in DMD patients. Indeed, preliminary studies show that loss of miR-206 in *mdx* mice shortens the time of onset of the disease and exacerbates the dystrophic phenotype.

Rhabdomyosarcoma

Rhabdomyosarcomas (RMS) are the most common soft tissue sarcomas in children and young adults (40). The defining characteristic of RMS is expression of myogenic differentiation markers (40,41). Although the exact etiology of RMS is unknown, based on the expression of myogenic differentiation markers, such as MyoD and desmin, it is surmised that the cell of origin is a myogenic progenitor cell that failed to undergo terminal differentiation.

Expression of miR-206 and miR-1 is suppressed in primary RMS and RMS cell lines (42,43). Forced overexpression of miR-206 in RMS cells promotes myogenic differentiation and blocks tumor growth (42,43). The action of miR-206 in RMS is postulated to be mediated by its repression of the product of the MET proto-oncogene, the Met tyrosine-kinase receptor, which is overexpressed in RMS and has been implicated in RMS pathogenesis (42,43). Furthermore, measuring miR-206 levels in RMS samples showed that miR-206 expression levels correlated with clinical behavior of RMS patients, implying a therapeutic potential of miR-206 in treatment of RMS (44).

miR-1 IN SKELETAL MUSCLE DEVELOPMENT, FUNCTION AND DISEASE

miR-1 is the most abundant miRNA in the heart, and it plays an important role in cardiomyocyte proliferation, development, and heart disease. miR-1 is also highly expressed in skeletal muscle and its involvement is skeletal muscle has only begun to be explored.

Myoblast Differentiation and Muscle Development

In cell culture, when myoblasts differentiate into myotubes, expression of miR-1 and miR-133 is upregulated. miR-1 promotes myoblast differentiation by targeting and repressing histone deacetylase 4 (HDAC4), a repressor of the transcription factor, MEF2 (Figure 61.4) (14). Thus, the interaction between miR-1 and HDAC4 provides a positive feed-forward loop in which MEF2 upregulates the expression of miR-1 causing repression of HDAC4 and ultimately increasing activity of MEF2, which drives myocyte differentiation. In *C. elegans*, miR-1 regulates

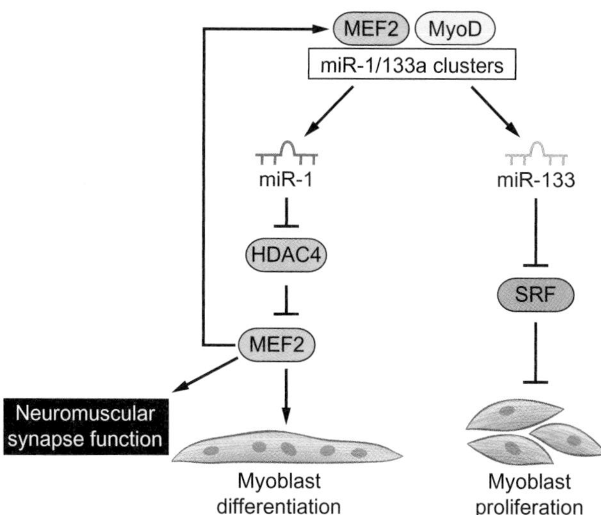

FIGURE 61.4 Regulation of myoblast proliferation and differentiation by miR-1 and miR-133. MyoD and MEF2 control expression of miR-1 and miR-133 in skeletal muscle. miR-1 promotes myoblast differentiation by repressing HDAC4. miR-133 promotes myoblast proliferation by repressing SRF.

aspects of both pre- and postsynaptic function at neuromuscular junctions by inhibition of MEF2 (45).

In *Drosophila*, miR-1 is expressed in most, if not all, the myogenic cells of the larval muscle system and its muscle-specific expression is controlled by Twist and MEF2 transcription factors (46,47). miR-1 is required for post-mitotic growth of larval muscle, and loss of miR-1 in *Drosophila* results in a severely deformed musculature (47,48). In zebrafish, downregulation of both miR-1 and miR-133 alters muscle gene expression and disrupts actin organization during sarcomere assembly, suggesting that miR-1 and miR-133 actively shape gene expression patterns in skeletal muscle by regulating sarcomeric actin organization (49).

Skeletal Muscle Function and Disease

miR-1 expression is dysregulated in many skeletal muscle stress and disease states. In a mouse model of skeletal muscle hypertrophy, miR-1 expression is decreased (50). However, it is unclear whether manipulation of miR-1 expression level has any consequence in skeletal muscle hypertrophy. Interestingly, a mutation that is responsible for the exceptional muscularity of Texel sheep has been mapped to a single G-to-A mutation in the 3′ UTR of the myostatin gene, which creates a binding site for miR-1 and miR-206 (51). Myostatin functions to repress muscle growth, and the translational repression of myostatin by miR-1/206 is believed to contribute to the muscular hypertrophy of Texel sheep (51). These findings implicate a role for miRNAs in skeletal muscle hypertrophy.

miR-1 is downregulated following muscle injury by cardiotoxin, in *mdx* mice and in DMD patients, implying that it might be a degenerating miRNA (52). It is worth noting that miR-206, on the other hand, is highly expressed in *mdx* mice and DMD patients. The difference between miR-1 and miR-206 expression levels in *mdx* mice can be explained by the differences in their chromatin remodeling. In *mdx* mice, miR-1, as well as miR-29, are repressed by HDAC2, which is a result of impaired nNOS activity and a decrease in HDAC2 nitrosylation (30). In contrast, miR-206 is independent of the nNOS-HDAC2 pathway, and instead is expressed in activated satellite cells and repressed by HDAC1 (30).

mir-133a IN SKELETAL MUSCLE BIOLOGY

Like miR-1, miR-133a is abundant in the heart and skeletal muscle and is involved in many aspects of cardiac and skeletal muscle development, function, and disease.

Myoblast Proliferation

Similar to miR-1 and miR-206, miR-133a expression is also upregulated upon C_2C_{12} myoblast differentiation (14). However, in contrast to these two miRNAs, miR-133a promotes myoblast proliferation, at least partly, by repressing SRF (14). Genetic deletion of both miR-133a-1 and miR-133a-2 showed that SRF is a direct target of miR-133a in cardiomyocytes and suggested that miR-133a suppresses cardiomyocyte proliferation (53). The genetic interaction between miR-133a and SRF constitutes a negative feedback loop in which the upregulation of miR-133a by SRF results in increased repression of SRF (Figure 61.2). Although the findings from myoblast and cardiomyocytes seem conflicting regarding a role for miR-133a in regulating proliferation, SRF has previously been shown to be capable of functioning as an activator of proliferation and differentiation (54).

Centronuclear Myopathy

Studies from mice lacking both miR-133a-1 and miR-133a-2 have revealed their important role in heart development and function. Interestingly, the skeletal muscle structure is normal in embryos and neonates of mice lacking miR-133a-1 and miR-133a-2 (dKO), indicating that miR-133a is dispensable for embryonic and neonatal skeletal muscle development (53). However, in adult skeletal muscle, dKO mice showed a high proportion of myofibers with centralized nuclei in fast (type II) fibers (Figure 61.5) (55). In addition, dKO mice were significantly smaller in body mass, muscle mass, as well as myofiber diameters. Accumulation of centralized nuclei is usually indicative of muscle regeneration in response to

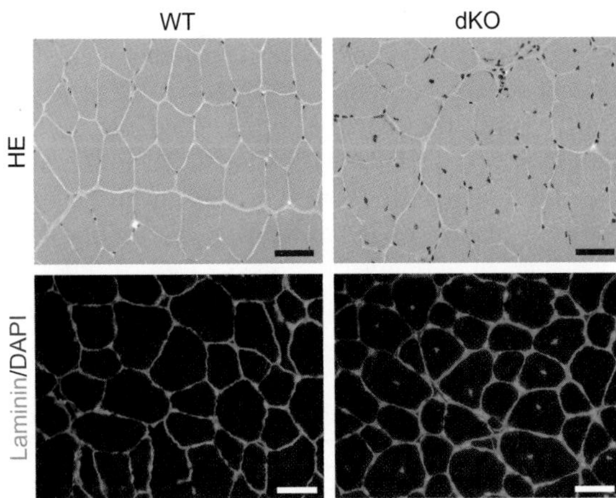

FIGURE 61.5 **Centronuclear myopathy in skeletal muscle of miR-133a dKO mice.** (Top panel) Hematoxylin and eosin (HE) stain showing centralized nuclei in TA myofibers of dKO mice. (Bottom panel) Immunostaining of TA muscle against laminin. Nuclei are stained with DAPI. dKO TA muscle shows central nuclei. *(Modified from Figure 2 of Liu et al., 2011 (55).)*

muscle damage or injury. However, dKO myofibers showed no sign of muscle damage and degeneration, inflammation, fibrosis or apoptosis (55). In addition, analysis of genes involved in skeletal muscle regeneration indicates that regeneration in dKO muscle is rare, which is insufficient to account for the extensive centronuclear fibers (55). dKO skeletal myofibers also showed disorganized triads where excitation–contraction (EC) coupling occurs, as well as, mitochondrial dysfunction and of fast-to-slow myofiber conversion (55).

The characteristics of the pathological phenotype of dKO mice is reminiscent of human centronuclear myopathy (CNM), which is a group of congenital myopathies characterized by muscle weakness and abnormal centralization of nuclei in muscle fibers (56). Several gene mutations in humans are linked to the disease. Among them, multiple missense mutations in the dynamin 2 locus, which encodes a ubiquitously expressed large GTPase, that has been linked to the autosomal dominant form of CNM (57). Most of these mutations do not affect dynamin 2 mRNA level, protein expression, or localization. In fact, it is now believed these dynamin 2 mutations function in a dominant negative form, or even a super-active form, in some cases (57). Interestingly, miR-133a is shown to target and repress dynamin 2 expression by binding to its 3′ UTR and dynamin 2 expression is upregulated at both mRNA and protein levels in dKO muscle (55). Moreover, elevated expression of dynamin 2 in skeletal muscle causes CNM, similar to the dKO muscle (55). These results demonstrate that the centronuclear myopathy observed in dKO muscle can be attributed, at least in part, to dysregulation of dynamin 2. Taken together, these findings highlight the important role of miR-133a in maintaining normal structure and function of adult skeletal muscle.

MyomiRs AND MYOFIBER TYPE SPECIFICATION

MyomiRs refer to a family of intronic miRNAs consisting of miR-208, miR-208b, and miR-499, which are embedded in the introns of three muscle-specific myosin genes (Myh6, Myh7, and Myh7b) (58). These three miRNAs share significant homology in seed sequences, implying that they may have overlapping functions by their regulation of the same set of targets. Among them, miR-208 is solely heart-specific, whereas miR-208b and miR-499 are expressed in both heart and slow (type I) skeletal muscle myofibers (58).

MyomiRs have important functions in regulating myosin content and stress-dependent cardiac remodeling (58,59). In skeletal muscle, miR-208b and miR-499 redundantly control muscle fiber identity by activating slow and repressing fast myofiber genes. Mice lacking both miR-208b and miR-499 showed a substantial loss of type I myofibers in the soleus muscle (58). Conversely, forced expression of miR-499 in skeletal muscle induces a complete conversion of all fast myofibers in soleus to slow (type I) fibers (58). The actions of MyomiRs in skeletal muscle are mediated by a collection of transcriptional repressors of slow muscle genes, including Sox6, Purß, and Sp3 (58). Among them, the transcription factor Sox6 is of special interest. Conditional deletion of Sox6 in neonatal skeletal muscle in mice leads to a fast to slow myofiber conversion, accompanied by changes in skeletal muscle mechanics and performance (60). Sox6 directly represses a collection of slow isoforms of sarcomeric and calcium regulatory proteins (60). These studies demonstrate the important roles of MyomiRs and Sox6 in regulating skeletal muscle gene program and muscle performance.

OTHER miRNAs IN SKELETAL MUSCLE BIOLOGY

In addition to the muscle-specific miRNAs, many other miRNAs are important regulators of skeletal muscle myogenesis and function. miR-27b is expressed in the differentiating myotome in embryos and in adult activated satellite cells (61). miR-27 promotes muscle stem cell differentiation by targeting and repressing Pax3, an essential protein for maintenance of skeletal muscle stem cell proliferation during development and adulthood (61).

miR-214 is expressed in skeletal muscle cell progenitors during zebrafish development and was shown to act as a positive regulator of the slow muscle phenotype by targeting suppressor of fused (sufu) expression, a negative regulator of Hedgehog signaling essential for proper specification of muscle cell types during somitogenesis (62). miR-214 is also shown to repress both myoblast proliferation and differentiation (63).

In addition, other miRNAs, such as miR-181, miR-322/424, miR-503, miR-214, and miR-29, are believed to promote myoblast differentiation by either repressing proliferation or inducing differentiation program (63–66). Conversely, other miRNAs, such as miR-221, miR-222, and miR-125b negatively regulate differentiation by promoting proliferation, which includes (67,68). Their function in skeletal muscle development *in vivo* remains to be determined.

Endurance exercise improves skeletal muscle function, by enhancing muscle energy metabolism and strength. Conversely, lack of exercise and immobilization induce skeletal muscle atrophy and decrease metabolic activity. In addition to changing the expression and activity of muscle enzymes and proteins, exercise also influences miRNA expression. For example, expression of miR-23 and miR-696 is decreased in skeletal muscle after endurance training in mice and is increased in the skeletal muscle of immobilized mice (69,70). Both of these miRNAs are shown to negatively regulate metabolism and mitochondrial biogenesis by repressing peroxisome proliferator-activated receptor-γ coactivator-α (PGC-1α), a key metabolic modulator in skeletal muscle (69,70). In addition, miRNA expression can be influenced by many factors, such as nutrition, hypertrophy, atrophy, and aging. While current studies mainly focus on miRNA expression profiling under different skeletal muscle conditions, it will be pivotal to understand whether any of these miRNAs play causal or protective roles in skeletal muscle.

Expression of miRNAs is dysregulated during skeletal muscle disease. Eisenberg and colleagues profiled miRNA expression in ten skeletal muscle disorders in humans, including the muscular dystrophies, inflammatory myopathies, and congenital myopathies. They discovered 185 miRNAs that are differentially expressed in diseased skeletal muscle. Of special interest among them are miR-146b, miR-155, miR-214, miR-221, and miR-222, which are increased in almost all of the samples (71). This observation suggests that these miRNAs are involved in a common underlying regulatory pathway among these skeletal muscle diseases. In addition, in myotonic dystrophy type I disease, miR-1 and miR-335 were upregulated, whereas miR-29b, -29c, and miR-33 were downregulated (72). It will be of further interest to examine whether these miRNAs contribute to the pathogenesis of these skeletal muscle diseases.

THERAPEUTIC IMPLICATIONS OF miRNAs IN SKELETAL MUSCLE DISORDERS

The distinct miRNA expression patterns in skeletal muscle myogenesis, function, and disease have opened up opportunities for miRNA-based therapeutics in diagnosing and treating skeletal muscle disease. miRNA profiling can be used diagnostically to determine the specific forms of skeletal muscle disorders. Remarkably, several miRNAs, including miR-206, miR-1, and miR-133, have been detected in the serum of *mdx* mice and patients with DMD and BMD (73,74). miR-206 is also found in serum of patients with RMS tumors (75). It is unknown how these miRNAs are released from injured tissues and secreted into blood. However, the detection of serum miRNAs provides new and valuable biomarkers for the diagnosis of DMD and RMS.

With a few exceptions, individual miRNAs seem to have minimal effect on basal level, unstressed adult tissues and appear to selectively contribute to cellular function under stress and disease states. These features make miRNAs attractive therapeutic targets, since strategies to inactivate disease-inducing miRNA may have minimal off-target effect on normal tissue. Drug therapies are being designed to repress pathological miRNAs, such as anti-miRs using locked nucleic acid (LNA)-modified oligonucleotides and seed-targeting tiny LNAs, or to overexpress protective miRNAs as miRNA mimics (76). Indeed, anti-miR-based studies against hepatitis C virus infection have proven their efficacy in non-human primates (77,78) and have been advanced to human clinical trials.

The application of miRNA-based therapies for skeletal muscle disorders in humans requires mechanistic understanding of the miRNA-based regulation of gene expression in normal and diseased muscle. It remains a great challenge to identify the mRNA targets that are relevant to a particular miRNA-regulated process among the many potential targets for each miRNA. It is also crucial to identify miRNAs that function cooperatively to regulate common or coordinated mRNA targets in skeletal muscle. This will provide important information in developing therapies such as anti-miR cocktails that may be more efficacious than targeting a single miRNA and can be used in conjunction with current therapies for treating skeletal muscle disease.

REFERENCES

1. Bartel DP. MicroRNAs: genomics, biogenesis, mechanism, and function. *Cell* 2004;**116**:281–97.
2. Cai X, Hagedorn CH, Cullen BR. Human microRNAs are processed from capped, polyadenylated transcripts that can also function as mRNAs. *RNA* 2004;**10**:1957–66.

3. Lee Y, Ahn C, Han J, Choi H, Kim J, Yim J, et al. The nuclear RNase III Drosha initiates microRNA processing. *Nature* 2003;**425**:415–9.
4. Denli AM, Tops BB, Plasterk RH, Ketting RF, Hannon GJ. Processing of primary microRNAs by the Microprocessor complex. *Nature* 2004;**432**:231–5.
5. Gregory RI, Yan KP, Amuthan G, Chendrimada T, Doratotaj B, Cooch N, et al. The Microprocessor complex mediates the genesis of microRNAs. *Nature* 2004;**432**:235–40.
6. Chendrimada TP, Gregory RI, Kumaraswamy E, Norman J, Cooch N, Nishikura K, et al. TRBP recruits the Dicer complex to Ago2 for microRNA processing and gene silencing. *Nature* 2005;**436**:740–4.
7. Filipowicz W, Bhattacharyya SN, Sonenberg N. Mechanisms of post-transcriptional regulation by microRNAs: are the answers in sight? *Nat Rev Genet* 2008;**9**:102–14.
8. Bartel DP. MicroRNAs: target recognition and regulatory functions. *Cell* 2009;**136**:215–33.
9. Gibbings DJ, Ciaudo C, Erhardt M, Voinnet O. Multivesicular bodies associate with components of miRNA effector complexes and modulate miRNA activity. *Nat Cell Biol* 2009;**11**:1143–9.
10. Valadi H, Ekstrom K, Bossios A, Sjostrand M, Lee JJ, Lotvall JO. Exosome-mediated transfer of mRNAs and microRNAs is a novel mechanism of genetic exchange between cells. *Nat Cell Biol* 2007;**9**:654–9.
11. Liu N, Olson EN. MicroRNA regulatory networks in cardiovascular development. *Dev Cell* 2010;**18**:510–25.
12. Small EM, Olson EN. Pervasive roles of microRNAs in cardiovascular biology. *Nature* 2011;**469**:336–42.
13. O'Rourke JR, Georges SA, Seay HR, Tapscott SJ, McManus MT, Goldhamer DJ, et al. Essential role for Dicer during skeletal muscle development. *Dev Biol* 2007;**311**:359–68.
14. Chen JF, Mandel EM, Thomson JM, Wu Q, Callis TE, Hammond SM, et al. The role of microRNA-1 and microRNA-133 in skeletal muscle proliferation and differentiation. *Nat Genet* 2006;**38**:228–33.
15. Liu N, Williams AH, Kim Y, McAnally J, Bezprozvannaya S, Sutherland LB, et al. An intragenic MEF2-dependent enhancer directs muscle-specific expression of microRNAs 1 and 133. *Proc Natl Acad Sci USA* 2007;**104**:20844–9.
16. Zhao Y, Samal E, Srivastava D. Serum response factor regulates a muscle-specific microRNA that targets Hand2 during cardiogenesis. *Nature* 2005;**436**:214–20.
17. Rao PK, Kumar RM, Farkhondeh M, Baskerville S, Lodish HF. Myogenic factors that regulate expression of muscle-specific microRNAs. *Proc Natl Acad Sci USA* 2006;**103**:8721–6.
18. Sanes JR, Lichtman JW. Induction, assembly, maturation and maintenance of a postsynaptic apparatus. *Nat Rev Neurosci* 2001;**2**:791–805.
19. Williams AH, Valdez G, Moresi V, Qi X, McAnally J, Elliott JL, et al. MicroRNA-206 delays ALS progression and promotes regeneration of neuromuscular synapses in mice. *Science* 2009;**326**:1549–54.
20. Bruijn LI, Miller TM, Cleveland DW. Unraveling the mechanisms involved in motor neuron degeneration in ALS. *Annu Rev Neurosci* 2004;**27**:723–49.
21. Dunckley T, Huentelman MJ, Craig DW, Pearson JV, Szelinger S, Joshipura K, et al. Whole-genome analysis of sporadic amyotrophic lateral sclerosis. *N Engl J Med* 2007;**357**:775–88.
22. Gurney ME, Pu H, Chiu AY, Dal Canto MC, Polchow CY, Alexander DD, et al. Motor neuron degeneration in mice that express a human Cu,Zn superoxide dismutase mutation. *Science* 1994;**264**:1772–5.
23. Son M, Puttaparthi K, Kawamata H, Rajendran B, Boyer PJ, Manfredi G, et al. Overexpression of CCS in G93A-SOD1 mice leads to accelerated neurological deficits with severe mitochondrial pathology. *Proc Natl Acad Sci USA* 2007;**104**:6072–7.
24. Charge SB, Rudnicki MA. Cellular and molecular regulation of muscle regeneration. *Physiol Rev* 2004;**84**:209–38.
25. Dhawan J, Rando TA. Stem cells in postnatal myogenesis: molecular mechanisms of satellite cell quiescence, activation and replenishment. *Trends Cell Biol* 2005;**15**:666–73.
26. Kuang S, Gillespie MA, Rudnicki MA. Niche regulation of muscle satellite cell self-renewal and differentiation. *Cell Stem Cell* 2008;**2**:22–31.
27. Buckingham M. Skeletal muscle progenitor cells and the role of Pax genes. *CR Biol* 2007;**330**:530–3.
28. Rudnicki MA, Le Grand F, McKinnell I, Kuang S. The molecular regulation of muscle stem cell function. *Cold Spring Harb Symp Quant Biol* 2008;**73**:323–31.
29. Chen JF, Tao Y, Li J, Deng Z, Yan Z, Xiao X, et al. microRNA-1 and microRNA-206 regulate skeletal muscle satellite cell proliferation and differentiation by repressing Pax7. *J Cell Biol* 2010;**190**:867–79.
30. Cacchiarelli D, Martone J, Girardi E, Cesana M, Incitti T, Morlando M, et al. MicroRNAs involved in molecular circuitries relevant for the Duchenne muscular dystrophy pathogenesis are controlled by the dystrophin/nNOS pathway. *Cell Metab* 2010;**12**:341–51.
31. Hirai H, Verma M, Watanabe S, Tastad C, Asakura Y, Asakura A. MyoD regulates apoptosis of myoblasts through microRNA-mediated down-regulation of Pax3. *J Cell Biol* 2010;**191**:347–65.
32. Yuasa K, Hagiwara Y, Ando M, Nakamura A, Takeda S, Hijikata T. MicroRNA-206 is highly expressed in newly formed muscle fibers: implications regarding potential for muscle regeneration and maturation in muscular dystrophy. *Cell Struct Funct* 2008;**33**:163–9.
33. Anderson C, Catoe H, Werner R. MIR-206 regulates connexin43 expression during skeletal muscle development. *Nucleic Acids Res* 2006;**34**:5863–71.
34. Kim HK, Lee YS, Sivaprasad U, Malhotra A, Dutta A. Muscle-specific microRNA miR-206 promotes muscle differentiation. *J Cell Biol* 2006;**174**:677–87.
35. Rosenberg MI, Georges SA, Asawachaicharn A, Analau E, Tapscott SJ. MyoD inhibits Fstl1 and Utrn expression by inducing transcription of miR-206. *J Cell Biol* 2006;**175**:77–85.
36. Davies KE, Nowak KJ. Molecular mechanisms of muscular dystrophies: old and new players. *Nat Rev Mol Cell Biol* 2006;**7**:762–73.
37. Hoffman EP, Fischbeck KH, Brown RH, Johnson M, Medori R, Loike JD, et al. Characterization of dystrophin in muscle-biopsy specimens from patients with Duchenne's or Becker's muscular dystrophy. *N Engl J Med.* 1988;**318**:1363–8.
38. Wallace GQ, McNally EM. Mechanisms of muscle degeneration, regeneration, and repair in the muscular dystrophies. *Annu Rev Physiol* 2009;**71**:37–57.
39. McCarthy JJ, Esser KA, Andrade FH. MicroRNA-206 is overexpressed in the diaphragm but not the hindlimb muscle of mdx mouse. *Am J Physiol Cell Physiol* 2007;**293**:C451–7.

40. Wachtel M, Runge T, Leuschner I, Stegmaier S, Koscielniak E, Treuner J, et al. Subtype and prognostic classification of rhabdomyosarcoma by immunohistochemistry. *J Clin Oncol* 2006;**24**:816–22.
41. Merlino G, Helman LJ. Rhabdomyosarcoma – working out the pathways. *Oncogene* 1999;**18**:5340–8.
42. Yan D, Dong Xda E, Chen X, Wang L, Lu C, Wang J, et al. MicroRNA-1/206 targets c-Met and inhibits rhabdomyosarcoma development. *J Biol Chem* 2009;**284**:29596–604.
43. Taulli R, Bersani F, Foglizzo V, Linari A, Vigna E, Ladanyi M, et al. The muscle-specific microRNA miR-206 blocks human rhabdomyosarcoma growth in xenotransplanted mice by promoting myogenic differentiation. *J Clin Invest* 2009;**119**:2366–78.
44. Missiaglia E, Shepherd CJ, Patel S, Thway K, Pierron G, Pritchard-Jones K, et al. MicroRNA-206 expression levels correlate with clinical behaviour of rhabdomyosarcomas. *Br J Cancer* 2010;**102**:1769–77.
45. Simon DJ, Madison JM, Conery AL, Thompson-Peer KL, Soskis M, Ruvkun GB, et al. The microRNA miR-1 regulates a MEF-2-dependent retrograde signal at neuromuscular junctions. *Cell* 2008;**133**:903–15.
46. Kwon C, Han Z, Olson EN, Srivastava D. MicroRNA1 influences cardiac differentiation in *Drosophila* and regulates Notch signaling. *Proc Natl Acad Sci USA* 2005;**102**:18986–91.
47. Sokol NS, Ambros V. Mesodermally expressed *Drosophila* microRNA-1 is regulated by Twist and is required in muscles during larval growth. *Genes Dev* 2005;**19**:2343–54.
48. Kwon YW, Manthena C, Oh JJ, Srivastava D. Vibrational characteristics of carbon nanotubes as nanomechanical resonators. *J Nanosci Nanotechnol* 2005;**5**:703–12.
49. Mishima Y, Abreu-Goodger C, Staton AA, Stahlhut C, Shou C, Cheng C, et al. Zebrafish miR-1 and miR-133 shape muscle gene expression and regulate sarcomeric actin organization. *Genes Dev* 2009;**23**:619–32.
50. McCarthy JJ, Esser KA. MicroRNA-1 and microRNA-133a expression are decreased during skeletal muscle hypertrophy. *J Appl Physiol* 2007;**102**:306–13.
51. Clop A, Marcq F, Takeda H, Pirottin D, Tordoir X, Bibe B, et al. A mutation creating a potential illegitimate microRNA target site in the myostatin gene affects muscularity in sheep. *Nat Genet* 2006;**38**:813–8.
52. Greco S, De Simone M, Colussi C, Zaccagnini G, Fasanaro P, Pescatori M, et al. Common micro-RNA signature in skeletal muscle damage and regeneration induced by Duchenne muscular dystrophy and acute ischemia. *FASEB J* 2009;**23**:3335–46.
53. Liu N, Bezprozvannaya S, Williams AH, Qi X, Richardson JA, Bassel-Duby R, et al. microRNA-133a regulates cardiomyocyte proliferation and suppresses smooth muscle gene expression in the heart. *Genes Dev* 2008;**22**:3242–54.
54. Pipes GC, Creemers EE, Olson EN. The myocardin family of transcriptional coactivators: versatile regulators of cell growth, migration, and myogenesis. *Genes Dev* 2006;**20**:1545–56.
55. Liu N, Bezprozvannaya S, Shelton JM, Frisard MI, Hulver MW, McMillan RP, et al. Mice lacking microRNA 133a develop dynamin 2–dependent centronuclear myopathy. *J Clin Invest* 2011;**121**:3258–68.
56. Romero NB. Centronuclear myopathies: a widening concept. *Neuromuscul Disord* **20**:223–8.
57. Durieux AC, Prudhon B, Guicheney P, Bitoun M. Dynamin 2 and human diseases. *J Mol Med* **88**:339–50.
58. van Rooij E, Quiat D, Johnson BA, Sutherland LB, Qi X, Richardson JA, et al. A family of microRNAs encoded by myosin genes governs myosin expression and muscle performance. *Dev Cell* 2009;**17**:662–73.
59. van Rooij E, Sutherland LB, Qi X, Richardson JA, Hill J, Olson EN. Control of stress-dependent cardiac growth and gene expression by a microRNA. *Science* 2007;**316**:575–9.
60. Quiat D, Voekler K, Pei J, Grishin N, Bassel-Duby R, Olson EN. Concerted regulation of myofiber specific gene expression and muscle performance by the transcriptional repressor Sox6. *Proc Natl Acad Sci USA* 2011;**108**:10196–201.
61. Crist CG, Montarras D, Pallafacchina G, Rocancourt D, Cumano A, Conway SJ, et al. Muscle stem cell behavior is modified by microRNA-27 regulation of Pax3 expression. *Proc Natl Acad Sci USA* 2009;**106**:13383–7.
62. Flynt AS, Li N, Thatcher EJ, Solnica-Krezel L, Patton JG. Zebrafish miR-214 modulates Hedgehog signaling to specify muscle cell fate. *Nat Genet* 2007;**39**:259–63.
63. Feng Y, Cao JH, Li XY, Zhao SH. Inhibition of miR-214 expression represses proliferation and differentiation of C2C12 myoblasts. *Cell Biochem Funct* 2011;**29**:378–83.
64. Naguibneva I, Ameyar-Zazoua M, Polesskaya A, Ait-Si-Ali S, Groisman R, Souidi M, et al. The microRNA miR-181 targets the homeobox protein Hox-A11 during mammalian myoblast differentiation. *Nat Cell Biol* 2006;**8**:278–84.
65. Sarkar S, Dey BK, Dutta A. MiR-322/424 and -503 are induced during muscle differentiation and promote cell cycle quiescence and differentiation by downregulation of Cdc25A. *Mol Biol Cell* 2010;**21**:2138–49.
66. Winbanks CE, Wang B, Beyer C, Koh P, White L, Kantharidis P, et al. TGF-β regulates miR-206 and miR-29 to control myogenic differentiation through regulation of HDAC4. *J Biol Chem* 2011;**286**:13805–14.
67. Cardinali B, Castellani L, Fasanaro P, Basso A, Alema S, Martelli F, et al. Microrna-221 and microrna-222 modulate differentiation and maturation of skeletal muscle cells. *PLoS One* 2009;**4**:e7607.
68. Ge Y, Sun Y, Chen J. IGF-II is regulated by microRNA-125b in skeletal myogenesis. *J Cell Biol* 2011;**192**:69–81.
69. Safdar A, Abadi A, Akhtar M, Hettinga BP, Tarnopolsky MA. miRNA in the regulation of skeletal muscle adaptation to acute endurance exercise in C57Bl/6J male mice. *PLoS One* 2009;**4**:e5610.
70. Aoi W, Naito Y, Mizushima K, Takanami Y, Kawai Y, Ichikawa H, et al. The microRNA miR-696 regulates PGC-1{alpha} in mouse skeletal muscle in response to physical activity. *Am J Physiol Endocrinol Metab* 2010;**298**:E799–806.
71. Eisenberg I, Eran A, Nishino I, Moggio M, Lamperti C, Amato AA, et al. Distinctive patterns of microRNA expression in primary muscular disorders. *Proc Natl Acad Sci USA* 2007;**104**:17016–21.
72. Perbellini R, Greco S, Sarra-Ferraris G, Cardani R, Capogrossi MC, Meola G, et al. Dysregulation and cellular mislocalization of specific miRNAs in myotonic dystrophy type 1. *Neuromuscul Disord* 2011;**21**:81–8.
73. Cacchiarelli D, Legnini I, Martone J, Cazzella V, D'Amico A, Bertini E, et al. miRNAs as serum biomarkers for Duchenne muscular dystrophy. *EMBO Mol Med* 2011;**3**:258–65.

74. Mizuno H, Nakamura A, Aoki Y, Ito N, Kishi S, Yamamoto K, et al. Identification of muscle-specific microRNAs in serum of muscular dystrophy animal models: promising novel blood-based markers for muscular dystrophy. *PLoS One* 2011;**6**: e18388.
75. Miyachi M, Tsuchiya K, Yoshida H, Yagyu S, Kikuchi K, Misawa A, et al. Circulating muscle-specific microRNA, miR-206, as a potential diagnostic marker for rhabdomyosarcoma. *Biochem Biophys Res Commun* 2010;**400**:89–93.
76. Stenvang J, Silahtaroglu AN, Lindow M, Elmen J, Kauppinen S. The utility of LNA in microRNA-based cancer diagnostics and therapeutics. *Semin Cancer Biol* 2008;**18**:89–102.
77. Elmen J, Lindow M, Schutz S, Lawrence M, Petri A, Obad S, et al. LNA-mediated microRNA silencing in non-human primates. *Nature* 2008;**452**:896–9.
78. Lanford RE, Hildebrandt-Eriksen ES, Petri A, Persson R, Lindow M, Munk ME, et al. Therapeutic silencing of microRNA-122 in primates with chronic hepatitis C virus infection. *Science* 2010;**327**:198–201.

Chapter 62

Musculoskeletal Tissue Injury and Repair: Role of Stem Cells, Their Differentiation, and Paracrine Effects

Burhan Gharaibeh[1,2,3], Bridget Deasy[1,2,3], Mitra Lavasani[1], James H. Cummins[1], Yong Li[1,2,3,4] and Johnny Huard[1,2,3,4,5]

[1]*Stem Cell Research Center, Department of Orthopaedic Surgery,* [2]*Department of Bioengineering,* [3]*McGowan Institute for Regenerative Medicine,* [4]*Department of Pathology,* [5]*Departments of Molecular Genetics and Biochemistry, Physical Medicine and Rehabilitation, University of Pittsburgh, Pittsburgh, PA*

PATHOPHYSIOLOGY OF SKELETAL MUSCLE INJURY

Skeletal muscle injuries are one of the most common complaints presented to general medical physicians and also account for a large majority of patients seen in orthopedic clinics (1). Investigations have demonstrated that the natural progression of muscle injury proceeds through a highly coordinated sequence of steps, leading to the restoration of normal tissue architecture and function. Unfortunately, the regenerative capacity of injured skeletal muscle is limited and commonly results in the formation of fibrotic tissue, which predisposes the muscle to recurrent injury and prolongs recovery of function (2). Clinical experience reveals a high recurrence rate of skeletal muscle strain injuries among athletes, approaching 30% in some professional-level athletes (3). Advances in the identification of molecular events and cellular transformations following muscle injury have flourished; however, the clinical treatment of this common condition still relies upon conventional therapies of rest, ice, and anti-inflammatory medications, which have a limited efficacy in preventing or treating the formation of post-traumatic muscle fibrosis (4–6). Injured muscle undergoes a sequential process of healing phases, including muscle degeneration/inflammation, regeneration, and fibrosis (7,8), which will be further discussed below. The development of different biological approaches to influence these phases of muscle healing has been extensively studied and will also be analyzed more in depth in this review.

Muscle Inflammation

Active muscle degeneration and inflammation occur within the first few days after injury (Figure 62.1). Non-steroidal anti-inflammatory drugs (NSAIDs) are often prescribed to relieve pain after muscle injury; however, the effect of this group of drugs on the muscle healing process remains largely controversial. To further examine the validity of using these drugs after muscle injury, we have performed two studies to determine the role that cyclooxygenase-2 (Cox-2) plays in the process of muscle healing (9,10). Our *in vitro* experiments showed that NS-398 (a Cox-2-specific inhibitor) hinders the proliferation and maturation of differentiated myogenic precursor cells. Similar results were obtained using the Cox-2 selective inhibitor SC-236 (11,12). Our data thus suggest that NS-398 may have a detrimental effect on skeletal muscle healing. Using a laceration model in mouse skeletal muscle, we analyzed the *in vivo* effect of NS-398 on muscle healing at time points up to 4 weeks after injury. Similar to the *in vitro* data, the *in vivo* results revealed delayed muscle regeneration at early time points after injury in the NS-398-treated mice. The lacerated muscles treated with NS-398 expressed higher levels of transforming growth factor-β1 (TGF-β1) than did the untreated control muscles, which also corresponded with increased fibrosis deposition. We also found fewer neutrophils and less macrophage infiltration in the treated muscles, which indicates that the delayed skeletal muscle healing observed after the injection of NS-398 could be due to the inhibitory effect of NS-398 on the inflammatory responses. In addition, we analyzed muscle healing following laceration injury on the tibialis anterior (TA) muscles of wild-type (Wt) and COX-$2^{-/-}$ mice (9). At 5 and 14 days after injury, we examined the TA muscles histologically and functionally. Histological and functional assessments of the TA muscles in the COX-$2^{-/-}$ mice revealed decreased regeneration relative to that observed

Muscle. DOI: http://dx.doi.org/10.1016/B978-0-12-381510-1.00062-4

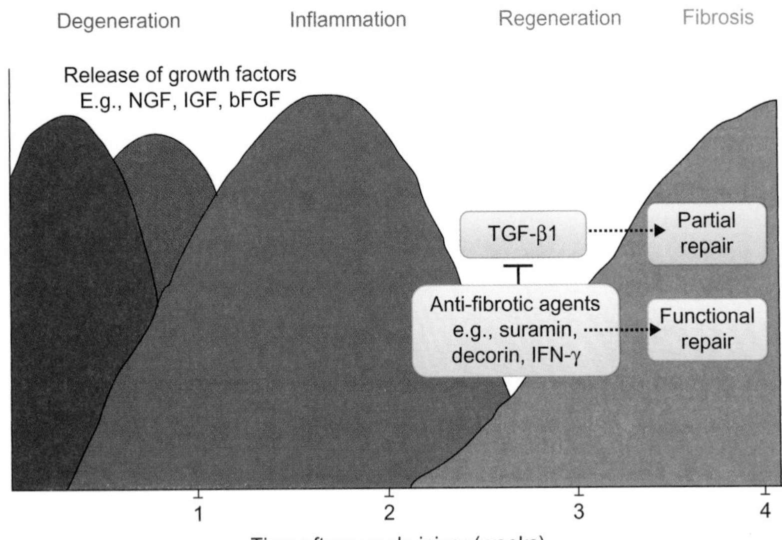

FIGURE 62.1 Healing process in the skeletal muscle. Several overlapping phases are accompanied by the release of growth factors that modulate regeneration and formation of fibrotic tissue. Use of antifibrotic agents minimizes muscle scarring and leads to better functional outcome.

in the Wt mice. The findings reported here demonstrate that the COX-2 pathway plays an important role in muscle healing and suggests that the decision to use NSAIDs to treat muscle injuries warrants critical evaluation, as NSAIDs might actually impair muscle healing.

Muscle Regeneration

Muscle regeneration usually begins during the first week after injury, peaks at 2 weeks, and then gradually slows 3–4 weeks after injury. Many reports have shown that growth factors play a variety of roles during muscle regeneration (13–49). In a mouse model, direct injections of insulin-like growth factor-1 (IGF-1), basic fibroblastic growth factor (bFGF), and, to a lesser extent, nerve growth factor (NGF), lead to enhanced muscle healing in lacerated, contused, and strain-injured muscle at 2, 5, and 7 days after injury (50). One advantage of using human recombinant growth factors to treat muscle injuries is the ease and safety of the injection; however, the efficacy of direct injection of recombinant proteins (growth factors) is limited by the high concentration of the factor typically required to elicit a measurable effect. Whereas growth factors have a dose-dependent effect on myoblast proliferation and differentiation *in vitro*, three consecutive injections of a relatively high concentration of NGF, IGF-1, or bFGF (100 ng/growth factor) are usually necessary to achieve detectable enhancement of skeletal muscle healing in mice (7,8,16,50–55). The bloodstream's rapid clearance of these molecules and their relatively short biological half-lives are the main reasons why such large concentrations of growth factors are typically required. Gene therapy may be an effective method by which to deliver high, maintainable concentrations of growth factor to injured muscle. Because previous studies had demonstrated IGF-1 to be a potent growth factor for stimulating muscle regeneration and improving muscle healing *in vivo* after injury (7,8,16,50–55), we engineered an adenovirus carrying the IGF-1 gene and evaluated its ability to improve muscle healing after injury (56). Myoblast-mediated *ex vivo* gene transfer of this adenovirus carrying the gene encoding for IGF-1 improved the healing of lacerated muscle in immunocompetent mice (56). Although we observed improved muscle healing, histology of the injected muscle revealed muscle fibrosis within the lacerated site, despite the production of a high level of IGF-1 (56). Taken together, these results suggest that, although we were able to achieve high levels of IGF-1 secretion mediated by the injected adenoviral vector, the functional recovery of the injured muscle remained incomplete. Some research suggests that the stimulatory action of IGF-1 on myofibroblast proliferation and the deposition of extra cellular matrix (ECM) – i.e. scar tissue – might interfere with the ability of this growth factor, even at high concentrations, to improve muscle healing after injury (20,34). Overall, these, and other results, indicate that the prevention of muscle fibrosis could be a better approach by which to improve muscle healing.

Muscle Fibrosis

Fibrosis (the formation of scar tissue) usually begins between the second and third week after injury, and scar tissue formation continues to increase in size over time (2,57). Our research findings strongly indicate that scar tissue formation precludes complete regeneration of injured muscle tissue. Although various studies have implicated TGF-β1 in the onset of fibrosis in various tissues (58–70), very few reports have examined the direct role of this cytokine in skeletal muscle fibrosis. Research has demonstrated that TGF-β1 is expressed at high levels and is associated with fibrosis in the skeletal muscle of Duchenne muscular dystrophy (DMD) patients (71–73). Studies also have revealed excess TGF-β1 in muscle biopsy specimens of patients with dermatomyositis (74,75). This excess TGF-β1 leads to chronic inflammation, the accumulation of ECM, and fibrosis (74,75). Using immunohistochemistry, we have observed strong expression of TGF-β1 in injured skeletal muscle (7,8). These results support the hypothesis that the expression of TGF-β1 in skeletal muscle plays an important role in the fibrotic cascade that occurs after the onset of muscle disease or trauma. Therefore, it is very feasible that neutralization of TGF-β1 expression in injured muscle could inhibit the formation of scar tissue (Figure 62.1).

Specifically, we have focused our recent efforts on agents that inhibit muscle fibrosis via the inhibition of TGF-β1. Using decorin, suramin, relaxin, and interferon-gamma (IFN-γ), we have demonstrated that therapies with these drugs can decrease fibrosis and increase regeneration following skeletal muscle injury (51–55,76). However, their use clinically is hampered by relatively severe side-effect profiles, lack of oral dosing formulations, and, in the case of decorin, lack of FDA approval for use in humans.

Modulating Fibrosis with Losartan

Fibrosis is a pathological process that is not unique to the skeletal muscle system. Observations have linked pathologic fibrosis in various organ systems to the local effects of a naturally-occurring molecule, angiotensin II, an end-product of the blood pressure-regulating renin-angiotensin system. The modulation of angiotensin II with angiotensin-converting enzyme inhibitors or angiotensin II receptor blockers has demonstrated decreased fibrosis and improved function in liver, kidney, lung tissue, and the aortic wall (77–81). Injured cardiac muscle, in diseases such as congestive heart failure, has also been demonstrated to be dysfunctional considering the amount of fibrosis present. Myocardium exposed to decreased levels of angiotensin II, either through the use of angiotensin converting enzyme inhibitors or angiotensin receptor blockers, has also demonstrated measurably improved function (81–83). Investigators have observed a relationship between the modulation of angiotensin II and skeletal muscle healing. Patients treated with angiotensin-modulating medications for the treatment of hypertension also displayed the unexpected side-effect of decreased rates of muscle wasting and a reduction in the relative amount of adipose tissue within their musculature (84). Moreover, treatment with angiotensin-converting enzyme (ACE) inhibitors and studies of persons carrying a deletion of ACE gene have shown that the skeletal muscle hypertrophic response to overloading is probably related to the renin-angiotensin system (84,85).

Recent experiments have been performed to elucidate the mechanism by which angiotensin II receptor blockade modulates TGF-β1, which has also been implicated in the prevention of muscle regeneration in murine models of chronic myopathic disease (86). These results indicate that by modulating the response to local and systemic angiotensin II, angiotensin receptor blocker therapy significantly reduced fibrosis and led to an increase in the number of regenerating myofibers in acutely injured skeletal muscle. These effects were apparent as early as 3 weeks after injury in mice treated with one-tenth of the anti-hypertensive dose of angiotensin receptor blocker used clinically. The clinical implications for this application of angiotensin receptor blockers are potentially far-reaching and include not only sports and military-related injuries, but also diseases like the muscular dystrophies. We believe that this treatment could be effective when instituting a non-invasive treatment after the injury has taken place, a more clinically relevant scenario in treating muscle injuries. Angiotensin receptor blockers may provide the ultimate safe, clinically available non-invasive treatment for improving healing following skeletal muscle injury. Additional studies prior to clinical translation to patients with sports- or military-related muscle injuries will need to be performed to determine proper dosing, timing of drug delivery and persistence of beneficial effects post injury.

MUSCLE STEM CELL-MEDIATED SKELETAL MUSCLE REPAIR

The use of a variety of muscle cell populations for cell therapy has been a focus of studies of cell transplantation for treating patients with Duchenne muscular dystrophy (DMD), a muscle disease characterized by the lack of dystrophin expression at the sarcolemma of muscle fibers (87). Transplantation of committed myoblasts into dystrophin-deficient muscle delivers normal myoblasts that fuse among themselves and/or with host muscle fibers and restores dystrophin; however, this approach is hindered by numerous limitations including immune responses, limited spreading and poor survival of the transplanted cells (88–93). Although the immune response and the low spreading capacity of the cells have been overcome, at least in part (94,95), the low survival of the transplanted cells is still a major limitation. Indeed, numerous studies report that only a small percentage of the transplanted cells (less than 1–5%) survive, therefore approaches to increase cell survival post-implantation are a major interest for myoblast transplantation in DMD (89,96,97).

Direct efforts to promote myoblast survival initially focused on overcoming the inflammatory response (97–99). Myoblasts genetically engineered to express an inhibitor of the inflammatory cytokine, IL-1, showed an improved survival rate compared to non-engineered cells (99). Treatment of the host with $CD4^+/CD8^+$-depleting antibodies enhanced donor myoblast survival in dystrophic animals (97), and death of the transplanted myoblasts could be reduced by treating the host animals with antibodies against leukocyte function-associated molecule 1 (LFA-1) (98).

Alternatively, other studies, including ours, focused their efforts on the identification of specific subsets of donor cells capable of surviving after transplantation (96,100,101). We have shown that muscle-derived cells contain a slowly adhering fraction that repairs muscle in a more effective manner than myoblasts, which tend to more rapidly adhere to collagen-coated flasks. The slowly adhering populations were characterized with stem cell markers and termed muscle derived stem cells (MDSCs) (102,103). It has been shown that a subpopulation of surviving cells, that are slowly dividing (refractory to [^{3}H] thymidine uptake) and undergo long-term proliferation in the skeletal muscle, are predominantly the cells that participate in the repair process (96). Similarly, Collins et al. showed that among aged muscle satellite cells, the majority of cells progress to apoptosis; however, there is also a subset of cells that survive and this minority population is responsible for muscle regeneration (101). A recent report by Wagers' group used FACS to isolate a specific population of skeletal muscle precursors (SMPs: $CD45^-Sca\text{-}1^-Mac\text{-}1^-CXCR4^+\beta1\text{-}integrin^+$) that show a high level of muscle cell repair, while non-SMPs ($CXCR4^-/\beta1\text{-}integrin^-$) were rarely identified in the muscles after transplantation (104). It would be interesting to determine if these subpopulations secrete factors, which act both via an autocrine and paracrine fashions, to support their own survival and enhance their participation in skeletal muscle repair. Indeed, our previous study involving *ex vivo* gene transfer has shown that the transplantation of MDSCs, either stimulated with or genetically engineered to express NGF, into the skeletal muscle of dystrophic mdx mice, resulted in the regeneration of significantly more dystrophin-positive myofibers than the transplantation of non-transduced MDSCs (105). Our observations of newly regenerated myofibers by the transplanted MDSCs, particularly the engineered MDSCs, suggest an autocrine function as well as paracrine effect on neighboring regenerated myofibers.

One factor that may be involved in cell survival and tissue regeneration is the cells' expression of antioxidants. Recent studies show that a reduction of antioxidant levels negatively affects the regeneration index of myoblasts and satellite cells (106–108) and hematopoietic stem cells (109), likely through the cells' increased ability to survive post-implantation. We recently showed that the MDSCs express high levels of the antioxidants glutathione (GSH) and superoxide dismutase (SOD, which likely plays a role in the cells' ability to better survive the harsh transplantation microenvironment better than myoblasts and hence increase their ability to more efficiently regenerate the tissue (103,108). A reduction of the antioxidant level of MDSCs was also shown to decrease their regeneration potential while an improvement in their regenerative potential could be observed by increasing their anti-oxidant levels prior to transplantation (108,110).

Although it is not well known what bioactive factors may be secreted by the cells nor whether they have any immunomodulatory activity, a few studies have shown that transplanted muscle cells may induce angiogenesis in the host tissue and vascular endothelial growth factor (VEGF) may be involved (46,111,112). Similarly, the phenotype of the host cells that may play a role in the repair process is unclear, but evidence that anti-inflammatory drugs delay muscle repair implicates inflammatory cells in the repair process (9,113–115). The following sections suggest that the paracrine effect of the surviving cells, particularly with regard to angiogenesis induction, is a determining factor in donor cells contribution to the regeneration of various tissues including the heart, bone, and cartilage.

MUSCLE STEM CELL-MEDIATED CARDIAC REPAIR

The importance of paracrine signaling for stem cell therapy has been well documented in the area of cardiac tissue repair. Indeed, from cardiac tissue engineering, we find examples of significant improvements in tissue repair following stem cell transplantation, yet the donor stem cells show little or no evidence of cell differentiation to the cardiac lineage. In this case, evidence supports a critical role for donor cell secretion of signaling molecules and trophic paracrine effects in the repair process.

Transplantation of exogenous cells into damaged myocardium – also known as cellular cardiomyoplasty (CCM) – is a possible cell therapy for the treatment of several cardiac diseases. A range of cell types have been examined for CCM, including embryonic stem cells (116,117), hematopoietic stem cells (HSCs) (118,119), bone marrow-derived mesenchymal stem cells (BM-MSCs) (120–123), skeletal myoblasts (124–128), endothelial progenitors (129–131), fibroblasts (121,132–136), and cardiac stem cells (137–139).

The results from transplantation studies of several stem cell types strongly support the notion that a stem cell's ability to differentiate into cardiomyocytes is not required for the stem cells to be capable of improving the repair of an injured heart (140–145). MSCs (142,146) have shown some level of differentiation, and HSCs (119,141,147–149) have shown variable results in terms of *in vivo* cardiomyocyte differentiation. Several other cell types, such as adipose-derived stem cells (140), myoblasts (143), and AC133$^+$ MSCs (144), have shown little capacity to differentiate; however, the donor cells still conveyed therapeutic benefits. If tissue repair occurs, yet donor cell differentiation is limited, the interesting biologic question is: What is the mechanism of action of the donor stem cells that leads to cardiac repair? The answer for the mechanism may not be completely clear; however, reported outcomes of these studies show a cell-mediated paracrine effect that involves angiogenesis, vasoprotection, vasculotropic activity or cytoprotection. The transplanted cells may act as a reservoir of secreting molecules that play a role in the repair process without actively differentiating toward a certain lineage or by fusing with host cells (145,150). Several studies have reported improved cardiac repair via neovascularization, reduced scarring, and reduced apoptosis at the infarct or injury (151).

Increased angiogenesis is particularly involved with transplanted cell-mediated improvements in cardiac function, and this appears to be modulated through donor cell secretion of VEGF, stromal-cell derived growth factor (SDF-1), Akt1, and granulocyte colony stimulating factors (G-CSF) among others. Transplanted MSCs stimulated an increase in VEGF, SDF-1 and bFGF-2 secretion that was associated with increased vascularity and blood flow, and a decrease in cell apoptosis of the host cells (142). MSCs genetically engineered with Akt1 to promote survival post-implantation also showed that this prevented remodeling and collagen deposition and nearly normalized cardiac performance in an infarct model (123). Further, we reported that inhibiting angiogenesis by injecting genetically engineered MDSCs that express the anti-angiogenic protein sFlt-1 (a soluble receptor to VEGF) reduces the regeneration capacity of the MDSCs in the injured heart (152). These findings suggested that most of the cells contributing to the repair process were chemo-attracted to the injury site by the transplanted MDSCs (152). Interestingly, overexpression of VEGF did not result in further significant improvement in cardiac repair, likely due to sufficient endogenous VEGF expression by the MDSCs (152). Since the cardiac differentiation of BM-MSCs and MDSCs is extremely low, the findings support the notion that their beneficial effect is likely due to the promotion of angiogenesis through the secretion of VEGF and other cytokines and not due to the differentiation capacity of the donor cells toward a cardiac phenotype.

Tightly linked with the cells ability to impart a paracrine effect on the host is their ability to survive post-transplantation. Indeed, several studies show that preconditioning the cells to survive also contributes to the repair of the tissue, and this occurs even in the absence of donor cell differentiation. A recent study showed that hypoxia preconditioning of BM-MSCs led to the upregulation of VEGF, hypoxia inducible factor 1 (HIF-1), B-cell lymphoma 2 (Bcl-2), and others that enhanced their capacity to repair infarcted myocardium; this was attributable to both an improved cell survival and an increase in angiogenesis and pro-angiogenic factors (153). Pasha et al. also reported that preconditioning cells with the chemokine SDF-1 could significantly enhance BM-MSCs survival, vascular density, engraftment, and myocardial function (154). In addition, MSCs derived from adult bone marrow and genetically modified to express the anti-apoptotic gene, Bcl-2, could improve cell survival, engraftment, revascularization, and functional improvement in a rat left anterior descending ligation model of myocardial infarction via intracardiac injection (155).

Although the paracrine action of donor stem cells is clearly demonstrated, the phenotype of the host cells that participate in the repair process remains largely unknown. Likely candidates for the host cells involved in the repair process include bone marrow-derived cells, vascular-derived endothelial progenitor cells, inflammatory cells, and resident tissue stem cells. Particularly when angiogenesis is part of the host response, the mobilization and incorporation of bone marrow-derived endothelial progenitor cells (156,157) or pericytes (158) may be involved in the repair process. Given that blood vessel walls may be the origin of a wide variety of stem cells (159–162), it is likely that these cells play an important role in tissue repair.

The question remains whether differentiating the stem cells toward a cardiac lineage prior to their implantation could further improve cardiac repair. It should also be considered that the cardiac differentiation of the stem cells could re-direct the cells' paracrine signaling by downregulating these signaling molecules while upregulating the differentiation cascade; this could influence their action in the cardiac repair process. Yet, stem cells with cardiomyocyte properties (such as cardiac stem cells, or genetically engineered cells with cardiomyocyte inducers) are presumably more likely to integrate effectively with the host myocardium and participate in functional heart activity than stem cells incapable of differentiating toward a cardiac lineage, although this has yet to be shown.

Taken together, the cells' ability to secrete paracrine factors that induce angiogenesis, inhibit apoptosis, increase proliferation, mobilize host cell migration, and modulate the immune response within the injured heart, all appear to be important determining factors for the regenerative capacity of the cells (Figure 62.2). It may be

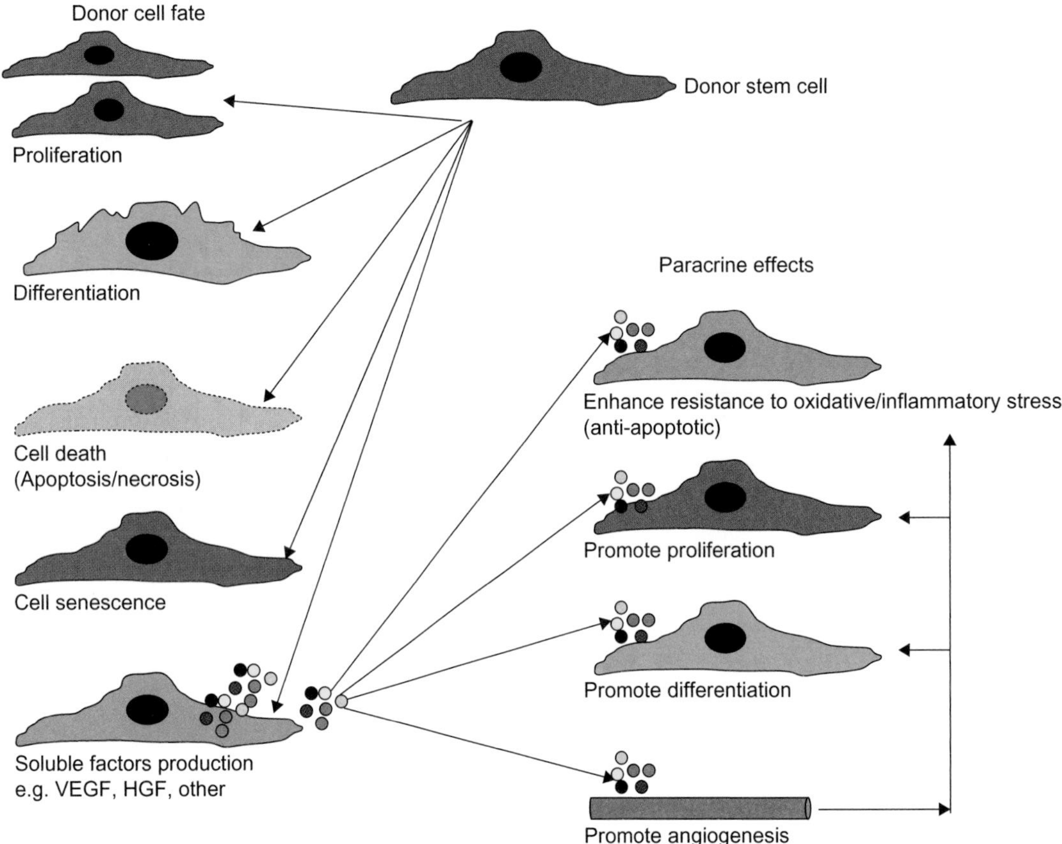

FIGURE 62.2 **Schematic of potential scenario of events taking place during cell therapy.** Donor stem cells proliferate, differentiate, apoptose, senesce or more importantly produce trophic factors that would have autocrine and paracrine effects on other donor and host cells. Furthermore, certain factors (e.g. VEGF) promote angiogenesis which can positively affect other processes.

that paracrine signaling is an alternative pathway for cells that do not differentiate, or cells that secrete bioactive molecules are engaged in paracrine signaling and do not readily move toward differentiation. The following sections will show that secretion of signaling molecules by donor stem cells also contributes to bone and articular cartilage repair. This does not preclude other fractions of donor cells from differentiating to osteogenic and chondrogenic lineages.

MUSCLE STEM CELL-MEDIATED BONE REPAIR

The importance of host cells chemo-attracted to the site of injury after implantation of stem cells has been well documented in the area of bone repair. Indeed, numerous reports also show a critical role for paracrine signaling and the influence of the host cells in stem cell therapies designed to treat bone injuries. In these studies, osteogenic differentiation is observed, yet donor cell signaling is also a significant contributor to tissue repair. Cell therapeutics for bone repair may provide benefits for devastating bone defects associated with delayed union or non-union injuries, and hence a variety of cell types have been explored in this regard. To promote bone healing, investigators have incorporated bone marrow stromal cells (163), adipose tissue-derived cells (164), fibrous tissue-derived cells (165,166), and skeletal muscle-derived cells (167,168) into regenerative medicine strategies. While several of these cell types demonstrate osteogenic differentiation capacity *in vitro*, it is often observed that it is the host cells that are predominantly involved in the *in vivo* repair even after cell transplantation.

Donor cell signaling via bone morphogenic proteins (BMPs), angiogenic factors, and other factors have been identified as contributing to improved bone healing. The normal process of bone healing involves a series of molecular events, including BMP expression (169), Noggin expression (170), and the induction of neovascularization by VEGF (171−173). Angiogenesis plays a role in bone formation, fracture healing, and endochondral ossification in the growth plate (171,174). An improvement of bone formation was reported with the transplantation of bone marrow stromal cells co-expressing the osteogenic factor BMP2 and the angiogenic factors angiopoietin-1 (Ang-1) and VEGF (175). The authors showed that the combination of multiple factors resulted in more efficient bone healing than when any of the factors were utilized alone. These results suggest neo-angiogenesis induced through donor cell signaling led to enhanced bone formation (175). Hausman and colleagues (176) also showed that when the angiogenesis inhibitor TNP-470 is used, bone fracture healing is inhibited in a rat injury model. Consequently, the combination of therapies that use stem cells and growth factor releasing scaffolds customized to promote angiogenesis and osteogenesis are under development for bone regeneration (177). We reported that VEGF acts synergistically with BMP4 to induce bone formation after stem cell therapy with MDSCs (178,179). Transplantation of BMP-expressing stem cells improves bone repair; however, the majority of the repair process is mediated by the chemo-attraction of host cells (180,181). Further, inhibiting angiogenesis by genetically engineering the MDSCs to express the anti-angiogenic protein sFlt-1 reduced the bone regeneration capacity of the MDSCs despite their inherent osteogenic potential, even when stimulated by BMP. The reduced regeneration may also be attributable to decreased viability of the transplanted cells in the hypoxic delivery site. In contrast, an improvement of bone healing was observed with stem cells over-expressing VEGF (179). These results demonstrated that the inhibition of donor cell paracrine signaling of pro-survival and angiogenic factors significantly reduced the bone tissue repair process of the cells despite the osteogenic potential of the cells. These findings support the notion that the multipotent behavior of stem cells is not the only factor involved in promoting significant tissue repair.

Other studies show paracrine signaling by transplanted human adipose-derived stromal cells (hASCs), possibly through sonic hedgehog signaling, was associated with regenerated murine calvarial bone defects (182). hASCs showed evidence of stimulation of host cell osteogenesis by increased expression of bone markers at the defect and increased host (murine) osteogenic gene expression (182). Finally, intravenous delivery of human BM-MSCs stimulated an increase in host bone density of patients with osteogenesis imperfecta despite the low differentiation of the donor cells toward osteogenesis (183).

As was described for cardiac repair above, however, a question remains unanswered: What is the phenotype of the host cells that participate in the bone repair process? It can be speculated that the improvement of tissue healing, via donor cell secretion of bioactive factors that also induce angiogenesis, could be due to the recruitment of blood vessel-derived cells (such as endothelial progenitors or pericytes) during the repair process; however, cells from the local micro-environment or from the circulatory system including inflammatory/immune cells and bone marrow-derived cells remain un-investigated and also could play a role in the regeneration process. In fact, it has been observed that blocking inflammation reduces bone repair, implicating the inflammatory cells in the cascade of events to improve bone healing (184). The studies using hASCs suggested that it was the mouse calvarial osteoblasts that responded to the donor cell signaling and participated in the repair process (182). The above studies highlight the systemic paracrine effect of transplanted stem cells and show that their role is likely through improved angiogenesis (Figure 62.3). However, with increased vascularity, the contribution of blood vessel wall cells and circulating blood cells and platelets is still unclear. The following section includes examples of cartilage repair that illustrate the effect that donor cell signaling has on the local micro-environment.

MUSCLE STEM CELL-MEDIATED CARTILAGE REPAIR

Contrary to most tissues, articular cartilage is an avascular tissue poorly supplied by blood vessels, nerves, and the lymphatic system (185). Transplantation of stem or progenitor cells with chondrogenic capacity has been widely examined to treat joint disorders such as chronic osteoarthritis (OA). While arthroplasty is a standard treatment, and autologous chondrocyte transplantation is becoming more common, new tissue engineering techniques using stem cells are being studied. Bone marrow MSCs have been the most extensively studied cell type for cartilage repair (186–188); however, stem cells from synovium, adipose tissue, skeletal muscle, and umbilical cord stroma have shown chondrogenic potential (189–192). Recently, stem cell-based therapies have been used clinically for cartilage repair (193,194), and many additional clinical trials are under way. Yet, there are few reports that describe the level of stem cell integration, and fewer that examine donor cell signaling after transplantation.

As described above for skeletal muscle, heart, and bone, trophic signaling of cytokines or growth factors by donor cells would also be expected to play an important role in cartilage repair. Gelse et al. reported that transplantation of chondrocytes that secrete BMP2 resulted in cartilage repair in osteochondral lesions; the repaired tissue included ingrowing host bone marrow-derived cells that may have responded to BMP2 secretion. In this same study, periosteal cells that did not secrete BMP2 led to a less pronounced repair (195). Other reports suggest that in the special case of cartilage, anti-angiogenic signaling with factors like troponin 1 (196) and chondromodulin 1 (197) is important for healthy articular cartilage. Since

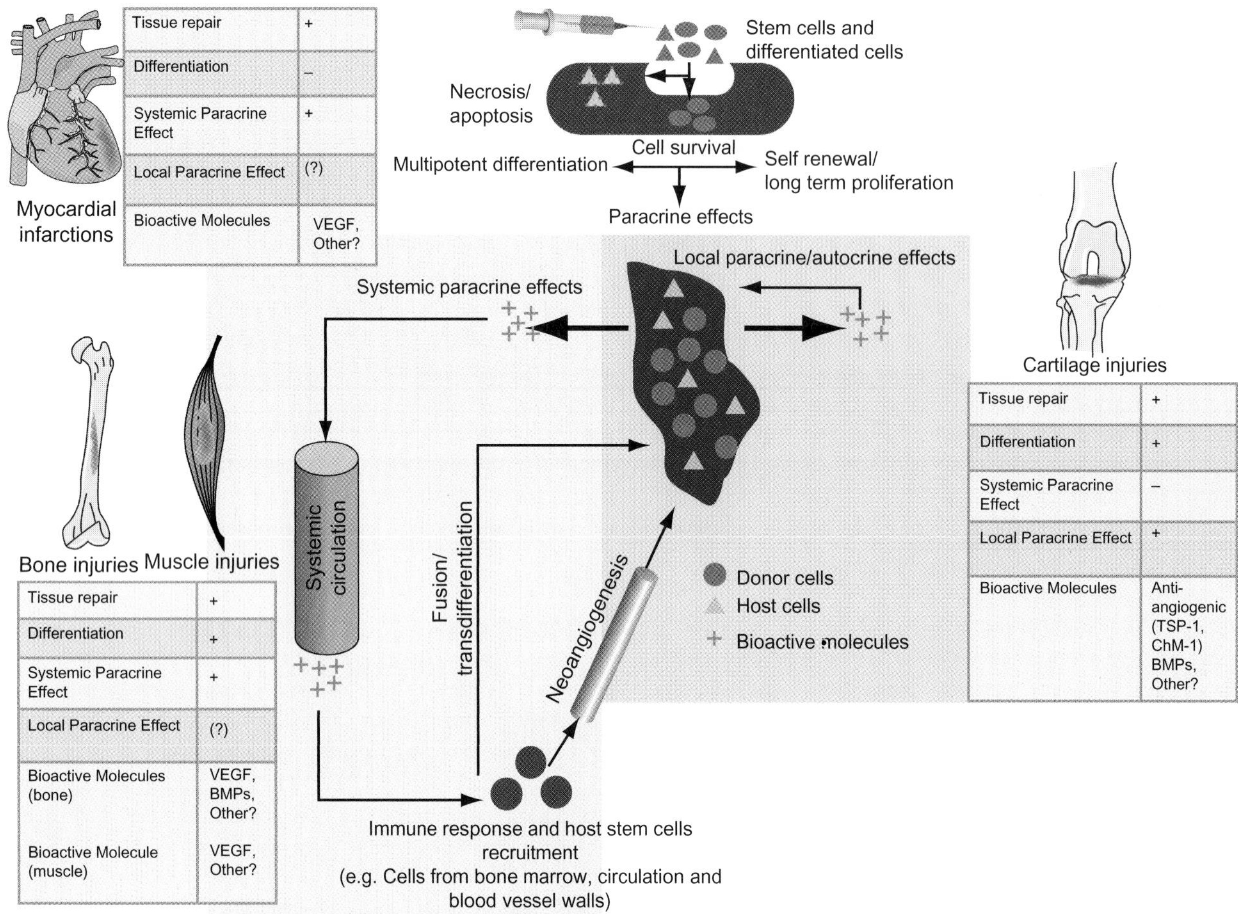

FIGURE 62.3 Paracrine effects of implanted stem cells on four examples of tissues. After implantation in the injured tissue, surviving cells secrete a battery of soluble molecules which can induce a variety of responses in donor and host cells. The paracrine effect can be local or systemic. In cartilage, soluble factors (such as TSP-1) in the microenvironment blocks angiogenesis and promote repair in articular cartilage. In the heart, VEGF increases angiogenesis at the injury site in myocardial infarction. Other factors likely travel via systemic circulation and aid in the healing process by attracting a multitude of stem cells to the injured tissues.

VEGF expression by chondrocytes is related to cartilage destruction and progressive breakdown of the extracellular matrix (198–200), osteocyte formation (201), and the induction of arthritis (202–204), molecules that block VEGF would provide a beneficial strategy to prevent or delay the progression of OA. Reports show that treatment with sFlt-1 blocks VEGF signaling and decreases the severity of arthritis in a murine model (205,206). We found that transplantation of MDSCs expressing both BMP4 and sFlt-1 improves AC repair more effectively than the expression of BMP4 alone (207). The sFlt-1/BMP4-transduced MDSCs, which were transplanted intra-capsularly into an OA rat model, enhanced cartilage regeneration via BMP4's autocrine/paracrine effects. These transduced MDSCs prevented host chondrocyte apoptosis while promoting proliferation, by blocking both the VEGF catabolic pathway and VEGF-induced vascular invasion (207).

The question arises again as to which host cells are participating in the repair process. In the regenerated cartilage, we reported that the host cells, rather than donor cells, are predominantly present at the injury site. Since it has been shown that the removal of the synovium prior to stem cell transplantation significantly reduced the repair process, and we observed that MDSC transplantation into the joint fluid leads to a massive attachment of the transplanted cells to the synovium (207); we posited that synovial-derived cells may be contributing to the repair process. Gelse and colleagues (195) also showed that host cells, specifically bone marrow-derived cells, respond to stimulatory cytokines released by cells transplanted into the joint. They found synergistic effects of transplanted chondrocytes and periosteal cells that induced the ingrowth and chondrogenic activity of bone marrow-derived cells of the host. Murphy et al. similarly transplanted MSCs by direct intra-articular injection in a goat model of OA, and reported that the MSCs both regenerated the meniscus and led to a reduction in degeneration of the articular cartilage, osteophytic remodeling, and subchondral sclerosis despite the poor participation of the MSCs in the regenerated tissue (208); however, the extent of signaling to host cells and which host cells contributed to the repair is not clear.

The mechanisms of how host cells are recruited and the beneficial effect of blocking angiogenesis in articular cartilage repair are still not fully elucidated; however, these results highlight the effect that donor cells have on the local micro-environment even in the absence of stem cell differentiation. Since blocking angiogenesis eliminates the systemic recruitment of blood vessel and circulation-derived progenitor cells, this suggests that in the case of direct implantation of stem cells to the joint, the cells exert their paracrine effects locally.

MUSCLE STEM CELL DIFFERENTIATION INTO HOST TISSUE IS NOT A MAJOR DETERMINANT OF SUCCESS OF REPAIR

Over the past decade, translational stem cell studies have extensively examined the multipotency and self-renewal as the defining characteristics of stem cells. Cell-based regenerative medicine particularly focuses on methods to induce cell differentiation to a specific lineage. Exciting results now show that stem cell-mediated repair may occur in the absence of cell differentiation. These benefits may be due to the less well-investigated characteristics of stem cells – cell survival and subsequent paracrine signaling (122,150,209). In fact, these characteristics may be unique to robust stem cells that contribute to tissue repair through their interaction with host cells and the environment. Further, the stem cells' intrinsic ability to survive cell transplantation may be directly related to the bioactive factors that they secrete to promote the healing of host tissue.

Several studies, including the ones described above, show that cell transplantation is associated with massive cell death; therefore cell survival after transplantation may be considered the first critical checkpoint in the *in vivo* pathway to tissue repair (Figure 62.3). Survival may entail overcoming immune rejection, inflammation, and the physical stresses of cell manipulation. Cells may survive by being immunoprotected, or by expressing higher levels of anti-oxidant or anti-apoptotic genes, or by modulating the host cells and environment. Whatever cellular mechanisms may be in place or tissue engineering approaches that may be used, the ability of cells to survive transplantation is a key factor in stem cell-mediated tissue repair.

Subsequently, at a second critical checkpoint, the surviving cells may contribute to tissue repair via various stem cell activities including self-renewal and multipotent differentiation, or the unique activity of paracrine signaling. An emerging finding among transplantation studies is that significant tissue repair is often observed despite low donor cell differentiation and integration within the regenerated tissue. Indeed, over the past decade, many studies that identify new stem cell sources often report on their ability to repair a given tissue without quantification of the frequency of donor cell differentiation, or it is reported that only a small fraction differentiate to the specific cell type of interest (for a review of the literature, see Table 1 in reference 150). It may be speculated that the low level of differentiation suggests that the cells are participating in other stem cell activities such as self-renewal or *in vivo* expansion. More recently, evidence suggests that donor stem cells may participate in repair by signaling with host cells.

Paracrine signaling by transplanted donor cells (either systemic or local), appears to represent a third critical checkpoint in the pathway to cell-mediated repair. The trophic signaling or release of cytokines or other signaling molecules may provide an impetus for host cells to participate in the repair, perhaps by having an effect in the local micro-environment and/or by inducing a systemic effect or by mediating an inflammatory response. Studies presented above show that transplanted donor cells may inhibit tissue damage (including cell death and/or fibrosis formation) at the site of injury, may stimulate proliferation of host cells that contribute to tissue repair, and may stimulate angiogenesis in some cases.

We discuss the role of cell survival and paracrine signaling in stem cell-mediated repair of injured tissues using examples from skeletal and cardiac muscles. We provided non-muscle examples of tissue repair (bone and articular cartilage) that further support this unique role for stem cells in the regenerative process. The role of cell survival was highlighted in stem cell-mediated skeletal muscle repair, while cardiac and bone repair demonstrate the role of donor cell paracrine signaling and systemic effects, particularly on neovascularization. Finally, the role of the local micro-environment was discussed in stem cell therapy for articular cartilage repair.

CONCLUSIONS

Although it has been speculated for numerous years that the regenerative potential of stem cells is due to their multipotentiality, current findings indicate that the cells' ability to survive implantation represents a critical step for tissue regeneration and repair. While the surviving cells may undergo different fates within the transplanted tissue, the findings that very few donor cells differentiate and participate in the regeneration of these injured tissues suggest that the repair process occurs by host-derived cells chemo-attracted to the site of injury through local and systemic paracrine effects imparted by the donor cells. This notion is supported by the results that show few donor cells within the regenerated tissue and the findings that when donor stem cell paracrine signaling is interrupted (e.g. blocking VEGF and neovascularization) there is a reduction in the regeneration and repair capacity of the injured tissues as is the case for well-vascularized tissues such as skeletal muscle, bone, and the heart. Other cell types, not discussed in detail here – such as endothelial and endothelial progenitor cells (210,211) and kidney-derived MSCs (212,213) – likewise show little cell differentiation yet therapeutic benefits have been attributed to signaling from these donor cells. Although it is still unclear which host cells are involved in the repair processes after stem cell transplantation, the role of blood vessel-derived cells, immune and inflammatory cells and resident cells at the injury site, appear to play a role in the regeneration process.

It is clear that the multipotentiality of the stem cells does not represent a major determinant for the success of stem cell therapy. This idea challenges current dogma that suggests that embryonic stem cells may have an advantage over adult-derived stem cells because of their higher level of multipotentiality. We speculate that it is the stem cell's high level of cell survival and paracrine signaling capacity that leads to their increased ability to attract host cells and it is this feature that is the key for successful stem cell therapy.

FUTURE DIRECTIONS IN STEM CELL THERAPY

The targeted regulation of cell differentiation will continue to be of valuable interest since the ultimate goal is to restore functionally differentiated cells within the regenerated tissue. Still, additional efforts to promote cell survival and identify the essential paracrine factors released by the stem cells that stimulate a host response are a necessary avenue of future investigation.

It is now tempting to include cell resistance to stress as an important stem cell characteristic that will play a critical role in stem cell therapy, in addition to self-renewal and multipotency. Indeed this characteristic may be used to isolate potent stem cells. For example, aldehyde dehydrogenase (ALDH), which usually confers a tolerance to oxidative stress (214), has been used to purify a variety of progenitor cells (215) with high regenerative potentials from various tissues including: hematopoietic, neural, endothelial and mesenchymal, and skeletal muscle tissues (216–219). It is perhaps possible that the current techniques that are used to isolate stem cells such as FACS, the preplate technique, and centrifugation rely on exposing stem cells to a stressful environment and that the resulting surviving cells represent a robust stem cell pool. Nevertheless, the emerging roles of cell survival and donor cell paracrine signaling on the success of stem cell therapy provides a potential means to identify and isolate future stem cell candidates for tissue regeneration and repair.

ACKNOWLEDGMENTS

This work was supported in part by the Department of Defense Contract (W81XWH-08-0076; AFIRM W81XWH-08-2-0032) the National Institute of Health (R01 DE013420-09), the William F. and Jean W. Donaldson Chair at the Children's Hospital of Pittsburgh, the Henry J. Mankin Endowed Chair in Orthopaedic Surgery at the University of Pittsburgh and the Orris C. Hirtzel and Beatrice Dewey Hirtzel Memorial Foundation.

REFERENCES

1. American Academy of Family Physicians. *ICD-9 Codes for Family Medicine 2005–2006*. Leawood, KS: AAFP.
2. Huard J, Li Y, Fu FH. Muscle injuries and repair: current trends in research. *J Bone Joint Surg Am* 2002;**84-A**:822–32.
3. Woods C, Hawkins RD, Maltby S, Hulse M, Thomas A, Hodson A. The Football Association Medical Research Programme: an audit of injuries in professional football – analysis of hamstring injuries. *Br J Sports Med* 2004;**38**:36–41.
4. Almekinders LC. Anti-inflammatory treatment of muscular injuries in sports. *Sports Med* 1993;**15**:139–45.
5. Jarvinen MJ, Lehto MU. The effects of early mobilisation and immobilisation on the healing process following muscle injuries. *Sports Med* 1993;**15**:78–89.
6. Worrell TW. Factors associated with hamstring injuries. An approach to treatment and preventative measures. *Sports Med* 1994;**17**:338–45.
7. Li Y, Huard J. Differentiation of muscle-derived cells into myofibroblasts in injured skeletal muscle. *Am J Pathol* 2002; **161**:895–907.
8. Li Y, Foster W, Deasy BM, Chan Y, Prisk V, Tang Y, et al. Transforming growth factor-beta1 induces the differentiation of myogenic cells into fibrotic cells in injured skeletal muscle: a key event in muscle fibrogenesis. *Am J Pathol* 2004;**164**:1007–19.
9. Shen W, Li Y, Tang Y, Cummins J, Huard J. NS-398, a cyclooxygenase-2-specific inhibitor, delays skeletal muscle healing by decreasing regeneration and promoting fibrosis. *Am J Pathol* 2005;**167**:1105–17.
10. Shen W, Prisk V, Li Y, Foster W, Huard J. Inhibited skeletal muscle healing in cyclooxygenase-2 gene-deficient mice: the role of PGE2 and PGF2alpha. *J Appl Physiol* 2006;**101**:1215–21.
11. Bondesen BA, Mills ST, Kegley KM, Pavlath GK. The COX-2 pathway is essential during early stages of skeletal muscle regeneration. *Am J Physiol Cell Physiol* 2004;**287**:C475–83.
12. Bondesen BA, Mills ST, Pavlath GK. The COX-2 pathway regulates growth of atrophied muscle via multiple mechanisms. *Am J Physiol Cell Physiol* 2006;**290**:C1651–9.

13. Allen RE, Boxhorn LK. Regulation of skeletal muscle satellite cell proliferation and differentiation by transforming growth factor-beta, insulin-like growth factor I, and fibroblast growth factor. *J Cell Physiol* 1989;**138**:311–5.
14. Anderson JE, Liu L, Kardami E. Distinctive patterns of basic fibroblast growth factor (bFGF) distribution in degenerating and regenerating areas of dystrophic (mdx) striated muscles. *Dev Biol* 1991;**147**:96–109.
15. Barnard W, Bower J, Brown MA, Murphy M, Austin L. Leukemia inhibitory factor (LIF) infusion stimulates skeletal muscle regeneration after injury: injured muscle expresses lif mRNA. *J Neurol Sci* 1994;**123**:108–13.
16. Barton-Davis ER, Shoturma DI, Musaro A, Rosenthal N, Sweeney HL. Viral mediated expression of insulin-like growth factor I blocks the aging-related loss of skeletal muscle function. *Proc Natl Acad Sci USA* 1998;**95**:15603–7.
17. Chambers RL, McDermott JC. Molecular basis of skeletal muscle regeneration. *Can J Appl Physiol* 1996;**21**:155–84.
18. Coleman ME, DeMayo F, Yin KC, Lee HM, Geske R, Montgomery C, et al. Myogenic vector expression of insulin-like growth factor I stimulates muscle cell differentiation and myofiber hypertrophy in transgenic mice. *J Biol Chem* 1995;**270**:12109–16.
19. Damon SE, Haugk KL, Birnbaum RS, Quinn LS. Retrovirally mediated overexpression of insulin-like growth factor binding protein 4: evidence that insulin-like growth factor is required for skeletal muscle differentiation. *J Cell Physiol* 1998;**175**:109–20.
20. De Deyne PG, Kinsey S, Yoshino S, Jensen-Vick K. The adaptation of soleus and edl in a rat model of distraction osteogenesis: IGF-1 and fibrosis. *J Orthop Res* 2002;**20**:1225–31.
21. Doumit ME, Cook DR, Merkel RA. Fibroblast growth factor, epidermal growth factor, insulin-like growth factors, and platelet-derived growth factor-BB stimulate proliferation of clonally derived porcine myogenic satellite cells. *J Cell Physiol* 1993; **157**:326–32.
22. Engert JC, Berglund EB, Rosenthal N. Proliferation precedes differentiation in IGF-I-stimulated myogenesis. *J Cell Biol* 1996; **135**:431–40.
23. Florini JR, Ewton DZ, Coolican SA. Growth hormone and the insulin-like growth factor system in myogenesis. *Endocr Rev* 1996;**17**:481–517.
24. Florini JR, Ewton DZ, Falen SL, Van Wyk JJ. Biphasic concentration dependency of stimulation of myoblast differentiation by somatomedins. *Am J Physiol* 1986;**250**:C771–8.
25. Floss T, Arnold HH, Braun T. A role for FGF-6 in skeletal muscle regeneration. *Genes Dev* 1997;**11**:2040–51.
26. Gospodarowicz D, Weseman J, Moran JS, Lindstrom J. Effect of fibroblast growth factor on the division and fusion of bovine myoblasts. *J Cell Biol* 1976;**70**:395–405.
27. Gowdak LH, Poliakova L, Wang X, Kovesdi I, Fishbein KW, Zacheo A, et al. Adenovirus-mediated VEGF(121) gene transfer stimulates angiogenesis in normoperfused skeletal muscle and preserves tissue perfusion after induction of ischemia. *Circulation* 2000;**102**:565–71.
28. Grounds MD. Towards understanding skeletal muscle regeneration. *Pathol Res Pract* 1991;**187**:1–22.
29. Harrington MA, Daub R, Song A, Stasek J, Garcia JG. Interleukin 1 alpha mediated inhibition of myogenic terminal differentiation: increased sensitivity of Ha-ras transformed cultures. *Cell Growth Differ* 1992;**3**:241–8.
30. Inselburg J, Applebaum B. Proteins synthesized in minicells containing plasmid ColE1 and its mutants. *J Bacteriol* 1978; **133**:1444–51.
31. Jennische E. Sequential immunohistochemical expression of IGF-I and the transferrin receptor in regenerating rat muscle in vivo. *Acta Endocrinol (Copenh)* 1989;**121**:733–8.
32. Jin P, Rahm M, Claesson-Welsh L, Heldin CH, Sejersen T. Expression of PDGF A-chain and beta-receptor genes during rat myoblast differentiation. *J Cell Biol* 1990;**110**:1665–72.
33. Johnson SE, Allen RE. Activation of skeletal muscle satellite cells and the role of fibroblast growth factor receptors. *Exp Cell Res* 1995;**219**:449–53.
34. Jones JI, Clemmons DR. Insulin-like growth factors and their binding proteins: biological actions. *Endocr Rev* 1995; **16**:3–34.
35. Keller St HL, Pierre Schneider B, Eppihimer LA, Cannon JG. Association of IGF-I and IGF-II with myofiber regeneration in vivo. *Muscle Nerve* 1999;**22**:347–54.
36. Kurek JB, Bower JJ, Romanella M, Koentgen F, Murphy M, Austin L. The role of leukemia inhibitory factor in skeletal muscle regeneration. *Muscle Nerve* 1997;**20**:815–22.
37. Lamberts SW, van den Beld AW, van der Lely AJ. The endocrinology of aging. *Science* 1997;**278**:419–24.
38. Lefaucheur JP, Sebille A. Muscle regeneration following injury can be modified in vivo by immune neutralization of basic fibroblast growth factor, transforming growth factor beta 1 or insulin-like growth factor I. *J Neuroimmunol* 1995;**57**:85–91.
39. Linkhart TA, Clegg CH, Hauschika SD. Myogenic differentiation in permanent clonal mouse myoblast cell lines: regulation by macromolecular growth factors in the culture medium. *Dev Biol* 1981;**86**:19–30.
40. McFarland DC, Pesall JE, Gilkerson KK. The influence of growth factors on turkey embryonic myoblasts and satellite cells in vitro. *Gen Comp Endocrinol* 1993;**89**:415–24.
41. Musaro A, Giacinti C, Borsellino G, Dobrowolny G, Pelosi L, Cairns L, et al. Stem cell-mediated muscle regeneration is enhanced by local isoform of insulin-like growth factor 1. *Proc Natl Acad Sci USA* 2004;**101**:1206–10.
42. Olson EN, Sternberg E, Hu JS, Spizz G, Wilcox C. Regulation of myogenic differentiation by type beta transforming growth factor. *J Cell Biol* 1986;**103**:1799–805.
43. Papadakis MA, Grady D, Black D, Tierney MJ, Gooding GA, Schambelan M, et al. Growth hormone replacement in healthy older men improves body composition but not functional ability. *Ann Intern Med* 1996;**124**:708–16.
44. Quinn LS, Haugk KL. Overexpression of the type-1 insulin-like growth factor receptor increases ligand-dependent proliferation and differentiation in bovine skeletal myogenic cultures. *J Cell Physiol* 1996;**168**:34–41.
45. Sheehan SM, Tatsumi R, Temm-Grove CJ, Allen RE. HGF is an autocrine growth factor for skeletal muscle satellite cells in vitro. *Muscle Nerve* 2000;**23**:239–45.
46. Springer ML, Chen AS, Kraft PE, Bednarski M, Blau HM. VEGF gene delivery to muscle: potential role for vasculogenesis in adults. *Mol Cell* 1998;**2**:549–58.

47. Tatsumi R, Anderson JE, Nevoret CJ, Halevy O, Allen RE. HGF/SF is present in normal adult skeletal muscle and is capable of activating satellite cells. *Dev Biol* 1998;**194**:114–28.
48. Yablonka-Reuveni Z, Balestreri TM, Bowen-Pope DF. Regulation of proliferation and differentiation of myoblasts derived from adult mouse skeletal muscle by specific isoforms of PDGF. *J Cell Biol* 1990;**111**:1623–9.
49. Zdanowicz MM, Moyse J, Wingertzahn MA, O'Connor M, Teichberg S, Slonim AE. Effect of insulin-like growth factor I in murine muscular dystrophy. *Endocrinology* 1995;**136**:4880–6.
50. Menetrey J, Kasemkijwattana C, Day CS, Bosch P, Vogt M, Fu FH, et al. Growth factors improve muscle healing in vivo. *J Bone Joint Surg Br* 2000;**82**:131–7.
51. Chan YS, Li Y, Foster W, Horaguchi T, Somogyi G, Fu FH, et al. Antifibrotic effects of suramin in injured skeletal muscle after laceration. *J Appl Physiol* 2003;**95**:771–80.
52. Foster W, Li Y, Usas A, Somogyi G, Huard J. Gamma interferon as an antifibrosis agent in skeletal muscle. *J Orthop Res* 2003;**21**:798–804.
53. Fukushima K, Badlani N, Usas A, Riano F, Fu F, Huard J. The use of an antifibrosis agent to improve muscle recovery after laceration. *Am J Sports Med* 2001;**29**:394–402.
54. Negishi S, Li Y, Usas A, Fu FH, Huard J. The effect of relaxin treatment on skeletal muscle injuries. *Am J Sports Med* 2005;**33**:1816–24.
55. Sato K, Li Y, Foster W, Fukushima K, Badlani N, Adachi N, et al. Improvement of muscle healing through enhancement of muscle regeneration and prevention of fibrosis. *Muscle Nerve* 2003;**28**:365–72.
56. Lee CW, Fukushima K, Usas A, Xin L, Pelinkovic D, Martinek V, et al. Biological intervention based on cell and gene therapy to improve muscle healing after laceration. *J Musculoskelet Res* 2000;**4**:265.
57. Li Y, Cummins J, Huard J. Muscle injury and repair. *Curr Opin Orthop* 2001;**12**:409–15.
58. Barcellos-Hoff MH, Derynck R, Tsang ML, Weatherbee JA. Transforming growth factor-beta activation in irradiated murine mammary gland. *J Clin Invest* 1994;**93**:892–9.
59. Barnes JL, Abboud HE. Temporal expression of autocrine growth factors corresponds to morphological features of mesangial proliferation in Habu snake venom-induced glomerulonephritis. *Am J Pathol* 1993;**143**:1366–76.
60. Brandes ME, Allen JB, Ogawa Y, Wahl SM. Transforming growth factor beta 1 suppresses acute and chronic arthritis in experimental animals. *J Clin Invest* 1991;**87**:1108–13.
61. Coimbra T, Wiggins R, Noh JW, Merritt S, Phan SH. Transforming growth factor-beta production in anti-glomerular basement membrane disease in the rabbit. *Am J Pathol* 1991;**138**:223–34.
62. Czaja MJ, Weiner FR, Flanders KC, Giambrone MA, Wind R, Biempica L, et al. In vitro and in vivo association of transforming growth factor-beta 1 with hepatic fibrosis. *J Cell Biol* 1989;**108**:2477–82.
63. Kagami S, Border WA, Miller DE, Noble NA. Angiotensin II stimulates extracellular matrix protein synthesis through induction of transforming growth factor-beta expression in rat glomerular mesangial cells. *J Clin Invest* 1994;**93**:2431–7.
64. Khalil N, Whitman C, Zuo L, Danielpour D, Greenberg A. Regulation of alveolar macrophage transforming growth factor-beta secretion by corticosteroids in bleomycin-induced pulmonary inflammation in the rat. *J Clin Invest* 1993;**92**:1812–8.
65. Logan A, Berry M, Gonzalez AM, Frautschy SA, Sporn MB, Baird A. Effects of transforming growth factor beta 1 on scar production in the injured central nervous system of the rat. *Eur J Neurosci* 1994;**6**:355–63.
66. Okuda S, Languino LR, Ruoslahti E, Border WA. Elevated expression of transforming growth factor-beta and proteoglycan production in experimental glomerulonephritis. Possible role in expansion of the mesangial extracellular matrix. *J Clin Invest* 1990;**86**:453–62.
67. Sporn MB, Roberts AB. A major advance in the use of growth factors to enhance wound healing. *J Clin Invest* 1993;**92**:2565–6.
68. Westergren-Thorsson G, Hernnas J, Sarnstrand B, Oldberg A, Heinegard D, Malmstrom A. Altered expression of small proteoglycans, collagen, and transforming growth factor-beta 1 in developing bleomycin-induced pulmonary fibrosis in rats. *J Clin Invest* 1993;**92**:632–7.
69. Wolf YG, Rasmussen LM, Ruoslahti E. Antibodies against transforming growth factor-beta 1 suppress intimal hyperplasia in a rat model. *J Clin Invest* 1994;**93**:1172–8.
70. Yamamoto T, Nakamura T, Noble NA, Ruoslahti E, Border WA. Expression of transforming growth factor beta is elevated in human and experimental diabetic nephropathy. *Proc Natl Acad Sci USA* 1993;**90**:1814–8.
71. Bernasconi P, Torchiana E, Confalonieri P, Brugnoni R, Barresi R, Mora M, et al. Expression of transforming growth factor-beta 1 in dystrophic patient muscles correlates with fibrosis. Pathogenetic role of a fibrogenic cytokine. *J Clin Invest* 1995;**96**:1137–44.
72. Yamazaki M, Minota S, Sakurai H, Miyazono K, Yamada A, Kanazawa I, et al. Expression of transforming growth factor-beta 1 and its relation to endomysial fibrosis in progressive muscular dystrophy. *Am J Pathol* 1994;**144**:221–6.
73. Zanotti S, Negri T, Cappelletti C, Bernasconi P, Canioni E, Di Blasi C, et al. Decorin and biglycan expression is differentially altered in several muscular dystrophies. *Brain* 2005;**128**:2546–55.
74. Amemiya K, Semino-Mora C, Granger RP, Dalakas MC. Downregulation of TGF-beta1 mRNA and protein in the muscles of patients with inflammatory myopathies after treatment with high-dose intravenous immunoglobulin. *Clin Immunol* 2000;**94**:99–104.
75. Confalonieri P, Bernasconi P, Cornelio F, Mantegazza R. Transforming growth factor-beta 1 in polymyositis and dermatomyositis correlates with fibrosis but not with mononuclear cell infiltrate. *J Neuropathol Exp Neurol* 1997;**56**:479–84.
76. Li Y, Negishi S, Sakamoto M, Usas A, Huard J. The use of relaxin improves healing in injured muscle. *Ann NY Acad Sci* 2005;**1041**:395–7.
77. Lim DS, Lutucuta S, Bachireddy P, Youker K, Evans A, Entman M, et al. Angiotensin II blockade reverses myocardial fibrosis in a transgenic mouse model of human hypertrophic cardiomyopathy. *Circulation* 2001;**103**:789–91.
78. Otsuka M, Takahashi H, Shiratori M, Chiba H, Abe S. Reduction of bleomycin induced lung fibrosis by candesartan cilexetil, an angiotensin II type 1 receptor antagonist. *Thorax* 2004;**59**:31–8.

79. Paizis G, Gilbert RE, Cooper ME, Murthi P, Schembri JM, Wu LL, et al. Effect of angiotensin II type 1 receptor blockade on experimental hepatic fibrogenesis. *J Hepatol* 2001;**35**:376–85.
80. Suga S, Mazzali M, Ray PE, Kang DH, Johnson RJ. Angiotensin II type 1 receptor blockade ameliorates tubulointerstitial injury induced by chronic potassium deficiency. *Kidney Int* 2002; **61**:951–8.
81. Habashi JP, Doyle JJ, Holm TM, Aziz H, Schoenhoff F, Bedja D, et al. Angiotensin II type 2 receptor signaling attenuates aortic aneurysm in mice through ERK antagonism. *Science* 2011;**332**:361–5.
82. Swedberg K, Kjekshus J. Effects of enalapril on mortality in severe congestive heart failure: results of the Cooperative North Scandinavian Enalapril Survival Study (CONSENSUS). *Am J Cardiol* 1988;**62**:60A–6A.
83. Gremmler B, Kunert M, Schleiting H, Ulbricht LJ. Improvement of cardiac output in patients with severe heart failure by use of ACE-inhibitors combined with the AT1-antagonist eprosartan. *Eur J Heart Fail* 2000;**2**:183–7.
84. Onder G, Vedova CD, Pahor M. Effects of ACE inhibitors on skeletal muscle. *Curr Pharm Des* 2006;**12**:2057–64.
85. Folland J, Leach B, Little T, Hawker K, Myerson S, Montgomery H, et al. Angiotensin-converting enzyme genotype affects the response of human skeletal muscle to functional overload. *Exp Physiol* 2000;**85**:575–9.
86. Bedair HS, Karthikeyan T, Quintero A, Li Y, Huard J. Angiotensin II receptor blockade administered after injury improves muscle regeneration and decreases fibrosis in normal skeletal muscle. *Am J Sports Med* 2008;**36**:1548–54.
87. Hoffman EP, Brown Jr. RH, Kunkel LM. Dystrophin: the protein product of the Duchenne muscular dystrophy locus. *Cell* 1987;**51**:919–28.
88. Huard J, Bouchard JP, Roy R, Labrecque C, Dansereau G, Lemieux B, et al. Myoblast transplantation produced dystrophin-positive muscle fibres in a 16-year-old patient with Duchenne muscular dystrophy. *Clin Sci (Lond)* 1991;**81**:287–8.
89. Fan Y, Maley M, Beilharz M, Grounds M. Rapid death of injected myoblasts in myoblast transfer therapy. *Muscle Nerve* 1996;**19**:853–60.
90. Karpati G, Pouliot Y, Zubrzycka-Gaarn E, Carpenter S, Ray PN, Worton RG, et al. Dystrophin is expressed in mdx skeletal muscle fibers after normal myoblast implantation. *Am J Pathol* 1989;**135**:27–32.
91. Morgan JE, Hoffman EP, Partridge TA. Normal myogenic cells from newborn mice restore normal histology to degenerating muscles of the mdx mouse. *J Cell Biol* 1990;**111**:2437–49.
92. Mendell JR, Kissel JT, Amato AA, King W, Signore L, Prior TW, et al. Myoblast transfer in the treatment of Duchenne's muscular dystrophy. *N Engl J Med* 1995;**333**:832–8.
93. Gussoni E, Blau HM, Kunkel LM. The fate of individual myoblasts after transplantation into muscles of DMD patients. *Nat Med* 1997;**3**:970–7.
94. Kinoshita I, Vilquin JT, Guerette B, Asselin I, Roy R, Tremblay JP. Very efficient myoblast allotransplantation in mice under FK506 immunosuppression. *Muscle Nerve* 1994;**17**:1407–15.
95. Vilquin JT, Guerette B, Kinoshita I, Roy B, Goulet M, Gravel C, et al. FK506 immunosuppression to control the immune reactions triggered by first-generation adenovirus-mediated gene transfer. *Hum Gene Ther* 1995;**6**:1391–401.
96. Beauchamp JR, Morgan JE, Pagel CN, Partridge TA. Dynamics of myoblast transplantation reveal a discrete minority of precursors with stem cell-like properties as the myogenic source. *J Cell Biol* 1999;**144**:1113–22.
97. Hodgetts SI, Beilharz MW, Scalzo AA, Grounds MD. Why do cultured transplanted myoblasts die in vivo? DNA quantification shows enhanced survival of donor male myoblasts in host mice depleted of $CD4^+$ and $CD8^+$ cells or $Nk1.1^+$ cells. *Cell Transplant* 2000;**9**:489–502.
98. Guerette B, Asselin I, Skuk D, Entman M, Tremblay JP. Control of inflammatory damage by anti-LFA-1: increase success of myoblast transplantation. *Cell Transplant* 1997;**6**:101–7.
99. Qu Z, Balkir L, van Deutekom JC, Robbins PD, Pruchnic R, Huard J. Development of approaches to improve cell survival in myoblast transfer therapy. *J Cell Biol* 1998;**142**:1257–67.
100. Baroffio A, Hamann M, Bernheim L, Bochaton-Piallat ML, Gabbiani G, Bader CR. Identification of self-renewing myoblasts in the progeny of single human muscle satellite cells. *Differentiation* 1996;**60**:47–57.
101. Collins CA, Zammit PS, Ruiz AP, Morgan JE, Partridge TA. A population of myogenic stem cells that survives skeletal muscle aging. *Stem Cells* 2007;**25**:885–94.
102. Gharaibeh B, Lu A, Tebbets J, Zheng B, Feduska J, Crisan M, et al. Isolation of a slowly adhering cell fraction containing stem cells from murine skeletal muscle by the preplate technique. *Nat Protoc* 2008;**3**:1501–9.
103. Qu-Petersen Z, Deasy B, Jankowski R, Ikezawa M, Cummins J, Pruchnic R, et al. Identification of a novel population of muscle stem cells in mice: potential for muscle regeneration. *J Cell Biol* 2002;**157**:851–64.
104. Cerletti M, Jurga S, Witczak CA, Hirshman MF, Shadrach JL, Goodyear LJ, et al. Highly efficient, functional engraftment of skeletal muscle stem cells in dystrophic muscles. *Cell* 2008;**134**:37–47.
105. Lavasani M, Lu A, Peng H, Cummins J, Huard J. Nerve growth factor improves the muscle regeneration capacity of muscle stem cells in dystrophic muscle. *Hum Gene Ther* 2006;**17**:180–92.
106. Lee S, Shin HS, Shireman PK, Vasilaki A, Van Remmen H, Csete ME. Glutathione-peroxidase-1 null muscle progenitor cells are globally defective. *Free Radic Biol Med* 2006;**41**:1174–84.
107. Fulle S, Di Donna S, Puglielli C, Pietrangelo T, Beccafico S, Bellomo R, et al. Age-dependent imbalance of the antioxidative system in human satellite cells. *Exp Gerontol* 2005; **40**:189–97.
108. Urish KL, Vella JB, Okada M, Deasy BM, Tobita K, Keller BB, et al. Antioxidant levels represent a major determinant in the regenerative capacity of muscle stem cells. *Mol Biol Cell* 2009;**20**:509–20.
109. Ito K, Hirao A, Arai F, Takubo K, Matsuoka S, Miyamoto K, et al. Reactive oxygen species act through p38 MAPK to limit the lifespan of hematopoietic stem cells. *Nat Med* 2006; **12**:446–51.
110. Drowley L, Okada M, Beckman S, Vella J, Keller B, Tobita K, et al. Cellular antioxidant levels influence muscle stem cell therapy. *Mol Ther* 2010;**18**:65–73.
111. Deasy BM, Feduska JM, Payne TR, Li Y, Ambrosio F, Huard J. Effect of VEGF on the regenerative capacity of muscle stem cells in dystrophic skeletal muscle. *Mol Ther* 2009;**17**:1788–98.

112. Springer ML, Ozawa CR, Banfi A, Kraft PE, Ip TK, Brazelton TR, et al. Localized arteriole formation directly adjacent to the site of VEGF-induced angiogenesis in muscle. *Mol Ther* 2003;**7**:441–9.
113. Almekinders LC, Gilbert JA. Healing of experimental muscle strains and the effects of nonsteroidal antiinflammatory medication. *Am J Sports Med* 1986;**14**:303–8.
114. Mishra DK, Friden J, Schmitz MC, Lieber RL. Anti-inflammatory medication after muscle injury. A treatment resulting in short-term improvement but subsequent loss of muscle function. *J Bone Joint Surg Am* 1995;**77**:1510–1.
115. Obremsky WT, Seaber AV, Ribbeck BM, Garrett Jr WE. Biomechanical and histologic assessment of a controlled muscle strain injury treated with piroxicam. *Am J Sports Med* 1994;**22**:558–61.
116. Klug MG, Soonpaa MH, Koh GY, Field LJ. Genetically selected cardiomyocytes from differentiating embronic stem cells form stable intracardiac grafts. *J Clin Invest* 1996;**98**:216–24.
117. Yamashita J, Itoh H, Hirashima M, Ogawa M, Nishikawa S, Yurugi T, et al. Flk1-positive cells derived from embryonic stem cells serve as vascular progenitors. *Nature* 2000;**408**:92–6.
118. Hirschi KK, Goodell MA. Hematopoietic, vascular and cardiac fates of bone marrow-derived stem cells. *Gene Ther* 2002;**9**:648–52.
119. Orlic D, Kajstura J, Chimenti S, Jakoniuk I, Anderson SM, Li B, et al. Bone marrow cells regenerate infarcted myocardium. *Nature* 2001;**410**:701–5.
120. Paul D, Samuel SM, Maulik N. Mesenchymal stem cell: present challenges and prospective cellular cardiomyoplasty approaches for myocardial regeneration. *Antioxid Redox Signal* 2009;**11**:1841–55.
121. Sakai T, Li RK, Weisel RD, Mickle DA, Kim EJ, Tomita S, et al. Autologous heart cell transplantation improves cardiac function after myocardial injury. *Ann Thorac Surg* 1999;**68**:2074–80 discussion 80-1.
122. Gnecchi M, He H, Liang OD, Melo LG, Morello F, Mu H, et al. Paracrine action accounts for marked protection of ischemic heart by Akt-modified mesenchymal stem cells. *Nat Med* 2005;**11**:367–8.
123. Mangi AA, Noiseux N, Kong D, He H, Rezvani M, Ingwall JS, et al. Mesenchymal stem cells modified with Akt prevent remodeling and restore performance of infarcted hearts. *Nat Med* 2003;**9**:1195–201.
124. Marelli D, Desrosiers C, el-Alfy M, Kao RL, Chiu RC. Cell transplantation for myocardial repair: an experimental approach. *Cell Transplant* 1992;**1**:383–90.
125. Kessler PD, Byrne BJ. Myoblast cell grafting into heart muscle: cellular biology and potential applications. *Annu Rev Physiol* 1999;**61**:219–42.
126. Reinecke H, Poppa V, Murry CE. Skeletal muscle stem cells do not transdifferentiate into cardiomyocytes after cardiac grafting. *J Mol Cell Cardiol* 2002;**34**:241–9.
127. Taylor DA, Atkins BZ, Hungspreugs P, Jones TR, Reedy MC, Hutcheson KA, et al. Regenerating functional myocardium: improved performance after skeletal myoblast transplantation. *Nat Med* 1998;**4**:929–33.
128. Menasche P, Hagege AA, Scorsin M, Pouzet B, Desnos M, Duboc D, et al. Myoblast transplantation for heart failure. *Lancet* 2001;**357**:279–80.
129. Asahara T, Murohara T, Sullivan A, Silver M, van der Zee R, Li T, et al. Isolation of putative progenitor endothelial cells for angiogenesis. *Science* 1997;**275**:964–7.
130. Shi Q, Rafii S, Wu MH, Wijelath ES, Yu C, Ishida A, et al. Evidence for circulating bone marrow-derived endothelial cells. *Blood* 1998;**92**:362–7.
131. Takahashi T, Kalka C, Masuda H, Chen D, Silver M, Kearney M, et al. Ischemia- and cytokine-induced mobilization of bone marrow-derived endothelial progenitor cells for neovascularization. *Nat Med* 1999;**5**:434–8.
132. Leor J, Patterson M, Quinones MJ, Kedes LH, Kloner RA. Transplantation of fetal myocardial tissue into the infarcted myocardium of rat. A potential method for repair of infarcted myocardium? *Circulation* 1996;**94**:II332–6.
133. Scorsin M, Marotte F, Sabri A, Le Dref O, Demirag M, Samuel JL, et al. Can grafted cardiomyocytes colonize peri-infarct myocardial areas? *Circulation* 1996;**94**:II337–40.
134. Watanabe E, Smith Jr DM, Delcarpio JB, Sun J, Smart FW, Van Meter Jr. CH, et al. Cardiomyocyte transplantation in a porcine myocardial infarction model. *Cell Transplant* 1998;**7**:239–46.
135. Koh GY, Soonpaa MH, Klug MG, Field LJ. Long-term survival of AT-1 cardiomyocyte grafts in syngeneic myocardium. *Am J Physiol* 1993;**264**:H1727–33.
136. Hutcheson KA, Atkins BZ, Hueman MT, Hopkins MB, Glower DD, Taylor DA. Comparison of benefits on myocardial performance of cellular cardiomyoplasty with skeletal myoblasts and fibroblasts. *Cell Transplant* 2000;**9**:359–68.
137. Beltrami AP, Barlucchi L, Torella D, Baker M, Limana F, Chimenti S, et al. Adult cardiac stem cells are multipotent and support myocardial regeneration. *Cell* 2003;**114**:763–76.
138. Martin CM, Meeson AP, Robertson SM, Hawke TJ, Richardson JA, Bates S, et al. Persistent expression of the ATP-binding cassette transporter, Abcg2, identifies cardiac SP cells in the developing and adult heart. *Dev Biol* 2004;**265**:262–75.
139. Oh H, Bradfute SB, Gallardo TD, Nakamura T, Gaussin V, Mishina Y, et al. Cardiac progenitor cells from adult myocardium: homing, differentiation, and fusion after infarction. *Proc Natl Acad Sci USA* 2003;**100**:12313–8.
140. Wang L, Deng J, Tian W, Xiang B, Yang T, Li G, et al. Adipose-derived stem cells are an effective cell candidate for treatment of heart failure: an MR imaging study of rat hearts. *Am J Physiol Heart Circ Physiol* 2009;**297**:H1020–31.
141. Ciulla MM, Montelatici E, Ferrero S, Braidotti P, Paliotti R, Annoni G, et al. Potential advantages of cell administration on the inflammatory response compared to standard ACE inhibitor treatment in experimental myocardial infarction. *J Transl Med* 2008;**6**:30.
142. Tang YL, Zhao Q, Qin X, Shen L, Cheng L, Ge J, et al. Paracrine action enhances the effects of autologous mesenchymal stem cell transplantation on vascular regeneration in rat model of myocardial infarction. *Ann Thorac Surg* 2005;**80**:229–36. discussion 36-7.
143. Perez-Ilzarbe M, Agbulut O, Pelacho B, Ciorba C, San Jose-Eneriz E, Desnos M, et al. Characterization of the paracrine effects of human skeletal myoblasts transplanted in infarcted myocardium. *Eur J Heart Fail* 2008;**10**:1065–72.
144. Agbulut O, Vandervelde S, Al Attar N, Larghero J, Ghostine S, Leobon B, et al. Comparison of human skeletal myoblasts and

bone marrow-derived CD133$^+$ progenitors for the repair of infarcted myocardium. *J Am Coll Cardiol* 2004;**44**:458–63.
145. Caplan AI, Dennis JE. Mesenchymal stem cells as trophic mediators. *J Cell Biochem* 2006;**98**:1076–84.
146. Jiang Y, Jahagirdar BN, Reinhardt RL, Schwartz RE, Keene CD, Ortiz-Gonzalez XR, et al. Pluripotency of mesenchymal stem cells derived from adult marrow. *Nature* 2002;**418**:41–9.
147. Balsam LB, Wagers AJ, Christensen JL, Kofidis T, Weissman IL, Robbins RC. Haematopoietic stem cells adopt mature haematopoietic fates in ischaemic myocardium. *Nature* 2004;**428**: 668–73.
148. Murry CE, Soonpaa MH, Reinecke H, Nakajima H, Nakajima HO, Rubart M, et al. Haematopoietic stem cells do not transdifferentiate into cardiac myocytes in myocardial infarcts. *Nature* 2004;**428**:664–8.
149. Kinnaird T, Stabile E, Burnett MS, Shou M, Lee CW, Barr S, et al. Local delivery of marrow-derived stromal cells augments collateral perfusion through paracrine mechanisms. *Circulation* 2004;**109**:1543–9.
150. Gharaibeh B, Lavasani M, Cummins J, Huard J. Terminal differentiation is not a major determinant to the success of stem cell therapy–cross talk between muscle derived stem cells and host cells. *Stem Cell Res Ther* 2011;**2**:31.
151. Maltais S, Tremblay JP, Perrault LP, Ly HQ. The paracrine effect: pivotal mechanism in cell-based cardiac repair. *J Cardiovasc Transl Res* 2010;**3**(6):652–62.
152. Payne TR, Oshima H, Okada M, Momoi N, Tobita K, Keller BB, et al. A relationship between vascular endothelial growth factor, angiogenesis, and cardiac repair after muscle stem cell transplantation into ischemic hearts. *J Am Coll Cardiol* 2007;**50**:1677–84.
153. Hu X, Yu SP, Fraser JL, Lu Z, Ogle ME, Wang JA, et al. Transplantation of hypoxia-preconditioned mesenchymal stem cells improves infarcted heart function via enhanced survival of implanted cells and angiogenesis. *J Thorac Cardiovasc Surg* 2008;**135**:799–808.
154. Pasha Z, Wang Y, Sheikh R, Zhang D, Zhao T, Ashraf M. Preconditioning enhances cell survival and differentiation of stem cells during transplantation in infarcted myocardium. *Cardiovasc Res* 2008;**77**:134–42.
155. Li W, Ma N, Ong LL, Nesselmann C, Klopsch C, Ladilov Y, et al. Bcl-2 engineered MSCs inhibited apoptosis and improved heart function. *Stem Cells* 2007;**25**:2118–27.
156. Matsumoto T, Kuroda R, Mifune Y, Kawamoto A, Shoji T, Miwa M, et al. Circulating endothelial/skeletal progenitor cells for bone regeneration and healing. *Bone* 2008;**43**:434–9.
157. Matsumoto T, Kawamoto A, Kuroda R, Ishikawa M, Mifune Y, Iwasaki H, et al. Therapeutic potential of vasculogenesis and osteogenesis promoted by peripheral blood CD34-positive cells for functional bone healing. *Am J Pathol* 2006;**169**:1440–57.
158. Sorrell JM, Baber MA, Caplan AI. Influence of adult mesenchymal stem cells on in vitro vascular formation. *Tissue Eng Part A* 2009;**15**:1751–61.
159. Cossu G, Bianco P. Mesoangioblasts – vascular progenitors for extravascular mesodermal tissues. *Curr Opin Genet De* 2003; **13**:537–42.
160. Caplan AI. All MSCs are pericytes? *Cell Stem Cell* 2008; **3**:229–30.
161. Crisan M, Yap S, Casteilla L, Chen CW, Corselli M, Park TS, et al. A perivascular origin for mesenchymal stem cells in multiple human organs. *Cell Stem Cell* 2008;**3**:301–13.
162. Zheng B, Cao B, Crisan M, Sun B, Li G, Logar A, et al. Prospective identification of myogenic endothelial cells in human skeletal muscle. *Nat Biotechnol* 2007;**25**:1025–34.
163. Chang SC, Chuang HL, Chen YR, Chen JK, Chung HY, Lu YL, et al. Ex vivo gene therapy in autologous bone marrow stromal stem cells for tissue-engineered maxillofacial bone regeneration. *Gene Ther* 2003;**10**:2013–9.
164. Zuk PA, Zhu M, Mizuno H, Huang J, Futrell JW, Katz AJ, et al. Multilineage cells from human adipose tissue: implications for cell-based therapies. *Tissue Eng* 2001;**7**:211–28.
165. Krebsbach PH, Gu K, Franceschi RT, Rutherford RB. Gene therapy-directed osteogenesis: BMP-7-transduced human fibroblasts form bone in vivo. *Hum Gene Ther* 2000;**11**:1201–10.
166. Rutherford RB, Moalli M, Franceschi RT, Wang D, Gu K, Krebsbach PH. Bone morphogenetic protein-transduced human fibroblasts convert to osteoblasts and form bone in vivo. *Tissue Eng* 2002;**8**:441–52.
167. Lee JY, Qu-Petersen Z, Cao B, Kimura S, Jankowski R, Cummins J, et al. Clonal isolation of muscle-derived cells capable of enhancing muscle regeneration and bone healing. *J Cell Biol* 2000;**150**:1085–100.
168. Lee JY, Musgrave D, Pelinkovic D, Fukushima K, Cummins J, Usas A, et al. Effect of bone morphogenetic protein-2-expressing muscle-derived cells on healing of critical-sized bone defects in mice. *J Bone Joint Surg Am* 2001;**83-A**:1032–9.
169. Nakase T, Nomura S, Yoshikawa H, Hashimoto J, Hirota S, Kitamura Y, et al. Transient and localized expression of bone morphogenetic protein 4 messenger RNA during fracture healing. *J Bone Miner Res* 1994;**9**:651–9.
170. Yoshimura Y, Nomura S, Kawasaki S, Tsutsumimoto T, Shimizu T, Takaoka K. Colocalization of noggin and bone morphogenetic protein-4 during fracture healing. *J Bone Miner Res* 2001;**16**:876–84.
171. Ferguson C, Alpern E, Miclau T, Helms JA. Does adult fracture repair recapitulate embryonic skeletal formation? *Mech Dev* 1999;**87**:57–66.
172. Gerber HP, Vu TH, Ryan AM, Kowalski J, Werb Z, Ferrara N. VEGF couples hypertrophic cartilage remodeling, ossification and angiogenesis during endochondral bone formation. *Nat Med* 1999;**5**:623–8.
173. Street J, Bao M, deGuzman L, Bunting S, Peale Jr FV, Ferrara N, et al. Vascular endothelial growth factor stimulates bone repair by promoting angiogenesis and bone turnover. *Proc Natl Acad Sci USA* 2002;**99**:9656–61.
174. Mori S, Yoshikawa H, Hashimoto J, Ueda T, Funai H, Kato M, et al. Antiangiogenic agent (TNP-470) inhibition of ectopic bone formation induced by bone morphogenetic protein-2. *Bone* 1998;**22**:99–105.
175. Hou H, Zhang X, Tang T, Dai K, Ge R. Enhancement of bone formation by genetically-engineered bone marrow stromal cells expressing BMP-2, VEGF and angiopoietin-1. *Biotechnol Lett* 2009;**31**:1183–9.
176. Hausman MR, Schaffler MB, Majeska RJ. Prevention of fracture healing in rats by an inhibitor of angiogenesis. *Bone* 2001;**29**:560–4.

177. Kanczler JM, Oreffo RO. Osteogenesis and angiogenesis: the potential for engineering bone. *Eur Cell Mater* 2008;**15**: 100–14.
178. Peng H, Usas A, Olshanski A, Ho AM, Gearhart B, Cooper GM, et al. VEGF improves, whereas sFlt1 inhibits, BMP2-induced bone formation and bone healing through modulation of angiogenesis. *J Bone Miner Res* 2005;**20**:2017–27.
179. Peng H, Wright V, Usas A, Gearhart B, Shen HC, Cummins J, et al. Synergistic enhancement of bone formation and healing by stem cell-expressed VEGF and bone morphogenetic protein-4. *J Clin Invest* 2002;**110**:751–9.
180. Musgrave DS, Pruchnic R, Bosch P, Ziran BH, Whalen J, Huard J. Human skeletal muscle cells in ex vivo gene therapy to deliver bone morphogenetic protein-2. *J Bone Joint Surg Br* 2002;**84**:120–7.
181. Lee JY, Peng H, Usas A, Musgrave D, Cummins J, Pelinkovic D, et al. Enhancement of bone healing based on ex vivo gene therapy using human muscle-derived cells expressing bone morphogenetic protein 2. *Hum Gene Ther* 2002;**13**:1201–11.
182. Levi B, James AW, Nelson ER, Li S, Peng M, Commons G, et al. Human adipose-derived stromal cells stimulate autogenous skeletal repair via paracrine hedgehog signaling with calvarial osteoblasts. *Stem Cells Dev* 2010;**20**:243–57.
183. Horwitz EM, Prockop DJ, Fitzpatrick LA, Koo WW, Gordon PL, Neel M, et al. Transplantability and therapeutic effects of bone marrow-derived mesenchymal cells in children with osteogenesis imperfecta. *Nat Med* 1999;**5**:309–13.
184. Darowish M, Rahman R, Li P, Bukata SV, Gelinas J, Huang W, et al. Reduction of particle-induced osteolysis by interleukin-6 involves anti-inflammatory effect and inhibition of early osteoclast precursor differentiation. *Bone* 2009;**45**:661–8.
185. Mow VC, Proctor CS, Kelly MA. Biomechanics of articular cartilage. In: Nordin M, Frankel VH, editors. *Basic biomechanics of the musculoskeletal system*. 2nd ed. Philadelphia: Lea & Febiger; 1989. p. 32.
186. Caplan AI, Koutroupas S. The control of muscle and cartilage development in the chick limb: the role of differential vascularization. *J Embryol Exp Morphol* 1973;**29**:571–83.
187. San Antonio JD, Tuan RS. Chondrogenesis of limb bud mesenchyme in vitro: stimulation by cations. *Dev Biol* 1986;**115**:313–24.
188. Barry F, Boynton RE, Liu B, Murphy JM. Chondrogenic differentiation of mesenchymal stem cells from bone marrow: differentiation-dependent gene expression of matrix components. *Exp Cell Res* 2001;**268**:189–200.
189. El Tamer MK, Reis RL. Progenitor and stem cells for bone and cartilage regeneration. *J Tissue Eng Regen Med* 2009;**3**:327–37.
190. Estes BT, Diekman BO, Gimble JM, Guilak F. Isolation of adipose-derived stem cells and their induction to a chondrogenic phenotype. *Nat Protoc* 2010;**5**:1294–311.
191. Kuroda R, Usas A, Kubo S, Corsi K, Peng H, Rose T, et al. Cartilage repair using bone morphogenetic protein 4 and muscle-derived stem cells. *Arthritis Rheum* 2006;**54**:433–42.
192. Schugar RC, Chirieleison SM, Wescoe KE, Schmidt BT, Askew Y, Nance JJ, et al. High harvest yield, high expansion, and phenotype stability of CD146 mesenchymal stromal cells from whole primitive human umbilical cord tissue. *J Biomed Biotechnol* 2009; **2009**:789526.
193. Wakitani S, Mitsuoka T, Nakamura N, Toritsuka Y, Nakamura Y, Horibe S. Autologous bone marrow stromal cell transplantation for repair of full-thickness articular cartilage defects in human patellae: two case reports. *Cell Transplant* 2004;**13**:595–600.
194. Kuroda R, Ishida K, Matsumoto T, Akisue T, Fujioka H, Mizuno K, et al. Treatment of a full-thickness articular cartilage defect in the femoral condyle of an athlete with autologous bone-marrow stromal cells. *Osteoarthritis Cartilage* 2007;**15**:226–31.
195. Gelse K, Brem M, Klinger P, Hess A, Swoboda B, Hennig F, et al. Paracrine effect of transplanted rib chondrocyte spheroids supports formation of secondary cartilage repair tissue. *J Orthop Res* 2009;**27**:1216–25.
196. Moses MA, Wiederschain D, Wu I, Fernandez CA, Ghazizadeh V, Lane WS, et al. Troponin I is present in human cartilage and inhibits angiogenesis. *Proc Natl Acad Sci USA* 1999;**96**:2645–50.
197. Shukunami C, Oshima Y, Hiraki Y. Chondromodulin-I and tenomodulin: a new class of tissue-specific angiogenesis inhibitors found in hypovascular connective tissues. *Biochem Biophys Res Commun* 2005;**333**:299–307.
198. Enomoto H, Inoki I, Komiya K, Shiomi T, Ikeda E, Obata K, et al. Vascular endothelial growth factor isoforms and their receptors are expressed in human osteoarthritic cartilage. *Am J Pathol* 2003;**162**:171–81.
199. Hashimoto S, Ochs RL, Komiya S, Lotz M. Linkage of chondrocyte apoptosis and cartilage degradation in human osteoarthritis. *Arthritis Rheum* 1998;**41**:1632–8.
200. Pufe T, Lemke A, Kurz B, Petersen W, Tillmann B, Grodzinsky AJ, et al. Mechanical overload induces VEGF in cartilage discs via hypoxia-inducible factor. *Am J Pathol* 2004;**164**:185–92.
201. Hashimoto S, Creighton-Achermann L, Takahashi K, Amiel D, Coutts RD, Lotz M. Development and regulation of osteophyte formation during experimental osteoarthritis. *Osteoarthritis Cartilage* 2002;**10**:180–7.
202. Afuwape AO, Kiriakidis S, Paleolog EM. The role of the angiogenic molecule VEGF in the pathogenesis of rheumatoid arthritis. *Histol Histopathol* 2002;**17**:961–72.
203. Matsumoto Y, Tanaka K, Hirata G, Hanada M, Matsuda S, Shuto T, et al. Possible involvement of the vascular endothelial growth factor-Flt-1-focal adhesion kinase pathway in chemotaxis and the cell proliferation of osteoclast precursor cells in arthritic joints. *J Immunol* 2002;**168**:5824–31.
204. Murakami M, Iwai S, Hiratsuka S, Yamauchi M, Nakamura K, Iwakura Y, et al. Signaling of vascular endothelial growth factor receptor-1 tyrosine kinase promotes rheumatoid arthritis through activation of monocytes/macrophages. *Blood* 2006;**108**:1849–56.
205. Afuwape AO, Feldmann M, Paleolog EM. Adenoviral delivery of soluble VEGF receptor 1 (sFlt-1) abrogates disease activity in murine collagen-induced arthritis. *Gene Ther* 2003;**10**:1950–60.
206. De Bandt M, Ben Mahdi MH, Ollivier V, Grossin M, Dupuis M, Gaudry M, et al. Blockade of vascular endothelial growth factor receptor I (VEGF-RI), but not VEGF-RII, suppresses joint destruction in the K/BxN model of rheumatoid arthritis. *J Immunol* 2003;**171**:4853–9.
207. Matsumoto T, Cooper GM, Gharaibeh B, Meszaros LB, Li G, Usas A, et al. Cartilage repair in a rat model of osteoarthritis through intraarticular transplantation of muscle-derived stem cells expressing bone morphogenetic protein 4 and soluble Flt-1. *Arthritis Rheum* 2009;**60**:1390–405.

208. Murphy JM, Fink DJ, Hunziker EB, Barry FP. Stem cell therapy in a caprine model of osteoarthritis. *Arthritis Rheum* 2003; **48**:3464–74.
209. Murry CE, Reinecke H, Pabon LM. Regeneration gaps: observations on stem cells and cardiac repair. *J Am Coll Cardiol* 2006;**47**:1777–85.
210. Santhanam AV, Smith LA, He T, Nath KA, Katusic ZS. Endothelial progenitor cells stimulate cerebrovascular production of prostacyclin by paracrine activation of cyclooxygenase-2. *Circ Res* 2007;**100**:1379–88.
211. Yoon CH, Hur J, Park KW, Kim JH, Lee CS, Oh IY, et al. Synergistic neovascularization by mixed transplantation of early endothelial progenitor cells and late outgrowth endothelial cells: the role of angiogenic cytokines and matrix metalloproteinases. *Circulation* 2005;**112**:1618–27.
212. Chen J, Park HC, Addabbo F, Ni J, Pelger E, Li H, et al. Kidney-derived mesenchymal stem cells contribute to vasculogenesis, angiogenesis and endothelial repair. *Kidney Int* 2008;**74**:879–89.
213. Togel F, Weiss K, Yang Y, Hu Z, Zhang P, Westenfelder C. Vasculotropic, paracrine actions of infused mesenchymal stem cells are important to the recovery from acute kidney injury. *Am J Physiol Renal Physiol* 2007;**292**:F1626–35.
214. Marchitti SA, Brocker C, Orlicky DJ, Vasiliou V. Molecular characterization, expression analysis, and role of ALDH3B1 in the cellular protection against oxidative stress. *Free Radic Biol Med* 2010;**49**:1432–43.
215. Moreb JS. Aldehyde dehydrogenase as a marker for stem cells. *Curr Stem Cell Res Ther* 2008;**3**:237–46.
216. Cai J, Cheng A, Luo Y, Lu C, Mattson MP, Rao MS, et al. Membrane properties of rat embryonic multipotent neural stem cells. *J Neurochem* 2004;**88**:212–26.
217. Povsic TJ, Zavodni KL, Vainorius E, Kherani JF, Goldschmidt-Clermont PJ, et al. Common endothelial progenitor cell assays identify discrete endothelial progenitor cell populations. *Am Heart J* 2009;**157**:335–44.
218. Gentry T, Foster S, Winstead L, Deibert E, Fiordalisi M, Balber A. Simultaneous isolation of human BM hematopoietic, endothelial and mesenchymal progenitor cells by flow sorting based on aldehyde dehydrogenase activity: implications for cell therapy. *Cytotherapy* 2007;**9**:259–74.
219. Vauchez K, Marolleau JP, Schmid M, Khattar P, Chapel A, Catelain C, et al. Aldehyde dehydrogenase activity identifies a population of human skeletal muscle cells with high myogenic capacities. *Mol Ther* 2009;**17**:1948–58.

Chapter 63

Immunological Responses to Muscle Injury

James G. Tidball[1,2,3] and Chiara Rinaldi[2]

[1]Molecular, Cellular & Integrative Physiology Program, [2]Department of Integrative Biology and Physiology, and Department of Pathology and Laboratory Medicine, [3]David Geffen School of Medicine at UCLA, University of California, Los Angeles, CA

GENERAL CHARACTERISTICS OF THE INFLAMMATORY RESPONSE TO ACUTE MUSCLE INJURY

The response of skeletal muscle to acute injury resembles the stereotypic inflammatory response of other tissues to trauma. In each tissue, the inflammatory response is dominated by an innate immune response in which neutrophils and macrophages are the major constituents of the inflammatory infiltrate. The early-invading, inflammatory cells are avidly phagocytic and remove debris produced by injury. Later-invading populations of inflammatory cells are associated with tissue repair rather than phagocytosis. However, these generic aspects of the inflammatory response to acute injury for all tissues can have additional importance and complications in skeletal muscle. First, skeletal muscle injuries are extremely common. The superficial location of many muscles and the large proportion of the body that is comprised of muscle leaves muscles frequently subjected to injuries from blunt trauma, lacerations, burns, freezing, toxin exposure, and puncture wounds. Thus, many muscles are subjected to injury on a routine basis throughout life. In addition, accumulating evidence shows that muscle inflammation serves an adaptive as well as a reparative function. Muscle inflammation that results from exercise or modified muscle use contributes to muscle regeneration and growth that occur in response to increased muscle use. This suggests that experimental or therapeutic manipulations of the inflammatory response in muscle can provide a means to increase muscle regeneration and growth in response to modified use.

THE Th1 INFLAMMATORY RESPONSE IN INJURED SKELETAL MUSCLE

Activation of Myeloid Cells in the Th1 Inflammatory Response to Muscle Injury

Neutrophils

The Th1 inflammatory response to muscle injury resembles the early inflammatory response to infection. The designation as "Th1" reflects the activation status of T-helper cells (Th cells) that generate many of the cytokines that typify this immune response. In the context of infection, naïve Th cells are activated by antigens presented by professional antigen-presenting cells, such as dendritic cells and macrophages, which enable them to reach an activated state as Th0 cells. These mature, activated Th0 cells can then be driven to a more specialized phenotype, Th1, when further stimulated with specific Th1 cytokines. The most potent Th1 cytokines are interferon-gamma (IFN-γ) and tumor necrosis factor-α (TNF-α) (1). Upon reaching Th1 activation, Th1 cells boost the Th1 inflammatory response by increased secretion of IFN-γ and TNF-α, which also act upon myeloid cells to influence their phenotype, promote their activation, and attract them to sites of injury or infection. The ability of Th1 cytokines to amplify the early immune response is the basis for their designation as "pro-inflammatory" cytokines.

Activation of neutrophils is an early and rapid feature of the Th1 inflammatory response to acute injury. For example, neutrophils can become activated and invade injured muscle within 45 minutes to 6 hours of the initial injury (2). However, Th1 cells are not typically a component of acute muscle injury so that mechanisms other than

Muscle. DOI: http://dx.doi.org/10.1016/B978-0-12-381510-1.00063-6

Th1 cell-derived cytokines must be in place to activate neutrophils in response to muscle injury. Although neutrophils can be activated by TNF-α *in vitro* and the administration of exogenous TNF-α to injured muscle *in vivo* can boost neutrophil-activation (3), no data are available to show that neutrophils are activated by endogenous TNF-α in acute muscle injuries. Lipopolysaccharides and N-formylmethionine leucyl-phenylalanine are also potent, well-characterized activators of neutrophils (4), but they are encountered in bacterial infections, not in the sterile injuries that typically occur in damaged muscle. However, other factors, such as platelet-activating factor (PAF), have been implicated in neutrophil-activation associated with muscle injury or increased loading *in vivo*. PAF is a biologically-active phosphoglyceride that can be generated in systemic inflammatory responses by phagocytes, endothelial cells, and platelets (5). PAF is a strong inducer of neutrophil activation and systemic levels of PAF can be elevated by exercise that causes muscle injury (6). Furthermore, the elevation of PAF in exercised subjects was associated with increased numbers of neutrophils in circulation (6). Thus, PAF may contribute to neutrophil activation during muscle inflammation associated with muscle injury, although the importance of the contribution of PAF in this context is unknown.

Neutrophils are also activated by the complement system (7), which may be a particularly important system for their activation following muscle injuries in the absence of infection. The complement system consists of a family of soluble proteins that are normally present in monomeric, inactive forms in the extracellular space. However, complement proteins can be cleaved into biologically-active fragments by proteases that are activated by injury or infection. Two of these proteolytic fragments, C3a and C5a, can be bound by complement receptors at the neutrophil surface, leading to the activation and chemoattraction of neutrophils to the site of injury (8). Complement activation results from acute muscle injury or prolonged exercise (9), but also occurs in some chronic muscle diseases, such as muscular dystrophy (10) and dermatomyositis (11). Furthermore, neutrophil activation by complement can promote muscle damage by neutrophils. For example, in a rodent model of modified muscle loading in which weight-bearing is removed from hindlimbs for a period of 10-days followed by return to normal weight-bearing (the unloading/reloading model of muscle injury), the complement system is activated early in the reloading process and complement activation is associated with neutrophil activation and muscle injury (12). Blocking complement activation with a soluble form of complement receptor-1, a ligand of C3b, reduced the numbers of neutrophils in the reloaded muscle and reduced muscle damage (12).

Although activation of the complement system is sufficient to cause neutrophil activation and thereby promote the Th1 inflammatory response to injured muscle, the mechanism of complement activation in acute muscle injury is not understood clearly. However, findings from investigations of tissue injuries caused by ischemia followed by periods of reperfusion (I/R injuries) collectively support a model in which natural antibodies that function in the innate immune response can trigger the complement cascade and initiate the Th1 inflammatory response to muscle injury. Natural antibodies are present in the circulatory systems of naïve animals, prior to exposure to foreign antigens (13). Most natural antibodies are immunoglobin-M (IgM) secreted by the B1 subset of B cells. Natural IgMs are reactive to phylogenetically-conserved structural motifs that are typically encountered on foreign, infectious substances; however, host antigens may display structurally similar motifs and thereby bind natural IgM. Remarkably, binding of a single IgM pentamer is sufficient to activate the complement system (14). Thus, the presence of natural IgMs in the circulation prior to infection and their ability to activate effector systems in the innate immune system by the binding of a single pentamer enables natural IgMs to serve as rapid and effective surveillance molecules in the innate immune system.

Natural immunoglobins have been implicated in neutrophil activation and muscle damage in several genetic models in which normal Ig production was perturbed. For example, mice that are RAG-2 mutants do not develop mature B or T cells and they display reduced muscle damage in I/R injuries, but injury levels are restored when wild-type serum is returned to the mutant mice (15). Similarly, administering natural, wild-type IgM to RAG-1-null mice subjected to myocardial I/R injury restores neutrophil numbers and tissue injury to levels that occur in wild-type mice experiencing I/R injury (16), suggesting a role for the natural IgM in neutrophil activation and a role for neutrophils in promoting tissue damage following I/R. Providing natural IgM to complement receptor-2 mutant mice that have reduced numbers of B1 cells also restores neutrophil numbers and tissue damage to wild-type levels following I/R (16,17). Furthermore, I/R injury of skeletal muscle causes deposition of IgM and C3 on muscle fibers, with IgM deposition appearing to occur before C3 deposition (18). Finally, a link between IgM-binding, complement activation and neutrophil activation is supported by *in vitro* studies that showed that IgM-coated surfaces bind C3, leading to neutrophil activation (19), implying that this sequence of events may occur *in vivo* in response to acute injury and leading to activation of the Th1 inflammatory response.

Monocytes and Macrophages

Soon after neutrophil extravasation into injured muscle, invasion by monocytes and macrophages begins, leading

M1 macrophages in injured muscle:
- are classically activated by Th1 cytokines (e.g., IFN-γ and TNF-α)
- are cytolytic and phagocytic
- invade injured fibers
- express pro-inflammatory cytokines
- express iNOS
- express receptors for oxidized phospholipids (e.g., CD68)
- express complement receptors

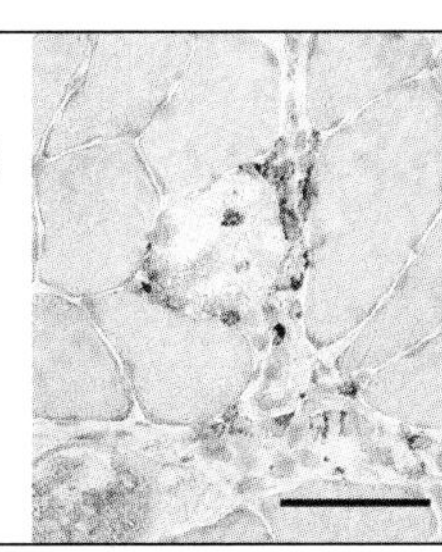

FIGURE 63.1 **M1 macrophages in injured muscle.** Micrograph shows a cross-section of rat soleus muscle that was reloaded by normal weight-bearing after a 10-day period of muscle unloading, causing muscle injury and inflammation. The muscle fiber in the center of the micrograph shows less blue staining with hematoxylin, indicating fiber damage. M1 macrophages are stained red with antibodies to CD68, a receptor for oxidized lipoproteins and phospholipids. Many $CD68^+$ M1 macrophages are distributed around the periphery of the injured fiber, while one M1 macrophage has invaded the injured fiber, to lie near its center. The granular, cytosolic staining for CD68 in M1 macrophages reflects its internalization in endosomes within phagocytic macrophages. Scale bar = 50 μm.

to significant elevation of their numbers in the injured tissue by 12–24 hours following acute injury (20,21). This rapidly-invading population of macrophages is designated as M1 macrophages (Figure 63.1), to reflect their activation by Th1 cytokines, especially TNF-α or IFN-γ. However, in the absence of Th1 cell activation in acute muscle injury, non-lymphoid cells appear to be the source of cytokines that drive M1 macrophage activation following acute muscle injury. Although few systematic studies have explored the mechanisms of activation of M1 macrophages in muscle injury, several sets of observations suggest that neutrophils play a role in promoting the M1 phenotype of macrophages that invade injured muscle. First, neutrophil activation and invasion precedes the increases in M1 macrophages in the muscle, suggesting that M1 macrophage activation may be a consequence of neutrophil activation following muscle injury. However, the sequential appearance of the two cell types in injured muscle is insufficient evidence to conclude one event causes the other. In addition, experimental manipulations that reduce neutrophil activation or invasion of injured muscle also reduce macrophage numbers (21). However, that correlation is not conclusive evidence for a role of neutrophils in M1 activation of macrophages in muscle injury; for example, reductions in macrophage numbers in injured tissues in which neutrophil numbers are reduced may reflect a loss of chemoattraction of monocytes into the injured muscle rather than impaired differentiation of monocytes to the M1 phenotype. Nevertheless, activated neutrophils express IFN-γ and TNF-α, showing that they have the capacity to drive M1 activation of macrophages. However, whether the ablation of TNF-α or IFN-γ expression by neutrophils affects M1 macrophage activation following muscle injury is unknown.

Neutrophils may also promote M1 activation of macrophages by a less direct mechanism than the release of Th1 cytokines. Upon arrival at a site of inflammation, activated neutrophils release granule proteins that can modulate the activation state of macrophages. In particular, α-defensins released by neutrophils can drive monocytes to increase expression of TNF-α and other Th1 cytokines, such as interleukin-1alpha (IL-1α) (22), which would have the potential to promote the M1 phenotype. Furthermore, activated neutrophils release serine proteinases that can modify the activity and availability of cytokines that affect M1 activation of macrophages. For example, proteinase-3, a neutrophil-derived proteinase, cleaves a precursor form of TNF-α on monocytes, leading to the release of an activated form of TNF-α (23), which may be sufficient to promote the M1 phenotype.

Function of Myeloid Cells in Injured Muscle in the Th1 Inflammatory Response

Neutrophils and M1 macrophages are both phagocytic cell populations. Clearing of infectious organisms by either phagocytic population can result from the specific recognition of particles that have been opsonized with immunoglobins or with complement-derived factors. Receptors on the phagocyte surface specifically recognize, bind and thereby initiate internalization of the opsonin and its coated cargo, leading to its proteolytic degradation by the phagocyte. Although tissue debris caused by muscle injury does not lead to opsonization of tissue fragments by IgG as would occur in a humoral inflammatory response, activated complement can bind the surface of injured muscle which may target its removal by phagocytic cells. Complement deposition on necrotic and injured muscle fibers following acute damage or disease occurs (12,24), supporting a potential role for opsonization of injured muscle by complement as a trigger for phagocytic removal of the debris.

Injured tissue debris can also be targeted for phagocytosis by oxidative modification. Phagocytosis of oxidatively modified substances by myeloid cells is primarily mediated by monocytes and macrophages that are equipped with specific receptors for oxidized phospholipids (PLs) or low-density lipoproteins (LDLs) (25). In contrast, neutrophils are relatively inept at phagocytosis of non-opsonized materials. Although the best characterized receptors for oxidized LDLs and PLs have been studied primarily in the context of binding and metabolizing of LDLs, especially the receptors CD36 and CD68, their binding can also mediate the recognition and phagocytosis of apoptotic cells and other cellular debris (25). M1 macrophages express high levels of CD36 (26) and CD68, suggesting that they play an especially significant role in the removal of debris produced by oxidative processes associated with the Th1 inflammatory response.

Both neutrophils and M1 macrophages express enzymes that generate high levels of oxidative, free radicals upon activation of the cells. Neutrophil activation induces the expression and activation of NADPH-oxidase, myeloperoxidase (MPO), and inducible nitric oxide synthetase (iNOS), each of which generates free radicals that can kill infectious organisms and target them for phagocytosis. However, production of these potentially cytotoxic substances may be less adaptive in the context of sterile tissue damage such as exercise-induced muscle injuries. While the oxidative modification of tissue debris by neutrophil-derived free radicals may have a beneficial effect in targeting debris for removal following muscle injury, the free radicals generated by these enzymes can amplify muscle damage by producing lesions in the cell membranes of muscle fibers. For example, in the unloading/reloading model of muscle damage, ablation of the MPO gene reduced muscle membrane damage during reloading by 52% (27). Similarly, null mutation of $gp91^{phox}$, the catalytic subunit of NADPH-oxidase, caused a 90% reduction of muscle membrane damage during muscle reloading (28). Both of these treatment effects are largely attributable to reducing neutrophil-mediated cytotoxicity because neutrophils primarily express these enzymes. Nitric oxide (NO) generated by iNOS is also cytotoxic in injured muscle and both neutrophils and M1 macrophages express iNOS upon activation. Ablation of iNOS in *mdx* mice, a genetic model of DMD, caused significant reductions in muscle membrane lysis during muscle inflammation (29). Furthermore, interactions between free radicals derived from NADPH-oxidase metabolism in neutrophils and from iNOS generated NO in M1 macrophages can interact to amplify tissue damage. *In vitro* studies show that the cytotoxicity of these two cell types is magnified in cell cultures where reactants of superoxide and NO can be generated (30). Thus, increased production of free radicals during the Th1 inflammatory response in muscle may be valuable for targeting cellular debris for phagocytosis, but those same free radicals or related intermediates also promote muscle damage that can worsen muscle injury.

The prominent phagocytic activities of myeloid cells that predominate in the Th1 inflammatory response to muscle injury have suggested that phagocytosis is an important and perhaps essential feature of muscle repair and regeneration following injury. Indeed, several studies have shown that perturbations of the immune response to muscle injury cause a slowing of phagocytosis and a slowing of muscle regeneration; those findings led to the expectation that phagocytosis is necessary for regeneration. While this may be true, there are not yet experimental data to show causation. Alternatively, phagocytosis and regeneration may be two independent functions mediated by the inflammatory cells.

THE Th2 INFLAMMATORY RESPONSE IN INJURED SKELETAL MUSCLE

Activation of Myeloid Cells in the Th2 Inflammatory Response to Muscle Injury

The Th1 inflammatory response, which is associated with phagocytosis and inducing further damage to host tissue, is followed by a Th2 inflammatory response that contributes to tissue repair and regeneration. The Th2 response in injured muscle is dominated by a population of macrophages designated as the M2 phenotype to reflect their selective activation by Th2 cytokines (Figure 63.2). M2 macrophages enter a state of alternative activation, in contrast to the classical activation that is experienced by M1 macrophages. Alternative activation is achieved by the binding of the Th2 cytokines interleukin-4 (IL-4), IL-10 or IL-13 by their specific receptors on the macrophage surface (31). More specifically, IL-4 and IL-13 binding drives macrophages to an M2a phenotype in which they express arginase and a cell-surface antigen CD206. IL-10 can strongly suppress the M1 macrophage phenotype by inhibiting the expression of IFN-γ and TNF-α (32) and drive macrophages to an M2c phenotype in which they express CD163 and CD206.

Alternative activation of macrophages to the M2a or M2c phenotype induces their production of Th2 cytokines that further promote alternative activation as well as deactivating M1 macrophages (31). Once the transition from an M1 to an M2 phenotype begins in a population of macrophages, the transition can be rapid. Injured muscle typically experiences a peak in M1 macrophages at 24–48 hours post-injury, but once that peak is reached M1 populations rapidly decline as M2 macrophage numbers increase in the injured muscle (33). Interestingly, the act of phagocytosis by M1 macrophages may be sufficient to initiate the transition from an M1 to M2 phenotype, depending on the identity

M2 macrophages in injured muscle:

- are alternatively activated by Th2 cytokines (IL-4, IL-10, IL-13)
- are non-cytolytic, non-phagocytic
- express Th2 cytokines that deactivate M1 macrophages
- express arginase and promote fibrosis
- express CD206 that can bind and target for degradation proteins that can worsen muscle damage (e.g., MPO)
- promote muscle repair, regeneration and growth

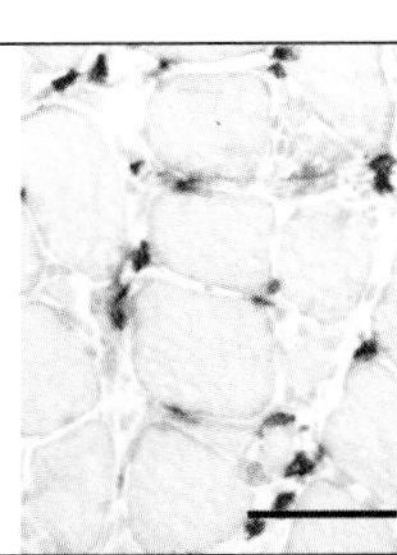

FIGURE 63.2 **M2 macrophages in injured muscle.** Micrograph shows a cross-section of rat soleus muscle that was reloaded by normal weight-bearing after a 10-day period of muscle unloading, causing muscle injury and inflammation. M2 macrophages are stained red with antibodies to CD163, a receptor for complexes of hemoglobin and haptoglobin, indicating the macrophages are more specifically of the M2c phenotype. Although M2 macrophages can lie in close association with the surface of muscle fibers, they do not invade injured fibers. Scale bar = 50 μm.

of the substance that is engulfed by the macrophage. For example, phagocytosis of apoptotic neutrophils, but not opsonized neutrophils, reduces the macrophage expression of Th1 cytokines such as TNF-α and increases expression of the Th2 cytokine, transforming growth factor-beta (TGF-β), which indicates a shift to the M2 phenotype (34). In contrast, phagocytosis of lyzed neutrophils, but not apoptotic neutrophils, increased TNF-α secretion by macrophages, suggesting a bias toward a M1 phenotype (35). Furthermore, macrophage phagocytosis of cellular debris produced by treating myoblasts with hydrogen peroxide produced decreases in TNF-α production with increases in TGF-β production (36). The possibility that the phagocytosis of apoptotic neutrophils or muscle debris provides a phenotypic switch for macrophages *in vivo* is supported by time-course data. Using the unloading/reloading model of muscle injury and inflammation, observations showed that apoptosis of inflammatory cells in the muscle peaked at day 2 of muscle reloading and returned to control levels by day 4 of reloading (37). In this same injury model, the rate of change of macrophages phenotypes from predominantly M1 to predominantly M2 is most rapid between days 2 and 4 of reloading.

Function of Myeloid Cells in Injured Muscle in the Th2 Inflammatory Response

M2 Macrophages Can Attenuate the Th1 Inflammatory Response and Reduce Tissue Damage by Neutrophils and M1 Macrophages

Phenotypic markers expressed by M1 and M2 macrophages play important roles in determining the functional capacities of specific populations of macrophages. For example, CD206 expression by M2a macrophages may contribute to the ability of M2 macrophages to attenuate muscle damage caused by M1 macrophages. CD206 is a mannose receptor that binds and internalizes sugar moieties on molecules present at high levels in inflamed tissue and its ligation elevates the expression of anti-inflammatory cytokines that contribute to the deactivation of M1 macrophages (38). In addition, CD206 binds MPO causing its internalization and degradation (39). This function is important in the context of reducing muscle damage by neutrophils because MPO released by neutrophils contributes significantly to muscle damage following injury (27). Likewise, arginase production by M2a macrophages contributes significantly to macrophage function in injured tissues. Arginase metabolizes arginine to produce profibrotic substances such as ornithine and polyamines that are necessary for normal wound healing and repair following acute injury (40,41). In fact, the availability of arginine for metabolism by arginase can be rate-limiting in the wound healing process. Although wound healing that involves arginine metabolism by arginase is a beneficial component of tissue repair following acute injury, the same metabolic processes can be detrimental in chronic muscle inflammations. For example, the *mdx* model of Duchenne muscular dystrophy (DMD) involves persistent elevations of M2a macrophages that can persist for years, which contributes to pathological fibrosis of the muscle (42,43).

CD163 expression by M2c macrophages plays a central role in their functional specialization, especially contributing to the capacity of M2c macrophages to attenuate muscle damage that can be caused by neutrophils and M1 macrophages during the Th1 inflammatory response. CD163 expression is inhibited by Th1 cytokines, such as TNF-α and IFN-γ (44) but is elevated by IL-10 (44,45). CD163 is a transmembrane receptor for complexes of hemoglobin and haptoglobin complexes that are subsequently internalized, targeted to the endosome and degraded following binding (46). The breakdown of the heme subunit of hemoglobin by heme oxygenase-1 leads to the production and release of bilirubin, carbon monoxide, and iron (47,48), all of which can function as anti-inflammatory substances, in addition to serving as anti-oxidants (49). Furthermore, CD163 ligation can increase the expression of IL-10 (48). Thus, CD163 activated signaling and

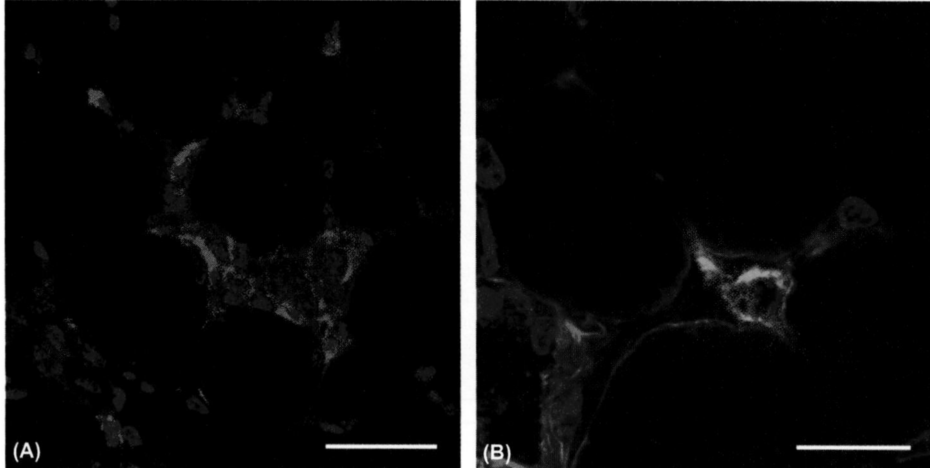

FIGURE 63.3 **Macrophages in *mdx* muscular dystrophy.** The inflammatory infiltrate in muscular dystrophy is also dominated by M1 and M2 macrophages. (A) An inflammatory lesion in 4-week-old *mdx* muscle containing numerous $CD68^+$ M1 macrophages (yellow) surrounded by a pathological accumulation of connective tissue proteins that includes laminin (red) between dystrophic muscle fibers (black). Nuclei show blue labeling with Hoechts stain. (Bar = 50 μm.) (B) $CD163^+$ M2c macrophages (yellow) are also present in *mdx* muscular dystrophy, lying in close apposition to the surface of dystrophic fibers (black) that are encircled with laminin-rich (red) basal lamina. Note the polarization distribution of CD163 on the macrophage cell surface that is not apposed to the muscle fiber surface. Bar = 25 μm.

metabolism by M2c macrophages can both attenuate the Th1 inflammatory response and reduce tissue damage caused by free radicals generated by neutrophils and M1 macrophages following muscle injury or in muscular dystrophy (Figure 63.3).

M2 Macrophages Promote Muscle Regeneration and Growth Following Injury

Macrophages have been associated with muscle repair and regeneration for decades, but only recently have experimental observations supported that expectation. Some of the important, early studies showed that muscle regeneration in recipients of whole muscle grafts was slower if the graft recipients were irradiated prior to transplantation. Those findings suggested that the activities of normally-proliferative cells in the recipient, such as monocytes and macrophages, were necessary for normal rates of muscle regeneration. *In vitro* findings supported that interpretation. For example, transfer of conditioned media from cultures of peritoneal macrophages or macrophage cell lines to muscle cell cultures increased the rate of proliferation of myoblasts and increased the number of muscle cells that expressed MyoD, a muscle transcription factor that is upregulated in muscle cells during early stages of differentiation (50–52).

Recently, the pro-regenerative effects of macrophages on muscle have been attributed more specifically to M2 macrophages. $CD163^+$ M2 macrophages tend to be closely associated with regenerative muscle fibers and the time at which their numbers increase in muscle following injury (about 2–4 days post-injury) coincides with stage at which muscle regeneration begins to proceed rapidly (53,54). The specific depletion of macrophage populations during the 2–4-day window of muscle regeneration post-injury prevented increases in the number of regenerative muscle fibers that normally occurs at this stage of regeneration (54). Also, macrophage depletion during this post-injury period prevented muscle membrane repair that normally occurs during this period and eliminated any significant growth of muscle fibers, in contrast to post-injury muscle in which macrophages were not depleted (54). Effects were also seen in patterns of expression of transcription factors that regulate muscle regeneration. Following macrophage depletion, MyoD levels remained high in muscle 4 days post-injury, while MyoD levels in injured muscles containing macrophages were significantly lower than in muscle at that stage of regeneration (54). This outcome parallels previous *in vitro* observations that showed that $CD163^+$ macrophages (called $ED2^+$ macrophages in rats) that were isolated from peritoneal exudates and co-cultured with muscle cells produced an increase in $MyoD^+$ myonuclei (52). Collectively, the observations support a significant role for M2 macrophages in modulating muscle growth, regeneration, repair and differentiation following acute injury.

Other injury models similarly indicate that disruption in the normal expansion of macrophage populations during this post-injury period leads to slower regeneration and growth of the injured muscle. For example, ablating the expression of chemokine receptor-2 (CCR2) or its ligand CCL2 in mice subjected to muscle injury by toxin injection (55) or ischemia (56,57) caused tremendous reductions in macrophages present in the muscle at 3–7 days post-injury. This reduction in macrophage numbers was accompanied by a delay in the appearance of regenerative fibers and slowing of fiber growth in injured areas. Although myoblasts express CCR2 constitutively and stimulation of myoblasts with CCL2 increases their proliferation *in vitro* (58), experimental findings suggest that the disruptions of macrophage function are more important in contributing to defects in muscle regeneration in CCR2-null or CCL2-null mice. The regenerative defects in muscles that were injured by toxin injection which were attributable to CCR2-null mutation were prevented by the transplantation of wild-type bone marrow to the mutant mice before injury (59).

INFLAMMATORY CELL-DERIVED CYTOKINES HAVE DIRECT EFFECTS ON MUSCLE GROWTH AND REGENERATION

Cytokines that are released by inflammatory cells play central roles in regulating the activation, phenotype, and movements of leukocytes to injured muscle. However, cytokines that act directly on myeloid cells to influence their functions can also have profound effects on muscle cells and the number of cytokines that are known to influence muscle cell activation, proliferation or differentiation has grown tremendously over the last decade. One of these, TNF-α, is emphasized here because it plays crucial roles in directing the phenotype of macrophages during muscle inflammation following injury and because it may play a central role in coordinating the processes of inflammation and regeneration by regulating differentiation of cells in both the myeloid and muscle compartments.

TNF-α plays a complex role in injured muscle. TNF-α levels reach their peak in injured muscle at about 24 hours after injury, when the Th1 inflammatory response is at its highest level and muscle membrane lesions are most extensive (60). Likely, these coinciding events are mechanistically related. TNF-α stimulation of macrophages activates the M1 phenotype and elevates the expression of iNOS by muscle macrophages, thereby increasing their cytotoxicity (42). However, TNF-α can also affect muscle repair and regeneration by affecting satellite cell proliferation and differentiation. *In vitro* studies show that treating myogenic cells with TNF-α increases cell proliferation (61) and inhibits fusion (62,63). Similarly, TNF-α null mutants and TNF-α receptor mutants showed lower levels of expression of transcripts associated with satellite cell activation and proliferation following an acute injury (60,64). Thus, TNF-α could promote apparently conflicting processes by increasing muscle damage by its actions through the myeloid compartment but promoting repair via actions on the muscle compartment.

TNF-α also plays conflicting, regulatory roles within the muscle compartment following injury because TNF-α binding by muscle cells can either inhibit or promote muscle differentiation. TNF-α binding by myoblasts activates the transcription factor NF-κB that increases proliferation and suppresses differentiation through several processes operating in parallel. NF-κB activation increases the expression of cyclin D1, which can contribute to increased cell proliferation (65,66). NF-κB activation also reduces the stability of MyoD mRNA (63,65). Because MyoD is a transcription factor that helps drive expression of muscle-specific genes that are activated as part of the differentiation program of muscle, the result of this NF-κB effect would also be to suppress differentiation. Finally, NF-κB also binds to the promoter of the transcriptional repressor YY1, which increases YY1 expression, which in turn suppresses the expression of several, muscle-specific genes that are upregulated in differentiation (67).

In contrast to the differentiation-suppressing effects of TNF-α on proliferative muscle cells that are mediated through NF-κB activation, TNF-α can promote differentiation of muscle cells that have exited the cell cycle, possibly by affecting the activation of p38 kinase. However, the relationship between TNF-α stimulation, p38 activation and muscle cell proliferation or differentiation is not yet clear. Although TNF-α stimulation of non-muscle cells increases p38 activation *in vitro* (68) and treatment of *mdx* mice with neutralizing antibodies to TNF-α reduces p38 activation in whole muscle extracts (69), there are no data to show whether the TNF-α stimulation directly affects p38 activation in muscle. However, several investigations have established downstream consequences of p38 activation in muscle that may be independent of TNF-α stimulation. Increased activation of p38 increases the activity of MyoD (70) which would contribute to early stages of muscle differentiation. Similarly, inhibition of p38 reduces the expression of other muscle specific transcription factors that drive muscle differentiation (myogenin and MEF2) and inhibits the formation of myotubes, which is a watershed event in the differentiation of mononucleated muscle cells into fully-differentiated muscle fibers. In part, these p38-mediated effects on muscle differentiation may reflect epigenetic regulation of muscle-specific transcription factors or other muscle-specific proteins – for example, p38 phosphorylates Ezh2, a methyltransferase that associates with YY1 to bind and suppress transcription of genes that promote muscle differentiation (69,71). However, whether the regulatory affects of p38 activation promote or suppress muscle differentiation may vary with the p38 isoform that is activated – for example, activated p38α phosphorylates E47 leading to E47 dimerization with MyoD to enable dimer binding to the E-box of muscle specific proteins (72) that promote muscle differentiation. In contrast, p38γ directly phosphorylates MyoD which leads to its assembly into a complex that represses the expression of muscle specific genes involved in muscle differentiation (73). The importance of this p38γ -mediated pathway in muscle regeneration following injury has been established. Muscles of p38γ null-mutant mice that were injured by toxin injection showed impaired expansion of myogenic cell populations following injury and fewer muscle fibers in regenerative area of the muscle (73). However, a definitive link between activation of the p38γ signaling pathway and TNF-α in injured muscle has not yet been demonstrated.

FUTURE DIRECTIONS

Our expanding understanding of the functional specializations of myeloid cells that invade injured muscle now shows that muscle inflammation can worsen muscle damage following acute injury, but also shows that myeloid cells can promote repair, regeneration, and growth (Figure 63.4). However, much needs to be learned concerning the mechanisms through which these processes are mediated. Although natural antibodies and activation of the complement system can activate the Th1

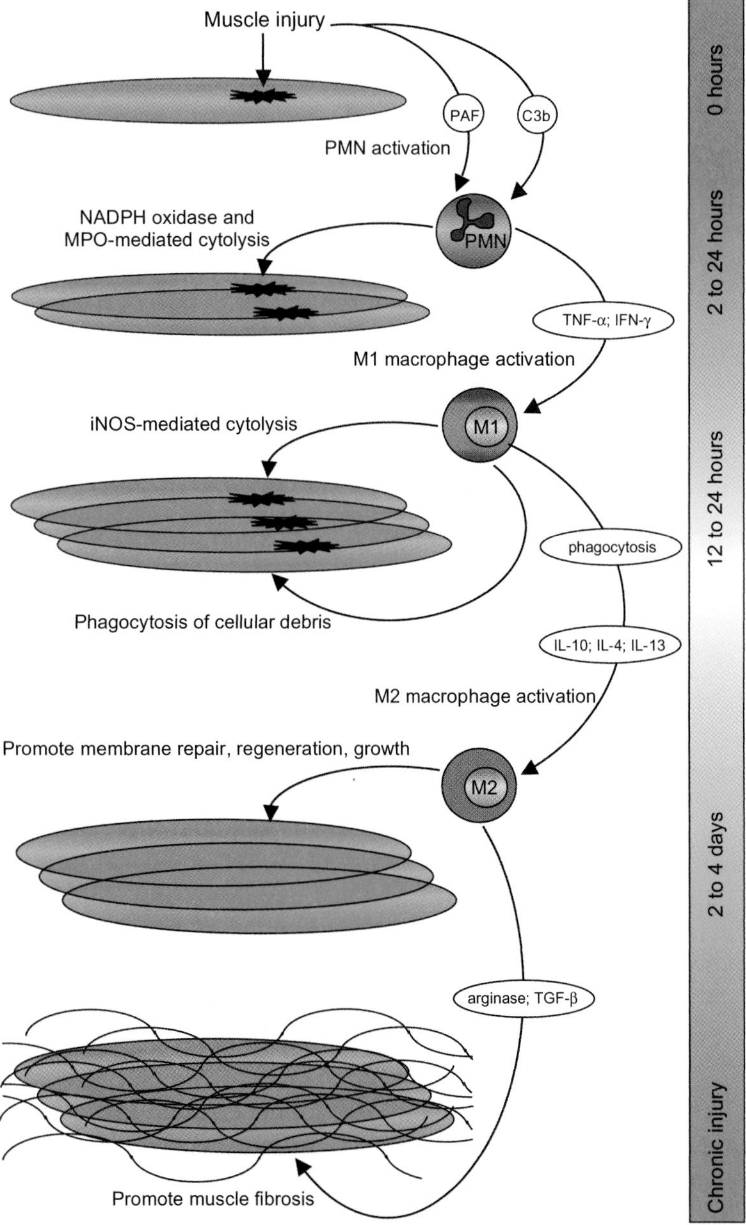

FIGURE 63.4 Schematic of the stages of involvement of myeloid cells in muscle injury, repair, growth, and fibrosis of skeletal muscle following injury. PMN = polymorphonuclear neutrophils.

inflammatory response in some specific injuries, such as I/R injuries or the unloading/reloading model of muscle injury, whether those processes contribute significantly to activation of the inflammatory response following other acute muscle injuries is unknown. Although phagocytosis precedes regeneration of injured muscle and perturbation of the inflammatory response can impede both phagocytosis and regeneration, whether regeneration and phagocytosis are mechanistically-linked in muscle inflammation has not been tested. Perhaps most basically, the importance of the inflammatory response to successful regeneration of muscle remains unknown. Although current findings show that perturbations of muscle inflammation can influence muscle regeneration, whether the perturbations affect the ultimate outcome of regeneration or merely influence the kinetics of the repair response has not been tested. Muscle growth and differentiation occur rapidly and successfully in the absence of inflammation during embryogenesis and early post-natal growth, so is muscle inflammation really required for successful regeneration following acute injury? If so, then manipulations of the inflammatory response may provide a valuable route for influencing muscle repair, regeneration, and growth following injury or disease.

ACKNOWLEDGMENTS

During the preparation of this article, support was received from the Muscular Dystrophy Association, USA (#157881 and #4031) and the National Institutes of Health (R01 AR47721, RO1 AR47855, R01 AR/AG054451).

REFERENCES

1. Szabo SJ, Sullivan BM, Peng SL, Glimcher LH. Molecular mechanisms regulating Th1 immune responses. *Annu Rev Immunol* 2003;**21**:713–58.
2. Fielding RA, Manfredi TJ, Ding W, Fiatarone MA, Evans WJ, Cannon JG. Acute phase response in exercise. III. Neutrophil and IL-1β accumulation in skeletal muscle. *Am J Physiol* 1993;**265**: R166–72.
3. Peterson JM, Feeback KD, Baas JH, Pizza FX. Tumor necrosis factor-alpha promotes the accumulation of neutrophils and macrophages in skeletal muscle. *J Appl Physiol* 2006;**101**:1394–9.
4. Lynn WA, Raetz CR, Qureshi N, Golenbock DT. Lipopolysaccharide-induced stimulation of CD11b/CD18 expression on neutrophils. Evidence of specific receptor-based response and inhibition by lipid A-based antagonists. *J Immunol* 1991;**147**:3072–9.
5. Hanahan DJ. Platelet activating factor: a biologically active phosphoglyceride. *Ann Rev Biochem* 1986;**55**:483–509.
6. Milias GA, Nomikos T, Fragopoulou E, Athanasopoulos S, Antonopoulou S. Effects of eccentric exercise-induced muscle injury on blood levels of platelet activating factor (PAF) and other inflammatory markers. *Eur J Appl Physiol* 2005;**95**:504–13.
7. Martin TR. Leukocyte migration and activation in the lungs. *Eur Respir J* 1997;**10**:770–1.
8. Kajita T, Hugli TE. C5a-induced neutrophilia: a primary humoral mechanism for recruitment of neutrophils. *Am J Pathol* 1990;**137**:467–77.
9. Dufaux B, Order U. Complement activation after prolonged exercise. *Clin Chim Acta* 1989;**179**:45–9.
10. Spuler S, Engel AG. Unexpected sarcolemmal complement membrane attack complex deposits on nonnecrotic muscle fibers in muscular dystrophies. *Neurol* 1998;**50**:41–6.
11. Kissel JT, Halterman RK, Rammohan KW, Mendell JR. The relationship of complement-mediated microvasculopathy to the histologic features and clinical duration of disease in dermatomyositis. *Arch Neurol* 1991;**48**:26–30.
12. Frenette J, Cai B, Tidball JG. Complement activation promotes muscle inflammation during modified muscle use. *Am J Pathol* 2000;**156**:2103–10.
13. Ochsenbein AF, Zinkernagel RM. Natural antibodies and complement link innate and acquired immunity. *Immunol Today* 2000;**21**:624–30.
14. Cooper NR. The classical complement pathway: activation and regulation of the first complement component. *Adv Immunol* 1985;**37**:151–216.
15. Weiser MR, Williams JP, Moore Jr FD, Kobzik L, Ma M, Hechtman HB, et al. Reperfusion injury of ischemic skeletal muscle is mediated by natural antibody and complement. *J Exp Med* 1996;**183**:2343–8.
16. Zhang M, Michael LH, Grosjean SA, Kelly RA, Carroll MC, Entman ML. The role of natural IgM in myocardial ischemia-reperfusion injury. *J Mol Cell Cardiol* 2006;**41**:62–7.
17. Austen Jr WG, Zhang M, Chan R, Friend D, Hechtman HB, Carroll MC, et al. Murine hindlimb reperfusion injury can be initiated by a self-reactive monoclonal IgM. *Surgery* 2004;**136**: 401–6.
18. Chan RK, Ding G, Verna N, Ibrahim S, Oakes S, Austen Jr WG, et al. IgM binding to injured tissue precedes complement activation during skeletal muscle ischemia-reperfusion. *J Surg Res* 2004;**122**:29–35.
19. Wetterö J, Bengtsson T, Tengvall P. C1q-independent activation of neutrophils by immunoglobulin M-coated surfaces. *J Biomed Mater Res* 2001;**57**:550–8.
20. Shireman PK, Contreras-Shannon V, Ochoa O, Karia BP, Michalek JE, McManus LM. MCP-1 deficiency causes altered inflammation with impaired skeletal muscle regeneration. *J Leukoc Biol* 2007;**81**:775–85.
21. Teixeira CF, Zamuner SR, Zuliani JP, Fernandes CM, Cruz-Hofling MA, Fernandes I, et al. Neutrophils do not contribute to local tissue damage, but play a key role in skeletal muscle regeneration, in mice injected with *Bothrops asper* snake venom. *Muscle Nerve* 2003;**28**:449–59.
22. Chaly YV, Paleolog EM, Kolesnikova TS, Tikhonov II, Petratchenko EV, Voitenok NN. Neutrophil alpha-defensin human neutrophil peptide modulates cytokine production in human monocytes and adhesion molecule expression in endothelial cells. *Eur Cytokine Netw* 2000;**11**:257–66.
23. Robache-Gallea S, Morand V, Bruneau JM, Schoot B, Tagat E, Réalo E, et al. In vitro processing of human tumor necrosis factor. *J Biol Chem* 1995;**270**:23688–92.

24. Orimo S, Hiyamuta E, Arahata K, Sugita H. Analysis of inflammatory cells and complement C3 in bupivacaine-induced myonecrosis. *Muscle Nerve* 1991;**14**:515–20.
25. Chang MK, Bergmark C, Laurila A, Hörkkö S, Han KH, Friedman P, et al. Monoclonal antibodies against oxidized low-density lipoprotein bind to apoptotic cells and inhibit their phagocytosis by elicited macrophages: evidence that oxidation-specific epitopes mediate macrophage recognition. *Proc Natl Acad Sci USA* 1999;**96**:6353–8.
26. Kennedy DJ, Kuchibhotla S, Westfall K, Silverstein R, Morton E, Febbraio M. A CD36-dependent pathway enhances macrophage and adipose tissue inflammation and impairs insulin signaling. *Cardiovasc Res* 2011;**89**:604–13.
27. Nguyen HX, Lusis AJ, Tidball JG. Null mutation of myeloperoxidase in mice prevents mechanical activation of neutrophil lysis of muscle cell membranes in vitro and in vivo. *J Physiol* 2005;**565**:403–13.
28. Nguyen HX, Tidball JG. Null mutation of gp91phox reduces muscle membrane lysis during muscle inflammation in mice. *J Physiol* 2003;**553**:833–41.
29. Nguyen HX, Tidball JG. Expression of a muscle-specific, nitric oxide synthase transgene prevents muscle membrane injury and reduces muscle inflammation during modified muscle use in mice. *J Physiol* 2003;**550**:347–56.
30. Nguyen HX, Tidball JG. Null mutation of gp91phox reduces muscle membrane lysis during muscle inflammation in mice. *J Physiol* 2003;**553**:833–41.
31. Gordon S. Alternative activation of macrophages. *Nature Rev* 2003;**3**:23–35.
32. Fiorentino DF, Zlotnik A, Mosmann TR, Howard M, O'Garra A. IL-10 inhibits cytokine production by activated macrophages. *J Immunol* 1991;**147**:3815–22.
33. St. Pierre BA, Tidball JG. Differential response of macrophage subpopulations to soleus muscle reloading after rat hindlimb suspension. *J Appl Physiol* 1994;**77**:290–7.
34. Fadok VA, Bratton DL, Konowal A, Freed PW, Westcott JY, Henson PM. Macrophages that have ingested apoptotic cells in vitro inhibit proinflammatory cytokine production through autocrine/paracrine mechanisms involving TGF-β, PGE2, and PAF. *J Clin Invest* 1998;**101**:890–8.
35. Fadok VA, Bratton DL, Guthrie L, Henson PM. Differential effects of apoptotic versus lysed cells on macrophage production of cytokines: role of proteases. *J Immunol* 2001;**166**:6847–54.
36. Arnold L, Henry A, Poron F, Baba-Amer Y, van Rooijen N, Plonquet A, et al. Inflammatory monocytes recruited after skeletal muscle injury switch into antiinflammatory macrophages to support myogenesis. *J Exp Med* 2007;**204**:1057–69.
37. Tidball St. JG, Pierre BA. Apoptosis of macrophages during the resolution of muscle inflammation. *J Leukoc Biol* 1996;**59**:380–8.
38. Chieppa M, Bianchi G, Doni A, Del Prete A, Sironi M, Laskarin G, et al. Cross-linking of the mannose receptor on monocyte-derived dendritic cells activates an anti-inflammatory immunosuppressive program. *J Immunol* 2003;**171**:4552–60.
39. Shepherd VL, Hoidal JR. Clearance of neutrophil-derived myeloperoxidase by the macrophage mannose receptor. *Am J Respir Cell Mol Biol* 1990;**2**:335–40.
40. Witte MB, Barbul A. Arginine physiology and its implication for wound healing. *Wound Repair Regen* 2003;**11**:419–23.
41. Curran JN, Winter DC, Bouchier-Hayes D. Biological fate and clinical implications of arginine metabolism in tissue healing. *Wound Repair Regen* 2006;**14**:376–86.
42. Villalta SA, Nguyen HX, Deng B, Gotoh T, Tidball JG. Shifts in macrophage phenotypes and macrophage competition for arginine metabolism affect the severity of muscle pathology in muscular dystrophy. *Human Molec Genetics* 2009;**18**:482–96.
43. Wehling-Henricks M, Jordan MC, Gotoh T, Grody WW, Roos KP, Tidball JG. Arginine metabolism by macrophages promotes cardiac and muscle fibrosis in mdx muscular dystrophy. *PLoS One* 2010;**5**: e10763.
44. Buechler C, Ritter M, Orso E, Langmann T, Klucken J, Schmitz G. Regulation of scavenger receptor CD163 expression in human monocytes and macrophages by pro- and anti-inflammatory stimuli. *J Leukoc Biol* 2000;**67**:97–103.
45. Villalta SA, Rinaldi C, Deng B, Liu G, Fedor B, Tidball JG. Interleukin-10 reduces the pathology of mdx muscular dystrophy by deactivating M1 macrophages and modulating macrophage phenotype. *Human Molec Genetics* 2011;**20**:790–805.
46. Schaer CA, Schoedon G, Imhof A, Kurrer MO, Schaer DJ. Constitutive endocytosis of CD163 mediates hemoglobin-heme uptake and determines the noninflammatory and protective transcriptional response of macrophages to hemoglobin. *Circ Res* 2006;**99**:943–50.
47. Schaer CA, Vallelian F, Imhof A, Schoedon G, Schaer DJ. Heme carrier protein (HCP-1) spatially interacts with the CD163 hemoglobin uptake pathway and is a target of inflammatory macrophage activation. *J Leukoc Biol* 2008;**83**:325–33.
48. Philippidis P, Mason JC, Evans BJ, Nadra I, Taylor KM, Haskard DO, et al. Hemoglobin scavenger receptor CD163 mediates interleukin-10 release and heme oxygenase-1 synthesis: anti-inflammatory monocyte-macrophage responses in vitro, in resolving skin blisters in vivo, and after cardiopulmonary bypass surgery. *Circ Res* 2004;**94**:119–26.
49. Otterbein LE, Soares MP, Yamashita K, Bach FH. Heme oxygenase-1: unleashing the protective properties of heme. *Trends Immunol* 2003;**24**:449–55.
50. Cantini M, Carraro U. Macrophage-released factor stimulates selectively myogenic cells in primary muscle culture. *J Neuropathol Exp Neurol* 1995;**54**:121–8.
51. Merly F, Lescaudron L, Rouaud T, Crossin F, Gardahaut MF. Macrophages enhance muscle satellite cell proliferation and delay their differentiation. *Muscle Nerve* 1999;**22**:724–32.
52. Massimino M, Rapizzi E, Cantini M, Libera L, Mazzoeni F, Arsian P, et al. $ED2^+$ macrophages increase selectively myoblast proliferation in muscle cultures. *Biochem Biophys Res Commun* 1997;**235**:754–9.
53. McLennan IS. Resident macrophages (ED2- and ED3-positive) do not phagocytose degenerating rat skeletal muscle fibres. *Cell Tissue Res* 1993;**272**:193–6.
54. Tidball JG, Wehling-Henricks M. Macrophages promote muscle membrane repair and muscle fibre growth and regeneration during modified muscle loading in mice in vivo. *J Physiol* 2007;**578**:327–36.
55. Ochoa O, Sun D, Reyes-Reyna SM, Waite LL, Michalek JE, McManus LM, et al. Delayed angiogenesis and VEGF production in $CCR2^{-/-}$ mice during impaired skeletal muscle regeneration. *Am J Physiol* 2007;**293**:R651–61.

56. Shireman PK, Contreras-Shannon V, Ochoa O, Karia BP, Michalek JE, McManus LM. MCP-1 deficiency causes altered inflammation with impaired skeletal muscle regeneration. *J Leukoc Biol* 2007;**81**:775–85.
57. Contreras-Shannon V, Ochoa O, Reyes-Reyna SM, Sun D, Michalek JE, Kuziel WA, et al. Fat accumulation with altered inflammation and regeneration in skeletal muscle of $CCR2^{-/-}$ mice following ischemic injury. *Am J Physiol* 2007;**292**:C953–67.
58. Yahiaoui L, Gvozdic D, Danialou G, Mack M, Petrof BJ. CC family chemokines directly regulate myoblast responses to skeletal muscle injury. *J Physiol* 2008;**586**:3991–4004.
59. Sun D, Martinez CO, Ochoa O, Ruiz-Willhite L, Bonilla JR, Centonze VE, et al. Bone marrow-derived cell regulation of skeletal muscle regeneration. *FASEB J* 2009;**23**:382–95.
60. Warren GL, Hulderman T, Jensen N, McKinstry M, Mishra M, Luster MI, et al. Physiological role of tumor necrosis factor alpha in traumatic muscle injury. *FASEB J* 2002;**16**:1630–2.
61. Li YP. TNF-alpha is a mitogen in skeletal muscle. *Am J Physiol* 2003;**285**:C370–6.
62. Langen RC, Schols AM, Kelders MC, Wouters EF, Janssen-Heininger YM. Inflammatory cytokines inhibit myogenic differentiation through activation of nuclear factor-kappaB. *FASEB J* 2001;**15**:1169–80.
63. Langen RC, Van Der Velden JL, Schols AM, Kelders MC, Wouters EF, Janssen-Heininger YM. Tumor necrosis factor-alpha inhibits myogenic differentiation through MyoD protein destabilization. *FASEB J* 2004;**18**:227–37.
64. Chen SE, Gerken E, Zhang Y, Zhan M, Mohan RK, Li AS, et al. Role of TNF-α signaling in regeneration of cardiotoxin-injured muscle. *Am J Physiol* 2005;**289**:C1179–87.
65. Guttridge DC, Albanese C, Reuther JY, Pestell RG, Baldwin Jr AS. NF-κB controls cell growth and differentiation through transcriptional regulation of cyclin D1. *Mol Cell Biol* 1999;**19**:5785–99.
66. Hinz M, Krappmann D, Eichten A, Heder A, Scheidereit C, Strauss M. NF-κB function in growth control: regulation of cyclin D1 expression and G0/G1-to-S-phase transition. *Mol Cell Biol* 1999;**19**:2690–8.
67. Wang H, Hertlein E, Bakkar N, Sun H, Acharyya S, Wang J, et al. NF-κB regulation of YY1 inhibits skeletal myogenesis through transcriptional silencing of myofibrillar genes. *Mol Cell Biol* 2007;**27**:4374–87.
68. Raingeaud J, Gupta S, Rogers JS, Dickens M, Han J, Ulevitch RJ, et al. Pro-inflammatory cytokines and environmental stress cause p38 mitogen-activated protein kinase activation by dual phosphorylation on tyrosine and threonine. *J Biol Chem* 1995;**270**: 7420–6.
69. Palacios D, Mozzetta C, Consalvi S, Caretti G, Saccone V, Proserpio V, et al. TNF/p38α/polycomb signaling to Pax7 locus in satellite cells links inflammation to the epigenetic control of muscle regeneration. *Cell Stem Cell* 2010;**7**:455–69.
70. Zetser A, Gredinger E, Bengal E. p38 mitogen-activated protein kinase pathway promotes skeletal muscle differentiation. Participation of the Mef2c transcription factor. *J Biol Chem* 1999;**274**:5193–200.
71. Caretti G, Di Padova M, Micales B, Lyons GE, Sartorelli V. The Polycomb Ezh2 methyltransferase regulates muscle gene expression and skeletal muscle differentiation. *Genes Dev* 2004; **18**:2627–38.
72. Lluís F, Ballestar E, Suelves M, Esteller M, Muñoz-Cánoves P. E47 phosphorylation by p38 MAPK promotes MyoD/E47 association and muscle-specific gene transcription. *EMBO J* 2005;**24**:974–84.
73. Gillespie MA, Le Grand F, Scimè A, Kuang S, von Maltzahn J, Seale V, et al. p38-gamma-dependent gene silencing restricts entry into the myogenic differentiation program. *J Cell Biol* 2009;**187**:991–1005.

Chapter 64

Skeletal Muscle Adaptation to Exercise

John J. McCarthy and Karyn A. Esser
Center for Muscle Biology, Department of Physiology, College of Medicine, University of Kentucky, Lexington, KY

Adult skeletal muscle has a significant capacity for altering its physical makeup (phenotype) in response to changes in contractile activity. This phenotypic plasticity is highly specific, with the terminal phenotype being defined by the pattern of muscle activity. Moreover, the ability of a muscle to adapt to a chronic, consistent change in activity appears to be intrinsic to the muscle and not secondary to other systemic changes known to occur with exercise (1,2). A bout of exercise can be described by the intensity, duration, and frequency of muscle activity with the summation of these components broadly defining two types of exercise: high-resistance exercise and endurance exercise. High-resistance exercise (RE) typically involves some form of weightlifting performed at a high-intensity (70–90% one-repetition maximum) for a short duration (three sets of 8–12 repetitions) with modest frequency (2–3 days per week) which ultimately results in greater muscle mass and strength. Alternatively, endurance exercise is performed at a relatively low-intensity for a longer duration (30–60 minutes) on almost a daily basis (5 days per week) leading to increased muscular endurance. The distinct phenotypic transformations brought about by these different forms of exercise have been well described in both humans and animal models. Throughout the last two decades, there have been significant advances in our understanding of the molecules and signaling networks involved in regulating the specific adaptations that occur in skeletal muscle following RE or EE. The purpose of this chapter is to provide an overview of the current state of knowledge regarding the molecular mechanisms underlying the adaptation of skeletal muscle to RE and EE and conclude with a brief discussion on the future direction of the field. We acknowledge, however, that due to space limitations, we were not able to cover all aspects of exercise adaptations in this chapter.

SPECIFICITY OF SIGNALING

Relying on the principles of exercise specificity, Nader and Esser provided early molecular evidence that different forms of exercise would activate unique signaling responses (3). These authors used different electrical stimulation patterns to mimic either RE or EE and reported that only high-frequency RE stimulation caused a prolonged activation of ribosomal protein S6 kinase 1 (S6K1), a finding consistent with increased protein synthesis required for muscle hypertrophy (3,4). Using a similar protocol, Atherton and colleagues confirmed and extended these finding by showing high- and low-frequency stimulation-activated distinct signaling pathways, Akt/mTOR (thymoma viral proto-oncogene 1/mammalian target of rapamycin) and AMPK/PGC-1α (AMP-activated protein kinase/peroxisome proliferative activated receptor γ, coactivator 1α), respectively, and that protein synthesis was only elevated after high-frequency stimulation, mimicking RE (5). In humans, the specificity of the adaptive response appears to become more refined after training such that RE only stimulated myofibrillar protein synthesis whereas EE stimulated just the synthesis of mitochondrial proteins (6). The identification of key molecules and characterization of the signaling pathways involved in regulating the specific adaptation of skeletal muscle are discussed in the following sections.

ADAPTATION OF SKELETAL MUSCLE TO RESISTANCE EXERCISE

Milo of Crotona, a famous ancient Greek wrestler, was reputed to have achieved his great strength by carrying a bull on his back every day since the time it was a calf. This legendary tale demonstrates what has been known intuitively for a long time – skeletal muscle is capable of adapting to a progressive, high-resistance exercise regime by increasing its size and strength. Modern day high-resistance exercise protocols prescribe three sets of 8–12 repetitions, performed three times per week (on alternating days) for each major muscle group (7). After approximately 8–12 weeks, a high-resistance exercise program of this nature will produce a 10–14% increase in muscle size and strength, with the results being influenced by training status, muscle group, sex and age (8). The gain in muscle size and strength follows a linear progression

Muscle. DOI: http://dx.doi.org/10.1016/B978-0-12-381510-1.00064-8

during the first six months of training, after which further size and strength gains begin to plateau. In addition to the change in muscle size, neurological adaptations occur which contribute to the early increase in strength observed following the initiation of a resistance exercise program. The exact neurological factors thought to contribute to enhanced strength remain to be clearly established but the latest findings support a role for greater neural drive leading to increased motor discharge rate (9).

Hypertrophy vs. Hyperplasia

The increase in mammalian skeletal muscle size in response to RE is primarily caused by an increase in the size of individual muscle cells (fibers) with little to no contribution from an increase in the number of muscle fibers (10,11). This cellular hypertrophy, as opposed to hyperplasia, is largely brought about by a net accretion of both sarcoplasmic and myofibrillar proteins (12). The view that hypertrophy is the sole mechanism underlying muscle growth in response to resistance exercise, however, is not without controversy. There are both human and animal studies that have reported observing both fiber hypertrophy as well as fiber hyperplasia following increased mechanical loading (13,14). Changes in muscle morphology (angle of pennation), appearance of small "regenerative" fibers and limitations imposed by small muscle biopsy samples (in the case of human studies) have prevented this issue from being completely resolved but the weight of the evidence supports a minor role for hyperplasia in skeletal muscle adaptation to resistance exercise (15).

Mechanism of Muscle Hypertrophy: Increased Protein Synthesis

Hypertrophy in skeletal muscle is characterized, in large part, by increased content of the proteins that comprise the sarcomere, with total protein content of the skeletal muscle increasing but the concentration of protein (mg protein/g muscle mass) not changing. This type of adaptation requires the muscle to shift protein metabolism such that there is a sustained, net increase in the rate of protein synthesis over the rate of degradation. For the purpose of this review we will focus on the regulation of protein synthesis following RE as there has been little known about whether regulation of protein degradation contributes to strength gains and muscle hypertrophy.

Regulation of Protein Synthesis by mTOR Signaling Pathway

The signaling pathway most established as a regulator of protein synthesis, especially during cellular growth, is the mTOR signaling pathway (see Figure 64.1). The mTOR pathway acts as a master regulator of protein synthesis within all cell types by integrating diverse input such as mechanical strain, growth factors, nutrition and energy status (16). In mammalian cells, mTOR is the catalytic subunit of two distinct multi-protein complexes designated mTOR complex 1 (TORC1) and mTOR complex 2 (TORC2). TORC1 is comprised of mTOR, regulatory associated protein of mTOR (Raptor), and G-protein β-subunit-like (Gβl/also known as mLST8) whereas TORC2 contains mTOR, rapamycin-insensitive companion of mTOR (Rictor), stress-activated-protein-kinase-interacting protein 1 (SIN1), and Gβl. For the purpose of this review, we will focus on TORC1 regulation of protein synthesis given that TORC2 has been shown to be involved in regulating the cytoskeleton, cell cycle progression, and cell survival (16).

Resistance Exercise Activates mTOR Signaling

Early studies clearly showed in humans and animal models that high-resistance contractions produce an elevation in the rate of protein synthesis in skeletal muscle (17–20). Baar and Esser (4) provided the first mechanistic data showing that high-resistance contractions caused an increase in both the polysomal RNA fraction and phosphorylation of S6K1, findings consistent with the idea that increased translational efficiency was responsible for the elevation in protein synthesis (4). Interestingly, the level of S6K1 phosphorylation (Thr389) at 6 hours after the initial training bout was predictive of the degree of muscle hypertrophy following a six-week training program (4). Building on these pioneering studies, Bodine and co-workers used pharmacological and genetic tools to demonstrate that the TORC1 signaling pathway was necessary for skeletal muscle hypertrophy through regulation of its downstream effectors S6K1 and 4E-BP1 (21). Furthermore, this same group showed that regulation of muscle hypertrophy by TORC1 signaling could be mediated through IGF-1 activation of the PI3K/Akt pathway and that Akt activation was sufficient to drive hypertrophy (see Figure 64.1) (21,22).

The findings from animal studies have been extended to humans such that we now know the increase in protein synthesis following RE is primarily regulated by the TORC1 signaling pathway and is highly influenced by the intensity (percentage of one-repetition maximum, % 1-RM), volume (number of sets), mode (concentric vs. eccentric contraction) of the exercise as well as fiber-type and the ingestion of amino acids post-exercise (23–29).

Terzis et al. reported the percent increase in leg muscle size, 1-RM, and cross-sectional area of type IIa fibers

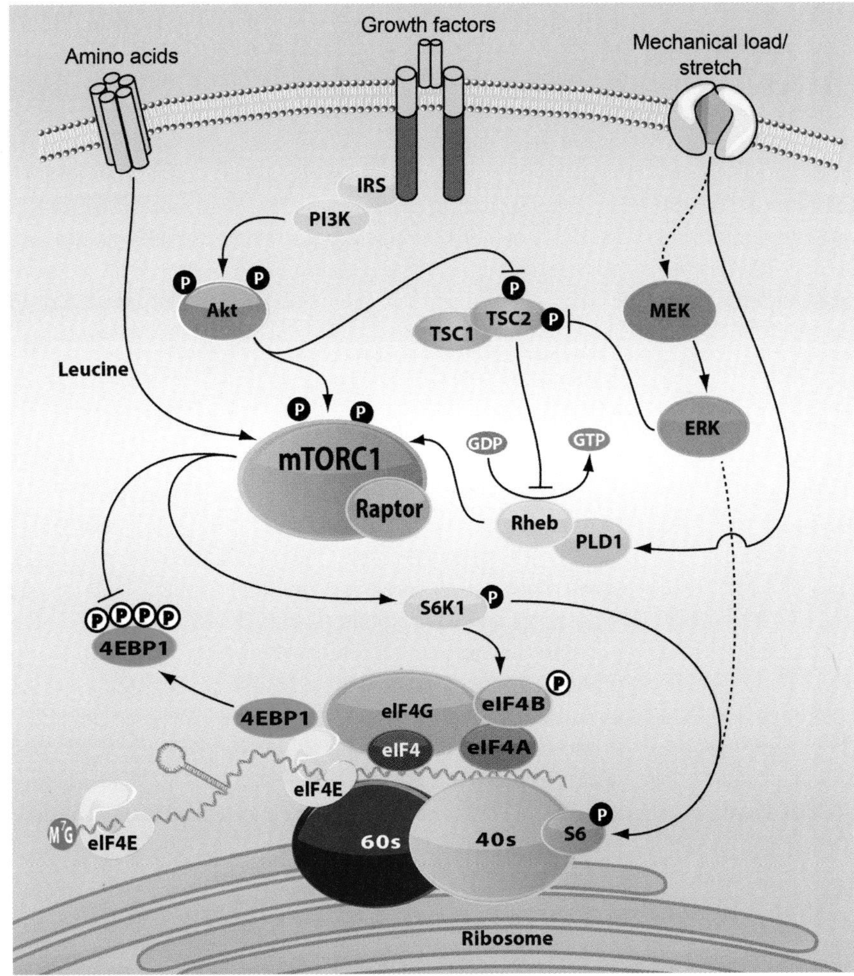

FIGURE 64.1 **Resistance exercise activates TORC1 signaling through different upstream factors.** Amino acids (primarily leucine), growth factors such as IGF-1 or mechanical load/stretch can all contribute to activation of mTORC1 (mammalian target of rapamycin complex 1) signaling. Growth factor binding activates Akt via IRS (insulin receptor substrate)/ PI3K (phosphatidylinositol 3-kinase) interaction; phosphorylation of Akt leads to inhibition of TSC complex (tuberous sclerosis complex 1 and 2) and activation of TORC1 by phosphorylation events. TSC1/2 is a negative regulator of TORC1 through inhibition of Rheb (Ras homolog enriched in brain) by promoting a GDP-bound state. Mechanical overload or stretch can activate TORC1 through inhibition of the TSC complex, likely through MEK, or through Rheb activation via PLD1 (phospholipase D1). TORC1 activation increases protein synthesis by enhancing translational efficiency through the phosphorylation of S6K1 (ribosomal protein S6 kinase) and 4EBP1 (eukaryotic translation initiation factor 4E binding protein 1). S6K1 phosphorylation promotes translation initiation complex formation by phosphorylation of eIF4B (eukaryotic translation initiation factor 4B) and Rps6 (ribosomal protein small 6). Phosphorylation of 4EBP1 causes the release of eIF4E (eukaryotic translation initiation factor 4E) allowing for the formation of the initiation complex by binding to the cap structure. The increase in protein synthesis as the result of TORC1 signaling ultimately leads to muscle hypertrophy through the net accretion of myofibrillar proteins.

was closely correlated to S6K1 phosphorylation after the first training session, confirming the original finding of Baar and Esser in the rat (4,25). In a somewhat surprising result, Burd and co-workers found a single bout of RE performed at 30% 1-RM to failure was more effective in stimulating myofibrillar protein synthesis than exercise performed at 90% 1-RM to failure (26). This finding was supported by earlier work reporting the same level of stimulation of S6K1 activity and myofibrillar protein synthesis following 60% 1-RM or 90% 1-RM resistance exercise (30). It will be of great interest to determine if the increase in protein synthesis observed in response to a low-load, high-volume exercise protocol as described by Burd et al. will translate into an increase in muscle mass and strength (26).

Upstream Regulators of mTOR Signaling

While there is little doubt that insulin-like growth factor 1 (IGF-1) is a potent growth factor capable of promoting muscle hypertrophy through TORC1 activation, Spangenburg and colleagues showed IGF-1 signaling was not necessary for muscle hypertrophy in response to mechanical loading (31). Interestingly, the level of Akt and S6K1 activation was not diminished in the absence of IGF-1 signaling indicating additional upstream factors involved in TORC1 activation during muscle growth (31). This finding is supported by a recent study by Miyazaki et al., in which the early activation of TORC1 signaling in response to mechanical overload was independent of PI3K/Akt signaling (32). Hornberger et al. showed that TORC1 could be activated independent of IGF-1 signaling by a pathway involving phospholipase D (PLD) via its metabolite, the lipid second messenger phosphatidic acid (PA) (33). More recently, the activation of mTOR by eccentric contractions required PLD synthesis of PA that was demonstrated to be independent of PI3K-Akt activity (34). While the exact mechanism through which PA activates mTOR remains to be elucidated, there is intriguing evidence indicating PLD1 physically interacts with Rheb (Ras homolog enriched in brain) in a GTP-dependent manner to activate TORC1 signaling (see Figure 64.1) (35,36). The overexpression of Rheb in skeletal muscle demonstrated TORC1 activity, independent of PI3K/Akt signaling, was sufficient to drive fiber hypertrophy through a cell autonomous mechanism (37). A role for PLD or Rheb regulation of TORC1 in human skeletal muscle adaptation to RE remains to be explored but Drummond et al. showed that Rheb transcript levels increased following an anabolic stimulus that included exercise and amino acids (38).

There is emerging evidence that the mitogen-activated protein kinase (MAPK) signaling pathway may also have a role in regulation protein synthesis in response to resistance exercise. Miyazaki et al. performed a time course analysis following mechanical overload and found the initial phosphorylation of ribosomal protein small 6 (Rps6) was paralleled by an increase in MAPK signaling (as indicated by increased phosphorylation of MEK1/2, ERK1/2, and RSK) that was independent of Akt activation and not blocked by rapamycin treatment (32). Furthermore, this same study reported that MAPK signaling could activate TORC1 signaling by targeting TSC2, a repressor of TORC1 signaling (32). These findings are consistent with results from an earlier human study in which rapamycin was used to block the initial increase in protein synthesis following resistance exercise (39). From these findings, the authors proposed that full activation of protein synthesis required both TORC1 and MAPK signaling (39).

Satellite Cells in Skeletal Muscle Hypertrophy

Within his original description of satellite cells, Mauro showed remarkable insight when he proposed that these cells may have a role in skeletal muscle adaptability (40). Since then, a great deal of effort has gone into characterizing and understanding the role of satellite cells in skeletal muscle adaptability (41). As a result of these efforts, satellite cells are now considered to be the primary stem cell of skeletal muscle and are thought to have an essential role in skeletal muscle regeneration, growth (hypertrophy and re-growth following atrophy), and maintenance (42). The necessity of satellite cells for skeletal muscle hypertrophy is based on the concept of nuclear domain which posits that each nucleus in a multinucleated muscle fiber is responsible for "overseeing" a certain volume of cytoplasm (43). The current model postulates that quiescent satellite cells once activated following RE, proliferate and their progeny fuse to a muscle fiber during hypertrophy to contribute their nuclei for the maintenance of greater cytoplasmic volume (43). In support of this idea, studies using gamma-irradiation to prevent satellite cell proliferation have reported a lack or severely blunted hypertrophic response (44–46). More recent studies, however, have provided intriguing evidence that muscle hypertrophy occurred independent of satellite cell activity following inactivation of myostatin or overexpression of Akt (47,48). The use of currently available genetic mouse models to specifically ablate satellite cells in adult skeletal muscle will permit a more critical assessment of the necessity of satellite cells in skeletal muscle hypertrophy.

Myostatin

Myostatin (Mstn) is a secreted protein of the TGF-β superfamily that functions as a potent negative regulator of skeletal muscle growth by inhibiting Akt/TORC1 signaling (49–52). As such, the modulation of myostatin levels through exercise or pharmacological means has been proposed as a potential therapeutic strategy for the prevention and/or restoration of muscle mass following prolonged inactivity or with such muscle-wasting diseases as muscular dystrophy and cachexia (53). The challenge in the coming years will be to determine if exercise does indeed represent a viable therapeutic strategy for reducing myostatin expression and thereby promoting muscle growth.

ADAPTATION TO ENDURANCE EXERCISE

Muscle activity that is performed at a moderate level of intensity for a relatively long duration (30–60 minutes) can be defined as EE. Endurance exercise repeated on a regular basis over a few months will lead to greater exercise capacity primarily resulting from metabolic and vascular changes within the muscle that allow for greater oxygen utilization (54–56). In particular, endurance training brings about a shift to a more oxidative metabolism as a consequence of an increase in the mitochondrial content and capillary density of the muscle (56). The metabolic shift allows a trained individual, at the same relative intensity, to rely more heavily on lipid oxidation for energy than carbohydrates, thus improving exercise capacity and performance by sparing glycogen (57–59). During the last decade, great strides have been made in deciphering the signaling molecules and pathways that are involved in regulating mitochondrial biogenesis in response to EE, as discussed in the following section.

Regulation of Mitochondrial Biogenesis

The cellular mechanism regulating the complex process of mitochondrial biogenesis in response to muscle activity remained unknown until the exciting discovery of

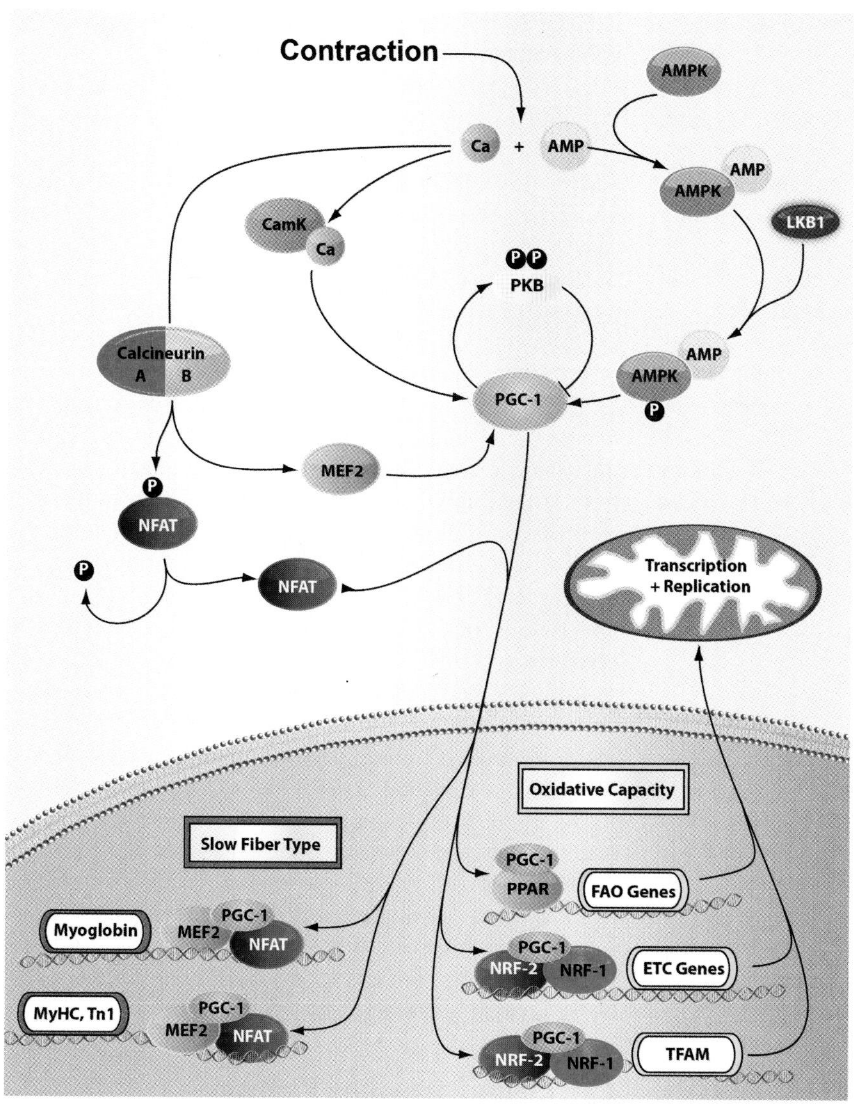

FIGURE 64.2 PGC-1α regulation of skeletal muscle adaptation to endurance exercise. Endurance exercise activates PGC-1α (peroxisome proliferative activated receptor, gamma, coactivator 1 beta) signaling through changes in upstream factors: a change intracellular Ca^{2+} levels activates calcium/calmodulin-dependent protein kinase (CamK) and calcineurin, a Ca^{2+}-activated phosphatase; increased AMP levels activates AMP-activated kinase. CamK, AMPK, and Akt regulate the expression and/or activity of PGC-1α which in turn drives mitochondrial biogenesis and the slow twitch fiber phenotype. PGC-1α cooperates with PPAR (peroxisome proliferator activated receptor) and NRFs (nuclear respiratory factor) to upregulate the expression of genes involved in fatty acid oxidative (FAO), electron transport chain (ETC) and mitochondrial biogenesis via Tfam (transcription factor A, mitochondrial) expression. PGC-1α also cooperates with NFAT (nuclear factor of activated T cells) and MEF2 (myocyte enhancer factor) transcription factors to regulate expression of slow twitch genes such as myoglobin, slow myosin heavy chain (MyHC) and slow troponin I (Tn1). PGC-1α regulation of mitochondrial biogenesis enhances muscle endurance by increasing the oxidative capacity of the muscle.

PGC-1α. PGC-1α is PPARγ-interacting protein that functions as a co-activator of transcription. Studies demonstrated that overexpression of PGC-1α in muscle cells *in vitro* promoted mitochondrial biogenesis through activation of the nuclear respiratory factors (NRF-1 and NRF-2) with subsequent transcription of mitochondrial transcription factor A (Tfam) (see Figure 64.2) (60,61).

PGC-1α: Master Regulator of Mitochondrial Biogenesis

Researchers in the field quickly realized the central role PGC-1α might have in skeletal muscle adaptation to EE and in short time confirmed increased expression of PGC-1α following exercise (a single bout and following training) in rodents and humans (62–68). Consistent with the original description, increased PGC-1α expression was associated with upregulation of the NRFs, Tfam, and mitochondrial genes in response to exercise (63,64). The constitutive overexpression of PGC-1α in type II fibers caused a shift to a type I phenotype as evidenced by increased expression of mitochondrial genes, myoglobin, slow isoforms of troponin, and increased endurance capacity both voluntary and forced (low and high intensity, respectively) (69–71). In contrast, Wende et al. found that induced overexpression of PGC-1α in adult mice resulted in no change in exercise capacity at low intensity and a decrease in capacity at high intensity treadmill exercise, despite having greater mitochondrial content and increased glycogen storage (72). The germline deletion of the PGC-1α gene caused a loss of type I fibers and reduced mitochondrial content which translated into the soleus muscle being less fatigue-resistant and lower exercise capacity (73). However, a separate study in which PGC-1α was deleted in mice reported no change in muscle mitochondria content or fiber type in the knockout compared to wild-type (74). To resolve this disparity, Handschin et al. generated a skeletal muscle-specific PGC-1α knockout and reported a shift to more glycolytic fibers and a reduced exercise capacity (75).

While these gain- and loss-of-function studies generally confirmed the ability of PGC-1α to regulate mitochondrial biogenesis, and by extension exercise capacity, they still did not address the primary question of whether or not PGC-1α is necessary for the metabolic adaptation of skeletal muscle to endurance exercise. Leick et al. addressed this question directly using the germline PGC-1α knockout strain with treadmill running and they found no difference between the PGC-1α knockout and wild-type strains in the adaptive response to exercise training as assessed by expression of mitochondrial and metabolic genes following five weeks of training (76). Collectively, the findings from these studies indicate PGC-1α is capable of driving mitochondrial biogenesis in skeletal muscle but is not essential in mediating the adaptations that occur in response to endurance exercise training.

Upstream Regulators of PGC-1α Expression

Wright and colleagues provided evidence showing that it was the initial nuclear translocation of PGC-1α that was important for the early change in mitochondrial gene expression with the later upregulation in PGC-1α expression necessary for the sustained increase in mitochondrial biogenesis (77). A number of different upstream kinases, which are known to be activated with muscle activity, have been shown to regulate PGC-1α expression such as Ca^{2+}/calmodulin-dependent kinase (CaMK), AMPK and p38 MAPK (see Figure 64.2) (78,79). The notion that a CaMK might have a role in mediating muscle adaptation to exercise was supported by the work of Wu et al. that reported the overexpression of a constitutively-activated CaMK IV in skeletal muscle was sufficient to increase PGC-1α expression and mitochondrial content (80). The importance of CaMK IV for exercise adaptation has been called into question though because mice harboring a germline deletion of CaMK IV show similar adaptation to 4 weeks of wheel-running as wild-type mice and electrical stimulation is still capable of increasing PGC-1α expression (81). Furthermore, based on the work of Zong and co-workers, it appears that AMPK, and not CaMK, is the critical upstream kinase responsible for regulating mitochondrial biogenesis (82). Mice expressing a dominant negative form of AMPK failed to show the normal increase in PGC-1α and CaMK IV expression and mitochondrial biogenesis when treated with the creatine analog beta-guanidinopropionic acid (β-GPA) to reduce the AMP:ATP ratio (activating AMPK) (82). These findings indicate AMPK is the primary kinase regulating the metabolic adaptation of skeletal muscle to EE.

AMPK: Metabolic Sensor

AMPK is a Ser/Thr kinase that detects the energy status of the cell by responding to changes in the AMP:ATP ratio caused by metabolic stress such as that induced by contractile exercise (83). Winder and Hardie provided the first evidence of a rapid and sustained increase in AMPK activity following EE (84). Numerous studies in humans and rodents have confirmed and extended these initial findings by showing the level of AMPK activation is sensitive to intensity and duration of muscle contraction (85,86). In transgenic mice, overexpression of a dominant negative form of the catalytic α2 subunit of AMPK blunted the shift in fiber-type following 6 weeks of running, though there was still a significant increase in markers of mitochondrial biogenesis (87). AMPK-activating mutations in the α-subunit (α1, R70Q; α3, R225Q) resulted in greater muscle glycogen and a two-fold increase in exercise capacity consistent with the increase in PGC-1α expression and mitochondrial biogenesis (88–90). Somewhat surprising, the inactivation of α1 or α2 catalytic subunits, however, did not prevent the increase in PGC-1α expression in response to 90 minutes of treadmill running (91). Together, the results from these genetic mouse models indicate that enhanced AMPK activity can mediate many of the adaptive responses to endurance exercise but that AMPK activity is not essential, suggesting other pathways are involved, or can compensate for the loss of AMPK activity, in regulating skeletal muscle plasticity.

Calcineurin Signaling Pathway

There is evidence that in addition to AMPK signaling, the calcineurin/NFAT pathway may also have a role in regulating skeletal muscle adaptation to EE (see Figure 64.2). Calcineurin is a Ca^{2+}/calmodulin-dependent protein phosphatase that promotes nuclear translocation of the NFAT (nuclear factor of activated T cells) transcription factor and activation of target genes. Naya and colleagues (92) reported overexpression of constitutively active form of calcineurin in type II fibers caused a modest increase in the number of type I fibers, confirming an earlier *in vitro* study by Chin et al. (93). It is now well established that the calcineurin/NFAT pathway is important for the maintenance of the slow twitch phenotype, is responsive to tonic, low frequency nerve stimulation, and required for fast-to-slow fiber-type transformation (94–99). Blocking calcineurin activity with cyclosporine A treatment during EE training did not, however, prevent the upregulation of markers of mitochondrial biogenesis (PGC-1α, NRF-2, and Tfam) indicating that the AMPK pathway operates in parallel to calcineurin/NFAT signaling (100,101). More recent though, Jiang et al. found that mice expressing a constitutively active form of calcineurin in skeletal muscle were more fatigue-resistant, as assessed by treadmill running, than wild-type mice, likely due to glycogen sparing as a result of greater oxidative capacity (102). These findings are consistent with a study by Guerfali et al. showing that calcineurin/NFAT pathway directly regulates the expression of PGC-1α (103). While the results from both gain-of-function and pharmacological studies support a role for calcineurin/NFAT signaling in muscle adaptation, loss-of-function studies using conditional knockout technology would provide more definitive evidence for the necessity of this pathway in skeletal muscle adaptation to EE.

FUTURE DIRECTIONS

There has been enormous progress in defining the distinct molecules and signaling pathways that underlie the adaptation of skeletal muscle to RE and EE. Not surprisingly, evidence is emerging showing crosstalk between these pathways, providing a possible mechanistic explanation for the limitations of concurrent RE and EE training (104,105). Future studies will surely continue to enhance our understanding of the aforementioned pathways as well as begin to explore the role of epigenetic modifications and microRNAs in skeletal muscle adaptation to exercise. This former point is highlighted by the results of a recent study by Davidsen and co-workers (106) that identified a set of microRNAs that were differentially expressed between high- and low-responders to RE training, suggesting microRNAs regulation of gene expression may help to explain the variability in adaptation to exercise. Beyond the intellectual satisfaction, our better understanding of the mechanisms underlying skeletal muscle adaptation to exercise has important clinical implications by allowing for the development of more effective therapies to prevent or restore muscle function with aging, disease, and prolonged inactivity.

ACKNOWLEDGMENTS

We would like to acknowledge the important work of our colleagues which we were unable to cite because of the strict space limitations of this chapter.

REFERENCES

1. West DW, Kujbida GW, Moore DR, Atherton P, Burd NA, Padzik JP, et al. Resistance exercise-induced increases in putative anabolic hormones do not enhance muscle protein synthesis or intracellular signalling in young men. *J Physiol* 2009;**587**:5239–47.
2. West DW, Burd NA, Staples AW, Phillips SM. Human exercise-mediated skeletal muscle hypertrophy is an intrinsic process. *Int J Biochem Cell Biol* 2010;**42**:1371–5.
3. Nader GA, Esser KA. Intracellular signaling specificity in skeletal muscle in response to different modes of exercise. *J Appl Physiol* 2001;**90**:1936–42.
4. Baar K, Esser K. Phosphorylation of p70(S6k) correlates with increased skeletal muscle mass following resistance exercise. *Am J Physiol* 1999;**276**:C120–7.
5. Atherton PJ, Babraj J, Smith K, Singh J, Rennie MJ, Wackerhage H. Selective activation of AMPK-PGC-1alpha or PKB-TSC2-mTOR signaling can explain specific adaptive responses to endurance or resistance training-like electrical muscle stimulation. *FASEB J* 2005;**19**:786–8.
6. Wilkinson SB, Phillips SM, Atherton PJ, Patel R, Yarasheski KE, Tarnopolsky MA, et al. Differential effects of resistance and endurance exercise in the fed state on signalling molecule phosphorylation and protein synthesis in human muscle. *J Physiol* 2008;**586**:3701–17.
7. Hass CJ, Feigenbaum MS, Franklin BA. Prescription of resistance training for healthy populations. *Sports Med* 2001;**31**:953–64.
8. Folland JP, Williams AG. The adaptations to strength training: morphological and neurological contributions to increased strength. *Sports Med* 2007;**37**:145–68.
9. Duchateau J, Semmler JG, Enoka RM. Training adaptations in the behavior of human motor units. *J Appl Physiol* 2006; **101**:1766–75.
10. Snow MH, Chortkoff BS. Frequency of bifurcated muscle fibers in hypertrophic rat soleus muscle. *Muscle Nerve* 1987;**10**: 312–7.
11. MacDougall JD, Sale DG, Alway SE, Sutton JR. Muscle fiber number in biceps brachii in bodybuilders and control subjects. *J Appl Physiol* 1984;**57**:1399–403.
12. Goldberg AL. Protein turnover in skeletal muscle. I. Protein catabolism during work-induced hypertrophy and growth induced with growth hormone. *J Biol Chem* 1969;**244**:3217–22.
13. Larsson L, Tesch PA. Motor unit fibre density in extremely hypertrophied skeletal muscles in man. Electrophysiological signs of muscle fibre hyperplasia. *Eur J Appl Physiol Occup Physiol* 1986;**55**:130–6.
14. Giddings CJ, Gonyea WJ. Morphological observations supporting muscle fiber hyperplasia following weight-lifting exercise in cats. *Anat Rec* 1992;**233**:178–95.
15. Kelley G. Mechanical overload and skeletal muscle fiber hyperplasia: a meta-analysis. *J Appl Physiol* 1996;**81**:1584–8.
16. Zoncu R, Efeyan A, Sabatini DM. mTOR: from growth signal integration to cancer, diabetes and ageing. *Nat Rev Mol Cell Biol* 2011;**12**:21–35.
17. Goldspink DF, Garlick PJ, McNurlan MA. Protein turnover measured in vivo and in vitro in muscles undergoing compensatory growth and subsequent denervation atrophy. *Biochem J* 1983;**210**:89–98.
18. Chesley A, MacDougall JD, Tarnopolsky MA, Atkinson SA, Smith K. Changes in human muscle protein synthesis after resistance exercise. *J Appl Physiol* 1992;**73**:1383–8.
19. Wong TS, Booth FW. Protein metabolism in rat tibialis anterior muscle after stimulated chronic eccentric exercise. *J Appl Physiol* 1990;**69**:1718–24.

20. Wong TS, Booth FW. Protein metabolism in rat gastrocnemius muscle after stimulated chronic concentric exercise. *J Appl Physiol* 1990;**69**:1709–17.
21. Bodine SC, Stitt TN, Gonzalez M, Kline WO, Stover GL, Bauerlein R, et al. Akt/mTOR pathway is a crucial regulator of skeletal muscle hypertrophy and can prevent muscle atrophy in vivo. *Nat Cell Biol* 2001;**3**:1014–9.
22. Rommel C, Bodine SC, Clarke BA, Rossman R, Nunez L, Stitt TN, et al. Mediation of IGF-1-induced skeletal myotube hypertrophy by PI(3)K/Akt/mTOR and PI(3)K/Akt/GSK3 pathways. *Nat Cell Biol* 2001;**3**:1009–13.
23. Karlsson HK, Nilsson PA, Nilsson J, Chibalin AV, Zierath JR, Blomstrand E. Branched-chain amino acids increase p70S6k phosphorylation in human skeletal muscle after resistance exercise. *Am J Physiol Endocrinol Metab* 2004;**287**:E1–7.
24. Koopman R, Zorenc AH, Gransier RJ, Cameron-Smith D, van Loon LJ. Increase in S6K1 phosphorylation in human skeletal muscle following resistance exercise occurs mainly in type II muscle fibers. *Am J Physiol Endocrinol Metab* 2006;**290**: E1245–52.
25. Terzis G, Spengos K, Mascher H, Georgiadis G, Manta P, Blomstrand E. The degree of p70 S6k and S6 phosphorylation in human skeletal muscle in response to resistance exercise depends on the training volume. *Eur J Appl Physiol* **110**:835–843.
26. Burd NA, West DW, Staples AW, Atherton PJ, Baker JM, Moore DR, et al. Low-load high volume resistance exercise stimulates muscle protein synthesis more than high-load low volume resistance exercise in young men. *PLoS One* 2010;**5**:e12033.
27. Tannerstedt J, Apro W, Blomstrand E. Maximal lengthening contractions induce different signaling responses in the type I and type II fibers of human skeletal muscle. *J Appl Physiol* 2009;**106**:1412–8.
28. Dreyer HC, Drummond MJ, Glynn EL, Fujita S, Chinkes DL, Volpi E, et al. Resistance exercise increases human skeletal muscle AS160/TBC1D4 phosphorylation in association with enhanced leg glucose uptake during postexercise recovery. *J Appl Physiol* 2008;**105**:1967–74.
29. Eliasson J, Elfegoun T, Nilsson J, Kohnke R, Ekblom B, Blomstrand E. Maximal lengthening contractions increase p70 S6 kinase phosphorylation in human skeletal muscle in the absence of nutritional supply. *Am J Physiol Endocrinol Metab* 2006;**291**: E1197–205.
30. Kumar V, Selby A, Rankin D, Patel R, Atherton P, Hildebrandt W, et al. Age-related differences in the dose-response relationship of muscle protein synthesis to resistance exercise in young and old men. *J Physiol* 2009;**587**:211–7.
31. Spangenburg EE, Le Roith D, Ward CW, Bodine SC. A functional insulin-like growth factor receptor is not necessary for load-induced skeletal muscle hypertrophy. *J Physiol* 2008;**586**:283–91.
32. Miyazaki M, McCarthy JJ, Fedele MJ, Esser KA. Early activation of mTORC1 in response to mechanical overload is independent of PI3K/Akt signaling. *J Physiol.* ePub ahead of print February 7, 2011, doi: 10.1113/jphysiol.2011.205658.
33. Hornberger TA, Chu WK, Mak YW, Hsiung JW, Huang SA, Chien S. The role of phospholipase D and phosphatidic acid in the mechanical activation of mTOR signaling in skeletal muscle. *Proc Natl Acad Sci USA* 2006;**103**:4741–6.
34. O'Neil TK, Duffy LR, Frey JW, Hornberger TA. The role of phosphoinositide 3-kinase and phosphatidic acid in the regulation of mammalian target of rapamycin following eccentric contractions. *J Physiol* 2009;**587**:3691–701.
35. Toschi A, Lee E, Xu L, Garcia A, Gadir N, Foster DA. Regulation of mTORC1 and mTORC2 complex assembly by phosphatidic acid: competition with rapamycin. *Mol Cell Biol* 2009;**29**:1411–20.
36. Sun Y, Fang Y, Yoon MS, Zhang C, Roccio M, Zwartkruis FJ, et al. Phospholipase D1 is an effector of Rheb in the mTOR pathway. *Proc Natl Acad Sci USA* 2008;**105**:8286–91.
37. Goodman CA, Miu MH, Frey JW, Mabrey DM, Lincoln HC, Ge Y, et al. A phosphatidylinositol 3-kinase/protein kinase B-independent activation of mammalian target of rapamycin signaling is sufficient to induce skeletal muscle hypertrophy. *Mol Biol Cell* 2010;**21**:3258–68.
38. Drummond MJ, Miyazaki M, Dreyer HC, Pennings B, Dhanani S, Volpi E, et al. Expression of growth-related genes in young and older human skeletal muscle following an acute stimulation of protein synthesis. *J Appl Physiol* 2009;**106**:1403–11.
39. Drummond MJ, Fry CS, Glynn EL, Dreyer HC, Dhanani S, Timmerman KL, et al. Rapamycin administration in humans blocks the contraction-induced increase in skeletal muscle protein synthesis. *J Physiol* 2009;**587**:1535–46.
40. Mauro A. Satellite cell of skeletal muscle fibers. *J Biophys Biochem Cytol* 1961;**9**:493–5.
41. Shi X, Garry DJ. Muscle stem cells in development, regeneration, and disease. *Genes Dev* 2006;**20**:1692–708.
42. Zammit PS, Partridge TA, Yablonka-Reuveni Z. The skeletal muscle satellite cell: the stem cell that came in from the cold. *J Histochem Cytochem* 2006;**54**:1177–91.
43. Allen DL, Roy RR, Edgerton VR. Myonuclear domains in muscle adaptation and disease. *Muscle Nerve* 1999;**22**:1350–60.
44. Rosenblatt JD, Parry DJ. Gamma irradiation prevents compensatory hypertrophy of overloaded mouse extensor digitorum longus muscle. *J Appl Physiol* 1992;**73**:2538–43.
45. Rosenblatt JD, Parry DJ. Adaptation of rat extensor digitorum longus muscle to gamma irradiation and overload. *Pflugers Arch* 1993;**423**:255–64.
46. Fleckman P, Bailyn RS, Kaufman S. Effects of the inhibition of DNA synthesis on hypertrophying skeletal muscle. *J Biol Chem* 1978;**253**:3320–7.
47. Blaauw B, Canato M, Agatea L, Toniolo L, Mammucari C, Masiero E, et al. Inducible activation of Akt increases skeletal muscle mass and force without satellite cell activation. *FASEB J* 2009;**23**:3896–905.
48. Amthor H, Otto A, Vulin A, Rochat A, Dumonceaux J, Garcia L, et al. Muscle hypertrophy driven by myostatin blockade does not require stem/precursor-cell activity. *Proc Natl Acad Sci USA* 2009;**106**:7479–84.
49. McPherron AC, Lawler AM, Lee SJ. Regulation of skeletal muscle mass in mice by a new TGF-beta superfamily member. *Nature* 1997;**387**:83–90.
50. Amirouche A, Durieux AC, Banzet S, Koulmann N, Bonnefoy R, Mouret C, et al. Down-regulation of Akt/mammalian target of rapamycin signaling pathway in response to myostatin overexpression in skeletal muscle. *Endocrinology* 2009;**150**: 286–94.

51. Trendelenburg AU, Meyer A, Rohner D, Boyle J, Hatakeyama S, Glass DJ. Myostatin reduces Akt/TORC1/p70S6K signaling, inhibiting myoblast differentiation and myotube size. *Am J Physiol Cell Physiol* 2009;**296**:C1258–70.
52. Welle S, Burgess K, Mehta S. Stimulation of skeletal muscle myofibrillar protein synthesis, p70 S6 kinase phosphorylation, and ribosomal protein S6 phosphorylation by inhibition of myostatin in mature mice. *Am J Physiol Endocrinol Metab* 2009;**296**: E567–72.
53. Lee SJ. Regulation of muscle mass by myostatin. *Annu Rev Cell Dev Biol* 2004;**20**:61–86.
54. Andersen P, Henriksson J. Training induced changes in the subgroups of human type II skeletal muscle fibres. *Acta Physiol Scand* 1977;**99**:123–5.
55. Armstrong RB, Laughlin MH. Exercise blood flow patterns within and among rat muscles after training. *Am J Physiol* 1984;**246**: H59–68.
56. Holloszy JO. Adaptation of skeletal muscle to endurance exercise. *Med Sci Sports* 1975;**7**:155–64.
57. Hurley BF, Nemeth PM, Martin 3rd WH, Hagberg JM, Dalsky GP, Holloszy JO. Muscle triglyceride utilization during exercise: effect of training. *J Appl Physiol* 1986;**60**:562–7.
58. Kiens B, Essen-Gustavsson B, Christensen NJ, Saltin B. Skeletal muscle substrate utilization during submaximal exercise in man: effect of endurance training. *J Physiol* 1993;**469**:459–78.
59. Phillips SM, Green HJ, Tarnopolsky MA, Heigenhauser GF, Hill RE, Grant SM. Effects of training duration on substrate turnover and oxidation during exercise. *J Appl Physiol* 1996;**81**:2182–91.
60. Puigserver P, Wu Z, Park CW, Graves R, Wright M, Spiegelman BM. A cold-inducible coactivator of nuclear receptors linked to adaptive thermogenesis. *Cell* 1998;**92**:829–39.
61. Wu Z, Puigserver P, Andersson U, Zhang C, Adelmant G, Mootha V, et al. Mechanisms controlling mitochondrial biogenesis and respiration through the thermogenic coactivator PGC-1. *Cell* 1999;**98**:115–24.
62. Goto M, Terada S, Kato M, Katoh M, Yokozeki T, Tabata I, et al. cDNA cloning and mRNA analysis of PGC-1 in epitrochlearis muscle in swimming-exercised rats. *Biochem Biophys Res Commun* 2000;**274**:350–4.
63. Baar K, Wende AR, Jones TE, Marison M, Nolte LA, Chen M, et al. Adaptations of skeletal muscle to exercise: rapid increase in the transcriptional coactivator PGC-1. *FASEB J* 2002; **16**:1879–86.
64. Bengtsson J, Gustafsson T, Widegren U, Jansson E, Sundberg CJ. Mitochondrial transcription factor A and respiratory complex IV increase in response to exercise training in humans. *Pflugers Arch* 2001;**443**:61–6.
65. Pilegaard H, Saltin B, Neufer PD. Exercise induces transient transcriptional activation of the PGC-1alpha gene in human skeletal muscle. *J Physiol* 2003;**546**:851–8.
66. Terada S, Goto M, Kato M, Kawanaka K, Shimokawa T, Tabata I. Effects of low-intensity prolonged exercise on PGC-1 mRNA expression in rat epitrochlearis muscle. *Biochem Biophys Res Commun* 2002;**296**:350–4.
67. Russell AP, Feilchenfeldt J, Schreiber S, Praz M, Crettenand A, Gobelet C, et al. Endurance training in humans leads to fiber type-specific increases in levels of peroxisome proliferator-activated receptor-gamma coactivator-1 and peroxisome proliferator-activated receptor-alpha in skeletal muscle. *Diabetes* 2003;**52**: 2874–81.
68. Terada S, Tabata I. Effects of acute bouts of running and swimming exercise on PGC-1alpha protein expression in rat epitrochlearis and soleus muscle. *Am J Physiol Endocrinol Metab* 2004;**286**:E208–216.
69. Lin J, Wu H, Tarr PT, Zhang CY, Wu Z, Boss O, et al. Transcriptional co-activator PGC-1 alpha drives the formation of slow-twitch muscle fibres. *Nature* 2002;**418**:797–801.
70. Miura S, Kai Y, Ono M, Ezaki O. Overexpression of peroxisome proliferator-activated receptor gamma coactivator-1alpha down-regulates GLUT4 mRNA in skeletal muscles. *J Biol Chem* 2003;**278**:31385–90.
71. Calvo JA, Daniels TG, Wang X, Paul A, Lin J, Spiegelman BM, et al. Muscle-specific expression of PPARgamma coactivator-1alpha improves exercise performance and increases peak oxygen uptake. *J Appl Physiol* 2008;**104**:1304–12.
72. Wende AR, Schaeffer PJ, Parker GJ, Zechner C, Han DH, Chen MM, et al. A role for the transcriptional coactivator PGC-1alpha in muscle refueling. *J Biol Chem* 2007;**282**:36642–51.
73. Leone TC, Lehman JJ, Finck BN, Schaeffer PJ, Wende AR, Boudina S, et al. PGC-1alpha deficiency causes multi-system energy metabolic derangements: muscle dysfunction, abnormal weight control and hepatic steatosis. *PLoS Biol* 2005;**3**:e101.
74. Arany Z, He H, Lin J, Hoyer K, Handschin C, Toka O, et al. Transcriptional coactivator PGC-1 alpha controls the energy state and contractile function of cardiac muscle. *Cell Metab* 2005;**1**:259–71.
75. Handschin C, Choi CS, Chin S, Kim S, Kawamori D, Kurpad AJ, et al. Abnormal glucose homeostasis in skeletal muscle-specific PGC-1alpha knockout mice reveals skeletal muscle-pancreatic beta cell crosstalk. *J Clin Invest* 2007;**117**:3463–74.
76. Leick L, Wojtaszewski JF, Johansen ST, Kiilerich K, Comes G, Hellsten Y, et al. PGC-1alpha is not mandatory for exercise- and training-induced adaptive gene responses in mouse skeletal muscle. *Am J Physiol Endocrinol Metab* 2008;**294**:E463–74.
77. Wright DC, Han DH, Garcia-Roves PM, Geiger PC, Jones TE, Holloszy JO. Exercise-induced mitochondrial biogenesis begins before the increase in muscle PGC-1alpha expression. *J Biol Chem* 2007;**282**:194–9.
78. Ojuka EO, Jones TE, Han DH, Chen M, Holloszy JO. Raising Ca^{2+} in L6 myotubes mimics effects of exercise on mitochondrial biogenesis in muscle. *FASEB J* 2003;**17**:675–81.
79. Rose AJ, Kiens B, Richter EA. Ca^{2+}-calmodulin-dependent protein kinase expression and signalling in skeletal muscle during exercise. *J Physiol* 2006;**574**:889–903.
80. Wu H, Kanatous SB, Thurmond FA, Gallardo T, Isotani E, Bassel-Duby R, Williams RS. Regulation of mitochondrial biogenesis in skeletal muscle by CaMK. *Science* 2002;**296**: 349–52.
81. Akimoto T, Ribar TJ, Williams RS, Yan Z. Skeletal muscle adaptation in response to voluntary running in Ca^{2+}/calmodulin-dependent protein kinase IV-deficient mice. *Am J Physiol Cell Physiol* 2004;**287**:C1311–9.
82. Zong H, Ren JM, Young LH, Pypaert M, Mu J, Birnbaum MJ, et al. AMP kinase is required for mitochondrial biogenesis in skeletal muscle in response to chronic energy deprivation. *Proc Natl Acad Sci USA* 2002;**99**:15983–7.

83. Hardie DG. Energy sensing by the AMP-activated protein kinase and its effects on muscle metabolism. *Proc Nutr Soc* **70**:92–99.
84. Winder WW, Hardie DG. Inactivation of acetyl-CoA carboxylase and activation of AMP-activated protein kinase in muscle during exercise. *Am J Physiol* 1996;**270**:E299–304.
85. Frosig C, Jorgensen SB, Hardie DG, Richter EA, Wojtaszewski JF. 5′-AMP-activated protein kinase activity and protein expression are regulated by endurance training in human skeletal muscle. *Am J Physiol Endocrinol Metab* 2004;**286**:E411–7.
86. Jensen TE, Wojtaszewski JF, Richter EA. AMP-activated protein kinase in contraction regulation of skeletal muscle metabolism: necessary and/or sufficient? *Acta Physiol (Oxf)* 2009;**196**:155–74.
87. Rockl KS, Hirshman MF, Brandauer J, Fujii N, Witters LA, Goodyear LJ. Skeletal muscle adaptation to exercise training: AMP-activated protein kinase mediates muscle fiber type shift. *Diabetes* 2007;**56**:2062–9.
88. Barnes BR, Marklund S, Steiler TL, Walter M, Hjalm G, Amarger V, et al. The 5'-AMP-activated protein kinase gamma3 isoform has a key role in carbohydrate and lipid metabolism in glycolytic skeletal muscle. *J Biol Chem* 2004;**279**:38441–7.
89. Barre L, Richardson C, Hirshman MF, Brozinick J, Fiering S, Kemp BE, et al. Genetic model for the chronic activation of skeletal muscle AMP-activated protein kinase leads to glycogen accumulation. *Am J Physiol Endocrinol Metab* 2007;**292**: E802–811.
90. Garcia-Roves PM, Osler ME, Holmstrom MH, Zierath JR. Gain-of-function R225Q mutation in AMP-activated protein kinase gamma3 subunit increases mitochondrial biogenesis in glycolytic skeletal muscle. *J Biol Chem* 2008;**283**:35724–34.
91. Jorgensen SB, Wojtaszewski JF, Viollet B, Andreelli F, Birk JB, Hellsten Y, et al. Effects of alpha-AMPK knockout on exercise-induced gene activation in mouse skeletal muscle. *FASEB J* 2005;**19**:1146–8.
92. Naya FJ, Mercer B, Shelton J, Richardson JA, Williams RS, Olson EN. Stimulation of slow skeletal muscle fiber gene expression by calcineurin in vivo. *J Biol Chem* 2000;**275**:4545–8.
93. Chin ER, Olson EN, Richardson JA, Yang Q, Humphries C, Shelton JM, et al. A calcineurin-dependent transcriptional pathway controls skeletal muscle fiber type. *Genes Dev* 1998;**12**:2499–509.
94. Dunn SE, Simard AR, Bassel-Duby R, Williams RS, Michel RN. Nerve activity-dependent modulation of calcineurin signaling in adult fast and slow skeletal muscle fibers. *J Biol Chem* 2001;**276**:45243–54.
95. Serrano AL, Murgia M, Pallafacchina G, Calabria E, Coniglio P, Lomo T, et al. Calcineurin controls nerve activity-dependent specification of slow skeletal muscle fibers but not muscle growth. *Proc Natl Acad Sci U S A* 2001;**98**:13108–13.
96. Parsons SA, Wilkins BJ, Bueno OF, Molkentin JD. Altered skeletal muscle phenotypes in calcineurin Aalpha and Abeta gene-targeted mice. *Mol Cell Biol* 2003;**23**:4331–43.
97. Parsons SA, Millay DP, Wilkins BJ, Bueno OF, Tsika GL, Neilson JR, et al. Genetic loss of calcineurin blocks mechanical overload-induced skeletal muscle fiber type switching but not hypertrophy. *J Biol Chem* 2004;**279**:26192–200.
98. McCullagh KJ, Calabria E, Pallafacchina G, Ciciliot S, Serrano AL, Argentini C, et al. NFAT is a nerve activity sensor in skeletal muscle and controls activity-dependent myosin switching. *Proc Natl Acad Sci USA* 2004;**101**:10590–5.
99. Miyazaki M, Hitomi Y, Kizaki T, Ohno H, Haga S, Takemasa T. Contribution of the calcineurin signaling pathway to overload-induced skeletal muscle fiber-type transition. *J Physiol Pharmacol* 2004;**55**:751–64.
100. Garcia-Roves PM, Jones TE, Otani K, Han DH, Holloszy JO. Calcineurin does not mediate exercise-induced increase in muscle GLUT4. *Diabetes* 2005;**54**:624–8.
101. Garcia-Roves PM, Huss J, Holloszy JO. Role of calcineurin in exercise-induced mitochondrial biogenesis. *Am J Physiol Endocrinol Metab* 2006;**290**:E1172–9.
102. Jiang, LQ, Garcia-Roves PM, de Castro Barbosa T, Zierath JR. Constitutively active calcineurin in skeletal muscle increases endurance performance and mitochondrial respiratory capacity. *Am J Physiol Endocrinol Metab* **298**:E8–E16.
103. Guerfali I, Manissolle C, Durieux AC, Bonnefoy R, Bartegi A, Freyssenet D. Calcineurin A and CaMKIV transactivate PGC-1alpha promoter, but differentially regulate cytochrome c promoter in rat skeletal muscle. *Pflugers Arch* 2007;**454**:297–305.
104. Baar K. Training for endurance and strength: lessons from cell signaling. *Med Sci Sports Exerc* 2006;**38**:1939–44.
105. Pruznak AM, Kazi AA, Frost RA, Vary TC, Lang CH. Activation of AMP-activated protein kinase by 5-aminoimidazole-4-carboxamide-1-beta-D-ribonucleoside prevents leucine-stimulated protein synthesis in rat skeletal muscle. *J Nutr* 2008;**138**:1887–94.
106. Davidsen PK, Gallagher IJ, Hartman JW, Tarnopolsky MA, Dela F, Helge JW, et al. High responders to resistance exercise training demonstrate differential regulation of skeletal muscle microRNA expression. *J Appl Physiol* **110:**309–17.

Chapter 65

Skeletal Muscle Regeneration

Denis C. Guttridge

Department of Molecular Virology, Immunology, and Medical Genetics, Human Cancer Genetics Program, The Ohio State University, Columbus, OH

INTRODUCTION

Skeletal muscle is the most abundant tissue in the human body and performs what seemingly appears to be an unlimited number of tasks, which we take for granted, such as standing, running, swallowing, and even blinking. Thus, it is easy to understand why the integrity of this tissue is so vital to maintain. Skeletal muscle, only second to bone marrow, possesses a tremendous capacity to regenerate in response to trauma, which can occur acutely due to toxin exposure or strenuous exercise, or more chronically, as in the case of muscular dystrophies. The thrust of this regenerative capacity derives from a specialized cellular population called satellite cells that function as resident stem cells. Satellite cells were first identified in frog muscles using electron microscopy. Mauro described the location of these cells as being "wedged" between the basement membrane and sarcolemma of a muscle fiber, and containing a high nuclear to cytoplasmic ratio (1). Mauro also accurately noted that satellite cells are rare, but at that time was not able to properly estimate their frequency. More advanced techniques that rely on the cellular markings of satellite cells now indicate that these cells represent 2–5% of all myofiber nuclei in adult hindlimb muscle (2). This range depends on factors such as age and muscle type, as aging may cause the decline in satellite cell number, whereas satellite cell density is greater in oxidative fibers. Findings also demonstrate that satellite cells tend to reside in close proximity to blood capillaries (3). The presence of a vascular system is likely to influence the niche that maintains satellite cell homeostasis in response to muscle injury.

The regeneration program has been modeled most accurately and reproducibly using acute injury conditions, typically administered with freezing, or chemical agents such as cardiotoxin, neotoxin, and barium chloride (for detailed reviews, see 2, 4–9). Following trauma, myofibers are lysed and subsequently stimulate an inflammatory immune response that causes the recruitment mainly of macrophages to regulate the phagocytosis of injured myofibers. During this process, quiescent satellite cells are activated by expressing the basic helix loop helix transcription factor, MyoD, and subsequently re-enter the cell cycle to promote an expansion of cells and commit to becoming myoblasts. These myogenic cells progress through the regeneration program by migrating to the site of injury, withdrawing from the cell cycle, and inducing the expression of another basic helix loop helix transcription factor, myogenin, which acts in concert with MyoD and other transcription factors and chromatin remodeling complexes to regulate the terminal stages of myogenic differentiation. In response to severe injury and complete myofiber degeneration, these stages are characterized by the fusion of myoblasts into newly formed myofibers that contain centrally positioned nuclei and expression of myofibrillar proteins that form contractile sarcomeres. With less severe injury, myoblasts instead complete terminal stages of differentiation by fusing with surrounding damaged myofibers to restore myonuclear domain and stimulate muscle growth and repair (Figure 65.1). Generally, regeneration is complete within a 2-week period. During this regeneration program, a fraction of activated satellite cells can also exit from cell cycle to re-establish a quiescent state within their specialized niche. In this way, satellite cells are able to self-renew, which ensures the maintenance of a resident stem cell pool, available for subsequent rounds of regeneration and muscle repair.

Successful regeneration is dependent on multiple factors emanating from a variety of cell types. Because of this complexity, specific aspects of the regeneration program involving immune cells and the nervous system will not be covered here, as these topics are discussed in depth in related chapters in this textbook. The focus in this chapter will instead be placed on the regulation and function of satellite cells, with additional emphasis given to specific signaling pathways that participate in orchestrating the activation of these cells and their differentiation into newly formed myotubes. Because of an increasing appreciation for the study of non-satellite progenitor cells in the muscle environment, additional discussion will also be given to progenitor cell types that contribute to

Muscle. DOI: http://dx.doi.org/10.1016/B978-0-12-381510-1.00065-X

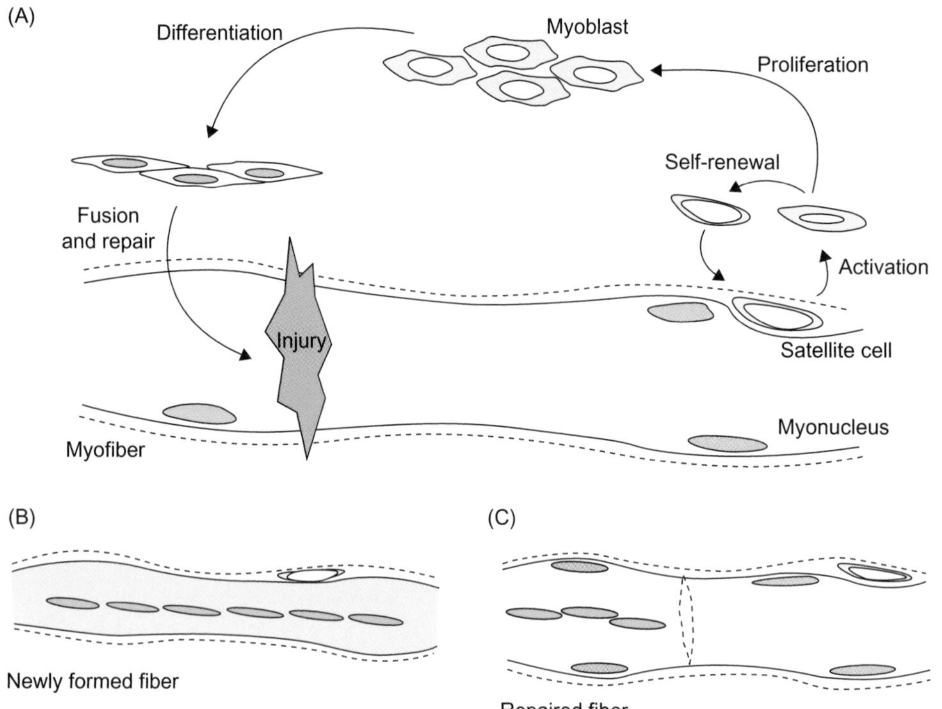

FIGURE 65.1 Skeletal muscle regeneration involves the activation of satellite cells and myoblast differentiation. (A) Upon injury, muscle-resident satellite cells are activated and subsequently undergo proliferation. These cells then either self-renew to replenish the stem cell pool, or instead commit to a myoblast and proceed through differentiation. Myoblasts expand by proliferating and migrate to the sites of injury and then exit the cell cycle. These cells subsequently align and fuse to form nascent myotubes, which can repopulate the injured area as newly formed myotubes, characterized by their centrally-located nuclei and smaller diameter (B), or if the initial damage is not extensive, fuse into the existing injured myofibers to contribute to repair and myofiber growth (C).

skeletal muscle regeneration. Although the origin and hierarchy of these progenitors continue to be examined, significant progress has been made to identify these cell types and ascertain their myogenic potential and therapeutic value for the treatment of degenerative muscle diseases.

REQUIREMENT OF SATELLITE CELLS IN REGENERATION

Identification of the Satellite Cell

From ultrastructural studies, myogenic satellite cells were first identified anatomically, as rare cells located between the sarcolemma and basal lamina that contained a high nuclear to cytoplasmic ratio. The chromatin of these cells was also found to be highly condensed, which indicated a transcriptionally inactivate state, consistent with quiescence. Today, protein markers are widely used to simplify the identification and isolation of satellite cells. These markers are expressed on the cell surface or reside as nuclear factors. Surface proteins used in this analysis include the glycoprotein and vascular stem cell marker, CD34, the c-Met receptor, adhesion molecules M-cadherin, neural cell adhesion molecule (NCAM), vascular adhesion molecule-1 (VCAM-1), heparin sulfate proteoglycans, syndecan-3 and syndecan-4, chemokine receptor, CXCR4, and the extracellular matrix binding protein, integrin α-7. For nuclear proteins, paired box transcription factors Pax3 and Pax7 are commonly used. Whereas Pax7 is expressed in a majority of satellite cells, Pax3 is less common and limited to satellite cells of specific muscle groups (10).

The Origin of Satellite Cells

Accumulating evidence over the years has strengthened the argument that satellite cells derive from mesodermal cells within the somite. Early fate mapping studies supported this notion using somites from quail embryos that were transplanted into host chick embryos (11,12). As chicks developed, quail cells could be seen contributing to the satellite cell compartment in chick postnatal muscles. Later, genetic studies were performed using the green fluorescent protein (GFP) reporter gene targeted into the Pax3 locus (13). By following GFP expression, investigators observed that Pax3 positive cells were highly represented in the myotome of the somites. These cells could also express Pax7, but were negative for the committed myogenic marker MyoD, demonstrating that GFP^+ cells maintained a precursor phenotype. As development proceeded to fetal stage and then postnatal skeletal muscle, Pax3-expressing cells assumed a satellite cell position between the myofiber sarcolemma and basal lamina. Analogous lineage tracing methods to assess the origins of Pax3 and Pax7 myogenic precursor cells have recently been performed using the Cre recombinase gene that, similar to GFP described above, was targeted into

Pax3 and Pax7 genes (14). These mice were bred with other mice containing the β-galactosidase (LacZ) reporter gene that was engineered in the Rosa26 genomic locus under the control of a Lox-Stop-Lox cassette (15). Transcriptional activation of Pax3 or Pax7 expresses Cre, which functions in the recombination of the LoxP sites to induce LacZ. Results with this reporter system confirmed a hierarchical expression pattern between Pax3 and Pax7 during skeletal muscle development and formation of satellite cells. Pax3 is expressed in the somites at E9.5 and contributes to the majority of primary myogenesis during embryo development, while Pax7 expression in somites is slightly delayed and coincides with precursor cells that give rise to secondary fibers during fetal development. As a modification to this lineage tracing genetic system, investigators adopted a Pax7 reporter system that relied on additional temporal tracing of embryonic Pax7-expressing cells. This system utilized a tamoxifen-inducible form of the Cre recombinase estrogen receptor fusion protein (ERCre) under the control of the Pax7 locus (16). By controlling the timing of the reporter, investigators elucidated that Pax7 was expressed in non-myogenic precursors as early at E9.5 in the dermomyotome, but consistent with earlier work, was restricted to a myogenic fate when expressed at a later developmental stage at E11.5. In all, these results support the somatic origin of satellite cells.

However, studies have also proposed an alternative scenario suggesting that multipotential progenitor cells of non-somitic origin exist as precursors to satellite cells. Analogous to somite transplantation studies discussed above, the grafting of myogenic cells derived from the dorsal aorta into newborn mice led to a contribution of these cells to postnatal muscle growth and muscle regeneration (17). In addition, $CD45^+$ hematopoietic cells can be coaxed into a myogenic lineage whose presence in skeletal muscle is dependent on the satellite cell marker, Pax7 (18,19). Moreover, bone marrow has been described as another source of satellite cells. By marking bone marrow cells with GFP, investigators discovered that these cells could be converted to satellite cells that contributed to the formation of labeled myofibers (20). Other non-somitic progenitor cell types have been identified whose contribution to muscle regeneration will be described further below. These studies emphasize the plasticity of progenitor cells that under proper conditions can adopt a myogenic fate, which may include a transitional stage into the satellite cell.

The Role of Pax7 in Muscle Regeneration

The combination of immunohistochemical analysis with more recent transgenic reporter systems established that Pax7 expression associates with a subpopulation of muscle precursor cells in embryogenesis that gives rise to fetal myofibers and later in development adopts the characteristics of satellite cells. In fact, perhaps more than any other protein, Pax7 serves as an unequivocal marker for identifying satellite cells in postnatal skeletal muscle. At the functional level, complete genetic ablation of Pax7 in mice showed that this paired box transcription factor was dispensable for embryonic myogenesis (21,22). A similar conclusion was drawn with a ERCre inducer under the control of the Pax7 locus, which when crossed with mice containing diphtheria toxin (DTA) in the Rosa26 locus under control of a Lox-Stop-Lox expression cassette, allowed the selected rapid cell death of Pax7 expressing cells (14). Use of this genetic system revealed that loss of Pax7 positive cells in embryogenesis led to a normal muscle pattern, confirming results from $Pax7^{-/-}$ mice. However, a similar strategy to deplete Pax7 expressing cells immediately prior to birth produced muscles smaller in size with a reduced number of myofibers. These data supported that Pax7 is required for proper differentiation of fetal myofibers.

Consistent with this phenotype, $Pax7^{-/-}$ mice are viable, but develop severe skeletal muscle defects and fail to thrive (21,22). Although the numbers of satellite cells between $Pax7^{+/+}$ and $Pax7^{-/-}$ mice are approximately equivalent at birth, these numbers rapidly decline in developing neonates and juvenile $Pax7^{-/-}$ mice, correlating with reduced muscle size. These young $Pax7^{-/-}$ mice challenged with cardiotoxin exhibit impaired regeneration, which worsens with age as the number of satellite cells continues to decline. Since Pax7 expression in postnatal skeletal muscle is predominantly restricted to satellite cells, such phenotypes in $Pax7^{-/-}$ mice suggests that this transcription factor plays a critical role in maintaining the regenerative capacity of satellite cells. To determine whether this function was cell autologous, investigators engineered an ingenious genetic model whereby a conditional floxed allele for the Pax7 gene was generated in mice and crossed with other mice containing a knockin of ERCre in the Pax7 locus that creates a null mutation. The result of these crosses produced progeny that in the presence of tamoxifen deleted Pax7 specifically in satellite cells (23). Similar to the total knockout, skeletal muscles from young mice conditionally depleted of Pax7 exhibited poor regeneration in response to cardiotoxin treatment. Such studies highlight the functional importance of Pax7 in muscle regeneration specific to satellite cells.

In vitro experimentation was performed to ascertain the mechanism by which Pax7 functions in satellite cells to regulate muscle regeneration. Results showed that $Pax7^{-/-}$ satellite cells exhibited a pronounced proliferative defect and an increased propensity to undergo apoptosis (24,25). Presumably during a regenerative response, Pax7 functions by stimulating satellite cell growth and viability to both ensure the expansion of committed myoblasts to complete differentiation and muscle repair, and secure the self-renewing process of satellite cells to maintain a steady pool of myogenic progenitors, available for subsequent rounds of regeneration.

As appealing as this model is to explain the requirement of Pax7 in postnatal muscle regeneration, provocative results were recently provided in adult skeletal muscle that challenges the model and forces alternative interpretations. These data generated from the same genetic system described above, to conditionally delete Pax7 specifically in satellite cells, showed that this transcription factor was dispensable for successful regeneration in adult skeletal muscle (23). Although Pax3 functions in a analogous manner *in vitro* to promote satellite cell growth and viability, investigators showed that normal muscle regeneration in adult mice specifically lacking Pax7 in satellite cells was not due to a functional compensation by Pax3, as mice generated lacking both Pax7 and Pax3 in satellite cells also exhibited normal muscle regeneration (23). Thus, although Pax7 plays a key role in fetal and early postnatal muscle development, it appears that its role in regeneration and self-renewal is less critical in adult satellite cells. Why this occurs is not known, but since non-satellite cell progenitors in the muscle compartment have been shown to enter a myogenic lineage in response to trauma (see below), one possible scenario is that these same cells that induce Pax7 might compensate in the regenerative response for satellite cells lacking Pax3 and Pax7 transcription factors. This interesting aspect of muscle regeneration will certainly warrant further investigation.

SIGNALING PATHWAYS IN SKELETAL MUSCLE REGENERATION

As described above, satellite cells represent the key component to a successful regeneration program. How satellite cells are cued to activate, proliferate, and subsequently commit to becoming myoblasts, which differentiate into multinucleated myotubes, are processes regulated by signaling factors that emanate from the surrounding satellite cell niche. These mediators derive from multiple cellular sources such as immune cells, vascular endothelium, motor neurons, myofibers, and the satellite cells themselves. The communication of this signaling network is highly complex, involving multiple paracrine and autocrine factors that act through selective cellular receptors to transduce signals that activate satellite cells and fine-tune their differentiation. These include growth factors and cytokines such as, fibroblast growth factors (FGFs), platelet-derived growth factor (PDGF), transforming growth factor-beta (TGF-β) and the TGF-β family member myostatin, tumor necrosis factor-alpha (TNF-α), interleukins IL-4 and IL-6, and others discussed in greater detail below, whose functions regulate discrete stages of the regenerative program (Figure 65.2).

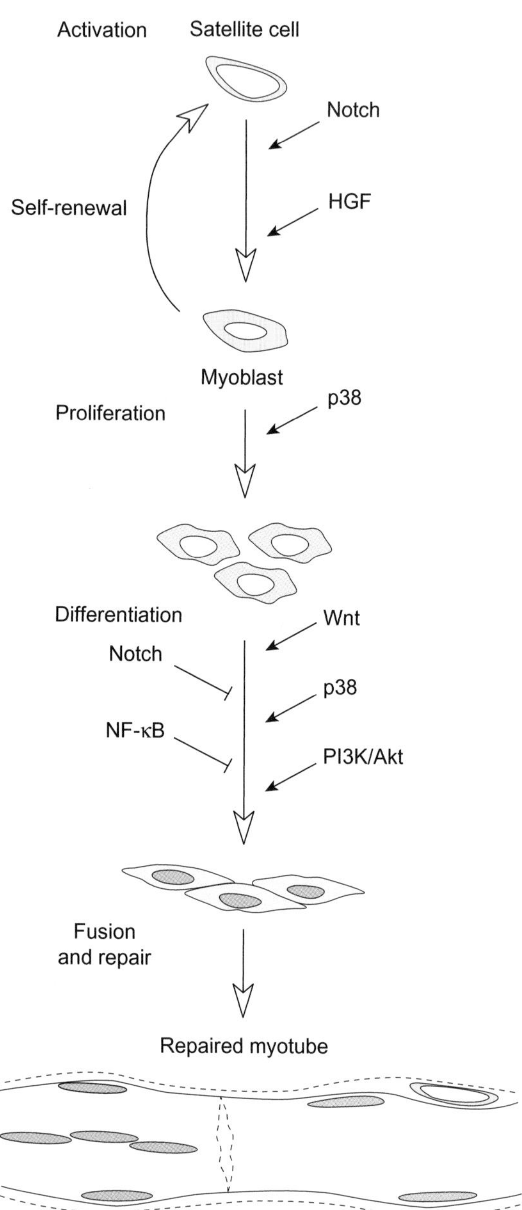

FIGURE 65.2 Signaling pathways contribute to skeletal muscle regeneration. Injury signals activate satellite cells, a process mediated in part through the positive feedback by Notch and HGF. A portion of these cells self-renew and replenish the muscle-resident stem cell population, while the others proceed through the differentiation program. MAPK/p38 functions during the activation phase to stimulate proliferation of satellite cells that commit to myoblasts from muscle precursors. Signaling pathways active in myoblasts coordinate their positive (p38, Wnt, PI3K/Akt) and negative (Notch, NF-κB) activities that influence the temporal expression and levels of myogenic genes needed to differentiate myoblasts into newly synthesized or repaired myofibers.

Hepatocyte Growth Factor (HGF)

HGF, or otherwise-called scatter factor, is the ligand for the c-met receptor, which is often used as a satellite cell marker. Mice deleted in c-met are unable to properly develop embryonic muscle due to impaired migration of muscle progenitor cells (26). During muscle injury or in response to mechanical stretch, HGF is released from the extracellular matrix of the myofiber by a nitric oxide (NO)-dependent mechanism (27,28). Active HGF then binds to the c-met receptor of quiescent satellite cells causing their subsequent activation by stimulating cell cycle and cellular division (29–31). The mechanisms by which HGF induces proliferation of satellite cells is less established, although signaling mediators PI3K and mitogen activated protein kinases (MAPK) p38 are involved (32,33). In addition, HGF appears to further direct the early steps of regeneration by negatively regulating the differentiation potential of myoblasts (34) through inhibition of myogenic transcription factors, MyoD and myogenin (35).

Insulin-Like Growth Factor (IGF) Phosphatidylinositol 3′-Kinase (PI3K)/AKT

IGF is synthesized as alternative transcript forms, IGF-I and IGF-II from skeletal muscle cells. In contrast to the inhibitory differentiation activities of growth factors, TGF-β, myostatin, and FGF, IGF-1 stimulates proliferation as well as differentiation of cultured satellite cells (36). In addition, neutralization of IGF-1 following acute muscle injury reduces the number of regenerating fibers (37), supporting earlier *in vitro* findings that IGF-1 functions as a promoter of skeletal muscle regeneration. Results suggest that IGF-1 is produced during muscle injury to stimulate proliferation of activated satellite cells. Studies further revealed that this stimulatory activity was mediated through the PI3K/AKT pathway, which can promote G1/S cell cycle progression through inhibition of the cyclin-dependent kinase inhibitor, p27Kip1 (38). Repression of p27 occurs at the transcriptional level, mediated through the AKT inhibitory target FoxO1 (39).

AKT is expressed in three forms, AKT1, AKT2, and AKT3, which share a common structure and are activated in parallel by the upstream kinase signaling molecule, PI3K (40). Although AKT2 is induced during skeletal muscle differentiation, studies in cultured muscle cells indicate that this form of AKT is dispensable, whereas AKT1 is essential for muscle differentiation (41). AKT1 mediates this process by promoting cell survival (42), and by stimulating myogenic gene expression through activation of MyoD transcriptional activity (41,43). IGF-1 stimulation of AKT is also an important regulator of skeletal muscle hypertrophy (44,45). AKT mediates this function by activating the mammalian target of rapamycin (mTOR), which phosphorylates downstream targets to induce protein synthesis (46). In contrast to IGF-I, less is known about how IGF-II participates in skeletal muscle regeneration. IGF-II is expressed endogenously during myoblast differentiation and is required to stimulate mTOR activity in maturing myofibers to regulate myoblast fusion (47).

Notch/Wnt

The Notch and Wnt signaling pathways function in antagonist fashions and are temporally regulated to control the switch point in activated satellite cells to a commitment of differentiation. For this reason, these pathways will be jointly discussed. Notch is a transmembrane receptor that in muscle cells becomes activated predominantly in response to binding to its ligand, Delta. Ligand binding leads to an enzymatic cleavage in the intracellular portion of the receptor, otherwise referred to the NICD (Notch intracellular domain) (48). NICD translocates to the nucleus where it binds to a family of transcriptional repressors, converting them to activators of transcription. The most recognizable form of this family is RBP-J. The target genes of this molecular interaction in vertebrates are the HES and HEY genes.

In postnatal skeletal muscle, Notch signaling plays a critical role in satellite cell activation (see Note following References below). Shortly after injury, Delta expression is increased in both satellite cells as well as uninjured myofibers proximal to the injury site (49). In conjunction with Delta, Notch receptor levels also increase, and functions to stimulate proliferation of activated satellite cells in order to generate a large number of intermediate progenitor cells. Following this expansion phase, Notch levels decline to allow committed myoblasts to complete differentiation and skeletal muscle repair (49). Reduction of Notch during muscle regeneration is required, as maintained levels in cultured myoblast studies strongly indicate that Notch functions as a repressor of myogenesis (50,51). Mechanistically, Notch represses differentiation through HES expression that impedes MyoD activity indirectly by inhibiting the MyoD binding partner, E47 (52,53). In addition, MyoD can be directly targeted through repressive interactions with RBP-J (54). How Notch signaling is downregulated during regeneration to allow the completion of differentiation involves potentially multiple mechanisms. The number of cell surface receptors of Notch decline through endocytosis during embryogenesis (55) so a parallel mechanism may exist in postnatal skeletal muscle. Likewise, studies suggest that Notch turnover is regulated through ubiquitin-dependent proteolysis (56). More recently, the inflammatory cytokine TNF-α was found to repress Notch gene expression through an epigenetic mechanism involving histone and DNA methylation (57).

Whether this latter mechanism occurs in activated satellite cells during a physiological injury response remains to be tested.

In contrast, canonical Wnt signaling functions as a potent inducer of skeletal muscle differentiation and its function is vital in muscle regeneration in response to injury or physiological stress factors (58). Wnt proteins are soluble ligands that induce signaling through frizzled receptors and low-density lipoprotein receptor-related protein co-receptors (LRP). These interactions inactivate GSK3β to promote stabilization of the transcription factor, beta-catenin, which translocates to the nucleus, and upon binding to TCF/LEF1 transcription factors, induces genes acting in multiple cellular processes. Several days after an acute muscle injury, Wnt5a, 5b, 7a, and 7b ligands are induced, followed by a corresponding increase in TCF transcriptional activity (59). The induction of Wnt signaling promotes muscle regeneration, but this activity is thought to occur late in the repair program when myoblasts undergo fusion and terminal differentiation. *In vitro*, inhibition of Wnt signaling with antagonists of frizzled receptor proteins strongly abrogate myogenesis, while *in vivo*, administration of Wnt3a to freeze-injured muscles stimulates premature myogenic differentiation (59). Recent evidence also indicates that Wnt7a acting through the noncanonical Fzd7 receptor regulates expansion of satellite cells in response to injury, and similar to Wnt3a, Wnt7a also stimulates muscle regeneration to produce increases in myofiber number and size (60).

Investigators showed that Notch and Wnt signaling pathways intersect at a switch point during the regeneration process. While Notch is active during progenitor cell expansion, Wnt activity is silent during this period, but rises later in the differentiation process precisely when Notch activity declines (59). This relationship between temporal expression and activity of Notch and Wnt pathways are well supported by inhibitor studies confirming their respective anti- and pro-myogenic activities at precise stages of the regeneration program.

MAPK/p38

p38 belongs to the MAPK family, which include other signaling mediators, extracellular signal-regulated kinases (ERKs) and c-jun NH_3-terminal kinases/stress activated protein kinase (JNK). In mammals, four forms of p38 exist, p38α, p38β, p38γ, and p38δ, which are activated by phosphorylation by MAPK kinases MKK3/6 (61). Although each of these forms of p38 at the mRNA level are expressed in skeletal muscle, the majority of studies have focused on the role of p38α, as both pharmacological inhibition *in vitro* using the compounds SB203580 and SB202190 (which also block p38β), or genetic ablation *in vivo* of p38α, severely impairs myogenic differentiation (43,62–69). In culture, p38α is activated early during the differentiation program. Similarly, in freshly isolated myofibers, p38α is rapidly activated and localized to the nuclei demonstrating that this MAPK is an early marker of satellite cell activation (70). Functionally, p38α activation in satellite cells, as modeled in cultured myoblasts, is considered vital to regulate MyoD and MEF2 activity (67,68,70,71). Early in satellite cell activation, p38α is thought to promote proliferation (70), whereas later in the regeneration program p38α regulates cell cycle exit by antagonizing the activity of JNK, which stimulates cyclin D1 expression (64). In addition, in myoblasts p38α activation acts in a unique fashion by signaling to chromatin modeling complexes to stimulate myogenic gene expression. Specifically, activated p38α stimulates recruitment of the SWI-SNF complex to myogenic genes by promoting interaction with MyoD and MEF2 with the enzymatic subunits of SWI-SNF (66). This interaction was shown to function cooperatively on myogenic promoters with the IGF-1/PI3K/AKT pathway, which phosphorylates the p300 acetyltransferase protein to promote MyoD/p300 interaction and subsequent MyoD acetylation by another acetyltransferase protein, PCAF, thereby stimulating differentiation gene expression.

In vivo studies show that in contrast to p38α, p38β and p38δ are dispensable in skeletal muscle regeneration, most likely due to a compensatory function by p38α (72). Although similar acute injury performed with hindlimb muscles of p38γ knockout mice reported no difference in muscle regeneration compared to wild type (72), closer analysis looking at longer time points (>21 days) revealed a phenotype consistent with impaired regeneration (73). In keeping with a possible role for p38γ in regeneration, both p38α and p38γ mRNA are induced during acute skeletal muscle injury (72,73). However, in cultured myoblasts undergoing differentiation, p38α is induced while p38γ is downregulated, suggesting that these MAPK have contrasting functions in muscle repair. Indeed, recent work using p38γ-deficient mice demonstrated that in contrast to the pro-myogenic activity of p38α, the gamma form of p38 negatively regulates muscle regeneration by phosphorylating MyoD, which enhances MyoD occupancy on the myogenin promoter causing histone methylation and repression of myogenin transcription (73).

NF-κB

NF-κB is a transcription factor that is synthesized as either a homo- or heterodimer from the combination of five gene-coding subunits, RelA/p65, c-Rel, RelB, p50, and p52. The most common forms of NF-κB are the p50/p65 heterodimer and the p50/p50 homodimer. Whereas p65, c-Rel, and RelB contain transactivation domains in their carboxyl terminus to drive gene expression, p50 and p52 subunits lack these domains, but are capable of DNA binding similar to p65, c-Rel, and RelB (74). The majority of NF-κB acts through a pathway referred to as the canonical or classical signaling pathway. This pathway is activated typically by injury-related factors such as inflammatory cytokines or by bacterial and viral products. These factors activate the I-κB kinase (IKK) complex that functions to phosphorylate an inhibitor protein called I κB, which binds to NF-κB and masks its nuclear localization signal, thereby maintaining NF-κB in the cytoplasm as an inactive transcription factor (75). Phosphorylation of I κB by IKK causes the polyubiquitination of I κB, thus signaling its degradation by the 26S proteasome complex and allowing NF-κB to move into the nucleus where it binds DNA and stimulates gene expression. In contrast to this classical activation scheme operating mainly through p50/p65 dimers, NF-κB is also activated in a non-canonical or alternative pathway (76). This pathway is triggered by lymphoid factors involved in B cell development that activate a different IKK complex leading to nuclear translocation of a p52/RelB dimer, that like p50/p65 binds DNA, but is thought to regulate a different set of genes in comparison to classical NF-κB signaling.

In recent years NF-κB has emerged as a relevant signaling pathway in the regulation of skeletal muscle regeneration. Earlier studies were controversial as to how NF-κB functioned in muscle differentiation, but there is now wider acceptance that myoblasts contain a constitutive activity of NF-κB derived from the classical pathway, which functions to repress differentiation. NF-κB mediates this repressive activity through multiple mechanisms, acting on the one hand to stimulate cell proliferation through cyclin D1 (77,78) and on the other to function indirectly to repress the synthesis of MyoD (79–81). TRAF7, which activates NF-κB, is under the transcriptional control of MyoD in myoblasts (82) and is thought to form a feedback loop to prevent excessive NF-κB signaling. Moreover, NF-κB stimulates expression of the transcription factor Yin Yang1 (YY1) (83) that recruits members of the Polycomb group, as well as the histone deacetylase, HDAC-1, to repress transcription of myofibrillar genes in myoblasts when they are not meant to be expressed (83,84). Through YY1, NF-κB also epigenetically silences the pro-myogenic microRNA, miR-29 in proliferating myoblasts (85). Negative regulation of muscle regeneration by classical NF-κB signaling is thought to contribute to the pathology of Duchenne muscular dystrophy (57,86,87) and rhabdomyosarcoma (85), and even under physiological conditions of muscle injury, the negative effect on muscle regeneration by NF-κB appears to be maintained (83).

CONTRIBUTION TO MUSCLE REGENERATION BY OTHER STEM CELLS

Although satellite cells possess a substantial self-renewing capacity that unequivocally qualifies these cells as the main contributors to skeletal muscle growth and repair (88), an expanding list of additional progenitor cells have been described that are thought on the hierarchical scale to act upstream of satellite cells to contribute to the regenerative program (reviewed in 89). The location and origins of these cell types continue to be a point of discussion, and their potential to efficiently propagate in culture and commit to a myogenic lineage, even when delivered systemically in a host, make these non-satellite populations intriguing to pursue, especially from the standpoint of transplanting such stem cells in cell-based therapies for the treatment of muscular dystrophy disorders.

Side Population (SP) Cells

SP cells were first identified as bone marrow-derived hematopoietic progenitor cells that later were also isolated from skeletal muscle (90–94). These cells express the Sca1 marker and are absent for CD45 and c-kit, making their identification and isolation using a combined antibody and fluorescence-activated cell sorting (FACS) strategy particularly challenging. Instead, SP cells are identified and isolated by FACS, based on their ability to efflux the Hoechst33342 dye, which occurs due to expression of the Abcg2 multidrug resistance protein (90,91,95–97). Similar to satellite cells, muscle-resident SPs are heterogeneous and rare (88,98), compromising 1–5% of total hindlimb cells (96). Most SP cells in normal non-regenerating muscle express CD31 and are endothelial in nature, but a minor $CD31^-$, $CD45^-$ fraction actively expand in injured muscle and express myogenic genes, and on their own can engraft to give rise to differentiated myofibers, or in combination can also increase the transplantation efficiency of myoblasts (99,100). Transplantation of wild-type SPs were also shown to be successful in reconstituting dystrophin expression and occupying the satellite cell niche in *mdx* mice (101). These results are consistent with the notion that SP cells on their own are not myogenic but can initiate myogenesis when cultured with satellite cells or other skeletal muscle cell lines (102). Another more recently described minor fraction of SPs were shown to remarkably express the satellite cell markers, syndecan-4 and Pax7, suggesting that SP cells possess the ability to exist as a hybrid phenotype with satellite cells pre-committed to a myogenic lineage (103). These cells are capable of forming myotubes in culture, and following transplantation, predominantly engraft into the satellite cell niche, implying their role as satellite cell precursors.

Mesoangioblasts/Pericytes

Mesoangioblasts were first identified in the wall of embryonic dorsal aortas in mice (17,104). These blood vessel-associated stem cells share characteristics with endothelial and pericyte cells, and in culture exhibit a robust proliferative potential capable of differentiating into multiple cell types of mesenchymal origin. In postnatal skeletal muscle, mesoangioblasts closely resemble pericytes and their *in vitro* activities, with respect to proliferation, are similar to their embryonic counterpart. An advantage of using mesoangioblasts for cell-based therapies is their ability to be delivered intra-arterially and to successfully engraft in skeletal muscle. This technique was used to rescue mice with a primary defect in α-sarcoglycan that underlies limb-girdle muscular dystrophy (105), and whose engraftment could be significantly improved by stimulating mesoangioblast migration with administration of selective cytokine and adhesion factors (106). A highly favorable response was also observed with respect to dystrophin expression and improved skeletal muscle function when wild-type mesoangioblasts were systemically administered in a golden retriever model of Duchenne muscular dystrophy (107). These findings are highly promising and have far-reaching therapeutic implications.

Related pericytes are located on the periphery of blood vessels and therefore can also be isolated from the vascular system, and like mesoangioblasts, are efficiently expanded in culture and display a high propensity to differentiate into myotubes (108). Human tissue pericytes can be isolated by their cellular surface markings NG2, CD146, and alkaline phosphatase. In uninjured skeletal muscle, pericytes are negative for Pax7, but adopt a myogenic fate when prompted by injury factors *in vivo* or under differentiation conditions *in vitro* (108). Furthermore, expression of a human mini-dystrophin transgene in pericytes isolated from patients with Duchenne muscular dystrophy was successfully expanded in culture and subsequently transplanted in immunocompromised *mdx* mice to produce a significant degree of dystrophin positive myofibers.

Muscle Derived Stem Cells (MDSC)

In common with pericytes, MDSCs are located within the blood vessel wall (109). MDSCs were discovered by culturing mouse post-natal muscle mononuclear cells by a pre-plating technique to isolate various populations based on their adherence to collagen-coated flasks (110,111). MDSCs reside in the late pre-plate fraction, which distinguishes them by their cell surface markings from satellite cells present in an earlier pre-plate fraction. Murine MDSCs share CD34 expression with satellite cells, but are positive for Sca1, which is absent in quiescent satellite cells. In culture, MDSCs commit to a myogenic lineage based on their MyoD expression profile and are efficient at differentiating into myotubes (111), but possess a remarkable capacity to differentiate into multiple other cell types (111,112), including cells from all three germ layers, mesodermal, ectoderm, and endoderm (113). This evidence supports the notion that MDSCs may functionally behave as precursors to satellite cells. *In vivo* transplantation experiments in *mdx* mice show that MDSCs display an improved regeneration and cell survival activity compared to myoblasts (111). This is indicative that MDSCs have a strong self-renewing capacity. Indeed MDSCs can be passaged in culture for over 300 population doublings without showing signs of replicative senescence (114). In addition, *in vivo* they exhibit a unique capability to stimulate angiogenesis (115), which may be another mechanism to favor muscle repair.

Hematopoietic/Bone Marrow Cells

Previous studies identified a population of cells positive for the hematopoietic marker CD45 that, upon muscle injury and activation of the Wnt pathway, expressed Pax7 and exhibited myogenic potential (18,19). Hematopoietic cells derive from the bone marrow, which is another source of stem cells connected to skeletal muscle regeneration. Using nLacZ reporter mice, labeled bone marrow cells were shown to be recruited to injured skeletal muscle and possess the ability to reconstitute fully differentiated myotubes (116). Consistent with this notion, using GFP-labeled bone marrow-derived cells and other genetically engineered systems, progenitor cells were shown to home to skeletal muscle in response to injury or stress, and contribute to regeneration by occupying the satellite cell niche (20,117–119). The degree to which bone marrow contributes to a regenerative program in injured muscle has been debated (120–123) and additional studies await to better comprehend the myogenic fate of such populations.

Interstitial Cells

More recently, a population of stem cells was discovered that occupied the skeletal muscle interstitium (124). The cells expressed a zinc finger gene named PW1, which is not restricted to muscle cells, but is tightly associated with skeletal muscle differentiation in both embryogenesis and postnatal muscle development (125,126). PW1 positive cells are also positive for Sca1 and CD34, and, similar to many other precursor cells described above, are able to differentiate into multiple cell lineages (124). Skeletal muscle interstitial PW1 positive cells, referred to as PICs, are absent for Pax7 expression in unperturbed conditions, and require the induction of Pax7 in order to enter a satellite cell lineage and contribute to skeletal muscle regeneration upon muscle injury. Interestingly, in resting conditions, Pax7 positive satellite cells also express PW1, suggesting that PICs represent an additional progenitor population that is hierarchically upstream of satellite cells (124).

CONCLUDING REMARKS

We are currently celebrating the half-century mark since Mauro's discovery of the satellite cell. From those initial ultrastructural observations an amazing biological process has been revealed that brings with it an immense appreciation for the dynamics of skeletal muscle. Although much has been learned, much also remains to be discovered. Modern cellular, molecular and genetic tools have facilitated the identification and, importantly, the isolation of satellite cells to study their regulation and function, yet with these advanced technologies have come the realization that satellite cells are heterogeneous in nature for reasons we do not yet understand, and although significant progress has been made in elucidating their origin during skeletal muscle development, the temporal and spatial regulatory mechanisms that underlie their heterogeneity remain to be resolved. In addition, through the combination of *in vitro* and *in vivo* studies in animal models of acute and chronic muscle injury, a much clearer picture of the "life cycle" of satellite cells in postnatal muscle has emerged. From beginning to end of the regeneration program, the fate of satellite cells can be followed, and the process whereby these cells when activated in response to injury either commit to a myoblast cell and proceed through differentiation to repair damaged tissue, or instead return back to a protected satellite cell niche is now well understood. Mechanistically, insight has also been gained in understanding which extracellular factors are responsible for contributing to the activation and maturation phases of satellite cells and how these factors transduce their activities through defined signaling pathways that modulate gene expression and protein function within the regeneration program. Some of the phases of muscle regeneration, such as the transition from myoblasts to myotubes are better resolved as compared to extracellular factors and signaling pathways that regulate satellite cell quiescence and the self-renewal process. Furthermore, although some level of understanding has been gained with regards to the importance of factors that serve in a communication network between the satellite cell niche and surrounding cells, such as the adjacent myofiber, endothelial, neuronal, immune, and other cells in the stroma, there remains a wide gap in elucidating the identity of these factors and their cellular origins. Genetic models that allow tissue-specific expression and deletion of genes that encode these factors will certainly help advance this understanding, but improved techniques to reconstitute the three-dimensional surroundings of satellite cells *in vitro* are also vital to this effort.

Not only will this knowledge increase our appreciation for the biology of skeletal muscle regeneration, but it can also be translated into improving therapies to combat skeletal muscle disorders where impaired muscle regeneration is considered an underlying cause, such as in Duchenne muscular dystrophy (DMD) and age-related sarcopenia. Elucidating extracellular factors and intracellular signaling pathways that are intrinsic to impaired satellite cell function, such as TGF-β (127) and NF-κB (86) in DMD and Notch in sarcopenia (128), identifies new classes of therapeutic targets. In addition, we now recognize that satellite cells are not the only cell population residing in postnatal skeletal muscle tissue possessing the capacity to contribute to regeneration (89). Therefore, efforts to isolate and propagate these cells and achieve their successful systemic delivery provide further therapeutic strategies in aging and skeletal muscle-related disorders.

ACKNOWLEDGMENTS

I am grateful to Nadine Bakkar, Katherine Ladner, and Jennifer Peterson for their helpful comments, as well as Nadine Bakkar for assistance with the figures. Support was provided by the National Institutes of Heath project, R01AR052787.

REFERENCES

1. Mauro A. Satellite cell of skeletal muscle fibers. *J Biophys Biochem Cytol* 1961;**9**:493–5.
2. Hawke TJ, Garry DJ. Myogenic satellite cells: physiology to molecular biology. *J Appl Physiol* 2001;**91**:534–51.
3. Christov C, Chretien F, Abou-Khalil R, Bassez G, Vallet G, et al. Muscle satellite cells and endothelial cells: close neighbors and privileged partners. *Mol Biol Cell* 2007;**18**:1397–409.
4. Charge SB, Rudnicki MA. Cellular and molecular regulation of muscle regeneration. *Physiol Rev* 2004;**84**:209–38.
5. Dhawan J, Rando TA. Stem cells in postnatal myogenesis: molecular mechanisms of satellite cell quiescence, activation and replenishment. *Trends Cell Biol* 2005;**15**:666–73.
6. Kuang S, Gillespie MA, Rudnicki MA. Niche regulation of muscle satellite cell self-renewal and differentiation. *Cell Stem Cell* 2008;**2**:22–31.
7. Sartorelli V, Caretti G. Mechanisms underlying the transcriptional regulation of skeletal myogenesis. *Curr Opin Genet Dev* 2005;**15**:528–35.
8. Shi X, Garry DJ. Muscle stem cells in development, regeneration, and disease. *Genes Dev* 2006;**20**:1692–708.
9. Tidball JG. Inflammatory processes in muscle injury and repair. *Am J Physiol Regul Integr Comp Physiol* 2005;**288**: R345–353.

10. Buckingham M, Bajard L, Chang T, Daubas P, Hadchouel J, Meilhac S, et al. The formation of skeletal muscle: from somite to limb. *J Anat* 2003;**202**:59–68.
11. Christ B, Jacob HJ, Jacob M. Origin of wing musculature. Experimental studies on quail and chick embryos. *Experientia* 1974;**30**:1446–9.
12. Le Douarin N, Barq G. Use of Japanese quail cells as "biological markers" in experimental embryology. *C R Acad Sci Hebd Seances Acad Sci D* 1969;**269**:1543–6.
13. Relaix F, Rocancourt D, Mansouri A, Buckingham M. A Pax3/Pax7-dependent population of skeletal muscle progenitor cells. *Nature* 2005;**435**:948–53.
14. Hutcheson DA, Zhao J, Merrell A, Haldar M, Kardon G. Embryonic and fetal limb myogenic cells are derived from developmentally distinct progenitors and have different requirements for beta-catenin. *Genes Dev* 2009;**23**:997–1013.
15. Soriano P. Generalized lacZ expression with the ROSA26 Cre reporter strain. *Nat Genet* 1999;**21**:70–1.
16. Lepper C, Fan CM. Inducible lineage tracing of Pax7-descendant cells reveals embryonic origin of adult satellite cells. *Genesis* 2010;**48**:424–36.
17. De Angelis L, Berghella L, Coletta M, Lattanzi L, Zanchi M, Cusella-De Angelis MG, et al. Skeletal myogenic progenitors originating from embryonic dorsal aorta coexpress endothelial and myogenic markers and contribute to postnatal muscle growth and regeneration. *J Cell Biol* 1999;**147**:869–78.
18. Polesskaya A, Seale P, Rudnicki MA. Wnt signaling induces the myogenic specification of resident $CD45^+$ adult stem cells during muscle regeneration. *Cell* 2003;**113**:841–52.
19. Seale P, Ishibashi J, Scime A, Rudnicki MA. Pax7 is necessary and sufficient for the myogenic specification of CD45+ :Sca1+ stem cells from injured muscle. *PLoS Biol* 2004;**2**:E130.
20. LaBarge MA, Blau HM. Biological progression from adult bone marrow to mononucleate muscle stem cell to multinucleate muscle fiber in response to injury. *Cell* 2002;**111**:589–601.
21. Oustanina S, Hause G, Braun T. Pax7 directs postnatal renewal and propagation of myogenic satellite cells but not their specification. *EMBO J* 2004;**23**:3430–9.
22. Seale P, Sabourin LA, Girgis-Gabardo A, Mansouri A, Gruss P, Rudnicki MA. Pax7 is required for the specification of myogenic satellite cells. *Cell* 2000;**102**:777–86.
23. Lepper C, Conway SJ, Fan CM. Adult satellite cells and embryonic muscle progenitors have distinct genetic requirements. *Nature* 2009;**460**:627–31.
24. Kuang S, Charge SB, Seale P, Huh M, Rudnicki MA. Distinct roles for Pax7 and Pax3 in adult regenerative myogenesis. *J Cell Biol* 2006;**172**:103–13.
25. Relaix F, Montarras D, Zaffran S, Gayraud-Morel B, Rocancourt D, Tajbakhsh S, et al. Pax3 and Pax7 have distinct and overlapping functions in adult muscle progenitor cells. *J Cell Biol* 2006;**172**:91–102.
26. Bladt F, Riethmacher D, Isenmann S, Aguzzi A, Birchmeier C. Essential role for the c-met receptor in the migration of myogenic precursor cells into the limb bud. *Nature* 1995;**376**:768–71.
27. Tatsumi R, Liu X, Pulido A, Morales M, Sakata T, Dial S, et al. Satellite cell activation in stretched skeletal muscle and the role of nitric oxide and hepatocyte growth factor. *Am J Physiol Cell Physiol* 2006;**290**:C1487–94.
28. Wozniak AC, Anderson JE. Nitric oxide-dependence of satellite stem cell activation and quiescence on normal skeletal muscle fibers. *Dev Dyn* 2007;**236**:240–50.
29. Allen RE, Sheehan SM, Taylor RG, Kendall TL, Rice GM. Hepatocyte growth factor activates quiescent skeletal muscle satellite cells in vitro. *J Cell Physiol* 1995;**165**:307–12.
30. Anastasi S, Giordano S, Sthandier O, Gambarotta G, Maione R, Comoglio P, et al. A natural hepatocyte growth factor/scatter factor autocrine loop in myoblast cells and the effect of the constitutive Met kinase activation on myogenic differentiation. *J Cell Biol* 1997;**137**:1057–68.
31. Tatsumi R, Anderson JE, Nevoret CJ, Halevy O, Allen RE. HGF/SF is present in normal adult skeletal muscle and is capable of activating satellite cells. *Dev Biol* 1998;**194**:114–28.
32. Lluis F, Perdiguero E, Nebreda AR, Munoz-Canoves P. Regulation of skeletal muscle gene expression by p38 MAP kinases. *Trends Cell Biol* 2006;**16**:36–44.
33. Wozniak AC, Kong J, Bock E, Pilipowicz O, Anderson JE. Signaling satellite-cell activation in skeletal muscle: markers, models, stretch, and potential alternate pathways. *Muscle Nerve* 2005;**31**:283–300.
34. Miller KJ, Thaloor D, Matteson S, Pavlath GK. Hepatocyte growth factor affects satellite cell activation and differentiation in regenerating skeletal muscle. *Am J Physiol Cell Physiol* 2000;**278**:C174–81.
35. Gal-Levi R, Leshem Y, Aoki S, Nakamura T, Halevy O. Hepatocyte growth factor plays a dual role in regulating skeletal muscle satellite cell proliferation and differentiation. *Biochim Biophys Acta* 1998;**1402**:39–51.
36. Allen RE, Boxhorn LK. Regulation of skeletal muscle satellite cell proliferation and differentiation by transforming growth factor-beta, insulin-like growth factor I, and fibroblast growth factor. *J Cell Physiol* 1989;**138**:311–5.
37. Lefaucheur JP, Sebille A. Muscle regeneration following injury can be modified in vivo by immune neutralization of basic fibroblast growth factor, transforming growth factor beta 1 or insulin-like growth factor I. *J Neuroimmunol* 1995;**57**:85–91.
38. Chakravarthy MV, Abraha TW, Schwartz RJ, Fiorotto ML, Booth FW. Insulin-like growth factor-I extends in vitro replicative life span of skeletal muscle satellite cells by enhancing G1/S cell cycle progression via the activation of phosphatidylinositol 3′-kinase/Akt signaling pathway. *J Biol Chem* 2000;**275**:35942–52.
39. Machida S, Spangenburg EE, Booth FW. Forkhead transcription factor FoxO1 transduces insulin-like growth factor's signal to p27Kip1 in primary skeletal muscle satellite cells. *J Cell Physiol* 2003;**196**:523–31.
40. Woodgett JR. Recent advances in the protein kinase B signaling pathway. *Curr Opin Cell Biol* 2005;**17**:150–7.
41. Wilson EM, Rotwein P. Selective control of skeletal muscle differentiation by Akt1. *J Biol Chem* 2007;**282**:5106–10.
42. Lawlor MA, Rotwein P. Insulin-like growth factor-mediated muscle cell survival: central roles for Akt and cyclin-dependent kinase inhibitor p21. *Mol Cell Biol* 2000;**20**:8983–95.
43. Serra C, Palacios D, Mozzetta C, Forcales SV, Morantte I, Ripani M, et al. Functional interdependence at the chromatin level between the MKK6/p38 and IGF1/PI3K/AKT pathways during muscle differentiation. *Mol Cell* 2007;**28**:200–13.

44. Musaro A, McCullagh K, Paul A, Houghton L, Dobrowolny G, Molinaro M, et al. Localized Igf-1 transgene expression sustains hypertrophy and regeneration in senescent skeletal muscle. *Nat Genet* 2001;**27**:195–200.
45. Rommel C, Bodine SC, Clarke BA, Rossman R, Nunez L, et al. Mediation of IGF-1-induced skeletal myotube hypertrophy by PI (3)K/Akt/mTOR and PI(3)K/Akt/GSK3 pathways. *Nat Cell Biol* 2001;**3**:1009–13.
46. Han B, Tong J, Zhu MJ, Ma C, Du M. Insulin-like growth factor-1 (IGF-1) and leucine activate pig myogenic satellite cells through mammalian target of rapamycin (mTOR) pathway. *Mol Reprod Dev* 2008;**75**:810–7.
47. Park IH, Chen J. Mammalian target of rapamycin (mTOR) signaling is required for a late-stage fusion process during skeletal myotube maturation. *J Biol Chem* 2005;**280**:32009–17.
48. Luo D, Renault VM, Rando TA. The regulation of Notch signaling in muscle stem cell activation and postnatal myogenesis. *Semin Cell Dev Biol* 2005;**16**:612–22.
49. Conboy IM, Rando TA. The regulation of Notch signaling controls satellite cell activation and cell fate determination in postnatal myogenesis. *Dev Cell* 2002;**3**:397–409.
50. Nofziger D, Miyamoto A, Lyons KM, Weinmaster G. Notch signaling imposes two distinct blocks in the differentiation of C2C12 myoblasts. *Development* 1999;**126**:1689–702.
51. Shawber C, Nofziger D, Hsieh JJ, Lindsell C, Bogler O, Hayward D, Weinmaster G. Notch signaling inhibits muscle cell differentiation through a CBF1-independent pathway. *Development* 1996;**122**:3765–73.
52. Ordentlich P, Lin A, Shen CP, Blaumueller C, Matsuno K, Artavanis-Tsakonas S, Kadesch T. Notch inhibition of E47 supports the existence of a novel signaling pathway. *Mol Cell Biol* 1998;**18**:2230–9.
53. Sasai Y, Kageyama R, Tagawa Y, Shigemoto R, Nakanishi S. Two mammalian helix-loop-helix factors structurally related to Drosophila hairy and Enhancer of split. *Genes Dev* 1992;**6**:2620–34.
54. Kuroda K, Tani S, Tamura K, Minoguchi S, Kurooka H, Honjo T. Delta-induced Notch signaling mediated by RBP-J inhibits MyoD expression and myogenesis. *J Biol Chem* 1999;**274**:7238–44.
55. Le Borgne R, Bardin A, Schweisguth F. The roles of receptor and ligand endocytosis in regulating Notch signaling. *Development* 2005;**132**:1751–62.
56. Lai EC. Protein degradation: four E3s for the Notch pathway. *Curr Biol* 2002;**12**:R74–8.
57. Acharyya S, Sharma SM, Cheng AS, Ladner KJ, He W, Kline W, et al. TNF inhibits Notch-1 in skeletal muscle cells by Ezh2 and DNA methylation mediated repression: implications in duchenne muscular dystrophy. *PLoS One* 2010;**5**:e12479.
58. Tsivitse S. Notch and Wnt signaling, physiological stimuli and postnatal myogenesis. *Int J Biol Sci* 2010;**6**:268–81.
59. Brack AS, Conboy IM, Conboy MJ, Shen J, Rando TA. A temporal switch from Notch to Wnt signaling in muscle stem cells is necessary for normal adult myogenesis. *Cell Stem Cell* 2008;**2**:50–9.
60. Le Grand F, Jones AE, Seale V, Scime A, Rudnicki MA. Wnt7a activates the planar cell polarity pathway to drive the symmetric expansion of satellite stem cells. *Cell Stem Cell* 2009;**4**:535–47.
61. Nebreda AR, Porras A. p38 MAP kinases: beyond the stress response. *Trends Biochem Sci* 2000;**25**:257–60.
62. Briata P, Forcales SV, Ponassi M, Corte G, Chen CY, Karin M, et al. p38-dependent phosphorylation of the mRNA decay-promoting factor KSRP controls the stability of select myogenic transcripts. *Mol Cell* 2005;**20**:891–903.
63. Lluis F, Ballestar E, Suelves M, Esteller M, Munoz-Canoves P. E47 phosphorylation by p38 MAPK promotes MyoD/E47 association and muscle-specific gene transcription. *EMBO J* 2005;**24**:974–84.
64. Perdiguero E, Ruiz-Bonilla V, Gresh L, Hui L, Ballestar E, Sousa-Victor P, et al. Genetic analysis of p38 MAP kinases in myogenesis: fundamental role of p38alpha in abrogating myoblast proliferation. *EMBO J* 2007;**26**:1245–56.
65. Rampalli S, Li L, Mak E, Ge K, Brand M, Tapscott SJ, et al. p38 MAPK signaling regulates recruitment of Ash2L-containing methyltransferase complexes to specific genes during differentiation. *Nat Struct Mol Biol* 2007;**14**:1150–6.
66. Simone C, Forcales SV, Hill DA, Imbalzano AN, Latella L, Puri PL. p38 pathway targets SWI-SNF chromatin-remodeling complex to muscle-specific loci. *Nat Genet* 2004;**36**:738–43.
67. Wu Z, Woodring PJ, Bhakta KS, Tamura K, Wen F, Feramisco JR, et al. p38 and extracellular signal-regulated kinases regulate the myogenic program at multiple steps. *Mol Cell Biol* 2000;**20**:3951–64.
68. Zetser A, Gredinger E, Bengal E. p38 mitogen-activated protein kinase pathway promotes skeletal muscle differentiation. Participation of the Mef2c transcription factor. *J Biol Chem* 1999;**274**:5193–200.
69. Zhao M, New L, Kravchenko VV, Kato Y, Gram H, di Padova F, et al. Regulation of the MEF2 family of transcription factors by p38. *Mol Cell Biol* 1999;**19**:21–30.
70. Jones NC, Tyner KJ, Nibarger L, Stanley HM, Cornelison DD, Fedorov YV, et al. The p38alpha/beta MAPK functions as a molecular switch to activate the quiescent satellite cell. *J Cell Biol* 2005;**169**:105–16.
71. Puri PL, Wu Z, Zhang P, Wood LD, Bhakta KS, Han J, et al. Induction of terminal differentiation by constitutive activation of p38 MAP kinase in human rhabdomyosarcoma cells. *Genes Dev* 2000;**14**:574–84.
72. Ruiz-Bonilla V, Perdiguero E, Gresh L, Serrano AL, Zamora M, Sousa-Victor P, et al. Efficient adult skeletal muscle regeneration in mice deficient in p38beta, p38gamma and p38delta MAP kinases. *Cell Cycle* 2008;**7**:2208–14.
73. Gillespie MA, Le Grand F, Scime A, Kuang S, von Maltzahn J, Seale V, et al. p38-γ-dependent gene silencing restricts entry into the myogenic differentiation program. *J Cell Biol* 2009;**187**:991–1005.
74. Hayden MS, Ghosh S. Shared principles in NF-kappaB signaling. *Cell* 2008;**132**:344–62.
75. Zandi E, Rothwarf DM, Delhase M, Hayakawa M, Karin M. The IkappaB kinase complex (IKK) contains two kinase subunits, IKKalpha and IKKbeta, necessary for IkappaB phosphorylation and NF-kappaB activation. *Cell* 1997;**91**:243–52.
76. Senftleben U, Cao Y, Xiao G, Greten FR, Krahn G, Bonizzi G, et al. Activation by IKKalpha of a second, evolutionary conserved, NF-kappa B signaling pathway. *Science* 2001;**293**:1495–9.
77. Dahlman JM, Wang J, Bakkar N, Guttridge DC. The RelA/p65 subunit of NF-kappaB specifically regulates cyclin D1 protein stability: implications for cell cycle withdrawal and skeletal myogenesis. *J Cell Biochem* 2009;**106**:42–51.

78. Guttridge DC, Albanese C, Reuther JY, Pestell RG, Baldwin Jr. AS. NF-kappaB controls cell growth and differentiation through transcriptional regulation of cyclin D1. *Mol. Cell. Biol.* 1999;**19**:5785–99.
79. Dogra C, Changotra H, Mohan S, Kumar A. Tumor necrosis factor-like weak inducer of apoptosis inhibits skeletal myogenesis through sustained activation of nuclear factor-kappaB and degradation of MyoD protein. *J Biol Chem* 2006;**281**:10327–36.
80. Guttridge DC, Mayo MW, Madrid LV, Wang C-Y, Baldwin Jr. AS. NF-kB-induced loss of MyoD messenger RNA: possible role in muscle decay and cachexia. *Science* 2000;**289**:2363–6.
81. Langen RC, Van Der Velden JL, Schols AM, Kelders MC, Wouters EF, Janssen-Heininger YM. Tumor necrosis factor-alpha inhibits myogenic differentiation through MyoD protein destabilization. *FASEB J* 2004;**18**:227–37.
82. Tsikitis M, Acosta-Alvear D, Blais A, Campos EI, Lane WS, Sanchez I, et al. Traf7, a MyoD1 transcriptional target, regulates nuclear factor-kappaB activity during myogenesis. *EMBO Rep* 2010;**11**:969–76.
83. Wang H, Hertlein E, Bakkar N, Sun H, Acharyya S, Wang J, et al. NF-kappaB regulation of YY1 inhibits skeletal myogenesis through transcriptional silencing of myofibrillar genes. *Mol Cell Biol* 2007;**27**:4374–87.
84. Caretti G, Di Padova M, Micales B, Lyons GE, Sartorelli V. The Polycomb Ezh2 methyltransferase regulates muscle gene expression and skeletal muscle differentiation. *Genes Dev* 2004;**18**:2627–38.
85. Wang H, Garzon R, Sun H, Ladner KJ, Singh R, Dahlman J, et al. NF-kappaB-YY1-miR-29 regulatory circuitry in skeletal myogenesis and rhabdomyosarcoma. *Cancer Cell* 2008;**14**:369–81.
86. Acharyya S, Villalta SA, Bakkar N, Bupha-Intr T, Janssen PM, Carathers M, et al. Interplay of IKK/NF-kappaB signaling in macrophages and myofibers promotes muscle degeneration in Duchenne muscular dystrophy. *J Clin Invest* 2007;**117**:889–901.
87. Tubaro C, Arcuri C, Giambanco I, Donato R. S100B protein in myoblasts modulates myogenic differentiation via NF-kappaB-dependent inhibition of MyoD expression. *J Cell Physiol* 2010;**223**:270–82.
88. Collins CA, Olsen I, Zammit PS, Heslop L, Petrie A, Partridge TA, et al. Stem cell function, self-renewal, and behavioral heterogeneity of cells from the adult muscle satellite cell niche. *Cell* 2005;**122**:289–301.
89. Peault B, Rudnicki M, Torrente Y, Cossu G, Tremblay JP, Partridge T, et al. Stem and progenitor cells in skeletal muscle development, maintenance, and therapy. *Mol Ther* 2007;**15**:867–77.
90. Goodell MA, Brose K, Paradis G, Conner AS, Mulligan RC. Isolation and functional properties of murine hematopoietic stem cells that are replicating in vivo. *J Exp Med* 1996;**183**:1797–806.
91. Goodell MA, Rosenzweig M, Kim H, Marks DF, DeMaria M, Paradis G, et al. Dye efflux studies suggest that hematopoietic stem cells expressing low or undetectable levels of CD34 antigen exist in multiple species. *Nat Med* 1997;**3**:1337–45.
92. Jackson KA, Mi T, Goodell MA. Hematopoietic potential of stem cells isolated from murine skeletal muscle. *Proc Natl Acad Sci USA* 1999;**96**:14482–6.
93. Meeson AP, Hawke TJ, Graham S, Jiang N, Elterman J, Hutcheson K, et al. Cellular and molecular regulation of skeletal muscle side population cells. *Stem Cells* 2004;**22**:1305–20.
94. Rivier F, Alkan O, Flint AF, Muskiewicz K, Allen PD, Leboulch P, et al. Role of bone marrow cell trafficking in replenishing skeletal muscle SP and MP cell populations. *J Cell Sci* 2004;**117**:1979–88.
95. Martin CM, Meeson AP, Robertson SM, Hawke TJ, Richardson JA, Bates S, et al. Persistent expression of the ATP-binding cassette transporter, Abcg2, identifies cardiac SP cells in the developing and adult heart. *Dev Biol* 2004;**265**:262–75.
96. Montanaro F, Liadaki K, Schienda J, Flint A, Gussoni E, Kunkel LM. Demystifying SP cell purification: viability, yield, and phenotype are defined by isolation parameters. *Exp Cell Res* 2004;**298**:144–54.
97. Zhou S, Schuetz JD, Bunting KD, Colapietro AM, Sampath J, Morris JJ, et al. The ABC transporter Bcrp1/ABCG2 is expressed in a wide variety of stem cells and is a molecular determinant of the side-population phenotype. *Nat Med* 2001;**7**:1028–34.
98. Kuang S, Kuroda K, Le Grand F, Rudnicki MA. Asymmetric self-renewal and commitment of satellite stem cells in muscle. *Cell* 2007;**129**:999–1010.
99. Motohashi N, Uezumi A, Yada E, Fukada S, Fukushima K, Imaizumi K, et al. Muscle CD31(-) CD45(-) side population cells promote muscle regeneration by stimulating proliferation and migration of myoblasts. *Am J Pathol* 2008;**173**:781–91.
100. Uezumi A, Ojima K, Fukada S, Ikemoto M, Masuda S, Miyagoe-Suzuki Y, et al. Functional heterogeneity of side population cells in skeletal muscle. *Biochem Biophys Res Commun* 2006;**341**:864–73.
101. Gussoni E, Soneoka Y, Strickland CD, Buzney EA, Khan MK, Flint AF, et al. Dystrophin expression in the mdx mouse restored by stem cell transplantation. *Nature* 1999;**401**:390–4.
102. Asakura A, Rudnicki MA. Side population cells from diverse adult tissues are capable of in vitro hematopoietic differentiation. *Exp Hematol* 2002;**30**:1339–45.
103. Tanaka KK, Hall JK, Troy AA, Cornelison DD, Majka SM, Olwin BB. Syndecan-4-expressing muscle progenitor cells in the SP engraft as satellite cells during muscle regeneration. *Cell Stem Cell* 2009;**4**:217–25.
104. Minasi MG, Riminucci M, De Angelis L, Borello U, Berarducci B, Innocenzi A, et al. The meso-angioblast: a multipotent, self-renewing cell that originates from the dorsal aorta and differentiates into most mesodermal tissues. *Development* 2002;**129**:2773–83.
105. Sampaolesi M, Torrente Y, Innocenzi A, Tonlorenzi R, D'Antona G, Pellegrino MA, et al. Cell therapy of alpha-sarcoglycan null dystrophic mice through intra-arterial delivery of mesoangioblasts. *Science* 2003;**301**:487–92.
106. Galvez BG, Sampaolesi M, Brunelli S, Covarello D, Gavina M, Rossi B, et al. Complete repair of dystrophic skeletal muscle by mesoangioblasts with enhanced migration ability. *J Cell Biol* 2006;**174**:231–43.
107. Sampaolesi M, Blot S, D'Antona G, Granger N, Tonlorenzi R, Innocenzi A, et al. Mesoangioblast stem cells ameliorate muscle function in dystrophic dogs. *Nature* 2006;**444**:574–9.
108. Dellavalle A, Sampaolesi M, Tonlorenzi R, Tagliafico E, Sacchetti B, Perani L, et al. Pericytes of human skeletal muscle are myogenic precursors distinct from satellite cells. *Nat Cell Biol* 2007;**9**:255–67.
109. Tavian M, Zheng B, Oberlin E, Crisan M, Sun B, Huard J, et al. The vascular wall as a source of stem cells. *Ann NY Acad Sci* 2005;**1044**:41–50.

110. Gharaibeh B, Lu A, Tebbets J, Zheng B, Feduska J, Crisan M, et al. Isolation of a slowly adhering cell fraction containing stem cells from murine skeletal muscle by the preplate technique. *Nat Protoc* 2008;**3**:1501–9.
111. Qu-Petersen Z, Deasy B, Jankowski R, Ikezawa M, Cummins J, Pruchnic R, et al. Identification of a novel population of muscle stem cells in mice: potential for muscle regeneration. *J Cell Biol* 2002;**157**:851–64.
112. Cao B, Zheng B, Jankowski RJ, Kimura S, Ikezawa M, Deasy B, et al. Muscle stem cells differentiate into haematopoietic lineages but retain myogenic potential. *Nat Cell Biol* 2003;**5**:640–6.
113. Deasy BM, Li Y, Huard J. Tissue engineering with muscle-derived stem cells. *Curr Opin Biotechnol* 2004;**15**:419–23.
114. Deasy BM, Gharaibeh BM, Pollett JB, Jones MM, Lucas MA, Kanda Y, et al. Long-term self-renewal of postnatal muscle-derived stem cells. *Mol Biol Cell* 2005;**16**:3323–33.
115. Deasy BM, Feduska JM, Payne TR, Li Y, Ambrosio F, Huard J. Effect of VEGF on the regenerative capacity of muscle stem cells in dystrophic skeletal muscle. *Mol Ther* 2009;**17**:1788–98.
116. Ferrari G, Cusella-De Angelis G, Coletta M, Paolucci E, Stornaiuolo A, Cossu G, et al. Muscle regeneration by bone marrow-derived myogenic progenitors. *Science* 1998;**279**:1528–30.
117. Corbel SY, Lee A, Yi L, Duenas J, Brazelton TR, Blau HM, et al. Contribution of hematopoietic stem cells to skeletal muscle. *Nat Med* 2003;**9**:1528–32.
118. Dreyfus PA, Chretien F, Chazaud B, Kirova Y, Caramelle P, Garcia L, et al. Adult bone marrow-derived stem cells in muscle connective tissue and satellite cell niches. *Am J Pathol* 2004;**164**:773–9.
119. Palermo AT, Labarge MA, Doyonnas R, Pomerantz J, Blau HM. Bone marrow contribution to skeletal muscle: a physiological response to stress. *Dev Biol* 2005;**279**:336–44.
120. Lapidos KA, Chen YE, Earley JU, Heydemann A, Huber JM, Chien M, et al. Transplanted hematopoietic stem cells demonstrate impaired sarcoglycan expression after engraftment into cardiac and skeletal muscle. *J Clin Invest* 2004;**114**:1577–85.
121. Sherwood RI, Christensen JL, Conboy IM, Conboy MJ, Rando TA, Weissman IL, et al. Isolation of adult mouse myogenic progenitors: functional heterogeneity of cells within and engrafting skeletal muscle. *Cell* 2004;**119**:543–54.
122. Wernig G, Janzen V, Schafer R, Zweyer M, Knauf U, Hoegemeier O, et al. The vast majority of bone-marrow-derived cells integrated into mdx muscle fibers are silent despite long-term engraftment. *Proc Natl Acad Sci USA* 2005;**102**: 11852–7.
123. Zammit PS, Partridge TA, Yablonka-Reuveni Z. The skeletal muscle satellite cell: the stem cell that came in from the cold. *J Histochem Cytochem* 2006;**54**:1177–91.
124. Mitchell KJ, Pannerec A, Cadot B, Parlakian A, Besson V, Gomes ER, et al. Identification and characterization of a non-satellite cell muscle resident progenitor during postnatal development. *Nat Cell Biol* 2010;**12**:257–66.
125. Relaix F, Weng X, Marazzi G, Yang E, Copeland N, Jenkins N, et al. Pw1, a novel zinc finger gene implicated in the myogenic and neuronal lineages. *Dev Biol* 1996;**177**:383–96.
126. Schwarzkopf M, Coletti D, Sassoon D, Marazzi G. Muscle cachexia is regulated by a p53-PW1/Peg3-dependent pathway. *Genes Dev* 2006;**20**:3440–52.
127. Cohn RD, van Erp C, Habashi JP, Soleimani AA, Klein EC, Lisi MT, et al. Angiotensin II type 1 receptor blockade attenuates TGF-beta-induced failure of muscle regeneration in multiple myopathic states. *Nat Med* 2007;**13**:204–10.
128. Conboy IM, Conboy MJ, Smythe GM, Rando TA. Notch-mediated restoration of regenerative potential to aged muscle. *Science* 2003;**302**:1575–7.
129. Bjornson CR, Cheung TH, Liu L, Tripathi PV, Steeper KM, Rando, TA. Notch signaling is necessary to maintain quiescence in adult muscle stem cells. *Stem Cells* 2012;**30**:232–42.
130. Mourikis P, Sambasivan R, Castel D, Rocheteau P, Bizzarro V, Tajbakhsh, S. A critical requirement for notch signaling in maintenance of the quiescent skeletal muscle stem cell state. *Stem Cells* 2012;**30**:243–52.

Chapter 66

Skeletal Muscle Dystrophin-Glycoprotein Complex and Muscular Dystrophy

Yvonne M. Kobayashi and Kevin P. Campbell
Howard Hughes Medical Institute, Department of Molecular Physiology and Biophysics, Department of Neurology, Department of Internal Medicine, Roy J. and Lucille A. Carver College of Medicine, The University of Iowa, Iowa City, IA

INTRODUCTION

Duchenne muscular dystrophy (DMD) is a lethal neuromuscular disorder that is characterized by progressive muscle weakness (1). It is caused by mutations that lie within the DMD gene and lead to the complete absence of dystrophin in the sarcolemma of skeletal muscle (2–6). Biochemical and cell biological research on dystrophin led to the discovery of the skeletal muscle dystrophin–glycoprotein complex (7–11, for reviews see 12,13), which spans the muscle-cell membrane and links the actin cytoskeleton to the surrounding basement membrane. Mutations in genes that encode either components of the complex itself (14–19) or mediators of its requisite post-translational modifications lead to distinct forms of muscular dystrophy (20–26). This chapter focuses on the structure and function of the dystrophin-glycoprotein complex in skeletal muscle, and its role in the pathogenesis of muscular dystrophy.

THE DYSTROPHIN-GLYCOPROTEIN COMPLEX IN SKELETAL MUSCLE

Efforts to understand the function of dystrophin in skeletal muscle led to the identification and purification of the dystrophin-glycoprotein complex, a multimeric protein complex embedded in the sarcolemma (7–10) (Figure 66.1). The central protein of this complex is dystroglycan, which consists of α- and β-dystroglycan subunits (27). The subsarcolemma subcomplex is composed of dystrophin, the syntrophins (α, β), and dystrobrevin (DTNA). Stabilizing the dystrophin-glycoprotein complex at the membrane is the sarcoglycan–sarcospan subcomplex, which is composed of α-, β-, γ-, and δ-sarcoglycan, and sarcospan (SSPN). Although these proteins represent the "core" dystrophin-glycoprotein complex, additional proteins (i.e. neuronal nitric oxide synthase, nNOS) associate with it but are removed during purification (28,29). The primary structures of all of the integral components of the dystrophin-glycoprotein complex are known (14–18,30–32). Biochemical experiments show that α-dystroglycan binds to laminin-2 (also called merosin, the laminin isoform found in muscle) with high affinity in a calcium-dependent manner (9,27). However, β-dystroglycan anchors dystrophin to the sarcolemma membrane via its C-terminus (33). Thus, the dystroglycan-mediated linkage between the cytoskeleton and the extracellular matrix provides an important mechanism for anchoring the muscle sarcolemma to the surrounding basement membrane (Figure 66.1). The overall organization and high density of the dystrophin-glycoprotein complex at the sarcolemma strongly suggest that this complex has a structural role in skeletal muscle. One proposed function of the dystrophin-glycoprotein complex is that it confers stability to the muscle cell membrane, protecting muscle fibers from contraction-induced damage.

The dystrophin–glycoprotein complex also plays a role in scaffolding signaling molecules such as nNOS. In the absence of dystrophin or its central rod domain (as found in Becker muscular dystrophy patients) nNOS is lost from the sarcolemma (34–36). Loss of nNOS from the sarcolemma is also identified with limb-girdle muscular dystrophies associated with the sarcoglycans (36,37). In various mouse models this loss of sarcolemmal nNOS leads to a deficiency in the normal contraction-induced cGMP-dependent attenuation of local vasoconstriction, resulting in post-exercise narrowing of the muscle vasculature (36). Functional muscle ischemia is also reported in DMD patients (35). The decrease in blood flow manifests as an exaggerated fatigue response to mild activity, and in dystrophic muscle, causes exercise-induced muscle

Muscle. DOI: http://dx.doi.org/10.1016/B978-0-12-381510-1.00066-1

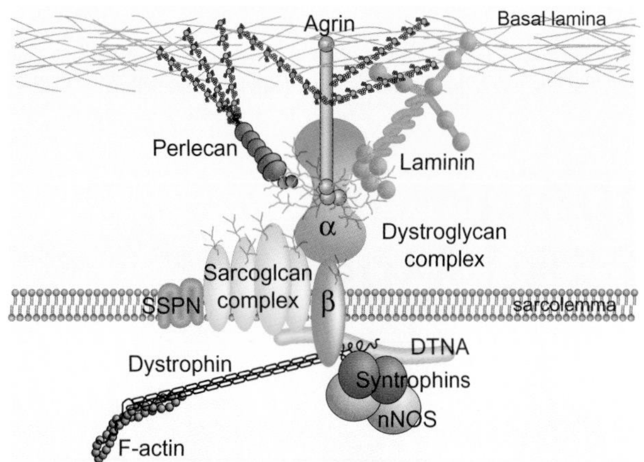

FIGURE 66.1 **Molecular organization of integral and peripheral components of the dystrophin-glycoprotein complex.** The core of the complex is the dystroglycan subcomplex (α, β), which links proteins of the basal lamina (including laminin, agrin, and perlecan) to F-actin of the subsarcolemmal cytoskeleton. The subsarcolemmal subcomplex is composed of dystrophin, the syntrophins (α, β), and dystrobrevin (DTNA). Additionally, nNOS is linked to the subsarcolemmal subcomplex through interactions with both the syntrophins and dystrophin. Stabilizing the dystrophin-glycoprotein complex at the membrane is the sarcoglycan-sarcospan subcomplex, which is composed of sarcospan (SSPN) and α-, β-, γ-, and δ-sarcoglycan.

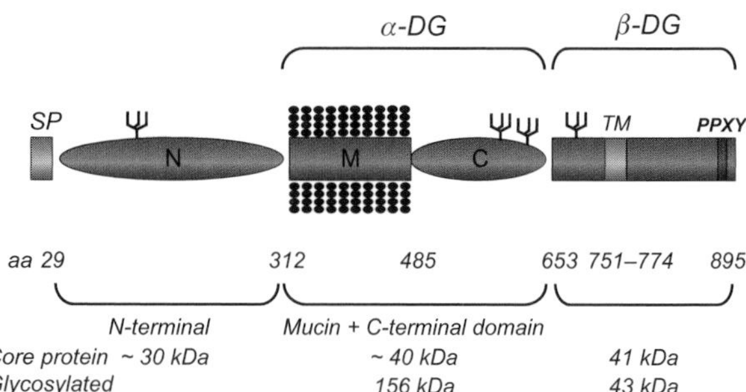

FIGURE 66.2 **Domain organization of dystroglycan.** Dystroglycan is synthesized as a precursor with a signal peptide (SP), an N-terminal domain (N), a mucin domain (M), a C-terminal domain (C), and a transmembrane polypeptide. Following proteolytic processing, mature dystroglycan consists of α-dystroglycan (mucin plus C-terminal domain) and β-dystroglycan (features a single transmembrane domain (TM) and the dystrophin binding site (PPXY)). Circles indicate O-linked sugar chains on the mucin domain. Branches indicate N-linked sugar chains. Molecular masses refer to the protein mass in the absence (core protein) or presence of glycosyl groups.

edema. In mouse models with mislocalized nNOS, exercise-induced fatigue and muscle edema can be relieved pharmacologically by enhancing nitric oxide-cGMP signaling from active muscle (36).

DYSTROGLYCAN: POST-TRANSLATIONAL PROCESSING AND FUNCTION

The transmembrane protein dystroglycan, which is ultimately cleaved into an α and a β component (Figure 66.2), is a key link between the cytoskeleton and extracellular-matrix proteins that bear laminin globular domains (e.g., laminin-2). Mature α-dystroglycan consists solely of a mucin domain and C-terminal domain since the N-terminal domain is removed by furin cleavage (38). This mucin domain is modified with numerous O-linked oligosaccharides that are essential for its normal function as an extracellular-matrix receptor in various tissues (27,38). Dystrophin is anchored to the sarcolemma membrane by interacting with the C-terminal 15 amino acids of β-dystroglycan (33), whereas β-dystroglycan binds to the second half of a region on dystrophin that has a cysteine-rich domain (33). This cysteine-rich domain is present in all known dystrophin isoforms and is well conserved in the dystrophin homolog utrophin. The proline-rich motif in β-dystroglycan interacts directly with Grb2, an adapter protein involved in signal transduction and cytoskeletal organization (39). Thus, through its interactions with laminin and dystrophin, dystroglycan acts as a transmembrane link for the extracellular matrix and the cytoskeleton. Moreover, this linkage may play an important role in extracellular matrix-mediated signal transduction and/or cytoskeleton organization in muscle.

In addition to binding to laminin-2, α-dystroglycan binds to agrin, a protein that mediates the formation of neuromuscular junctions (40). In this binding capacity, α-dystroglycan may functionally be important for agrin activity and neuromuscular junction formation (41). Dystroglycan can also undergo clustering within the membrane in response to the cytoskeletal protein rapsyn; this clustering may mediate an association between dystroglycan and acetylcholine receptors (41). Thus, dystroglycan may be an important part of a specialized extracellular matrix-cytoskeletal complex at the neuromuscular junction.

Dystroglycan expression extends to many call types other than muscle, particularly those associated with basement membranes (42). During mouse development, dystroglycan is expressed in several epithelial tissues (42). Its expression is essential for early embryonic development, as evidenced by the results of gene disruption in mouse (43,44). Homozygous mutant embryos exhibit early lethality, and do not progress beyond 5.5 days of development. Analysis of the mutant phenotype revealed a disruption of Reichert's membrane, an extra-embryonic basement membrane essential for early development. Thus dystroglycan is required for the development of Reichert's membrane and perhaps other basement membranes in epithelia, nerve, and muscle.

The structural basis for the high-affinity binding of laminin globular domains to α-dystroglycan is extensively being investigated. Notably, a growing number of putative and known glycotransferases (POMT1, POMT2, POMGnT1, LARGE, Fukutin, and FKRP) are involved in post-translational processing of dystroglycan (20–25), producing a complex O-linked glycoprotein structure. POMT1/2 are known to add mannose to the mucin domain of dystroglycan, whereas POMGnT1 adds GlyNAc (21,23). Dystroglycan is also post-translationally processed by the novel glycosyltransferase, LARGE, and this modification is essential for its function (38). Recognition by LARGE is dependent on the N-terminal domain of α-dystroglycan (38); the enzyme-substrate recognition motif within this domain is critical for the post-translational modification of dystroglycan and is necessary for its functional maturation into a matrix receptor. Notably, this motif is proteolytically processed later in the post-translational modification pathway. The unique pathway is significant *in vivo*, as gene transfer into muscle-specific gene knockout mice rescues the domain-specific functions of dystroglycan in the whole animal. Thus, molecular recognition by LARGE along the biosynthetic pathway is essential to producing functional dystroglycan. Recently, it was shown that maturation of α-dystroglycan to its laminin-binding form requires a novel biosynthetic pathway involving phosphorylation on O-mannosyl glycans, and that LARGE is crucial for further modification of phosphorylated O-mannosyl glycans on α-dystroglycan (45). NMR-based analysis identified the novel phosphorylated O-glycan as GalNAc-β-1,3-GlcNAc-β-1,4-[PO_4-6-Man]. This mannosyl phosphorylation occurs in the Golgi, independently of the known mannose-6-phosphate synthetic pathway to which the UDP-GlcNAc:lysosomal enzyme GlcNAc-1-phosphotransferase and GlcNAc-1-phosphodiester α-N-acetylglucos-aminidase contribute. Biochemical and viral rescue studies of myodystrophy mice (*Large*^{myd}) demonstrate that LARGE assembles the laminin-binding moiety onto the phosphate residue of the O-mannosyl glycan. In addition, immobilized metal-affinity chromatography reveal that cells from patients with muscle-eye-brain disease and Fukuyama congenital muscular dystrophy, which are characterized by genetically distinct abnormalities, are similarly deficient in modifying the phosphoryl branch chain of the O-mannosyl glycan. Overall, these findings indicate that α-dystroglycan receptor function requires phosphorylation of the O-mannosyl glycan, and that laminin-binding is dependent on the formation of a phosphodiester linkage.

SARCOGLYCAN-SARCOSPAN SUBCOMPLEX

The sarcoglycan complex is composed of four transmembrane glycoproteins (α-, β-, γ-, and δ-sarcoglycan) that form a distinct subcomplex within the dystrophin-glycoprotein complex (46). The functional importance of this complex was first demonstrated by the deficiency of α-sarcoglycan (adhalin) in autosomal-recessive muscular dystrophy patients from Arabic countries (14). The cDNA encoding α-sarcoglycan was initially isolated from a rabbit skeletal muscle library (30). In contrast to dystroglycan, which is expressed in a wide variety of muscle and non-muscle tissues, α-sarcoglycan is expressed only in skeletal and cardiac muscle (14,30). Since the cloning of α-sarcoglycan, additional sarcoglycans were identified that also participate in the dystrophin-glycoprotein complex (15–18). As a group, the sarcoglycans have no homology to any other known proteins. All four skeletal-muscle sarcoglycans have single transmembrane domains, relatively small intracellular domains, and large extracellular domains, and their primary structures are highly conserved across mammalian species.

Sarcospan is a 25 kDa membrane protein that co-localizes with the dystrophin-glycoprotein complex at the sarcolemma, co-purifies with the dystrophin-glycoprotein complex, and is an integral part of the sarcoglycan complex. These unique aspects demonstrate that sarcospan is an integral component of the dystrophin-glycoprotein complex (31,47). Sarcospan contains four transmembrane spanning helices with both N-and C-termini located intracellularly (31). The topology of sarcospan and its primary structure are similar to that of a superfamily of proteins called tetraspans, which are thought to play important roles in mediating transmembrane protein interactions. Biochemical analyses demonstrate that α-, β-, γ-, and δ-sarcoglycan and sarcospan are present at equal stoichiometry in the skeletal muscle sarcoglycan–sarcospan complex (47). Thus, membrane stability or the targeting of each sarcoglycan protein is dependent on the integrity of the sarcoglycan–sarcospan complex as a whole (47).

DUCHENNE MUSCULAR DYSTROPHY AND DISRUPTION OF THE DYSTROPHIN-GLYCOPROTEIN COMPLEX

Defects occur in genes encoding either proteins of the dystrophin-glycoprotein complex or enzymes necessary for its post-translational processing lead to various forms of muscular dystrophy, including Duchenne muscular dystrophy, limb-girdle and congenital muscular dystrophies (Figure 66.3). The absence of dystrophin expression from skeletal muscle of DMD patients perturbs the integrity of the dystrophin-glycoprotein complex and results in reduced sarcolemmal expression of dystroglycan, the sarcoglycan-sarcospan complex, and the other components, thereby disrupting the link between the extracellular matrix and the subsarcolemma cytoskeleton (18,48)

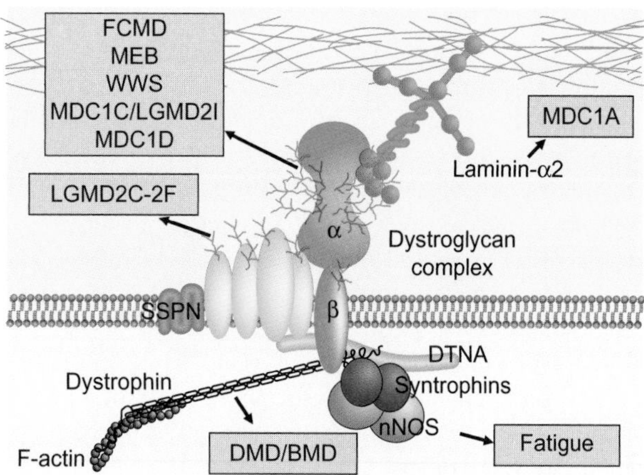

FIGURE 66.3 Muscular dystrophies associated with the dystrophin-glycoprotein complex. Several forms of muscular dystrophy arise from primary mutations in genes encoding components of the dystrophin-glycoprotein complex. Duchenne and Becker muscular dystrophies (DMD/BMD), a subset of limb-girdle muscular dystrophies (LGMD2C-2F), and merosin-deficient muscular dystrophy (MDCIA) are caused by mutations in the dystrophin-, sarcoglycan- or laminin-α2 chain-encoding genes. In addition, several forms of congenital muscular dystrophy (CMD) and LGMD (FCMD, MEB, WWS, MDCIC/LGMD2I, MDCID) are caused by mutations in genes responsible for the glycosylation of α-dystroglycan.

(Figure 66.4). Like DMD patients, the *mdx* mouse has a naturally occurring mutation in dystrophin that leads to the perturbation of the dystrophin-glycoprotein complex and development of muscular dystrophy. Loss of the dystrophin-glycoprotein complex in different animal models has been used to test the hypothesis that the role of this complex is to protect the sarcolemma. Tracer molecules, like Evans blue dye (a low molecular weight diazo dye that binds serum albumin), do not cross into skeletal muscle fibers in normal mice. With the *mdx* mouse, there is significant intracellular Evans blue dye accumulation in skeletal muscle fibers, indicating that a loss of sarcolemmal integrity results from plasma membrane disruptions (49–51). These findings support the hypothesis that the dystrophin-glycoprotein complex provides mechanical reinforcement for the sarcolemma.

SARCOGLYCAN-DEFICIENT LIMB-GIRDLE MUSCULAR DYSTROPHY

Limb-girdle muscular dystrophy (LGMD) types 2C, 2D, 2E, and 2F are caused by mutations in γ-, α-, β-, and δ-sarcoglycan genes, respectively, and are characterized by shoulder and girdle skeletal muscle weakness and often cardiomyopathy (14–18) (see Figure 66.3). Missense mutations in α-sarcoglycan were first identified in a European family (14). A homozygous missense mutation in β-sarcoglycan was later identified in a large Amish pedigree with autosomal recessive limb-girdle muscular dystrophy (15). Extensive analysis of LGMD families has resulted in the identification of many distinct mutations that cause disease ranging in clinical phenotype from mild impairment with slow progression to severe disability and rapid deterioration. However, it is possible that the consequences of these mutations lie not in specific perturbations of function, but rather in the ability of the newly synthesized protein or complex to be correctly processed and translocated to the cell surface. Consistent with this hypothesis is the loss or significant reduction of all sarcoglycan components from the sarcolemma in sarcoglycan-deficient LGMD patients. This concomitant loss of sarcoglycan complex components demonstrates that the membrane targeting of each sarcoglycan is dependent on the integrity of the sarcoglycan complex (see Figure 66.4). In addition, α-dystroglycan is destabilized at the extracellular surface of sarcoglycan-deficient muscle fibers, suggesting that α-dystroglycan depends on the sarcoglycan complex for its anchorage to the sarcolemma (50–52).

The molecular pathogenesis of sarcoglycan-deficient muscular dystrophies was investigated by the generation of genetically engineered mice deficient for α-sarcoglycan, β-sarcoglycan, γ-sarcoglycan or δ-sarcoglycan (50–53). These mouse models develop progressive muscular dystrophy with pathology similar to that seen in human sarcoglycanopathy patients, and like patients, exhibit a loss or significant reduction of the sarcoglycan–sarcospan complex at the sarcolemma. Biochemical analyses of skeletal muscle from these mice show that the sarcoglycan–sarcospan complex is responsible for anchoring α-dystroglycan to the sarcolemma. In addition, assembly of the sarcoglycan complex in cultured cells show that all four sarcoglycans are required for proper targeting to the cell membrane (46,54). These findings provided biochemical evidence in support of the hypothesis that the molecular defects in sarcoglycan-deficient muscular dystrophy are aberrant assembly and trafficking of the sarcoglycan complex.

The exploration of the structure of the sarcoglycan complex has been facilitated by the use of gene transfer in animal models of muscular dystrophy, such as the BIO 14.6 hamster, which is deficient for δ-sarcoglycan (55). The skeletal muscle phenotype in the BIO 14.6 hamster can be corrected via direct intramuscular injection of an adenovirus that contains a cDNA encoding the normal human δ-sarcoglycan. High levels of expression can be generated from a single injection, which restores all sarcoglycan proteins to the sarcolemma. Importantly, restoration of the sarcoglycan complex results in stabilization of dystroglycan at the extracellular face. The restoration of the dystrophin–glycoprotein complex has clear functional effects. First, using Evans blue dye as a marker for

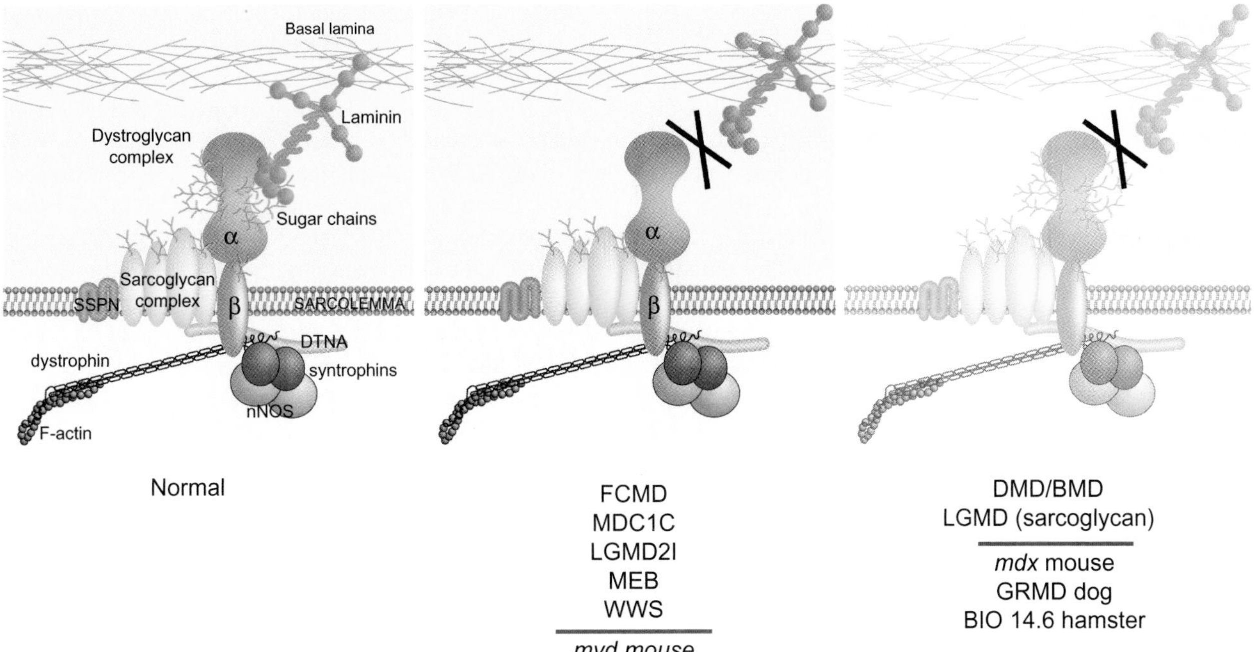

FIGURE 66.4 **Disruption of the subsarcolemma cytoskeleton-extracellular matrix link in dystrophin-glycoprotein complex-related muscular dystrophies.** The left panel depicts normal skeletal muscle with an intact dystrophin-glycoprotein complex that links F-actin of the subsarcolemmal cytoskeleton to laminin-2α within the basal lamina of the extracellular matrix. The middle panel illustrates the defect in congenital muscular dystrophies associated with deficiencies in the α-dystroglycan glycosylation, in which case the link to the extracellular matrix is disrupted. These include: FKTN, associated with mutations in Fukutin; MDCIC and LGMD2I, which are associated with mutations in Fukutin-related protein; and muscle-eye-brain disease (MEB) and Walker-Warburg syndrome (WWS). An animal model used to study these congenital muscular dystrophies is the myodystrophy mouse (myd), which has a naturally occurring mutation in the gene that encodes LARGE, a putative glycosyltransferase. The right panel illustrates muscular dystrophies associated with defects in dystrophin and the sarcoglycans, in which case the link from the subsarcolemmal cytoskeleton to the extracellular matrix is broken. These include: Duchenne and Becker muscular dystrophies (DMD/BMD) and limb-girdle muscular dystrophies (LGMD, defect in sarcoglycans). Animal models used to study these muscular dystrophies include the DMD^{mdx} (mdx) mouse and the Golden Retriever muscular dystrophy dog (GRMD), both of which have naturally occurring mutations in the dystrophin gene, *Dmd*. The BIO 14.6 hamster is also used for such studies, and it has a naturally occurring mutation in the gene for δ-sarcoglycan.

sarcolemmal damage, adenoviral delivery of δ-sarcoglycan was found to result in a dramatic restoration of membrane integrity. Second, early administration of δ-sarcoglycan adenovirus reduced the level of central nucleation, a hallmark of progressive muscle degeneration, of transduced fibers. This functional effect indicates that the continual cycle of muscle-fiber degeneration and regeneration was averted. The most remarkable finding of this recent study is the long-term expression that was achieved: a single injection of an adenoviral construct carrying δ-sarcoglycan into a 3-week-old hamster resulted in persistent expression of δ-sarcoglycan for as long as 9 months, with very little evidence of a host-immune response. Prevention of limb-girdle muscular dystrophy by adenovirus-mediated gene transfer of human α-sarcoglycan is demonstrated using the α-sarcoglycan-deficient mouse (50,56). In this case, a single intramuscular injection of a first-generation adenovirus into the skeletal muscle of α-sarcoglycan-deficient neonatal mice led to sustained expression of α-sarcoglycan at the sarcolemma of transduced myofibers. The morphology of the transduced muscles was consequently preserved. Contrast agent-enhanced magnetic resonance imaging demonstrated that sarcolemmal integrity was maintained in the transduced myofibers. These studies provide evidence that early virus-mediated gene transfer of a sarcoglycan protein constitutes a promising therapeutic strategy for limb-girdle muscular dystrophies.

DYSTROGLYCANOPATHIES: LIMB-GIRDLE TO CONGENITAL MUSCULAR DYSTROPHY

In the past ten years, novel insights have been obtained into the role of dystroglycan in the pathogenesis of Fukuyama congenital muscular dystrophy, muscle-eye-brain disease, and Walker-Warburg syndrome, each of which are congenital muscular dystrophies with associated developmental brain defects (see Figure 66.3, for review see 57). Genetic data show that mutations in proteins with homology to glycosyltransferases (20–26) are linked to these congenital muscular dystrophies. The *fukutin* gene in Fukuyama congenital muscular dystrophy was the first to be identified, and encodes a protein with homology to glycoconjugate modifying enzymes (20). Actual glycosyltransferase activity has been demonstrated for proteins mutated in muscle-eye-brain disease and Walker-Warburg syndrome, the *O*-mannosyl-β1, 2-*N*-acetylglucosaminyl-transferase (POMGnT1) and putative *O*-mannosyltransferase (POMT1), respectively (21,23). Biochemical analysis of muscle biopsies revealed a convergent role for these proteins in the glycosylation of α-dystroglycan, a process required for functional activity. The abnormal glycosylation of dystroglycan in disease disrupts the normal binding activity for each of its major extracellular matrix ligands in muscle and brain. In turn, the disruption of dystroglycan ligand binding results in loss of the functional link between the cytoskeleton and the extracellular matrix, and leads to severe muscular dystrophy (see Figure 66.4). Dystroglycanopathy is also found in milder forms of limb-girdle muscular dystrophy, with or without brain involvement. Unlike the more severe cases, which are characterized by a nearly complete lack of functional glycosylation, milder cases of LGMD feature only reduced glycosylation.

A convergent phenotype in the spontaneous mutant myodystrophy mouse (*Large^{myd}*) and human congenital muscular dystrophy type 1D is now identified. The mutation in the myodystrophy gene, LARGE, results in abnormal glycosylation of dystroglycan in muscle and brain, and a loss of ligand binding activity for laminin, neurexin, and agrin (58). In addition to a severe muscular dystrophy phenotype, the *Large^{myd}* mouse exhibits significant abnormal neuronal migration in the cerebral cortex, cerebellum, and hippocampus.

The function of dystroglycan in muscle has also been examined by specific targeted deletion of the dystroglycan gene in differentiated skeletal muscle (59). A surprisingly mild phenotype was observed in these mice. However, the creatine kinase promoter used to express cre-recombinase in these studies does not target the dystroglycan gene deletion in satellite cells, and these mice displayed a remarkable ability to regenerate muscle compared to other mouse models of dystrophin-glycoprotein complex-associated dystrophies. These findings suggest that dystroglycan plays an important role in satellite-cell function and/or muscle fiber regeneration. Brain-selective deletion of dystroglycan is sufficient to cause congenital muscular dystrophy-like brain malformations, including disarray of cerebral cortical layering, fusion of cerebral hemispheres, and discontinuities in the pial surface basal lamina (glia limitans) (60). Thus, disruption of dystroglycan function is sufficient for the development of brain abnormalities in the glycosyltransferase-deficient congenital muscular dystrophies.

An increased expression of LARGE has been investigated as a potential treatment for glycosyltransferase-deficient muscular dystrophies (61). Overexpression of LARGE is able to modify the sugar moieties of α-dystroglycan, and to prevent muscular dystrophy in *Large^{myd}* mice. Importantly, high levels of LARGE expression restore the function of α-dystroglycan and modulate its glycosylation in myoblasts and fibroblasts from patients affected with Fukuyama congenital muscular dystrophy, muscle-eye-brain disease and Walker-Warburg syndrome. LARGE-dependent glycosylation of α-dystroglycan is required for dystroglycan function, and the induction of LARGE expression restores α-dystroglycan function regardless of the type of glycosyltransferase mutated in patients.

A mutation in the dystroglycan gene in a patient with muscular dystrophy and cognitive impairment was recently discovered (19). Analyses reveal that this missense mutation causes hypoglycosylation of α-dystroglycan, and thereby impairs binding between α-dystroglycan and the extracellular matrix protein laminin. Surprisingly, the affected residue is not a site of O-glycosylation but lies in the dystroglycan N-terminal domain, and disrupts the association of dystroglycan with the putative glycosyltransferase LARGE. Disruption of the glycosyltransferase-targeting required to initiate functional dystroglycan O-glycosylation is a novel pathogenic mechanism that underlies certain forms of muscular dystrophy.

THE MECHANISTIC BASIS OF MAINTAINING MUSCLE MEMBRANE INTEGRITY

Compromised integrity of the muscle sarcolemma has been proposed to initiate muscle fiber pathology in muscular dystrophy, yet the molecular underpinning of this membrane disruption has never been clearly established. Recently, a novel *in situ* laser damage assay was developed to study a role of dystroglycan in maintaining sarcolemmal integrity, and to measure muscle damage induced by lengthening contractions (62). To directly test the function of the dystroglycan-mediated link between the basal lamina and the sarcolemma, we examined the sarcolemmal integrity of the muscle fibers from the *Large^{myd}* mouse which is an animal model for dystroglycan hypoglycosylation that lacks only the laminin globular (LG) domain-binding O-glycan that is present in wild-type counterparts. Despite maintaining an intact dystrophin–glycoprotein complex, *Large^{myd}* muscle fibers have reduced sarcolemmal integrity and exhibit detachment from the basal lamina. This detachment makes *Large^{myd}* muscles highly susceptible to lengthening contraction-induced injury. Furthermore, recombinant glycosylated α-dystroglycan can restore sarcolemma integrity of the

Large^{myd} muscle fibers. Therefore, dystroglycan-dependent, tight physical attachment of the basal lamina to the sarcolemma is important for transmission of the basal lamina's structural strength to the sarcolemma, providing resistance to mechanical stress (see Figure 66.4). These findings establish a mechanism that accounts for the increased susceptibility of patients with hypoglycosylated dystroglycan to contraction-induced muscle injury, and highlights the importance of this protective basic cellular mechanism in the context of mechanical damage.

REFERENCES

1. Walton JN, Gardner-Medwin D. Progressive muscular dystrophy and the myotonic disorders. In: Walton SJ, editor. *Disorders of voluntary muscle*. Edinburgh: Churchill Livingstone; 1981. p. 481–524.
2. Hoffman EP, Brown RH, Kunkel LM. Dystrophin: the protein product of the Duchenne muscular dystrophy locus. *Cell* 1987;**51**:919–28.
3. Zubrzycka-Caarn EE, Bulman DE, Karpati G, Burghes AHM, Belfall B, Klamut HJ, et al. The Duchenne muscular dystrophy gene product is localized in sarcolemma of human skeletal muscle. *Nature* 1988;**333**:466–9.
4. Arahata K, Ishiura S, Ishiguro T, Tsukahara T, Suhara Y, Eguchi C, et al. Immunostaining of skeletal and cardiac muscle surface membrane with antibody against duchenne muscular dystrophy peptide. *Nature* 1988;**333**:861–3.
5. Watkins SC, Hoffman EP, Slayter HS, Kunkel LM. Immunoelectron microscopic localization of dystrophin in myofibres. *Nature* 1988;**333**:863–6.
6. Hoffman EP, Fischbeck KH, Brown RH, Johnson M, Medori R, Loire JD, et al. Characterization of Dystrophin in muscle-biopsy specimens from patients with Duchenne's or Becker's muscular dystrophy. *N Eng J Med* 1988;**318**:1363–8.
7. Campbell KP, Kahl SD. Association of dystrophin and an integral membrane glycoprotein. *Nature* 1989;**338**:259–62.
8. Ervasti JM, Ohlendieck K, Kahl SD, Gaver MG, Campbell KP. Deficiency of a glycoprotein component of the dystrophin complex in dystrophic muscle. *Nature* 1990;**345**:315–9.
9. Ervasti JM, Campbell KP. Membrane organization of the dystrophin–glycoprotein complex. *Cell* 1991;**66**:1121–31.
10. Ervasti JM, Campbell KP. A role for the dystrophin–glycoprotein complex as a transmembrane linker between laminin and actin. *J Cell Biol* 1993;**122**:809–23.
11. Yoshida M, Ozawa E. glycoprotein complex anchoring dystrophin to sarcolemma. *J Biochem* 1990;**108**:748–52.
12. Campbell KP. Three muscular dystrophies: loss of cytoskeleton-extracellular matrix linkage. *Cell* 1995;**80**:675–9.
13. Durbeej M, Campbell KP. Muscular dystrophies involving the dystrophin–glycoprotein complex: an overview of current mouse models. *Curr Opin Genet Dev* 2002;**12**:349–61.
14. Roberds SL, Leturcq F, Allamand V, Piccolo F, Jeanpierre M, Anderson RD, et al. Missense mutations in the adhalin gene linked to autosomal recessive muscular dystrophy. *Cell* 1994;**78**:625–33.
15. Lim LE, Duclos F, Broux O, Bourg N, Sunada Y, Allamand V, et al. β-sarcoglycan: characterization and role in limb-girdle muscular dystrophy linked to 4q12. *Nature Genet* 1995;**11**:257–65.
16. Bonnemann CG, Modi R, Noguchi S, Mizuno Y, Yoshida M, Gussoni E, et al. Beta-sarco-glycan (A3b) mutations cause autosomal recessive muscular dystrophy with loss of the sarcoglycan complex. *Nat Genet* 1995;**11**:266–73.
17. Noguchi S, McNally EM, Ben Othmane K, Hagiwara Y, Mizuno Y, Yoshida M, et al. Mutations in the dystrophin-associated protein γ-sarcoglycan in chromosome 13 muscular dystrophy. *Science* 1995;**270**:819–22.
18. Nigro V, de Sa Moreira E, Piluso G, Vainzof M, Belsito A, Politano L, et al. Autosomal recessive limb-girdle muscular dystrophy, LGMD2F, is caused by a mutation in the δ–sarcoglycan gene. *Nat Genet* 1996;**14**:195–8.
19. Hara Y, Balci B, Kanagawa M, et al. A dystroglycan missense mutation associated with mild muscular dystrophy and cognitive impairment. *N Engl J Med* 2011;**364**:939–46.
20. Kobayashi K, Nakahori Y, Miyake M, Matsumura K, Kondo-Iida E, Nomura Y, et al. An ancient retrotransposal insertion causes Fukuyama-type congenital muscular dystrophy. *Nature* 1998;**394**: 388–92.
21. Yoshida A, Kobayashi K, Manya H, Taniguchi K, Kano H, Mizuno M, et al. Muscular dystrophy and neuronal migration disorder caused by mutations in a glycosyltransferase, POMGnT1. *Dev Cell* 2001;**1**:717–24.
22. Brockington M, Blake DJ, Prandini P, Brown SC, Torelli S, Benson MA, et al. Mutations in the fukutin-related protein gene (FKRP) cause a form of congenital muscular dystrophy with secondary laminin α2 deficiency and abnormal glycosylation of α-dystroglycan. *Am J Hum Genet* 2001;**69** 11981–209.
23. Beltran-Valero de Bernabe D, Currier S, Steinbrecher A, Celli J, van Beusekom E, van der Zwaag B, et al. Mutations in the O-mannosyltransferase gene POMT1 give rise to the severe neuronal migration disorder Walker–Warburg syndrome. *Am J Hum Genet* 2002;**71**:1033–43.
24. Longman C, Brockington M, Torelli S, Jimenez-Mallebrera C, Kennedy C, Khalil N, et al. Mutations in the human LARGE gene cause MDC1D, a novel form of congenital muscular dystrophy with severe mental retardation and abnormal glycosylation of α-dystroglycan. *Hum Mol Genet* 2003;**12**:2853–61.
25. van Reeuwijk J, Janssen M, van den Elzen C, Beltran-Valero de Bernabé D, Sabatelli P, et al. POMT2 mutations cause α-dystroglycan hypoglycosylation and Walker–Warburg syndrome. *J Med Genet* 2005;**42**:907–12.
26. van Reeuwijk J, Grewal PK, Salih MA, Beltrán-Valero de Bernabé D, McLaughlan JM, Michielse CB, et al. Intragenic deletion in the LARGE gene causes Walker–Warburg syndrome. *Hum Genet* 2007;**121**:685–90.
27. Ibraghimov-Beskrovnaya O, Ervasti JM, Leveille CJ, Slaughter CA, Sernett SW, Campbell KP. Primary structure of the 43 K and 156 K dystrophin-associated glycoproteins linking dystrophin to the extracellular matrix. *Nature* 1992;**355**:696–702.
28. Crosbie RH, Straub V, Yun HY, Lee JC, Rafael JA, Chamberlain JS, et al. *mdx* Muscle pathogenesis is independent of nNOS perturbation. *Hum Mol Genet* 1998;**7**:823–9.
29. Crosbie RH, Yamada H, Venzke DP, Lisanti MP, Campbell KP. Caveolin-3 is not an integral component of the dystrophin–glycoprotein complex. *FEBS Lett* 1998;**427**:279–82.
30. Roberds SL, Anderson RD, Ibraghimov-Beskrovnaya O, Campbell KP. Primary structure and muscle-specific expression of the 50-kDa

dystrophin-associated glycoprotein (adhalin). *J Biol Chem* 1993;**268**:23739–42.
31. Crosbie RH, Heighway J, Venzke DP, Lee JC, Campbell KP. Sarcospan, the 25-kDa transmembrane component of the dystrophin–glycoprotein complex. *J Biol Chem* 1997;**272**:31221–4.
32. Jung D, Duclos F, Apostol B, Straub V, Lee JC, Allamand V, et al. Characterization of δ-sarcoglycan, a novel component of the oligomeric sarcoglycan complex involved in limb-girdle muscular dystrophy. *J Biol Chem* 1996;**271**:32321–9.
33. Jung D, Yang B, Meyer J, Chamberlain JS, Campbell KP. Identification and characterization of the dystrophin anchoring site on β-dystroglycan. *J Biol Chem* 1995;**270**:27305–10.
34. Torelli S, Brown SC, Jimenez-Mallebrera C, Feng L, Muntoni F, Sewry CA. Absence of neuronal nitric oxide synthase (nNOS) as a pathological marker for the diagnosis of Becker muscular dystrophy with rod domain deletions. *Neuropathol Appl Neurobiol* 2004;**30**:540–5.
35. Sander M, Chavoshan B, Harris SA, Iannaccone ST, Stull JT, Thomas GD, et al. Functional muscle ischemia in neuronal nitric oxide synthase-deficient skeletal muscle of children with Duchenne muscular dystrophy. *Proc Natl Acad Sci USA* 2000;**97**:13818–23.
36. Kobayashi YM, Rader EP, Crawford RW, Iyengar NK, Thedens DR, Faulkner JA, et al. Sarcolemma-localized nNOS is required to maintain activity after mild exercise. *Nature* 2008;**456**:511–5.
37. Crosbie RH, Barresi R, Campbell KP. Loss of sarcolemma nNOS in sarcoglycan-deficient muscle. *FASEB J* 2002;**16**:1786–91.
38. Kanagawa M, Saito F, Kunz S, Yoshida-Moriguchi T, Barresi R, Kobayashi YM, et al. Molecular recognition by LARGE is essential for expression of functional dystroglycan. *Cell* 2004;**117**:953–64.
39. Yang B, Jung D, Motto D, Meyer J, Koretzky G, Campbell KP. SH3 Domain-mediated interaction of dystroglycan and Grb2. *J Biol Chem* 1995;**270**:11711–4.
40. Campanelli JT, Roberds SL, Campbell KP, Scheller RH. A role for dystrophin-associated glycoproteins and utrophin in agrin-induced AChR clustering. *Cell* 1994;**77**:663–74.
41. Apel ED, Roberds SL, Campbell KP, Merlie JP. Rapsyn may function as a link between the acetylcholine receptor and the agrin-binding dystrophin-associated glycoprotein complex. *Neuron* 1995;**15**:115–26.
42. Durbeej M, Larsson E, Ibraghimov-Beskrovnaya O, Roberds SL, Campbell KP, Ekblom P. Non-muscle α-dystroglycan is involved in epithelial development. *J Cell Biol* 1995;**130**:79–91.
43. Williamson RA, Henry MD, Daniels KJ, Hrstka RF, Lee JC, Sunada Y, et al. Dystroglycan is essential for early embryonic development: disruption of Reichert's membrane in Dag1-null mice. *Hum Mol Gen* 1997;**6**:831–41.
44. Henry MD, Campbell KP. A role for dystroglycan in basement membrane assembly. *Cell* 1998;**95**:859–70.
45. Yoshida-Moriguchi T, Yu L, Stalnaker SH, Davis S, Kunz S, Madson M, et al. O-Mannosyl phosphorylation of alpha-dystroglycan is required for laminin binding. *Science* 2010;**327**:88–92.
46. Holt KH, Campbell KP. Assembly of the sarcoglycan complex: insights for muscular dystrophy. *J Biol Chem* 1998;**273**:34667–70.
47. Crosbie RH, Lim LE, Moore SA, Hirano M, Hays AP, Maybaum SW, et al. Molecular and genetic characterization of sarcospan: insights into sarcoglycan-sarcospan domains. *Hum Mol Genet* 2000;**9**:2019–27.
48. Ohlendieck K, Matsumura K, Ionasescu VV, Towbin JA, Bosch EP, Weinstein SL, et al. Duchenne muscular dystrophy: deficiency of dystrophin-associated proteins in the sarcolemma. *Neurol* 1993;**43**:795–800.
49. Straub V, Rafael JA, Chamberlain JS, Campbell KP. Animal models for muscular dystrophy show different patterns of sarcolemmal disruption. *J Cell Biol* 1997;**139**:375–85.
50. Duclos F, Straub V, Moore SA, Venzke DP, Hrstka RF, Crosbie RH, et al. Progressive muscular dystrophy in α-sarcoglycan deficient mice. *J Cell Biol* 1998;**142**:1461–71.
51. Durbeej M, Cohn RD, Hrstka RF, Moore SA, Allamand V, Davidson BL, et al. Disruption of the β-sarcoglycan gene reveals pathogenetic complexity of limb-girdle muscular dystrophy type 2E. *Mol Cell* 2000;**5**:141–51.
52. Coral-Vazquez R, Cohn RD, Moore SA, Hill JA, Weiss RM, Davisson R, et al. Disruption of the sarcoglycan-sarcospan complex in vascular smooth muscle: a novel mechanism in the pathogenesis of cardiomyopathy and muscular dystrophy. *Cell* 1999;**98**:465–74.
53. Hack AA, Ly CT, Jiang F, Clendenin CJ, Sigrist KS, Wollmann RL, et al. Gamma-sarcoglycan deficiency leads to muscle membrane defects and apoptosis independent of dystrophin. *J Cell Biol* 1998;**142**:1279–87.
54. Holt KH, Crosbie RH, Venzke DP, Campbell KP. Biosynthesis of dystroglycan: processing of a precursor propeptide. *FEBS Lett* 2000;**468**:79–83.
55. Holt KH, Lim LE, Straub V, Venzke DP, Duclos F, Anderson RD, et al. Functional rescue of the sarcoglycan complex in the BIO 14.6 hamster using δ-sarcoglycan gene transfer. *Mol Cell* 1998;**1**:841–8.
56. Allamand V, Donahue KM, Straub V, Davisson RL, Davidson BL, Campbell KP. Early adenovirus-mediated gene transfer effectively prevents muscular dystrophy in αlpha-sarcoglycan-deficient mice. *Gene Ther* 2000;**7**:1385–91.
57. Michele DE, Campbell KP. Dystrophin–glycoprotein complex: post-translational processing and dystroglycan function. *J Biol Chem* 2003;**278**:15457–60.
58. Michele DE, Barresi R, Kanagawa M, Saito F, Cohn RD, Satz JS, et al. Post-translational disruption of dystroglycan-ligand interactions in congenital muscular dystrophies. *Nature* 2002;**418**:417–22.
59. Cohn RD, Henry MD, Michele DE, Barresi R, Saito F, Moore SA, et al. Disruption of Dag1 in dfferentiated skeletal muscle reveals a role for dystroglycan in muscle regeneration. *Cell* 2002;**110**:639–48.
60. Moore SA, Saito F, Chen J, Michele DE, Henry M, Messing A, et al. Deletion of brain dystroglycan recapitulates aspects of congenital muscular dystrophy. *Nature* 2002;**418**:422–5.
61. Barresi R, Michele DE, Kanagawa M, Harper HA, Dovico SA, Satz JS, et al. LARGE can functionally bypass α-dystroglycan glycosylation defects in distinct congenital muscular dystrophies. *Nat Med* 2004;**10**:696–703.
62. Han R, Kanagawa M, Yoshida-Moriguchi T, Rader E, Ng. RA, Michele DE, et al. Basal lamina strengthens cell membrane integrity via the laminin G domain binding of α-dystroglycan. *Proc Natl Acad Sci USA* 2009;**31**:12573–9.

Section C

Skeletal Muscle Disease

Chapter 67

Statin-Induced Muscle Toxicity: Clinical and Genetic Determinants of Risk

QiPing Feng and Russell A. Wilke
Department of Medicine, Division of Clinical Pharmacology, Vanderbilt University Medical Center, Nashville, TN

CLINICAL ASPECTS

Scope of the Problem

Cholesterol is synthesized from acetyl-coenzyme A, through a linear series of enzymatic steps (Figure 67.1) (1,2). The rate-limiting enzyme is HMG coenzyme A reductase (HMGCR). Multiple large clinical trials have demonstrated that statins (HMGCR inhibitors) reduce the incidence of both primary and secondary coronary artery disease in patients at risk (3–6). Primary prevention trials have demonstrated that statin use can reduce the risk of first major coronary event by 20–30% (5,7). Secondary prevention trials reveal a risk reduction of similar magnitude (4,8,9), and aggressive intervention (greater lipid lowering) is associated with even further reduction in risk (8,10).

Statins are among the most commonly prescribed drugs in the industrialized world, and there are seven statins currently available within this class. The first statin to be approved by the US Food and Drug Administration was lovastatin in 1987, followed by simvastatin, 1988; pravastatin, 1991; fluvastatin, 1994; atorvastatin, 1997; rosuvastatin, 2003; and pitavastatin, 2009 (11,12). One additional agent, cerivastatin, was released in 1998 but was subsequently withdrawn from the market due to increased frequency of muscle toxicity. Between 1998 and 2001, 40 reported cases of muscle toxicity due to cerivastatin use were fatal (13).

Skeletal muscle toxicity is the primary adverse drug reaction (ADR) associated with this class of drugs (14,15). Over the past two decades, statin use has expanded dramatically, and statin-induced muscle toxicity is becoming more fully characterized (12,16,17). The clinical presentation of this ADR varies widely, from mild myalgias (focal or diffuse) to rhabdomyolysis (severe skeletal muscle damage accompanied by acute kidney injury). In the context of clinical practice, statin-induced myotoxicity is diagnosed based upon two variables: muscle pain and circulating levels of a relatively non-specific muscle enzyme, creatine kinase (CK). CK level is often used as a marker for severity (14,15). Because CK levels can occasionally be elevated in the absence of pain, accurate risk prediction models are needed for preventing rhabdomyolysis.

Even in the absence of elevated circulating CK levels, myalgias can be accompanied by measurable decrements in muscle strength, and these functional changes have been accompanied by histological evidence of sarcomere disruption (18). Ultrastructural studies in experimental animal models typically show mitochondrial disruption (Figure 67.2). Similar findings have been reported in humans by Troseid and colleagues (19), who studied four related patients with statin-induced myalgias in the context of normal serum CK levels. Two of the four subjects had electromyographic findings suggestive of skeletal muscle pathology, accompanied by histological evidence for mitochondrial changes. A third subject had similar findings, although milder and non-diagnostic. In all subjects evaluated in this case series, the myalgias resolved clinically following cessation of the statin (19).

Overall Event Frequency

The literature currently supports at least four diagnostic strata, based solely upon CK level: (1) *intermediate myotoxicity*, defined as CK above upper limit of normal (ULN) but less than three-fold ULN; (2) *incipient myopathy*, defined as CK above three-fold ULN but less than 10-fold ULN; (3) *myopathy*, defined as CK above 10-fold ULN but less than 50-fold ULN; and (4) *rhabdomyolysis*, defined as CK above 50-fold ULN. As noted above, it is important to recognize that these strata are only weakly associated with myopathic symptoms (20). Due to this phenotypic heterogeneity, it has been difficult to quantify the true frequency of statin-related muscle damage. Although systematic reviews have attempted to survey the problem, randomized clinical trials often

Muscle. DOI: http://dx.doi.org/10.1016/B978-0-12-381510-1.00067-3

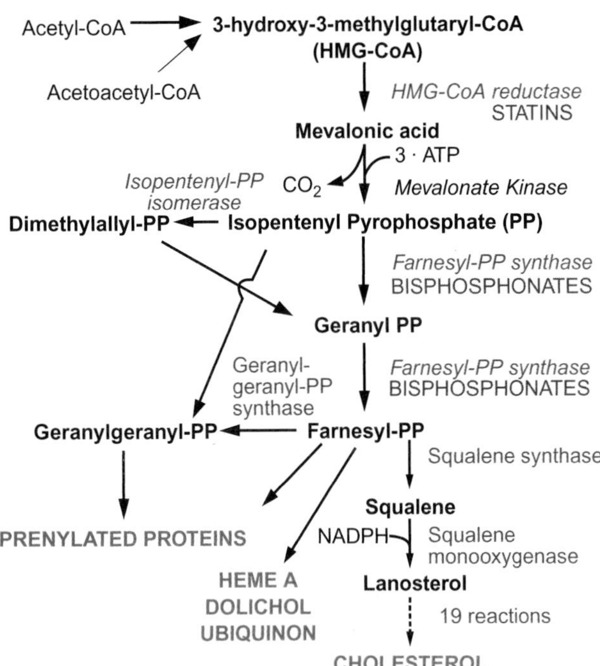

FIGURE 67.1 Cholesterol synthesis pathway/pharmacodynamic pathway of statin metabolism. *(Reproduced under the terms of the GNU Free Documentation License, Version 1.2 or any later version published by the Free Software Foundation, http://www.gnu.org/copyleft/)*

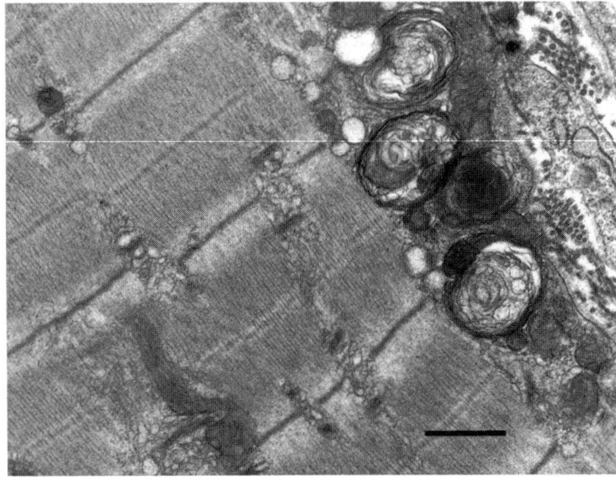

FIGURE 67.2 **Rosuvastatin-induced ultrastructural changes in type II muscle fiber.** Early ultrastructural changes in type II muscle fiber from the biceps femoris of a rosuvastatin-dosed rat (150 mg/kg/day for two weeks). Enlarged degenerating mitochondria are present in subsarcolemmal areas. Other components of the sarcoplasm show no abnormalities. Bar = 1 μm. *(Reproduced by permission of SAGE Publications. Westwood FR, Scott RC, Marsden AM, Bigley A, Randall K. Toxicologic Pathology 36(2):345–52. Copyright © 2008 by Society of Toxicologic Pathology.)*

underestimate the frequency of this ADR because patients with symptoms of intolerance are typically excluded during the run-in period (21,22). Frequency estimates derived from databases maintained by regulatory agencies (e.g., FDA) also tend to underestimate the problem because such event-reporting is voluntary (23). As such, large observational databases linked to electronic medical records may represent the most accurate way of quantifying statin-induced muscle toxicity within the community (Figure 67.3) (24).

Mild myalgias related to statin use are quite common (25). In the context of statin monotherapy, myalgias have been reported to occur at a frequency of approximately 1% (16), and this number approaches 10% in the context of specific concomitant medications (discussed later). Myalgias accompanied by elevation in serum CK level occur at a much lower frequency (26,27). The Health Improvement Network (THIN) and MediPlus databases report an annual incidence approaching 700 per million exposed per year for intermediate myotoxicity (28). If the definition of myotoxicity is restricted to include an elevation in CK level > 10-fold ULN (true myopathy), the frequency appears to be 0.1% or less for all currently available statins (17,26,29). Event rates appear to be similar for atorvastatin and rosuvastatin, the two most potent agents within the class (30). Event rates also appear to be dose-dependent (20,25,27).

Rhabdomyolysis represents the most severe and potentially lethal form of this ADR (14,15), and many clinicians consider an elevation in serum CK level > 50-fold ULN both necessary and sufficient to make the diagnosis. For research purposes, Graham and colleagues have published a now widely accepted step-wise approach for the identification of muscle toxicity cases in hospitalized patients (based on procedural codes for hospital admission, discharge diagnoses and clinical laboratory data beyond CK level) (31). When applied to the medical records of more than 250,000 statin-exposed patients, this algorithm generated combined myopathy and rhabdomyolysis rates of 0.000044 events per person-year (31). Similar rates have been observed for more than 100,000 first-time statin users followed in the United Kingdom over a course of 20 months (32).

Factors Influencing Severity

Statin-induced muscle toxicity is dose-dependent. McClure and colleagues quantified the frequency of this ADR in one of the largest managed care populations in the United States (27). Using a relatively stringent definition of "myopathy" (CK level ≥ 10,000 Units per liter, plus a relevant ICD-9 diagnostic code), they observed that the incidence rate for myotoxicity was roughly 10-fold higher in patients on high-dose statin therapy (i.e., defined as a dose equivalent to 40 mg of lovastatin daily

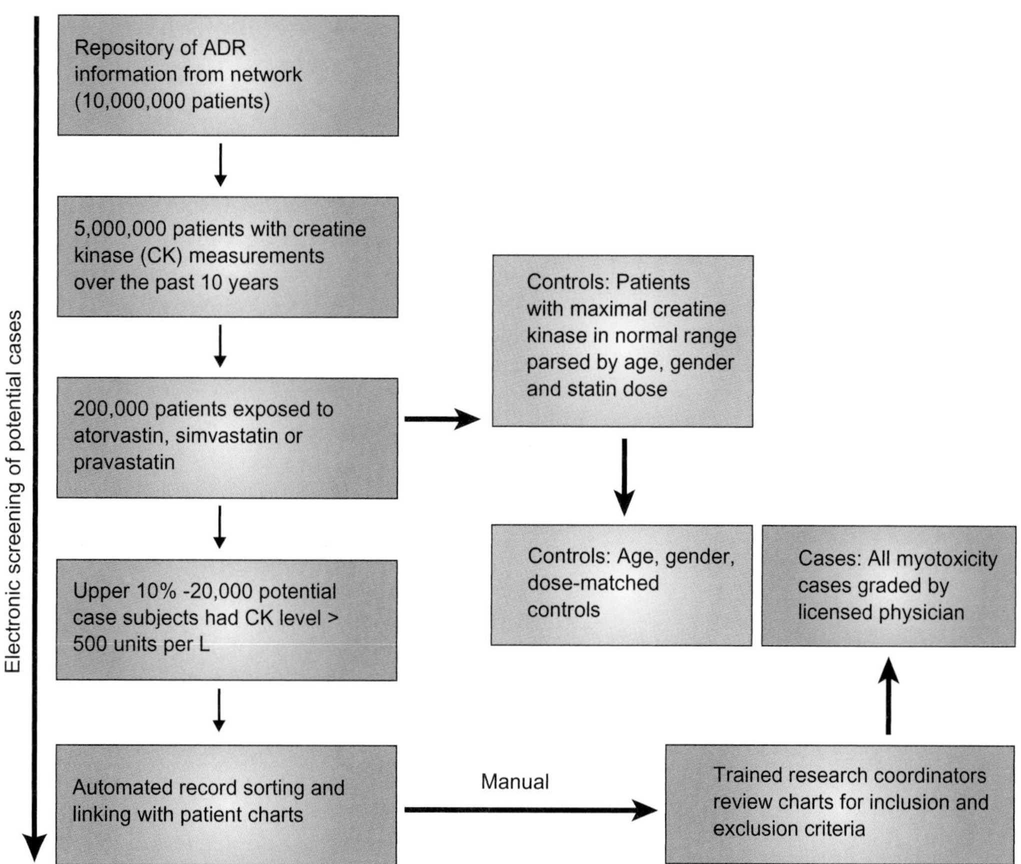

FIGURE 67.3 **An example of automated screening for statin adverse drug reaction cases.** In this example of automated case screening, a search of a comprehensive electronic medical record (EMR) database resulted in 5,000,000 patients with creatine kinase (CK) measurements and 200,000 of those patients were exposed to statins. These cases include 20,000 patients with elevated CK levels (over 500 units/per liter), which were subsequently screened for inclusion and exclusion criteria by trained research coordinators and, lastly, by a physician content expert. Age and gender matched controls can be selected in a similar fashion. *(Reprinted from Wilke et al. (24) by permission of Nature Publishing Group, © 2008.)*

or greater). A recent meta-analyses of four large randomized trials (10,33–35) also revealed a 10-fold increased risk of myopathy associated with intensive statin treatment (36). Because simvastatin is often prescribed at higher doses than other statins, it has been associated with a slightly higher incidence of myotoxicity (37). This observation has been replicated in an independent clinical practice-based cohort (20). From the records of nearly 2,000,000 unique individuals served by a single comprehensive system of care, 213 validated cases of statin-induced muscle toxicity were enrolled in a population-based study of genetic risk determinants (www.pharmgkb.org/contributors/pgrn/parc_profile.jsp). Within this observational cohort, the relationship between simvastatin dose and severity of myotoxicity was dose-dependent (20).

The clinical severity of this ADR is also increased by co-morbid liver or kidney disease (27,38). In their initial assessment of dose–response, McClure and colleagues also observed that the relative risk for statin-related muscle toxicity was 4.3 (95% CI = 1.5–13) in the context of liver disease and 2.5 (95% CI = 1.3–5.0) in the context of kidney disease (27). This increased risk is thought to be due to perturbations in the clearance of parent drug and/or statin metabolite (reviewed in detail below) (38–41). Additional clinical risk determinants include advanced age, small body mass index, Asian ancestry, female gender, metabolic co-morbidities (e.g., hypothyroidism), and vigorous physical exercise (20,24). Even in the absence of statin exposure (i.e., in healthy volunteers on no medications), strenuous exercise can increase circulating CK level to more than 4,000 Units/liter, an effect that remains evident 96 hours after exercise (42). A large fraction of statin ADRs are preceded by exercise or skeletal muscle trauma.

PHARMACOKINETIC FACTORS

Oxidation (Phase I Metabolism)

The clinical severity of statin-induced muscle toxicity is also influenced by drug–drug interactions, particularly

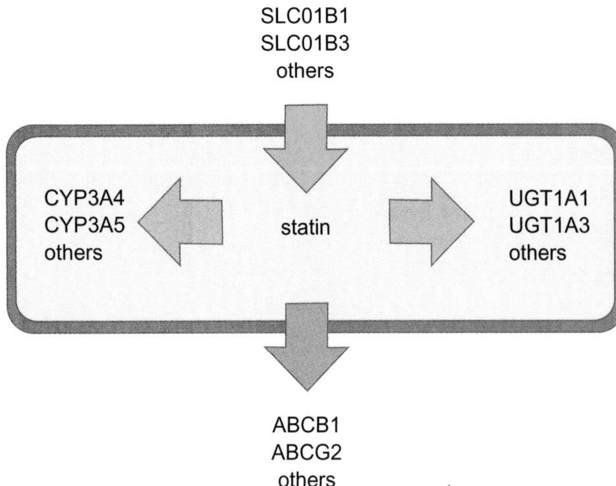

FIGURE 67.4 Statin disposition. A general cellular schematic highlights several pharmacokinetic candidate gene products impacting uptake, oxidation, conjugation, and efflux of statins.

within the context of agents altering statin disposition (absorption, distribution, metabolism, and elimination, ADME) (Figure 67.4) (43). Pharmacokinetic handling of statins differs on a drug-by-drug basis (44). For example, while many statins undergo a great deal of phase I oxidation (atorvastatin, fluvastatin, lovastatin, simvastatin), the impact of phase I oxidation on others (pitavastatin, pravastatin, rosuvastatin) is very limited (45). Correspondingly, drugs known to inhibit cytochrome P450 (CYP) enzyme activity (e.g., CYP3A inhibitors such as the macrolide antibacterials or azole antifungals) have been associated with increased myotoxicity severity for many of the statins (46). Within the FDA's Adverse Event Reporting System (AERS) database, there are 38.4 cases of rhabdomyolysis for every 10 million simvastatin users simultaneously exposed to a CYP3A4 inhibitor, compared to only 6 cases for every 10 million patients using simvastatin alone (47). No such discrepancy was observed in the same database for pravastatin, a drug that is known to be excreted through renal mechanisms.

Genetic variability in phase I oxidation also appears to influence the severity of this ADR (48). In a small retrospective observational cohort study, a splice variant in CYP3A5 was associated with the degree of CK elevation. However, the strength of the association was dependent on the presence or absence of concomitant medications known to interact with statins through mechanisms other than phase I oxidation (48). Many statins undergo additional modification through phase II conjugation by isoforms of the UDP-glucuronosyltransferase-1 (UGT1) family, a process that can be disrupted by concomitant administration of fibric acid (49).

Conjugation (Phase II Metabolism)

Following oxidative phase I drug metabolism, many statins form hydroxyl intermediates (e.g., atorvastatin is converted to 2-OH atorvastatin and 4-OH atorvastatin (50)). These hydroxy-statin derivatives then undergo further modification, through UGT1-dependent processes (Figure 67.4) (49). Gemfibrozil, a commonly prescribed fibric acid derivative, is known to alter the kinetic handling of a variety of statins (31). For example, by inhibiting the glucuronidation of simvastatin hydroxy acid (51), gemfibrozil is known to attenuate the biliary excretion of simvastatin and place patients at increased risk for development of statin-related muscle toxicity.

It is therefore tempting to speculate that genetic variability in the UGT1 enzyme family would contribute to myopathy risk as well. The entire family of UGT1 gene products (UGT1A1-12) is derived from the same locus. Different exons 1, are combined with four common exons 2–5, and polymorphisms (particularly promoter variants) at this locus have been associated with clinical outcome in the context of cancer drugs (52). Since experiments conducted using human liver microsomes reveal that common variants in UGT1A3 alter the lactonization of atorvastatin (53), studies are now under way to determine if these variants influence the severity of atorvastatin-induced myopathy in a clinical practice-based setting (www.PharmGKB.org).

Cellular Uptake

As noted earlier, cerivastatin was withdrawn from the market a decade ago, due to a high rate of skeletal muscle toxicity, a risk profile driven in part by a pharmacokinetic interaction with gemfibrozil at the level of UGT1A1. Statins also interact with gemfibrozil at the level of cellular uptake (54–56). Organic anion transporting polypeptide OATP-1B1 (gene name SLCO1B1) facilitates the hepatic uptake of most statins. Other relevant hepatic uptake transporters include OATP1B3, OATP2B1, OATP1A2, and the sodium-dependent taurocholate co-transporting polypeptide, NTCP (57,58). Genetic variability in membrane transport clearly influences statin-related clinical outcome. Polymorphisms in candidate solute transporter genes are associated with the altered hepatic uptake of simvastatin (59) and pravastatin (60). Much of this variability can be attributed to two coding variants in the SLCO1B1 gene, Asn130Asp and Val174Ala (61).

One of the most widely cited examples of a successful genome-wide association study (GWAS) within the field of pharmacogenomics has involved the characterization of this gene. In 2008, the SEARCH Collaborative Group applied a 317 K SNP scan to 85 cases of incipient myopathy and 90 frequency-matched drug exposed controls, to identify markers of muscle toxicity specifically within the context of high dose simvastatin (80 mg daily) (62). A single variant survived statistical correction for multiple testing: a base substitution in the SLCO1B1 gene (62). After genomic re-sequencing of SLCO1B1, the putative causative allele (Val174Ala) was retested for association in a subset of definite myopathy cases from the original study cohort, revealing an odds ratio for myopathy of 4.5 per copy of the variant allele (95% CI = 2.6–7.7) (62).

This association has since been replicated in four independent study populations (62–65). In HPS, 24 cases of incipient myopathy were identified in 10,269 participants receiving primary prevention with a lower dose of simvastatin (40 mg daily); 21 were genotyped retrospectively for the variant identified in SEARCH (62), and the relative risk was 2.6 per copy of the variant allele (95% CI = 1.3–5.0). In a practice-based setting, where the definition of intolerance includes discontinuation of the drug for any reason, the relative risk appears to be closer to 1.5 (63–65). Efforts are now being made to move this pharmacogenetic association into routine clinical practice through the application of novel decision-support mechanisms (66).

Cellular Efflux

As shown in Figure 67.4, other transporters can also influence the development and severity of statin-induced muscle toxicity. Many statins are substrates for efflux transporters such as multidrug resistance protein MDR1 (gene name ABCB1) or multidrug resistance-associated protein MRP2 (gene name ABCC2) (67). Located on the canalicular membrane of hepatocytes, these ATP-binding cassette proteins mediate the final step in hepatobiliary clearance of statins. It therefore seems plausible (and in fact likely) that variability in the activity of these transporters would alter the course of statin-related clinical events. The pharmacokinetics of most statins are markedly altered by changes in the activity of ABCG2 (68,69). This is particularly true for atorvastatin and rosuvastatin, the two most potent drugs in the class (68,69). Because a common variant in ABCG2 (Gln141Lys) is known to affect its transporter function *in vitro* (70), risk prediction models are being developed for assessment of this variant in the clinical arena (70).

Given the fact that drug half-life is strongly associated with both statin efficacy and toxicity, any factor that influences the disposition of these drugs – uptake, oxidation, conjugation, and efflux – would conceivably alter the severity of statin-induced skeletal muscle toxicity. Yet, this only represents part of the story (i.e., what the body does to the drug). To fully understand the risk mechanism and risk determinants underlying this clinically important ADR, one must also consider pharmacodynamic factors (i.e., what the drug does to the body). The final section of this chapter surveys these factors, and explores ongoing efforts to understand them further.

PHARMACODYNAMIC FACTORS

Cholesterol Synthesis

Statins inhibit HMGCR and reduce the production of mevalonic acid, a critical step in cholesterol biosynthesis. Because cholesterol is a key determinant of cell membrane fluidity, it is conceivable that statins directly disturb membrane stability. Support for this claim comes from the observation that fibrates (71,72) and niacin (73) can also cause myotoxicity. It is unlikely, however, that alterations in membrane fluidity alone are sufficient to induce this ADR. Although patients with inborn errors of metabolism within the cholesterol biosynthetic pathway have been shown to have very low cholesterol levels, they do not appear to develop myopathy (74).

As shown in Figure 67.1, mevalonic acid is an early intermediate in this linear biosynthetic pathway (2), and many distal intermediates are known to impact important cellular functions. All are attenuated by the inhibition of HMGCR. After the generation of mevalonic acid, the pathway subsequently produces geranyl pyrophosphate (10 carbons), farnesyl pyrophosphate (15 carbons), and geranylgeranyl pyrophosphate (20 carbons). The isoprenoid side chains of these biosynthetic intermediates can transfer farnesyl or geranyl moieties to C-terminal cysteine(s) of target proteins, through a process call protein prenylation. There are three enzymes that carry out prenylation within the cell: farnesyl transferase, CAAX protease, and methyl transferase (75). Farnesyl transferase inhibitors have been shown to modulate apoptosis (discussed further below). The observation that the inhibition of cholesterol biosynthesis distal to these critical isoprenoid intermediates (e.g., at the level of squalene synthase) can lower cholesterol without causing myotoxicity underscores the importance of prenylation (76).

Mitochondrial Dysfunction

Because prenylation is necessary for synthesizing the side chain within ubiquinone (coenzyme Q10), statins may disturb the integrity of electron transport within the mitochondria (Figure 67.1). The claim that mitochondrial dysfunction is responsible for statin-related myopathy is further supported by extensive pathological evidence (18,77,78). Vladutiu and colleagues have demonstrated that 52% of muscle biopsies from patients with statin-related myalgias reveal mitochondrial abnormalities, and 31% of these biopsies revealed multiple defects (78). Similar observations have been published independently by Gambelli and colleagues (77). It has also been reported that high-dose simvastatin decreases skeletal muscle mitochondrial DNA (79).

Skeletal muscle biopsies have also been used to assess mitochondrial respiratory chain enzyme activity in statin-treated subjects (80). For simvastatin, respiratory chain enzyme activity was reduced even though these patients had normal serum CK levels and no myalgias. It is therefore tempting to speculate that subtle changes in mitochondrial function occur very early in the development of myotoxicity. As noted above, isoprenoids derived from mevalonic acid are necessary for the production of coenzyme Q10. Because cellular deprivation of this critical component in the mitochondrial electron transport system is likely to disrupt oxidative phosphorylation, some investigators have advocated for co-administration of coenzyme Q10 in patients taking statins (81). The efficacy of such an approach remains unclear, in part because the clinical trials testing this hypothesis have been of very limited sample size. While at least one randomized controlled trial suggested a 40% reduction in the severity of pain for patients taking supplemental coenzyme Q10 (versus patients talking supplemental vitamin E) (82), this trial involved only 32 individuals, and two subsequent trials of similar size and design failed to find any benefit in terms of pain reduction (83), hepatic transaminases or serum CK levels (81).

Although statins appear to lower serum levels of endogenous coenzyme Q10 (84), serum levels are not consistently associated with levels of coenzyme Q10 in skeletal muscle (80,85,86). Again, this effect may be dose-dependent. While levels of coenzyme Q10 within skeletal muscle appear to increase in response to low dose simvastatin (10 mg daily) (86), high dose simvastatin (80 mg daily) appears to decrease levels (80). It is conceivable that subclinical perturbations in the maintenance of mitochondrial electron transport do not become clinically evident until challenged with exogenous drug. Two variants in COQ2, a gene product involved in the production of coenzyme Q10, are more common in myopathy cases than controls (87).

Apoptosis

As noted above, inhibitors of protein prenylation have been shown to modulate apoptosis. Because statins also attenuate protein prenylation (by decreasing the pool of available isoprenoid substrates), it seems likely that statin-induced skeletal muscle damage may be partly attributable to the activation of programmed cell death. Statin-induced apoptosis has been demonstrated in various relevant cell culture model systems, including myotubes (88), myoblasts (89,90), and differentiated primary human skeletal muscle cells (91). Statins also induce apoptosis in cancer cells (92), although epidemiological data reported to date have not consistently revealed a reduction in cancer incidence (or death) in subjects exposed to statins in clinical trials (93).

Multiple statins have been shown to induce apoptosis in a novel myotube culture model (measured by caspase-3 activation and TUNEL nuclei staining), through a mechanism that appears to be independent of statin structure (i.e., not related to partition coefficient) (88). This effect can be reproduced by geranylgeranyl transferase inhibitors, and rescued by replacement of mevalonic acid (88). Because statins clearly induce apoptosis at concentrations that suppress the prenylation of Rap1a (a 21kD GTPase and substrate for geranylation), statin-induced apoptosis in skeletal muscle may be transduced via altered prenylation of critical signaling proteins (88).

Small G-proteins, such as Rho (89) and Rab (94), require prenylation to optimally function in signal transduction. They are involved in a wide range of signaling pathways, including mitogen-activated protein kinase (MAPK) signaling. After treating myoblasts with simvastatin or fluvastatin, Itagaki and colleagues reported an apoptotic cell death accompanied by redistribution of small G-proteins, an effect that can be reproduced by treating the myoblasts with a selective Rho inhibitor (95). Changes in geranylation also alter expression of atrogin-1, an important molecular marker during the early muscle atrophy process (96,97). The importance of this protein in the maintenance of skeletal muscle integrity is underscored by the observation that atrogin-1 knockout mice are resistant to muscle atrophy following denervation (98).

Systems biology (network-based) approaches are therefore being developed to further characterize *integration* of the mechanisms leading to apoptosis in skeletal muscle following statin exposure. Gene-expression data are being combined with lipidomic data to identify candidate pathways that warrant further study (i.e., rather than candidate genes) (2,99,100). Regression of lipidomic data on gene expression data for pathway-based signaling networks (multiple genes in combination, based upon prior expert knowledge in annotated databases) has confirmed the involvement of lipid-derived signaling pathways (e.g., prostanoid biosynthesis), and suggested a role for Ca^{2+}-dependent pathways known to modulate apoptosis (e.g., phospholipase C) (99,100). Similar studies conducted in statin-treated patients exposed to vigorous physical exercise have documented altered expression of genes involved in protein folding and apoptosis (101), highlighting the importance of environment in this specific ADR.

Outlook

Mild myalgias occur in up to 10% of patients exposed to statins, but the occurrence of rhabdomyolysis is extremely rare. Both phenotypes are clinically relevant. Rhabdomyolysis represents the most severe form of statin-induced skeletal muscle toxicity, and it can be life-threatening. In the absence of severe muscle toxicity, myalgias can still impact clinical outcome, particularly if patients opt to discontinue statin therapy altogether (14,15). Statins are highly efficacious in reducing atherosclerotic coronary artery disease, and nonadherence to therapy has unequivocally been shown to increase morbidity and mortality in patients who discontinue their use (102). Insight into the molecular mechanisms underlying statin-induced muscle complications will allow the development and implementation of accurate risk prediction models for myopathy.

REFERENCES

1. Mangravite LM, Wilke RA, Zhang J, Krauss RM. Pharmacogenomics of statin response. *Curr Opin Mol Ther* 2008;**10**:555–61.
2. Wilke RA, Mareedu RK, Moore JH. The pathway less traveled: moving from candidate genes to candidate pathways in the analysis of genome-wide data from large scale pharmacogenetic association studies. *Curr Pharmacogenomics Person Med* 2008;**6**:150–9.
3. The Lipid Research Clinics Coronary Primary Prevention. Trial results. I. Reduction in incidence of coronary heart disease. *JAMA* 1984;**251**:351–64.
4. Scandinavian Simvastatin Survival Study Group. Randomised trial of cholesterol lowering in 4444 patients with coronary heart disease: the Scandinavian Simvastatin Survival Study (4S). *Lancet* 1994;**344**:1383–9.
5. Shepherd J, Cobbe SM, Ford I, Isles CG, Lorimer AR, MacFarlane PW, et al. Prevention of coronary heart disease with pravastatin in men with hypercholesterolemia. West of scotland coronary prevention study group. *N Engl J Med* 1995;**333**:1301–7.
6. Yee HS, Fong NT. Atorvastatin in the treatment of primary hypercholesterolemia and mixed dyslipidemias. *Ann Pharmacother* 1998;**32**:1030–43.
7. Ridker PM, Danielson E, Fonseca FA, Genest J, Gotto Jr AM, Kastelein JJ, et al. Rosuvastatin to prevent vascular events in men and women with elevated C-reactive protein. *N Engl J Med* 2008;**359**:2195–207.
8. Baigent C, Blackwell L, Emberson J, Holland LE, Reith C, Bhala N, *et al.* Efficacy and safety of more intensive lowering of LDL cholesterol: a meta-analysis of data from 170,000 participants in 26 randomised trials. *Lancet*; **376**:1670–81.
9. Baigent C, Keech A, Kearney PM, Blackwell L, Buck G, Pollicino C, et al. Efficacy and safety of cholesterol-lowering treatment: prospective meta-analysis of data from 90,056 participants in 14 randomised trials of statins. *Lancet* 2005;**366**:1267–78.
10. LaRosa JC, Grundy SM, Waters DD, Shear C, Barter P, Fruchart JC, et al. Intensive lipid lowering with atorvastatin in patients with stable coronary disease. *N Engl J Med* 2005;**352**:1425–35.
11. Ahmad H, Cheng-Lai A. Pitavastatin: a new HMG-CoA reductase inhibitor for the treatment of hypercholesterolemia. *Cardiol Rev*; **18**:264–7.
12. Tobert JA. Lovastatin and beyond: the history of the HMG-CoA reductase inhibitors. *Nat Rev Drug Discov* 2003;**2**:517–26.
13. Ballantyne CM, Corsini A, Davidson MH, Holdaas H, Jacobson TA, Leitersdorf E, et al. Risk for myopathy with statin therapy in high-risk patients. *Arch Intern Med* 2003;**163**:553–64.
14. Thompson PD, Clarkson PM, Rosenson RS. An assessment of statin safety by muscle experts. *Am J Cardiol* 2006;**97**:69C–76C.
15. McKenney JM, Davidson MH, Jacobson TA, Guyton JR. Final conclusions and recommendations of the national lipid association statin safety assessment task force. *Am J Cardiol* 2006;**97**:89C–94C.
16. Thompson PD, Clarkson P, Karas RH. Statin-associated myopathy. *JAMA* 2003;**289**:1681–90.
17. Waters DD. Safety of high-dose atorvastatin therapy. *Am J Cardiol* 2005;**96**:69F–75F.
18. Phillips PS, Haas RH, Bannykh S, Hathaway S, Gray NL, Kimura BJ, et al. Statin-associated myopathy with normal creatine kinase levels. *Ann Intern Med* 2002;**137**:581–5.
19. Trøseid M, Henriksen OA, Lindal S. Statin-associated myopathy with normal creatine kinase levels. Case report from a Norwegian family. *Apmis* 2005;**113**:635–7.
20. Mareedu RK, Modhia FM, Kanin EI, Linneman JG, Kitchner T, McCarty CA, et al. Use of an electronic medical record to characterize cases of intermediate statin-induced muscle toxicity. *Prev Cardiol* 2009;**12**:88–94.
21. Harper CR, Jacobson TA. The broad spectrum of statin myopathy: from myalgia to rhabdomyolysis. *Curr Opin Lipidol* 2007;**18**:401–8.
22. Psaty BM, Vandenbroucke JP. Opportunities for enhancing the FDA guidance on pharmacovigilance. *JAMA* 2008;**300**:952–4.
23. Law M, Rudnicka AR. Statin safety: a systematic review. *Am J Cardiol* 2006;**97**:52C–60C.
24. Wilke RA, Lin DW, Roden DM, Watkins PB, Flockhart D, Zineh I, et al. Identifying genetic risk factors for serious adverse drug reactions: current progress and challenges. *Nat Rev Drug Discov* 2007;**6**:904–16.
25. Bruckert E, Hayem G, Dejager S, Yau C, Begaud B. Mild to moderate muscular symptoms with high-dosage statin therapy in hyperlipidemic patients – the PRIMO study. *Cardiovasc Drugs Ther* 2005;**19**:403–14.
26. Chan J, Hui RL, Levin E. Differential association between statin exposure and elevated levels of creatine kinase. *Ann Pharmacother* 2005;**39**:1611–6.
27. McClure DL, Valuck RJ, Glanz M, Murphy JR, Hokanson JE. Statin and statin-fibrate use was significantly associated with increased myositis risk in a managed care population. *J Clin Epidemiol* 2007;**60**:812–8.
28. Molokhia M, McKeigue P, Curcin V, Majeed A. Statin induced myopathy and myalgia: time trend analysis and comparison of risk associated with statin class from 1991–2006. *PLoS ONE* 2008;**3**:e2522.
29. Pasternak RC, Smith SC, Bairey-Merz CN, Grundy SM, Cleeman JI, Lenfant C. ACC/AHA/NHLBI clinical advisory on the use and safety of statins. *Circulation* 2002;**106**:1024–8.
30. Wlodarczyk J, Sullivan D, Smith M. Comparison of benefits and risks of rosuvastatin versus atorvastatin from a meta-analysis of

head-to-head randomized controlled trials. *Am J Cardiol* 2008;**102**:1654–62.
31. Graham DJ, Staffa JA, Shatin D, Andrade SE, Schech SD, La Grenade L, et al. Incidence of hospitalized rhabdomyolysis in patients treated with lipid-lowering drugs. *JAMA* 2004;**292**:2585–90.
32. Garcia-Rodriguez LA, Masso-Gonzalez EL, Wallander MA, Johansson S. The safety of rosuvastatin in comparison with other statins in over 100,000 statin users in UK primary care. *Pharmacoepidemiol Drug Saf* 2008;**17**:943–52.
33. Cannon CP, Braunwald E, McCabe CH, Rader DJ, Rouleau JL, Belder R, et al. Intensive versus moderate lipid lowering with statins after acute coronary syndromes. *N Engl J Med* 2004;**350**:1495–504.
34. de Lemos JA, Blazing MA, Wiviott SD, Lewis EF, Fox KA, White HD, et al. Early intensive vs a delayed conservative simvastatin strategy in patients with acute coronary syndromes: phase Z of the A to Z trial. *JAMA* 2004;**292**:1307–16.
35. Pedersen TR, Faergeman O, Kastelein JJ, Olsson AG, Tikkanen MJ, Holme I, et al. High-dose atorvastatin vs usual-dose simvastatin for secondary prevention after myocardial infarction: the IDEAL study: a randomized controlled trial. *JAMA* 2005;**294**:2437–45.
36. Silva M, Matthews ML, Jarvis C, Nolan NM, Belliveau P, Malloy M, et al. Meta-analysis of drug-induced adverse events associated with intensive-dose statin therapy. *Clin Ther* 2007;**29**:253–60.
37. Backes JM, Howard PA, Ruisinger JF, Moriarty PM. Does simvastatin cause more myotoxicity compared with other statins? *Ann Pharmacother* 2009;**43**:2012–20.
38. Kasiske BL, Wanner C, O'Neill WC. An assessment of statin safety by nephrologists. *Am J Cardiol* 2006;**97**:82C–5C.
39. Bottorff MB. Statin safety and drug interactions: clinical implications. *Am J Cardiol* 2006;**97**:27C–31C.
40. Sica DA, Gehr TW. 3-Hydroxy-3-methylglutaryl coenzyme A reductase inhibitors and rhabdomyolysis: considerations in the renal failure patient. *Curr Opin Nephrol Hypertens* 2002;**11**:123–33.
41. Singhvi SM, Pan HY, Morrison RA, Willard DA. Disposition of pravastatin sodium, a tissue-selective HMG-CoA reductase inhibitor, in healthy subjects. *Br J Clin Pharmacol* 1990;**29**:239–43.
42. Yamin C, Amir O, Sagiv M, Attias E, Meckel Y, Eynon N, et al. ACE ID genotype affects blood creatine kinase response to eccentric exercise. *J Appl Physiol* 2007;**103**:2057–61.
43. Wilke RA, Reif DM, Moore JH. Combinatorial pharmacogenetics. *Nat Rev Drug Discov* 2005;**4**:911–8.
44. Kirchheiner J, Brockmoller J. Clinical consequences of cytochrome P450 2C9 polymorphisms. *Clin Pharmacol Ther* 2005;**77**:1–16.
45. Neuvonen PJ, Niemi M, Backman JT. Drug interactions with lipid-lowering drugs: mechanisms and clinical relevance. *Clin Pharmacol Ther* 2006;**80**:565–81.
46. Mazzu AL, Lasseter KC, Shamblen EC, Agarwal V, Lettieri J, Sundaresen P. Itraconazole alters the pharmacokinetics of atorvastatin to a greater extent than either cerivastatin or pravastatin. *Clin Pharmacol Ther* 2000;**68**:391–400.
47. Rowan C, Brinker AD, Nourjah P, Chang J, Mosholder A, Barrett JS, et al. Rhabdomyolysis reports show interaction between simvastatin and CYP3A4 inhibitors. *Pharmacoepidemiol Drug Saf* 2009;**18**:301–9.
48. Wilke RA, Moore JH, Burmester JK. Relative impact of CYP3A genotype and concomitant medication on the severity of atorvastatin-induced muscle damage. *Pharmacogenet Genomics* 2005;**15**:415–21.
49. Jemal M, Ouyang Z, Chen BC, Teitz D. Quantitation of the acid and lactone forms of atorvastatin and its biotransformation products in human serum by high-performance liquid chromatography with electrospray tandem mass spectrometry. *Rapid Commun Mass Spectrom* 1999;**13**:1003–15.
50. Bullen WW, Miller RA, Hayes RN. Development and validation of a high-performance liquid chromatography tandem mass spectrometry assay for atorvastatin, ortho-hydroxy atorvastatin, and para-hydroxy atorvastatin in human, dog, and rat plasma. *J Am Soc Mass Spectrom* 1999;**10**:55–66.
51. Prueksaritanont T, Tang C, Qiu Y, Mu L, Subramanian R, Lin JH. Effects of fibrates on metabolism of statins in human hepatocytes. *Drug Metab Dispos* 2002;**30**:1280–7.
52. Perera MA, Innocenti F, Ratain MJ. Pharmacogenetic testing for uridine diphosphate glucuronosyltransferase 1A1 polymorphisms: are we there yet? *Pharmacotherapy* 2008;**28**:755–68.
53. Riedmaier S, Klein K, Hofmann U, Keskitalo JE, Neuvonen PJ, Schwab M, et al. UDP-glucuronosyltransferase (UGT) polymorphisms affect atorvastatin lactonization in vitro and in vivo. *Clin Pharmacol Ther* 2010;**87**:65–73.
54. Davidson MH. Controversy surrounding the safety of cerivastatin. *Expert Opin Drug Saf* 2002;**1**:207–12.
55. Schneck DW, Birmingham BK, Zalikowski JA, Mitchell PD, Wang Y, Martin PD, et al. The effect of gemfibrozil on the pharmacokinetics of rosuvastatin. *Clin Pharmacol Ther* 2004;**75**:455–63.
56. Shitara Y, Hirano M, Sato H, Sugiyama Y. Gemfibrozil and its glucuronide inhibit the organic anion transporting polypeptide 2 (OATP2/OATP1B1:SLC21A6)-mediated hepatic uptake and CYP2C8-mediated metabolism of cerivastatin: analysis of the mechanism of the clinically relevant drug-drug interaction between cerivastatin and gemfibrozil. *J Pharmacol Exp Ther* 2004;**311**:228–36.
57. Matsushima S, Maeda K, Kondo C, Hirano M, Sasaki M, Suzuki H, et al. Identification of the hepatic efflux transporters of organic anions using double-transfected Madin-Darby canine kidney II cells expressing human organic anion-transporting polypeptide 1B1 (OATP1B1)/multidrug resistance-associated protein 2, OATP1B1/multidrug resistance 1, and OATP1B1/breast cancer resistance protein. *J Pharmacol Exp Ther* 2005;**314**:1059–67.
58. Ho RH, Tirona RG, Leake BF, Glaeser H, Lee W, Lemke CJ, et al. Drug and bile acid transporters in rosuvastatin hepatic uptake: function, expression, and pharmacogenetics. *Gastroenterology* 2006;**130**:1793–806.
59. Pasanen MK, Neuvonen M, Neuvonen PJ, Niemi M. SLCO1B1 polymorphism markedly affects the pharmacokinetics of simvastatin acid. *Pharmacogenet Genomics* 2006;**16**:873–9.
60. Mwinyi J, Johne A, Bauer S, Roots I, Gerloff T. Evidence for inverse effects of OATP-C (SLC21A6) 5 and 1b haplotypes on pravastatin kinetics. *Clin Pharmacol Ther* 2004;**75**:415–21.
61. Niemi M. Transporter pharmacogenetics and statin toxicity. *Clin Pharmacol Ther* 2010;**87**:130–3.
62. Link E, Parish S, Armitage J, Bowman L, Heath S, Matsuda F, et al. SLCO1B1 variants and statin-induced myopathy – a genomewide study. *N Engl J Med* 2008;**359**:789–99.

63. Voora D, Shah SH, Spasojevic I, Ali S, Reed CR, Salisbury BA, et al. The SLCO1B1*5 genetic variant is associated with statin-induced side effects. *J Am Coll Cardiol* 2009;**54**:1609–16.
64. Donnelly LA, Doney AS, Tavendale R, Lang CC, Pearson ER, Colhoun HM, et al. Common nonsynonymous substitutions in SLCO1B1 predispose to statin intolerance in routinely treated individuals with type 2 diabetes: a go-DARTS study. *Clin Pharmacol Ther* 2011;**89**:210–6.
65. Peters BJM. Methodological approaches to the pharmacogenomics of statins. Thesis, Utrecht University 2010. ISBN/EAN 978-90-8559-277-8.
66. Wilke RA, Xu H, Denny JC, Roden DM, Krauss RM, McCarty CA, et al. The emerging role of electronic medical records in pharmacogenomics. *Clin Pharmacol Ther* 2011;**89**:379–86.
67. Ho RH, Kim RB. Transporters and drug therapy: implications for drug disposition and disease. *Clin Pharmacol Ther* 2005;**78**:260–77.
68. Keskitalo JE, Zolk O, Fromm MF, Kurkinen KJ, Neuvonen PJ, Niemi M. ABCG2 polymorphism markedly affects the pharmacokinetics of atorvastatin and rosuvastatin. *Clin Pharmacol Ther* 2009;**86**:197–203.
69. Keskitalo JE, Pasanen MK, Neuvonen PJ, Niemi M. Different effects of the ABCG2 c.421C > A SNP on the pharmacokinetics of fluvastatin, pravastatin and simvastatin. *Pharmacogenomics* 2009;**10**:1617–24.
70. Robey RW, To KK, Polgar O, Dohse M, Fetsch P, Dean M, Bates SE. ABCG2: a perspective. *Adv Drug Deliv Rev* 2009;**61**:3–13.
71. Langer T, Levy RI. Acute muscular syndrome associated with administration of clofibrate. *N Engl J Med* 1968;**279**:856–8.
72. Smals AG, Beex LV, Kloppenborg PW. Clofibrate-induced muscle damage with myoglobinuria and cardiomyopathy. *N Engl J Med* 1977;**296**:942.
73. Gharavi AG, Diamond JA, Smith DA, Phillips RA. Niacin-induced myopathy. *Am J Cardiol* 1994;**74**:841–2.
74. Baker SK, Tarnopolsky MA. Statin-associated neuromyotoxicity. *Drugs Today (Barc)* 2005;**41**:267–93.
75. Maurer-Stroh S, Eisenhaber F. Refinement and prediction of protein prenylation motifs. *Genome Biol* 2005;**6**:R55.
76. Flint OP, Masters BA, Gregg RE, Durham SK. Inhibition of cholesterol synthesis by squalene synthase inhibitors does not induce myotoxicity in vitro. *Toxicol Appl Pharmacol* 1997;**145**:91–8.
77. Gambelli S, Dotti MT, Malandrini A, Mondelli M, Stromillo ML, Gaudiano C, et al. Mitochondrial alterations in muscle biopsies of patients on statin therapy. *J Submicrosc Cytol Pathol* 2004;**36**:85–9.
78. Vladutiu GD, Simmons Z, Isackson PJ, Tarnopolsky M, Peltier WL, Barboi AC, et al. Genetic risk factors associated with lipid-lowering drug-induced myopathies. *Muscle Nerve* 2006;**34**:153–62.
79. Schick BA, Laaksonen R, Frohlich JJ, Paiva H, Lehtimaki T, Humphries KH, et al. Decreased skeletal muscle mitochondrial DNA in patients treated with high-dose simvastatin. *Clin Pharmacol Ther* 2007;**81**:650–3.
80. Paiva H, Thelen KM, Van Coster R, Smet J, De Paepe B, Mattila KM, et al. High-dose statins and skeletal muscle metabolism in humans: a randomized, controlled trial. *Clin Pharmacol Ther* 2005;**78**:60–8.
81. Mabuchi H, Nohara A, Kobayashi J, Kawashiri MA, Katsuda S, Inazu A, et al. Effects of CoQ10 supplementation on plasma lipoprotein lipid, CoQ10 and liver and muscle enzyme levels in hypercholesterolemic patients treated with atorvastatin: a randomized double-blind study. *Atherosclerosis* 2007;**195**:e182–189.
82. Caso G, Kelly P, McNurlan MA, Lawson WE. Effect of coenzyme q10 on myopathic symptoms in patients treated with statins. *Am J Cardiol* 2007;**99**:1409–12.
83. Young JM, Florkowski CM, Molyneux SL, McEwan RG, Frampton CM, George PM, et al. Effect of coenzyme Q(10) supplementation on simvastatin-induced myalgia. *Am J Cardiol* 2007;**100**:1400–3.
84. Tomasetti M, Alleva R, Solenghi MD, Littarru GP. Distribution of antioxidants among blood components and lipoproteins: significance of lipids/CoQ10 ratio as a possible marker of increased risk for atherosclerosis. *Biofactors* 1999;**9**:231–40.
85. Laaksonen R, Jokelainen K, Laakso J, Sahi T, Harkonen M, Tikkanen MJ, et al. The effect of simvastatin treatment on natural antioxidants in low-density lipoproteins and high-energy phosphates and ubiquinone in skeletal muscle. *Am J Cardiol* 1996;**77**:851–4.
86. Laaksonen R, Jokelainen K, Sahi T, Tikkanen MJ, Himberg JJ. Decreases in serum ubiquinone concentrations do not result in reduced levels in muscle tissue during short-term simvastatin treatment in humans. *Clin Pharmacol Ther* 1995;**57**:62–6.
87. Oh J, Ban MR, Miskie BA, Pollex RL, Hegele RA. Genetic determinants of statin intolerance. *Lipids Health Dis* 2007;**6**:7.
88. Johnson TE, Zhang X, Bleicher KB, Dysart G, Loughlin AF, Schaefer WH, et al. Statins induce apoptosis in rat and human myotube cultures by inhibiting protein geranylgeranylation but not ubiquinone. *Toxicol Appl Pharmacol* 2004;**2004**:237–50.
89. Matzno S, Yasuda S, Juman S, Yamamoto Y, Nagareya-Ishida N, Tazuya-Murayama K, et al. Statin-induced apoptosis linked with membrane farnesylated Ras small G protein depletion, rather than geranylated Rho protein. *J Pharm Pharmacol* 2005;**57**: 1475–84.
90. Mutoh T, Kumano T, Nakagawa H, Kuriyama M. Involvement of tyrosine phosphorylation in HMG-CoA reductase inhibitor-induced cell death in L6 myoblasts. *FEBS Lett* 1999;**444**:85–9.
91. Sacher J, Weigl L, Werner M, Szegedi C, Hohenegger M. Delineation of myotoxicity induced by 3-hydroxy-3-methylglutaryl CoA reductase inhibitors in human skeletal muscle cells. *J Pharmacol Exp Ther* 2005;**314**:1032–41.
92. Graaf MR, Richel DJ, van Noorden CJ, Guchelaar HJ. Effects of statins and farnesyltransferase inhibitors on the development and progression of cancer. *Cancer Treat Rev* 2004;**30**:609–41.
93. Kuoppala J, Lamminpää A, Pukkala E. Statins and cancer: a systematic review and meta-analysis. *Eur J Cancer* 2008;**44**:2122–32.
94. Sakamoto K, Honda T, Yokoya S, Waguri S, Kimura J. Rab-small GTPases are involved in fluvastatin and pravastatin-induced vacuolation in rat skeletal myofibers. *FASEB J* 2007;**21**:4087–94.
95. Itagaki M, Takaguri A, Kano S, Kaneta S, Ichihara K, Satoh K. Possible mechanisms underlying statin-induced skeletal muscle toxicity in L6 fibroblasts and in rats. *J Pharmacol Sci* 2009;**109**:94–101.
96. Hanai JI, Cao P, Tanksale P, Imamura S, Koshimizu E, Zhao J, et al. The muscle-specific ubiquitin ligase atrogin-1/MAFbx mediates statin-induced muscle toxicity. *J Clin Invest* 2007;**117**:3940–51.

97. Cao P, Hanai J, Tanksale P, Imamura S, Sukhatme VP, Lecker SH. Statin-induced muscle damage and atrogin-1 induction is the result of a geranylgeranylation defect. *FASEB J* 2009;**23**:2844–54.
98. Bodine SC, Latres E, Baumhueter S, Lai VK, Nunez L, Clarke BA, et al. Identification of ubiquitin ligases required for skeletal muscle atrophy. *Science* 2001;**294**:1704–8.
99. Laaksonen R. On the mechanisms of statin-induced myopathy. *Clin Pharmacol Ther* 2006;**79**:529–31.
100. Laaksonen R, Katajamaa M, Paiva H, Sysi-Aho M, Saarinen L, Junni P, et al. A systems biology strategy reveals biological pathways and plasma biomarker candidates for potentially toxic statin-induced changes in muscle. *PLoS ONE* 2006;**1**:e97.
101. Urso ML, Clarkson PM, Hittel D, Hoffman EP, Thompson PD. Changes in ubiquitin proteasome pathway gene expression in skeletal muscle with exercise and statins. *Arterioscler Thromb Vasc Biol* 2005;**25**:2560–6.
102. Caro J, Klittich W, McGuire A, Ford I, Pettitt D, Norrie J, et al. International economic analysis of primary prevention of cardiovascular disease with pravastatin in WOSCOPS. West of scotland coronary prevention study. *Eur Heart J* 1999;**20**:263–8.

Chapter 68

Myotonic Dystrophy

Charles Thornton
Department of Neurology, University of Rochester, Rochester, NY

Myotonic dystrophy (dystrophia myotonica, DM) is a dominantly inherited degenerative disease affecting skeletal, cardiac, and smooth muscle. DM is one of the commonest hereditary muscle disorders that causes major disability and premature death [estimated frequency in European populations is 1 in 7,400 to 9,400 (1,2)]. The median survival is to age 55, mainly limited by respiratory failure or cardiac arrhythmia (3). The disorder was first described in 1909 by the German clinician Steinert, who described the core features of myotonia, weakness, and muscle wasting (1). In 1918 Fleischer observed that some parents or grandparents of DM1-affected individuals had premature cataracts as the sole manifestation – the first example in human genetics of anticipation, in which genetic disease becomes more severe in successive generations (4,5). Owing to anticipation, the symptoms of DM1 are extremely variable in affected members of a family. The genetic basis for myotonic type 1 (DM1) was revealed by the 1992 discovery of an unstable expansion of CTG repeats in the 3′ untranslated region of the *dystrophia myotonica protein kinase* (*DMPK*) gene (6). A second form of DM was recognized in 1994, when genetic analysis revealed that a subset of individuals who carried the diagnosis did not have the DM1 mutation (7,8). DM type 2 (DM2) was subsequently shown to result from an unstable expansion of tandem repeats at a different locus, involving a CCTG tetramer repeat in the first intron of *zinc finger 9 (ZNF9)*. Studies in both types of DM have shown that the synthesis of RNA with an expanded repeat has a deleterious effect. These disorders provided the first example of RNA dominance, in which mutant RNA exerts a toxic gain-of-function. In additional to muscle symptoms, both types of DM are multisystem diseases that lead to cataracts, gonadal atrophy, premature balding, and CNS effects. However, this chapter will focus on pathophysiology of the muscle component.

GENETICS AND MECHANISM OF REPEAT EXPANSION

The human genome contains 1.1 million simple tandem repeats (STRs) in which di-, tri-, or tetra-nucleotide repeat sequences are arranged in head-to-tail arrays (9). The number of STRs is much greater than expected by chance alone, suggesting that they provide a selective advantage or that a mechanism exists for propagating them in the genome. Because of their repetitive nature, STRs are inherently prone to replication slippage during DNA synthesis (10,11). Most slippage errors are recognized and correctly repaired by proteins in the mismatch repair pathway. However, errors that are not repaired result in extension or contraction of a repeat tract by one or more units (12). By this mechanism STRs have mutation frequencies that are elevated 10^2- to 10^5-fold above the genomic background, with longer repeats having higher frequencies (13,14). In the absence of selective pressure, STR mutability will inevitably lead to the generation of allelic series, in which a spectrum of different repeat lengths is observed at a particular locus in the general population. For STRs that lie within genes or regulatory regions, these differences may have subtle effects on gene function (15). One potential role of STRs, therefore, is to engineer flexibility into the genome at particular sites, consisting of changes in repeat length, with functional consequences that are modulatory rather than catastrophic. Flexibility of this type may confer the benefits of rapid adaptation and increased evolvability (15,16).

The putative advantages of STRs, however, may come at the expense of diseases associated with unstable repeat expansions (UREs). DM1, DM2, and more than 15 other genetic disorders are caused by STRs that become highly expanded and extremely unstable. This behavior is only exhibited by a tiny fraction of STRs, suggesting that the transition from STR to URE is conditioned by local features of the genome landscape. Studies of population genetics suggest that UREs arise from uncommon mutational events in which "large normal" STRs, having more than 20 repeats, expand to an abnormal range, with more than 40 or 50 repeats (17). Having reached this size, and depending on the specific biophysical properties of the repeat sequence, the nascent URE may then become highly unstable. Most UREs involve CTG:CAG or CCG:CGG repeats, which are GC-rich sequences that exhibit a

Muscle. DOI: http://dx.doi.org/10.1016/B978-0-12-381510-1.00068-5

propensity to form hairpins of single-stranded DNA, stabilized by G•C and C•G basepairs in the hairpin stem (11). Formation of hairpins, as extra-helical loop-outs of repetitive DNA, is stimulated by processes that involve strand separation, such as DNA repair, DNA replication, or transcription. Current data suggest that the basic mechanism that drives instability of expanded repeats is the incorrect repair, by normal proteins in the mismatch repair pathway, of these looped-out structures. This counterintuitive concept is suggested by studies in which components of the mismatch repair pathway were eliminated. For example, ablation of mismatch repair proteins MSH2 or MSH3 had the expected effect of increasing the frequency of STR mutations throughout the genome, because replication slippage errors went unrepaired. However, at UREs the opposite effect was observed – expanded repeats were stabilized (18,19). The instability of UREs was also affected by transcription. Instability of CTG•CAG repeats was enhanced by transcription across the repeat tract in one direction (20), and further aggravated by transcription in both directions (21,22), a process known to occur at the DM1 locus in muscle cells (23). The coupling of transcription with incorrect DNA repair can produce CTG•CAG instability even in non-dividing cells (20), which presumably accounts for the remarkable instability of the DM1 expansion in skeletal and cardiac muscle. Individuals with classical DM1 typically inherit an allele with several hundred CTG repeats, but they go on to develop expansions of 2000–5000 repeats in skeletal muscle and heart, the tissues that express *DMPK* most highly (24–27).

In DM1, as in other repeat expansion disorders, the age of onset and disease severity depends on the size of the expanded repeat (28,29). Unaffected individuals have 5–37 CTG repeats in *DMPK*. Expansions of 50–100 CTG repeats are associated with mild disease and late-onset symptoms. Expansions of more than 1000 repeats are associated with severe disease that usually begins in utero (congenital DM1). Most DM1 mutations, however, lie between these extremes. For individuals with expansions of 100 to 600 repeats there is a rough correlation of repeat length with disease severity, but the predictive power of repeat size is relatively poor. Upon intergenerational transmission, the size of the expansion will typically increase by more than 100 CTG repeats in a single generation – the genetic event that underlies anticipation (29). It is important to note, however, that the correlations of repeat length with disease severity were established using DNA from circulating leukocytes, a tissue that is not representative of skeletal or cardiac muscle. Studies of skeletal or cardiac muscle have shown that expansions are 2- to 13-fold larger than those found in blood samples (24,25). Currently there are no studies that address the relationship between disease severity and expansion length in DNA from muscle tissue.

The length threshold for CCTG repeats causing DM2 is less well defined. Almost all affected individuals have more than 1000 CCTG repeats in *ZNF9*, the median repeat length is around 5000 repeats, and some individuals have expansions of more than 10,000 repeats (30). As in DM1, the expanded CCTG repeat is unstable in somatic cells, becoming larger in muscle than in peripheral blood (26).

In summary, the instability of the CTG repeat expansion results in extreme variability of the DM1 phenotype. The genetic circumstances that led to the initial expansion, which likely include bidirectional transcription and other as-yet-undiscovered features at the DM1 locus, cause ongoing CTG repeat instability in somatic cells throughout the life of an affected individual. Growth of the expansion can occur in non-dividing cells, and is particularly dramatic in skeletal muscle and heart, which may prove to be a key determinant of symptom onset and disease progression.

SKELETAL MUSCLE IN DM1

DM1 was initially recognized for its effects on skeletal muscle, the core features being muscle weakness, wasting, and delayed relaxation. Serum levels of creatine kinase (CK), a marker of sarcolemmal integrity, are normal or mildly elevated (less than 10-fold above normal). In contrast to other dystrophies, DM has little tendency to cause muscle contracture. The most common initial symptoms are muscle stiffness and delayed relaxation. Affected individuals typically report "locking up" of fingers when gripping the hand, or stiffness of the tongue and jaw when speaking or chewing – the symptoms of action myotonia. Action myotonia is most pronounced after a period of rest and then improves with continued muscle activity, the so-called "warm up" phenomenon. Myotonia does not occur in cardiac or smooth muscle.

Physiological studies have shown that muscle activation in DM1 triggers involuntary runs of action potentials, thereby distinguishing myotonia from other causes of delayed relaxation, such as ATP depletion or slowing of calcium reuptake. Myotonia can also be triggered by direct mechanical stimulation of muscle fibers ("percussion myotonia"), and it persists after neuromuscular blockade, proving that the repetitive action potentials are muscle-generated and independent of neural input. Myotonic discharges are also provoked by insertion of an extracellular recording electrode into muscle, which previously led to the use of electromyography (EMG) as a diagnostic test. The resulting electrical discharge shows a characteristic pattern of waxing and waning frequency, firing up to 80 Hz and lasting up to 30 seconds. In non-dystrophic hereditary myotonia, similar electrical discharges are caused by point mutations in genes encoding the *CLCN1* chloride channel or *SCN4* sodium channel (31,32). However, direct analysis of chloride conductance and sodium gating failed to show a consistent defect in DM1 muscle (33,34), which led to a concept that myotonia in DM1 results from changes in the membrane environment rather than a specific ion channel defect. As discussed below, resolution of this question awaited the generation of mouse models, which established the central role of *CLCN1* chloride channels.

Muscle weakness and wasting in DM1 is first apparent and most pronounced in the distal limbs, and in muscles of the face, tongue, and anterior neck. The selective vulnerability of these muscle groups is striking, in that limb-girdle muscles often display normal strength at a time when the ankle or finger movements are extremely weak. In the later stages, however, the proximal muscle groups are also affected. The selective pattern of muscle involvement, together with myotonia, is highly characteristic of DM1, making the clinical distinction from other forms of muscular dystrophy relatively straightforward. Weakness in DM1 generally appears proportional to muscle wasting, suggesting that it mainly results from loss of contractile units. However, in some individuals particular muscles may exhibit weakness that is disproportionate to wasting, raising the possibility of a concurrent defect of neuromuscular transmission or excitation–contraction coupling. Survival in DM1 is limited mainly by involvement of the oropharyngeal and respiratory muscles, especially the diaphragm.

The relationship between myotonia and weakness in DM1 is complex. In contrast to generalized myotonia in individuals who carry inactivating mutations in *CLCN1,* the myotonia in DM1 selectively involves specific muscle groups (35). In the upper limbs the myotonia is most prominent in the forearm and hand muscles, the same muscles that are preferentially affected by weakness. In those muscles the myotonia precedes weakness or develops concurrently with weakness. The association of grip myotonia with weakness has an important functional significance because the combined effect leads to marked impairment of manual dexterity, a major source of disability in this population. The combination may also have a mechanistic significance because repetitive action potentials may impose a mechanical or metabolic stress that accelerates the muscle degeneration. However, the distal leg muscles present a different picture, in which the progressive muscle wasting is not accompanied by action myotonia, although myotonic discharges can be detected by EMG. Yet another view emerges in congenital DM1, in which muscle weakness is present from birth although myotonia generally is not apparent until 4–10 years later (36). Finally, it is important to note that chloride channelopathy itself causes transient weakness as well as myotonia, because fibers are depolarized to the point of inexcitability (37). While transient weakness is conspicuous in individuals with inactivating mutations in *CLCN1* it is rarely observed in DM1 (38), presumably because residual chloride conductance is sufficient to maintain fiber excitability.

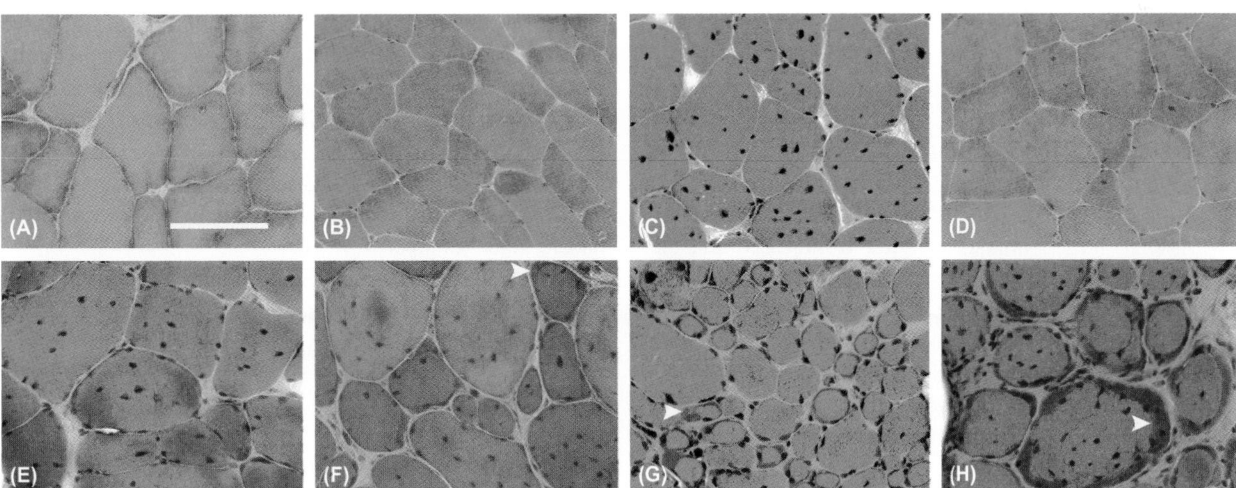

FIGURE 68.1 Frozen sections of tibialis anterior (TA) muscle from eight individuals with DM1, illustrating the variable extent of muscle histopathology. Sections are ordered from A to H according to increasing weakness of ankle dorsiflexion. Variable atrophy and hypertrophy of muscle fibers, central nucleation, and increased endomysial connective tissue is apparent. Arrows show sarcoplasmic masses. All images are displayed at the same magnification (bar in (A) = 100 μm). CTG repeat length, age, and weakness are as follows: (A) 90 repeats, 46 yrs, normal strength; (B) 37 years, 92 repeats, normal strength; (C) 41 years, 200 repeats, slight weakness; (D), 60 years, 140 repeats, slight weakness; (E) 52 years, 700 repeats, moderate weakness; (F) 52 years, 200 repeats, moderate weakness; (G) 30 years, 440 repeats, marked weakness; (H) 48 years, 820 repeats, marked weakness. Except for (A) and (B), all muscles showed active electromyographic myotonia.

The histopathology of DM1 shows muscle fiber atrophy and degeneration with little inflammation or cell necrosis (Figure 68.1). The earliest change is an increase in the overall number of myonuclei and central nuclei (39). While the pathophysiological basis for this finding is unknown, it implies an early effect on the regulation of myonuclear domains, the volume of cytoplasm served by single myonuclei. In the mid- to late stages the histologic picture is dominated by fiber atrophy and disorganization of cytoarchitecture. In some muscles there is selective atrophy of type I fibers, but this is not a constant feature (40). Commonly there are "nuclear clumps", fibers that contain numerous myonuclei but scant cytoplasm, and an increase of the endomysial connective tissue. The organization of myofibrils is severely affected, with areas of cytoplasm that are devoid of myofibrils (sarcoplasmic masses), or fibers in which myofibrils are mis-oriented, following a circular or spiral course (ring fibers).

Around 10% of affected individuals have congenital onset, associated with a phenotype that is qualitatively different from classical DM1 (41). The transmission of congenital DM1 (CDM) shows a strong parent-of-origin effect. Almost every case is inherited from an affected mother, which reflects gender differences in the dynamics of repeat instability. CDM is associated with large *DMPK* alleles, usually above 1000 repeats, and the generation of these large expansions is more likely during oogenesis than spermatogenesis (42,43). Mothers of infants with CDM usually report decreased fetal movement, indicating onset *in utero*. Reduced muscle tone is noted at birth. Oropharyngeal weakness causes difficulties with neonatal feeding, and later it interferes with development of speech. Affected infants may have respiratory insufficiency that requires temporary or long-term ventilatory support (44). The mortality in infancy is 25–40% (45,46). Histologic findings of reduced muscle fiber diameter, poor definition of fiber types, and chains of central nuclei suggested an arrest or slowing of muscle maturation (47–49). This concept was supported by observations that myoblasts isolated from CDM muscle displayed incomplete or delayed differentiation *in vitro* (50). Individuals who survive infancy will subsequently display functional gains, accompanied by histologic improvement, suggesting that maturation can finally be achieved. However, as teenagers these individuals will begin to develop the degenerative features of DM1.

SKELETAL MUSCLE IN DM2

The myotonic myopathy in DM2 is similar to DM1 in many respects, although the overall functional impairment is less severe. In limb muscles the weakness in DM2 is first apparent in proximal rather than distal muscles. The earliest and most affected muscles are in the shoulder and hip girdle, neck flexors, and elbow extensors. Muscle wasting is less conspicuous than in DM1, and there is less involvement of the cranial and respiratory muscles. The extent of myotonia is variable. In some individuals it is difficult to observe clinically or detect by EMG (30). When present, however, the myotonia can be more generalized than in DM1, often generating signs and symptoms in the trunk, legs, and arms. An important distinction is that DM2 is not associated with a congenital phenotype, and is not known to affect muscle development or myogenic differentiation (51,52). Histologic features of DM2 are similar to DM1, except that muscle atrophy selectively affects fibers expressing fast myosin heavy chain, and fiber hypertrophy is more prominent (53).

CARDIAC MUSCLE IN DM1

The cardiac conduction system is selectively vulnerable to the effects of DM1. Surface electrocardiograms (ECGs) show an increase of the PR interval or prolongation of QRS duration in 65% of affected individuals (54). Slowing can occur at any point along the conduction pathway but is most commonly localized to the His–Purkinje system (55). The effects on the conduction system are progressive over time, with an average increase of 5 msec/yr for the PR interval and 2 msec/yr for QRS duration (56). Eventually this can lead to atrioventricular block, resulting in severe bradycardia or asystole, complications that are largely preventable by insertion of a pacemaker (57). DM1 also predisposes to atrial and, less commonly, ventricular tachycardia (57). Cardiac dysrhythmia ranks second after respiratory failure among causes of death in DM1 (3). In a large prospective study the risk of sudden death was 1.1% per year in adults (56). Cardiac histology shows focal areas of fibrosis and fatty infiltration in the conduction system (58). However, it is not known whether these changes can account for the physiologic defect, or whether functional changes, perhaps resembling the chloride channelopathy in skeletal muscle, may be superimposed.

The effects of DM1 on cardiac contractility are much less profound. Conventional echocardiography has shown normal ventricular size and systolic function in most individuals (59,60). In a study of 406 affected individuals, 10% had clinically evident heart failure or echocardiographic changes suggesting left ventricular systolic dysfunction (LVSD) (61). The frequency of LVSD increased after age 40, reaching levels as high as 30% by the eighth decade.

CARDIAC MUSCLE IN DM2

Few studies have addressed the cardiac manifestations of DM2, but qualitatively the effects are similar to DM1.

Compared to DM1, individuals with DM2 were less likely to have major disease of the conduction system and more likely to have LVSD (62). In a group of 297 patients, four experienced sudden death prior to age 45 (63). On postmortem examination these individuals exhibited dilated cardiomyopathy and fibrosis of the conduction system.

PATHOPHYSIOLOGY OF DM

Four different pathogenic mechanisms, each involving a distinct biological effect of expanded repeats, have been proposed in DM. These are DNA toxicity, protein toxicity, RNA toxicity, and haploinsufficiency. Current evidence suggests that RNA toxicity is the predominant mechanism, reflecting a deleterious gain-of-function by transcripts having expanded repeats. Each mechanism will be discussed, with detailed consideration given to the RNA-mediated effects.

DNA Toxicity

Studies of cell models have shown that factors involved in sensing DNA damage are recruited to expanded CTG•CAG repeats, especially when there is bidirectional transcription or DNA replication across the repeat tract (21,64,65). These events lead to activation of signaling pathways indicative of DNA damage, such as phosphorylation of p53, causing growth arrest and apoptosis. These observations raise the possibility that in *DMPK*-expressing tissues the expanded repeat is a direct stimulus for chronic cellular stress, independent of its RNA or protein products. As yet, however, there is no evidence for activation of the DNA damage response in DM1 cells *in vivo*.

Protein Toxicity

Initial studies of repeat expansion disorders supported the concept that expansions in protein-coding-regions led to gain-of-function by mutant protein, whereas expansions in non-coding sequence led to gene silencing, RNA toxicity, or, in the case of DM1, both. More recently this distinction has begun to fray. Evidence was presented that coding-region expansions may lead to RNA as well as protein toxicity (66). However, the converse proposition, that the non-coding expansion in DM1 could give rise to protein toxicity, was not considered for the simple reason that the repeat expansion was located in the 3′ UTR. Since the expansion did not impact the processing of upstream exons (67), the only conceivable translation product was the wild-type DMPK protein. However, the possibility of protein toxicity must now be reconsidered in light of observations that translation can initiate within tracts of expanded CUG or CAG repeats, by a mechanism that resembles cap-independent translation initiation at internal ribosomal entry sequences (68). This process of repeat-associated, non-ATG-dependent (RAN) translation could potentially occur from the expanded CUG repeat of the *DMPK* sense transcript, or from the expanded CAG repeat in the antisense transcript. Depending on which strand and reading frame was translated, RAN translation could create homopolymeric proteins with polyglutamine, polyserine, polyalanine, polycysteine, or polyleucine tracts. Such proteins would likely be toxic but are difficult to detect, due to insolubility and paucity of epitopes. An initial study suggested that a small fraction of DM1 cardiomyocytes and circulating monocytes did indeed express proteins from RAN translation (68). However, it is also possible that the nuclear retention of transcripts with highly expanded repeats (discussed below) may largely protect against RAN translation. Studies of RAN translation are at an early stage and the significance of this mechanism for DM1 pathogenesis is presently unclear.

Haploinsufficiency of *DMPK* or *SIX5*

DM1 is associated with reduced expression of genes on 19q13.2, through *cis* effects on genes adjacent to the expanded repeat. The best-studied examples concern *DMPK* itself and its neighboring gene, *SIX5*. The effect on *DMPK* is posttranscriptional, due to nuclear retention of mRNA containing an expanded CUG repeat (69,70). The reduced translation of mutant mRNA is not compensated by upregulation of the wild-type allele, resulting in a 30–50% reduction of DMPK protein (71). By contrast, *SIX5* silencing is transcriptional and the mechanism is epigenetic (72,73). The position of the CTG repeat is immediately upstream from the regulatory elements that control *SIX5* expression (Figure 68.2). When expanded, the repeat triggers epigenetic changes in the *SIX5* enhancer-promoter, creating patterns of cytosine and histone methylation that are characteristic of heterochromatin (23). Similar epigenetic modifications and silencing effects have been observed when repetitive DNA sequences were inserted at other genomic sites (74). The epigenetic effect does not silence transcription of *DMPK* itself (67), whose promoter is 12 kilobases distant from the CTG repeat, suggesting that it may not act over long distances.

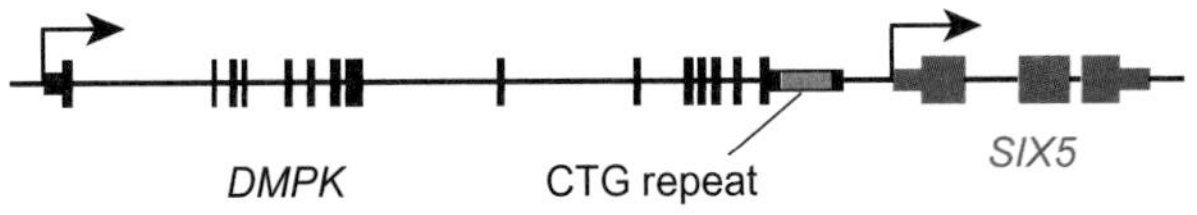

FIGURE 68.2 Scale diagram of the DM1 locus on chromosome 19, showing location of the expanded repeat in the final exon of *DMPK*, close to the 5′ end of *SIX5*.

While these *cis*-acting effects on gene expression have been documented in patient-derived cells and tissue, their role in DM1 pathogenesis remains unclear. DMPK is a serine–threonine kinase expressed mainly in skeletal, cardiac, and smooth muscle (6,75). DMPK isoforms are localized in the cytosol or associated with membranes, depending on alternative splicing at the carboxyl terminus (76). This kinase is expressed in myoblasts and muscle fibers, with highest levels of protein accumulation at the neuromuscular and myotendinous junction (77,78). In cardiac cells DMPK localizes to the intercalated disc (75). While the physiological substrates of this kinase have not been determined, several candidates have been identified (79). DMPK, like several other closely-related kinases, is able to modulate organization of the actomyosin cytoskeleton, thereby regulating cell motility, formation of stress fibers, and membrane trafficking (76,79,80).

The requirement of DMPK in striated muscle was evaluated by targeted deletion of the murine gene (81,82). Homozygous *Dmpk* knockout mice developed a mild, late-onset skeletal myopathy in sternomastoid (82), a muscle that is selectively affected in DM1. However, the histologic features did not closely resemble DM1, and the changes in limb muscle were subtle. The knockout mice did not exhibit myotonia or defects of neuromuscular transmission. Whereas sternomastoid force generation was normal in young *Dmpk*$^{-/-}$ mice, in older mice (8 to 11 months) the tetanic tension was reduced by 38% (82). However, muscle in the heterozygous knockout mice displayed normal histology and specific force. In cardiac muscle the *Dmpk* knockout mice developed progressive disease of the conduction system, occasionally leading to complete atrioventricular block (83). Similar to human DM1, the conduction defect was not accompanied by histologic or echocardiographic evidence of cardiomyopathy. However, in heterozygous knockout mice the conduction defect did not progress beyond mild prolongation of the PR interval (83). Absence of DMPK also caused a decrease of insulin signaling in cardiac and skeletal muscle (80). This effect was manifested by reduced recruitment of insulin receptor to the surface membrane, decreased glucose disposal, and failure of insulin stimulated translocation of the GLUT4 glucose transporter to the surface membrane. In summary, while the exact role and physiological substrates of DMPK are not fully defined, there are clear indications that this kinase is required for normal function of striated muscle. Most impressively, atrioventricular conduction is sensitive to DMPK gene dose, raising the possibility that haploinsufficiency may contribute to the cardiac features of human DM1. However, in the heterozygous knockout mice, which appear to be the most appropriate genetic model for DMPK reduction in DM1, studies of striated muscle have shown normal development, contractility, metabolism, and maintenance, suggesting that DMPK deficiency has a limited role, at most, in DM1 pathogenesis.

SIX5 encodes a homeodomain transcription factor expressed in striated muscle and many other tissues (84). Although CTG expansion causes silencing of the DM1-linked allele (72,73,85), the total (bi-allelic) level of SIX5 mRNA in DM1 muscle was normal in some (85,86) but not all studies (87), suggesting a mechanism for dosage compensation. Studies of *SIX5* knockout mice indicate that this factor is dispensable for muscle and cardiac development in rodents (88). Although heterozygous knockout mice displayed slight prolongation of QRS duration, this finding was only apparent on ECGs under general anesthesia (89). Thus, while CTG expansion causes allele-specific silencing of *SIX5*, there is little evidence that this contributes to the muscle phenotypes of DM1, though it may have relevance for the development of premature cataracts (72,90).

In summary, targeted inactivation of DM1 region genes has failed to reproduce DM1 in mice, except possibly in a fragmentary fashion. Furthermore, extensive genetic testing has failed to uncover a single instance in which deletion at 19q13.2, or any mutation other than repeat expansion, has produced a phenocopy or partial reproduction of DM1. Taken together, these observations argue that haploinsufficiency is not a key mechanism for DM1, though it may have a contributory role when coupled with gain-of-function by RNA, protein, or DNA.

Haploinsufficiency in DM2

ZNF9 regulates translation of specific mRNAs by binding to conserved elements in the 5′ UTR (91,92). Initial reports indicated that expansion of the intronic CCTG repeat had no effect on expression of *ZNF9* mRNA or protein (93,94). Even in rare individuals who were homozygous for the DM2 mutation, levels of ZNF9 expression were not reduced, and the clinical features were indistinguishable from heterozygotes (94,95). In cells from homozygotes the ZNF9 transcript was correctly processed and the RNA in nuclear foci was comprised purely of CCUG repeats, stripped of other sequences from the *ZNF9* locus, indicating that the retained RNA was a trapped decay intermediate of the excised intron (94). Furthermore, *ZNF9* knockout mice diplayed major CNS and cranial malformations (96), whereas developmental phenotypes are absent in DM2. Taken together, these findings supported the concept that phenotypic similarities of DM1 and DM2 reflected a shared RNA-mediated pathogenic mechanism, with little role for abnormal expression of ZNF9 protein (97). However, subsequent studies found decreased levels of ZNF9 protein in DM2 muscle cells, accompanied by an overall reduction of

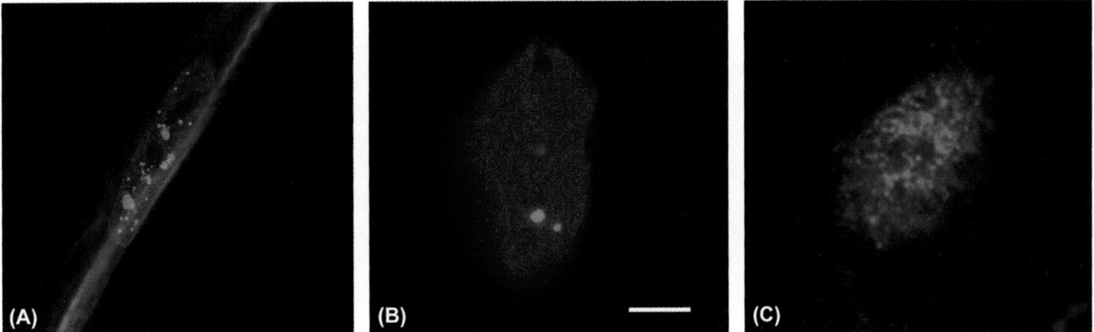

FIGURE 68.3 Nuclear foci of CUG^{exp} RNA and MBNL1 protein in muscle cells. (A) Fluorescence *in situ* hybridization showing nuclear foci of mutant DMPK mRNA (red) in the nucleus (blue) of a DM1 myotube. Myosin heavy chain is stained in green. (B,C) High powered views of single cardiomyocyte nuclei (blue) show sequestration of MBNL1 protein (green) in nuclear foci in postmortem DM1 cardiac muscle (B), as compared to diffuse MBNL1 distribution in a non-disease control (C). Images were obtained and thresholded under the same conditions.

protein synthesis, suggesting that muscle weakness results partly from global suppression of translation (92,98,99). The explanation for these discrepant findings is unclear. At this time the role of ZNF9 deficiency in DM2 remains an open question.

RNA Toxicity

Elements in the 3′ UTR are known to regulate stability, translation, and cytoplasmic localization of mRNA. To determine whether CUG repeats have such an activity the metabolic and biophysical properties of mutant *DMPK* mRNA were examined. Analysis of patient-derived cells and tissue showed that expanded repeats had no effect on the synthesis, processing, or stability of *DMPK* mRNA (67,69). However, cell fractionation studies and *in situ* hybridization revealed that mutant *DMPK* transcripts were quantitatively retained in the nucleus, where they accumulate in discrete foci (Figure 68.3A) (69,70,100). This abnormal metabolic behavior was a direct consequence of CUG expansion, because insertion of a CUG^{exp} tract in other transcripts induced the same effect (101,102). Moreover, expanded CUG repeats (CUG^{exp}), when synthesized *in vitro* and examined in the absence of binding proteins, had unusual biophysical properties. These sequences formed extended hairpins, in which the stem resembled a long RNA duplex that was stabilized by intramolecular C•G and G•C base pairing (103,104). The periodic U•U mismatch had a relatively minor effect on the stability or structure of the double-stranded RNA helix (105). As yet there is no conclusive evidence that CUG^{exp} tracts form hairpin structures *in vivo*, but their high stability makes it likely that they do so. These metabolic and structural features focused attention on the possibility that mutant *DMPK* transcripts may affect nuclear function. The discovery of nuclear CCUG-repeat foci in DM2 provided further evidence for RNA gain-of-function (97), the most parsimonious explanation for the phenotypic similarity from non-coding mutations in two unrelated genes. Other examples of RNA gain-of-function were subsequently uncovered, and interestingly all arise from unstable expansions of tandem repeats, leading to the designation of "RNA dominance" for this genetic mechanism (106).

Experimental support for RNA toxicity comes from studies of transgenic models that express CUG^{exp} RNA in myoblasts, mice, or flies (101,102,107–110). Across several studies, the major conclusion was that non-coding expansions of CUG repeats could inhibit myogenic differentiation and induce degenerative changes in several organs, including skeletal and cardiac muscle. The models exhibited hallmark features of DM1, such as myotonic myopathy (102,110), or, delay of cardiac conduction (109), arguing that RNA level effects were disease-specific. When physiological perturbations, such as chloride channelopathy, were observed in models and subsequently confirmed in human DM1 (111), this provided an additional layer of validation. While numerous models have been generated, notably absent is a model having targeted insertion of a highly expanded CTG repeat at the murine locus, or a model of any design that has fully replicated the multisystemic features of DM1, or even provided a full recapitulation in a single tissue. Nevertheless the current models have been useful for dissecting biochemical mechanisms and therapeutic development.

Current data suggest that the major molecular consequence of expressing CUG^{exp} RNA is to induce extensive alterations of the muscle transcriptome, comprising misregulation of alternative splicing and changes in the level of mRNA expression, that result from perturbations in the function of RNA binding proteins (112–115). The first protein shown to have CUG-repeat binding activity was designated CUG binding protein 1 (CUGBP1), a multifunctional protein that has diverse effects on alternative splicing, RNA decay, and translation (112,116–118). Although named for its ability to bind short CUG repeat fragments *in vitro*, subsequent studies have shown a stronger binding preference for other RNA sequences (118) and a relatively weak affinity for expanded CUG repeats (119–121). Presently there is no conclusive evidence that CUGBP1 interacts with mutant *DMPK* mRNA *in vivo*, nor does it colocalize with nuclear CUG- or CCUG-foci in cells (109,119,122–125), and its expression is not affected in DM2 (52,113). Nevertheless, this protein may have an important role in DM1 pathogenesis. CUGBP1 is upregulated in human DM1 muscle (126,127) and in some (109,110), but not all (102) CUG^{exp}-expressing mouse models. The mechanism for CUGBP1 upregulation is post-translational and is mediated by activation of protein kinase C (PKC), which leads to phosphorylation and stabilization of CUGBP1 (128). The stimulus for PKC activation is unknown, but this signaling event occurs within hours of inducing CUG^{exp} expression in mice (109). This effect was modeled by generating transgenic mice with overexpression of CUGBP1. Modest (two-fold) overexpression appeared to be well tolerated, but strong (eight-fold) overexpression resulted in cardiomyopathy (129) and extensive muscle degeneration (130).

A second group of RNA-binding proteins implicated in DM pathogenesis are homologs of the *Drosophila* muscleblind protein, required for muscle and retinal development in flies (131). The human Muscleblind-like (MBNL) proteins were initially isolated as the major CUG^{exp}-binding proteins in the mammalian nucleus (132). Of three family members, MBNL1 predominates in skeletal muscle and is best characterized, MBNL1 and MBNL2 are expressed in heart, and MBNL3 is expressed in muscle precursor cells (133). MBNL proteins regulate alternative splicing by binding to conserved sequence elements in primary transcripts (134). MBNL1, for example, represses the splicing of exons when it binds to the upstream intron, or promotes the inclusion of exons when it binds to the downstream intron (115,135). In rodent muscle MBNL1 orchestrates a group of splicing changes in the first three weeks of postnatal life, thereby contributing to the final steps of muscle and heart maturation (113,136). Other MBNL family members may function at earlier stages of muscle development, or in non-muscle tissue. Currently the functional distinctions among different MBNL proteins are unclear because in overexpression studies they exhibit overlapping specificities of target regulation (134). Although MBNL proteins have been studied mainly in the context of their splicing regulatory activity, these proteins are also distributed to the cytoplasm where they regulate stability and localization of mRNA (114,137) and biogenesis of microRNA (138).

In carrying out its splicing regulatory functions, MBNL1 recognizes conserved sequence elements having a YGCY sequence motif (where Y is a C or U) (115,135). The binding affinity is much greater for transcripts having two or more YGCA motifs in close proximity (135). As this motif is enormously reiterated in expanded CUG or CCUG repeats, the affinity of MBNL1 for mutant DM1 or DM2 RNA is very high (dissociation constant of 5 nM for CUG^{exp} RNA (139)). Furthermore, structural data indicate that MBNL1 has four RNA-binding domains, through which it can synchronously engage more than one YCGY motif (135,140). In the case of CUG^{exp} RNA, this property may lead to formation of cross-links between different transcripts. This possibility, coupled with observations that MBNL1 knockdown in DM1 cells leads to marked reduction of nuclear foci (141), suggests that the CUG^{exp}-MBNL1 interaction is in fact the primary molecular event that nucleates the formation of RNA foci. As a consequence, MBNL1 is recruited into foci so heavily that the levels of unbound protein in the nucleus are markedly depleted (Figure 68.3B,C) (113,125), raising the possibility that loss of MBNL1 function may contribute to symptoms of DM1 (132). Consistent with a sequestration model, homozygous MBNL1 knockout mice displayed DM1-like splicing alterations, myotonia, cataracts, and cardiac arrhythmia (142). In studies that directly compared the effects of CUG^{exp} expression or MBNL1 ablation in mice, more than 200 CUG^{exp}-induced splicing alterations were detected in muscle, of which > 80% could be attributed to MBNL1 sequestration, and several hundred non-splicing changes of gene expression were detected, of which more than 70% could be attributed to MBNL1 sequestration (113,115). However, while MBNL1 knockout mice exhibit histologic changes in muscle, the myopathy is not severe and the extent of fiber atrophy, hyper-nucleation, and disruption of myofibrillar architecture is much less than in human DM1 (142). Taken together these observations suggest that sequestration of MBNL1 is an important contributing factor but not a unitary explanation for the complex phenotype. At present there is less information about the functional consequences of MBNL2 or MBNL3 sequestration, or the combinatorial effects of losing several MBNL family members.

Considering that CUG^{exp} expression can modulate the function of several RNA binding proteins, each having its particular downstream consequences on gene expression, a major challenge has been to determine which alterations of the transcriptome are responsible for different aspects of the phenotype. The clearest example of a functional connection between misregulated splicing and physiological impairment relates to the pathogenesis of myotonia. Studies determined that myotonia in CUG^{exp}-expressing or MBNL1 knockout mice was associated with marked reduction of chloride conductance and CLCN1 chloride channels (111,143). Both models showed increased inclusion of CLCN1 alternative exon 7a (111), an exon normally repressed by MBNL1 (144). Inclusion of this exon leads to expression of truncated CLCN1 protein that has no ion channel activity (145). This same derangement was confirmed in DM1 and DM2 muscle (111,146). CLCN1 splicing was corrected in mouse models by viral-mediated overexpression of MBNL1 (147) or splice-shifting oligonucleotides that blocked the inclusion of exon 7a (148), resulting in complete elimination of the myotonia. Myotonia is therefore a discrete feature of DM, arising from sequestration of a specific splicing factor, that is rescued by correction of a single splicing defect. Evidence suggests that other endophenotypes of DM1 can result from abnormal regulation of other MBNL1 or CUGBP1 targets. Misregulated alternative splicing of the insulin receptor, resulting from upregulation of CUGBP1 and sequestration of MBNL1, may contribute to the insulin resistance that occurs in many people with DM1 (126). Altered splicing of bridging integrator-1 (BIN1), also a direct target of MBNL1 regulation, may contribute to weakness and changes in the morphology of the transverse tubule system (149). A particularly intriguing observation is that MBNL1 recognizes a YGCY element in the microRNA-1 (miR-1) precursor (138). This recognition event facilitates processing of the miR-1precursor by Dicer, which is necessary to generate functional microRNA. When MBNL1 is sequestered, the levels of miR-1 are reduced, and miR-1 targets, such as connexin43 and calcium channel $Ca_v1.2$, are upregulated in cardiomyocytes. This finding may have direct implications for cardiac conduction in DM1, because miR-1 knockout mice have sudden death and widening of the QRS complex (150). Whether metabolism of other microRNAs is similarly affected has not been determined.

Other mechanisms for RNA toxicity have been proposed. CUG^{exp} hairpins can be cleaved by Dicer, leading to short CUG fragments that may inhibit expression of genes containing CAG repeats (151). Expression of the toxic RNA was also associated with upregulation of transcription factor NKX2-5 in DM1 cardiac muscle (152). Finally, the mutant DMPK RNA was also reported to cause "leaching" of transcription factors from chromatin (153).

THERAPEUTIC IMPLICATIONS

Presently there is no treatment that can reverse DM or slow its progression. However, the elucidation of RNA toxicity has opened up several lines of therapeutic development. Targeting the mutant RNA with antisense oligonucleotides or antisense RNA has lead to impressive phenotypic correction in DM1 cells and mouse models (154–156). Significant progress has also been made in developing small molecules that inhibit CUG^{exp}-MBNL1 binding (157,158). Another promising strategy is to inhibit PKC activation, which ameliorates the CUGBP1 upregulation and cardiac phenotype in mouse models (159). Taken together, these initial studies suggest that DM may prove to be surprisingly reversible, and that RNA-mediated disease mechanisms may be unusually susceptible to therapeutic intervention.

REFERENCES

1. Harper PS. *Myotonic dystrophy*. London: W.B. Saunders; 2001.
2. Norwood FL, Harling C, Chinnery PF, Eagle M, Bushby K, Straub V. Prevalence of genetic muscle disease in Northern England: in-depth analysis of a muscle clinic population. *Brain* 2009;**132**:3175–86.
3. de Die-Smulders CE, Howeler CJ, Thijs C, Mirandolle JF, Anten HB, Smeets HJ, et al. Age and causes of death in adult-onset myotonic dystrophy. *Brain* 1998;**121**:1557–63.
4. Fleischer B. Uber myotonische dystrophie mit katarakt. *Albrecht von Graefes Arch Kin Exp Opthalmol* 1918;**96**:91–133.
5. Harper PS, Harley HG, Reardon W, Shaw DJ. Anticipation in myotonic dystrophy: new light on an old problem. *Am J Hum Genet* 1992;**51**:10–6.
6. Brook JD, McCurrach ME, Harley HG, Buckler AJ, Church D, Aburatani H, et al. Molecular basis of myotonic dystrophy: expansion of a trinucleotide (CTG) repeat at the 3′ end of a transcript encoding a protein kinase family member. *Cell* 1992;**68**:799–808.
7. Thornton CA, Griggs RC, Moxley RT. Myotonic dystrophy with no trinucleotide repeat expansion. *Ann Neurol* 1994;**35**:269–72.
8. Ricker K, Koch MC, Lehmann-Horn F, Pongratz D, Otto M, Heine R, et al. Proximal myotonic myopathy: a new dominant disorder with myotonia, muscle weakness, and cataracts. *Neurology* 1994;**44**:1448–52.
9. Kelkar YD, Tyekucheva S, Chiaromonte F, Makova KD. The genome-wide determinants of human and chimpanzee microsatellite evolution. *Genome Res* 2008;**18**:30–8.
10. Ellegren H. Microsatellites: simple sequences with complex evolution. *Nat Rev Genet* 2004;**5**:435–45.
11. Pearson CE, Nichol EK, Cleary JD. Repeat instability: mechanisms of dynamic mutations. *Nat Rev Genet* 2005;**6**:729–42.
12. Kruglyak S, Durrett RT, Schug MD, Aquadro CF. Equilibrium distributions of microsatellite repeat length resulting from a balance between slippage events and point mutations. *Proc Natl Acad Sci USA* 1998;**95**:10774–8.
13. Ellegren H. Heterogeneous mutation processes in human microsatellite DNA sequences. *Nat Genet* 2000;**24**:400–2.
14. Lynch M, Sung W, Morris K, Coffey N, Landry CR, Dopman EB, et al. A genome-wide view of the spectrum of spontaneous mutations in yeast. *Proc Natl Acad Sci USA* 2008;**105**:9272–7.
15. Vinces MD, Legendre M, Caldara M, Hagihara M, Verstrepen KJ. Unstable tandem repeats in promoters confer transcriptional evolvability. *Science* 2009;**324**:1213–6.
16. Fondon JW, Garner HR. Molecular origins of rapid and continuous morphological evolution. *Proc Natl Acad Sci USA* 2004;**101**:18058–63.

17. Martorell L, Monckton DG, Sanchez A, Lopez dM, Baiget M. Frequency and stability of the myotonic dystrophy type 1 premutation. *Neurology* 2001;**56**:328–35.
18. Manley K, Shirley TL, Flaherty L, Messer A. Msh2 deficiency prevents in vivo somatic instability of the CAG repeat in Huntington disease transgenic mice. *Nat Genet* 1999;**23**:471–3.
19. Savouret C, Brisson E, Essers J, Kanaar R, Pastink A, te Riele H, et al. CTG repeat instability and size variation timing in DNA repair-deficient mice. *EMBO J* 2003;**22**:2264–73.
20. Lin Y, Dion V, Wilson JH. Transcription promotes contraction of CAG repeat tracts in human cells. *Nat Struct Mol Biol* 2006;**13**:179–80.
21. Lin Y, Leng M, Wan M, Wilson JH. Convergent transcription through a long CAG tract destabilizes repeats and induces apoptosis. *Mol Cell Biol* 2010;**30**:4435–51.
22. Nakamori M, Pearson CE, Thornton CA. Bidirectional transcription stimulates expansion and contraction of expanded (CTG)* (CAG) repeats. *Hum Mol Genet* 2011;**20**:580–8.
23. Cho DH, Thienes CP, Mahoney SE, Analau E, Filippova GN, Tapscott SJ. Antisense transcription and heterochromatin at the DM1 CTG repeats are constrained by CTCF. *Mol Cell* 2005;**20**:483–9.
24. Ashizawa T, Dubel JR, Harati Y. Somatic instability of CTG repeat in myotonic dystrophy. *Neurology* 1993;**43**:2674–8.
25. Thornton CA, Johnson K, Moxley RT. Myotonic dystrophy patients have larger CTG expansions in skeletal muscle than in leukocytes. *Ann Neurol* 1994;**35**:104–7.
26. Nakamori M, Sobczak K, Moxley RT, Thornton CA. Scaled-down genetic analysis of myotonic dystrophy type 1 and type 2. *Neuromuscul Disord* 2009;**19**:759–62.
27. Zatz M, Passos-Bueno MR, Cerqueira A, Marie SK, Vainzof M, Pavanello RC. Analysis of the CTG repeat in skeletal muscle of young and adult myotonic dystrophy patients: when does the expansion occur? *Hum Mol Genet* 1995;**4**:401–6.
28. Harley HG, Rundle SA, MacMillan JC, Myring J, Brook JD, Crow S, et al. Size of the unstable CTG repeat sequence in relation to phenotype and parental transmission in myotonic dystrophy. *Am J Hum Genet* 1993;**52**:1164–74.
29. Redman JB, Fenwick Jr RG, Fu YH, Pizzuti A, Caskey CT. Relationship between parental trinucleotide GCT repeat length and severity of myotonic dystrophy in offspring. *JAMA* 1993;**269**:1960–5.
30. Day JW, Ricker K, Jacobsen JF, Rasmussen LJ, Dick KA, Kress W, et al. Myotonic dystrophy type 2: molecular, diagnostic and clinical spectrum. *Neurology* 2003;**60**:657–64.
31. Koch MC, Steinmeyer K, Lorenz C, Ricker K, Wolf F, Otto M, et al. The skeletal muscle chloride channel in dominant and recessive human myotonia. *Science* 1992;**257**:797–800.
32. Ptacek LJ, George Jr AL, Griggs RC, Tawil R, Kallen RG, Barchi RL, et al. Identification of a mutation in the gene causing hyperkalemic periodic paralysis. *Cell* 1991;**67**:1021–7.
33. Lipicky RJ, Rowland LP. Studies of human myotonic dystrophy. In: Rowland LP, editor. *Pathogenesis of Muscular Dystrophies*. Amsterdam: Excerpta Medica; 1977. p. 729–34.
34. Franke C, Hatt H, Iaizzo PA, Lehmann-Horn F. Characteristics of Na^+ channels and Cl- conductance in resealed muscle fibre segments from patients with myotonic dystrophy. *J Physiol* 1990;**425**:391–405.
35. Logigian EL, Ciafaloni E, Quinn LC, Dilek N, Pandya S, Moxley RT, et al. Severity, type, and distribution of myotonic discharges are different in type 1 and type 2 myotonic dystrophy. *Muscle Nerve* 2007;**35**:479–85.
36. Roig M, Balliu PR, Navarro C, Brugera R, Losada M. Presentation, clinical course, and outcome of the congenital form of myotonic dystrophy. *Pediatr Neurol* 1994;**11**:208–13.
37. Rudel R, Ricker K, Lehmann-Horn F. Transient weakness and altered membrane characteristic in recessive generalized myotonia (Becker). *Muscle Nerve* 1988;**11**:202–11.
38. Zwarts MJ, van Weerden TW. Transient paresis in myotonic syndromes. A surface EMG study. *Brain* 1989;**112**:665–80.
39. Vassilopoulos D, Lumb EM. Muscle nuclear changes in myotonic dystrophy. *Eur Neurol* 1980;**19**:237–40.
40. Brooke MH, Engel WK. The histographic analysis of human muscle biopsies with regard to fiber types. 3. Myotonias, myasthenia gravis, and hypokalemic periodic paralysis. *Neurology* 1969;**19**:469–77.
41. Dyken PR, Harper PS. Congenital dystrophia myotonica. *Neurology* 1973;**23**:465–73.
42. Jansen G, Willems P, Coerwinkel M, Nillesen W, Smeets H, Vits L, et al. Gonosomal mosaicism in myotonic dystrophy patients: involvement of mitotic events in (CTG)n repeat variation and selection against extreme expansion in sperm. *Am J Hum Genet* 1994;**54**:575–85.
43. De Temmerman N, Sermon K, Seneca S, De Rycke M, Hilven P, Lissens W, et al. Intergenerational instability of the expanded CTG repeat in the DMPK gene: studies in human gametes and preimplantation embryos. *Am J Hum Genet* 2004;**75**:325–9.
44. Campbell C, Sherlock R, Jacob P, Blayney M. Congenital myotonic dystrophy: assisted ventilation duration and outcome. *Pediatrics* 2004;**113**:811–6.
45. Reardon W, Newcombe R, Fenton I, Sibert J, Harper PS. The natural history of congenital myotonic dystrophy: mortality and long term clinical aspects. *Arch Dis Child* 1993;**68**:177–81.
46. Hageman AT, Gabreels FJ, Liem KD, Renkawek K, Boon JM. Congenital myotonic dystrophy; a report on thirteen cases and a review of the literature. *J Neurol Sci* 1993;**115**:95–101.
47. Karpati G, Carpenter S, Watters GV, Eisen AA, Andermann F. Infantile myotonic dystrophy. Histochemical and electron microscopic features in skeletal muscle. *Neurology* 1973;**23**:1066–77.
48. Farkas E, Tome FM, Fardeau M, Arsenio-Nunes ML, Dreyfus P, Diebler MF. Histochemical and ultrastructural study of muscle biopsies in 3 cases of dystrophia myotonica in the newborn child. *J Neurol Sci* 1974;**21**:273–88.
49. Sarnat HB, Silbert SW. Maturational arrest of fetal muscle in neonatal myotonic dystrophy. A pathologic study of four cases. *Arch Neurol* 1976;**33**:466–74.
50. Furling D, Lemieux D, Taneja K, Puymirat J. Decreased levels of myotonic dystrophy protein kinase (DMPK) and delayed differentiation in human myotonic dystrophy myoblasts. *Neuromuscul Disord* 2001;**11**:728–35.
51. Cardani R, Baldassa S, Botta A, Rinaldi F, Novelli G, Mancinelli E, et al. Ribonuclear inclusions and MBNL1 nuclear sequestration do not affect myoblast differentiation but alter gene splicing in myotonic dystrophy type 2. *Neuromuscul Disord* 2009;**19**:335–43.
52. Pelletier R, Hamel F, Beaulieu D, Patry L, Haineault C, Tarnopolsky M, et al. Absence of a differentiation defect in muscle satellite cells from DM2 patients. *Neurobiol Dis* 2009;**36**:181–90.

53. Vihola A, Bassez G, Meola G, Zhang S, Haapasalo H, Paetau A, et al. Histopathological differences of myotonic dystrophy type 1 (DM1) and PROMM/DM2. *Neurology* 2003;**60**:1854–7.
54. Groh WJ, Lowe MR, Zipes DP. Severity of cardiac conduction involvement and arrhythmias in myotonic dystrophy type 1 correlates with age and CTG repeat length. *J Cardiovasc Electrophysiol* 2002;**13**:444–8.
55. Lazarus A, Varin J, Ounnoughene Z, Radvanyi H, Junien C, Coste J, et al. Relationships among electrophysiological findings and clinical status, heart function, and extent of DNA mutation in myotonic dystrophy. *Circulation* 1999;**99**:1041–6.
56. Groh WJ, Groh MR, Saha C, Kincaid JC, Simmons Z, Ciafaloni E, et al. Electrocardiographic abnormalities and sudden death in myotonic dystrophy type 1. *N Engl J Med* 2008;**358**:2688–97.
57. Laurent V, Pellieux S, Corcia P, Magro P, Pierre B, Fauchier L, et al. Mortality in myotonic dystrophy patients in the area of prophylactic pacing devices. *Int J Cardiol* 2011;**150**:54–8.
58. Nguyen HH, Wolfe III JT, Holmes Jr DR, Edwards WD. Pathology of the cardiac conduction system in myotonic dystrophy: a study of 12 cases. *J Am Coll Cardiol* 1988;**11**:662–71.
59. Morner S, Lindqvist P, Mellberg C, Olofsson BO, Backman C, Henein M, et al. Profound cardiac conduction delay predicts mortality in myotonic dystrophy type 1. *J Intern Med* 2010;**268**:59–65.
60. Badano L, Autore C, Fragola PV, Picelli A, Antonini G, Vichi R, et al. Left ventricular myocardial function in myotonic dystrophy. *Am J Cardiol* 1993;**71**:987–91.
61. Bhakta D, Groh MR, Shen C, Pascuzzi RM, Groh WJ. Increased mortality with left ventricular systolic dysfunction and heart failure in adults with myotonic dystrophy type 1. *Am Heart J* 2010;**160**:1137–41.
62. Wahbi K, Meune C, Becane HM, Laforet P, Bassez G, Lazarus A, et al. Left ventricular dysfunction and cardiac arrhythmias are frequent in type 2 myotonic dystrophy: a case control study. *Neuromuscul Disord* 2009;**19**:468–72.
63. Schoser BG, Ricker K, Schneider-Gold C, Hengstenberg C, Durre J, Bultmann B, et al. Sudden cardiac death in myotonic dystrophy type 2. *Neurology* 2004;**63**:2402–4.
64. Lin Y, Wilson JH. Transcription-induced DNA toxicity at trinucleotide repeats: double bubble is trouble. *Cell Cycle* 2011;**10**:611–8.
65. Sundararajan R, Freudenreich CH. Expanded CAG/CTG repeat DNA induces a checkpoint response that impacts cell proliferation in *Saccharomyces cerevisiae*. *PLoS Genet* 2011;**7**:e1001339.
66. Li LB, Bonini NM. Roles of trinucleotide-repeat RNA in neurological disease and degeneration. *Trends Neurosci* 2010;**33**:292–8.
67. Krahe R, Ashizawa T, Abbruzzese C, Roeder E, Carango P, Giacanelli M, et al. Effect of myotonic dystrophy trinucleotide repeat expansion on DMPK transcription and processing. *Genomics* 1995;**28**:1–14.
68. Zu T, Gibbens B, Doty NS, Gomes-Pereira M, Huguet A, Stone MD, et al. Non-ATG-initiated translation directed by microsatellite expansions. *Proc Natl Acad Sci USA* 2011;**108**:260–5.
69. Davis BM, McCurrach ME, Taneja KL, Singer RH, Housman DE. Expansion of a CUG trinucleotide repeat in the 3′ untranslated region of myotonic dystrophy protein kinase transcripts results in nuclear retention of transcripts. *Proc Natl Acad Sci USA* 1997;**94**:7388–93.
70. Hamshere M, Newman E, Alwazzan M, Brook JD. Nuclear retenton of DMPK transcripts in myotonic dystrophy. *Am J Hum Genet* 1996;**59**:A262.
71. Maeda M, Taft CS, Bush EW, Holder E, Bailey WM, Neville H, et al. Identification, tissue-specific expression, and subcellular localization of the 80- and 71-kDa forms of myotonic dystrophy kinase protein. *J Biol Chem* 1995;**270**:20246–9.
72. Klesert TR, Otten AD, Bird TD, Tapscott SJ. Trinucleotide repeat expansion at the myotonic dystrophy locus reduces expression of the DMAHP gene. *Nat Genet* 1997;**16**:402–6.
73. Thornton CA, Wymer JP, Simmons Z, McClain C, Moxley RT. Expansion of the myotonic dystrophy CTG repeat reduces expression of the flanking DMAHP gene. *Nat Genet* 1997;**16**:407–9.
74. Saveliev A, Everett C, Sharpe T, Webster Z, Festenstein R. DNA triplet repeats mediate heterochromatin-protein-1-sensitive variegated gene silencing. *Nature* 2003;**422**:909–13.
75. Lam LT, Pham YC, Nguyen TM, Morris GE. Characterization of a monoclonal antibody panel shows that the myotonic dystrophy protein kinase, DMPK, is expressed almost exclusively in muscle and heart. *Hum Mol Genet* 2000;**9**:2167–73.
76. Mulders SA, van Horssen R, Gerrits L, Bennink MB, Pluk H, de Boer-van Huizen RT, et al. Abnormal actomyosin assembly in proliferating and differentiating myoblasts upon expression of a cytosolic DMPK isoform. *Biochim Biophys Acta* 2011;**1813**:867–77.
77. van der Ven PF, Jansen G, van Kuppevelt TH, Perryman MB, Lupa M, Dunne PW, et al. Myotonic dystrophy kinase is a component of neuromuscular junctions. *Hum Mol Genet* 1993;**2**:1889–94.
78. Wheeler TM, Krym MC, Thornton CA. Ribonuclear foci at the neuromuscular junction in myotonic dystrophy type 1. *Neuromuscul Disord* 2007;**17**:242–7.
79. Kaliman P, Llagostera E. Myotonic dystrophy protein kinase (DMPK) and its role in the pathogenesis of myotonic dystrophy 1. *Cell Signal* 2008;**20**:1935–41.
80. Llagostera E, Carmona MC, Vicente M, Escorihuela RM, Kaliman P. High-fat diet induced adiposity and insulin resistance in mice lacking the myotonic dystrophy protein kinase. *FEBS Lett* 2009;**583**:2121–5.
81. Jansen G, Groenen PJTA, Bachner D, Jap PH, Coerwinkel M, Oerlemans F, et al. Abnormal myotonic dystrophy protein kinase levels produce only mild myopathy in mice. *Nat Genet* 1996;**13**:316–24.
82. Reddy S, Smith DBJ, Rich MM, Leferovich JM, Reilly P, Davis BM, et al. Mice lacking the myotonic dystrophy protein kinase develop a late onset progressive myopathy. *Nat Genet* 1996;**13**:325–34.
83. Berul CI, Maguire CT, Aronovitz MJ, Greenwood J, Miller C, Gehrmann J, et al. DMPK dosage alterations result in atrioventricular conduction abnormalities in a mouse myotonic dystrophy model. *J Clin Invest* 1999;**103**:R1–7.
84. Boucher CA, King SK, Carey N, Krahe R, Winchester CL, Rahman S, et al. A novel homeodomain-encoding gene is associated with a large CpG island interrupted by the myotonic dystrophy unstable (CTG)n repeat. *Hum Mol Genet* 1995;**4**:1919–25.
85. Korade-Mirnics Z, Tarleton J, Servidei S, Casey RR, Gennarelli M, Pegoraro E, et al. Myotonic dystrophy: tissue-specific effect of

somatic CTG expansions on allele-specific DMAHP/SIX5 expression. *Hum Mol Genet* 1999;**8**:1017–23.
86. Eriksson M, Ansved T, Edstrom L, Anvret M, Carey N. Simultaneous analysis of expression of the three myotonic dystrophy locus genes in adult skeletal muscle samples: the CTG expansion correlates inversely with DMPK and 59 expression levels, but not DMAHP levels. *Hum Mol Genet* 1999;**8**:1053–60.
87. Inukai A, Doyu M, Kato T, Liang Y, Kuru S, Yamamoto M, et al. Reduced expression of DMAHP/SIX5 gene in myotonic dystrophy muscle. *Muscle and Nerve* 2000;**23**:1421–6.
88. Klesert TR, Cho DH, Clark JI, Maylie J, Adelman J, Snider L, et al. Mice deficient in Six5 develop cataracts: implications for myotonic dystrophy. *Nat Genet* 2000;**25**:105–9.
89. Wakimoto H, Maguire CT, Sherwood MC, Vargas MM, Sarkar PS, Han J, et al. Characterization of cardiac conduction system abnormalities in mice with targeted disruption of Six5 gene. *J Interv Card Electrophysiol* 2002;**7**:127–35.
90. Sarkar PS, Appukuttan B, Han J, Ito Y, Ai CW, Tsai WL, et al. Heterozygous loss of Six5 in mice is sufficient to cause ocular cataracts. *Nat Genet* 2000;**25**:110–4.
91. Gerbasi VR, Link AJ. The myotonic dystrophy type 2 protein ZNF9 is part of an ITAF complex that promotes cap-independent translation. *Mol Cell Proteomics* 2007;**6**:1049–58.
92. Huichalaf C, Schoser B, Schneider-Gold C, Jin B, Sarkar P, Timchenko L. Reduction of the rate of protein translation in patients with myotonic dystrophy 2. *J Neurosci* 2009;**29**:9042–9.
93. Botta A, Caldarola S, Vallo L, Bonifazi E, Fruci D, Gullotta F, et al. Effect of the [CCTG]n repeat expansion on ZNF9 expression in myotonic dystrophy type II (DM2). *Biochim Biophys Acta* 2006;**1762**:329–34.
94. Margolis JM, Schoser BG, Moseley ML, Day JW, Ranum LP. DM2 intronic expansions: evidence for CCUG accumulation without flanking sequence or effects on ZNF9 mRNA processing or protein expression. *Hum Mol Genet* 2006;**15**:1808–15.
95. Schoser BG, Kress W, Walter MC, Halliger-Keller B, Lochmuller H, Ricker K. Homozygosity for CCTG mutation in myotonic dystrophy type 2. *Brain* 2004;**127**:1868–77.
96. Chen W, Liang Y, Deng W, Shimizu K, Ashique AM, Li E, et al. The zinc-finger protein CNBP is required for forebrain formation in the mouse. *Development* 2003;**130**:1367–79.
97. Liquori CL, Ricker K, Moseley ML, Jacobsen JF, Kress W, Naylor SL, et al. Myotonic dystrophy type 2 caused by a CCTG expansion in intron 1 of ZNF9. *Science* 2001;**293**:864–7.
98. Raheem O, Olufemi SE, Bachinski LL, Vihola A, Sirito M, Holmlund-Hampf J, et al. Mutant (CCTG)n expansion causes abnormal expression of zinc finger protein 9 (ZNF9) in myotonic dystrophy type 2. *Am J Pathol* 2010;**177**:3025–36.
99. Sammons MA, Antons AK, Bendjennat M, Udd B, Krahe R, Link AJ. ZNF9 activation of IRES-mediated translation of the human ODC mRNA is decreased in myotonic dystrophy type 2. *PLoS One* 2010;**5**: e9301.
100. Taneja KL, McCurrach M, Schalling M, Housman D, Singer RH. Foci of trinucleotide repeat transcripts in nuclei of myotonic dystrophy cells and tissues. *J Cell Biol* 1995;**128**:995–1002.
101. Amack JD, Paguio AP, Mahadevan MS. Cis and trans effects of the myotonic dystrophy (DM) mutation in a cell culture model. *Hum Mol Genet* 1999;**8**:1975–84.
102. Mankodi A, Logigian E, Callahan L, McClain C, White R, Henderson D, et al. Myotonic dystrophy in transgenic mice expressing an expanded CUG repeat. *Science* 2000;**289**:1769–73.
103. Napierala M, Krzyzosiak WJ. CUG repeats present in myotonin kinase RNA form metastable slippery hairpins. *J Biol Chem* 1997;**272**:31079–85.
104. Tian B, White RJ, Xia T, Welle S, Turner DH, Mathews MB, et al. Expanded CUG repeat RNAs form hairpins that activate the double-stranded RNA-dependent protein kinase PKR. *RNA* 2000;**6**:79–87.
105. Mooers BH, Logue JS, Berglund JA. The structural basis of myotonic dystrophy from the crystal structure of CUG repeats. *Proc Natl Acad Sci USA* 2005;**102**:16626–31.
106. Osborne RJ, Thornton CA. RNA-dominant diseases. *Hum Mol Genet* 2006;**15**:R162–9.
107. de Haro M, Al Ramahi I, De Gouyon B, Ukani L, Rosa A, Faustino NA, et al. MBNL1 and CUGBP1 modify expanded CUG-induced toxicity in a Drosophila model of myotonic dystrophy type 1. *Hum Mol Genet* 2006;**15**:2138–45.
108. Seznec H, Agbulut O, Sergeant N, Savouret C, Ghestem A, Tabti N, et al. Mice transgenic for the human myotonic dystrophy region with expanded CTG repeats display muscular and brain abnormalities. *Hum Mol Genet* 2001;**10**:2717–26.
109. Wang GS, Kearney DL, De Biasi M, Taffet G, Cooper TA. Elevation of RNA-binding protein CUGBP1 is an early event in an inducible heart-specific mouse model of myotonic dystrophy. *J Clin Invest* 2007;**117**:2802–11.
110. Orengo JP, Chambon P, Metzger D, Mosier DR, Snipes GJ, Cooper TA. Expanded CTG repeats within the DMPK 3′ UTR causes severe skeletal muscle wasting in an inducible mouse model for myotonic dystrophy. *Proc Natl Acad Sci USA* 2008;**105**:2646–51.
111. Mankodi A, Takahashi MP, Jiang H, Beck CL, Bowers WJ, Moxley RT, et al. Expanded CUG repeats trigger aberrant splicing of ClC-1 chloride channel pre-mRNA and hyperexcitability of skeletal muscle in myotonic dystrophy. *Mol Cell* 2002;**10**:35–44.
112. Philips AV, Timchenko LT, Cooper TA. Disruption of splicing regulated by a CUG-binding protein in myotonic dystrophy. *Science* 1998;**280**:737–41.
113. Lin X, Miller JW, Mankodi A, Kanadia RN, Yuan Y, Moxley RT, et al. Failure of MBNL1-dependent postnatal splicing transitions in myotonic dystrophy. *Hum Mol Genet* 2006;**15**:2087–97.
114. Osborne RJ, Lin X, Welle S, Sobczak K, O'Rourke JR, Swanson MS, et al. Transcriptional and post-transcriptional impact of toxic RNA in myotonic dystrophy. *Hum Mol Genet* 2009;**18**:1471–81.
115. Du H, Cline MS, Osborne RJ, Tuttle DL, Clark TA, Donohue JP, et al. Aberrant alternative splicing and extracellular matrix gene expression in mouse models of myotonic dystrophy. *Nat Struct Mol Biol* 2010;**17**:187–93.
116. Timchenko LT, Miller JW, Timchenko DR, DeVore KV, Datar KV, Lin L, et al. Identification of a (CUG)n triplet repeat RNA-binding protein and its expression in myotonic dystrophy. *Nucleic Acids Res* 1996;**24**:4407–14.
117. Timchenko NA, Iakova P, Cai ZJ, Smith JR, Timchenko LT. Molecular basis for impaired muscle differentiation in myotonic dystrophy. *Mol Cell Biol* 2001;**21**:6927–38.
118. Vlasova IA, Tahoe NM, Fan D, Larsson O, Rattenbacher B, Sternjohn JR, et al. Conserved GU-rich elements mediate mRNA

decay by binding to CUG-binding protein 1. *Mol Cell* 2008;**29**:263–70.

119. Michalowski S, Miller JW, Urbinati CR, Paliouras M, Swanson MS, Griffith J. Visualization of double-stranded RNAs from the myotonic dystrophy protein kinase gene and interactions with CUG-binding protein. *Nucleic Acids Res* 1999;**27**:3534–42.
120. Kino Y, Mori D, Oma Y, Takeshita Y, Sasagawa N, Ishiura S. Muscleblind protein, MBNL1/EXP, binds specifically to CHHG repeats. *Hum Mol Genet* 2004;**13**:495–507.
121. Mori D, Sasagawa N, Kino Y, Ishiura S. Quantitative analysis of CUG-BP1 binding to RNA repeats. *J Biochem* 2008;**143**: 377–83.
122. Fardaei M, Larkin K, Brook JD, Hamshere MG. In vivo co-localisation of MBNL protein with DMPK expanded-repeat transcripts. *Nucleic Acids Res* 2001;**29**:2766–71.
123. Mankodi A, Teng-umnuay P, Krym M, Henderson D, Swanson M, Thornton CA. Ribonuclear inclusions in skeletal muscle in myotonic dystrophy types 1 and 2. *Ann Neurol* 2003;**54**:760–8.
124. Jiang H, Mankodi A, Swanson MS, Moxley RT, Thornton CA. Myotonic dystrophy type 1 associated with nuclear foci of mutant RNA, sequestration of muscleblind proteins, and deregulated alternative splicing in neurons. *Hum Mol Genet* 2004;**13**:3079–88.
125. Mankodi A, Lin X, Blaxall BC, Swanson MS, Thornton CA. Nuclear RNA foci in the heart in myotonic dystrophy. *Circ Res* 2005;**97**:1152–5.
126. Savkur RS, Philips AV, Cooper TA. Aberrant regulation of insulin receptor alternative splicing is associated with insulin resistance in myotonic dystrophy. *Nat Genet* 2001;**29**:40–7.
127. Timchenko NA, Cai ZJ, Welm AL, Reddy S, Ashizawa T, Timchenko LT. RNA CUG repeats sequester CUGBP1 and alter protein levels and activity of CUGBP1. *J Biol Chem* 2001;**276**:7820–6.
128. Kuyumcu-Martinez NM, Wang GS, Cooper TA. Increased steady-state levels of CUGBP1 in myotonic dystrophy 1 are due to PKC-mediated hyperphosphorylation. *Mol Cell* 2007;**28**: 68–78.
129. Koshelev M, Sarma S, Price RE, Wehrens XH, Cooper TA. Heart-specific overexpression of CUGBP1 reproduces functional and molecular abnormalities of myotonic dystrophy type 1. *Hum Mol Genet* 2010;**19**:1066–75.
130. Ward AJ, Rimer M, Killian JM, Dowling JJ, Cooper TA. CUGBP1 overexpression in mouse skeletal muscle reproduces features of myotonic dystrophy type 1. *Hum Mol Genet* 2010;**19**:3614–22.
131. Artero R, Prokop A, Paricio N, Begemann G, Pueyo I, Mlodzik M, et al. The muscleblind gene participates in the organization of Z-bands and epidermal attachments of Drosophila muscles and is regulated by Dmef2. *Dev Biol* 1998;**195**:131–43.
132. Miller JW, Urbinati CR, Teng-umnuay P, Stenberg MG, Byrne BJ, Thornton CA, et al. Recruitment of human muscleblind proteins to (CUG)(n) expansions associated with myotonic dystrophy. *EMBO J* 2000;**19**:4439–48.
133. Kanadia RN, Urbinati CR, Crusselle VJ, Luo D, Lee YJ, Harrison JK, et al. Developmental expression of mouse muscleblind genes Mbnl1, Mbnl2 and Mbnl3. *Gene Expr Patterns* 2003;**3**:459–62.
134. Ho TH, Charlet B, Poulos MG, Singh G, Swanson MS, Cooper TA. Muscleblind proteins regulate alternative splicing. *EMBO J* 2004;**23**:3103–12.
135. Goers ES, Purcell J, Voelker RB, Gates DP, Berglund JA. MBNL1 binds GC motifs embedded in pyrimidines to regulate alternative splicing. *Nucleic Acids Res* 2010;**38**:2467–84.
136. Kalsotra A, Xiao X, Ward AJ, Castle JC, Johnson JM, Burge CB. A postnatal switch of CELF and MBNL proteins reprograms alternative splicing in the developing heart. *Proc Natl Acad Sci USA* 2008;**105**:20333–8.
137. Adereth Y, Dammai V, Kose N, Li R, Hsu T. RNA-dependent integrin alpha3 protein localization regulated by the Muscleblind-like protein MLP1. *Nat Cell Biol* 2005;**7**:1240–7.
138. Rau F, Freyermuth F, Fugier C, Villemin JP, Fischer MC, Jost B, et al. Misregulation of miR-1 processing is associated with heart defects in myotonic dystrophy. *Nat Struct Mol Biol* 2011;**18**:840–5.
139. Yuan Y, Compton SA, Sobczak K, Stenberg MG, Thornton CA, Griffith JD, et al. Muscleblind-like 1 interacts with RNA hairpins in splicing target and pathogenic RNAs. *Nucleic Acids Res* 2007;**35**:5474–86.
140. Teplova M, Patel DJ. Structural insights into RNA recognition by the alternative-splicing regulator muscleblind-like MBNL1. *Nat Struct Mol Biol* 2008;**15**:1343–51.
141. Dansithong W, Paul S, Comai L, Reddy S. MBNL1 is the primary determinant of focus formation and aberrant insulin receptor splicing in DM1. *J Biol Chem* 2005;**280**:5773–80.
142. Kanadia RN, Johnstone KA, Mankodi A, Lungu C, Thornton CA, Esson D, et al. A muscleblind knockout model for myotonic dystrophy. *Science* 2003;**302**:1978–80.
143. Lueck JD, Mankodi A, Swanson MS, Thornton CA, Dirksen RT. Muscle chloride channel dysfunction in two mouse models of myotonic dystrophy. *J Gen Physiol* 2007;**129**:79–94.
144. Kino Y, Washizu C, Oma Y, Onishi H, Nezu Y, Sasagawa N, et al. MBNL and CELF proteins regulate alternative splicing of the skeletal muscle chloride channel CLCN1. *Nucleic Acids Res* 2009;**37**:6477–90.
145. Berg J, Jiang H, Thornton CA, Cannon SC. Truncated ClC-1 mRNA in myotonic dystrophy exerts a dominant-negative effect on the Cl current. *Neurology* 2004;**63**:2371–5.
146. Charlet-B N, Savkur RS, Singh G, Philips AV, Grice EA, Cooper TA. Loss of the muscle-specific chloride channel in type 1 myotonic dystrophy due to misregulated alternative splicing. *Mol Cell* 2002;**10**:45–53.
147. Kanadia RN, Shin J, Yuan Y, Beattie SG, Wheeler TM, Thornton CA, et al. Reversal of RNA missplicing and myotonia after muscleblind overexpression in a mouse poly(CUG) model for myotonic dystrophy. *Proc Natl Acad Sci USA* 2006;**103**:11748–53.
148. Wheeler TM, Lueck JD, Swanson M, Dirksen RT, Thornton CA. Correction of ClC-1 splicing eliminates chloride channelopathy and myotonia in mouse models of myotonic dystrophy. *J Clin Invest* 2007;**117**:3952–7.
149. Fugier C, Klein AF, Hammer C, Vassilopoulos S, Ivarsson Y, Toussaint A, et al. Misregulated alternative splicing of BIN1 is associated with T tubule alterations and muscle weakness in myotonic dystrophy. *Nat Med* 2011;**17**:720–5.
150. Zhao Y, Ransom JF, Li A, Vedantham V, von Drehle M, Muth AN, et al. Dysregulation of cardiogenesis, cardiac conduction, and cell cycle in mice lacking miRNA-1-2. *Cell* 2007;**129**:303–17.
151. Krol J, Fiszer A, Mykowska A, Sobczak K, de Mezer M, Krzyzosiak WJ. Ribonuclease dicer cleaves triplet repeat hairpins

into shorter repeats that silence specific targets. *Mol Cell* 2007;**25**:575−86.

152. Yadava RS, Frenzel-McCardell CD, Yu Q, Srinivasan V, Tucker AL, Puymirat J, et al. RNA toxicity in myotonic muscular dystrophy induces NKX2-5 expression. *Nat Genet* 2008;**40**:61−8.
153. Ebralidze A, Wang Y, Petkova V, Ebralidse K, Junghans RP. RNA leaching of transcription factors disrupts transcription in myotonic dystrophy. *Science* 2004;**303**:383−7.
154. Wheeler TM, Sobczak K, Lueck JD, Osborne RJ, Lin X, Dirksen RT, et al. Reversal of RNA dominance by displacement of protein sequestered on triplet repeat RNA. *Science* 2009;**325**:336−9.
155. Mulders SA, van den Broek WJ, Wheeler TM, Croes HJ, van Kuik-Romeijn P, de Kimpe SJ, et al. Triplet-repeat oligonucleotide-mediated reversal of RNA toxicity in myotonic dystrophy. *Proc Natl Acad Sci USA* 2009;**106**:13915−20.
156. Francois V, Klein AF, Beley C, Jollet A, Lemercier C, Garcia L, et al. Selective silencing of mutated mRNAs in DM1 by using modified hU7-snRNAs. *Nat Struct Mol Biol* 2011;**18**:85−7.
157. Warf MB, Nakamori M, Matthys CM, Thornton CA, Berglund JA. Pentamidine reverses the splicing defects associated with myotonic dystrophy. *Proc Natl Acad Sci USA* 2009;**106**:18551−6.
158. Pushechnikov A, Lee MM, Childs-Disney JL, Sobczak K, French JM, Thornton CA, et al. Rational design of ligands targeting triplet repeating transcripts that cause RNA dominant disease: application to myotonic muscular dystrophy type 1 and spinocerebellar ataxia type 3. *J Am Chem Soc* 2009;**131**:9767−79.
159. Wang GS, Kuyumcu-Martinez MN, Sarma S, Mathur N, Wehrens XH, Cooper TA. PKC inhibition ameliorates the cardiac phenotype in a mouse model of myotonic dystrophy type 1. *J Clin Invest* 2009;**119**:3797−806.

Chapter 69

Facioscapulohumeral Muscular Dystrophy: Unraveling the Mysteries of a Complex Epigenetic Disease

Charis L. Himeda and Charles P. Emerson, Jr
Boston Biomedical Research Institute, Watertown, MA

CLINICAL AND HISTOLOGICAL FEATURES

Facioscapulohumeral muscular dystrophy (FSHD) is the third most common inherited neuromuscular disorder, and poses both a unique clinical challenge and an intriguing biological problem. Inheritance in FSHD is autosomal dominant, with a high frequency of sporadic cases. Approximately half of sporadic cases result from a post-zygotic mutation that leads to mosaicism (1). The disease is characterized by progressive and often asymmetric weakness and atrophy of muscles of the face, upper arms, and shoulder girdle, progressing to muscles of the pelvic girdle and lower extremities (2). Patients usually develop symptoms in their twenties, while the most severely affected individuals are confined to a wheelchair in their early teens (3). The clinical manifestation of FSHD (age of onset, severity, and range of affected muscles) is highly variable, both between and within families. Although primarily a disorder of skeletal muscle, FSHD is also associated with retinal vasculopathy and high-tone deafness, as well as epilepsy and mental retardation in the most extreme cases (4–6).

There is a large phenotypic heterogeneity among FSHD families and individuals. Even within an individual, symptoms are highly variable, with some muscles highly affected (shoulder muscles, biceps), others only slightly affected (deltoid), and many anatomical muscles apparently healthy (1). Compounding this difficulty, histological changes in affected FSHD muscles tend to be relatively minor and non-specific to the disease. Early-affected muscles display abnormal variation in fiber size and increased central nuclei, while end-stage muscles are characterized by fiber necrosis, fibrosis, and inflammatory infiltrates (1). As these histological changes are general features of muscular dystrophies, they offer no clues as to the disease-specific mechanisms of FSHD.

GENETIC FEATURES

The most common form of FSHD (FSHD1, OMIM 158900, hereafter referred to as FSHD) is linked to contractions of a macrosatellite repeat array in the subtelomere of chromosome 4 at 4q35.2 (7–9). Each repeat consists of a 3.3 kb DNA unit termed D4Z4. In the general population, this repeat array varies between 11 and 100 D4Z4 units, whereas in FSHD patients, it is contracted to 1–10 units (Figure 69.1). This telomeric region exists as two prominent alleles distal to the array: 4qA, which contains a 6.2 kb β-satellite region distal to D4Z4, and 4qB. Only contractions on specific disease-permissive haplotypes of 4qA (the common 4qA161 variant and the rare 4qA159 and 4qA168 variants) are associated with FSHD (10–12) (Figure 69.1). In general, there is an inverse correlation between size of the residual D4Z4 region and severity of the disease. Interestingly, less than 5% of cases (known as phenotypic FSHD or FSHD2, OMIM 158901) show no contraction of the D4Z4 repeats on chromosome 4, although these patients still carry at least one permissive 4qA161 allele (13,14) (Figure 69.1). As the result of an ancient gene duplication, the subtelomere of chromosome 10q contains an almost identical D4Z4 repeat array, but contractions in this region are non-pathogenic (15,16). Adding to the complexity of the disease, translocated copies of D4Z4 repeats from chromosomes 4 and 10 are frequently encountered on either chromosome end, with variable pathological consequences (17,18).

EPIGENETIC FEATURES

In addition to the genetic lesion, FSHD is associated with a number of epigenetic alterations in the D4Z4 region (Figure 69.2). The D4Z4 repeat is highly GC-rich, with characteristics of a CpG island. There is a general

Muscle. DOI: http://dx.doi.org/10.1016/B978-0-12-381510-1.00069-7

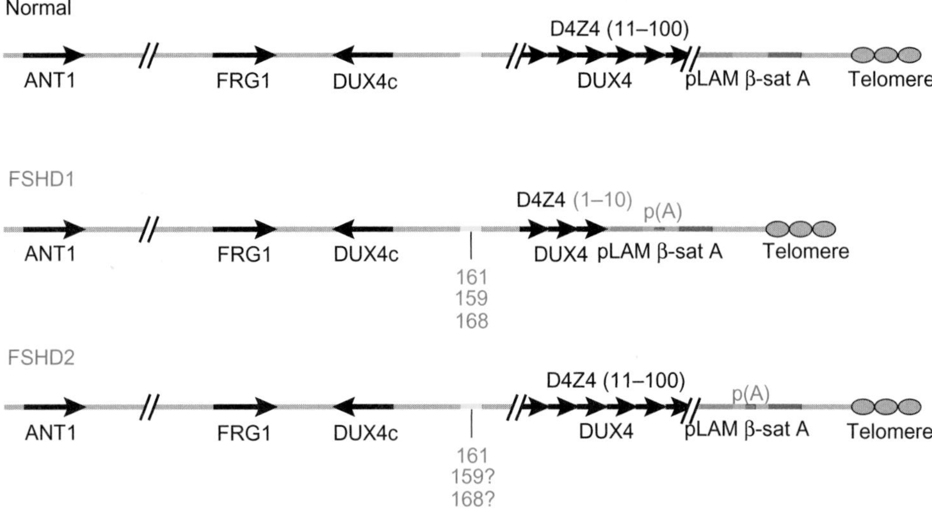

FIGURE 69.1 The FSHD locus. Diagram of the chromosome 4qA subtelomere, with FSHD candidate genes shown as black arrows. Normal individuals possess 11–100 units of the D4Z4 macrosatellite repeat (each of which contains the DUX4 ORF). In FSHD1 patients, the D4Z4 region is contracted to 1–10 units on specific permissive haplotypes of 4qA (161, 159, and 168; SSLP shown in yellow). By contrast, FSHD2 patients show no contraction of D4Z4, although they still carry at least one permissive allele (4qA161). The 4qA allele (blue) contains a pLAM region (turquoise) and β-satellite region (green) downstream of D4Z4. On permissive alleles of 4qA, the β-satellite region contains a poly(A) site for the distal DUX4 transcript.

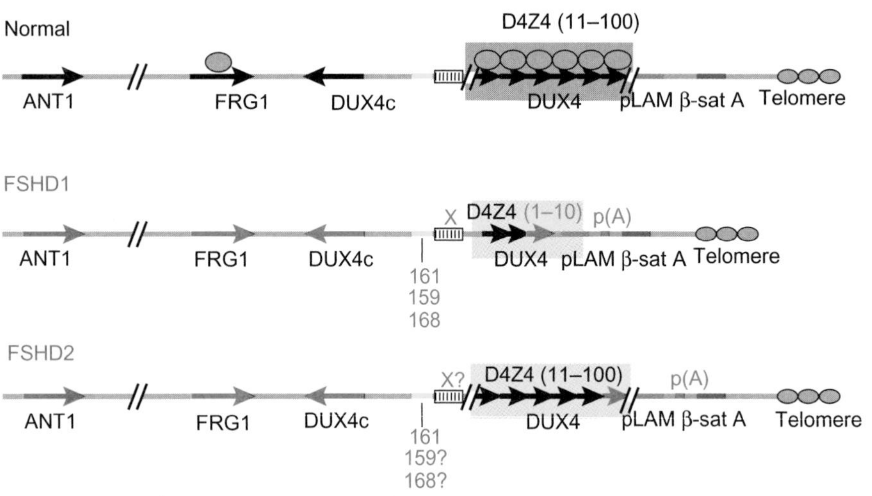

FIGURE 69.2 Epigenetic models of FSHD. In normal individuals, the D4Z4 region on chromosome 4qA is in a relatively closed chromatin configuration (grey shaded box), whereas in FSHD1 and 2 it is in a more open chromatin configuration (pink shaded box). D4Z4 contraction (FSHD1) or a separate mechanism (FSHD2) might result in decreased binding for a repressor complex (dark grey circles) or decreased attachment to the nuclear matrix (S/MAR site shown as striped box), causing aberrant overexpression of nearby genes (red arrows). On permissive alleles of 4qA, the β-satellite region downstream of D4Z4 contains a poly(A) site for the distal DUX4 transcript, allowing inappropriate, stable production of the full-length DUX4 mRNA. Refer to text for more details.

hypomethylation of the contracted allele, although DNA methylation levels vary widely among affected individuals, and asymptomatic gene carriers also show reduced methylation (19). Since DNA methylation is associated with gene silencing, this finding suggested that FSHD might be caused by the aberrant upregulation of genes in the D4Z4 region. Histone modifications at D4Z4 in FSHD vs. control cells are also more consistent with unexpressed euchromatin than with facultative heterochromatin, indicative of a chromatin environment that is poised for gene expression (20,21). Interestingly, cases of phenotypic FSHD also display D4Z4 hypomethylation

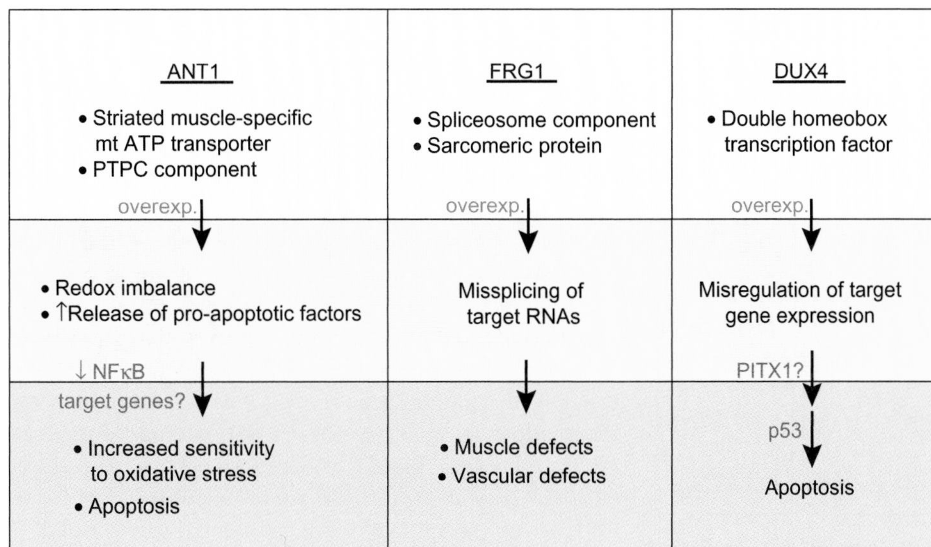

FIGURE 69.3 **Models for FSHD candidate gene activity.** In FSHD, D4Z4 contraction or a separate mechanism is thought to lead to changes in chromatin structure on permissive alleles of 4qA that result in overexpression of the nearby genes. The three major FSHD candidate genes are shown, along with the likely results of their overexpression and consequent FSHD pathology. Refer to text for more details. PTPC: Permeability Transition Pore Complex; mt: mitochondrial.

(19), lending further support to an epigenetic model of the disease.

Several models have been proposed involving derepression of candidate genes in the region of D4Z4. Gabellini et al. demonstrated that a transcriptional repressor complex consisting of high-mobility group box 2 (HMGB2), nucleolin, and the transcription factor YY1 binds an element within D4Z4 (22). Bodega et al. have also reported binding of YY1 and the repressive Polycomb Group protein EZH2 to D4Z4 and the FRG1 promoter, and a reduction in an EZH2-mediated repressive histone mark in these regions in FSHD myoblasts (23). It has been proposed that contraction of D4Z4 results in decreased binding sites for these repressive factors, leading to inappropriate overexpression of candidate genes in the region (22,24). In the case of phenotypic FSHD, this model would suggest that hypomethylation of D4Z4 (rather than contraction) prevents repressor binding, but this remains to be demonstrated.

Petrov et al. identified a nuclear scaffold/matrix attachment region (S/MAR) just proximal to D4Z4, and showed that attachment to the nuclear matrix was greatly diminished in FSHD muscles compared to controls (25). Whereas the D4Z4 region and neighboring genes normally lie in two chromatin loops, loss of nuclear matrix attachment in FSHD resulted in formation of a single loop (25). These authors later showed that D4Z4 contains a strong transcriptional enhancer, and the matrix attachment site can block the activity of this enhancer; thus, loss of the boundary in FSHD may cause derepression of the proximal genes (26). In a contrasting study, Ottaviani et al. have shown that a single D4Z4 unit behaves as a transcriptional insulator, and this activity is lost upon multimerization (27). In this model, FSHD is caused by a gain-of-function insulator at contracted D4Z4 repeats, which blocks normal repression of the proximal genes (27).

Unlike most telomeres, the FSHD region at 4q is localized to the nuclear envelope (through a region proximal to D4Z4), and the nuclear lamina component lamin A/C is required for this localization (28). Interestingly, several other neuromuscular disorders (Emery–Dreifuss muscular dystrophy, limb-girdle muscular dystrophy 1B, and dilated cardiomyopathy) are caused by defects in the nuclear envelope, either through a disruption of nuclear structural integrity or through an alteration of signaling pathways and gene expression (29). In the model proposed by Masny et al. contractions in D4Z4 and the presence of the β-satellite in 4qA might lead to altered recruitment of transcription factors or chromatin modifiers at the nuclear envelope, resulting in a dystrophic phenotype (28).

CANDIDATE GENES AND AFFECTED PATHWAYS

There is at least one gene located within the D4Z4 array, double homeobox 4 (*DUX4*), and several genes directly proximal to D4Z4 on chromosome 4, including: adenine nucleotide translocator 1 (*ANT1*), FSHD region gene 1 (*FRG1*), and *DUX4c* (Figures 69.1, 69.2). While some studies have demonstrated abnormal expression of these genes in FSHD muscles and cells (22,30,31), many other studies have failed to confirm this (21,28,32–37). Nonetheless, all of these genes have intriguing links to FSHD pathology (Figure 69.3).

ANT1

ANT1 serves as a cardiac and skeletal muscle-specific ATP transporter involved in mitochondrial DNA maintenance and apoptosis. ANT1 has been shown to stimulate recruitment of IκB–NFκB complexes into the mitochondria (38), and overexpression in FSHD muscles was shown to correlate with a redox imbalance (31). This suggests a model in which overexpression of ANT1 in FHSD causes inappropriate recruitment of IκB–NFκB complexes into the mitochondria, reducing the expression of nuclear NF-κB gene targets involved in stress response and anti-apoptosis (31). ANT1 is also a component of the Permeability Transition Pore Complex in the mitochondrial membrane (39); thus, increased expression of ANT1 might facilitate the release of pro-apoptotic factors into the cytosol (40). Taken together, these data implicate ANT1 as a likely candidate to explain the increased sensitivity of FSHD muscle cells to oxidative stress (see below). Furthermore, in the three reports showing elevation of ANT1 protein in FSHD muscles, this effect was shown to be specific (compared to muscles from patients with other muscular dystrophies), suggesting that the impaired stress response/enhanced apoptosis in FSHD muscles is a primary defect (22,30,31).

FRG1

FRG1 is a highly conserved component of the human spliceosome (41), and muscle-specific mRNAs were shown to be misspliced in FRG1-overexpressing mice and cells, and in FSHD myoblasts (41–43). FRG1 is also a sarcomeric protein, capable of binding and promoting the bundling of F-actin (44,45). Overexpression of FRG1 in mice, frogs, and worms causes muscle defects (43,44,46–48), and recent evidence suggests that FRG1 plays critical roles in both skeletal muscle and vasculature, the two most prominent tissues affected in FSHD (43,46,47).

DUX4

Each D4Z4 repeat contains a conserved ORF for the *DUX4* retrogene, encoding a double homeobox protein thought to be derived from retrotransposition of the *DUXC* gene (49) (Figures 69.1, 69.2). *DUX4* also has homology to the mouse Duxbl gene, a member of the DUXA family that is expressed in mouse germline cells and in the early phases of myogenesis (50). *DUX4* mRNA and protein have been selectively detected in FSHD patient-derived muscle cells (35,51), and overexpression of the protein in C2C12 myoblasts and in mouse, frog, and zebrafish muscles results in an apoptotic/dystrophic phenotype (51–55).

The distal 4q35 D4Z4 unit produces a *DUX4* transcript containing a unique third exon encoding a 3′ UTR from the adjacent pLAM region (7,35,56). Recently, Lemmers et al. demonstrated that this pLAM region selectively encodes a polyadenylation signal for the *DUX4* mRNA on FSHD-permissive chromosomes (including a hybrid repeat array on chromosome 10 that ends with chromosome 4-type units), but not on non-permissive 4qB or 10qA chromosomes. If non-permissive 4qA variants are also found to lack the *DUX4* poly(A) signal, this would account for the exclusive linkage of FSHD to particular 4qA haplotypes and provide strong evidence that stabilization of the Dux4 transcript by polyadenylation is required for FSHD pathogenesis (12). Interestingly, the pLAM region and poly(A) signal are intact in patients with a proximal deletion of D4Z4, as well as in phenotypic FSHD patients, who display a relaxed chromatin configuration on 4qA161 without D4Z4 contraction (12,14,57).

In a follow-up study, Snider et al. showed that a C-terminal truncated transcript of *DUX4* (DUX4-s) was present in control muscle biopsies and some FSHD samples, whereas the full-length transcript (DUX4-fl) was present only in muscle biopsies and cells from patients with FSHD (including two with phenotypic FSHD) (58). DUX4-fl is normally expressed in testis, whereas a subset of differentiated tissues, including skeletal muscle, express only DUX4-s (58). The authors showed that control fibroblasts, which express only DUX4-s, switch to production of DUX4-fl upon iPS induction. Importantly, iPS cells from control fibroblasts switch back to production of DUX4-s upon differentiation, whereas iPS cells from FSHD fibroblasts continue to express DUX4-fl (58). Finally, expression of DUX4-s vs. DUX4-fl correlated with higher levels of a repressive chromatin marker, which might favor the use of a cryptic splice donor site (58). Taken together, these data led to the proposal of a new disease model in which DUX4-fl is produced in germ cells and pluripotent cells during development. As cells differentiate, the chromatin in this region condenses, repressing DUX4 expression and favoring the use of an alternate splice donor site and the switch to production of DUX4-s in cells that escape repression. On FSHD permissive chromosomes (which contain a poly(A) signal to stabilize DUX4 transcripts), either D4Z4 contraction or a separate mechanism maintains the local chromatin in an open state, leading to inappropriate expression of DUX4-fl. Although only ~0.1% of FSHD muscle nuclei express DUX4, the protein aggregates in nuclear foci characteristic of DUX4-induced apoptosis (58). It will be important to assess the expression of DUX4 isoforms in FSHD2 patients. If the open chromatin configuration of D4Z4 in these patients is sufficient to allow expression of DUX4-fl, it is possible that two separate mechanisms (contraction in FSHD1 and an unknown mechanism in FSHD2) result in pathology caused by the same downstream effector.

Although the biological roles of DUX4 during development and in FSHD pathology have yet to be elucidated, DUX4 has been shown to transactivate the paired-like homeodomain transcription factor Pitx1, likely through a conserved homeodomain motif in the *Pitx1* promoter (35). Importantly, PITX1 is specifically upregulated in muscles of FSHD patients, indicative of an early role in FSHD pathogenesis (35). As *Pitx1* is required for anterior–posterior limb specification and left–right symmetry during development (59–64), it is interesting to speculate on its potential role in the asymmetric manifestation of FSHD. Interestingly, even low-level overexpression of either DUX4 or Pitx1 in the *Xenopus laevis* model caused gross developmental abnormalities and massive apoptosis (47), and PITX1 overexpression also induced apoptosis in two human cancer cell lines (65). In addition to its developmental role, PITX1 has been reported to regulate aspects of inflammation (66), induce tumorigenicity by inhibiting the RAS pathway (67), and transactivate the p53 tumor suppressor (65). Since DUX4-mediated toxicity appears to require p53 (54), PITX1 could be downstream of DUX4 in activating p53-dependent apoptosis.

The current body of data warrants further characterization of DUX4 and its gene targets, including PITX1. In particular, determining the normal spatiotemporal pattern of DUX4 expression *in vivo* should help to clarify our understanding of this transcription factor and its role in FSHD progression. If DUX4 is abnormally expressed in FSHD muscle satellite cells, its toxic effects could manifest as a regeneration defect over time, which would be useful to assess in an *in vivo* regeneration model. It would also be interesting to investigate a potential regeneration role for DUX4 in normal muscle injury and in other muscle disorders. Since the *DUX4* retrogene has been retained in primates, whereas the parental *DUXC* gene has not, it has been speculated that DUX4 serves to prevent hypermuscularity of the face and upper extremity in primates, and leaky expression results in a progressive toxicity that gives rise to FSHD (58). However, it remains to be seen whether DUX4 is preferentially expressed in the most severe areas of FSHD pathology (muscles of the face and shoulder girdle, retinal vasculature, etc).

DUX4c

Interestingly, the DUX4 homologue *DUX4c* (located 42 kb centromeric from the D4Z4 region on 4q) is also upregulated in FSHD primary myoblasts and muscle biopsies (68). Overexpression of *DUX4c* has been reported to cause muscle differentiation defects and inhibition of *Myf5* and *MyoD* expression (69), while another study reported *Myf5* induction, enhanced proliferation, and decreased differentiation, consistent with a role for *DUX4c* in muscle regeneration (68). While the occurrence of FSHD in families with a proximal deletion encompassing *DUX4c* indicates that this gene is not likely to be a causal factor, it may nonetheless contribute to disease heterogeneity and progression (70).

Affected Pathways

Unfortunately, due to anatomical heterogeneity as well as experimental variability (e.g., heterogeneity of source material and different cell culture parameters), the FSHD literature embodies a number of conflicting reports regarding the morphology, behavioral characteristics, and gene expression profiles of FSHD muscle cells (32,34,71–73). However, even within a single study demonstrating deregulation of MyoD gene targets in FSHD muscles, different subsets of targets appear to be altered in different patients (32). By contrast, multiple studies support a role for oxidative stress in contributing to FSHD pathology (30–32,34,73,74). Increased sensitivity to oxidative stress appears to be specific to FSHD vs. other muscular dystrophies (30,31,34), and mu-crystallin, a protein with links to oxidative stress (as well as retinal and inner ear functions), was reported to be specifically upregulated in FSHD muscles (75). Interestingly, 62 miRNAs were found to be specifically increased in FSHD vs. other muscular dystrophies (76), while their predicted targets, mostly genes involved in histone acetylation and GPI anchor synthesis, were shown to be downregulated in FSHD patients vs. asymptomatic carriers (37). Collectively, while lacking in consensus, these findings suggest that global alterations in transcription, signaling, and the response to oxidative stress may underlie the pathogenesis of FSHD.

THERAPEUTIC STRATEGIES

Pharmacological Intervention and Surgical Techniques

The lack of a consensus FSHD target gene has prevented the generation of a faithful and reproducible animal model, thus severely hampering the development of therapeutic strategies. To date, pilot studies in FSHD patients (testing the effects of anti-inflammatory or anabolic drugs, creatine, calcium-entry blockers, and DNA methylating agents) have produced inconsistent or disappointing results (77). Likewise, the results of randomized trials show no significant benefits of surgical intervention (i.e., scapular fixation) for FSHD patients (78).

Cell Therapy

Despite the lack of an established model system, efforts have been made to test the engraftment potential of FSHD cells. Both myoblasts and mesoangioblasts (muscle-derived pericytes) from unaffected FSHD muscles are able to integrate and participate in significant muscle regeneration in immunocompromised mice (71,79). Intra-arterial delivery of mesoangioblasts was shown to ameliorate the dystrophic phenotype in other muscle disease models (i.e., the α-sarcoglycan null mouse model of limb-girdle muscular dystrophy and the Golden Retriever model of Duchenne muscular dystrophy) (80,81). Thus, systemic delivery of these cells represents a possible avenue of autologous cell therapy for FSHD; however, the primary genetic lesion in these cells might eventually lead to a pathological phenotype if left uncorrected.

Manipulation of Gene Expression

Transcripts that are specifically overexpressed in FSHD (such as *DUX4-fl*) represent viable candidates for knockdown strategies, and the identification of suppressor/modifier genes should also provide new therapeutic targets. Additionally, recent efforts have focused on improving muscle strength in FSHD patients by inhibiting myostatin, a transforming growth factor-beta family member that serves as a negative regulator of muscle growth. Mutations in myostatin cause a hypermuscular phenotype, and in the *mdx* mouse model of Duchenne muscular dystrophy, myostatin inhibition leads to functional improvement in the dystrophic muscles (82). Recently, the myostatin neutralizing antibody MYO-029 was shown to improve single muscle fiber contractile properties in 4 out of 5 patients with muscular dystrophy, including 2 with FSHD (83). Myostatin recognizes activin Type IIB receptors, and a soluble activin receptor (ActRIIB-Fc) is currently in clinical trials for the treatment of muscle wasting disorders. Inhibition of myostatin by ActRIIB-Fc led to changes in gene expression that were similar to those in myostatin null mice, validating its specificity as a potential therapeutic agent (84).

OUTLOOK AND FUTURE DIRECTIONS

The establishment of animal or cell culture models that accurately recapitulate FSHD pathology would greatly aid studies of disease mechanisms and the testing of novel therapies. However, FSHD-specific biomarkers will be required to validate any model and to provide a benchmark for clinical trials. While the plethora of studies aimed at identifying such biomarkers has yielded no obvious candidates, as Parkinson's disease illustrates, even relatively modest changes in gene expression can produce a severe phenotype over time. It is also possible that large-scale screens mask significant changes in a small proportion of cells. The expression of the Dux4-fl isoform in a mere 0.1% of FSHD muscle nuclei, and the subtle and heterogeneous defects in FSHD muscle give hope that the disease can be ameliorated by targeting only a small percentage of cells. Also, the fact that heterozygous and mosaic individuals have a much milder phenotype is promising for eventual therapy.

As changes in gene expression appear to be largely specific to an FSHD family or individual, it is clear that samples from a large number of families will be required to identify biomarkers. Thus, efforts are under way to identify genes that are consistently altered in FSHD muscle from large patient cohorts via microarray and proteomic approaches. Well-controlled comparisons of gene expression patterns in early affected vs. unaffected vs. control muscles should shed light on the initial mechanisms involved in FSHD pathogenesis. The need for carefully controlled studies cannot be overemphasized, as much of the controversy in the field can be attributed to differences in source material, handling, and experimental parameters. There is also a pressing need for a comprehensive analysis of the physiological characteristics of affected FSHD muscles, as this has not been well-studied (e.g., there is only a single published report of normal calcium homeostasis in FSHD myoblast cultures, and the source of these cells is unclear) (85). Likewise, careful studies of muscle satellite cell characteristics in FSHD muscle will be required to determine whether defects in satellite cell proliferation, survival, differentiation, or self-renewal are involved in the progression of the disease. As FSHD is primarily a disease of muscle weakness, it is tempting to speculate that calcium pathways or contractile proteins may be affected (86), and that efforts to improve muscle strength may yield beneficial results.

It was suggested by Cabianca et al. that heterogeneity in FSHD might reflect heterogeneity in the expression of multiple genes, based on different epigenetic alterations among families and individuals (24). Indeed, the presence of multiple candidate genes with links to FSHD-associated defects (Figure 69.3), as well as the involvement of non-muscle tissues in FSHD pathology, certainly supports such a model. Since the discovery of the genetic lesion 18 years ago, rapid progress has been made in characterizing the epigenetic defects in FSHD and identifying candidate disease/modifier genes. It remains to be seen whether the manipulation of any one candidate or pathway will be sufficient to correct the disease in a majority of patients.

ACKNOWLEDGMENTS

We acknowledge the many important studies that have regretfully had to be omitted here due to space limitations, and we thank

Marietta Barro, Jennifer Chen, and Peter Jones for critical reading of the manuscript. This work was supported by a Senator Paul D. Wellstone Muscular Dystrophy Cooperative Research Center grant to the Boston Biomedical Research Institute (HD060848).

REFERENCES

1. Upadhyaya M, Cooper DN. *Facioscapulohumeral muscular dystrophy (FSHD): clinical medicine and molecular cell biology.* Abingdon: Garland/BIOS Scientific Publishers;2004.
2. van der Maarel SM, Frants RR, Padberg GW. Facioscapulohumeral muscular dystrophy. *Biochim Biophys Acta* 2007;**1772**:186–94.
3. Klinge L, Eagle M, Haggerty ID, Roberts CE, Straub V, Bushby KM. Severe phenotype in infantile facioscapulohumeral muscular dystrophy. *Neuromusc Disord* 2006;**16**:553–8.
4. Funakoshi M, Goto K, Arahata K. Epilepsy and mental retardation in a subset of early onset 4q35-facioscapulohumeral muscular dystrophy. *Neurology* 1998;**50**:1791–4.
5. Padberg GW, Brouwer OF, de Keizer RJ, Dijkman G, Wijmenga C, Grote JJ, et al. On the significance of retinal vascular disease and hearing loss in facioscapulohumeral muscular dystrophy. *Muscle Nerve* 1995;**2**:S73–80.
6. Fitzsimons RB, Gurwin EB, Bird AC. Retinal vascular abnormalities in facioscapulohumeral muscular dystrophy. A general association with genetic and therapeutic implications. *Brain* 1987;**110**(Pt 3):631–48.
7. van Deutekom JC, Wijmenga C, van Tienhoven EA, Gruter AM, Hewitt JE, Padberg GW, et al. FSHD associated DNA rearrangements are due to deletions of integral copies of a 3.2 kb tandemly repeated unit. *Hum Mol Genet* 1993;**2**:2037–42.
8. Wijmenga C, Frants RR, Brouwer OF, Moerer P, Weber JL, Padberg GW. Location of facioscapulohumeral muscular dystrophy gene on chromosome 4. *Lancet* 1990;**336**:651–3.
9. Wijmenga C, Sandkuijl LA, Moerer P, van der Boorn N, Bodrug SE, Ray PN, et al. Genetic linkage map of facioscapulohumeral muscular dystrophy and five polymorphic loci on chromosome 4q35-qter. *Am J Hum Genet* 1992;**51**:411–5.
10. Lemmers RJ, de Kievit P, Sandkuijl L, Padberg GW, van Ommen GJ, Frants RR, et al. Facioscapulohumeral muscular dystrophy is uniquely associated with one of the two variants of the 4q subtelomere. *Nat Genet* 2002;**32**:235–6.
11. Lemmers RJ, Wohlgemuth M, van der Gaag KJ, van der Vliet PJ, van Teijlingen CM, de Knijff P, et al. Specific sequence variations within the 4q35 region are associated with facioscapulohumeral muscular dystrophy. *Am J Hum Genet* 2007;**81**:884–94.
12. Lemmers RJ, van der Vliet PJ, Klooster R, Sacconi S, Camano P, Dauwerse JG, et al. A unifying genetic model for facioscapulohumeral muscular dystrophy. *Science* 2010;**329**:1650–3.
13. Gilbert JR, Stajich JM, Wall S, Carter SC, Qiu H, Vance JM, et al. Evidence for heterogeneity in facioscapulohumeral muscular dystrophy (FSHD). *Am J Hum Genet* 1993;**53**:401–8.
14. de Greef JC, Lemmers RJ, van Engelen BG, Sacconi S, Venance SL, Frants RR, et al. Common epigenetic changes of D4Z4 in contraction-dependent and contraction-independent FSHD. *Hum Mutat* 2009;**30**:1449–59.
15. Lemmers RJL, de Kievit P, van Geel M, van der Wielen MJ, Bakker E, Padberg GW, et al. Complete allele information in the diagnosis of facioscapulohumeral muscular dystrophy by triple DNA analysis. *Ann Neurol* 2001;**50**:816–9.
16. Zhang Y, Forner J, Fournet S, Jeanpierre M. Improved characterization of FSHD mutations. *Ann Genet* 2001;**44**:105–10.
17. van Deutekom JC, Bakker E, Lemmers RJ, van der Wielen MJ, Bik E, Hofker MH, et al. Evidence for subtelomeric exchange of 3.3 kb tandemly repeated units between chromosomes 4q35 and 10q26: implications for genetic counselling and etiology of FSHD1. *Hum Mol Genet* 1996;**5**:1997–2003.
18. Lemmers RJ, van der Maarel SM, van Deutekom JC, van der Wielen MJ, Deidda G, Dauwerse HG, et al. Inter- and intrachromosomal sub-telomeric rearrangements on 4q35: implications for facioscapulohumeral muscular dystrophy (FSHD) aetiology and diagnosis. *Hum Mol Genet* 1998;**7**:1207–14.
19. van Overveld PG, Lemmers RJ, Sandkuijl LA, Enthoven L, Winokur ST, Bakels F, et al. Hypomethylation of D4Z4 in 4q-linked and non-4q-linked facioscapulohumeral muscular dystrophy. *Nat Genet* 2003;**35**:315–7.
20. Yang F, Shao C, Vedanarayanan V, Ehrlich M. Cytogenetic and immuno-FISH analysis of the 4q subtelomeric region, which is associated with facioscapulohumeral muscular dystrophy. *Chromosoma* 2004;**112**:350–9.
21. Jiang G, Yang F, van Overveld PG, Vedanarayanan V, van der Maarel S, Ehrlich M. Testing the position-effect variegation hypothesis for facioscapulohumeral muscular dystrophy by analysis of histone modification and gene expression in subtelomeric 4q. *Hum Mol Genet* 2003;**12**:2909–21.
22. Gabellini D, Green MR, Tupler R. Inappropriate gene activation in FSHD: a repressor complex binds a chromosomal repeat deleted in dystrophic muscle. *Cell* 2002;**110**:339–48.
23. Bodega B, Ramirez GD, Grasser F, Cheli S, Brunelli S, Mora M, et al. Remodeling of the chromatin structure of the facioscapulohumeral muscular dystrophy (FSHD) locus and upregulation of FSHD-related gene 1 (FRG1) expression during human myogenic differentiation. *BMC Biol* 2009;**7**:41.
24. Cabianca DS, Gabellini D. The cell biology of disease: FSHD: copy number variations on the theme of muscular dystrophy. *J Cell Biol* 2010;**191**:1049–60.
25. Petrov A, Pirozhkova I, Carnac G, Laoudj D, Lipinski M, Vassetzky YS. Chromatin loop domain organization within the 4q35 locus in facioscapulohumeral dystrophy patients versus normal human myoblasts. *Proc Natl Acad Sci USA* 2006;**103**: 6982–7.
26. Petrov A, Allinne J, Pirozhkova I, Laoudj D, Lipinski M, Vassetzky YS. A nuclear matrix attachment site in the 4q35 locus has an enhancer-blocking activity in vivo: implications for the facio-scapulo-humeral dystrophy. *Genome Res* 2008;**18**:39–45.
27. Ottaviani A, Rival-Gervier S, Boussouar A, Foerster AM, Rondier D, Sacconi S, et al. The D4Z4 macrosatellite repeat acts as a CTCF and A-type lamins-dependent insulator in facio-scapulo-humeral dystrophy. *PLoS Genet* 2009;**5**:e1000394.
28. Masny PS, Bengtsson U, Chung SA, Martin JH, van Engelen B, van der Maarel SM, et al. Localization of 4q35.2 to the nuclear periphery: is FSHD a nuclear envelope disease? *Hum Mol Genet* 2004;**13**:1857–71.
29. Maraldi NM, Capanni C, Cenni V, Fini M, Lattanzi G. Laminopathies and lamin-associated signaling pathways. *J Cell Biochem* 2011;**112**:979–92.

30. Laoudj-Chenivesse D, Carnac G, Bisbal C, Hugon G, Bouillot S, Desnuelle C, et al. Increased levels of adenine nucleotide translocator 1 protein and response to oxidative stress are early events in facioscapulohumeral muscular dystrophy muscle. *J Mol Med* 2005;**83**:216–24.
31. Macaione V, Aguennouz M, Rodolico C, Mazzeo A, Patti A, Cannistraci E, et al. RAGE-NF-kappaB pathway activation in response to oxidative stress in facioscapulohumeral muscular dystrophy. *Acta Neurol Scand* 2007;**115**:115–21.
32. Celegato B, Capitanio D, Pescatori M, Romualdi C, Pacchioni B, Cagnin S, et al. Parallel protein and transcript profiles of FSHD patient muscles correlate to the D4Z4 arrangement and reveal a common impairment of slow to fast fibre differentiation and a general deregulation of MyoD-dependent genes. *Proteomics* 2006;**6**:5303–21.
33. Osborne RJ, Welle S, Venance SL, Thornton CA, Tawil R. Expression profile of FSHD supports a link between retinal vasculopathy and muscular dystrophy. *Neurology* 2007;**68**:569–77.
34. Winokur ST, Chen YW, Masny PS, Martin JH, Ehmsen JT, Tapscott SJ, et al. Expression profiling of FSHD muscle supports a defect in specific stages of myogenic differentiation. *Hum Mol Genet* 2003;**12**:2895–907.
35. Dixit M, Ansseau E, Tassin A, Winokur S, Shi R, Qian H, et al. DUX4, a candidate gene of facioscapulohumeral muscular dystrophy, encodes a transcriptional activator of PITX1. *Proc Natl Acad Sci USA* 2007;**104**:18157–62.
36. Klooster R, Straasheijm K, Shah B, Sowden J, Frants R, Thornton C, et al. Comprehensive expression analysis of FSHD candidate genes at the mRNA and protein level. *Eur J Hum Genet* 2009;**17**:1615–24.
37. Arashiro P, Eisenberg I, Kho AT, Cerqueira AM, Canovas M, Silva HC, et al. Transcriptional regulation differs in affected facioscapulohumeral muscular dystrophy patients compared to asymptomatic related carriers. *Proc Natl Acad Sci USA* 2009;**106**:6220–5.
38. Zamora M, Merono C, Vinas O, Mampel T. Recruitment of NF-kappaB into mitochondria is involved in adenine nucleotide translocase 1 (ANT1)-induced apoptosis. *J Biol Chem* 2004;**279**:38415–23.
39. Zhivotovsky B, Galluzzi L, Kepp O, Kroemer G. Adenine nucleotide translocase: a component of the phylogenetically conserved cell death machinery. *Cell Death Differ* 2009;**16**:1419–25.
40. Brenner C, Grimm S. The permeability transition pore complex in cancer cell death. *Oncogene* 2006;**25**:4744–56.
41. van Koningsbruggen S, Straasheijm KR, Sterrenburg E, de Graaf N, Dauwerse HG, Frants RR, et al. FRG1P-mediated aggregation of proteins involved in pre-mRNA processing. *Chromosoma* 2007;**116**:53–64.
42. Davidovic L, Sacconi S, Bechara EG, Delplace S, Allegra M, Desnuelle C, et al. Alteration of expression of muscle specific isoforms of the fragile X related protein 1 (FXR1P) in facioscapulohumeral muscular dystrophy patients. *J Med Genet* 2008;**45**:679–85.
43. Gabellini D, D'Antona G, Moggio M, Prelle A, Zecca C, Adami R, et al. Facioscapulohumeral muscular dystrophy in mice overexpressing FRG1. *Nature* 2006;**439**:973–7.
44. Liu Q, Jones TI, Tang VW, Brieher WM, Jones PL. Facioscapulohumeral muscular dystrophy region gene-1 (FRG-1) is an actin-bundling protein associated with muscle-attachment sites. *J Cell Sci* 2010;**123**:1116–23.
45. Hanel ML, Sun CY, Jones TI, Long SW, Zanotti S, Milner D, et al. Facioscapulohumeral muscular dystrophy (FSHD) region gene 1 (FRG1) is a dynamic nuclear and sarcomeric protein. *Differentiation* 2010;**81**:107–18 2011
46. Hanel ML, Wuebbles RD, Jones PL. Muscular dystrophy candidate gene FRG1 is critical for muscle development. *Dev Dyn* 2009;**238**:1502–12.
47. Wuebbles RD, Hanel ML, Jones PL. FSHD region gene 1 (FRG1) is crucial for angiogenesis linking FRG1 to facioscapulohumeral muscular dystrophy-associated vasculopathy. *Dis Model Mech* 2009;**2**:267–74.
48. D'Antona G, Brocca L, Pansarasa O, Rinaldi C, Tupler R, Bottinelli R. Structural and functional alterations of muscle fibres in the novel mouse model of facioscapulohumeral muscular dystrophy. *J Physiol* 2007;**584**:997–1009.
49. Clapp J, Mitchell LM, Bolland DJ, Fantes J, Corcoran AE, Scotting PJ, et al. Evolutionary conservation of a coding function for D4Z4, the tandem DNA repeat mutated in facioscapulohumeral muscular dystrophy. *Am J Hum Genet* 2007;**81**:264–79.
50. Wu SL, Tsai MS, Wong SH, Hsieh-Li HM, Tsai TS, Chang WT, et al. Characterization of genomic structures and expression profiles of three tandem repeats of a mouse double homeobox gene: Duxbl. *Dev Dyn* 2010;**239**:927–40.
51. Kowaljow V, Marcowycz A, Ansseau E, Conde CB, Sauvage S, Matteotti C, et al. The DUX4 gene at the FSHD1A locus encodes a pro-apoptotic protein. *Neuromuscul Disord* 2007;**17**:611–23.
52. Bosnakovski D, Xu Z, Gang EJ, Galindo CL, Liu M, Simsek T, et al. An isogenetic myoblast expression screen identifies DUX4-mediated FSHD-associated molecular pathologies. *EMBO J* 2008;**27**:2766–79.
53. Bosnakovski D, Daughters RS, Xu Z, Slack JM, Kyba M. Biphasic myopathic phenotype of mouse DUX, an ORF within conserved FSHD-related repeats. *PLoS One* 2009;**4**:e7003.
54. Wallace LM, Garwick SE, Mei W, Belayew A, Coppee F, Ladner KJ, et al. DUX4, a candidate gene for facioscapulohumeral muscular dystrophy, causes p53-dependent myopathy in vivo. *Ann Neurol* 2010;**69**:540–52 2011
55. Wuebbles RD, Long SW, Hanel ML, Jones PL. Testing the effects of FSHD candidate gene expression in vertebrate muscle development. *Int J Clin Exp Pathol* 2010;**3**:386–400.
56. Snider L, Asawachaicharn A, Tyler AE, Geng LN, Petek LM, Maves L, et al. RNA transcripts, miRNA-sized fragments and proteins produced from D4Z4 units: new candidates for the pathophysiology of facioscapulohumeral dystrophy. *Hum Mol Genet* 2009;**18**:2414–30.
57. Zeng W, de Greef JC, Chen YY, Chien R, Kong X, Gregson HC, et al. Specific loss of histone H3 lysine 9 trimethylation and HP1gamma/cohesin binding at D4Z4 repeats is associated with facioscapulohumeral dystrophy (FSHD). *PLoS Genet* 2009;**5**: e1000559.
58. Snider L, Geng LN, Lemmers RJ, Kyba M, Ware CB, Nelson AM, et al. Facioscapulohumeral dystrophy: incomplete suppression of a retrotransposed gene. *PLoS Genet* 2010;**6**(10):e1001181.
59. Lanctot C, Moreau A, Chamberland M, Tremblay ML, Drouin J. Hindlimb patterning and mandible development require the Ptx1 gene. *Development* 1999;**126**:1805–10.

60. Szeto DP, Rodriguez-Esteban C, Ryan AK, O'Connell SM, Liu F, Kioussi C, et al. Role of the bicoid-related homeodomain factor Pitx1 in specifying hindlimb morphogenesis and pituitary development. *Genes Dev* 1999;**13**:484–94.
61. Cole NJ, Tanaka M, Prescott A, Tickle C. Expression of limb initiation genes and clues to the morphological diversification of threespine stickleback. *Curr Biol* 2003;**13**:R951–2.
62. Shapiro MD, Marks ME, Peichel CL, Blackman BK, Nereng KS, Jonsson B, et al. Genetic and developmental basis of evolutionary pelvic reduction in threespine sticklebacks. *Nature* 2004;**428**:717–23.
63. Tanaka M, Hale LA, Amores A, Yan YL, Cresko WA, Suzuki T, et al. Developmental genetic basis for the evolution of pelvic fin loss in the pufferfish Takifugu rubripes. *Dev Biol* 2005;**281**:227–39.
64. Gurnett CA, Alaee F, Kruse LM, Desruisseau DM, Hecht JT, Wise CA, et al. Asymmetric lower-limb malformations in individuals with homeobox PITX1 gene mutation. *Am J Hum Genet* 2008;**83**:616–22.
65. Liu DX, Lobie PE. Transcriptional activation of p53 by Pitx1. *Cell Death Differ* 2007;**14**:1893–907.
66. Island ML, Mesplede T, Darracq N, Bandu MT, Christeff N, Djian P, et al. Repression by homeoprotein pitx1 of virus-induced interferon a promoters is mediated by physical interaction and trans repression of IRF3 and IRF7. *Mol Cell Biol* 2002;**22**:7120–33.
67. Kolfschoten IG, van Leeuwen B, Berns K, Mullenders J, Beijersbergen RL, Bernards R, et al. A genetic screen identifies PITX1 as a suppressor of RAS activity and tumorigenicity. *Cell* 2005;**121**:849–58.
68. Ansseau E, Laoudj-Chenivesse D, Marcowycz A, Tassin A, Vanderplanck C, Sauvage S, et al. DUX4c is up-regulated in FSHD. It induces the MYF5 protein and human myoblast proliferation. *PLoS One* 2009;**4**:e7482.
69. Bosnakovski D, Lamb S, Simsek T, Xu Z, Belayew A, Perlingeiro R, et al. DUX4c, an FSHD candidate gene, interferes with myogenic regulators and abolishes myoblast differentiation. *Exp Neurol* 2008;**214**:87–96.
70. Lemmers RJ, Osborn M, Haaf T, Rogers M, Frants RR, Padberg GW, et al. D4F104S1 deletion in facioscapulohumeral muscular dystrophy: phenotype, size, and detection. *Neurology* 2003;**61**:178–83.
71. Vilquin JT, Marolleau JP, Sacconi S, Garcin I, Lacassagne MN, Robert I, et al. Normal growth and regenerating ability of myoblasts from unaffected muscles of facioscapulohumeral muscular dystrophy patients. *Gene Ther* 2005;**12**:1651–62.
72. Morosetti R, Mirabella M, Gliubizzi C, Broccolini A, Sancricca C, Pescatori M, et al. Isolation and characterization of mesoangioblasts from facioscapulohumeral muscular dystrophy muscle biopsies. *Stem Cells* 2007;**25**:3173–82.
73. Barro M, Carnac G, Flavier S, Mercier J, Vassetzky Y, Laoudj-Chenivesse D. Myoblasts from affected and non-affected FSHD muscles exhibit morphological differentiation defects. *J Cell Mol Med* 2010;**14**:275–89.
74. Winokur ST, Barrett K, Martin JH, Forrester JR, Simon M, Tawil R, et al. Facioscapulohumeral muscular dystrophy (FSHD) myoblasts demonstrate increased susceptibility to oxidative stress. *Neuromuscul Disord* 2003;**13**:322–33.
75. Reed PW, Corse AM, Porter NC, Flanigan KM, Bloch RJ. Abnormal expression of mu-crystallin in facioscapulohumeral muscular dystrophy. *Exp Neurol* 2007;**205**:583–6.
76. Eisenberg I, Eran A, Nishino I, Moggio M, Lamperti C, Amato AA, et al. Distinctive patterns of microRNA expression in primary muscular disorders. *Proc Natl Acad Sci USA* 2007;**104**:17016–21.
77. Tawil R, Van Der Maarel SM. Facioscapulohumeral muscular dystrophy. *Muscle Nerve* 2006;**34**:1–15.
78. Orrell RW, Copeland S, Rose MR. Scapular fixation in muscular dystrophy. *Cochrane Database Syst Rev* 2010; [CD003278.]
79. Morosetti R, Gidaro T, Broccolini A, Gliubizzi C, Sancricca C, Tonali PA, et al. Mesoangioblasts from facioscapulohumeral muscular dystrophy display in vivo a variable myogenic ability predictable by their in vitro behavior. Cell Transplant ePub ahead of print December 22, 2010, PMID: 21176400.
80. Sampaolesi M, Torrente Y, Innocenzi A, Tonlorenzi R, D'Antona G, Pellegrino MA, et al. Cell therapy of alpha-sarcoglycan null dystrophic mice through intra-arterial delivery of mesoangioblasts. *Science* 2003;**301**:487–92.
81. Sampaolesi M, Blot S, D'Antona G, Granger N, Tonlorenzi R, Innocenzi A, et al. Mesoangioblast stem cells ameliorate muscle function in dystrophic dogs. *Nature* 2006;**444**:574–9.
82. Bogdanovich S, Krag TO, Barton ER, Morris LD, Whittemore LA, Ahima RS, et al. Functional improvement of dystrophic muscle by myostatin blockade. *Nature* 2002;**420**:418–21.
83. Krivickas LS, Walsh R, Amato AA. Single muscle fiber contractile properties in adults with muscular dystrophy treated with MYO-029. *Muscle Nerve* 2009;**39**:3–9.
84. Rahimov F, King OD, Warsing LC, Powell RE, Emerson Jr. CP, Kunkel LM, et al. Gene expression profiling of skeletal muscles treated with a soluble activin type IIB receptor. *Physiol Genomics* 2011;**43**:398–407.
85. Vandebrouck C, Imbert N, Constantin B, Duport G, Raymond G, et al. Normal calcium homeostasis in dystrophin-expressing facioscapulohumeral muscular dystrophy myotubes. *Neuromuscul Disord* 2002;**12**:266–72.
86. Reed P, Porter NC, Strong J, Pumplin DW, Corse AM, Luther PW, et al. Sarcolemmal reorganization in facioscapulohumeral muscular dystrophy. *Ann Neurol* 2006;**59**:289–97.

Chapter 70

ECM-Related Myopathies and Muscular Dystrophies

Carsten G. Bönnemann[1] and Nicol C. Voermans[2]

[1]*Neuromuscular and Neurogenetic Disorders of Childhood Section, National Institute of Neurological Disorders and Stroke/NIH, Porter Neuroscience Research Center, Bethesda, MD,* [2]*Department of Neurology, Radboud University Nijmegen Medical Center, Nijmegen, The Netherlands*

INTRODUCTION

The extracellular matrix (ECM) of muscle is an essential component of muscle as a tissue and organ (1). The ECM is part of the connective tissue, which refers to the entire network of extracellular material, consisting of the ECM and of the nerve branches, capillaries, fibroblasts, and macrophages that are embedded within this matrix (2). As outlined in Chapter 53 the muscle matrix has roles as a longitudinal and lateral transmitter of the force generated by the muscle fibers, as a mechanical support system, a regulator of signaling, and a modulator of regenerative and inflammatory activity in the muscle. It is also becoming clear that the ECM in muscle is not a static molecular compartment but a highly adaptable and changing part of the tissue. The matrix reacts to many pathological conditions that can affect muscle. Such conditions include acute injury or infection/inflammation, or the induction of muscle atrophy, such as occurs in denervation or immobilization (Chapters 64, 65). Importantly, the matrix also actively participates in generating the more chronic changes associated with genetic disorders of muscle such as in the muscular dystrophies. In most of these situations the amount of matrix increases while at the same time it is changing its molecular composition, resulting in a state of fibrosis, which can then be detrimental to muscle function and regeneration in its own right (see Chapter 53) (3–5). In contrast to such secondary ECM reactions to another disease process, the current chapter is concerned with myopathies that arise from primary genetic mutations in components of the ECM itself or its receptors on the muscle membrane/sarcolemma. However, the downstream effects on the matrix will frequently also include fibrosis similar to muscle disorders without primary mutations in components of the matrix (6). Disorders that are commonly subsumed as predominantly disorders of muscle will be discussed first, followed by discussion of disorders that are primarily classified as disorders of the ECM (and generally considered as heritable/inherited connective tissue disorders) but that can also have a clear skeletal muscle component (see Table 70.1 for summary). Some of the relevant disorders are covered in other chapters and will be referred to at the appropriate places throughout this chapter (see Table 70.2 for summary).

MYOPATHIES OF THE ECM

It is of interest to note that a number of the major conditions caused by mutations in components of the ECM and its receptors fall into the broad realm of the congenital muscular dystrophies. Congenital muscular dystrophies (CMDs) are a heterogeneous group of genetic disorders that typically manifest at birth or in early infancy with muscle weakness and a muscle biopsy compatible with a dystrophic or myopathic process (7). To be subsumed under the CMD category the muscle biopsy should show no features that would be diagnostic of another specific diagnosis, for instance a congenital myopathy with defining histological features (such as nemaline rods, central cores, predominant central nuclei, etc.), a metabolic myopathy or a motor neuron disease such as spinal muscular atrophy. Even though the onset for the CMDs typically is in infancy, all of the conditions in the CMD category encompass a much wider phenotypic spectrum, extending into adulthood with milder and later onset presentations. The CMDs that are caused by defects of molecules located in the ECM and its receptors include the alpha dystroglycanopathies, the integrinopathy (ITGA7), LAMA2-related CMD, and the collagen VI-related myopathies (8). Following the ultrastructural anatomical subdivisions of the ECM immediately around muscle, the matrix myopathies discussed in this chapter can be classified as (i) disorders of ECM receptors at the sarcolemma, (ii) disorders of the basal lamina, and (iii) disorders of reticular lamina (see Figure 70.1).

Muscle. DOI: http://dx.doi.org/10.1016/B978-0-12-381510-1.00070-3

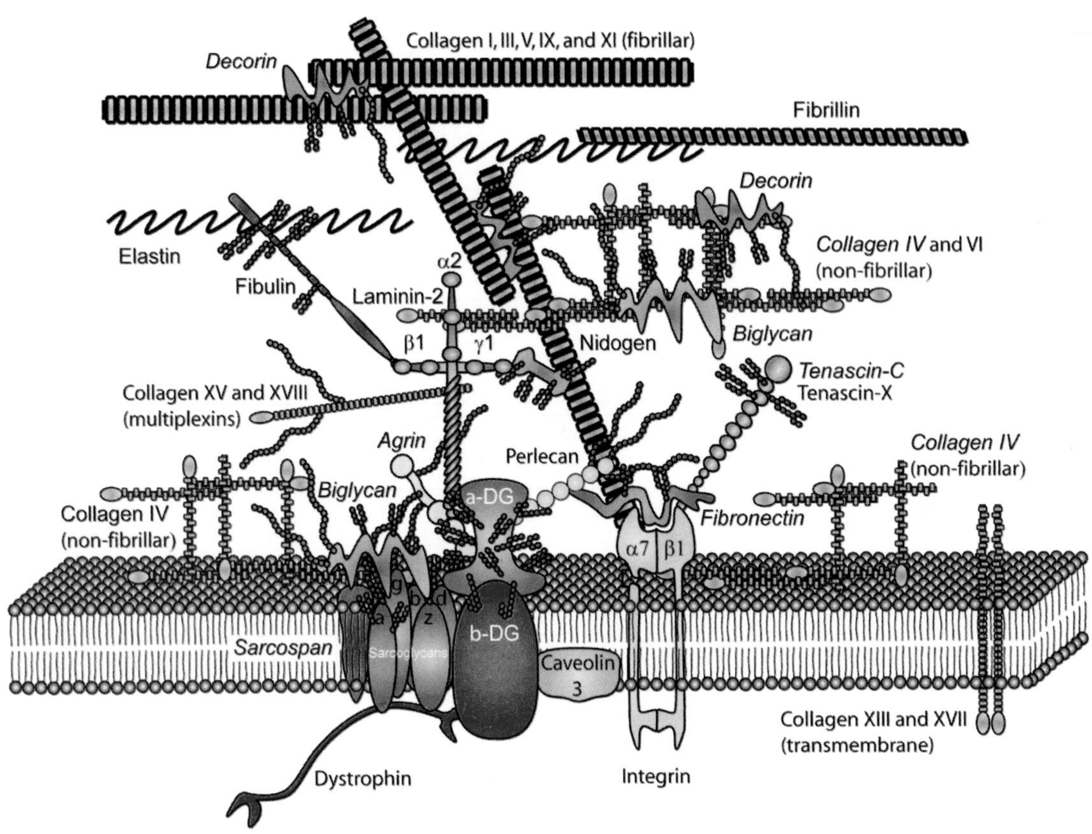

FIGURE 70.1 Schematic of the muscle extracellular matrix adjacent to the muscle fiber. This cartoon is not attempting to depict all interactions between the various molecules but rather provide an overview of the various molecular components in the matrix. *Modified from Voermans et al., 2008 (2).*

Disorders of ECM Receptors at the Sarcolemma

There are two myopathies that affect the most important matrix receptors on muscle, alpha-dystroglycan and integrin. Both alpha-dystroglycan as well as integrin alpha7/beta1 can function as the receptor for laminin 211 (formerly known as M-merosin or merosin; the numbers in the new laminin terminology refer to the chain composition of the laminin heterotrimer, i.e. laminin 211 contains an alpha2, a beta1, and a gamma1 chain (9)) on muscle.

The molecular defects in the alpha-dystroglycanopathies as a group result in an abnormal glycoepitope on alpha-dystroglycan, which then severely interferes with alpha-dystroglycan's function as a matrix receptor. The most important result of this is decreased binding of laminin 211 to muscle. This decreased binding is at the basis of the pathophysiology of these disorders and also results in a deficiency of the laminin 211 on immunostaining of muscle – hence the designation as secondary laminin 211 (merosin) deficiency. The alpha-dystroglycanopathies (primary and secondary) are comprehensively covered in Chapter 66 and will not be discussed here further. The second laminin 211 receptor on muscle is integrin alpha7/beta1. Mutations in integrin alpha7 are also a cause of myopathy.

Integrin alpha7

Laminin-binding integrins are composed of a large alpha chain in conjunction with a smaller beta1 chain (10). On muscle, integrin alpha7/beta1 is able to bind the laminins 211 and 111 (the latter however is not a physiological ligand in postnatal muscle) but also collagen type IV and fibronectin (11,12). Integrin alpha7/beta1 associates with various components of the integrin-associated adhesion protein complex on the intracellular site. During development the fibronectin receptor integrin alpha5/beta1 predominates, while in postnatal muscle integrin alpha7 replaces alpha5 and in association with the beta1 subunit is found both at the neuromuscular junction as well as prominently at the myotendinous junction, and to a lesser degree along the extra-junctional membrane (12,13). Integrin alpha7/beta1's functions as a laminin receptor are particularly important in lateral and longitudinal force transmission (12,14). Functions in signaling are likely also but have been less well defined. Inactivation of integrin alpha7 in the mouse causes a dystrophic myopathy (15). Human mutations in the gene coding for the alpha7 subunit (*ITGA7*) in muscle are recessive but are very rare and have so far only been described in two patients in Japan with congenital onset of muscle weakness (16). Both patients achieved the ability to walk at 2 and 2.5 years respectively but were unable to run. Other patients with an apparent deficiency of integrin alpha7 by biochemical methods did not have detectable mutations in the *ITGA7* gene, indicating that there likely are causes for a secondary integrin alpha7 deficiency (17). In the mouse model the muscle disease is most manifest at the myotendinous junction (MTJ) in muscle (14,15). This suggests a major mechanical role for this integrin at/in the MTJ and may also help explain that the rather mild findings seen in the biopsies from the two patients as biopsies are typically taken away from the MTJ. The mouse also shows a vascular phenotype that was not described in the human patients. Double inactivation of dystrophin together with *itga7* in the mouse leads to significantly more severe disease, confirming that there is an ITGA7-mediated mechanical transmembrane link to laminin 211 in addition to the dystrophin-associated glycoprotein complex (see Chapter 66) that partially compensates in the absence of dystrophin (18). Thus, forced overexpression of *itga7* is able to ameliorate the disease in dystrophin deficiency by establishing a mechanical link at extra-junctional membranes also (19).

Disorders of the Basal Lamina

The main molecular components of the lamina densa part of the basal lamina of the muscle basement membrane are laminin 211, perlecan, nidogen, and collagen type IV (20). There are two genetic disorders known to be associated with components of this part of muscle basement membrane – laminin 211-deficient congenital muscular dystrophy and Schwartz–Jampel syndrome and the allelic Silverman–Handmaker skeletal dysplasia.

LAMA2-Related CMD (MDC1A)

LAMA2 is the gene coding for the large alpha2 chain that is the defining component of both laminin 211 (former M-merosin) and laminin 221 (former S-merosin) (9). Primary mutations in *LAMA2* therefore cause a deficiency in both laminin 211 and 221. This condition was the first CMD for which the molecular basis was clarified by discovering the deficiency of laminin 211 with immunohistochemistry followed by the finding of causative mutations in the *LAMA2* gene on chromosome 6 (21). The disease is inherited as an autosomal recessive trait (22).

Most patients identified show a complete deficiency of laminin 211 on immunohistochemical analysis of the muscle biopsy (23,24). The typical disease presents in the newborn with significant weakness and hypotonia and elevated creatine kinase. Patients with complete deficiency of laminin 211 usually do not achieve the ability to ambulate independently but may achieve standing with support (24–26). Over the ensuing years there is a plateau in motor strength, followed by later slow additional loss of strength. Joint contractures affecting proximal as well as distal joints as well as scoliosis will be increasingly evident. In patients with incomplete deficiency of laminin 211 as judged by immunohistochemical examination symptoms can be milder in that ambulation may be achieved, although some patients with partial deficiency will be just as severe as the patients with complete deficiency are. In the largest series reported so far 5/13 patients with partial deficiency were able to ambulate, compared to only 2/33 patients with complete deficiency (24). The development of respiratory insufficiency is particularly common in the patients with complete laminin 211 deficiency and maybe manifest before 5 years of life or develop over the first 10–15 years of life. There also is a 30% incidence of seizures in patients with laminin 211-deficient CMD, suggesting that there is neo-cortical involvement in some patients. Consistent with this assumption there is a subgroup of patients (about 5%) who show abnormalities of cortical formation by MRI, usually affecting the occipital lobe (see below, Figure 70.3A,B, arrows), while other patients may show malformations in the posterior fossa, including cerebellar hypoplasia (27). A distinctive finding in all patients with complete or partial deficiency of laminin 211 is an abnormal signal on T_2-weighted MRI in regions of the white matter of the brain, while more compact white matter tracts such as the corpus callosum and the internal capsule are spared (see below, Figure 70.3A) (28). This is not a leukodystrophic change but rather appears to correspond to a higher water content in the white matter (29), although its precise pathophysiology remains to be worked out in detail. Since laminin 211 is also expressed in peripheral nerves there is evidence for the presence of a neuropathy predominantly of motor nerves, which however is clinically much less relevant compared to the muscular dystrophy (30).

Patients with complete deficiency have null mutations on both alleles, while patients with incomplete deficiency usually have compound heterozygous mutations of a missense or an in-frame mutation in conjunction with a null mutation on the other allele (24,26,31). Loss of laminin 211 around muscle leads to an abnormal lamina basalis as evidenced by ultrastructural examination (32). This seems to also result in an increase in sarcolemmal disruption as evidenced by the elevated CK that is found in all patients. A number of laminin 211 deficient mouse models has been identified, allowing for more detailed investigations of the pathophysiology of this condition (33).

The fundamental basis of the major disease manifestations lies in the loss of connection between alpha-dystroglycan and the basement membrane, which when re-established corrects the disease manifestations. For instance, laminin 111 containing the developmentally expressed alpha1 laminin chain is also capable of binding to alpha-dystroglycan as well as to alpha7 integrin via its G-domain (34). Proof of concept has been provided that laminin 111 is able to compensate for the absence of laminin 211 in transgenic experiments in laminin 211-deficient mouse models (35). Attempts at upregulation of the endogenous laminin alpha1 chain to make up for the deficiency of the alpha2 chain therefore have validity as a potential treatment strategy. Another strategy to re-establish a linkage between alpha-dystroglycan and the components of the basement membrane that has been shown to have effect in the animal model involves the use of a mini-agrin (36). Agrin includes an alpha-dystroglycan binding G-domain as well as a laminin binding domain able to link to laminin 411 which is present in the basement membrane of laminin 211-deficient muscle but is not itself capable of binding to alpha-dystroglycan. The presence of both these domains in the mini-agrin therefore allows for a re-establishment of a linkage between alpha-dystroglycan and the basement membrane. The mini-agrin construct dispenses much of the intervening agrin domains, resulting in a molecule that would be small enough for AAV-mediated gene therapy or even protein therapy.

Muscle in laminin 211-deficient muscle shows evidence for increased myofiber apoptosis as well as increased inflammation (37,38). Counteracting apoptosis in the animal model genetically (by expressing bcl2 or by inactivating bax) or pharmacologically (for instance with omigapil) has improved histology, function, and the lifespan of the animals (38). Another potentially important disease driver in laminin 211-deficient muscle is inflammation, which is evident both in the animal model as well as in patients. The degree of inflammation in the muscle biopsy can be so prominent as to suggest a primary inflammatory myopathy. Recent data in the dy3 mouse model of laminin alpha2 deficiency suggests that there also is increased activity of the muscle proteasome, inhibition of which prolonged life span, and improved histology and locomotion (39).

Transforming growth factor-beta upregulation has also been noted in the muscle of laminin 211-deficient animals and patients (40), providing another therapeutic target with significant translational potential, as has been shown for other conditions in which TGF-β upregulation plays an important role, such as Marfan syndrome (41), and in mdx mice (42). Regenerative activity in the muscle of laminin 211-deficient animals can also be improved by muscle-specific overexpression of an IGF1 transgene activating Akt and Erk1/2 signaling (43).

Perlecan (Schwartz–Jampel Syndrome)

Perlecan is the major multidomain heparan-sulphate-proteoglycan located within the basal lamina. In the basement membrane it interacts with laminin 211, nidogen, and collagen IV, and on the cell surface with integrin and alpha-dystroglycan (44). Perlecan also binds various growth factors and can be found in non-basement membrane extracellular matrices such as the matrix forming around chondrocytes. The perlecan gene (*HSGP2*) is located on chromosome 1 and mutations in it act in an autosomal recessive fashion. The clinical phenotype resulting from mutations in *HSGP2* consists of a combination of a myotonic myopathy and a chondrodysplasia (44,45). Complete deficiency of perlecan leads to a phenotype referred to as dyssegmental dysplasia, Silverman–Handmaker type (46). In this very severe disease resulting in neonatal lethality, the skeletal chondrodysplasia is associated with short limbs, vertebral segmentation defects, small thorax, and sometimes encephalocele. Survival time may be too limited for a clear muscle phenotype to become evident.

In contrast, Schwartz–Jampel syndrome results from an incomplete deficiency of perlecan. Patients present with a milder degree of chondrodysplasia as well as with signs of significant muscle stiffness, affecting the body muscles as well as muscles of the face. The facial involvement results in a typical appearance with blepharophimosis and a mask-like face (47). The disease may be evident in the newborn period (type 1B) or become evident somewhat later in childhood (type 1A). The muscle stiffness in conjunction with the skeletal dysplasia results in short stature as well as significant motor disability. Kyphoscoliosis, bowing of the long bones, and deformity of the ribcage are common skeletal manifestations. Weakness is not prominent and most of the disability results from the stiffness of the muscles. In adolescence and early adulthood there is some improvement of clinical features.

The physiological basis for the muscle stiffness appears to be electrical myotonia of the muscle, suggesting a secondary dysfunction of ion-channels on/at the sarcolemma. EMG reveals continuous high frequency low voltage discharge of the muscle fibers. However, no clear link between ion channel function and perlecan has been established so far. There is a known interaction between perlecan and the collagen Q tail of acetylcholinesterase (AchE) in the synaptic cleft, so that a deficiency in perlecan would lead to a secondary deficiency of AChE.

However, there are no clinical or electrophysiological signs of a disorder of the neuromuscular junction in perlecan deficiency. A direct interaction of perlecan with ion channels has thus been postulated but has not yet been directly shown. In contrast, primary mutations in the ColQ anchor of AChE result in a deficiency of AChE in the synaptic cleft, which leads to a form of congenital myasthenia (48).

Treatment has been attempted with carbamazepine, which has led to some improvement in the stiffness, presumably via its action at sodium channels, while treatment with a variety of other medications that are acting on ion channels including mexilitene and phenytoin has had only limited success (49).

A more severe and frequently lethal condition known as Schwartz–Jampel syndrome 2 or Struve–Wiedemann syndrome has been shown to be genetically distinct from Schwartz–Jampel syndrome 1 in that the former is caused by mutations in Leukemia Inhibitory Factor Receptor (LIFR) (50). Muscle myotonia has not been reported as being a major factor in this condition, although the facial features are very reminiscent. The skeletal dysplasia is prominent and progressive. Another group of disorders to consider in the larger differential diagnosis are the Crisponi syndrome/cold-induced sweat syndrome caused by mutations in the *CRLF1* and the *CLCF1* gene.

DISORDERS OF THE RETICULAR LAMINA AND BEYOND

Collagen VI-Associated Myopathies: Ullrich Congenital Muscular Dystrophy (UCMD)/ Bethlem Myopathy (BM) Spectrum

Collagen VI is a microfibrillar, non-fibril-forming collagen with short triple helical domains and larger globular domains. Collagen VI forms a basic heterotrimer that is composed of three polypeptides in equal stoichiometry, in its most common form involving the alpha1(VI), alpha2 (VI), and alpha3(VI) chains encoded by the smaller *COL6A1* and *COL6A2* genes on chromosome 21 and the *COL6A3* gene on chromosome 2 (51). While the collagenous triple helical domains are of similar length, the *COL6A3* gene encodes for a larger N-terminal domain that is the subject of alternative splicing and a larger C-terminal domain, which undergoes further proteolytic processing (52). The heterotrimer then undergoes an assembly process within the cell in which it forms an antiparallel dimer, two of these dimers in turn associate to form a tetramer, which is then secreted. In the matrix the tetramer forms extensive microfibrillar structures by end-to-end association of the globular domains, resulting in a bead-on-string appearance on ultrastructural examination (53). Collagen VI has been shown to interact with a variety of binding partners in the matrix, including biglycan, decorin, fibronectin, hyaluronic acid matrilin, and also collagen types I, II, and XIV. In the basement membrane collagen VI possibly interacts with collagen IV, perlecan, and indirectly with the dystroglycan complex via biglycan. Additional possible binding sites on the cell surface include the integrins and the surface proteoglycan NG2. Recently three additional collagen VI chain genes have been identified in the mouse (*col6a4*, *col6a5*, *col6a6*), of which two are functional in the human (*COL6A5* and *COL6A6*) (54,55). These chains appear to be able to substitute for the alpha3(VI) chain in the collagen VI heterotrimer, however, no disease-causing mutations have been identified in the genes for these new chains.

Disease-causing mutations in the three major collagen VI genes *COL6A1*, *COL6A2*, and *COL6A3* can be inherited in a recessive as well as dominant (negative) mode of action and have been associated with a disease that ranges from the severe congenital muscular dystrophy type Ullrich (UCMD) via phenotypes of intermediate severity to the milder Bethlem myopathy (BM) (56,57).

The congenital muscular dystrophy type Ullrich typically is evident at birth with significant hypotonia and weakness, as well as very significant distal joint hypermobility (Figure 70.2A), particularly affecting the hands and feet. In contrast, joint contractures may be present in the larger proximal joint (knees, hips, elbows, shoulders), ankles, and in the neck and spine (torticollis and kyphoscoliosis). Congenital hip dislocation is also present in a significant portion of patients (58,59). The contractures that are present at birth may initially show some improvement (although not always), but contractures will usually recur and become relentlessly progressive. The associated muscle weakness may be as severe as to preclude independent ambulation altogether. More commonly children reach the ability to ambulate after some delay, albeit with difficulty. As the disease progresses, ambulation will be lost again after a variable period of ambulation in the first decade of life or in the early teenage years due to increase of weakness and contractures. In addition there is worsening of the respiratory insufficiency in all patients usually leading to the need for non-invasive night-time ventilation in the first decade or in early teenage years (59). This respiratory insufficiency results from a combination of weakness of the diaphragm and other muscles of respiration in combination with an increasing stiffness of the ribcage, impairing its expandability.

In patients with a phenotype intermediate between Ullrich and Bethlem onset also is at birth or in the first year of life with muscle hypotonia, weakness and delay of motor milestones (60). However, the period of ambulation is longer, often extending into late teenage years and young adulthood. The concomitant decline in pulmonary

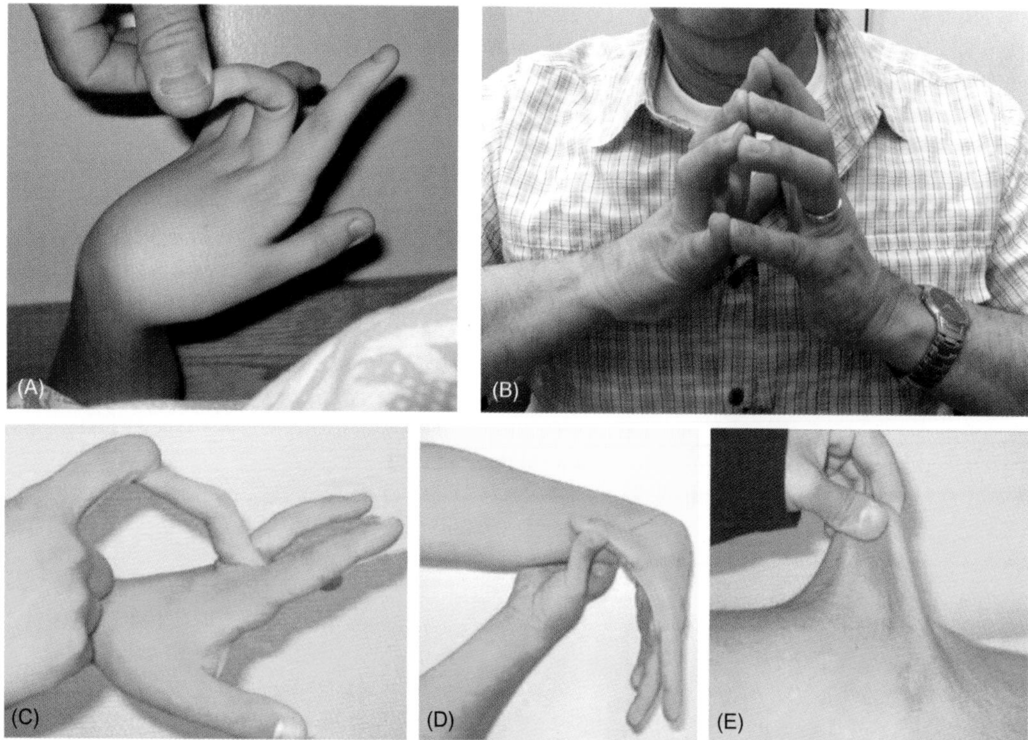

FIGURE 70.2 (A) Fingers of a patient with Ullrich CMD with striking hypermobility of the finger joints. The same patient has significant proximal contractures of the elbows and shoulders (not shown). (B) Hands of a patient with Bethlem myopathy, showing evidence for contractures of the long finger flexors, resulting in what has been referred to as the Bethlem sign. (C,D) The fingers of a patient with the TNX-deficient type of Ehlers–Danlos syndrome, with a hypermobility of the phalangeal joints that is very similar to the hyperlaxity seen in the Ullrich patient in (A). However, the patient with the EDS has no evidence for proximal contractures and the weakness is much more pronounced in the patient with Ullrich type CMD. (E) Skin hyperextensibility in the same patient with EDS, a phenomenon that is not seen in patients with collagen VI-related myopathies (Ullrich and Bethlem).

function also sets in later compared to the typical Ullrich phenotype, so that the onset of clinically relevant respiratory insufficiency is also delayed by about 5 years (59,60). In both the Ullrich and intermediate phenotypes the distal joint laxity tends to persist even in the face of increasing contractures. Both recessive loss of function mutations in the three disease relevant collagen VI genes (*COL6A1-3*) as well as de novo dominant negatively acting mutations can cause this early onset spectrum of collagen VI-associated muscle disease (60,61). Recessive mutations leading to complete absence of collagen VI have a tendency to underlie the more severe presentations of the Ullrich phenotype (62), such as the cases in which ambulation is precluded, while the dominant negative mutations (in-frame triple helical exon skipping mutations and triple helical glycine missense mutations) tend to be slightly less severe, i.e. allowing for ambulation for a period of time or falling into the intermediate range of severity (63,64). Glycine missense mutations affect the glycine of the collagenous Gly-Xaa-Yaa at the N-terminal end of the triple helical domain, with consequences on the triple helical domain the severity of which depend on their exact sequence context. This type of mutation is particularly prevalent in this intermediate range of severity. In general, for the dominantly acting mutations the consequences are more severe the more effective the mutations that are carried forward in the assembly process.

Bethlem myopathy is often also evident in early childhood with mild weakness and joint hypermobility (65). Ambulation in achieved and maintained into adulthood, although half of the patients need assistance with ambulation later in life. Characteristically there is development of contractures of the long finger flexors (Figure 70.2B), the elbows, shoulders and Achilles tendons (66). Respiratory involvement is seen in this group also, but later in the disease and to a milder degree. Typical dermatological findings, in particular keloid formation, can be seen in many patients. In Bethlem myopathy dominantly acting mutations are the predominant mutation type, and while recessive mutations can occur, they are rare (67). The dominant mutations seen in Bethlem have less dramatic consequences on the tetramer and microfibrillar assembly compared to the ones seen in the Ullrich and intermediate spectrum. In contrast to some other collagens, haploinsufficiency for a collagen VI gene is not associated with a disease phenotype.

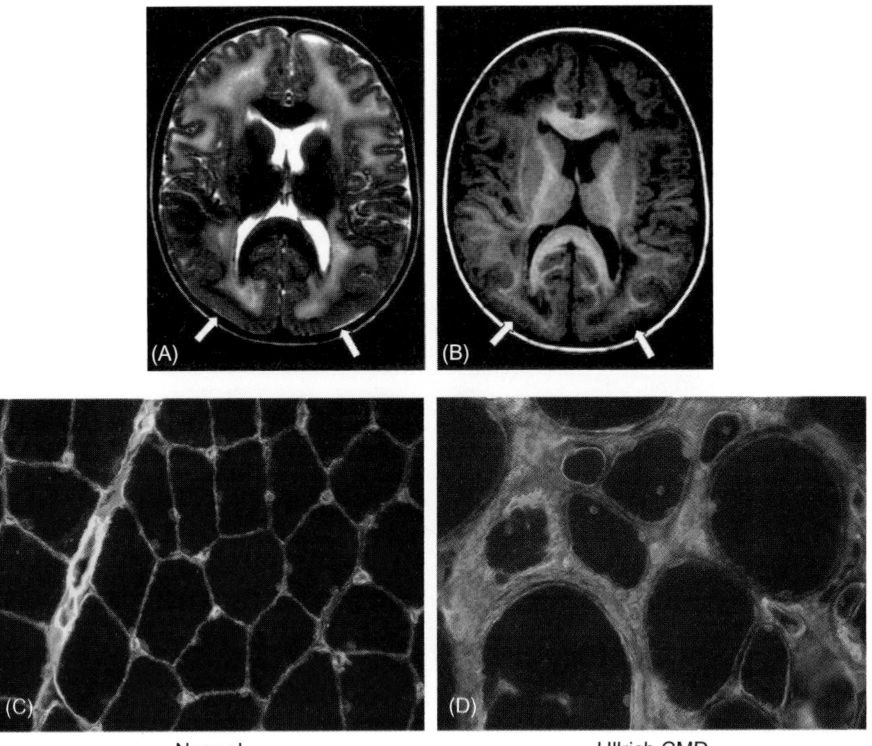

FIGURE 70.3 (A,B) MRI scan from a patient with LAMA2-related CMD depicting typical elevated T2 signal in the white matter, sparing compacted white matter tracts such as the corpus callosum and the internal capsule (A). There also is a malformation of the occipital cortex with lack of gyration, broadened cortical band, and an extra thin layer of heterotopic grey matter underlying the abnormal occipital cortex (B). While the white matter abnormalities are seen in all patients, a cortical malformation is seen only in a subgroup of about 5% of patients. (C,D) Immunohistochemical appearance of collagen VI in a typical case of dominantly acting mutation on one of the collagen VI chains. Collagen VI is labeled in red and laminin gamma1 as a marker of the basement membrane in labeled in green. In the normal case (C) there is direct overlap of collagen VI and the basement membrane resulting in the yellow color at the level of the basement membrane, whereas in the case of the mutation (D) the overlap between the two is lost, indicating that the mutant collagen VI is secreted into the matrix but incapable of making normal connections. *A and B reproduced with permission from Leite CC, Lucato LT, Martin MGM, Ferreira LG, Resende MBD, Carvalho MS, et al. Merosin-deficient congenital muscular dystrophy (CMD): a study of 25 Brazilian patients using MRI. Ped Radiol 2005;**35**:572–9.*

One of the most consistent findings seen in muscle biopsies from patients with collagen VI mutations is that collagen VI loses its normal connection with the lamina densa of the basement membrane (Figure 70.3C,D), which is obvious in the cases of total absence of collagen VI in patients with recessive mutations but is also prominently seen in biopsies from patients with dominant mutations (68). In the latter situation mutant collagen VI is secreted into the matrix, but the immunoreactivity is sparse at the lamina reticularis and does not overlap with the lamina densa of the basement membrane, while in the normal case there is a consistent overlap. Thus this connection to the muscle basement membrane likely is of great importance for the normal effects of collagen VI in skeletal muscle. Possible functions that have been put forward for collagen VI in various cell types have included roles in differentiation, adhesion, and cell survival (57). In a mouse model of collagen VI deficiency and also in patients there is evidence that myofiber apoptosis is one of the consequences of abnormal or absent collagen VI. The increased apoptosis as evidenced by an increase in TUNEL positive nuclei appears to be mediated by mitochondria via an inappropriate increase in breakdown of potential across the permeability transition pore when primed with oligomycin (69). As is evident from laminin 211 deficiency, increased myofiber apoptosis is not unique to collagen VI deficiency and it remains unclear how exactly the collagen VI deficiency leads to this phenomenon. However, this apoptotic mechanism lends itself as a potential target for pharmacological strategies. Cyclophilin D is a natural facilitator of the mitochondrial transition permeability pore, thus inactivating cyclophilin D will make the pore less susceptible to breakdown of the potential. Cyclosporine B in addition to its immunosuppressive effect via calcineurin also is an inhibitor of cyclophilin D and appears to decrease apoptosis and improve the disease in the mouse model (70). It has also been given to five patients in an uncontrolled study in which it also decreased apoptosis although its effect on the clinical manifestations of the disease was not clear (71). Other pharmacological strategies aimed at this apoptotic mechanism are under investigation. More recent data from the same group also showed that there appears to be decreased autophagic flux in the muscle of the collagen VI-deficient mouse model and of patients (72). The conclusion from this study was that there was also an impairment of mitophagy in the muscle, likely leading to a backup of the already dysfunctional mitochondria, thus worsening the mitochondrially mediated apoptosis.

Inherited Disorders of the ECM with Muscle Involvement

There is growing evidence for neuromuscular involvement in patients affected by disorders that are classically subsumed under inherited disorders of connective tissue. Many of the molecules involved in these disorders can also be found in the muscle ECM (2). One important pathophysiological theme emerging in a subgroup of these disorders involves the regulation of TGF-β signaling, which is particularly relevant in Marfan syndrome and related conditions (73) and as we have seen is also involved in some of the congenital muscular dystrophies described earlier. Muscle atrophy and weakness has been mentioned in the very first description of Marfan syndrome as well as subsequently (74,75). Fibrillin 1, the gene product involved in Marfan syndrome, is similar to collagen VI in that it is a microfibrillar ECM component (76). Marfan syndrome, Beal syndrome with its prominent contractural phenotype and Loeys Dietz syndrome are covered in Chapter 71.

Mutations in the fibulin genes coding for the elastic fiber-associated fibulins 4 and 5 are associated with cutis laxa syndromes. The clinical picture in patients is dominated by the cutis laxa and internal organ involvement (vascular occlusion and aneurysma formation), as well as pulmonary emphysema in the case of recessive fibulin 5 mutations. In addition, significant hypotonia often occurs. Both fibulin 4 and 5 interact with fibrillin 1 and help regulate TGF-β signaling via modulating LTBP1and LTBP 4 interactions with fibrillin 1. Beyond the clinical hypotonia seen in some patients there has been no systematic clinical or histological study of neuromuscular involvement in autosomal recessive cutis laxa patients (77).

Camurati Engelmann Syndrome (Progressive Diaphyseal Dysplasia)

While the genetic mutations in Marfan syndrome and other related conditions affect matrix components that regulate TGF-β signaling, in Camurati Engelmann syndrome the mutations affect the TGF-β precursor itself. Camurati Engelmann syndrome is a form of progressive diaphyseal dysplasia in which muscle involvement plays an early and important role (78). Frequently the initial clinical complaint before the skeletal dysplasia is obvious is of extremity pain (in 68% of patients) (79). The pain can become quite disabling and is frequently thought of as bone pain, but it seems possible also as it partly originates in muscle. A waddling gait is reported in 48% of patients, fatigability in 44%, and extremity weakness in 39%. The typical radiological features include conspicuous thickening of the bone cortex in the diaphyseal region of the long bones and also in the skull base, on the basis of a progressive osteosclerotic process. The muscle weakness, however, does not seem to be progressive (79). Muscles may appear to be atrophic but muscle biopsy findings are nonspecific (80).

The dominantly acting mutations in the TGF-β molecule are located in the latency-associated peptide region of the precursor, which mediates the interaction between the mature TGF-β peptide and LTBP. As a result of the mutation, mature TGF-β is released more easily, resulting in TGF-β overactivity. This overactivity leads to increased activity of the osteoblasts, but likely decreased satellite cell function and muscle regenerative potential. The mainstay of therapy has been the use of corticosteroids, which is partially effective against the pain (81). More recently, antagonists of TGF-β activity (including losartan) have been considered as well (42). Camurati Engelmann disease thus ties into the group of disorders in which TGF-β overactive signaling is involved at the level of the primary disease mechanism, the other one being Marfan syndrome. The causes for the clinical differences between these disorders are unclear but may in part be attributable to the distribution of the abnormal signaling directed by fibrillin in the case of Marfan syndrome, and perhaps also additional functions of fibrillin that are not fully explained by the LTBP anchoring defect alone.

OTHER SKELETAL DYSPLASIAS

Multiple Epiphyseal Dysplasia

The multiple epiphyseal dysplasias are a genetically heterogeneous group of disorders characterized by epiphyseal changes of variable severity. Mutations in collagen IX, cartilage oligomeric matrix protein (*COMP*), and matrilin 3 have been reported to underlie this group of conditions (82). Patients have often been noted to have mild muscle weakness and a waddling gait, even if the hips are not significantly affected by the dysplasia. Coexistence of a mild myopathy has been positively confirmed for collagen IX-related MED (83) and for COMP-related MED. In the latter case a mouse model of a human COMP mutation (associated with the related PSACH) has also been generated, replicating clinical findings of muscle weakness seen in patients (84). There was a strength deficit in the mice with only mild changes in the muscle itself, but clear evidence of abnormalities at the myotendinous junction, where COMP is also expressed. Collagen IX is found at the bone–tendon junction, suggesting that the phenotype attributable to muscle in these disorders is attributable to the muscle–tendon–bone interface rather than to an intrinsic muscle disease.

Osteogenesis Imperfecta

Osteogenesis imperfecta (OI) is an inherited connective tissue disorder characterized by small stature, reduced bone mineral density, and frequent fractures (85). More than 85% of patients with OI fall into four (types I–IV OI) of nine potential subtypes, due to predominantly dominant mutations in either of the type I collagen genes, *COL1A1* and *COL1A2* (86). Of the four classical types, type I OI is the mildest clinically and is characterized by blue sclerae, premature deafness, and mild to moderate bone fragility. Type II is perinatal lethal and type III OI (the most severe viable form) is characterized by short stature, deformity of the long bones and spine due to fractures, as well as premature hearing loss. Type IV OI has a moderate variable phenotype between types I and III.

Besides brittle bones, the clinical characteristics of OI subtypes are variable and include muscle weakness, exercise intolerance, hearing loss, and fatigue (87–89). Although clinically well defined, the pathophysiology of muscle weakness in OI has only recently been studied in more detail in a mouse model (90). The muscles of the OI mice were generally smaller, contained less fibrillar collagen, and had decreased muscle strength, with the homozygous mice being more severely affected than the heterozygous carriers (90).

The Ehlers–Danlos Syndromes

The Ehlers–Danlos syndromes are a group of genetic disorders of the ECM that are defined by the common feature of joint hypermobility, skin hyperextensibility, and tissue fragility. Important subtypes for the context of potential muscle involvement include the classical type, the hypermobility type, the vascular type, the Tenascin-X-deficient type, and the kyphoscoliotic type. Clinical features attributable to the neuromuscular system have been reported to a varying degree in the various EDS types (91,92). One of the most consistent complaints reported is excessive muscle fatigue, and physical examination also reveals muscle weakness (91,93). Peripheral nerve involvement has been detected in a number of EDS patients but will not be discussed further in the context of this chapter (90). The important theme emerging from the discussion of this group is the reinforcement of a concept of altered force transmission via tendon (longitudinal or myotendinous force transmission) and via the surrounding matrix (lateral or myofascial force transmission) due to the altered physical properties of the matrix (94).

Classical and Hypermobility EDS

The classical and hypermobility type together account for approximately 90% of the cases (95). In the classic type of EDS the joint hypermobility is associated with skin hyperextensibility and atrophic scar formation (96). Dominant mutations and haploinsufficiency have been reported in the *COL5A1* gene in about 50% of the patients fitting this phenotype. While the occurrence of a peripheral polyneuropathy has been described in some patients, complaints of muscle fatigue and weakness are more common and clinically relevant (91,93). The hypermobility type of EDS lacks the skin hyperextensibility seen in the patients with the classic EDS, but can be accompanied by a smooth velvety skin. Joint hypermobility is the dominant clinical manifestation, and certain joints, such as the shoulder, patella, and temporomandibular joints, dislocate frequently (96). Here the neuromuscular complaints are milder consisting mainly of muscle fatigue, weakness, and cramping.

The tenascin-X-deficient type is caused by a deficiency in the ECM protein tenascin X due to recessive loss of function mutations in *TNXB* (97). The phenotype is similar to that in the classical type, but inheritance is autosomal recessive and scars are generally less atrophic. Muscle involvement seems to be consistent in this type, with features reminiscent of Bethlem myopathy in one patient (91,98). In addition nerve conduction studies and electromyography show the presence of an axonal polyneuropathy in 40% of patients of this type, which could also play a role in the establishment of the weakness via diminished proprioceptive feedback from the muscles (91). A mild secondary deficiency of collagen VI in the muscle of a tenascin-X-deficient patient and in *Tnxb* knockout mice has been observed also (99,100). Physiological examination of muscle strength in the tenascin-X-deficient patients and in *Tnxb* knockout mice shows a considerable deficit in torque production, suggesting a deficit of force transmission from the muscle to the neighboring muscles and the surrounding connective tissue (myofascial force transmission) (94,99).

Tenascin-X is a complex ECM glycoprotein with a multimodular structure. It is found in the ECMs of skin, muscle, the digestive tract, peripheral nerves, and cornea (101). It is part of a larger family of tenascin molecules and interacts with a number of other ECM molecules and notably is involved in the regulation of collagen VI deposition and together with collagen VI in the fibrillogenesis of larger collagens (102,103). Together with the physiological data in the patients these molecular roles support a resulting force transmission deficit both laterally as well via the tendon.

Vascular and Arthrochalasia Type

Collagen type I and III belong to the large fibrillar collagens, and can frequently be found together. Both are found in the endo-, epi-, and perimyseum in muscle. Collagen I is found in virtually all extracellular matrices, including bone, skin, and tendons while collagen III also is an important component of blood vessels and hollow organs (1). Mutations in collagen type III underlie the vascular type of EDS (EDS type IV). The arterial, intestinal, and uterine fragility or rupture in this type often cause severe morbidity. Other typical features are a thin, translucent skin, extensive bruising, and a characteristic facial appearance. In addition, muscle cramps and pain as well as distal atrophy, and abnormal muscle imaging findings have been described (91).

The arthrochalasia type of EDS (EDS type VIIA and B) is also caused by mutations in collagen I and characterized by skin hyperextensibility, osteopenia and frequent joint dislocations that are a result of the joint hypermobility. Muscle hypotonia has been reported as an important part of the phenotype (95,96). The mechanism by which abnormalities of the large fibrillar collagens cause weakness are again likely related to a deficit in lateral force as well as possibly also longitudinal (i.e. tendon-mediated) force transmission.

Kyphoscoliotic EDS Type

The kyphoscoliotic type of EDS (former EDS type VI) is characterized by generalized joint hypermobility and often severe muscular hypotonia and weakness at birth. The defining feature is an early onset severe kyphoscoliotic deformity of the spine. In addition there is general tissue fragility, leading to atrophic scars as well as fragility of the sclera, which can lead to rupture of the ocular globe and fragility of the larger arteries. Muscle hypotonia and weakness can be very conspicuous, raising the strong suspicion of a congenital disorder of muscle (91,92,104). Ancillary investigations show signs of mild myopathy and polyneuropathy (92).

The kyphoscoliotic type A is caused by recessive mutations in the gene coding for lysyl hydroxylase 1 (procollagenlysine, 2-oxogluterate 5-dioxygenase 1). Lysyl hydroxylase is involved in the hydroxylation of lysyl residues at the second position of the Xaa-Lys-Gly collagenous amino acid triplet. The resulting hydroxylysine is important for both intermolecular crosslinking as well as for the addition of carbohydrate groups to ensure optimal lateral packing of the collagens. Both of these functions are crucial for the formation of higher order collagenous assemblies.

Recently a second type of kyphoscoliotic EDS (referred to as type B) has been found to be caused by recessive mutations in *CHST14* encoding carbohydrate sulfotransferase 14/dermatan-4-sulfotranserase 1 (105). Mutations in the same gene also cause the related adducted thumb clubfoot syndrome (ATCS) (106). Patients are also described as hypotonic and weak with a delay in gross motor development in addition to the early

TABLE 70.1 The ECM-Related Congenital Muscular Dystrophies (CMD)

Disease Entity	Locus Protein Product Gene Symbol Inheritance	Helpful Clinical Features	CNS Involvement	Laboratory Testing
Alpha-dystroglycanopathies – secondary merosin/laminin 211 deficiency				
Fukutin-related proteinopathy (MDC1C)	19q13.3 Fukutin-related protein *FKRP* AR	Often reminiscent of MDC 1A, but severity more variable, from severe CMD to LGMD as well as to WWS (q.v.), generally normal mental development, cases with structural brain involvement and mental retardation increasingly recognized, including MEB and WWS	Range from normal to significant structural abnormalities, ranging from cerebellar cysts to typical MEB and WWS	α-DG with diminished MW on WB, or reduction of IH using antibodies against glycosylated isotopes, secondary reductions in laminin-α_2 on IH/WB, mutation analysis
LARGE-related CMD (MDC1D)	22q12.3 Acetylglucosaminyltransferase-like protein *LARGE* AR	So far only one patient described. Congenital muscular dystrophy with profound mental retardation may eventually blend with the MEB/WWS spectrum	White matter changes, hypoplastic brain stem, mild pachygyria (similar to MEB)	IH/WB comparable to MDC1C, mutation analysis

(Continued)

TABLE 70.1 (Continued)

Disease Entity	Locus Protein Product Gene Symbol Inheritance	Helpful Clinical Features	CNS Involvement	Laboratory Testing
Fukuyama CMD (FCMD)	9q31 Fukutin *FCMD* AR	Frequent in Japanese population, never walk, mental retardation, epilepsy common – clinical overlap to MEB (q.v.)	Lissencephaly type II/ pachygyria, hypoplastic brain stem cerebellar abnormalities	IH/WB comparable to MDC1C, mutation analysis
Muscle–eye–brain disease (MEB)	1q32-q34 *POMGnT1* *FKRP, FKTN.* AR	Severe weakness and mental retardation, large head, prominent forehead, flat midface, walking rarely achieved, ocular involvement (e.g. severe myopia, retinal hypoplasia), deterioration because of spasticity	Lissencephaly type II/ pachygyria, eye malformations, brain stem and cerebellar abnormalities	IH/WB comparable to MDC1C, mutation analysis (genetic heterogeneity!)
Walker–Warburg syndrome (WWS)	9q34.1 *POMT1* *POMT2, FKRP, FKTN* AR	Severe, often lethal within first years of life because of severe CNS involvement	Lissencephaly type II, pachygyria, hydrocephalus, encephalocele, hypoplastic brain stem, cerebellar abnormalities, eye malformations	IH/WB comparable to MDC1C, mutation analysis (genetic heterogeneity!)
CMD with partial laminin 211 deficiency (MDC1B)	1q42 Not known AR	Rare, variety of severity, delayed onset possible, proximal girdle weakness, generalized muscle hypertrophy, early respiratory failure possible	Abnormal white matter and structural changes possible	Partial deficiency of laminin-α_2 on IH/WB, α-DG significantly reduced on IH, linkage analysis
Other ECM-related CMD				
CMD with primary laminin 211 (merosin) deficiency (MDC1A)	6q22-q23 Laminin-α_2 *LAMA2* AR	Sitting and standing with support as maximal motor ability if complete deficiency, neuropathy, epilepsy in about 30%, possible subclinical cardiomyopathy, generally normal mental development	Abnormal white matter signal (T2 MRI), 5% occipital pachy- or agyria, pontocerebellar atrophy (rare)	Mostly complete laminin-α_2 deficiency on IH/WB, secondary reduction of integrin α7 possible, mutation analysis.
Collagen VI related myopathies (Ullrich, Bethlem, intermediate)	21q22.3 and 2q37 *COL6A1, COL6A2, COL6A3* AD and AR	Distal joint hyperextensibility, proximal contractures, motor abilities variable, precludes independent ambulation in severe cases, soft palmar skin	No	IH for collagen VI with severe to mild deficiency, mutation analysis
Integrin α7	12q13 Integrin α7 *ITGA7* AR	Very rare, delayed motor milestones, walking with 2–3 yearss	No	Absence of integrin α7 on IH (secondary reduction possible), mutation analysis

**Schwartz-Jampel syndrome is not included in this table.*
IH, immunohistochemistry; AR, autosomal recessive; AD, autosomal dominant.

TABLE 70.2 Some Inherited Connective Tissue Disorders

Disease Entity	Locus Protein Product Gene Symbol Inheritance	Helpful Clinical Features	CNS Involvement	Laboratory Testing
Ehlers–Danlos syndrome (see Beighton et al. [96])				
Classic type (former type I and II)	9q34.2-q34.3 / 2q14-q32 *COL5A1 / COL5A2* AD 17q21.33 collagen 1 *COL1A1* AD	Skin hyperextensibility, widened atrophic scars (manifestation of tissue fragility), joint hypermobility, muscle hypotonia, mild proximal and distal weakness, severe fatigue, mild axonal polyneuropathy	No	Disturbed collagen fibrillogenesis ("cauliflower" deformity of collagen fibrils) on electron microscopy of a skin biopsy Abnormal electrophoresis' mobility of the proa1(V) or proa2(V) chains of collagen type V on fibroblasts Mutation analysis
Hypermobility type (former type III)	Not known (majority of cases) 6p21.3 *TNXB* Haploinsufficiency Tenascin-X (<5%) AD 2q31 *COL3A1* AD	Skin involvement (hyperextensibility and/or smooth, velvety skin), generalized joint hypermobility, musculoskeletal pain, muscle cramps, mild proximal and distal weakness, severe fatigue and pain	No	Measurement of TNX serum levels. Mutation analysis. Structurally abnormal collagen type III produced by fibroblasts: defective secretion, post-translational overmodification, thermal instability, and/or sensitivity to proteases Mutation analysis
Vascular type (former type IV)	2q31 *COL3A* (50%) AD	Thin, translucent skin, arterial/intestinal/uterine fragility or rupture, extensive bruising, characteristic facial appearance, muscle rupture, mild proximal and distal weakness, mild axonal polyneuropathy, muscle cramps	Aneurysms, parenchymal infarcts, caroticocavernous fistula	Structurally abnormal collagen type III produced by fibroblasts: defective secretion, posttranslational over modification, thermal instability, and/or sensitivity to proteases
Arthrochalasia type (former type VII)	Type A: 17q21.33 *COL1A1* AD Type B: 7q22.1 *COL1A2* AD	Severe generalized joint hypermobility, with recurrent subluxations, congenital bilateral hip dislocation, skin hyperextensibility, tissue fragility, including atrophic scars, easy bruising, muscle hypotonia, kyphoscoliosis, radiologically mild osteopenia	No	Electrophores of pNa1(I) or pNa2(I) chains extracted from dermal collagen or harvested from fibroblasts Mutation analysis
Kyphoscoliotic type (former type VI)	Type A: 1p36.22 *PLOD* AR Type B: 15q14 *CHST14* AR	Generalized joint laxity, severe muscle hypotonia at birth, scoliosis at birth, progressive; scleral fragility and rupture of the ocular globe, tissue fragility, including atrophic scars, easy bruising, arterial rupture, marfanoid habitus, microcornea, radiologically considerable osteopenia (both types Distinct craniofacial characteristics and multiple congenital contractures (type B)	No	Reduced enzyme activity in cultured skin fibroblasts, altered urinary ratio of lysyl pyridinoline:hydroxylysyl pyridinoline Mutation analysis
Tenascin-X deficient type {Schalkwijk 2001}	6p21.3 *TNXB* Tenascin-X AR	Generalized joint hypermobility, skin hyperextensibility, easy bruising without atrophic scarring, mild proximal and distal weakness, mild axonal polyneuropathy	No	Absence of TNX in serum Mutation analysis

** Marfan syndrome is not included in this table. AD, autosomal dominant; AR, autosomal recessive.*

kyphoscoliois (107,108). The 4-O-sulfation step is crucial to generate a final stable dermatan sulfate. Dermatan sulfate is crucial for the formation of dermatan proteoglycans, including decorin and biglycan. Both decorin and biglycan interact with collagen VI and decorin interacts with tenascin X. As a result, defects in collagen assembly and spacing can be observed, while there may be other additional effects on the regulation of growth factor signaling. This mechanism again appears to fit into a molecular framework in the ECM involving collagen VI, tenascin X, and small associated proteoglycans as well as their involvement in regulating larger collagen fibrillogenesis and organization (109).

This discussion of EDS types is not exhaustive, as we have selected types with some evidence for muscle involvement and new types are currently being recognized.

SUMMARY

This chapter has discussed both disorders that are commonly subsumed as predominantly disorders of muscle and others that are primarily classified as disorders of the ECM but also can have a clear skeletal muscle component (Table 70.1). For completeness, some disorders that are covered in detail in other chapters have also been referred to as appropriate (Table 70.2).

REFERENCES

1. Bosman FT, Stamenkovic I. Functional structure and composition of the extracellular matrix. *J Pathol* 2003;**200**:423–8.
2. Voermans NC, Bonnemann CG, Huijing PA, Hamel BC, van Kuppevelt TH, de Haan A, et al. Clinical and molecular overlap between myopathies and inherited connective tissue diseases. *Neuromuscul Disord* 2008;**18**:843–56.
3. Hantai D, Labat-Robert J, Grimaud JA, Fardeau M. Fibronectin, laminin, type I, III and IV collagens in Duchenne's muscular dystrophy, congenital muscular dystrophies and congenital myopathies: an immunocytochemical study. *Connect Tissue Res* 1985;**13**:273–81.
4. Serrano AL, Munoz-Canoves P. Regulation and dysregulation of fibrosis in skeletal muscle. *Exp Cell Res* 2010;**316**:3050–8.
5. Zhou L, Lu H. Targeting fibrosis in duchenne muscular dystrophy. *J Neuropathol Exp Neurol* 2010;**69**:771–6.
6. Taniguchi M, Kurahashi H, Noguchi S, Sese J, Okinaga T, Tsukahara T, et al. Expression profiling of muscles from Fukuyama-type congenital muscular dystrophy and laminin-alpha 2 deficient congenital muscular dystrophy; is congenital muscular dystrophy a primary fibrotic disease? *Biochem Biophys Res Commun* 2006;**342**:489–502.
7. Bönnemann CG. Congenital muscular dystrophy. In: Squire LR, editor. *Encyclopedia of neuroscience*. London: Academic Press;2008. p. 67–74.
8. Schessl J, Zou Y, Bonnemann CG. Congenital muscular dystrophies and the extracellular matrix. *Semin Pediatr Neurol* 2006;**13**:80–9.
9. Durbeej M. Laminins. *Cell Tissue Res* 2010;**339**:259–68.
10. Barczyk M, Carracedo S, Gullberg D. Integrins. *Cell Tissue Res* 2010;**339**:269–80.
11. Burkin DJ, Kaufman SJ. The alpha7beta1 integrin in muscle development and disease. *Cell Tissue Res* 1999;**296**:183–90.
12. Paul AC, Sheard PW, Kaufman SJ, Duxson MJ. Localization of alpha 7 integrins and dystrophin suggests potential for both lateral and longitudinal transmission of tension in large mammalian muscles. *Cell Tissue Res* 2002;**308**:255–65.
13. Vachon PH, Xu H, Liu L, Loechel F, Hayashi Y, Arahata K, et al. Integrins (alpha7beta1) in muscle function and survival. Disrupted expression in merosin-deficient congenital muscular dystrophy. *J Clin Invest* 1997;**100**:1870–81.
14. Welser JV, Rooney JE, Cohen NC, Gurpur PB, et al. Myotendinous junction defects and reduced force transmission in mice that lack alpha7 integrin and utrophin. *Am J Pathol* 2009;**175**:1545–54.
15. Mayer U, Saher G, Fässler R, Bornemann A, Echtermeyer F, von der Mark H, et al. Absence of integrin alpha 7 causes a novel form of muscular dystrophy. *Nature Genetics* 1997;**17**:318–23.
16. Hayashi YK, Chou FL, Engvall E, Ogawa M, Matsuda C, Hirabayashi S, et al. Mutations in the integrin alpha7 gene cause congenital myopathy. *Nat Genet* 1998;**19**:94–7.
17. Pegoraro E, Cepollaro F, Prandini P, Marin A, Fanin M, Trevisan CP, et al. Integrin alpha 7 beta 1 in muscular dystrophy/myopathy of unknown etiology. *Am J Pathol* 2002;**160**:2135–43.
18. Rooney JE, Welser JV, Dechert MA, Flintoff-Dye NL, Kaufman SJ, Burkin DJ, et al. Severe muscular dystrophy in mice that lack dystrophin and alpha7 integrin. *J Cell Sci* 2006;**119**:2185–95.
19. Burkin DJ, Wallace GQ, Nicol KJ, Kaufman DJ, Kaufman SJ. Enhanced expression of the alpha 7 beta 1 integrin reduces muscular dystrophy and restores viability in dystrophic mice. *J Cell Biol* 2001;**152**:1207–18.
20. Yurchenco PD. Basement membranes: cell scaffoldings and signaling platforms. *Cold Spring Harb Perspect Biol* 2011;**3**.
21. Hayashi YK, Koga R, Tsukahara T, Ishii H, Matsuishi T, Yamashita Y, et al. Deficiency of laminin alpha 2-chain mRNA in muscle in a patient with merosin-negative congenital muscular dystrophy. *Muscle Nerve* 1995;**18**:1027–30.
22. Allamand V, Guicheney P. Merosin-deficient congenital muscular dystrophy, autosomal recessive (MDC1A, MIM#156225, LAMA2 gene coding for alpha2 chain of laminin). *Eur J Hum Genet* 2002;**10**:91–4.
23. Tomé FM, Evangelista T, Leclerc A, Sunada Y, Manole E, Estornet B, et al. Congenital muscular dystrophy with merosin deficiency. *C R Acad Sci Paris* 1994;**317**:251–357.
24. Geranmayeh F, Clement E, Feng LH, Sewry C, Pagan J, Mein R, et al. Genotype-phenotype correlation in a large population of muscular dystrophy patients with LAMA2 mutations. *Neuromuscul Disord* 2010;**20**:241–50.
25. Philpot J, Sewry C, Pennock J, Dubowitz V. Clinical phenotype in congenital muscular dystrophy: correlation with expression of merosin in skeletal muscle. *Neuromuscul Disord* 1995;**5**:301–5.
26. Pegoraro E, Marks H, Garcia CA, Crawford T, Mancias P, Connolly AM, et al. Laminin alpha2 muscular dystrophy: genotype/phenotype studies of 22 patients. *Neurology* 1998;**51**:101–10.
27. Philpot JCOMP: Please continue reversing author surnames and initials from here on, Cowan F, Pennock J, Sewry C, Dubowitz V,

Bydder G, Muntoni F, et al. Merosin-deficient congenital muscular dystrophy: the spectrum of brain involvement on magnetic resonance imaging. *Neuromuscul Disord* 1999;**9**:81–5.

28. van der Knaap MS, Smit LM, Barth PG, Catsman-Berrevoets CE, Brouwer OF, Begeer JH. Magnetic resonance imaging in classification of congenital muscular dystrophies with brain abnormalities. *Ann Neurol* 1997;**42**:50–9.
29. Brockmann K, Dechent P, Bonnemann C, Schreiber G, Frahm J, Hanefeld F. Quantitative proton MRS of cerebral metabolites in laminin alpha2 chain deficiency. *Brain Dev* 2007;**29**:357–64.
30. Quijano-Roy S, Renault F, Romero N, Guicheney P, Fardeau M, Estournet. B. EMG and nerve conduction studies in children with congenital muscular dystrophy. *Muscle Nerve* 2004;**29**:292–9.
31. Di Blasi C, He Y, Morandi L, Cornelio F, Guicheney P, Mora M. Mild muscular dystrophy due to a nonsense mutation in the LAMA2 gene resulting in exon skipping. *Brain* 2001;**124**:698–704.
32. Shibuya S, Wakayama Y, Inoue M, Kojima H, Oniki H. Merosin (laminin-2) localization in basal lamina of normal skeletal muscle fibers and changes in plasma membrane of merosin-deficient skeletal muscle fibers. *Med Electron Microsc* 2003;**36**:213–20.
33. Guo LT, Zhang XU, Kuang W, Xu H, Liu LA, Vilquin JT, et al. Laminin alpha2 deficiency and muscular dystrophy; genotype-phenotype correlation in mutant mice. *Neuromuscul Disord* 2003;**13**:207–15.
34. Gawlik KI, Akerlund M, Carmignac V, Elamaa H, Durbeej M. Distinct roles for laminin globular domains in laminin alpha1 chain mediated rescue of murine laminin alpha2 chain deficiency. *PLoS One* 2010;**5**:e11549.
35. Gawlik K, Miyagoe-Suzuki Y, Ekblom P, Takeda S, Durbeej M. Laminin alpha1 chain reduces muscular dystrophy in laminin alpha2 chain deficient mice. *Hum Mol Genet* 2004;**13**:1775–84.
36. Moll J, Barzaghi P, Lin S, Bezakova G, Lochmuller H, Engvall E, Muller U. An agrin minigene rescues dystrophic symptoms in a mouse model for congenital muscular dystrophy. *Nature* 2001;**413**:302–7.
37. Mukasa T, Momoi T, Momoi MY. Activation of caspase-3 apoptotic pathways in skeletal muscle fibers in laminin alpha2-deficient mice. *Biochem Biophys Res Commun* 1999;**260**:139–42.
38. Girgenrath M, Dominov JA, Kostek CA, Miller JB. Inhibition of apoptosis improves outcome in a model of congenital muscular dystrophy. *J Clin Invest* 2004;**114**:1635–9.
39. Carmignac V, Quere R, Durbeej M. Proteasome inhibition improves the muscle of laminin alpha2 chain-deficient mice. *Hum Mol Genet* 2011;**20**:541–52.
40. Bernasconi P, Di Blasi C, Mora M, Morandi L, Galbiati S, Confalonieri P, et al. Transforming growth factor-beta1 and fibrosis in congenital muscular dystrophies. *Neuromuscul Disord* 1999;**9**:28–33.
41. Habashi JP, Judge DP, Holm TM, Cohn RD, Loeys BL, Cooper TK, et al. Losartan, an AT1 antagonist, prevents aortic aneurysm in a mouse model of marfan syndrome. *Science* 2006;**312**:117–21.
42. Cohn RD, van Erp C, Habashi JP, Soleimani AA, Klein EC, Lisi. MT. Angiotensin II type 1 receptor blockade attenuates TGF-beta-induced failure of muscle regeneration in multiple myopathic states. *Nat Med* 2007;**13**:204–10.
43. Kumar A, Yamauchi J, Girgenrath T, Girgenrath M. Muscle-specific expression of insulin-like growth factor 1 improves outcome in Lama2Dy-w mice, a model for congenital muscular dystrophy type 1A. *Hum Mol Genet* 2011;**20**:2333–43.
44. Nicole S, Davoine CS, Topaloglu H, Cattolico L, Barral D, Beighton P, et al. Perlecan, the major proteoglycan of basement membranes, is altered in patients with Schwartz–Jampel syndrome (chondrodystrophic myotonia). *Nat Genet* 2000;**26**:480–3.
45. Stum M, Davoine CS, Vicart S, Guillot-Noel L, Topaloglu H, Carod-Artal FJ. Spectrum of HSPG2 (Perlecan) mutations in patients with Schwartz–Jampel syndrome. *Hum Mutat* 2006;**27**:1082–91.
46. Arikawa-Hirasawa E, Wilcox WR, Le AH, Silverman N, Govindraj P, Hassell JR, et al. Dyssegmental dysplasia, silverman–handmaker type, is caused by functional null mutations of the perlecan gene. *Nat Genet* 2001;**27**:431–4.
47. Stum M, Davoine CS, Fontaine B, Nicole S. Schwartz–Jampel syndrome and perlecan deficiency. *Acta Myol* 2005;**24**:89–92.
48. Mihaylova V, Muller JS, Vilchez JJ, Salih MA, Kabiraj MM, D'Amico A, et al. Clinical and molecular genetic findings in COLQ-mutant congenital myasthenic syndromes. *Brain* 2008;**131**:747–59.
49. Reed UC, Reimao R, Espindola AA, Kok F, Ferreira LG, Resende MB, et al. Schwartz–Jampel syndrome: report of five cases. *Arq Neuropsiquiatr* 2002;**60**:734–8.
50. Dagoneau N, Scheffer D, Huber C, Al-Gazali LI, Di Rocco M, Godard A, et al. Null leukemia inhibitory factor receptor (LIFR) mutations in Stuve–Wiedemann/Schwartz–Jampel type 2 syndrome. *Am J Hum Genet* 2004;**74**:298–305.
51. Timpl R, Chu ML. Microfibrillar collagen type VI. In: Mecham RP, editor. *Extracellular matrix assembly and structure*. Orlando, FL: Academic Press;1994. p. 207–42.
52. Aigner T, Hambach L, Soder S, Schlotzer-Schrehardt U, Poschl E. The C5 domain of Col6A3 is cleaved off from the Col6 fibrils immediately after secretion. *Biochem Biophys Res Commun* 2002;**290**:743–8.
53. Baldock C, Sherratt MJ, Shuttleworth CA, Kielty CM. The supramolecular organization of collagen VI microfibrils. *J Mol Biol* 2003;**330**:297–307.
54. Gara SK, Grumati P, Urciuolo A, Bonaldo P, Kobbe B, Koch M, et al. Three novel collagen VI chains with high homology to the alpha3 chain. *J Biol Chem* 2008;**283**:10658–70.
55. Fitzgerald J, Rich C, Zhou FH, Hansen U. Three novel collagen VI chains, alpha4(VI), alpha5(VI), and alpha6(VI). *J Biol Chem* 2008;**283**:20170–80.
56. Lampe AK, Bushby KM. Collagen VI related muscle disorders. *J Med Genet* 2005;**42**:673–85.
57. Bönnemann CG. The collagen VI-related myopathies: muscle meets its matrix. *Nature Rev Neurol* 2011;**7**:379–90.
58. Bertini E, Pepe G. Collagen type VI and related disorders: bethlem myopathy and ullrich scleroatonic muscular dystrophy. *Eur J Paediatr Neurol* 2002;**6**:193–8.
59. Nadeau A, Kinali M, Main M, Jimenez-Mallebrera C, Aloysius A, Clement E, et al. Natural history of Ullrich congenital muscular dystrophy. *Neurology* 2009;**73**:25–31.
60. Brinas L, Richard P, Quijano-Roy S, Gartioux C, Ledeuil C, Lacene E, et al. Early onset collagen VI myopathies: genetic and clinical correlations. *Ann Neurol* 2010;**68**:511–20.
61. Lampe AK, Zou Y, Sudano D, O'Brien KK, Hicks D, Laval, et al. Exon skipping mutations in collagen VI are common and are

predictive for severity and inheritance. *Hum Mutat* 2008;**29**: 809–22.

62. Camacho Vanegas O, Bertini E, Zhang RZ, Petrini S, Minosse C, Sabatelli, et al. *Ullrich scleroatonic muscular dystrophy is caused by recessive mutations in collagen type VI. Proc Natl Acad Sci USA* 2001;**98**:7516–21.
63. Lucioli S, Giusti B, Mercuri E, Vanegas OC, Lucarini L, Pietroni V, et al. Detection of common and private mutations in the COL6A1 gene of patients with Bethlem myopathy. *Neurology* 2005;**64**:1931–7.
64. Allamand V, Merlini L, Bushby K. 166th ENMC International Workshop on Collagen type VI-related Myopathies, 22–24 May 2009, Naarden, The Netherlands. *Neuromuscul Disord* 2010;**20**: 346–54.
65. Jöbsis GJ, Boers JM, Barth PG, de Visser M. Bethlem myopathy: a slowly progressive congenital muscular dystrophy with contractures. *Brain* 1999;**122**:649–55.
66. Merlini L, Morandi L, Granata C, Ballestrazzi A. Bethlem myopathy: early-onset benign autosomal dominant myopathy with contractures. Description of two new families. *Neuromuscul Disord* 1994;**4**:503–11.
67. Foley AR, Hu Y, Zou Y, Columbus A, Shoffner J, Dunn DM, et al. Autosomal recessive inheritance of classic Bethlem myopathy. *Neuromuscul Disord* 2009;**19**:813–7.
68. Pan TC, Zhang RZ, Sudano DG, Marie SK, Bonnemann CG, Chu ML. New molecular mechanism for Ullrich congenital muscular dystrophy: a heterozygous in-frame deletion in the COL6A1 gene causes a severe phenotype. *Am J Hum Genet* 2003;**73**:355–69.
69. Irwin WA, Bergamin N, Sabatelli P, Reggiani C, Megighian A, Merlini, et al. Mitochondrial dysfunction and apoptosis in myopathic mice with collagen VI deficiency. *Nat Genet* 2003;**35**:367–71.
70. Angelin A, Tiepolo T, Sabatelli P, Grumati P, Bergamin N, Golfieri C, et al. Mitochondrial dysfunction in the pathogenesis of Ullrich congenital muscular dystrophy and prospective therapy with cyclosporins. *Proc Natl Acad Sci USA* 2007;**104**:991–6.
71. Merlini L, Angelin A, Tiepolo T, Braghetta P, Sabatelli P, Zamparelli, et al. Cyclosporin A corrects mitochondrial dysfunction and muscle apoptosis in patients with collagen VI myopathies. *Proc Natl Acad Sci USA* 2008;**105**:5225–9.
72. Grumati P, Coletto L, Sabatelli P, Cescon M, Angelin A, Bertaggia, et al. Autophagy is defective in collagen VI muscular dystrophies, and its reactivation rescues myofiber degeneration. *Nat Med* 2010;**16**:1313–20.
73. Dietz HC, Loeys B, Carta L, Ramirez F. Recent progress towards a molecular understanding of Marfan syndrome. *Am J Med Genet C Semin Med Genet* 2005;**139C**:4–9.
74. Behan WM, Longman C, Petty RK, Boxer M, Foskett P, Harriman DG. Muscle fibrillin deficiency in Marfan's syndrome myopathy. *J Neurol Neurosurg Psychiatry* 2003;**74**:633–8.
75. Voermans N, Timmermans J, van Alfen N, Pillen S, op den Akker J, Lammens M, et al. Neuromuscular features in Marfan syndrome. *Clin Genet* 2009;**76**:25–37.
76. Ramirez F, Dietz HC. Marfan syndrome: from molecular pathogenesis to clinical treatment. *Curr Opin Genet Dev* 2007;**17**:252–8.
77. Morava E, Wopereis S, Coucke P, Gillessen-Kaesbach G, Voit T, Smeitink, et al. Defective protein glycosylation in patients with cutis laxa syndrome. *Eur J Hum Genet* 2005;**13**:414–21.
78. Stenzler S, Grogan DP, Frenchman SM, McClelland S, Ogden JA. Progressive diaphyseal dysplasia presenting as neuromuscular disease. *J Pediatr Orthop* 1989;**9**:463–7.
79. Janssens K, Vanhoenacker F, Bonduelle M, Verbruggen L, Van Maldergem L, Ralston, et al. Camurati–Engelmann disease: review of the clinical, radiological, and molecular data of 24 families and implications for diagnosis and treatment. *J Med Genet* 2006;**43**:1–11.
80. Naveh Y, Ludatshcer R, Alon U, Sharf B. Muscle involvement in progressive diaphyseal dysplasia. *Pediatrics* 1985;**76**:944–9.
81. Naveh Y, Alon U, Kaftori JK, Berant M. Progressive diaphyseal dysplasia: evaluation of corticosteroid therapy. *Pediatrics* 1985;**75**:321–3.
82. Pirog KA, Briggs MD. Skeletal dysplasias associated with mild myopathy – a clinical and molecular review. *J Biomed Biotechnol* 2010;:686457 Epub May 24, 2010.
83. Bönnemann CG, Cox GF, Shapiro F, Wu JJ, Feener CA, Thompson TG, et al. A mutation in the alpha 3 chain of type IX collagen causes autosomal dominant multiple epiphyseal dysplasia with mild myopathy. *Proc Natl Acad Sci USA* 2000;**97**:1212–7.
84. Pirog KA, Jaka O, Katakura Y, Meadows RS, Kadler KE, Boot-Handford, et al. A mouse model offers novel insights into the myopathy and tendinopathy often associated with pseudoachondroplasia and multiple epiphyseal dysplasia. *Hum Mol Genet* 2010;**19**:52–64.
85. Steiner RD, Pepin MG, Byers PH. Osteogenesis imperfecta. In: Pagon RA, Bird TD, Dolan CR, Stephens K, editors. *GeneReviews* [Internet]. Seattle, WA: University of Washington;2005.
86. Basel D, Steiner RD. Osteogenesis imperfecta: recent findings shed new light on this once well-understood condition. *Genet Med* 2009;**11**:375–85.
87. Rauch F, Glorieux FH. Osteogenesis imperfecta. *Lancet* 2004;**363**:1377–85.
88. Engelbert RH, Uiterwaal CS, Gerver WJ, van der Net JJ, Pruijs HE, Helders PJ. Osteogenesis imperfecta in childhood: impairment and disability. A prospective study with 4-year follow-up. *Arch Phys Med Rehabil* 2004;**85**:772–8.
89. Takken T, Terlingen HC, Helders PJ, Pruijs H, Van der Ent CK, Engelbert RH. Cardiopulmonary fitness and muscle strength in patients with osteogenesis imperfecta type I. *J Pediatr* 2004;**145**:813–8.
90. Gentry BA, Ferreira JA, McCambridge AJ, Brown M, Phillips CL. Skeletal muscle weakness in osteogenesis imperfecta mice. *Matrix Biol* 2010;**29**:638–44.
91. Voermans NC, van Alfen N, Pillen S, Lammens M, Schalkwijk J, Zwarts, et al. Neuromuscular involvement in various types of Ehlers–Danlos syndrome. *Ann Neurol* 2009;**65**:687–97.
92. Voermans NC, Bonnemann CG, Lammens M, van Engelen BG, Hamel BC. Myopathy and polyneuropathy in an adolescent with the kyphoscoliotic type of Ehlers–Danlos syndrome. *Am J Med Genet A* 2009;**149A**:2311–6.
93. Voermans NC, Knoop H, van de Kamp N, Bleijenberg G, van Engelen BG. Fatigue is a frequent and clinically relevant problem in Ehlers–Danlos syndrome. *Semin Arthritis Rheum* 2010;**40**:267–74.
94. Huijing PA, Voermans NC, Baan GC, Buse TE, van Engelen BG, de Haan A. Muscle characteristics and altered myofascial force

transmission in tenascin-X-deficient mice, a mouse model of Ehlers–Danlos syndrome. *J Appl Physiol* 2010;**109**:986–95.

95. Steinmann B, Royce PM, Superti-Furga A. The Ehlers–Danlos syndromes. In: Steinmann B, Royce PM, editors. *Connective tissue and its heritable disorders*. New York: Wiley–Liss Inc;2002. p. 431–523.

96. Beighton P, De Paepe A, Steinmann B, Tsipouras P, Wenstrup RJ. Ehlers–danlos syndromes: revised nosology, villefranche, 1997. Ehlers–danlos national foundation (USA) and ehlers–danlos support group (UK). *Am J Med Genet* 1998;**77**:31–7.

97. Schalkwijk J, Zweers MC, Steijlen PM, Dean WB, Taylor G, van Vlijmen IM, et al. A recessive form of the Ehlers–Danlos syndrome caused by tenascin-X deficiency. *N Engl J Med* 2001;**345**:1167–75.

98. Voermans NC, Altenburg TM, Hamel BC, de Haan A, van Engelen BG. Reduced quantitative muscle function in tenascin-X deficient Ehlers–Danlos patients. *Neuromuscul Disord* 2007;**17**:597–602.

99. Voermans NC, Jenniskens GJ, Hamel BC, Schalkwijk J, Guicheney P, van Engelen BG. Ehlers–Danlos syndrome due to tenascin-X deficiency: muscle weakness and contractures support overlap with collagen VI myopathies. *Am J Med Genet A* 2007;**143A**:2215–9.

100. Voermans NC, Verrijp K, Eshuis L, Balemans MC, Egging D, Sterrenburg E, et al. Mild muscular features in tenascin-X knockout mice: a model of Ehlers–Danlos syndrome. *Connect Tissue Res* 2011;**52**:422–32.

101. Chiquet-Ehrismann R, Tucker RP. Connective tissues: signalling by tenascins. *Int J Biochem Cell Biol* 2004;**36**:1085–9.

102. Minamitani T, Ariga H, Matsumoto K. Deficiency of tenascin-X causes a decrease in the level of expression of type VI collagen. *Exp Cell Res* 2004;**297**:49–60.

103. Minamitani T, Ikuta T, Saito Y, Takebe G, Sato M, Sawa H, et al. Modulation of collagen fibrillogenesis by tenascin-X and type VI collagen. *Exp Cell Res* 2004;**298**:305–15.

104. Yis U, Dirik E, Chambaz C, Steinmann B, Giunta C. Differential diagnosis of muscular hypotonia in infants: the kyphoscoliotic type of Ehlers–Danlos syndrome (EDS VI). *Neuromuscul Disord* 2008;**18**:210–4.

105. Miyake N, Kosho T, Mizumoto S, Furuichi T, Hatamochi A, Nagashima Y, et al. Loss-of-function mutations of CHST14 in a new type of Ehlers–Danlos syndrome. *Hum Mutat* 2010;**31**:966–74.

106. Malfait F, Syx D, Vlummens P, Symoens S, Nampoothiri S, Hermanns-Le T, et al. Musculocontractural Ehlers–Danlos syndrome (former EDS type VIB) and adducted thumb clubfoot syndrome (ATCS) represent a single clinical entity caused by mutations in the dermatan-4-sulfotransferase 1 encoding CHST14 gene. *Hum Mutat* 2010;**31**:1233–9.

107. Kosho T, Takahashi J, Ohashi H, Nishimura G, Kato H, Fukushima Y. Ehlers–Danlos syndrome type VIB with characteristic facies, decreased curvatures of the spinal column, and joint contractures in two unrelated girls. *Am J Med Genet A* 2005;**138A**:282–7.

108. Kosho T, Miyake N, Hatamochi A, Takahashi J, Kato H, Miyahara T, et al. A new Ehlers–Danlos syndrome with craniofacial characteristics, multiple congenital contractures, progressive joint and skin laxity, and multisystem fragility-related manifestations. *Am J Med Genet A* 2010;**152A**:1333–46.

109. Voermans NC, Kempers M, Lammens M, van Alfen N, Janssen MC, Bönnemann C, et al. Myopathy in a 20-year-old female patient with D4ST-1 deficient Ehlers–Danlos syndrome due to a homozygous CHST14 mutation. *Am J Med Genet A*; **158A**: 850–5.

Chapter 71

Molecular Pathogenesis of Skeletal Muscle Abnormalities in Marfan Syndrome

Ronald D. Cohn[1] and Harry C. Dietz III[2]

[1]*McKusick–Nathans Institute of Genetic Medicine and Johns Hopkins Center for Hypotonia,* [2]*Institute of Genetic Medicine, Departments of Pediatrics, Medicine, and Molecular Biology & Genetics, Johns Hopkins University School of Medicine, and Howard Hughes Medical Institute, Baltimore, MD*

INTRODUCTION

It has been more than 100 years since French pediatrician Antoine Marfan made the original observation of extraordinary musculoskeletal abnormalities in a 5-year-old girl, which laid the foundation for the description of Marfan syndrome (MFS). MFS is a common autosomal dominant systemic disorder of connective tissue with an estimated prevalence of 1 in 5000–10,000 individuals (1). It is caused by mutations in *FBN1*, the gene encoding the extracellular matrix protein fibrillin-1 (2). Clinical manifestations of MFS include bone overgrowth, ocular lens dislocation, emphysema, and cardiac complications such as aortic aneurysm. *FBN1* encodes fibrillin-1, a widely distributed major component of microfibrils in the extracellular matrix with an important role for elastin deposition in elastic tissues.

A large subset of patients with MFS exhibits a significant decrease in muscle mass, which is often associated with hypotonia, particularly during early childhood. In addition, joint hypermobility is a common physical finding, most pronounced in distal joints and often accompanied by arachnodactyly. Congenital joint contractures, particularly of the elbow, occur with moderate frequency (3). Marfan patients frequently report muscle fatigue, and to a lesser extent muscle weakness, muscle hypoplasia, myalgia, and cramps (4–8). The majority of patients with MFS experience a life-long inability to increase muscle mass despite adequate nutrition and physical exercise. Fibrillin-1 is abundantly expressed in the skeletal muscle endomysium and perimysium, suggesting a causal link between muscle symptoms and the primary fibrillin-1 abnormality (9).

INCREASED ACTIVITY OF TGF-β SIGNALING IN MARFAN SYNDROME

Fibrillin-1 is a 350 kDa glycoprotein comprised of multiple epidermal growth factor (EGF)-like motifs that are arranged in tandem. There are 47 motifs in all, 43 of which contain a calcium-binding sequence and are termed calcium-binding EGF-like (cbEGF) domains (10). The cbEGF modules participate in multiple functions, including stabilization of an extended configuration for fibrillin-1 monomers, promotion of lateral packing of monomers within microfibrils, inhibition of proteolysis and protein–protein interactions (11,12). The tandem arrays of cbEGF motifs (1–12 repeats) are separated by seven 8-cys/TB modules, which have high homology to the latent transforming growth factor binding proteins (LTBPs) (10,12). Tropoelastin deposits on a meshwork of microfibrils during elastic fiber development and maturation. Microfibrils also participate in matrix-cell attachments, at least in part through direct interactions between fibrillin-1 and integrins expressed on the cell surface. Thus, it was initially speculated that fibrillin-1 mutations within the aorta lead to aneurysm due to aberrant formation of the lamellar unit composed of elastic fibers and neighboring smooth muscle cells and consequent structural weakness of the tissue (13).

Recent evidence has suggested that fibrillin-1 and microfibrils regulate the bioavailability, activation, and local activity of transforming growth factor-beta (TGF-β). TGF-β is synthesized as a prepropolypeptide that is cleaved in a post-Golgi compartment to yield a mature growth factor molecule and an inactive cleavage fragment, termed latency-associated peptide (LAP). Homodimers of TGF-β and LAP interact to form a biologically inactive complex called the small latent complex (SLC). Subsequently, the SLC binds covalently to one of three latent transforming growth factor-binding proteins (LTBPs 1, 3, or 4) to form the large latent complex (LLC) (11,14). This large latent complex (LLC) is then secreted from the cell and targets latent TGF-β to the extracellular matrix (ECM), with documented interactions with both fibrillin-1 and fibronectin (15,16). TGF-β must subsequently be released from the LLC (TGF-β activation) to activate its

Muscle. DOI: http://dx.doi.org/10.1016/B978-0-12-381510-1.00071-5

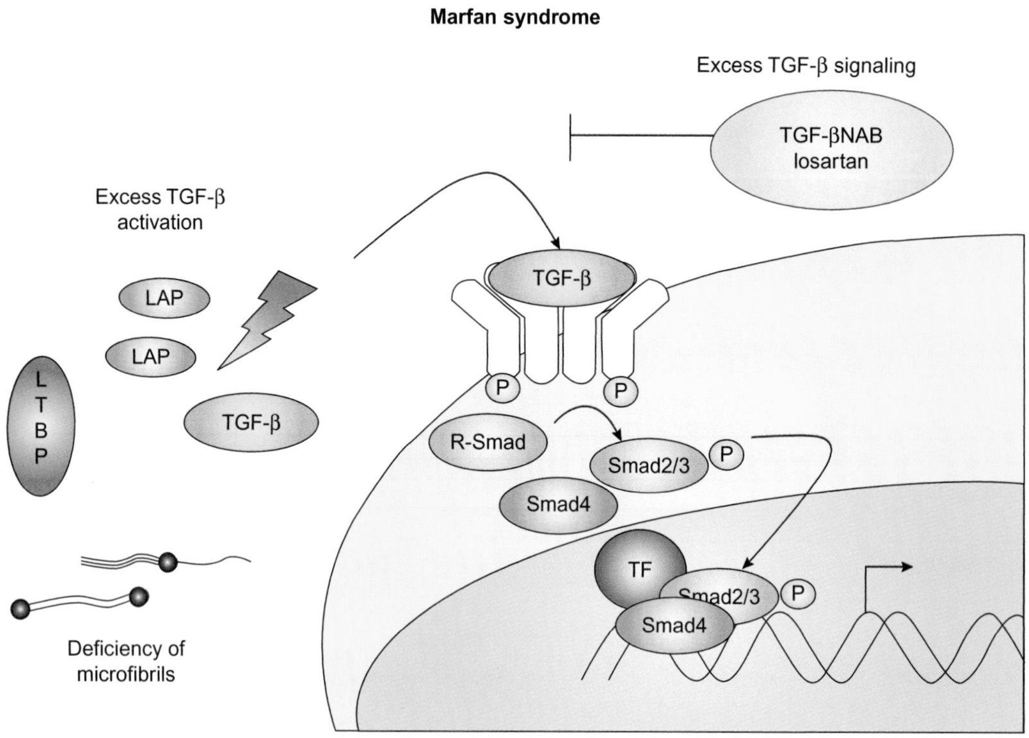

FIGURE 71.1 Increased TGF-β signaling contributes to the pathogenesis of Marfan syndrome.

cell surface receptor and initiate signaling. The long list of physiologic activators includes proteases (e.g. matrix metalloproteinases and plasmin), matricellular proteins (e.g. thrombospondin-1), integrins (e.g. αvβ6 and αvβ8), extremes of pH, reactive oxygen species, and mechanical traction.

Matrix binding of latent TGF-β has been proposed to serve multiple functions with both complementary and divergent consequences for TGF-β signaling. First, extracellular storage of TGF-β in a stable latent form allows for a rapid signaling response to a wide variety of cues in the microenvironment. Second, matrix sequestration provides a means to concentrate TGF-β – an event that may be particularly critical for attainment of signaling thresholds during tissue morphogenesis. Finally, dynamic variation in matrix abundance, composition, and integrity likely influences TGFβ presentation and/or other aspects of bioavailability for activation.

The first evidence for altered TGF-β signaling in Marfan syndrome occurred while studying developmental emphysema in fibrillin-1-deficient mice. Neptune et al. demonstrated that perinatal failure of distal alveolar septation associated with increased free and active TGF-β and increased TGF-β signaling in the developing lung. A coincident reduction in latent TGF-β suggested enhanced TGF-β activation as the primary event. Remarkably, systemic delivery of a pan-specific TGF-β neutralizing antibody improved alveolar septation in fibrillin-1-deficient mice in a dose-dependent manner, thus establishing a contribution of enhanced TGF-β signaling to the pathogenesis of Marfan syndrome (17). Subsequent studies in mice heterozygous for a missense mutation in *Fbn1* ($Fbn1^{C1039G/+}$) revealed evidence for increased TGF-β signaling in other affected tissues such as the mitral valve, dura mater and ascending aorta. This included nuclear accumulation of phosphorylated Smad2 and increased output of TGF-β-driven gene products such as collagens and connective tissue growth factor. Once again, TGF-β neutralizing antibody was able to attenuate or prevent important manifestations of Marfan syndrome including myxomatous degeneration of the mitral valve and progressive aortic root dilation (18). Habashi and colleagues demonstrated that treatment with the angiotensin II type 1 receptor blocker (ARB) losartan decreased TGF-β signaling, preserved aortic wall architecture and prevented aortic aneurysm in Marfan mice (19). Similar protection was seen in a small observational cohort of children with severe Marfan syndrome that was treated with losartan. Together, these studies suggest a strong causal link between enhanced TGF-β signaling and the clinical manifestations of MFS (see Figure 71.1).

FUNCTIONAL ROLE OF TGF-β SIGNALING IN SKELETAL MUSCLE

TGF-β1 is expressed during myogenesis and its spatial and temporal expression is correlated with the fiber-type

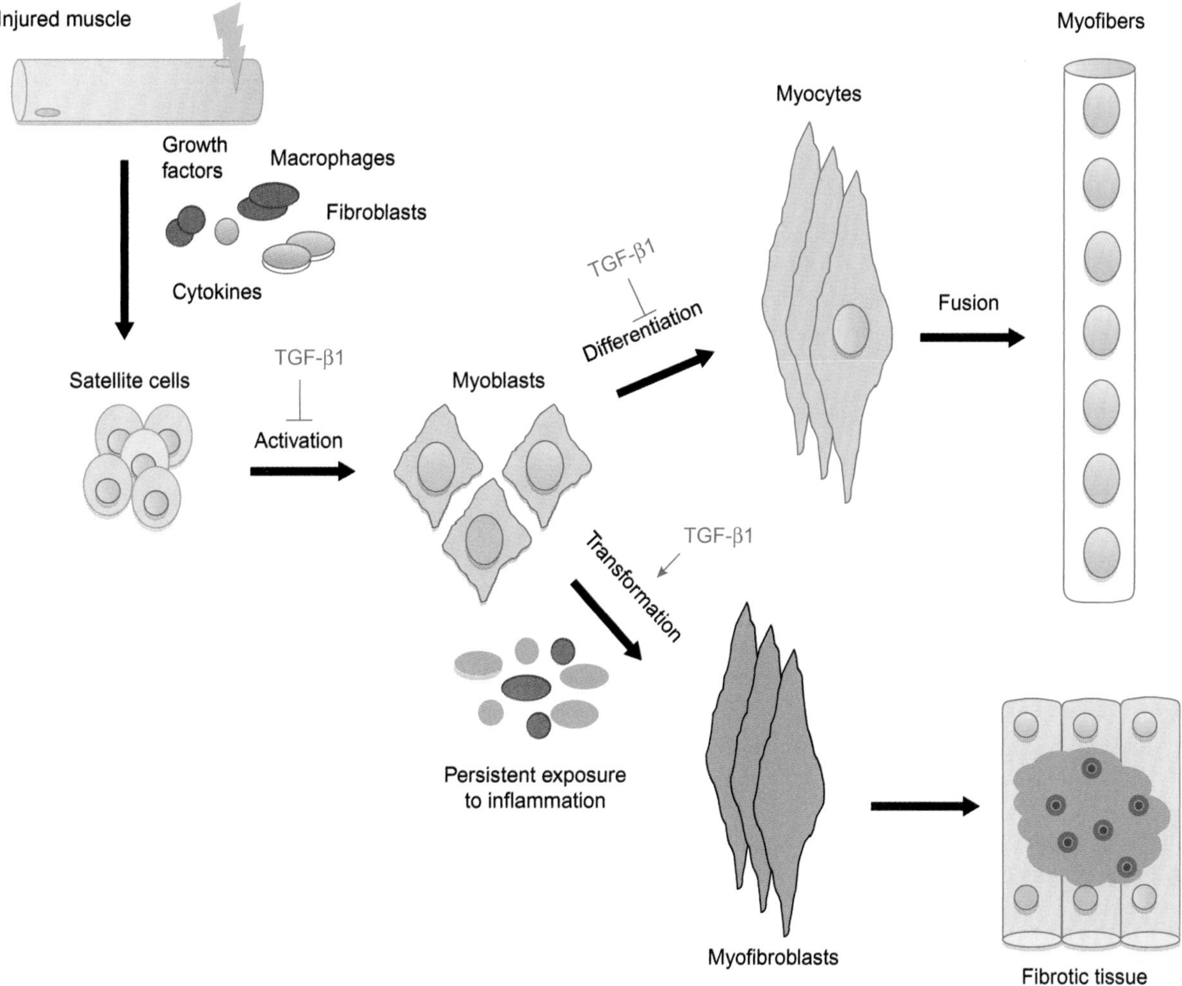

FIGURE 71.2 Excessive TGF-β signaling inhibits satellite cell proliferation and myocyte differentiation.

composition of the surrounding myotubes (20). In mature adult muscle, TGF-β has been shown to have a negative impact on skeletal muscle regeneration by inhibiting satellite cell proliferation, myofiber fusion and the expression of muscle-specific genes critical for the differentiation of myofibers (21). Furthermore, TGF-β1 induces the transformation of myogenic cells into fibrotic cells following injury (22). Following skeletal muscle injury, a well-coordinated repair process orchestrated by satellite cells occurs. This process includes the release of growth factors and cytokines as well as the migration and proliferation of macrophages and fibroblasts that increase the production of ECM components; these components are degraded as normal regeneration proceeds (23). The inflammatory response serves to clear myofiber debris and modulate regeneration (23). TGF-β1, a potent regulator of tissue wound healing and fibrosis, is physiologically upregulated in regenerating skeletal muscle following injury and exercise and is thought to participate in a transient inflammatory response to muscle damage (23). The persistent exposure of the inflammatory response leads to an altered ECM and elevated levels of growth factors and cytokines including TGF-β1 that contribute to the formation of fibrotic tissue (23). Therefore, TGF-β1 is one of the major factors promoting the transformation of myoblasts into fibrotic tissue following injury (see Figure 71.2). Interestingly, reducing the levels of TGF-β1 in various physiological and pathological conditions associated with muscle homeostasis and regeneration has proven to be beneficial for several myopathic conditions (24).

TGF-β SIGNALING IN SKELETAL MUSCLE OF MARFAN SYNDROME (5)

Mice heterozygous for a targeted missense mutation (cysteine to arginine at codon 1039; C1039G) in exon 25 of the mouse *Fbn1* gene were used for most of the studies assessing skeletal muscle dysfunction in MFS (25). Mice homozygous for the C1039G mutation (*Fbn1*$^{C1039G/C1039G}$) die between 10 and 14 days of age secondary to aortic dissection (25). Analysis of 10-day-old wild-type and homozygous mutant litter-mates showed a significant discrepancy in body weight that correlates with architectural abnormalities in all skeletal muscle groups examined (M. quadriceps, diaphragm, gastrocnemius, tibialis anterior, soleus and biceps). These abnormalities included a marked decrease in muscle fiber size and fiber number as well as increased amounts of connective tissue and fat between muscle fiber bundles, providing evidence of marked muscle hypotrophy as well as muscle hypoplasia. Mice heterozygous for the C1039G mutation (*Fbn1*$^{C1039G/+}$) exhibited significant variation in fiber size and endomysial fibrosis, which can also be observed in skeletal muscle of patients with MFS (25). Furthermore, immunohistochemical staining for fibrillin-1 revealed decreased endomysial expression in skeletal muscle from *Fbn1*$^{C1039G/+}$ mice and patients with MFS.

Given previous evidence for aberrant TGF-β signaling in other tissues, further experiments assessed skeletal muscle of fibrillin-1-deficient mice for increased TGF-β signaling by immunohistochemical staining for phosphorylated Smad2/3 (pSmad2/3). Ligand-activated TGFβ receptors induce phosphorylation of Smads 2 and 3 which form heteromeric complexes with Smad4 that translocate to the nucleus and mediate target gene responses (26). Immunofluorescent assessment exhibited nuclear accumulation of pSmad2/3 in myofibers of *Fbn1*$^{C1039G/+}$ mice. Further evidence of increased TGF-β signaling derived from analyses of the expression of periostin, a protein known to be induced by TGF-β in muscle (27). In contrast to wild-type mice, *Fbn1*$^{C1039G/+}$ animals demonstrated sarcolemmal expression of periostin in mature and uninjured skeletal muscle.

To assess for a cause-and-effect relationship between excess TGF-β signaling and development of myopathy in *Fbn1*$^{C1039G/+}$ mice, systemic TGF-β antagonism was accomplished *in vivo* by intraperitoneal injections of 1 mg/kg or 10 mg/kg TGF-β neutralizing antibody (TGF-β NAb) every two weeks, beginning at 7 weeks of age. Both TGF-β isoforms 1 and 2 are neutralized *in vivo* and *in vitro* by this antibody (17,19,25). The subsequent histologic and morphometric assessments revealed rescue of abnormal muscle morphology in mutant animals after 2 months of treatment with TGF-β NAb, independent of the dosage used. Moreover, neither nuclear accumulation of pSmad2/3 nor sarcolemmal periostin staining was observed in TGFβ NAb-treated *Fbn1*$^{C1039G/+}$ mice.

One interesting observation in Marfan mouse and patient muscle biopsies was the presence of multiple atrophic and split fibers suggestive for abnormal and/or incomplete muscle regeneration. As TGF-β signaling exerts a negative impact on muscle development and regeneration, it was proposed that an abnormal muscle regeneration response might be a contributing factor to the myopathic phenotype in Marfan syndrome. Detailed analysis of the regeneration response of *Fbn1*$^{C1039G/+}$ mice after injection of the snake venom cardiotoxin, showed delay in regeneration and only scattered newly formed muscle fibers 4 days after injury. Furthermore, at 18 days after cardiotoxin injection, when wild-type mice successfully complete muscle remodeling, *Fbn1*$^{C1039G/+}$ mice demonstrated multiple atrophic and small fibers with focal areas of fibrosis indicative of abnormal muscle repair. All animal groups showed nuclear accumulation of pSmad2/3 and sarcolemmal expression of periostin 4 days after cardiotoxin injection, which is consistent with the prior observation of a transient increase in expression of TGFβ1 and periostin within the first five days of muscle regeneration (27). In contrast, nuclear accumulation of pSmad 2/3 and periostin expression persisted in *Fbn1*$^{C1039G/+}$ mice 18 days after injury, which was not observed in wild-type or TGFβ Nab-treated *Fbn1*$^{C1039G/+}$ mice. Systemic administration of TGF-β NAb at the time of and two weeks after cardiotoxin injection significantly improved the muscle regeneration capacity of *Fbn1*$^{C1039G/+}$ mice. These data indicate that exaggeration and/or prolongation of the physiologic spike in TGF-β signaling that attends muscle injury and repair can limit regeneration and culminate in a myopathic phenotype in Marfan syndrome.

Given the inability to sufficiently repopulate damaged muscle fibers in response to injury, it was suggested that increased TGF-β signaling alters the performance of satellite cells. In the course of muscle regeneration, satellite cells exit their normal quiescent state and begin proliferating. After several rounds of proliferation, the majority of satellite cells differentiate and fuse to either form new myofibers or to repair damaged fibers. Immunohistochemical assessment of M-cadherin (a marker for proliferating satellite cells (28) and Pax7 at 48 h after injury revealed a dramatic decrease in satellite cells stained for these markers in serial sections of tibialis anterior muscle of *Fbn1*$^{C1039G/+}$ mice when compared to wild-type or TGFβ NAb-treated *Fbn1*$^{C1039G/+}$ mice. Furthermore, expression of myogenin, a myocyte regulatory factor involved in the late stage differentiation process of myofiber formation (29), exhibited a similar decrease in the tibialis anterior muscle of *Fbn1*$^{C1039G/+}$ mice 5 days after cardiotoxin challenge, as compared to wild-type or TGFβ NAb-treated *Fbn1*$^{C1039G/+}$ mice.

As mentioned above, previous evidence demonstrated that losartan, an angiotensin II type 1 receptor (AT1) antagonist causes a clinically relevant antagonism of TGF-β in MFS (19) and other disease states including chronic renal disease and cardiomyopathy (30,31). Losartan was therefore investigated as a potential treatment option for skeletal muscle abnormalities in fibrillin-1-deficient mice. Indeed, long-term treatment with losartan fully normalized steady state muscle architecture in *Fbn1*$^{C1039G/+}$ mice, which correlated with abrogation of TGF-β signaling in mature skeletal muscle. Moreover, administration of losartan prior to cardiotoxin-induced injury markedly improved muscle regeneration in *Fbn1*$^{C1039G/+}$ mice.

Taken together, these findings indicate that augmented TGF-β signaling causes impaired muscle repair by inhibiting satellite cell proliferation and differentiation in a mouse model of MFS. These observations are of significance as they likely explain both the congenital myopathy and the life-long inability to increase muscle mass in MFS. In the immediate perinatal period, skeletal muscle undergoes significant enhancement of mass mainly by an increase in muscle fiber number, a process regulated by satellite cells (32). Thereafter, skeletal muscle becomes differentiated and satellite cells only become activated in response to physiological and non-physiological demands such as exercise or injury. The physiologic satellite cell-mediated neonatal expansion of muscle mass therefore represents a time of particular vulnerability to the inhibitory effects of TGF-β. This serves as a likely explanation for the increased incidence and severity of both muscle hypoplasia and myopathy in young children with MFS, often with gradual improvement over time. Later in life, satellite cells may still not be able to respond adequately to physiological stimuli such as exercise given the ongoing increased activity of TGF-β.

The data derived from skeletal muscle studies in MFS represented the first evidence for a primary contribution of increased TGF-β activity to impaired muscle regeneration and a myopathic phenotype. Previously, there has been descriptive evidence for increased TGF-β activity associated with fibrosis in various genetic and acquired muscle disorders (33,34). An important mechanism in the pathogenesis of various degenerative myopathies including some forms of muscular dystrophy is a decline in satellite cell performance and muscle regeneration and subsequent development of fibrosis over time. TGF-β has therefore emerged as an attractive candidate mediator of these effects and subsequent studies have demonstrated that increased TGF-β signaling indeed plays an important role in various forms of muscular dystrophies (5,35,36). In keeping with this hypothesis, increased nuclear accumulation of pSmad2/3 and sarcolemmal expression of periostin in skeletal muscle of dystrophin-deficient *mdx* mice, an animal model for Duchenne muscular dystrophy, has been demonstrated. One complicating factor in interpretation of these data is that myostatin, another member of the TGF-β superfamily, also signals through the pSmad2/3 cascade (37). This variable was removed by showing ongoing increased nuclear pSmad2/3 and periostin expression in *myostatin-null/mdx* animals (5). Myostatin is a negative regulator of satellite cell activity and loss of function causes significant muscle hypertrophy in animals and humans (for review see 37). While myostatin antagonism has been shown to ameliorate the muscle phenotype in dystrophin-deficient *mdx* mice, there is evidence that the recovery is incomplete (38,39). Moreover, in contrast to TGF-β, evidence suggests that myostatin expression is decreased in muscular dystrophy, perhaps as a component of an inadequate physiologic attempt at compensation. Recent studies in fly models of muscular dystrophies support the findings that SMAD signaling is an important TGF-β signaling downstream target involved in the pathogenesis of muscular dystrophies (36). Using flies deficient for δ-sarcoglycan, the authors demonstrated increased TGF-β activity associated with skeletal and cardiac muscle injury. Haploinsufficient alleles were used to decrease SMAD signaling which was sufficient to rescue skeletal and cardiac muscle dysfunction in this mutant. Thus, while therapeutic strategies aimed at myostatin antagonism may provide some benefit by targeting a parallel pathway, TGF-β antagonism targets a pathway that appears directly involved in the pathogenesis of disease. Further evidence for a significant role for TGF-β signaling in the pathogenesis of muscular dystrophies has derived from studies of modifier genes in murine forms of muscular dystrophy (35). These studies identified that *Ltbp4*, a gene encoding a TGF-β-sequestering protein, serves as a genetic modifier of muscular dystrophy, demonstrating that reduced TGF-β signaling was associated with reduced membrane leakage and reduced fibrosis (35).

Given the significant role of TGF-β signaling in the pathogenesis of muscular dystrophy, several studies have analyzed the potential benefit of TGF-β anatagonism in the dystrophin-negative *mdx* mouse. Administration of TGF-β NAb improved the regenerative capacity of 9-month-old *mdx* mice (5). Additional studies using TGF-β NAb demonstrated reduced fibrosis but also produced an unfavorable cytokine profile in *mdx* diaphragm muscle (40). Subsequent studies explored losartan as a therapeutic agent to antagonize TGF-β signaling in mdx mice. Long-term administration of losartan decreased skeletal muscle fibrosis (5,41) and improved *in vivo* and *in vitro* skeletal muscle function in *mdx* mice (5). Furthermore, it was demonstrated that losartan improved cardiac muscle fibrosis and function in *mdx* mice (41). Taken together, these cumulative data indicate that increased TGF-β activity does not simply drive late fibrosis in dystrophin-deficient *mdx* mice, as previously inferred, but more importantly is both necessary and sufficient to impede the physiologic response of satellite cells to regenerate muscle in multiple genetically-defined forms of myopathy, a process essential for the preservation of muscle architecture and performance. Recent evidence demonstrated that increased TGF-β signaling also plays a critical role in acquired myopathic states. In particular, increased TGF-β signaling drives the fibrotic response in a model of severe muscle injury induced by laceration (42) and has also been shown to play a role in age-related decline of muscle regeneration and loss of muscle mass (sarcopenia) (43). These data suggest that TGF-β antagonism via the Food and Drug Administration-approved drug losartan may represent a productive treatment strategy for inherited forms of myopathy such as MFS and Duchenne muscular dystrophy, and also for acquired myopathic states.

REFERENCES

1. Pyeritz RE. The Marfan syndrome. *Annu Rev Med* 2000;**51**:481–510.
2. Dietz HC, Cutting GR, Pyeritz RE, Maslen CL, Sakai LY, Corson GM, et al. Marfan syndrome caused by a recurrent de novo missense mutation in the fibrillin gene. *Nature* 1991;**352**:337–9.
3. De Paepe A, Devereux RB, Dietz HC, Hennekam RC, Pyeritz RE. Revised diagnostic criteria for the Marfan syndrome. *Am J Med Genet* 1996;**62**:417–26.
4. Behan WM, Longman C, Petty RK, Comeglio P, Child AH, Boxer M, et al. Muscle fibrillin deficiency in Marfan's syndrome myopathy. *J Neurol Neurosurg Psychiatry* 2003;**74**:633–8.
5. Cohn RD, van Erp C, Habashi JP, Soleimani AA, Klein EC, Lisi MT, et al. Angiotensin II type 1 receptor blockade attenuates TGF-beta-induced failure of muscle regeneration in multiple myopathic states. *Nat Med* 2007;**13**:204–10.
6. Giske L, Stanghelle JK, Rand-Hendrikssen S, Strom V, Wilhelmsen JE, Roe C. Pulmonary function, working capacity and strength in young adults with Marfan syndrome. *J Rehabil Med* 2003;**35**:221–8.
7. Hasan A, Poloniecki J, Child A. Ageing in Marfan syndrome. *Int J Clin Pract* 2007;**61**:1308–20.
8. Percheron G, Fayet G, Ningler T, Le Parc JM, Denot-Ledunois S, Leroy M, et al. Muscle strength and body composition in adult women with Marfan syndrome. *Rheumatology (Oxford)* 2007;**46**:957–62.
9. Zhang H, Hu W, Ramirez F. Developmental expression of fibrillin genes suggests heterogeneity of extracellular microfibrils. *J Cell Biol* 1995;**129**:1165–76.
10. Yuan X, Downing AK, Knott V, Handford PA. Solution structure of the transforming growth factor beta-binding protein-like module, a domain associated with matrix fibrils. *EMBO J* 1997;**16**:6659–66.
11. Ramirez F, Dietz HC. Therapy insight: aortic aneurysm and dissection in Marfan's syndrome. *Nat Clin Pract Cardiovasc Med* 2004;**1**:31–6.
12. Ramirez F, Pereira L. Mutations of extracellular matrix components in vascular disease. *Ann Thorac Surg* 1999;**67**:1857–8 discussion 1868–70.
13. Pereira L, Lee SY, Gayraud B, Andrikopoulos K, Shapiro SD, Bunton T, et al. Pathogenetic sequence for aneurysm revealed in mice underexpressing fibrillin-1. *Proc Natl Acad Sci USA* 1999;**96**:3819–23.
14. Annes JP, Munger JS, Rifkin DB. Making sense of latent TGFbeta activation. *J Cell Sci* 2003;**116**:217–24.
15. Charbonneau NL, Ono RN, Corson GM, Keene DR, Sakai LY. Fine tuning of growth factor signals depends on fibrillin microfibril networks. *Birth Defects Res C Embryo Today* 2004;**72**:37–50.
16. Isogai Z, Ono RN, Ushiro S, Keene DR, Chen Y, Mazzieri R, et al. Latent transforming growth factor beta-binding protein 1 interacts with fibrillin and is a microfibril-associated protein. *J Biol Chem* 2003;**278**:2750–7.
17. Neptune ER, Frischmeyer PA, Arking DE, Myers L, Bunton TE, Gayraud B, et al. Dysregulation of TGF-beta activation contributes to pathogenesis in Marfan syndrome. *Nat Genet* 2003;**33**:407–11.
18. Ng CM, Cheng A, Myers LA, Martinez-Murillo F, Jie C, Bedja D, et al. TGF-beta-dependent pathogenesis of mitral valve prolapse in a mouse model of Marfan syndrome. *J Clin Invest* 2004;**114**:1586–92.
19. Habashi JP, Judge DP, Holm TM, Cohn RD, Loeys BL, Cooper TK, et al. Losartan, an AT1 antagonist, prevents aortic aneurysm in a mouse model of Marfan syndrome. *Science* 2006;**312**:117–21.
20. McLennan IS. Localisation of transforming growth factor beta 1 in developing muscles: implications for connective tissue and fiber type pattern formation. *Dev Dyn* 1993;**197**:281–90.
21. Allen RE, Boxhorn LK. Inhibition of skeletal muscle satellite cell differentiation by transforming growth factor-beta. *J Cell Physiol* 1987;**133**:567–72.
22. Li Y, Foster W, Deasy BM, Chan Y, Prisk V, Tang Y, et al. Transforming growth factor-beta1 induces the differentiation of myogenic cells into fibrotic cells in injured skeletal muscle: a key event in muscle fibrogenesis. *Am J Pathol* 2004;**164**:1007–19.
23. Serrano AL, Munoz-Canoves P. Regulation and dysregulation of fibrosis in skeletal muscle. *Exp Cell Res* 2010;**316**:3050–8.
24. Burks TN, Cohn RD. Role of TGF-β signaling in inherited and acquired myopathies. *Skeletal Muscle* 2011;**1**:19.
25. Judge DP, Biery NJ, Keene DR, Geubtner J, Myers L, Huso DL, et al. Evidence for a critical contribution of haploinsufficiency in the complex pathogenesis of Marfan syndrome. *J Clin Invest* 2004;**114**:172–81.
26. Heldin CH, Miyazono K, ten Dijke P. TGF-beta signalling from cell membrane to nucleus through SMAD proteins. *Nature* 1997;**390**:465–71.
27. Goetsch SC, Hawke TJ, Gallardo TD, Richardson JA, Garry DJ. Transcriptional profiling and regulation of the extracellular matrix during muscle regeneration. *Physiol Genomics* 2003;**14**:261–71.
28. Reimann J, Irintchev A, Wernig A. Regenerative capacity and the number of satellite cells in soleus muscles of normal and mdx mice. *Neuromuscul Disord* 2000;**10**:276–82.
29. Jin Y, Murakami N, Saito Y, Goto Y, Koishi K, Nonaka I. Expression of MyoD and myogenin in dystrophic mice, mdx and dy, during regeneration. *Acta Neuropathol (Berl)* 2000;**99**:619–27.
30. Lavoie P, Robitaille G, Agharazii M, Ledbetter S, Lebel M, Lariviere R. Neutralization of transforming growth factor-beta attenuates hypertension and prevents renal injury in uremic rats. *J Hypertens* 2005;**23**:1895–903.
31. Lim DS, Lutucuta S, Bachireddy P, Youker K, Evans A, Entman M, et al. Angiotensin II blockade reverses myocardial fibrosis in a transgenic mouse model of human hypertrophic cardiomyopathy. *Circulation* 2001;**103**:789–91.
32. Charge SB, Rudnicki MA. Cellular and molecular regulation of muscle regeneration. *Physiol Rev* 2004;**84**:209–38.

33. Salvadori C, Peters IR, Day MJ, Engvall E, Shelton GD. Muscle regeneration, inflammation, and connective tissue expansion in canine inflammatory myopathy. *Muscle Nerve* 2005;**31**:192–8.
34. Gosselin LE, Williams JE, Deering M, Brazeau D, Koury S, Martinez DA. Localization and early time course of TGF-beta 1 mRNA expression in dystrophic muscle. *Muscle Nerve* 2004;**30**:645–53.
35. Heydemann A, Ceco E, Lim JE, Hadhazy M, Ryder P, Moran JL, et al. Latent TGF-beta-binding protein 4 modifies muscular dystrophy in mice. *J Clin Invest* 2009;**119**:3703–12.
36. Goldstein JA, Kelly SM, LoPresti PP, Heydemann A, Earley JU, Ferguson EL, et al. SMAD signaling drives heart and muscle dysfunction in a Drosophila model of muscular dystrophy. *Hum Mol Genet* 2011;**20**:894–904.
37. Lee SJ. Regulation of muscle mass by myostatin. *Annu Rev Cell Dev Biol* 2004;**20**:61–86.
38. Wagner KR, McPherron AC, Winik N, Lee SJ. Loss of myostatin attenuates severity of muscular dystrophy in mdx mice. *Ann Neurol* 2002;**52**:832–6.
39. Bogdanovich S, Krag TO, Barton ER, Morris LD, Whittemore LA, Ahima RS, et al. Functional improvement of dystrophic muscle by myostatin blockade. *Nature* 2002;**420**:418–21.
40. Andreetta F, Bernasconi P, Baggi F, Ferro P, Oliva L, Arnoldi E, et al. Immunomodulation of TGF-beta 1 in mdx mouse inhibits connective tissue proliferation in diaphragm but increases inflammatory response: implications for antifibrotic therapy. *J Neuroimmunol* 2006;**175**:77–86.
41. Spurney CF, Sali A, Guerron AD, Iantorno M, Yu Q, Gordish-Dressman H, et al. Losartan decreases cardiac muscle fibrosis and improves cardiac function in dystrophin-deficient mdx mice. *J Cardiovasc Pharmacol Ther* 2011;**16**:87–95.
42. Bedair HS, Karthikeyan T, Quintero A, Li Y, Huard J. Angiotensin II receptor blockade administered after injury improves muscle regeneration and decreases fibrosis in normal skeletal muscle. *Am J Sports Med* 2008;**36**:1548–54.
43. Carlson ME, Hsu M, Conboy IM. Imbalance between pSmad3 and Notch induces CDK inhibitors in old muscle stem cells. *Nature* 2008;**454**:528–32.

Chapter 72

Diseases of the Nucleoskeleton

Anne T. Bertrand[1,2], Rabah Ben Yaou[1,2,3] and Gisèle Bonne[1,2,4]

[1]Inserm, UMR S974, [2]Université Pierre et Marie Curie-Paris 6, UM 76; CNRS, UMR 7215; Institut de Myologie, IFR14, [3]Association Institut de Myologie, [4]AP-HP, Groupe Hospitalier Pitié-Salpêtrière, UF Cardiogénétique et Myogénétique Moléculaire, Service de Biochimie Métabolique; Paris, France

INTRODUCTION

In 1994, mutations of a new gene encoding a protein that was called *emerin* have been reported in the X-linked forms of Emery–Dreifuss muscular dystrophy (EDMD) (1). Two years later, emerin was demonstrated to be a protein of the nuclear envelope. Shortly after, the first mutations of the *LMNA* gene encoding A-type lamins, proteins of the nuclear envelope were reported to be responsible for the autosomal dominant forms of EDMD (2), thus making the EDMD the first neuromuscular disorder of the nuclear envelope. Since then, mutations of *LMNA* gene have been implicated in a wide range of diseases. This cascade of identification has 're-activated' investigations of the nuclear envelope both at the cellular biology and human genetic levels. This has led to the identification of numerous new components of the nuclear envelope together with detailed investigations of their roles and functions and of their potential implication in human pathologies.

The nuclear envelope (NE) is a specialized structure constituted of two layers of lipid membrane that separate the cytoplasm from the nucleoplasm. The outer nuclear membrane (ONM) and the inner nuclear membrane (INM) are connected at the nuclear pore complexes. The latter insure the communication between the two compartments. Underlying the INM, the nuclear lamina is a meshwork of intermediate filaments: the A- and B-type lamins that interface and connect the chromatin to the nuclear envelope. The INM and the nuclear lamina constitute the nucleoskeleton. Proteins of the nucleoskeleton are implicated in a broad variety of nuclear functions such as DNA replication, gene transcription, cell signaling, cell cycle progression, and chromatin segregation.

This chapter focuses on the structure and function of lamins and some of their associated proteins, the description of pathologies due to mutations in their genes and the pathophysiological mechanisms under investigation.

STRUCTURE AND FUNCTION OF THE NUCLEOSKELETON

The nucleus is the place where DNA is conserved, duplicated, and transcribed. The NE, constituted of two layers of lipid membrane, the ONM and the INM, separates the chromatin from the cytoplasmic components of eukaryotic cells. The ONM and INM are separated by a luminal space of approximately 100 nm in width. Nuclear pore complexes allow the communication between the cytoplasm and the nucleoplasm by the import and the export of macromolecules. The ONM is connected to the rough endoplasmic reticulum (RER). The INM is composed of numerous transmembrane proteins, among which are emerin, nesprins, and lamin-associated polypeptides 2 (LAP2). The type V intermediate filaments, A- and B-type lamins, form a protein meshwork underneath the INM, the nuclear lamina, and are the central component of the nucleoskeleton. A-type lamins are also found dispersed in the nucleoplasm where they interact with other proteins, mainly transcription factors, to modulate their activities (Figure 72.1).

A- and B-Type Lamins

Lamins are composed of an unfolded N-terminal head, a central α-helical rod domain and a long C-terminal domain containing an immunoglobulin-like domain (3). *In vitro*, lamins form homodimers in a head-to-tail fashion which further assemble to form protofilaments which then associate laterally into 10 nm filaments and paracrystals (4). *In vivo*, lamins form the nuclear lamina, in close association with the INM and chromatin, and mechanically enforce the nuclear morphology. Seven different lamin isoforms have been described, that are classified in two groups: A- and B-type lamins. Three B-type lamins are encoded by *LMNB1* and *LMNB2* genes. While lamin B3 is only expressed in spermatocytes, lamins B1 and B2

Muscle. DOI: http://dx.doi.org/10.1016/B978-0-12-381510-1.00072-7

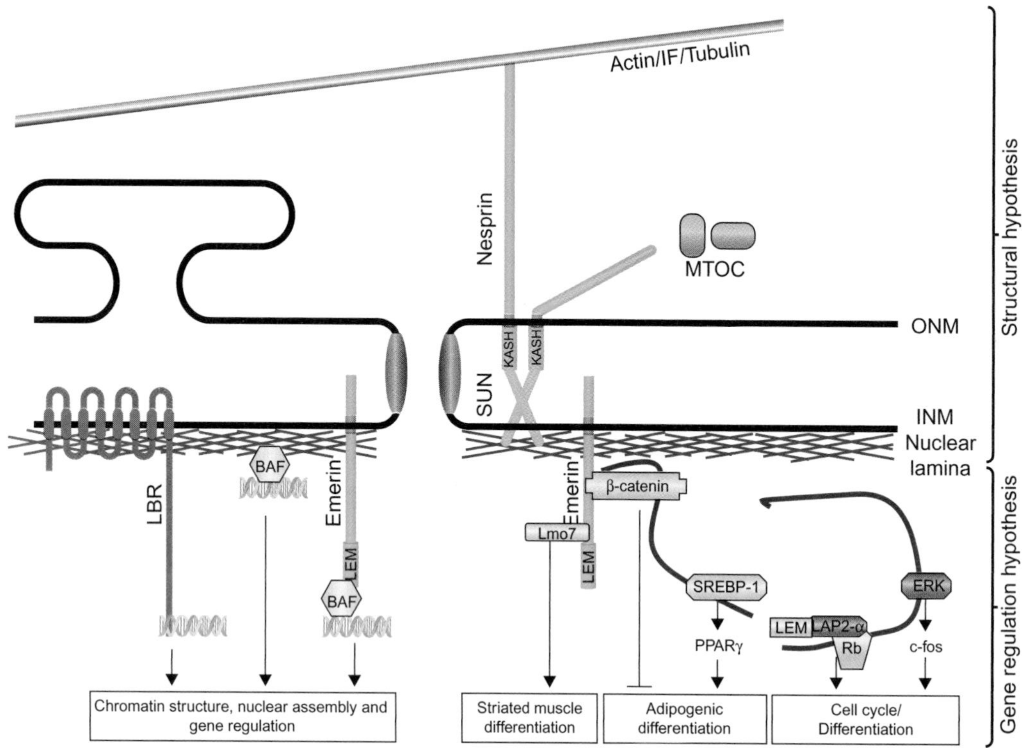

FIGURE 72.1 **Schematic representation of the nucleoskeleton.** A- and B-type lamins are shown in pink at the nuclear lamina, A-type lamins are also represented in the nucleoplasm. Lamin partners potentially involved in gene regulation are represented in blue with their main functions, while lamin partners implicated in nuclear structure and anchorage are depicted in green.

are essential for life, and expressed in all cells throughout development. In contrast, A-type lamins, encodes by the *LMNA* gene localized on chromosome 1q21, comprise two major isoforms, A and C, expressed at later stages of development and in most differentiated cells and two minor isoforms, AΔ10 and C2 expressed in tumor cells and in the germ line, respectively (3). Lamins A and B (but not lamin C) are translated as prelamins and undergo a sequence of processing steps at their C-terminal CaaX motif (where C is a cysteine, a is an aliphatic residue and X is undefined) (5). The first maturation step is the farnesylation of the cysteine residue, followed by an endopeptidase cleavage of the three last amino-acid aaX by ZMPSTE24 or RCE1. The last cysteine residue is then carboxymethylated. Whereas B-type lamins remain farnesylated, lamin A is cleaved further by the zinc metalloprotease ZMPSTE24, removing another 15 C-terminal residues with the farnesyl moiety. As a consequence, B-type lamins are tightly attached to the nuclear membrane even during mitosis, when the NE is disassembled, whereas lamins A and C are dispersed in the cell (3). A-type lamins interact with numerous INM transmembrane proteins, such as LEM domain proteins which have a major role in the structure and the anchorage of the chromatin to the NE. Lamins A/C also interact with LINC complex proteins that form a bridge between the nucleoskeleton and the cytoskeleton (6). Interaction of these proteins with lamins is thought to be necessary for their nuclear localization and sequestration (7). A-type lamins also interact with transcription factors such as the cell cycle regulator pRB, MOK2 a transcriptional repressor, SREBP-1 transcription factor involved in adipocyte differentiation, or more broad signaling pathways like SMADs or ERK/JNK (for a review see 8).

LEM Domain Proteins

This protein family is characterized by the presence of a LEM domain (acronym of the three first proteins identified with this domain: LAP2, emerin, MAN1, Figure 72.1) that mediates binding to BAF (barrier-to-autointegration factor), an essential protein with a role in chromatin structure, nuclear assembly and gene regulation (9). The *TMPO* gene encodes four alternatively spliced isoforms of LAP2 (lamin associated protein 2), three are integral membrane proteins that bind B-type lamins, while LAP2α has no transmembrane domain and forms complexes with the nucleoplasmic pool of lamin A/C and the retinoblastoma protein (pRb) to regulate cell cycle progression (10). The *EMD* gene encodes the INM integral protein emerin (1). Its nuclear localization is dependent on the presence of lamin at the nuclear periphery

(7). Emerin binds a broad variety of proteins, including β-catenin, and Lim domain only seven (Lmo7) (11). Beta-catenin is a component of the Wnt signaling pathway mainly implicated in specifying the fate of mesenchymal progenitor cells. Interaction of β-catenin with emerin prevents the transcriptional activation. Lmo7 is proposed to be a transcription activator, regulating a large number of genes. Many of these genes are muscle- or heart specific. As for β-catenin, interaction of Lmo7 with emerin inhibits its transcriptional activity (11).

LINC Complex Proteins

Another set of proteins are direct or indirect partners of lamins A/C and play a role in linking the nucleoskeleton to the cytoskeleton (LINC): the nesprin proteins, mainly found at the ONM and the SUN proteins, at the INM (Figure 72.1). *SYNE-1* and *SYNE-2* are two genes, constituted of more than 100 exons each, that encode for multiple nesprin isoforms by alternative splicing (12). Nesprin proteins are structured in spectrin repeats throughout the core of the protein, calponin homology domains in their N-terminal domain that mediates interaction with actin and a conserved KASH domain in their C-terminal end that anchor the proteins to the nuclear membranes by interacting with SUN proteins. Giant nesprin-1 and nesprin-2 isoforms localize to the ONM. Shorter isoforms such as nesprin-1α and nesprin-2α are found on the nucleoplasmic face of the INM where they interact with lamin A/C and emerin (13). Their localization to the NE is dependent on A-type lamin expression (14). Interestingly, nesprin-2 binds also to α- and β-catenin and regulates Wnt-signaling (15).

Identification of SUN (for Sad1 and UNC-84) proteins in the human followed their identification in *Caenorhabditis elegans*, where UNC-84 has been characterized for its nuclear membrane localization and its function in nuclear migration. In the human, four genes encode for SUN proteins, but only SUN1 and SUN2 have been documented as being integral proteins of the INM (6). They play a major role in nuclear-cytoplasmic connection by formation of a "bridge" across the NE, the LINC complex, via interaction with the conserved luminal KASH domain of nesprins in the lumen between the two NE and with emerin and lamin A at the nuclear lamina (13). Thus, the LINC complex is believed to contribute to cellular rigidity and nuclear positioning.

Other Lamins Interacting Partners

Among the multiple described interacting partners of lamins, LUMA is encoded by *TMEM43* gene. The protein forms homo-oligomers at the INM. It contains four transmembrane domains with a large hydrophilic domain between the two first transmembrane domains in the lumen between INM and ONM (16). While its INM localization is dependent on A-type lamin interaction, it has been shown that LUMA is important for emerin localization. LUMA also strongly interacts with lamin B2 (16).

DISEASES LINKED TO DEFECTS OF THE NUCLEOSKELETON

Since the first report in 1994, of *EMD* mutations responsible for X-linked EDMD (1), numerous diseases were linked to mutations in other genes encoding nuclear envelope proteins establishing the "nuclear connection" (17). This was particularly true after the implication of *LMNA* gene in several diseases collectively named laminopathies. This section will be devoted to the A- or B-type lamins-related diseases, as well as to diseases linked to other nuclear envelope proteins interacting with lamins with emphasis on those specifically affecting the striated muscle: emerin, nesprins, LUMA and LAP2α. Of note, more than 92% of mutations of genes encoding nucleoskeleton proteins related to human diseases are located in the *LMNA* and *EMD* genes (Table 72.1). The most frequently involved tissues are skeletal and cardiac muscles (*EMD, LMNA, TMEM43* and *TMPO*) and adipose tissue (*LMNA* and *LMNB2*). Peripheral or central nervous systems may be involved in *LMNA* and *LMNB1*-related diseases (Table 72.1).

Emerinopathies, the Emerin-Related Diseases

First described in the mid-1960s, the X-linked EDMD is characterized by the combination of a triple muscle–joint–heart involvement. The disease manifests in childhood with early joint contractures of the Achilles tendon, neck, and elbows, slowly progressive muscle weakness in a scapulo-humeroperoneal distribution, associated with a later cardiac disease characterized initially by arrhythmias, heart blocks with a substantial risk of sudden death in middle age, and finally dilated cardiomyopathy with chamber dilation and left ventricular dysfunction (18). Through a positional cloning strategy, mutations in a new gene (thereafter called *EMD)* were identified in X-linked EDMD families (1). The corresponding protein called emerin was later demonstrated to be an INM protein (19). Immunohistochemical and western blot analyses revealed that *EMD* mutations mainly result in the complete absence of emerin (20). *EMD* mutations may be also rarely associated with isolated cardiac disease (21,22) or limb-girdle muscular dystrophy (23). According to the UMD-*EMD* locus-specific database (www.umd.be/EMD/), the 86 different *EMD* mutations reported so far causing EDMD, are spread all along the gene, exon 2 and first ATG codon being the most frequently affected.

TABLE 72.1 Diseases of the Nucleoskeleton

Gene/Protein	Diseases	Inheritance	No. Families/No. Different Mutations
EMD/emerin	X-EDMD LGMD + cardiac disease Isolated cardiac disease	XL	158/86
LMNA/lamin A/C	Striated muscle laminopathies (EDMD, LGMD1B, congenital MD, dilated cardiomyopathy with conduction defects)	AD, AR	737/317
	Partial lipodystrophies	AD, AR	
	Peripheral nerve laminopathies	AR	
	Systemic laminopathies (premature ageing syndromes)	AD, AR	
	Overlapping laminopathies	AD, AR	
LMNB1/lamin B1	Adult-onset autosomal dominant leukodystrophy	AD	7/1
LMNB2/lamin B2	Barraquer–Simons syndrome	Sporadic	4/3
TMEM43/LUMA	Arrhythmogenic right ventricular cardiomyopathy type 5	AD	18/2
	Myopathies reminiscent of EDMD	AD	2/2
TMPO/*LAP2* α	Dilated cardiomyopathy	AD	1/1

MD, muscular dystrophy; EDMD, Emery–Dreifuss MD; LGMD, limb-girdle MD.

Laminopathies, the A-Type Lamin-Related Diseases

Twelve years after the description of the first mutations in *LMNA* gene in human disease (2), a galaxy of diseases collectively referred to as laminopathies were progressively linked to this gene. They fell into five classes affecting either specific tissue in an isolated way (striated muscles, peripheral nerves, adipose tissue) or in a systemic fashion (premature aging syndromes) (24). These different subgroups may sometimes coexist in a single patient thus defining the fifth subgroup: the "overlapping laminopathies". According to the UMD-*LMNA* locus-specific database (www.umd.be/LMNA/), more than 317 different mutations, spread all along the *LMNA* gene, have been reported so far in 737 families presenting one of these different laminopathies. Phenotype/genotype relations in laminopathies are not easy to display. Some mutations seem to lead to the same homogeneous phenotype. This is the case for the axonal form of Charcot–Marie–Tooth disease (mutation affecting of the Arg298 residue), partial lipodystrophy (Arg482), typical mandibuloacral dysplasia (Arg527 and Ala529) and typical progeria (Glu608). For others, an important intra- and interfamilial variability is observed making illusory any subtle correlation.

Striated Muscle Laminopathies (SML)

Isolated skeletal and/or cardiac muscle disorders account for 55% of the laminopathies (www.umd.be/LMNA/). Four clinical entities are found according to the presence or absence of skeletal muscle involvement, the age of onset, the distribution of muscle weakness/wasting, and joint contractures. The classical and most easily recognizable SML is the autosomal form of EDMD sharing the same clinical triad as the X-linked EDMD. By a positional cloning strategy, we identified the first *LMNA* gene mutation in autosomal dominant (2) as well as in autosomal recessive EDMD (25). Soon after, thanks to phenotypic similarities with EDMD and previous positional cloning to chromosome 1, the isolated dilated cardiomyopathy with conduction defects (DCM-CD) was linked to the *LMNA* gene (26,27). This latter disease is characterized by early occurrence of cardiac conduction defects and arrhythmias followed by ventricular dilation and reduced systolic function without skeletal muscle involvement. The limb-girdle muscular dystrophy type 1B (LGMD1B) is characterized by proximal muscle weakness and wasting associated with cardiac disease reminiscent of what is observed in DCM-CD or EDMD, rigid spine was absent, and elbow and Achilles tendon contractures were either minimal or late, distinguishing this disorder from EDMD. Thanks to previous positional cloning to chromosome 1q11-21 and phenotypic similarities with EDMD and DCM-CD, LGMD1B was linked to *LMNA* gene (28). More recently, another disease was added to the SML disease spectrum. Dominant *de novo LMNA* mutations were linked to a severe condition known as lamin A/C congenital muscular dystrophy (L-CMD) (29).

L-CMD is characterized by muscle weakness onset at birth or during the first year of life responsible for absence or delayed motor acquisitions. Affected subjects typically had selective weakness and wasting of cervico-axial, proximal in upper extremities and distal in lower extremities muscles, talipes feet, rigid spine with thoracic lordosis, later proximal limb contractures sparing the elbows, early respiratory involvement requiring ventilatory support, and cardiac arrhythmias. The invariable cardiac disease usually in adult life is the common denominator of SML. Its main characteristics are the presence of early conduction defects and arrhythmias followed by heart dysfunction. As a consequence, sudden death of cardiac origin due to extreme brady- or tachycardia arrhythmias is a frequent finding in these patients (27,30). Therefore, implantable cardioverter-defibrillators (ICD) set as a primary preventive device have been recommended to prevent lethal cardiac arrhythmias (31). However, ICD therapy does not alleviate cardiac disease progression and DCM often progresses toward heart failure and usually requires heart transplantation. *LMNA* mutations leading to SML are of all types and spread all along the gene (www.umd.be/LMNA/). Phenotype/genotype correlations are very limited as a single *LMNA* mutation may manifest by one of the SML or different types of SML may co-exist in the same family (27,32). The only exception seems to be mutations causing L-CMD as they co-segregate with particularly severe forms.

Adipose Tissue Laminopathies

These are mainly represented by the partial lipodystrophy of Dunnigan type (PLD), a condition characterized by selective and variable loss of adipose tissue associated with metabolic features. In PLD patients, fat distribution is normal in early childhood; with puberty they lose subcutaneous adipose tissue from limbs while it accumulates in axillae, intra-abdominal region and on the face and neck. Subsequently, insulin resistance, diabetes mellitus, hypertriglycideridemia, and liver steatosis develop after the second decade of life. By positional cloning, PLD was linked to chromosome 1q21 and *LMNA* mutations identified (33). So far, 80% of PLD patients carry a missense mutation affecting the Arg482 residue (p.R482W/Q/L, ww.umd.be/LMNA/).

Peripheral Nerve Laminopathies

They are mainly represented by a subgroup of autosomal recessive axonal form of Charcot–Marie–Tooth disease (CMT). CMT disease is a clinically and genetically heterogeneous group of inherited diseases affecting peripheral nerves characterized by progressive muscular and/or sensory loss in the distal extremities with chronic weakness of the distal limb muscles, deep tendons areflexia, and pes cavus. The axonal forms display normal nerve conduction velocity and reduced compound motor action potentials amplitudes. The CMT2B1 subgroup was characterized in North African autosomal recessive families, presenting classical axonal CMT features with additional proximal muscle involvement in some cases and linkage to 1q21. None had cardiac or adipose tissue diseases. *LMNA* was considered as a candidate as the *Lmna* null mice presented with axonal clinical and pathological phenotype highly similar to CMT2B1 patients. A unique homozygous p.Arg298Cys mutation was identified in all the studied families (34). To date, 15 families carrying this mutation were reported with a founder effect documented in some of these families (35).

Systemic Laminopathies: Premature Aging Syndromes

Mandibuloacral dysplasia (MAD) is a rare autosomal recessive disorder defined by postnatal growth retardation, mandibular and clavicular acroosteolysis, joint contractures, lipodystrophy, and mottled cutaneous pigmentation. Due to clinical similarities with PLD, MAD was linked to homozygous *LMNA* gene mutations (36). To date, homozygous mutations affecting Arg527 and Ala529 are responsible for all the reported MAD cases (www.umd.be/LMNA/). Hutchinson–Gilford progeria syndrome (HGPS) is an extremely rare and fatal genetic disorder (incidence <1 in 10^6 births). HGPS's clinical features appear within the first few years of life, and includes short stature, low weight, incomplete sexual maturation, widespread atherosclerosis, loss of subcutaneous fat, micrognathia, beaked nose, alopecia, restricted joint mobility, crowded dentition, thin and high-pitched voice, short and acroosteolytic clavicles, dystrophic nails, and acroosteolysis of terminal phalanges. Mental and emotional developments are normal. The whole clinical phenotype gives the appearance of senility at a striking degree. The median age of death is 13.4 years, frequently from coronary artery disease. By positional cloning and candidate gene approaches, *LMNA* mutations were identified in HGPS patients (37,38). The most frequent mutation (75% of the HGPS cases) is a *de novo* heterozygous single-base substitution resulting in a silent change (p.G608G) that activates a cryptic splice site within *LMNA* exon 11, resulting in an in-frame deletion of the last 50 amino acids within the C-terminal end of the prelamin A. The resulting abnormal prelamin A, named "progerin", lacks its ZMPSTE24 cleavage site, is not correctly post-translationally processed and therefore accumulates in tissue where it exerted toxic effect (5).

Werner syndrome (WS) is an adult onset premature aging syndrome. The main clinical features of WS are scleroderma-like skin changes, bilateral cataract, short stature, subcutaneous calcification, premature arteriosclerosis, diabetes mellitus, osteoporosis, soft tissue calcification, acroosteolysis of the distal phalanges of fingers and/or toes, neoplasms (sarcomas), abnormal voice, birdlike face, and premature graying hairs. Typical forms are due to homozygous mutations in the *WRN* gene encoding DNA helicase-like RECQL2 (39). As they share some phenotypic overlap with HGPS and MAD, a subset of not linked to *WRN* WS patients (atypical WS) were screened and found to carry *LMNA* mutations (40).

The last premature aging disease to be linked to *LMNA* gene is a neonatal condition named restrictive dermopathy (RD). Main clinical features of this extremely rare disorder are intrauterine growth retardation, tight and rigid skin with erosions, prominent superficial vasculature and epidermal hyperkeratosis, micrognathia, sparse or absent eyelashes and eyebrows, thin dysplastic clavicles, pulmonary hypoplasia, multiple joint contractures, and an early neonatal lethal course within the first hours of life. While most RD cases are linked to mutation in *ZMPSTE24* gene encoding the metalloproteinase involved in post-translational processing of the prelamin A, there is only 3 *LMNA* linked RD reported cases (5).

Overlapping Laminopathies

A growing number of patients presenting a combination of two or more of the laminopathies described above have been reported. The overlap frequently involves adipose and striated muscles tissues. Peripheral nerve involvement may rarely coexist with striated muscle disease with an autosomal dominant transmission in these cases. The more striking overlaps have been reported for the premature aging syndromes which may coexist with myopathy (for review see 24). Interestingly, the overlap may be absent at the first steps of the disease and appears later (41). These overlapping phenotypes may suggest that the different types of laminopathies may represent a unique multitissular disease with a variable marked tissular expression.

B-Type Lamins-Related Diseases

Lamin B1-Related Disease: Adult-Onset Autosomal Dominant Leukodystrophy (ADLD)

Leukodystrophies are rare hereditary disorders with widespread myelin loss affecting the white matter or myelin tracts of the central nervous system. Among leukodystrophies, ADLD is characterized by the occurrence within the fourth or fifth decade of life, of autonomic dysfunction (sweating, bowel and bladder dysfunction, postural hypotension), followed by motor dysfunction including cerebellar, pyramidal, and pseudobulbar signs. By a genome-wide linkage strategy, duplication of the *LMNB1* gene have been recognized as the underlying genetic defect resulting in increased gene dosage in brain tissue from individuals with ADLD (42).

Lamin B2-Related Disease: Acquired Partial Lipodystrophy

Among acquired partial lipodystrophies where no familial occurrence is observed, a subgroup also known as Barraquer–Simons syndrome is characterized by fat distribution "reverse" to what is observed in PLD with normal or decreased amount of fat in the upper part of the body and excess fat in the lower parts. These forms of lipodystrophy were suspected to be of autoimmune origin. However, using a candidate gene strategy, heterozygous variants in *LMNB2* gene encoding lamin B2, have been identified in 4 patients among 9 analyzed (43).

Nesprins-Related Diseases

Autosomal Recessive Cerebellar Ataxia

Hereditary ataxias are a group of disorders characterized by lack of coordination of gait and limbs. Additional neurological symptoms such as pyramidal features, peripheral neuropathy, extrapyramidal signs, cognitive loss or retinopathy may be associated. By a genome-wide linkage analysis in a group of 26 French-Canadian families with a pure cerebellar ataxia, named autosomal recessive cerebellar ataxia type 1 (ARCA1), Gros-Louis et al. identified five different mutations in the *SYNE1* gene involving the N-terminal regions of nesprin-1 proteins. Although immunohistochemical analysis of a patient muscle biopsy did not show any apparent structural defects in neuromuscular junctions, abnormal nuclear positioning at the neuromuscular junctions was observed (44).

Autosomal Recessive Arthrogryposis

Arthrogryposis is a group of disorders characterized by congenital joint contractures caused by reduced fetal movements. It can be secondary to a myopathic or neurogenic process, connective tissue disorders or to maternal diseases. The autosomal recessive form of myopathic arthrogryposis is characterized by decreased fetal movements, bilateral clubfoot, delay in motor milestones and progressive motor decline after the first decade. Attali et al. identified a locus on chromosome 6q in one family and then a homozygous mutation in *SYNE1* intron 136, resulting in the aberrant retention of the intron leading to premature stop codon and absence of the C-terminal transmembrane domain of nesprin-1 (45). Interestingly, mice lacking the C-terminal transmembrane domain of nesprin-1 display a myopathic phenotype similar to what is observed in patients (46).

SYNE1 and SYNE2 Genes and Myopathies Reminiscent of EDMD

By a candidate gene approach in a series of patients harboring cardiomuscular symptoms partially reminiscent of what is observed in EDMD, Zhang et al. identified additional *SYNE1* and *SYNE2* mutations occurring within the lamins A/C and emerin binding domains of nesprin-1 and -2 (47). The 7 affected subjects had either heterozygous *SYNE1* or *SYNE2* missense mutations or a double heterozygous *SYNE1* and *SYNE2* missense mutation. The clinical expression of the disease was variable, ranging from asymptomatic increased CK level to muscular dystrophy combined with severe dilated cardiomyopathy requiring heart transplantation in the doubly *SYNE1* and *SYNE2* mutated subject. However, contrary to typical EDMD syndrome, joint contractures were not one of the prominent features. Cellular analyses showed that fibroblasts and myoblasts from *SYNE1* and *SYNE2* mutated subjects had nuclear defects similar to what is described in *EMD* and *LMNA* patients and mislocalization of nesprin, emerin, and lamins A/C, all indicating loss of nuclear envelope integrity.

LUMA-Related Diseases

Arrhythmogenic Right Ventricular Cardiomyopathy Type 5 (ARVC5)

ARVC is a myocardial disorder characterized by ventricular arrhythmias, right- and/or left-ventricular involvement, heart failure, and fibrofatty infiltrations in the myocardium (48). Typical symptoms include palpitations, dizziness, syncope, and sudden cardiac death. ARVC is inherited in autosomal dominant or recessive fashions with incomplete penetrance and variable expressivity. Eleven genetic loci have been mapped and mutations in eight genes have been identified so far, five of them encoding desmosomal proteins, one the cardiac ryanodine receptor 2 and one the transforming growth factor-beta-3 (49). ARVC5 is due to mutations in the eighth reported gene, *TMEM43* encoding LUMA, with two mutations reported (p.Ser358Leu (50) and c.705 + 7G>A in intron 8 (51)). *TMEM43* mutated patients had distinctive features characterized by full penetrance, premature ventricular contractions, left ventricular dilation, and a lethal clinical course. Myocardium immunostaining studies in mutations carriers revealed abnormal LUMA signal levels with reduced desmosomal protein plakoglobin signal (50,51).

TMEM43 Gene and Myopathies Reminiscent of EDMD

More recently, two heterozygous *TMEM43* mutations have been identified in two unrelated patients (52). The first patient carrying the p.Glu85Lys substitution was diagnosed as EDMD as well as his son. The second patient carrying the p.Ile91Val substitution had muscle atrophy involving paraspinal, neck, upper arm, and thigh muscles, slowly progressive proximal muscle weakness over 64 years, and atrial fibrillation with bradycardia requiring pacemaker implantation. Evidence has been put forward arguing for the pathogenic effects of the variants (abnormal LUMA staining on skeletal muscle and failure in oligomerization for the p.Glu85Lys variant, reduced nuclear staining with or without aggregates of emerin and SUN2 together with a higher proportion of abnormally shaped nuclei in cells expressing mutant *TMEM43*).

LAP2α-Related Diseases

LAP2α encoded by the *TMPO* gene has been particularly incriminated in human disease. In a large series of patients presenting dilated cardiomyopathy, a unique missense *TMPO* mutation was identified in two brothers (53). Both had dilated cardiomyopathy beginning during the third or fourth decade and free of conduction defects. The mutation (p.Arg690Cys) is located in the C-terminal domain where LAP2α interacts with lamin A/C. It resulted in a low-level expression and abnormal nuclear localization of LAP2α in cardiac muscle. While there was no effect on peripheral and nucleoplasmic lamin A distribution observed in HeLa cells, the *in vitro* interaction of mutated LAP2α with the prelamin A C-terminus was significantly compromised.

PATHOPHYSIOLOGICAL MECHANISMS?

To date, apart from accumulation of toxic pre-lamin A that seems to be specific to HGPS and FPLD (5,62), two different hypotheses, not mutually exclusive, are proposed to explain the pathophysiology due to mutations in A-type lamins and in their partners: a structural/mechanical defect and a gene regulation defect.

Structural/Mechanical Defects

As part of the nucleoskeleton, nuclear lamina and associated partners are thought to have a predominant role in maintaining the structural integrity of nuclei and hence of cells (Figure 72.1). Mutations in lamins and some of their partners lead at least to a partial loss of function of the proteins and to the weakening of the nuclear lamina. This is evidenced by the high proportion of nuclei with abnormal-shaped NE in patient fibroblasts with mutations in A-type lamin and in some protein partners such as emerin or LUMA (3,16). The phenomenon is particularly exacerbated in cells subjected to mechanical stress such as skeletal and cardiac muscles and explains the high proportion of patients developing a muscular involvement when bearing a mutation in these genes. Proteins of the LINC complex are also thought to play a major role in maintaining the structural integrity of cells and in nuclear migration (6). As mentioned previously, expression of A-type lamins is required for the localization of SUN proteins at the INM and the localization of nesprin proteins at the ONM (13,14). Interestingly, two *Lmna* mouse models, the knock-out $Lmna^{-/-}$ and the knock-in $Lmna^{H222P/H222P}$, point to the importance of LINC complex proteins in the anchorage of myonuclei at the neuromuscular junction (NMJ). Analysis of nuclei at NMJ in these mice revealed an unequal distribution of SUN2 and nesprin-1 proteins at the NE and the displacement of nuclei beneath the synaptic plate (54). In addition, mutations in nesprin lead to mislocalization of SUN and emerin and to abnormal nuclear shape in humans (47). Here again, animal model knock-out for nesprin-1 helped demonstrating the importance of LINC complex proteins in nuclear positioning. Indeed, nesprin-$1^{-/-}$ mice have an increased proportion of nuclei positioned at the center of muscle fibers (55). Finally, if no mutations in SUN proteins have been identified in muscular dystrophies so far, knockdown experiments of SUN proteins induce an enlargement of the space between INM and ONM (56). Overall, these observations clearly indicate the interdependence of the proteins for their nuclear localization and for their function in maintaining the structural integrity of the NE and the cells.

Gene Expression/Signaling Defects

If the structural hypothesis is an attracting hypothesis to explain the pathophysiology of muscular dystrophies, it is less susceptible to clarify the development of the other diseases of the nucleoskeleton like lipodystrophies. Therefore, it has been proposed that altered gene expression due to mutations in A- or B-type lamins may be causal in these pathologies. The gene regulation hypothesis is based on the numerous transcription factors that interact with the proteins of the nucleoskeleton. Several of these interactions have been shown to induce a repression in the transcriptional activity (57,58) (Figure 72.1).

Adipogenesis is regulated by a number of genes including SREBP-1, peroxisome proliferator activator receptor gamma (PPAR-γ), and Rb (59). While Rb is required for cell cycle arrest and promotion of early differentiation events, PPAR-γ is pivotal to the activation of adipogenic genes. PPAR-γ is itself activated by SREBP-1. Interestingly, both Rb and SREBP-1 proteins have been identified as a lamin A-binding proteins (60,61). Accumulation of prelamin A in PLD has been shown to sequester SREBP-1 at the NE (62). More recently, the Wnt/β-catenin pathway has also been investigated during adipogenesis, as interaction with emerin inhibits β-catenin transcriptional activity (63) and suppression of the Wnt/β-catenin spontaneously promotes adipogenic conversion (64). This study has shown the importance of emerin expression in the degradation of beta-catenin prerequisite to adipogenesis (58). These different signaling pathways are certainly not restricted to lipodystrophies and might also be involved in some other types of diseases of the nucleoskeleton (8). Furthermore, other signaling pathways remain to be explored in the various disorders.

CONCLUSIONS AND PERSPECTIVES

The identification of mutations in genes encoding components of the nucleoskeleton has triggered a cascade of discoveries and opened widely both basic and clinical research linking the nucleoskeleton to neuromuscular disorders, cardiomyopathies, metabolic diseases and premature aging syndromes. The nucleoskeleton, primarily thought to have essentially structural functions, is actually a signaling platform; each of its components identified so far being implicated in various signaling pathways crucial for the different functions of the cells. Even if there are still numerous missing pieces in the puzzle of pathomechanisms involved in the different diseases linked so far to the nucleoskeleton, for some of them, promising therapeutic approaches are already emerging. Several compounds are tested in mouse models or even in patients to counteract PPAR-γ downregulation in lipodystrophy, prelamin A farnesylation in progeria, or Erk 1/2 hyperactivation in cardiac laminopathies (for review see 8). Thus, it is evident that new components of the nucleoskeleton remain to be discovered and with them potential related disorders. Their exploration will further feed and reinforce our knowledge and certainly reveal new targets for therapeutics strategies.

REFERENCES

1. Bione S, Maestrini E, Rivella S, Manchini M, Regis S, Romei G, et al. Identification of a novel X-linked gene responsible for Emery–Dreifuss muscular dystrophy. *Nature Genet* 1994;**8**:323–7.
2. Bonne G, Di Barletta MR, Varnous S, Becane H, Hammouda EH, Merlini L, et al. Mutations in the gene encoding lamin A/C cause autosomal dominant Emery–Dreifuss muscular dystrophy. *Nature Genet* 1999;**21**:285–8.
3. Broers J, Ramaekers F, Bonne G, Ben Yaou R, Hutchison C. The nuclear lamins: laminopathies and their role in premature ageing. *Physiol Rev* 2006;**86**:967–1008.
4. Ben-Harush K, Wiesel N, Frenkiel-Krispin D, Moeller D, Soreq E, Aebi U, et al. The supramolecular organization of the *C. elegans* nuclear lamin filament. *J Mol Biol* 2009;**386**:1392–402.
5. Navarro CL, Cau P, Levy N. Molecular bases of progeroid syndromes. *Hum Mol Genet* 2006;**15**(Spec No 2):R151–61.

6. Mejat A, Misteli T. LINC complexes in health and disease. *Nucleus* 2010;**1**:40–52.
7. Muchir A, van Engelen BG, Lammens M, Mislow JM, McNally E, Schwartz K, et al. Nuclear envelope alterations in fibroblasts from LGMD1B patients carrying nonsense Y259X heterozygous or homozygous mutation in lamin A/C gene. *Exp Cell Res* 2003;**291**:352–62.
8. Maraldi NM, Capanni C, Cenni V, Fini M, Lattanzi G. Laminopathies and lamin-associated signaling pathways. *J Cell Biochem* 2011;**112**:979–92.
9. Margalit A, Neufeld E, Feinstein N, Wilson KL, Podbilewicz B, Gruenbaum Y. Barrier to autointegration factor blocks premature cell fusion and maintains adult muscle integrity in *C. elegans*. *J Cell Biol* 2007;**178**:661–73.
10. Dechat T, Vlcek S, Foisner R. Review: lamina-associated polypeptide 2 isoforms and related proteins in cell cycle-dependent nuclear structure dynamics. *J Struct Biol* 2000;**129**:335–45.
11. Holaska JM. Emerin and the nuclear lamina in muscle and cardiac disease. *Circ Res* 2008;**103**:16–23.
12. Zhang Q, Skepper JN, Yang F, Davies JD, Hegyi L, Roberts RG, et al. Nesprins: a novel family of spectrin-repeat-containing proteins that localize to the nuclear membrane in multiple tissues. *J Cell Sci* 2001;**114**:4485–98.
13. Haque F, Mazzeo D, Patel JT, Smallwood DT, Ellis JA, Shanahan CM, et al. Mammalian SUN protein interaction networks at the inner nuclear membrane and their role in laminopathy disease processes. *J Biol Chem* 2010;**285**:3487–98.
14. Libotte T, Zaim H, Abraham S, Padmakumar VC, Schneider M, Lu W, et al. Lamin A/C-dependent localization of Nesprin-2, a giant scaffolder at the nuclear envelope. *Mol Biol Cell* 2005;**16**:3411–24.
15. Neumann S, Schneider M, Daugherty RL, Gottardi CJ, Eming SA, Beijer A, et al. Nesprin-2 interacts with α-catenin and regulates Wnt signaling at the nuclear envelope. *J Biol Chem* 2010;**285**:34932–8.
16. Bengtsson L, Otto H. LUMA interacts with emerin and influences its distribution at the inner nuclear membrane. *J Cell Sci* 2008;**121**:536–48.
17. Maidment SL, Ellis JA. Muscular dystrophies, dilated cardiomyopathy, lipodystrophy and neuropathy: the nuclear connection. *Expert Rev Mol Med* 2002;**4**:1–21.
18. Emery AEH. Emery–Dreifuss muscular dystrophy – a 40 year retrospective. *Neuromusc Disord* 2000;**10**:228–32.
19. Nagano A, Koga R, Ogawa M, Kurano Y, Kawada J, Okada R, et al. Emerin deficiency at the nuclear membrane in patients with Emery–Dreifuss muscular dystrophy. *Nature Genet* 1996;**12**:254–9.
20. Manilal S, Recan D, Sewry CA, Hoeltzenbein M, Llense S, Leturcq F, et al. Mutations in Emery–Dreifuss muscular dystrophy and their effects on emerin protein expression. *Hum Mol Genet* 1998;**7**:855–64.
21. Ben Yaou R, Toutain A, Arimura T, Demay L, Massart C, Peccate C, et al. Multitissular involvement in a family with LMNA and EMD mutations: Role of digenic mechanism? *Neurology* 2007;**68**:1883–94.
22. Karst ML, Herron KJ, Olson TM. X-linked nonsyndromic sinus node dysfunction and atrial fibrillation caused by emerin mutation. *J Cardiovasc Electrophysiol* 2008;**19**:510–5.
23. Ura S, Hayashi YK, Goto K, Astejada MN, Murakami T, Nagato M, et al. Limb-girdle muscular dystrophy due to emerin gene mutations. *Arch Neurol* 2007;**64**:1038–41.
24. Worman HJ, Bonne G. "Laminopathies": a wide spectrum of human diseases. *Exp Cell Res* 2007;**313**:2121–33.
25. di Barletta MR, Ricci E, Galluzzi G, Tonali P, Mora M, Morandi L, et al. Different mutations in the LMNA gene cause autosomal dominant and autosomal recessive Emery–Dreifuss muscular dystrophy. *Am J Hum Genet* 2000;**66**:1407–12.
26. Fatkin D, MacRae C, Sasaki T, Wolff MR, Porcu M, Frenneaux M, et al. Missense mutations in the rod domain of the lamin A/C gene as causes of dilated cardiomyopathy and conduction-system disease. *N Engl J Med* 1999;**341**:1715–24.
27. Bécane H-M, Bonne G, Varnous S, Muchir A, Ortega V, Hammouda EH, et al. High incidence of sudden death with conduction system and myocardial disease due to lamins A and C gene mutation. *Pacing Clin Electrophysiol* 2000;**23**:1661–6.
28. Muchir A, Bonne G, van der Kooi AJ, van Meegen M, Baas F, Bolhuis PA, et al. Identification of mutations in the gene encoding lamins A/C in autosomal dominant limb girdle muscular dystrophy with atrioventricular conduction disturbances (LGMD1B). *Hum Mol Genet* 2000;**9**:1453–9.
29. Quijano-Roy S, Mbieleu B, Bonnemann CG, Jeannet PY, Colomer J, Clarke NF, et al. De novo lmna mutations cause a new form of congenital muscular dystrophy. *Ann Neurol* 2008;**64**:177–86.
30. van Berlo JH, de Voogt WG, van der Kooi AJ, van Tintelen JP, Bonne G, Yaou RB, et al. Meta-analysis of clinical characteristics of 299 carriers of LMNA gene mutations: do lamin A/C mutations portend a high risk of sudden death? *J Mol Med* 2005;**83**:79–83.
31. Meune C, Van Berlo JH, Anselme F, Bonne G, Pinto YM, Duboc D. Primary prevention of sudden death in patients with lamin A/C gene mutations. *N Engl J Med* 2006;**354**:209–10.
32. Brodsky GL, Muntoni F, Miocic S, Sinagra G, Sewry C, Mestroni L. Lamin A/C gene mutation associated with dilated cardiomyopathy with variable skeletal muscle involvement. *Circulation* 2000;**101**:473–6.
33. Shackleton S, Lloyd DJ, Jackson SN, Evans R, Niermeijer MF, Singh BM, et al. LMNA, encoding lamin A/C, is mutated in partial lipodystrophy. *Nature Genet* 2000;**24**:153–6.
34. De Sandre-Giovannoli A, Chaouch M, Kozlov S, Vallat JM, Tazir M, Kassouri N, et al. Homozygous defects in *LMNA*, encoding lamin A/C nuclear-envelope proteins, cause autosomal recessive axonal neuropathy in human (Charcot–Marie–Tooth disorder Type 2) and mouse. *Am J Hum Genet* 2002;**70**:726–36.
35. Hamadouche T, Poitelon Y, Genin E, Chaouch M, Tazir M, Kassouri N, et al. Founder effect and estimation of the age of the c.892C > T (p.Arg298Cys) mutation in LMNA associated to Charcot–Marie–Tooth subtype CMT2B1 in families from North Western Africa. *Ann Hum Genet* 2008;**72**:590–7.
36. Novelli G, Muchir A, Sangiuolo F, Helbling-Leclerc A, Rosaria d'Apice M, Massart C, et al. Mandibuloacral dysplasia is caused by a mutation in LMNA encoding lamins A/C. *Am J Hum Genet* 2002;**71**:426–31.
37. De Sandre-Giovannoli A, Bernard R, Cau P, Navarro C, Amiel J, Boccacio I, et al. Lamin A truncation in Hutchinson-Gilford progeria. *Science* 2003;**300**:2055.
38. Eriksson M, Brown WT, Gordon LB, Glynn MW, Singer J, Scott L, et al. Recurrent de novo point mutations in lamin A cause Hutchinson–Gilford progeria syndrome. *Nature* 2003;**25**:25.

39. Yu C, Oshima J, Fu YH, Wijsman EM, Hisama F, Alisch R, et al. Positional cloning of the Werner's syndrome gene. *Science* 1996;**12**:258–62.
40. Chen L, Lee L, Kudlow B, Dos Santos H, Sletvold O, Shafeghati Y, et al. LMNA mutations in atypical Werner's syndrome. *Lancet* 2003;**362**:440–5.
41. Carboni N, Porcu M, Mura M, Cocco E, Marrosu G, Maioli MA, et al. Evolution of the phenotype in a family with an LMNA gene mutation presenting with isolated cardiac involvement. *Muscle Nerve* 2010;**41**:85–91.
42. Padiath QS, Saigoh K, Schiffmann R, Asahara H, Yamada T, Koeppen A, et al. Lamin B1 duplications cause autosomal dominant leukodystrophy. *Nat Genet* 2006;**38**:1114–23.
43. Hegele RA, Cao H, Liu DM, Costain GA, Charlton-Menys V, Rodger NW, et al. Sequencing of the reannotated LMNB2 gene reveals novel mutations in patients with acquired partial lipodystrophy. *Am J Hum Genet* 2006;**79**:383–9.
44. Gros-Louis F, Dupre N, Dion P, Fox MA, Laurent S, Verreault S, et al. Mutations in SYNE1 lead to a newly discovered form of autosomal recessive cerebellar ataxia. *Nat Genet* 2007;**39**: 80–5.
45. Attali R, Warwar N, Israel A, Gurt I, McNally E, Puckelwartz M, et al. Mutation of SYNE-1, encoding an essential component of the nuclear lamina, is responsible for autosomal recessive arthrogryposis. *Hum Mol Genet* 2009;**18**:3462–9.
46. Puckelwartz MJ, Kessler E, Zhang Y, Hodzic D, Randles KN, Morris G, et al. Disruption of nesprin-1 produces an Emery Dreifuss muscular dystrophy-like phenotype in mice. *Hum Mol Genet* 2009;**18**:607–20.
47. Zhang Q, Bethmann C, Worth NF, Davies JD, Wasner C, Feuer A, et al. Nesprin-1 and -2 are involved in the pathogenesis of Emery–Dreifuss muscular dystrophy and are critical for nuclear envelope integrity. *Hum Mol Genet* 2007;**16**:2816–33.
48. Marcus FI, McKenna WJ, Sherrill D, Basso C, Bauce B, Bluemke DA, et al. Diagnosis of arrhythmogenic right ventricular cardiomyopathy/dysplasia: proposed modification of the Task Force Criteria. *Eur Heart J* 2010;**31**:806–14.
49. Ghosh N, Haddad H. Recent progress in the genetics of cardiomyopathy and its role in the clinical evaluation of patients with cardiomyopathy. *Curr Opin Cardiol* 2011;**26**:155–64.
50. Merner ND, Hodgkinson KA, Haywood AF, Connors S, French VM, Drenckhahn JD, et al. Arrhythmogenic right ventricular cardiomyopathy type 5 is a fully penetrant, lethal arrhythmic disorder caused by a missense mutation in the TMEM43 gene. *Am J Hum Genet* 2008;**82**:809–21.
51. Christensen AH, Andersen CB, Tybjaerg-Hansen A, Haunso S, Svendsen JH. Mutation analysis and evaluation of the cardiac localization of TMEM43 in arrhythmogenic right ventricular cardiomyopathy. *Clin Genet* 2011;**80**:256–64.
52. Liang WC, Mitsuhashi H, Keduka E, Nonaka I, Noguchi S, Nishino I, et al. TMEM43 mutations in Emery–Dreifuss muscular dystrophy-related myopathy. *Ann Neurol* 2011;**69**:1003–15.
53. Taylor MR, Slavov D, Gajewski A, Vlcek S, Ku L, Fain PR, et al. Thymopoietin (lamina-associated polypeptide 2) gene mutation associated with dilated cardiomyopathy. *Hum Mutat* 2005;**26**:566–74.
54. Mejat A, Decostre V, Li J, Renou L, Kesari A, Hantai D, et al. Lamin A/C-mediated neuromuscular junction defects in Emery–Dreifuss muscular dystrophy. *J Cell Biol* 2009;**184**:31–44.
55. Zhang J, Felder A, Liu Y, Guo LT, Lange S, Dalton ND, et al. Nesprin 1 is critical for nuclear positioning and anchorage. *Hum Mol Genet* 2010;**19**:329–41.
56. Crisp M, Liu Q, Roux K, Rattner JB, Shanahan C, Burke B, et al. Coupling of the nucleus and cytoplasm: role of the LINC complex. *J Cell Biol* 2006;**172**:41–53.
57. Holaska JM, Rais-Bahrami S, Wilson KL. Lmo7 is an emerin-binding protein that regulates the transcription of emerin and many other muscle-relevant genes. *Hum Mol Genet* 2006;**15**:3459–72.
58. Tilgner K, Wojciechowicz K, Jahoda C, Hutchison C, Markiewicz E. Dynamic complexes of A-type lamins and emerin influence adipogenic capacity of the cell via nucleocytoplasmic distribution of beta-catenin. *J Cell Sci* 2009;**122**:401–13.
59. Fajas L, Fruchart JC, Auwerx J. Transcriptional control of adipogenesis. *Curr Opin Cell Biol* 1998;**10**:165–73.
60. Lloyd DJ, Trembath RC, Shackleton S. A novel interaction between lamin A and SREBP1: implications for partial lipodystrophy and other laminopathies. *Hum Mol Genet* 2002;**11**:769–77.
61. Frock RL, Kudlow BA, Evans AM, Jameson SA, Hauschka SD, Kennedy BK. Lamin A/C and emerin are critical for skeletal muscle satellite cell differentiation. *Genes Dev* 2006;**20**:486–500.
62. Capanni C, Mattioli E, Columbaro M, Lucarelli E, Parnaik VK, Novelli G, et al. Altered pre-lamin A processing is a common mechanism leading to lipodystrophy. *Hum Mol Genet* 2005;**14**:1489–502.
63. Markiewicz E, Tilgner K, Barker N, van de Wetering M, Clevers H, Dorobek M, et al. The inner nuclear membrane protein emerin regulates beta-catenin activity by restricting its accumulation in the nucleus. *EMBO J* 2006;**25**:3275–85.
64. Ross SE, Hemati N, Longo KA, Bennett CN, Lucas PC, Erickson RL, et al. Inhibition of adipogenesis by Wnt signaling. *Science* 2000;**289**:950–3.

Chapter 73

Channelopathies of Skeletal Muscle Excitability

Stephen C. Cannon
University of Texas Southwestern Medical Center, Dallas, TX

CLINICAL PHENOTYPES FROM CHANNEL MUTATIONS THAT ALTER SARCOLEMMAL EXCITABILITY

Voluntary contraction of skeletal muscle is rapid and highly reliable. To achieve this performance, the excitability of the muscle fiber must be robust such that the endplate potential at the neuromuscular junction (NMJ) will generate an action potential that propagates along the surface membrane and into the transverse tubules where depolarization triggers Ca^{2+} release from the sarcoplasmic reticulum (SR) and thereby initiates contraction. Myasthenic syndromes with fatiguable weakness result from disruption of NMJ that compromises the safety factor of neuromuscular transmission, wherein the amplitude of the endplate potential is reduced and does not reliably trigger an action potential in the fiber (1). In contrast, the ion channel disorders that disrupt the intrinsic excitability of the fiber cause myotonia and periodic paralysis (2).

Myotonia

Myotonia is caused by a pathological enhancement of muscle fiber excitability in which prolonged bursts of discharges persist for many seconds after the cessation of voluntary effort (3). These myotonic discharges elicit SR Ca^{2+} release and produce involuntary after-contractions that patients perceive as activity-dependent muscle stiffness. Symptoms fluctuate over time, with the myotonic stiffness being most severe with the first forceful movements after a period of rest and improvement during continued muscular effort (warm-up phenomenon). In paramyotonia, the myotonia paradoxically worsens with repeated activity and is usually exacerbated by muscle cooling.

The bursts of myotonic discharges originate from the muscle fiber, and are not dependent on persistent motor neuron activity. The needle electromyogram (EMG) shows repetitive after-discharges that persist for many seconds, with fluctuations in frequency that produce a musical "dive-bomber" pattern of discharges on the audio monitor (Figure 73.1). Latent myotonia may be detected by needle EMG in patients who are asymptomatic. Susceptibility to myotonia results from mutations of voltage-gated chloride channels or voltage-gated sodium channels.

Periodic Paralysis

Periodic paralysis is caused by a transient failure of muscle fiber excitability (4,5). During an attack of weakness, the fiber fails to maintain a normal resting potential and in this depolarized state the fiber is persistently refractory, unable to generate an action potential (Figure 73.1). The weakness may be focal or generalized, and attacks typically last for hours followed by spontaneous recovery, although return to full strength may take several days. The muscles for respiration are usually spared and ventilatory insufficiency is rare. The episodes of weakness do not have any regular periodicity, and instead are often triggered by provocative maneuvers. Familial periodic paralysis has been associated with mutations of voltage-gated sodium channels, the L-type calcium channels, or inward rectifier potassium channels (6).

Clinical subtypes of periodic paralysis have been defined on the basis of the serum potassium levels during an attack, associated provocative triggers, and the coexistence of myotonia (7). In hyperkalemic periodic paralysis (HyperPP), serum potassium is usually elevated at $>$5.5 mEq/L (3.5–5.5 mEq/L normal) during a spontaneous attack, although a normal value does not exclude HyperPP. Ingestion of potassium-rich foods, rest after exercise, or emotional stress may provoke an attack, whereas eating carbohydrates (which results in a shift of extracellular K^+ into muscle) may abort an attack. Myotonia may occur in a patient with HyperPP, especially just before an attack of weakness. Conversely, with hypokalemic periodic paralysis (HypoPP) the ictal potassium is low ($<$3.0 mEq/L), carbohydrate ingestion

Muscle. DOI: http://dx.doi.org/10.1016/B978-0-12-381510-1.00073-9

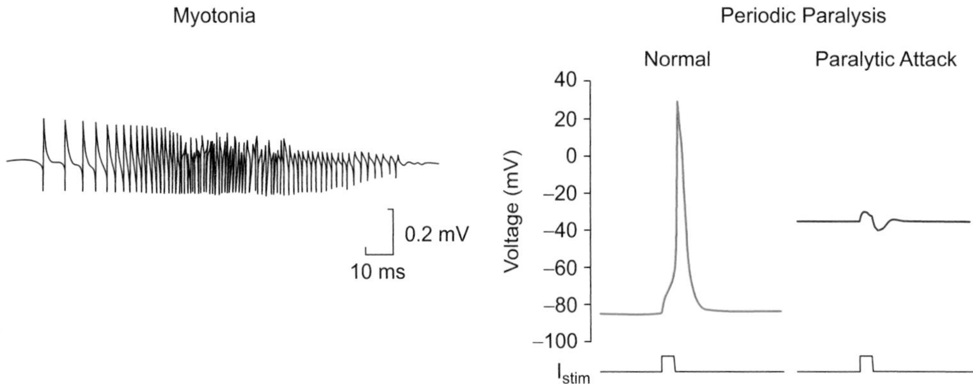

FIGURE 73.1 Derangements in fiber excitability caused by ion channelopathies of skeletal muscle. Needle electromyogram shows a sustained burst of myotonic discharges that wax and wane in frequency (*left*). Action potentials for a computer-simulated muscle fiber illustrate the loss of excitability that accompanies a depolarized shift of the resting potential (*right*).

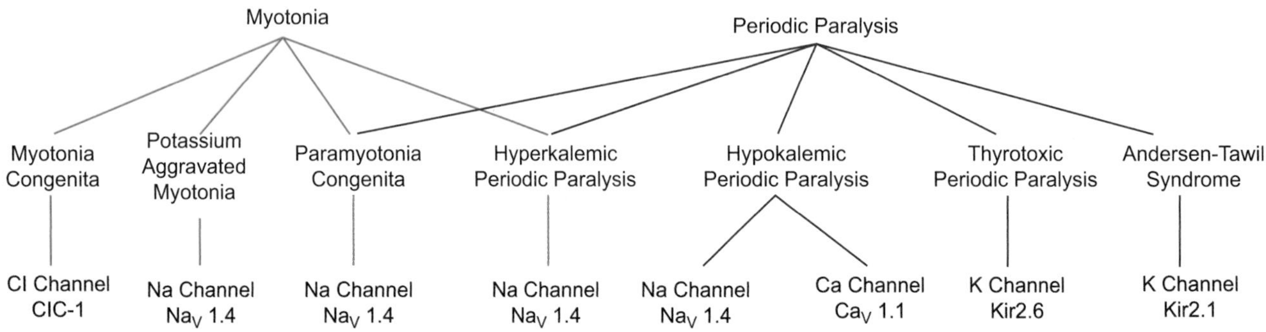

FIGURE 73.2 Spectrum of muscle disorders (*middle row*) and ion channel mutations (*bottom row*) associated with non-dystrophic myotonia and periodic paralysis. Myotonia and periodic paralysis may both occur in paramyotonia congenita and hyperkalemic periodic paralysis.

increases the risk of an attack and episodes of weakness may be prevented or foreshortened by oral potassium supplements. Rest after exercise and emotional stress may also provoke weakness in HypoPP. Myotonia does not occur in HypoPP.

The phenotypic variability of myotonia or periodic paralysis can be viewed as a continuum of overlapping symptoms that have been delineated clinically into specific disorders, with associated ion channel gene defects (Figure 73.2)

CHLORIDE CHANNEL LOSS-OF-FUNCTION DEFECTS CAUSE MYOTONIA

The sarcolemmal of resting skeletal muscle is highly permeable to chloride ions (8), which has a major influence on stabilizing the membrane potential at the resting value. Without this stabilizing influence, muscle becomes susceptible to self-sustained bursts of repetitive discharges, thereby resulting in myotonia (9).

The resting potential of skeletal muscle, V_{rest}, is determined primarily by the fiber permeability to K^+ ions that are conducted by inward rectifying K^+ channels. The ratio of extracellular to myoplasmic $[K^+]$ is about 4/155, which results in an equilibrium potential for K^+ of −98 mV. In skeletal muscle V_{rest} is −90 mV, slightly depolarized from the K^+ equilibrium potential because the sarcolemma is also slightly permeable to Na^+. Unlike the cations K^+ and Na^+, the chloride concentration gradient in muscle is not regulated by pumps. Consequently Cl^- flows in or out of the myoplasm until an internal Cl^- concentration is reached where Cl^- is in equilibrium at V_{rest}. There is no net Cl^- flow at V_{rest} and Cl^- ions do not set the value V_{rest}. The resting membrane is highly permeable to Cl^-, however, and therefore whenever the membrane potential deviates from V_{rest} , as occurs during an action potential, a large net Cl^- current will flow that tends to return the membrane potential to V_{rest}. In essence, the chloride conductance of resting muscle fibers functions as an electrical buffering mechanism to keep the membrane potential at V_{rest}. This critical role of the Cl^- conductance to stabilize V_{rest} of skeletal muscle was initially revealed by *in vitro* electrophysiological studies of fibers from goats with hereditary myotonia (9,10).

Normally, the resting conductance to Cl^- is four times larger than for K^+; whereas in fibers from myotonic goats the chloride conductance was virtually absent. Subsequent studies in fibers biopsied from patients with myotonia congenita also revealed a dramatic reduction in the resting chloride conductance (11). Indeed, normal muscle will become myotonic if the extracellular Cl^- is replaced by an impermeant anion. The myotonic after-discharges that continue beyond the cessation of motor neuron activity are triggered by activity-dependent K^+ accumulation in the transverse tubules (TT) (10). The efflux of K^+ during the repolarization phase of the action potential may transiently increase the $[K^+]$ in the TT to 10–15 mM during periods of intense voluntary contraction. This change in the transmembrane K^+ gradient produces a depolarized shift of the K^+ equilibrium potential by 20–30 mV. In the absence of the chloride conductance, V_{rest} will undergo a comparable depolarized shift, which may trigger action potentials. The normally high chloride conductance helps maintain the basal V_{rest} despite the depolarized shift in the K^+ equilibrium potential, thereby preventing after-discharges.

The major chloride channel of skeletal muscle is a homodimer of ClC-1, which is a member of the ClC family of voltage-dependent chloride channels and transporters (12). ClC-1 is expressed almost exclusively in skeletal muscle, and over 60 mutations in the gene *CLCN1* have been identified in families with myotonia congenita (13–15). The inheritance pattern is usually recessive (Becker myotonia congenita), with most patients being compound heterozygotes in which neither mutant allele encodes a functional channel. Many of these mutations are deletions or splice site mutations that cause a nonsense transcript with a premature termination codon. Family members with a single recessive mutant allele are asymptomatic or may have subclinical latent myotonia detectable only by EMG. Pharmacologic studies have shown that ~80% of ClC-1 channels must be blocked before muscle develops myotonia (16), which accounts for the recessive pattern of the phenotype for ClC-1 nonsense mutations; haploinsufficiency is clinically silent. In some families myotonia congenita has a dominant inheritance pattern (Thomsen's disease), resulting from missense mutations in ClC-1 that strongly shift the voltage dependence of channel opening to depolarized potentials (17). In wild-type channels, the opening probably is about 20% at V_{rest}. The depolarized shift of channel opening in homodimer mutant or heterodimeric ClC-1 channels produces a dominant-negative effect by drastically reducing the open probability at V_{rest}, resulting in myotonia.

The therapeutic approach for management of myotonia congenita is to avoid provocative maneuvers (slowly warm up before strenuous exercise, avoid cold environments) or as a preventive measure take Na^+ channel blockers (e.g. mexiletine) to reduce muscle excitability (18). Drugs that effectively increase the resting chloride conductance in muscle have not been identified. Moreover, these agents would likely be applicable only for the rarer Thomsen's myotonia congenita in which functional ClC-1 channels are expressed at the sarcolemma, since recessive myotonia congenita results from two non-functional mutant alleles.

SODIUM CHANNEL GAIN-OF-FUNCTION MUTATIONS CAUSE MYOTONIA OR PERIODIC PARALYSIS

The generation and propagation of action potentials in skeletal muscle are produced by the rapid opening of voltage-gated Na^+ channels. The major Na^+ channel in skeletal muscle is a heterodimer of the pore-forming α subunit, $Na_V1.4$ encoded by the *SCN4A* gene (19), and an accessory $\beta1$ subunit (20). Missense mutations in *SCN4A* have been associated with disorders in which the predominant manifestation is myotonia, periodic paralysis, or a combination of both symptoms in the same individual. Mutations of the $\beta1$ subunit have been associated with epilepsy and cardiac arrhythmia, but no skeletal muscle disease.

The sodium channel was first implicated as a possible cause for disorders of skeletal muscle excitability on the basis of microelectrode studies in fibers biopsied from patients with hyperkalemic periodic paralysis (HyperPP) and paramyotonia congenita (PMC). Recordings from affected fibers revealed an anomalous inward current that was blocked by tetrodotoxin, thereby suggesting a gain-of-function defect in the voltage-gated Na^+ channel (21,22). Both HyperPP and PMC are inherited as autosomal dominant traits with high penetrance. In HyperPP, the predominant symptom is episodic attacks of weakness associated with elevated serum K^+ (>5.5 mM) or triggered by ingestion of K^+-rich foods· Myotonia often occurs with the onset of or during the recovery from an episode of weakness. The acute attacks of weakness usually occur within the first decade of life, and may be followed by a late-onset slowly progressive permanent proximal weakness with vacuolar myopathy. In PMC, the predominant symptom is myotonic stiffness that paradoxically worsens with continued muscular exertion (paramyotonia) and is exacerbated by muscle cooling. Patients with PMC may also experience attacks of periodic paralysis. The clinical presentation of HyperPP or PMC has overlapping features, and symptoms typical of either disorder may co-exist in separate members of an affected family (23).

These electrophysiological studies implicated the voltage-gated sodium channel as a candidate disease gene for HyperPP, PMC, and possibly other disorders of skeletal muscle excitability (24). Genetic studies of patients with

HyperPP and PMC have identified over 50 mutations in the coding region of *SCN4A* (2,25). In all cases, the mutations cause missense substitutions, often located in critical transmembrane segments forming the voltage-sensor or vestibule of the pore. Many families with dominantly inherited myotonia, but no episodes of paralysis, were initially thought to have a form of myotonia congenita (Thomsen's disease), but no chloride channel mutation in ClC-1 could be detected. Secondary screening in these families revealed missense mutations in *SCN4A* (26). Several clinical subtypes were delineated within this group of myotonic patients with *SCN4A* mutations, and the disorders have been given descriptive names – potassium-aggravated myotonia, myotonia fluctuans, or myotonia permanans (27,28), often referred to collectively as PAM. For all of these myotonic disorders, as well as HyperPP and PMC, the mutant transcript is expressed at the plasma membrane and has a gain-of-function change.

The clinical delineation of four allelic disorders (PAM, PMC, HyperPP, and HypoPP) associated with over 70 missense mutations of *SCN4A*, suggests there are specific classes of biophysical defects among these Na^+ channel mutants, each of which causes a predilection for a specific clinical phenotype (29). Functional studies of mutant $Na_V1.4$ channels have revealed changes in channel behavior that can be mechanistically linked to susceptibility to myotonia, periodic paralysis, or both. These functional studies are based upon recording Na^+ currents from mutant channels expressed in immortalized (non-muscle) cell lines. Normally, Na^+ channels are closed at the resting potential, rapidly open within a fraction of a msec in response to depolarization, and then quickly inactivate within a few msec. The fiber is refractory from firing additional action potentials until the membrane has been hyperpolarized to the resting potential for several msec which allows recovery from inactivation. Mutations associated with the myotonia–HyperPP set of disorders (PAM, PMC, HyperPP) all produce gain-of-function defects that result in excessive inward Na^+ currents. The mutant channel inappropriately conducts current because of a change in the gating behavior that promotes channel opening, either through disruption of inactivation (30) or enhancement of activation (31).

The variety of clinical phenotypes in the $Na_V1.4$ channelopathies can be attributed to important differences in the details of these gain-of-function defects (Figure 73.3) (29,32). Mutations associated with myotonia only, for example PAM, slow the rate of channel inactivation about

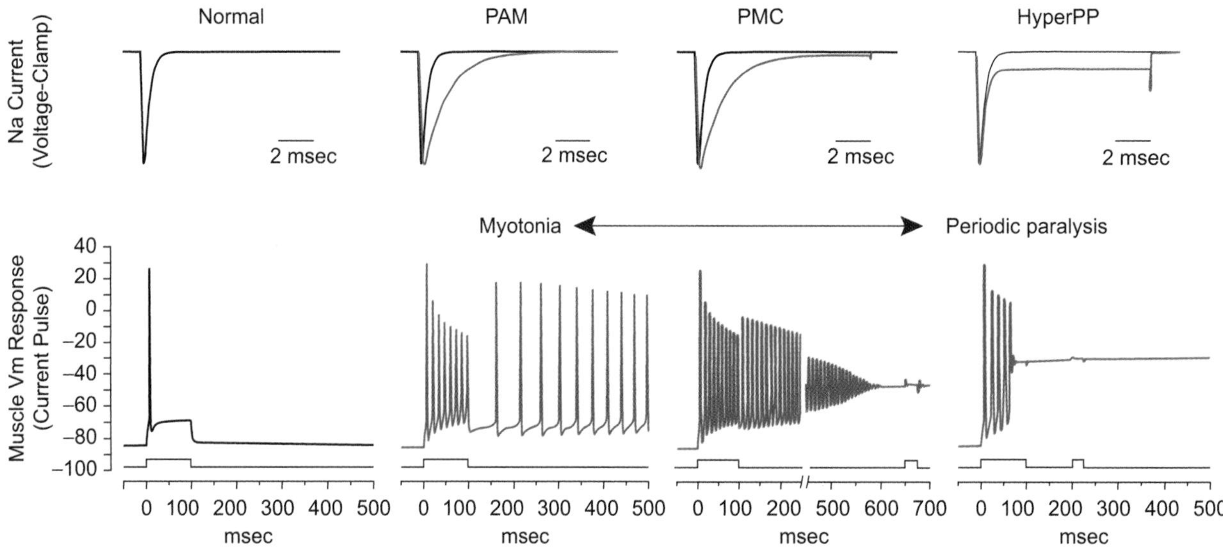

FIGURE 73.3 Gain-of-function changes in mutant $Na_V1.4$ channels may cause myotonia or periodic paralysis. Computer simulation was used to model defects in $Na_V1.4$ gating (*top row*, typical Na^+ currents that would be recorded under voltage clamp) and predict the consequences for muscle fiber excitability (*bottom row*). Left column simulates normal muscle with rapid activation and complete inactivation of the Na^+ channel that produces a brief inward Na^+ current (downward deflection) in response to depolarization (*top*). A simulated fiber with normal Na^+ channels responds with a single action potential in response to an injected stimulus current (*bottom*). Second column from left simulates a slower rate of inactivation (*top*, blue trace; black reference for normal) as occurs in potassium-aggravated myotonia (PAM). This kinetic defect of inactivation results in a burst of myotonic discharges that persist beyond the stimulus for the simulated fiber (*bottom*). Third column from left simulates the Na^+ channel defect in paramyotonia congenita (PMC) with a slower rate of inactivation and a small persistent current (*top*). The combined gating defects produce myotonic discharges and may cause paralysis if the membrane potential settles at a depolarized potential where Na^+ channels will be chronically inactivated (end of trace). Note the gap in traces between 300 and 500 msec. Right column simulates the large persistent Na^+ current conducted by mutant channels in hyperkalemic periodic paralysis (HyperPP, *top*). When incorporated into the simulated muscle fiber, the large persistent Na^+ current creates a strong susceptibility for a stable plateau depolarization with attendant inexcitability and paralysis (*bottom*). *(Modified from Cannon, 2006 (2).)*

five-fold (33). Because of this slower rate of inactivation, a fraction of mutant Na^+ channels will not have inactivated at the end of an action potential. The combination of this increased availability of Na channels (not – inactivated) plus the modest after-depolarization of V_{rest} from K^+ efflux into the transverse tubules may trigger bursts of myotonic discharges. In contrast, Na^+ channel mutations associated with HyperPP disrupt the completeness of inactivation (30) or may shift the voltage dependence of activation toward more hyperpolarized potentials (31). These changes result in an anomalous persistent inward Na^+ current whenever the membrane is depolarized. This persistent Na^+ current may chronically depolarize the fiber to about −50 mV, at which point all the normally behaving Na^+ channels (from the normal allele as well as the majority from the mutant allele) will be inactivated and the fiber therefore becomes inexcitable. The loss of excitability in depolarized fibers causes the flaccid weakness during an episode of periodic paralysis. The important distinction for these two gain-of-function examples is that the slower rate of inactivation in PAM produces a dynamic instability with a predilection for after-discharges, whereas the persistent Na^+ current in HyperPP is a steady-state change that may therefore produce a stable depolarization of V_{rest}, inexcitability, and paralysis. The persistent Na^+ current that underlies an attack of HyperPP is more prominent for channel mutations that disrupt slow inactivation (34,35), which operates over a course of seconds to minutes, in addition to the conventional fast inactivation that limits the duration of the action potential and produces the refractory period. For every member in the subset of $Na_V1.4$ mutations in which slow inactivation is impaired, the predominant clinical feature is periodic paralysis. Mutant channels associated with PMC typically display mixed biophysical defects with slowed inactivation plus a small persistent current, resulting in an intermediate clinical phenotype with myotonia and periodic paralysis. In general, for mutant channels with a larger persistent Na^+ current there will be a higher likelihood that the predominant symptom is periodic paralysis.

The management of myotonia and hyperkalemic periodic paralysis is based on symptomatic relief by avoiding provocative maneuvers (vigorous exercise, K^+-rich foods), by ingestion of carbohydrates to promote K^+ movement into muscle, or by pharmacologic intervention (7). Use-dependent Na^+ channel blockers, such as mexiletine, are effective at reducing the severity of myotonia by reducing fiber excitability. For unknown reasons, these agents are not also effective for ameliorating transient attacks of weakness. Carbonic anhydrase inhibitors, such as acetazolamide, reduce the frequency and severity of paralytic attacks when taken prophylactically (36). The mechanism by which acetazolamide is efficacious for ameliorating periodic paralysis is not understood, but effects on transmembrane pH gradients or activation of K^+ channels have been reported. There is no known therapy to prevent the late-onset permanent proximal weakness, nor does this late complication correlate well with the severity of acute transient attacks in early adulthood. Histologically, there is a shift to fast oxidative type IIa fiber predominance in myotonic muscle. Vacuolar myopathy is often seen, once permanent weakness ensues. Other changes may include internal nuclei, increased fiber size variability, and transverse tubular aggregates.

LEAKY MUTANT SODIUM CHANNELS CAUSE HYPOKALEMIC PERIODIC PARALYSIS

Familial hypokalemic periodic paralysis (HypoPP) has been linked to mutations in the L-type $Ca_V1.1$ calcium channel (37,38) encoded by *CACNL1AS* (60% of families), and the $Na_V.14$ sodium channel (39,40) encoded by *SCN4A* (20% of families). Curiously, 14 of 15 HypoPP missense mutations collectively found in $Na_V1.4$ or $Ca_V1.1$ occur at arginine residues in the voltage-sensor domains (41), formed by the fourth transmembrane segment (S4) in each of the homologous domains of the channel. The HypoPP mutations in $Na_V1.4$ cause a distinctly different class of functional defect, wherein the Na^+ current through the pore has only a mild loss-of-function defect, but more importantly mutant channels are "leaky" through an accessory pathway for ion flow (42,43). These HypoPP mutations create a "leak" in the crevasse between mobile S4 segment and the scaffolding of the channel protein, which allows an inward current to flow at V_{rest}. Upon depolarization of the membrane, the S4 segment translocates outward and thereby moves the arginine mutation out of the channel crevasse, and the current leak is abolished. Because movement of the S4 segment controls the "gates" for channel activation or inactivation, the cleft in the channel protein through which S4 moves has been called the "gating pore", and so the leakage current created by an arginine mutation is called the gating pore current. The gating pore current is carried by protons (H^+) for arginine to histidine mutations (44), whereas other missense mutations result in a non-selective leaky gating pore that conducts monovalent cations and even small organic molecules. The amplitude of the gating pore current at V_{rest} is small, on the order of 0.1 to 0.5 % of the peak Na^+ current conducted through the conventional pore during an action potential.

The mechanism by which the gating pore current causes susceptibility to HypoPP is revealed by a consideration of the balance of inward and outward ionic currents that set V_{rest} (Figure 73.4) (45–47). The resting potential

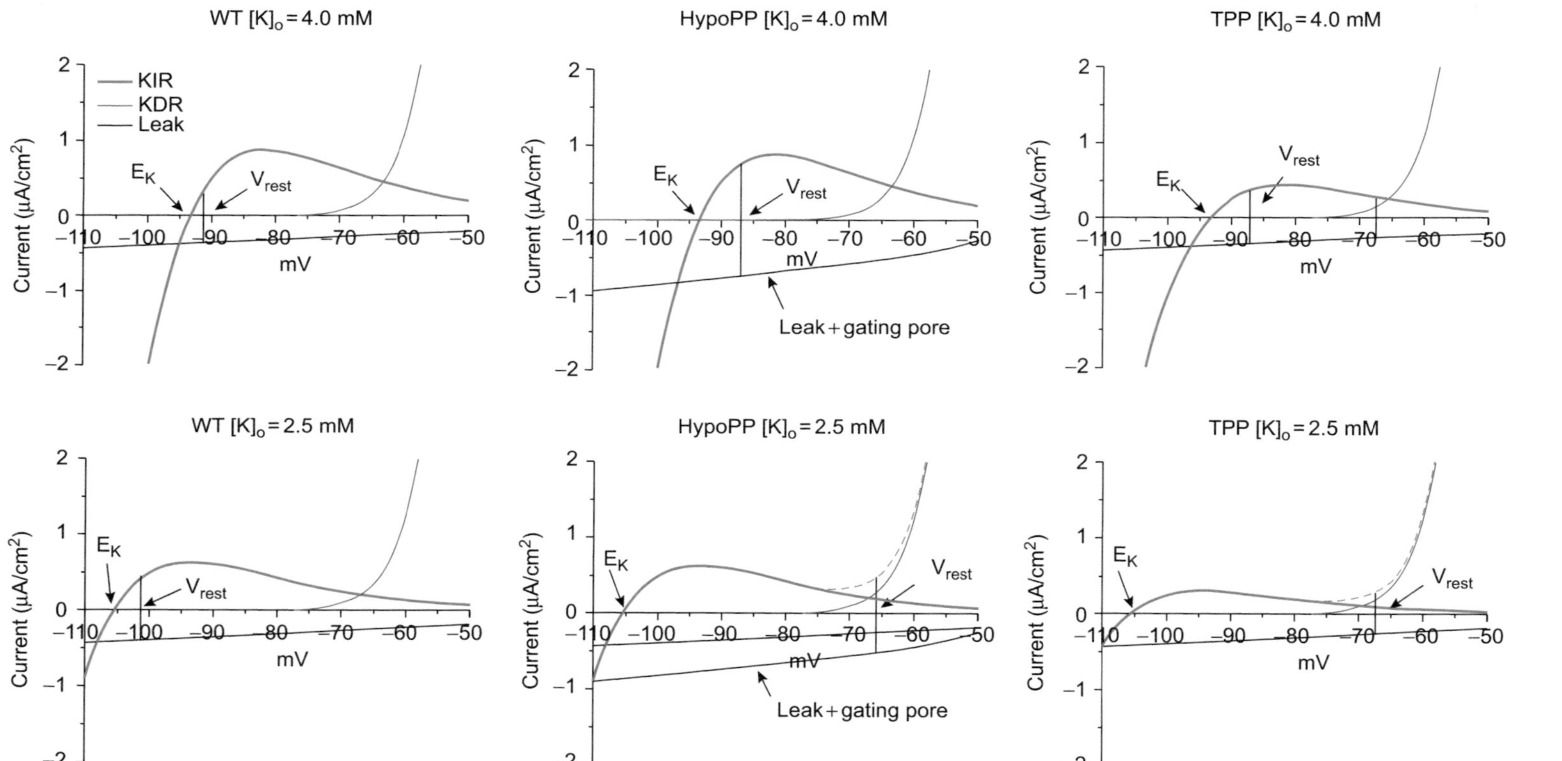

FIGURE 73.4 **Paradoxical depolarization of V_{rest} in low $[K^+]$ for familial HypoPP and TPP**. Each panel shows simulated current–voltage curves for K_{IR}, K_{DR}, Leak, or Leak+ Gating Pore currents. V_{rest} occurs where inward (negative) and outward (positive) currents balance for a net total current of zero. *Top row* shows simulated responses in 4.0 mM $[K^+]$ for wild-type, HypoPP, and TTP fibers. Compared to the wild-type V_{rest} −91 mV, a very small depolarization of the resting potential occurs in HypoPP (− 87 mV) or TPP (− 88 mV) fibers. Bottom row shows the effect of reducing $[K^+]$ to 2.5 mM. For wild-type fibers, Vrest hyperpolarizes to −102 mV; whereas HypoPP fibers depolarize to −65 mV and TPP to −68 mV. Paradoxical depolarization of V_{rest} occurs because the outward K_{IR} current is not able to balance the inward Leak + Gating Pore currents in HypoPP; whereas in TPP the reduced outward K_{IR} current is not able to balance the inward Leak current. At the paradoxical depolarized values of V_{rest}, the outward K_{DR} is required to balance the inward currents.

in normal muscle is about −90 mV and is determined by a balance of outward K^+ current through the inward rectifier channel (Kir), and inward current (mainly Na^+) through non-selective "leakage" channels. The addition of the anomalous inward gating pore current, from HypoPP mutant $Na_V1.4$, increases the total inward current and overwhelms the outward current conducted by K_{IR} channels. Consequently, the fiber will depolarize until voltage-activated delayed-rectifier K^+ channels (K_{DR}) open sufficiently to pass an outward K^+ current that balances the leak and gating pore currents. This new balance of inward and outward currents occurs at a membrane potential of about −50 mV, a voltage at which Na^+ channels will be inactivated, resulting in failure of excitation and paralysis. The sensitivity of attacks to hypokalemia occurs through the normal K^+-dependence of the inward rectified channel. As extracellular $[K^+]$ is lowered, the equilibrium potential for potassium (Nernst, E_K) shifts in the hyperpolarizing direction (more negative), and so the I−V curve for the K_{IR} channel moves negatively as well, which reduces the amplitude of outward K_{IR} current. Moreover, low external $[K^+]$ has a direct effect on the K_{IR} channels to reduce the K^+ conductance (48). The net result is that while the inward gating pore current produces only a modest depolarization of V_{rest} by 3−5 mV under normokalemic conditions in which the outward K_{IR} current is able to balance the net inward current, in hypokalemia the K_{IR} current is not able to balance total inward current and the fiber depolarizes to a stable membrane potential of −50 mV set by a balance with outward K currents from K_{DR} channels. In this way, the gating pore leak creates susceptibility to a paradoxical depolarized shift of V_{rest} in low external $[K^+]$, thereby resulting in a HypoPP phenotype.

The therapeutic approach for management of familial HypoPP is primarily through reduction of risk factors (avoid strenuous exercise or high carbohydrate meals), oral supplementation with K^+, or prophylactic use of carbonic anhydrase inhibitors. In principle, a selective blocker of the anomalous gating pore would be the ideal drug to eliminate the susceptibility to attacks of HypoPP.

CALCIUM CHANNEL MUTATIONS IN HYPOKALEMIC PERIODIC PARALYSIS

Missense mutations at arginine residues in the voltage-sensor S4 segments of $Ca_V1.1$ account for approximately 60% of cases of familial HypoPP (40,49). The L-type Ca^{2+} channel of skeletal muscle is a heteropentamer, with a main pore-forming α_1 subunit, $Ca_V1.1$, and four accessory subunits, β, γ, α_2, and δ. Mutations of only the α_1 $Ca_V1.1$ subunit have been identified in familial HypoPP. Conversely, mutations of $Ca_V1.1$ have also been reported in susceptibility to malignant hyperthermia.

As with other forms of periodic paralysis, the inciting event for an acute attack in $Ca_V1.1$ − HypoPP is a depolarization of V_{rest}, which inactivates Na^+ channels and renders the fiber inexcitable (4). The mechanism by which the depolarization-induced episodes of paralysis in HypoPP might be causally linked to missense mutations in $Ca_V1.1$ was a mystery for over 10 years. The L-type Ca^{2+} channel in skeletal muscle functions primarily as a voltage sensor that couples depolarization of the TT to ryanodine receptor opening and release of Ca^{2+} from the SR. The channel has no known role in stabilizing V_{rest}, and no defect of excitation−contraction coupling was detectable in biopsied fibers from patients with HypoPP. Insight into the pathomechanism of HypoPP for $Ca_V1.1$ mutations has been by analogy to defects caused by mutations in homologous regions of the S4 segments in $Na_V1.4$ (39,41). It has been proposed that a gating pore leak current, similar to that measured in HypoPP − $Na_V1.4$ mutant channels, is produced by the arginine mutations in S4 of $Ca_V1.1$. This anomalous inward current at V_{rest} would cause susceptibility to paradoxical depolarization with hypokalemia in $Ca_V1.1$-HypoPP. Experimental confirmation has not yet been possible, because the membrane expression of $Ca_V1.1$ is poor in heterologous expression systems. The hypothesis has received support from observations that (i) arginine mutations engineered into S4 segments of other channels (e.g. *Shaker* K channel) result in gating pore currents, (ii) five of the six known HypoPP mutations in $Ca_V1.1$ are missense mutations of arginines in S4, with the outlier being a valine to glutamate in an adjacent S3 segment that in principle could support a gating pore current, and (iii) six of the nine arginine mutations in S4 of $Na_V1.4$ have been tested experimentally and all six produce gating pore currents; whereas an S4 arginine to cysteine in $Na_V1.4$ associated with PMC does not cause a gating pore current (50).

INWARD RECTIFIER POTASSIUM CHANNEL LOSS-OF-FUNCTION DEFECTS IN THE ANDERSEN−TAWIL SYNDROME AND THYROTOXIC PERIODIC PARALYSIS

Mutations of two different inward rectifier K channels, Kir2.1 encoded by *KCNJ2* (51) and Kir2.6 encoded by *JCNJ18* (52), have been associated with periodic paralysis. The Andersen−Tawil Syndrome (ATS) is a triad of potassium-sensitive periodic paralysis, cardiac arrhythmia, and developmental abnormalities (51,53). The episodes of periodic paralysis are often associated with hypokalemia, although normal or even elevated K^+ have been reported. Myotonia does not occur in ATS. The cardiac manifestations are pleomorphic, with rhythm disturbances being far more common that structural abnormalities. ATS patients may have a prolonged QT interval (LQT7), pronounced U-waves on the electrocardiogram, or ventricular ectopy. The developmental abnormalities are similarly varied and have included syndactyly or clinodactyly, cleft palate, small mandible, low-set ears, wide-set eyes (hypertelorism), and scoliosis. Inheritance of ATS is autosomal dominant, with highly variable penetrance such that members of the same family may express different phenotypic features of the syndrome. In Kir2.1 mutation carriers, the frequency of periodic paralysis is about 65%, cardiac arrhythmia occurs in 70%, and developmental anomalies are present in 80% (54). Mutations of Kir2.1 account for 60% of patients with ATS. Thyrotoxic periodic paralysis (TPP) is the most prevalent form of periodic paralysis and presents with abrupt attacks of weakness and hypokalemia in the setting of hyperthyroidism. Affected individuals invariably have elevated levels of thyroid hormones and suppressed thyroid stimulating hormone, but there may not be overt clinical features of hyperthyroidism. Episodes of TTP resolve upon treatment of hyperthyroidism. Most cases of TTP are sporadic, with a high prevalence in Asian and Hispanic males for whom ~4% of patients with hyperthyroidism will have TTP (55), whereas in non-Hispanic male Caucasians in North America the prevalence is about 0.1% (56). The frequency of TTP in females is one-tenth of that in males. The clinical presentation suggested a genetic predisposition that was unmasked in the setting of hyperthyroidism. Screening of candidate ion channel genes expressed in skeletal muscle, revealed a previously unknown gene, given the name *KCNJ18*, that coded for an inward rectifying K^+ channel and has an upstream thyroid response element (52). In the original cohort of 30 patients with TTP, one-third had mutations in *KCNJ18* that were predicted to have a variety of consequences for the gene produce Kir2.6, resulting in frame-shift with premature termination, missense, or nonsense mutations. Subsequently, over 30 Kir2.1 mutations associated with TTP have been reported (57).

Inward rectifier K^+ channels have a vital role as a major determinant in setting V_{rest} of skeletal muscle. Several members of the Kir2.x subfamily of strong inward rectifiers are expressed in skeletal muscle (Kir2.1, Kir2.2, Kir2.3, Kir2.6), as well as the ATP-sensitive weakly rectifying Kir6.2/SUR2A channel (58). Kir2.x channels are tetrameric, and can be formed by hetero- or homo-multimeric combinations of subunits. While this family of channels is so-named for the ability to pass inward K^+ current more readily than outward, it is the small outward current at voltages depolarized relative to the equilibrium potential for K^+ (E_K) that is important for regulating the resting potential. Most ATS-mutations cause a dominant-negative suppression of Kir2.1 function. Mutant Kir2.1 subunits co-assemble with wild-type subunits and traffic to the membrane, but fail to conduct current, often due to a disruption of activation by phosphatidylinositol 4,5-bisphosphate (PIP_2) signaling (59). In the initial report of Kir6.2 mutations in TTP, the frameshift mutant did not form functional channels, and oocyte expression for four of the other five mutants resulted in a 20–50% reduction in K_{IR} current density (52). Overall, the Kir2.x mutations associated with periodic paralysis will reduce the K_{IR} current through dominant-negative effects on both homotetrameric and heterotetrameric channels.

The proposed mechanism by which ATS–Kir2.1 and TTP–Kir2.6 mutations produce a susceptibility to attacks of paralysis involves the same balance of inward and outward currents that was described above for the pathogenesis of HypoPP. While a predisposition to familial HypoPP is caused by an anomalous inward gating pore current, for ATS and TTP the defect is a reduction in the outward K_{IR} current. The consequences are the same. In the setting of reduced extracellular $[K^+]$, the K_{IR} current is overwhelmed by the net inward current. Therefore a balance of currents is achieved only after the fiber depolarizes sufficiently to activate voltage-gated K_{DR} channels. From this aberrantly depolarized V_{rest} of ~−50 mV, Na^+ channels are inactivated and flaccid paralysis ensues.

REFERENCES

1. Engel AG, Ohno K, Sine SM. Neurological diseases: sleuthing molecular targets for neurological diseases at the neuromuscular junction. *Nat Rev Neurosci* 2003;**4**:339–52.
2. Cannon SC. Pathomechanisms in channelopathies of skeletal muscle and brain. *Annu Rev Neurosci* 2006;**29**:387–415.
3. Rüdel R, Lehmann-Horn F. Membrane changes in cells from myotonia patients. *Physiol Rev* 1985;**65**:310–56.
4. Rüdel R, Lehmann-Horn F, Ricker K, Kuther G. Hypokalemic periodic paralysis: in vitro investigation of muscle fiber membrane parameters. *Muscle Nerve* 1984;**7**:110–20.
5. Creutzfeldt OD, Abbott PC, Fowler WM, Pearson CM. Muscle membrane potentials in episodica adynamia. *Electroenceph Clin Neurophysiol* 1963;**15**:508–15.
6. Cannon SC. An expanding view for the molecular basis of familial periodic paralysis. *Neuromuscul Disord* 2002;**12**:533–43.
7. Lehmann-Horn F, Rüdel R, Jurkat-Rott K. Nondystrophic myotonias and periodic paralyses. In: Engel AG, Franzini-Armstrong C, editors. *Myology*. New York: McGraw-Hill;2004. p. 1257–300.
8. Palade PT, Barchi RL. Characteristics of the chloride conductance in muscle fibers of the rat diaphragm. *J Gen Physiol* 1977;**69**:325–42.
9. Lipicky RJ, Bryant SH. Sodium, potassium, and chloride fluxes in intercostal muscle from normal goats and goats with hereditary myotonia congenita. *J Gen Physiol* 1966;**50**:89–111.
10. Adrian RH, Bryant SH. On the repetitive discharge in myotonic muscle fibres. *J Physiol* 1974;**240**:505–15.
11. Lipicky RJ, Bryant SH, Salmon JH. Cable parameters, sodium, potassium, chloride, and water content, and potassium efflux in

isolated external intercostal muscle of normal volunteers and patients with myotonia congenita. *J Clin Invest* 1971;**50**:2091–103.

12. Jentsch TJ. CLC chloride channels and transporters: from genes to protein structure, pathology and physiology. *Crit Rev Biochem Mol Biol* 2008;**43**:3–36.
13. Pusch M. Myotonia caused by mutations in the muscle chloride channel gene CLCN1. *Hum Mutat* 2002;**19**:423–34.
14. Steinmeyer K, Ortland C, Jentsch TJ. Primary structure and functional expression of a developmentally regulated skeletal muscle chloride channel. *Nature* 1991;**354**:301–4.
15. Koch MC, Steinmeyer K, Lorenz C, Ricker K, Wolf F, Otto M, et al. The skeletal muscle chloride channel in dominant and recessive human myotonia. *Science* 1992;**257**:797–800.
16. Furman RE, Barchi RL. The pathophysiology of myotonia produced by aromatic carboxylic acids. *Ann Neurol* 1978;**4**:357–65.
17. Pusch M, Steinmeyer K, Koch MC, Jentsch TJ. Mutations in dominant human myotonia congenita drastically alter the voltage dependence of the CIC-1 chloride channel. *Neuron* 1995;**15**:1455–63.
18. De Luca A, Pierno S, Natuzzi F, Franchini C, Duranti A, Lentini G, et al. Evaluation of the antimyotonic activity of mexiletine and some new analogs on sodium currents of single muscle fibers and on the abnormal excitability of the myotonic ADR mouse. *J Pharmacol Exp Ther* 1997;**282**:93–100.
19. George Jr. AL, Komisarof J, Kallen RG, Barchi RL. Primary structure of the adult human skeletal muscle voltage-dependent sodium channel. *Ann Neurol* 1992;**31**:131–7.
20. Isom LL, De Jongh KS, Patton DE, Reber BF, Offord J, Charbonneau H, et al. Primary structure and functional expression of the beta 1 subunit of the rat brain sodium channel. *Science* 1992;**256**:839–42.
21. Lehmann-Horn F, Rüdel R, Dengler R, Lorkovic H, Haass A, Ricker K. Membrane defects in paramyotonia congenita with and without myotonia in a warm environment. *Muscle Nerve* 1981;**4**:396–406.
22. Lehmann-Horn F, Rüdel R, Ricker K, Lorkovic H, Dengler R, Hopf HC. Two cases of adynamia episodica hereditaria: in vitro investigation of muscle cell membrane and contraction parameters. *Muscle Nerve* 1983;**6**:113–21.
23. DeSilva SM, Kuncl RW, Griffin JW, Cornblath DR, Chavoustie S. Paramyotonia congenita or hyperkalemic periodic paralysis? Clinical and electrophysiological features of each entity in one family. *Muscle Nerve* 1990;**13**:21–6.
24. Fontaine B, Khurana TS, Hoffman EP, Bruns GA, Haines JL, Trofatter JA, et al. Hyperkalemic periodic paralysis and the adult muscle sodium channel alpha-subunit gene. *Science* 1990;**250**:1000–2.
25. Lehmann-Horn F, Jurkat-Rott K. Voltage-gated ion channels and hereditary disease. *Physiol Rev* 1999;**79**:1317–72.
26. Lerche H, Heine R, Pika U, George Jr. AL, Mitrovic N, Browatzki M, et al. Human sodium channel myotonia: slowed channel inactivation due to substitutions for a glycine within the III-IV linker. *J Physiol* 1993;**470**:13–22.
27. Ricker K, Lehmann-Horn F, Moxley RT. Myotonia fluctuans. *Arch Neurol* 1990;**47**:268–72.
28. Kubota T, Kinoshita M, Sasaki R, Aoike F, Takahashi MP, Sakoda S, et al. New mutation of the Na channel in the severe form of potassium-aggravated myotonia. *Muscle Nerve* 2009;**39**:666–73.
29. Cannon SC. Spectrum of sodium channel disturbances in the nondystrophic myotonias and periodic paralyses. *Kidney Int* 2000;**57**:772–9.
30. Cannon SC, Brown Jr. RH, Corey DP. A sodium channel defect in hyperkalemic periodic paralysis: potassium-induced failure of inactivation. *Neuron* 1991;**6**:619–26.
31. Cummins TR, Zhou J, Sigworth FJ, Ukomadu C, Stephan M, Ptacek LJ, et al. Functional consequences of a Na^+ channel mutation causing hyperkalemic periodic paralysis. *Neuron* 1993;**10**:667–78.
32. Cannon SC, Brown Jr. RH, Corey DP. Theoretical reconstruction of myotonia and paralysis caused by incomplete inactivation of sodium channels. *Biophys J* 1993;**65**:270–88.
33. Yang N, Ji S, Zhou M, Ptacek LJ, Barchi RL, Horn R, et al. Sodium channel mutations in paramyotonia congenita exhibit similar biophysical phenotypes in vitro. *Proc Natl Acad Sci USA* 1994;**91**:12785–9.
34. Cummins TR, Sigworth FJ. Impaired slow inactivation in mutant sodium channels. *Biophys J* 1996;**71**:227–36.
35. Hayward LJ, Sandoval GM, Cannon SC. Defective slow inactivation of sodium channels contributes to familial periodic paralysis. *Neurology* 1999;**52**:1447–53.
36. Tawil R, McDermott MP, Brown Jr. R, Shapiro BC, Ptacek LJ, McManis PG, et al. Randomized trials of dichlorphenamide in the periodic paralyses. Working group on periodic paralysis. *Ann Neurol* 2000;**47**:46–53.
37. Fontaine B, Vale-Santos J, Jurkat-Rott K, Reboul J, Plassart E, Rime CS, et al. Mapping of the hypokalaemic periodic paralysis (HypoPP) locus to chromosome 1q31-32 in three European families. *Nature Genet* 1994;**6**:267–72.
38. Ptacek LJ, Tawil R, Griggs RC, Engel AG, Layzer RB, Kwiecinski H, et al. Dihydropyridine receptor mutations cause hypokalemic periodic paralysis. *Cell* 1994;**77**:863–8.
39. Bulman DE, Scoggan KA, van Oene MD, Nicolle MW, Hahn AF, Tollar LL, et al. A novel sodium channel mutation in a family with hypokalemic periodic paralysis. *Neurology* 1999;**53**:1932–6.
40. Sternberg D, Maisonobe T, Jurkat-Rott K, Nicole S, Launay E, Chauveau D, et al. Hypokalaemic periodic paralysis type 2 caused by mutations at codon 672 in the muscle sodium channel gene SCN4A. *Brain* 2001;**124**:1091–9.
41. Matthews E, Labrum R, Sweeney MG, Sud R, Haworth A, Chinnery PF, et al. Voltage sensor charge loss accounts for most cases of hypokalemic periodic paralysis. *Neurology* 2009;**72**:1544–7.
42. Sokolov S, Scheuer T, Catterall WA. Gating pore current in an inherited ion channelopathy. *Nature* 2007;**446**:76–8.
43. Struyk AF, Cannon SC. A Na^+ channel mutation linked to hypokalemic periodic paralysis exposes a proton-selective gating pore. *J Gen Physiol* 2007;**130**:11–20.
44. Struyk AF, Markin VS, Francis D, Cannon SC. Gating pore currents in DIIS4 mutations of NaV1.4 associated with periodic paralysis: saturation of ion flux and implications for disease pathogenesis. *J Gen Physiol* 2008;**132**:447–64.
45. Struyk AF, Cannon SC. Paradoxical depolarization of Ba^{2+}- treated muscle exposed to low extracellular K^+: insights into resting potential abnormalities in hypokalemic paralysis. *Muscle Nerve* 2008;**37**:326–37.
46. Cannon SC. Voltage-sensor mutations in channelopathies of skeletal muscle. *J Physiol* 2010;**588**:1887–95.

47. Jurkat-Rott K, Weber MA, Fauler M, Guo XH, Holzherr BD, Paczulla A, et al. K^+-dependent paradoxical membrane depolarization and Na^+ overload, major and reversible contributors to weakness by ion channel leaks. *Proc Natl Acad Sci USA* 2009;**106**:4036–41.
48. Chang HK, Lee JR, Liu TA, Suen CS, Arreola J, Shieh RC. The extracellular K^+ concentration dependence of outward currents through Kir2.1 channels is regulated by extracellular Na^+ and Ca^{2+}. *J Biol Chem* 2010;**285**:23115–25.
49. Elbaz A, Vale-Santos J, Jurkatt-Rott K, Lapie P, Ophoff RA, Bady B, et al. Hypokalemic periodic paralysis and the dihydropyridine receptor (CACNL1A3): genotype/phenotype correlations for two predominant mutations and evidence for the absence of a founder effect in 16 caucasian families. *Am J Hum Genet* 1995;**56**:374–80.
50. Francis D, Rybalchenko V, Struyk AF, Cannon SC. Sodium channel voltage sensor mutations in periodic paralysis, but not paramyotonia, produce a gating pore leak. *Neurology* 2011;**76**:1635–41.
51. Plaster NM, Tawil R, Tristani-Firouzi M, Canun S, Bendahhou S, Tsunoda A, et al. Mutations in Kir2.1 cause the developmental and episodic electrical phenotypes of Andersen's syndrome. *Cell* 2001;**105**:511–9.
52. Ryan DP, da Silva MR, Soong TW, Fontaine B, Donaldson MR, Kung AW, et al. Mutations in potassium channel Kir2.6 cause susceptibility to thyrotoxic hypokalemic periodic paralysis. *Cell* 2010;**140**:88–98.
53. Sansone V, Griggs RC, Meola G, Ptacek LJ, Barohn R, Iannaccone S, et al. Andersen's syndrome: a distinct periodic paralysis. *Ann Neurol* 1997;**42**:305–12.
54. Tristani-Firouzi M, Jensen JL, Donaldson MR, Sansone V, Meola G, Hahn A, et al. Functional and clinical characterization of KCNJ2 mutations associated with LQT7 (Andersen syndrome). *J Clin Invest* 2002;**110**:381–8.
55. Shizume K, Shishiba Y, Kuma K, Noguchi S, Tajiri J, Ito K, et al. Comparison of the incidence of association of periodic paralysis and hyperthyroidism in Japan in 1957 and 1991. *Endocrinol Jpn* 1992;**39**:315–8.
56. Kelley DE, Gharib H, Kennedy FP, Duda Jr. RJ, McManis PG. Thyrotoxic periodic paralysis. Report of 10 cases and review of electromyographic findings. *Arch Intern Med* 1989;**149**:2597–600.
57. Tristani-Firouzi M, Etheridge SP. Kir 2.1 channelopathies: the Andersen–Tawil syndrome. *Pflugers Arch* 2010;**460**:289–94.
58. Nichols CG, Lopatin AN. Inward rectifier potassium channels. *Annu Rev Physiol* 1997;**59**:171–91.
59. Donaldson MR, Jensen JL, Tristani-Firouzi M, Tawil R, Bendahhou S, Suarez WA, et al. PIP2 binding residues of Kir2.1 are common targets of mutations causing Andersen syndrome. *Neurology* 2003;**60**:1811–6.

Chapter 74

Thick and Thin Filament Proteins: Acquired and Hereditary Sarcomeric Protein Diseases

Julien Ochala and Lars Larsson

Department of Neuroscience, Clinical Neurophysiology, Uppsala University, Uppsala, Sweden

INTRODUCTION

Skeletal muscle comprises approximately 40% of the human body mass and loss of muscle mass and function associated with either primary neuromuscular disorders or secondary to critical illness, cancer, renal disease, HIV, postoperative trauma, chronic heart failure, obstructive pulmonary disease, aging and microgravity have a significant negative impact on morbidity, mortality and/or quality of life. The contractile proteins are the dominating proteins in skeletal muscle and myosin is probably the most amplified gene in the human body, but it is not until recently contractile proteins have been associated with specific skeletal muscle diseases. The increased awareness and interest in this disease entity has been triggered by the discovery of a direct link between cardiomyopathy and mutations in the *MYH7* gene encoding the type I/β-slow myosin heavy chain (MyHC) isoform expressed in both the myocardium and in slow skeletal muscle fibers. Cardiomyopathy-associated *MYH7* mutations have subsequently been shown to be associated with an impaired function of the type I/β-slow myosin in skeletal muscle fibers, but overshadowed by symptoms related to the cardiomyopathy (1).

A large number of patients with skeletal muscle weakness still fail to receive correct diagnosis or are given a descriptive diagnosis based on symptoms, electrophysiological measurements and histopathological examination of muscle biopsy samples. However, electrophysiology does not distinguish between different types of myopathies and histopathology describes structural abnormalities that need not reflect underlying mechanisms. The development of specific and increasingly sophisticated genetic and molecular diagnostic tools together with structure-function analyses at the cellular and subcellular levels has given us an unprecedented opportunity for improved diagnosis and understanding of underlying mechanisms.

This short review will focus on (i) acquired diseases and physiological conditions affecting contractile protein expression, as well as (ii) inherited conditions where mutations in genes encoding thick and/or thin filament proteins exist and induce myopathies.

ALTERED MYOSIN AND ACTIN PROTEIN EXPRESSION

Acute Quadriplegic Myopathy

Most muscle wasting conditions are characterized by a general loss of contractile proteins, such as the muscle wasting associated with prolonged bed rest (2). However, there are pathological and physiological conditions resulting in a preferential loss of either thick or thin filament proteins. The preferential complete or partial loss of myosin and myosin-associated thick filament proteins and maintained expression of actin and other thin filament proteins have been considered pathognomonic of the acute quadriplegia in intensive care unit (ICU) patients (3–5) and a significantly decreased myosin actin ratio is presently the most sensitive diagnostic marker for this type of acquired myopathy in ICU patients (4–6). This common complication of modern intensive care affects primarily limb and trunk muscles, leaving craniofacial muscles spared or less affected, and patients typically have intact sensory and cognitive functions. This disorder was originally given the name acute quadriplegic myopathy (AQM), but a number of different descriptive names have been given this disorder since then, such as critical illness myopathy, thick filament myosin myopathy, acute myopathy of severe asthma, myopathy of intensive care etc. (7). AQM is a potentially lethal complication that prolongs the recovery of critical care patients, increasing the median ICU treatment costs three-fold (8,9).

Muscle. DOI: http://dx.doi.org/10.1016/B978-0-12-381510-1.00074-0

Additional substantial costs can accrue with the subsequent extended rehabilitation requirements and often years of drastically impaired quality of life after hospital discharge (10–12). For many years, the AQM diagnosis was lumped together with muscle paralyses of neurogenic origin, such as the critical illness polyneuropathy and Guillain–Barré syndrome due to misinterpretation of electrophysiolocal signals (7). Conventional electrophysiological techniques have too low specificity and histopathological analyses of muscle tissue have too low sensitivity in the diagnosis of ICU patients with AQM (4,13). However, correct distinction between myopathy and neuropathy in the ICU is very important because: (i) prognosis differs significantly between the acquired neuropathy and myopathy, and (ii) systemic CS administration may be beneficial in the treatment of acute neuropathies, but this treatment has the opposite effect in ICU patients with the acquired myopathy. Mechanical ventilation, neuromuscular blockade (NMB), muscle unloading, sepsis, circulating active factors and/or corticosteroids have been proposed as triggering factors. The severe and rapid muscle wasting in patients with AQM has been suggested to be associated with activation of different proteolytic pathways (14,15), but it is also secondary to a dramatic downregulation of myosin synthesis at the transcriptional level according to *in situ* hybridization, real-time PCR, and microarray analyses (4,6).

Our poor understanding of basic mechanisms underlying AQM in the clinical setting is in part due to that the basic distinctions between myopathy and neuropathy have often not been clearly made and the complex clinical, electrophysiological, and histological abnormalities are often incompletely reported. Diagnosis and classification have frequently been based on clinical observations, electrophysiological measurements and muscle biopsy histopathology, but all are weak diagnostic indicators. The study of generalized muscle weakness is further complicated by the co-existence of more than one factor underlying muscle paralysis in the ICU patients. Different primary diseases, large variability in pharmacological treatment, and collection of muscle samples several weeks after admission to the ICU and exposure to causative agents are other factors complicating mechanistic studies of AQM in the clinical setting. There is, accordingly, compelling need for experimental animal models mimicking the ICU condition. A number of different experimental models have been used, but many of them lack key components of the ICU intervention such as mechanical ventilation and immobilization for long durations (weeks). Many contractile proteins have a very slow turnover and experimental models allowing long-term exposure to the ICU condition are critical for our understanding of how intracellular signaling and gene regulation influence protein expression and muscle fiber function.

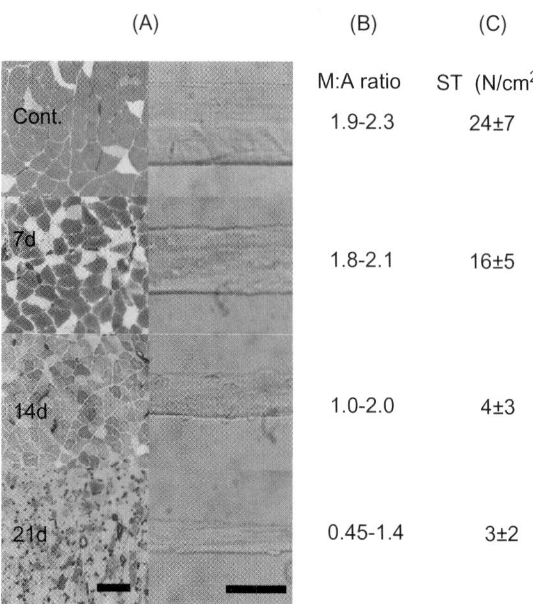

FIGURE 74.1 Enzyme-histochemically (mATPase) stained soleus cross-sections (horizontal bar = 200 μm) and single membrane permeabilized muscle fibers (horizontal bar = 100 μm) (A); myosin:actin (M:A) ratio (B); and specific tension (ST, maximum force normalized to cross-sectional area) at the single muscle fiber level (C) in the soleus muscle from control rats (Cont.) and rats exposed to the experimental ICU condition for 7, 14, and 21 days.

Dworkin and Dworkin (16) developed a unique experimental rat model to study blood pressure regulation where animals with NMB are mechanically ventilated and extensively monitored for very long durations (the longest duration to date is 93 days). This model offers a unique possibility to study the mechanisms underlying the loss of the motor protein myosin and myosin-associated proteins. Recent results using this model show that the downregulation of myosin synthesis at the transcriptional level and the enhanced degradation of contractile proteins parallels the complete mechanical silencing in ICU patients (Figure 74.1), i.e., the absence of weight-bearing and the lack of the internal strain that follows activation of contractile elements during muscle contraction (17). Detailed analyses of protein degradation pathways show that the ubiquitin proteasome pathway is highly involved in this process, i.e., the localization of MuRF1 and MuRF2 shows a sequential change in localization, with an initial relocalization from the sarcomere to the myonuclei in the first 4 days, and a later localization to the cytoplasm, where they co-localize with cytoplasmic SRF in the perinuclear space (17).

Cancer Cachexia

Although the preferential myosin loss has been forwarded to be a pathognomonic finding in ICU patients with

AQM, a series of other muscle wasting conditions have been shown to be associated with a preferential myosin loss such as cancer cachexia, chronic heart failure, chronic obstructive pulmonary disease and aging. More than 50% of patients with cancer suffer from cachexia and nearly a third of mortalities are estimated to result from cachexia rather than the tumor burden itself (18). Inflammatory cytokines such as tumor necrosis factor-alpha (TNF-α), interleukin(IL)-1β, IL-6, and interferon-γ have been associated with cancer cachexia, but none of these cytokines do alone induce cachexia, but in combination they promoted severe muscle wasting by selectively targeting myosin (19). *In vitro* experiments have shown that the combination of TNF-α and interferon-γ selectively and progressively deplete myosin both at the protein and mRNA level. A parallel decline in the expression of the MyoD nuclear transcription supports a significant role of transcriptional regulation of myosin synthesis in this type of muscle wasting (19). In the rodent cancer model, the myosin loss was not associated with a decrease in myosin mRNA levels, and the myosin loss was primarily related to an enhanced activation of the ubiquitin ligase-dependent proteasome pathway (19). Numerous cytokines, including TNF-α, IL-1, IL-6, and IL-8, are upregulated by the NF-κB transcriptional factor and Kawamura and co-workers have shown in experimental animal models that blocking NF-κB inhibits cancer cachexia, without affecting tumor growth (20,21). Further, a significant preferential loss of the motor protein myosin together with downregulation of protein synthesis at the transcriptional level has been reported in a patient developing rapid cachexia and paraplegia due to a lung cancer, and electromyography findings showed signs of a carcinomatous neuromyopathy in proximal and distal lower extremity muscles (22).

Other Conditions

The skeletal muscle weakness associated with both chronic heart failure and chronic obstructive pulmonary disease has been reported to be related to a decreased force generation capacity and a selective loss of myosin with no evidence for a generalized loss of myofibrillar proteins (23–25). A slight preferential loss of myosin also appears to be associated with the aging-related muscle wasting, i.e., sarcopenia, in rodents (26) and humans (27). Thus, a preferential loss of myosin has been reported in different muscle wasting conditions associated with increased morbidity and mortality, and a selective myosin loss cannot be regarded a pathognomonic finding of AQM. However, a severe to complete myosin loss has been observed in ICU patients with AQM and this preferential myosin loss exceeds (to our knowledge) the selective loss in any of the other conditions listed above.

Fitts and co-workers have reported a preferential loss of actin in human skeletal muscle in response to microgravity and prolonged space flight (28–30). There are accordingly muscle wasting conditions associated with selective myosin and actin loss, although most muscle atrophy models are characterized by a general myofibrillar protein loss. This indicates complex and coordinated signalling pathways regulating myofibrillar protein synthesis and degradation that are specific for different muscle wasting conditions, but our understanding of these signalling pathways remains incomplete.

HEREDITARY THICK AND THIN FILAMENT PROTEIN MYOPATHIES

Since the first discovery in 1990 (31), more than 300 different human mutations in 14 genes encoding thick and thin filament proteins have been identified and associated with skeletal muscle weakness and various disease phenotypes (Table 74.1), but the mechanisms underlying weakness remain unclear. Recent studies using multiple approaches from the single molecule to the whole-muscle level have given new important insights into these mechanisms. In this part of the chapter, we will highlight some of the results from these studies, and focus on the mechanisms by which mutations in genes encoding thick and thin filament proteins conduct to contractile dysfunction and skeletal muscle weakness.

Mutations in Genes Encoding Myosin and Related Proteins

Mutations in genes encoding isoforms expressed in adult muscles (*MYH2* and *MYH7*) are discussed, due to the lack of data concerning mutations in genes encoding isoforms present in the fetus, newborn, and child, such as *MYH8* and *MYH3* (perinatal and embryonic MyHCs, respectively). These defects are typically missense, modify one DNA nucleotide and induce the replacement of only one amino acid in various MyHC regions (32): in the actin-binding interface, near the nucleotide binding pocket, in the converter domain, close to the interface with the myosin light chain isoforms, or in the myosin rod. Unfortunately, only a few of these mutations have been functionally characterized.

Actin-Binding Interface

R403Q and R403W are the most studied defects (*MYH7* mutations). They induce skeletal muscle weakness as well as hypertrophic cardiomyopathy (Table 74.1). Because of their key location in the molecule, they tend to modify the kinetics of myosin head attachment to actin and the time spent in the strong binding state or duty ratio (33–35). Hence, R403Q and R403W alter the force-generating

TABLE 74.1 Diseases Associated with Mutations in Genes Encoding Thick and Thin Filament Proteins

Affected Gene	Affected Protein	Skeletal Muscle Weakness	Inherited Disease
MYH2	MyHC type IIa	Yes	Inclusion body myopathy
MYH3	Embryonic MyHC		Distal arthrogryposis syndrome
MYH7	MyHC type I	Yes	Laing early onset distal myopathy
		Yes	Hyaline body myopathy
		Yes	Myosin storage myopathy
		Yes	Distal myopathy
		Yes	Skeletal myopathy and hypertrophic cardiomyopathy
MYH8	Perinatal MyHC		Trismus and pseudocamtodactyly syndrome
			Distal arthrogryposis syndrome
MYBPC3	Myosin binding protein C	Yes	Skeletal myopathy and fatal cardiomyopathy
TNNI2	Fast troponin I		Distal arthrogryposis syndrome
TNNT1	Slow troponin T	Yes	Nemaline myopathy
TNNT3	Fast troponin T		Distal arthrogryposis syndrome
TPM2	Beta tropomyosin	Yes	Nemaline myopathy
		Yes	Cap disease
		Yes	Distal arthrogryposis syndrome
TPM3	Gamma tropomyosin	Yes	Nemaline myopathy
ACTA1	Skeletal alpha-actin	Yes	Nemaline myopathy
		Yes	Actin myopathy
		Yes	Congenital fiber type disproportion
		Yes	Rod–core myopathy
		Yes	Core myopathy
		Yes	Intranuclear rod myopathy
NEB	Nebulin	Yes	Nemaline myopathy
		Yes	Distal myopathy
		Yes	Core–rod myopathy
TTN	Titin	Yes	Hereditary myopathy with early respiratory failure
		Yes	Distal myopathy
			Limb-girdle muscular dystrophy

MyHC, myosin heavy chain.

capacity at the cell level (33,35,36). At the same time, they may change the rate of ATPase activity, leading to an inefficient ATP utilization and a higher energy cost to produce a given force. All together, these contractile dysfunctions, at the molecular and cellular levels, are thought to be primordial in the development of weakness and disease phenotype (36).

Nucleotide-Binding Pocket

R453C (other *MYH7* mutation) also conducts to skeletal muscle weakness and hypertrophic cardiomyopathy (Table 74.1). Unlike R403Q and R403W, R453C reduces the rate of ATPase activity (35,37,38). It also prolongs the duty ratio and increases the force production at the cell level (35,37). In R453C the motor activity is enhanced. This perturbs the balance of forces in the sarcomere and likely contributes to sarcomere disorganization, contractile dysregulation, and weakness (37).

Converter Domain

E706K, R719W, R723G, and F764L (*MYH7* and *MYH2* mutations) result in inclusion body myopathy or skeletal muscle weakness together with hypertrophic cardiomyopathy (Table 74.1). E706K and F764L disrupt myosin head detachment from actin by slowing down ATP hydrolysis (39). This increases the time spent in the strong binding state or duty ratio (39) and renders the sarcomere more susceptible to damages (35,40). In contrast, R719W and R723G do not modify ATP hydrolysis (41,42). Alternatively, they affect the elastic distortion of the converter region and probably the myosin head tilting process (41,42). At the cell level, this conducts to a stronger force-generating capacity (41,42). The unusual large forces on the sarcomere tend to facilitate disarray, contractile dysfunction, and weakness.

Myosin Rod

L908V, E1356K, R1500W, R1500P, L1793P, R1845W, E1886K, and H1901L (*MYH7* mutations) lead to a broad range of disease phenotypes (Table 74.1). Unlike the mutations described above, these particular substitutions alter myosin molecule formation and they destabilize the ability to form stable, functional bipolar thick filaments (43–45), preventing normal sarcomere genesis.

Apart from defects in *MYH2*, *MYH3*, *MYH7*, and *MYH8*, mutations in *MYBPC3* encoding for myosin binding protein C also exist but the characterization of the impairments at the molecular and cellular levels remain to be studied.

Mutations in Genes Encoding Thin Filament Proteins

The first mutation was identified in 1995 (46). Since then, many others have been discovered in *TNNI2*, *TNNT1*, *TNNT3*, *TPM2*, *TPM3*, *ACTA1*, and *NEB* (encoding for troponin I, troponin T isoforms, tropomyosin isoforms, actin and nebulin, respectively). However, links between most of these mutations and skeletal muscle weakness are still unknown and require further investigations. For this reason, here, we focus on the few existing studies on defects affecting *ACTA1*, *TPM2*, *TPM3*, and *NEB*.

Actin

More than 170 mutations in *ACTA1* causing disease phenotypes have been detected (Table 74.1). Some mutations are nonsense leading to a complete deficiency of skeletal actin and premature death within the first two years of life (47). Others are missense, as for *MYH2* and *MYH7*, and result in single amino acid changes in various actin regions. Unfortunately, to date, no direct correlations can be made between gene mutations, location of the amino acid replacements, functional alterations and weakness (48). In fact, M132V, D286G, and K336E tend to facilitate the strong binding of myosin heads to actin (48,49). Others, including D292V and P332S, located in similar regions, have no detectable contractile effects (48,50). Consequently, much remains to be done to decipher the mechanisms by which these mutations result in contractile dysfunction and skeletal muscle weakness.

Tropomyosin

Mutations in *TPM2* and *TPM3* encoding tropomyosin isoforms (β and γ, respectively) are usually missense and also result in the substitution of single amino acids along the protein. R133W leads to skeletal muscle weakness and distal arthrogryposis (Table 74.1). It lies in the mid-region of the tropomyosin molecule (51) and locally changes the stability of the coiled-coil dimer (52,53). As a consequence, tropomyosin movement over the thin filament is impaired. This changes the kinetics of myosin head attachment and detachment to/from actin, limiting the strong binding and duty ratio (54,55). At the cell level, this decreases the force-generating capacity and contributes to the development of weakness (55). R91P, R168H, and E241K are thought to behave similarly (56). Nevertheless, when replacements of amino acids occur at the N-terminus of the tropomyosin molecule, the functional deficits are significantly different. M9R and E41K associated with skeletal muscle weakness and nemaline myopathy (Table 74.1) do not induce the above cascade of events but rather deregulate the propagation of the calcium signal through the thin filament proteins (57,58). As M9R and E41K are located in a region close to the troponin complex binding, the information "relay" from troponin, the calcium sensor, to the myosin heads–actin interactions is likely to be disrupted. At the cell level, more calcium is needed to produce normal forces, resulting in an increased energy consumption and altered motor performance (58).

Nebulin

A large number of mutations in *NEB* have been reported (59,60). Among them, deletion of exon 55 is the most common and is related to a partial deficiency of nebulin as well as a reduction in thin filament length (61). This is not totally surprising considering that nebulin plays various important structural roles, notably stabilizing the thin filament (62,63). The shorter thin filament length does not allow a full overlap between thin and thick filaments and subsequently decreases the number of potential myosin heads strongly binding to actin (61). Hence, this alters the force-generating capacity at the cell level and leads to muscle weakness (61). Other *NEB* mutations also conduct to partial deficiencies of nebulin and weakness but are not always associated with decreases in thin filament length (64). Consequently, other molecular events may occur. For instance, skipping of exons 3 and 22 induces a dramatic decrease in the cycling rate of myosin heads attaching to actin and lowers the time spent in the strong binding state or duty ratio (64). Interestingly, at the same time, tropomyosin movement over the thin filament is partially limited, further preventing additional binding of myosin heads (64). At the cell level, as for the exon 55 deletion, this reduces the force-generating capacity (64).

Titin

In addition to mutations in *MYH2*, *MYH3*, *MYH7*, *MYH8*, *MYBPC3*, *TNNI2*, *TNNT1*, *TNNT3*, *TPM2*, *TPM3*, *ACTA1*, and *NEB*, a series of different mutations of the gene encoding the giant protein titin (*TTN*) have been reported in the past 15 years (65). Titin is not considered a thick or thin filament protein and is often referred to as the "third filament" spanning the entire length of the sarcomere from the Z-disc to the M-band (66). A number of mutations spanning from the Z-disc to the A-band region of the titin molecule have been reported to cause different cardiomyopathies. Interestingly, most titin mutations causing cardiomyopathies have no effect on skeletal muscle structure and function, and skeletal muscle titin mutations are not associated with heart failure (67). Heterozygous carriers of C-terminal region skeletal muscle titin mutations, i.e., in the M-band region, develop a late onset distal myopathy known as Udd's myopathy. Homozygous carriers, on the other hand, develop a severe early onset limb-girdle muscular dystrophy (LGMD2). Mutations in the titin kinase domain in another part of the C-terminal region are associated with complex phenotypes. Titin kinase interacts with a complex of different mechanosensitive proteins and is involved in regulation of muscle protein turnover (68). The R279W mutation in the titin kinase domain, originally described by Edström in 1990, leads to a hereditary myopathy with proximal upper and lower limb muscle weakness and early respiratory failure. The mutation disrupts the mechanosensing complex affecting muscle protein turnover and resulting in atrophy and weakness (68).

ACKNOWLEDGMENTS

We are grateful for the funding support from the Swedish Research Council, Association Française contre les Myopathies, Tore Nilson Stiftelse, Stiftelsen Apotekare Hedbergs fond för Medicinsk forskning, Rektors resebidrag från Wallenbergstiftelsen to J.O. and the Swedish Research Council (8651), the European Commission (MyoAge, EC Fp7 CT-223756 and COST CM1001), and King Gustaf V and Queen Victoria's Foundation to L.L.

REFERENCES

1. Cuda G, Fananapazir L, Zhu WS, Sellers JR, Epstein ND. Skeletal muscle expression and abnormal function of beta-myosin in hypertrophic cardiomyopathy. *J Clin Invest* 1993;**91**:2861–5.
2. Larsson L, Li X, Berg HE, Frontera WR. Effects of removal of weight-bearing function on contractility and myosin isoform composition in single human skeletal muscle cells. *Pflugers Arch* 1996;**432**:320–8.
3. Matsumoto N, Nakamura T, Yasui Y, Torii J. Analysis of muscle proteins in acute quadriplegic myopathy. *Muscle Nerve* 2000;**23**:1270–6.
4. Larsson L, Li X, Edstrom L, Eriksson LI, Zackrisson H, Argentini C, et al. Acute quadriplegia and loss of muscle myosin in patients treated with nondepolarizing neuromuscular blocking agents and corticosteroids: mechanisms at the cellular and molecular levels [see comments]. *Crit Care Med* 2000;**28**:34–45.
5. Stibler H, Edstrom L, Ahlbeck K, Remahl S, Ansved T. Electrophoretic determination of the myosin/actin ratio in the diagnosis of critical illness myopathy. *Intensive Care Med* 2003;**29**:1515–27.
6. Norman H, Zackrisson H, Hedstrom Y, Andersson P, Nordquist J, Eriksson LI, et al. Myofibrillar protein and gene expression in acute quadriplegic myopathy. *J Neurol Sci* 2009;**285**:28–38.
7. Larsson L. Acute quadriplegic myopathy: an acquired 'myosinopathy'. *Adv Exp Med Biol* 2008;**642**:92–8.
8. Rudis MI, Guslits BJ, Peterson EL, Hathaway SJ, Angus E, Beis S, et al. Economic impact of prolonged motor weakness complicating neuromuscular blockade in the intensive care unit. *Crit Care Med* 1996;**24**:1749–56.
9. Seneff MG, Wagner D, Thompson D, Honeycutt C, Silver MR. The impact of long-term acute-care facilities on the outcome and cost of care for patients undergoing prolonged mechanical ventilation. *Crit Care Med* 2000;**28**:342–50.
10. Cheung AM, Tansey CM, Tomlinson G, Diaz-Granados N, Matte A, Barr A, et al. Two-year outcomes, health care use and costs in survivors of ARDS. *Am J Respir Crit Care Med* 2006;**174**:538–44.
11. Herridge MS, Cheung AM, Tansey CM, Matte-Martyn A, Diaz-Granados N, Al-Saidi F, et al. One-year outcomes in survivors of the acute respiratory distress syndrome. *N Engl J Med* 2003;**348**:683–93.
12. van Mook WN, Hulsewe-Evers RP. Critical illness polyneuropathy. *Curr Opin Crit Care.* 2002;**8**:302–10.
13. Larsson L, Roland A. [Drug induced tetraparesis and loss of myosin. Mild types are probably overlooked]. *Lakartidningen* 1996;**93**:2249–54.
14. Di Giovanni S, Molon A, Broccolini A, Melcon G, Mirabella M, Hoffman EP, et al. Constitutive activation of MAPK cascade in acute quadriplegic myopathy. *Ann Neurol* 2004;**55**:195–206.
15. Lacomis D, Zochodne DW, Bird SJ. Critical illness myopathy. *Muscle Nerve* 2000;**23**:1785–8.

16. Dworkin BR, Dworkin S. Learning of physiological responses: I. Habituation, sensitization, and classical conditioning. *Behav Neurosci* 1990;**104**:298–319.
17. Ochala J, Gustafson AM, Diez ML, Renaud G, Li M, Aare S, et al. Preferential skeletal muscle myosin loss in response to mechanical silencing in a novel rat intensive care unit model: underlying mechanisms. *J Physiol* 2011;**589**:2007–26.
18. van Eys J. Nutrition and cancer: physiological interrelationships. *Annu Rev Nutr* 1985;**5**:435–61.
19. Acharyya S, Ladner KJ, Nelsen LL, Damrauer J, Reiser PJ, Swoap S, et al. Cancer cachexia is regulated by selective targeting of skeletal muscle gene products. *J Clin Invest* 2004;**114**:370–8.
20. Kawamura I, Morishita R, Tomita N, Lacey E, Aketa M, Tsujimoto S, et al. Intratumoral injection of oligonucleotides to the NF kappa B binding site inhibits cachexia in a mouse tumor model. *Gene Ther* 1999;**6**:91–7.
21. Kawamura I, Morishita R, Tsujimoto S, Manda T, Tomoi M, Tomita N, et al. Intravenous injection of oligodeoxynucleotides to the NF-kappaB binding site inhibits hepatic metastasis of M5076 reticulosarcoma in mice. *Gene Ther* 2001;**8**:905–12.
22. Banduseela V, Ochala J, Lamberg K, Kalimo H, Larsson L. Muscle paralysis and myosin loss in a patient with cancer cachexia. *Acta Myol* 2007;**26**:136–44.
23. Miller MS, Vanburen P, Lewinter MM, Lecker SH, Selby DE, Palmer BM, et al. Mechanisms underlying skeletal muscle weakness in human heart failure: alterations in single fiber myosin protein content and function. *Circ Heart Fail* 2009;**2**:700–6.
24. Ottenheijm CA, Heunks LM, Dekhuijzen PN. Diaphragm muscle fiber dysfunction in chronic obstructive pulmonary disease: toward a pathophysiological concept. *Am J Respir Crit Care Med* 2007;**175**:1233–40.
25. van Hees HW, van der Heijden HF, Ottenheijm CA, Heunks LM, Pigmans CJ, Verheugt FW, et al. Diaphragm single-fiber weakness and loss of myosin in congestive heart failure rats. *Am J Physiol Heart Circ Physiol* 2007;**293**:H819–28.
26. Thompson LV, Durand D, Fugere NA, Ferrington DA. Myosin and actin expression and oxidation in aging muscle. *J Appl Physiol* 2006;**101**:1581–7.
27. Cristea A, Vaillancourt DE, Larsson L. Aging-related changes in motor unit structure and function. In: Lynch G, editor. *Sarcopenia – age-related muscle wasting and weakness: mechanisms and treatments.* Dordrecht: Springer Science + Business Media;2010. p. 55–74.
28. Fitts RH, Riley DR, Widrick JJ. Physiology of a microgravity environment invited review: microgravity and skeletal muscle. *J Appl Physiol* 2000;**89**:823–39.
29. Fitts RH, Riley DR, Widrick JJ. Functional and structural adaptations of skeletal muscle to microgravity. *J Exp Biol* 2001;**204**:3201–8.
30. Riley DA, Bain JL, Thompson JL, Fitts RH, Widrick JJ, Trappe SW, et al. Decreased thin filament density and length in human atrophic soleus muscle fibers after spaceflight. *J Appl Physiol* 2000;**88**:567–72.
31. Geisterfer-Lowrance AA, Kass S, Tanigawa G, Vosberg HP, McKenna W, Seidman CE, et al. A molecular basis for familial hypertrophic cardiomyopathy: a beta cardiac myosin heavy chain gene missense mutation. *Cell* 1990;**62**:999–1006.
32. Rayment I, Holden HM, Sellers JR, Fananapazir L, Epstein ND. Structural interpretation of the mutations in the beta-cardiac myosin that have been implicated in familial hypertrophic cardiomyopathy. *Proc Natl Acad Sci USA* 1995;**92**:3864–8.
33. Keller DI, Coirault C, Rau T, Cheav T, Weyand M, Amann K, et al. Human homozygous R403W mutant cardiac myosin presents disproportionate enhancement of mechanical and enzymatic properties. *J Mol Cell Cardiol* 2004;**36**:355–62.
34. Palmiter KA, Tyska MJ, Haeberle JR, Alpert NR, Fananapazir L, Warshaw DM. R403Q and L908V mutant beta-cardiac myosin from patients with familial hypertrophic cardiomyopathy exhibit enhanced mechanical performance at the single molecule level. *J Muscle Res Cell Motil* 2000;**21**:609–20.
35. Debold EP, Schmitt JP, Patlak JB, Beck SE, Moore JR, Seidman JG, et al. Hypertrophic and dilated cardiomyopathy mutations differentially affect the molecular force generation of mouse alpha-cardiac myosin in the laser trap assay. *Am J Physiol Heart Circ Physiol* 2007;**293**:H284–91.
36. Belus A, Piroddi N, Scellini B, Tesi C, Amati GD, Girolami F, et al. The familial hypertrophic cardiomyopathy-associated myosin mutation R403Q accelerates tension generation and relaxation of human cardiac myofibrils. *J Physiol* 2008;**586**:3639–44.
37. Wang Q, Moncman CL, Winkelmann DA. Mutations in the motor domain modulate myosin activity and myofibril organization. *J Cell Sci* 2003;**116**:4227–38.
38. Palmer BM, Fishbaugher DE, Schmitt JP, Wang Y, Alpert NR, Seidman CE, et al. Differential cross-bridge kinetics of FHC myosin mutations R403Q and R453C in heterozygous mouse myocardium. *Am J Physiol Heart Circ Physiol* 2004;**287**:H91–9.
39. Zeng W, Conibear PB, Dickens JL, Cowie RA, Wakelin S, Malnasi-Csizmadia A, et al. Dynamics of actomyosin interactions in relation to the cross-bridge cycle. *Philos Trans R Soc Lond B Biol Sci* 2004;**359**:1843–55.
40. Li M, Lionikas A, Yu F, Tajsharghi H, Oldfors A, Larsson L. Muscle cell and motor protein function in patients with a IIa myosin missense mutation (Glu-706 to Lys). *Neuromuscul Disord* 2006;**16**:782–91.
41. Seebohm B, Matinmehr F, Kohler J, Francino A, Navarro-Lopez F, Perrot A, et al. Cardiomyopathy mutations reveal variable region of myosin converter as major element of cross-bridge compliance. *Biophys J* 2009;**97**:806–24.
42. Kohler J, Winkler G, Schulte I, Scholz T, McKenna W, Brenner B, et al. Mutation of the myosin converter domain alters cross-bridge elasticity. *Proc Natl Acad Sci USA* 2002;**99**:3557–62.
43. Armel TZ, Leinwand LA. A mutation in the beta-myosin rod associated with hypertrophic cardiomyopathy has an unexpected molecular phenotype. *Biochem Biophys Res Commun* 2010;**391**:352–6.
44. Armel TZ, Leinwand LA. Mutations at the same amino acid in myosin that cause either skeletal or cardiac myopathy have distinct molecular phenotypes. *J Mol Cell Cardiol* 2010;**48**:1007–13.
45. Armel TZ, Leinwand LA. Mutations in the beta-myosin rod cause myosin storage myopathy via multiple mechanisms. *Proc Natl Acad Sci USA* 2009;**106**:6291–6.
46. Laing NG, Wilton SD, Akkari PA, Dorosz S, Boundy K, Kneebone C, et al. A mutation in the alpha tropomyosin gene TPM3 associated with autosomal dominant nemaline myopathy NEM1. *Nat Genet* 1995;**10**:249.
47. Laing NG, Dye DE, Wallgren-Pettersson C, Richard G, Monnier N, Lillis S, et al. Mutations and polymorphisms of the skeletal muscle alpha-actin gene (ACTA1). *Hum Mutat* 2009;**30**:1267–77.

48. Feng JJ, Marston S. Genotype-phenotype correlations in ACTA1 mutations that cause congenital myopathies. *Neuromuscul Disord* 2009;**19**:6–16.
49. Marston S, Mirza M, Abdulrazzak H, Sewry C. Functional characterisation of a mutant actin (Met132Val) from a patient with nemaline myopathy. *Neuromuscul Disord* 2004;**14**:167–74.
50. Clarke NF, Ilkovski B, Cooper S, Valova VA, Robinson PJ, Nonaka I, et al. The pathogenesis of ACTA1-related congenital fiber type disproportion. *Ann Neurol* 2007;**61**:552–61.
51. Tajsharghi H, Kimber E, Holmgren D, Tulinius M, Oldfors A. Distal arthrogryposis and muscle weakness associated with a beta-tropomyosin mutation. *Neurology* 2007;**68**:772–5.
52. Moraczewska J, Greenfield NJ, Liu Y, Hitchcock-DeGregori SE. Alteration of tropomyosin function and folding by a nemaline myopathy-causing mutation. *Biophys J* 2000;**79**:3217–25.
53. Robinson P, Lipscomb S, Preston LC, Altin E, Watkins H, Ashley CC, et al. Mutations in fast skeletal troponin I, troponin T, and beta-tropomyosin that cause distal arthrogryposis all increase contractile function. *FASEB J* 2007;**21**:896–905.
54. Ochala J, Iwamoto H, Larsson L, Yagi N. A myopathy-linked tropomyosin mutation severely alters thin filament conformational changes during activation. *Proc Natl Acad Sci USA* 2010;**107**:9807–12.
55. Ochala J, Li M, Tajsharghi H, Kimber E, Tulinius M, Oldfors A, et al. Effects of a R133W beta-tropomyosin mutation on regulation of muscle contraction in single human muscle fibres. *J Physiol* 2007;**581**:1283–92.
56. Ottenheijm CA, Lawlor MW, Stienen GJ, Granzier H, Beggs AH. Changes in cross-bridge cycling underlie muscle weakness in patients with tropomyosin 3-based myopathy. *Hum Mol Genet* 2011;**20**:2015–25.
57. Michele DE, Albayya FP, Metzger JM. A nemaline myopathy mutation in alpha-tropomyosin causes defective regulation of striated muscle force production. *J Clin Invest* 1999;**104**:1575–81.
58. Ochala J, Li M, Ohlsson M, Oldfors A, Larsson L. Defective regulation of contractile function in muscle fibres carrying an E41K beta-tropomyosin mutation. *J Physiol* 2008;**586**:2993–3004.
59. Pelin K, Hilpela P, Donner K, Sewry C, Akkari PA, Wilton SD, et al. Mutations in the nebulin gene associated with autosomal recessive nemaline myopathy. *Proc Natl Acad Sci USA* 1999;**96**:2305–10.
60. Lehtokari VL, Pelin K, Sandbacka M, Ranta S, Donner K, Muntoni F, et al. Identification of 45 novel mutations in the nebulin gene associated with autosomal recessive nemaline myopathy. *Hum Mutat* 2006;**27**:946–56.
61. Ottenheijm CA, Witt CC, Stienen GJ, Labeit S, Beggs AH, Granzier H. Thin filament length dysregulation contributes to muscle weakness in nemaline myopathy patients with nebulin deficiency. *Hum Mol Genet* 2009;**18**:2359–69.
62. Castillo A, Nowak R, Littlefield KP, Fowler VM, Littlefield RS. A nebulin ruler does not dictate thin filament lengths. *Biophys J* 2009;**96**:1856–65.
63. Pappas CT, Krieg PA, Gregorio CC. Nebulin regulates actin filament lengths by a stabilization mechanism. *J Cell Biol* 2010;**189**:859–70.
64. Ochala J, Lehtokari VL, Iwamoto H, Li M, Feng HZ, Jin JP, et al. Disrupted myosin cross-bridge cycling kinetics triggers muscle weakness in nebulin-related myopathy. *FASEB J* 2011;**25**:1903–13.
65. Ottenheijm CA, Granzier H. Role of titin in skeletal muscle function and disease. *Adv Exp Med Biol* 2010;**682**:105–22.
66. Labeit S, Kolmerer B, Linke WA. The giant protein titin. Emerging roles in physiology and pathophysiology. *Circ Res* 1997;**80**:290–4.
67. Udd B. Third filament diseases. In: Laing NG, editor. *The sarcomere and skeletal muscle disease*. Austin, TX: Landes Bioscience;2008. p. 99–115.
68. Lange S, Xiang F, Yakovenko A, Vihola A, Hackman P, Rostkova E, et al. The kinase domain of titin controls muscle gene expression and protein turnover. *Science* 2005;**308**:1599–603.

Metabolic and Mitochondrial Myopathies

Ronald G. Haller[1] and Salvatore DiMauro[2]

[1]Department of Neurology, University of Texas Southwestern Medical Center and North Texas VA Medical Center, and Neuromuscular Center, Institute for Exercise and Environmental Medicine, Texas Health Presbyterian Hospital, Dallas, TX, [2]H. Houston Merritt Clinical Research Center for Muscular Dystrophy and Related Diseases, Columbia University Medical Center, New York, NY

MUSCLE FAT METABOLISM AND DISORDERS (FIGURE 75.1)

Fatty Acid Defects Causing Recurrent Myalgia, Rhabdomyolysis and Myoglobinuria

Carnitine Palmitoyltransferase (CPT) 2 Deficiency

The adult or myopathic form of CPT2 deficiency is the most common fatty acid oxidation defect affecting skeletal muscle and the most common metabolic cause of recurrent rhabdomyolysis and myoglobinuria (1). Attacks typically are triggered by prolonged submaximal exercise, especially when activity is undertaken while fasting (2). As exercise is sustained, patients experience aching in active muscles that worsens and becomes widespread. In sharp contrast to individuals with muscle glycolytic disorders, these patients easily tolerate brief maximal exercise. The vulnerability of skeletal muscle to exercise-induced injury in adult CPT2 deficiency may be explained by the presence of 15–20% residual enzyme activity, which is sufficient to support fat oxidation at rest but does not allow the increase in fat oxidation needed to supply muscle energy during exercise (3). An infantile form is due to mutations in CPT2 that result in more severe enzyme deficiency and cause recurrent liver failure, hypoketotic hypoglycemia, encephalopathy, and sudden death. The diagnosis of CPT2 deficiency is supported by one or more of the following laboratory changes: increased long chain (C-18, 18:1, 16) acylcarnitines in blood after an overnight fast or in fibroblasts incubated with long chain fatty acids; decreased CPT2 enzyme activity in fibroblasts, lymphocytes or skeletal muscle; or the identification of pathogenic mutations. More than 30 pathogenic mutations have been identified, but the Ser113Leu missense mutation accounts for more than 60% of mutant alleles in Europe and North America (4). The focus of treatment involves optimizing alternative fuel availability by providing sufficient carbohydrate in the diet and carbohydrate-rich snacks between meals when patients are physically active. Medium chain triglycerides (MCT) as sources of medium chain fatty acids, which diffuse into mitochondria independently of the carnitine/CPT system, may also increase fuel availability (4). Another approach to therapy is to increase mitochondrial biogenesis to augment net enzymatic capacity. Bezafibrate, a peroxisome proliferator-activated receptor (PPAR) agonist, has been shown to increase enzymatic activity and ameliorate symptoms in patients with adult CPT2 deficiency (5).

Other Fatty Acid Oxidation Defects Causing Recurrent Rhabdomyolysis

Very Long chain Acyl-CoA Dehydrogenase (VLCAD) Deficiency

Null mutations in very long chain acyl Co-A dehydrogenase (VLCAD) cause severe, often fatal multisystem disease in infancy whereas missense mutations that maintain some residual enzyme activity cause recurrent rhabdomyolysis and myoglobinuria that mimics adult CPT2 deficiency. The diagnosis is reached by tandem mass spectroscopy-detection of long chain acylcarnitines (especially C14:1) in blood or in fibroblasts incubated with long chain acylcarnitine (6). There are diverse pathogenic mutations and treatment is based on a high carbohydrate, low fat diet, and/or MCT supplements. The benefit of increasing mitochondrial mass utilizing bezafibrate may also apply to VLCAD deficiency (7).

Trifunctional Protein (TP)/Long Chain 3-hydroxy-acyl-CoA Dehydrogenase (LCHAD) Deficiency

As the name implies, TP encompasses three enzyme reactions, enoyl-CoA hydratase, LCHAD, and acyl thiolase,

Muscle. DOI: http://dx.doi.org/10.1016/B978-0-12-381510-1.00075-2

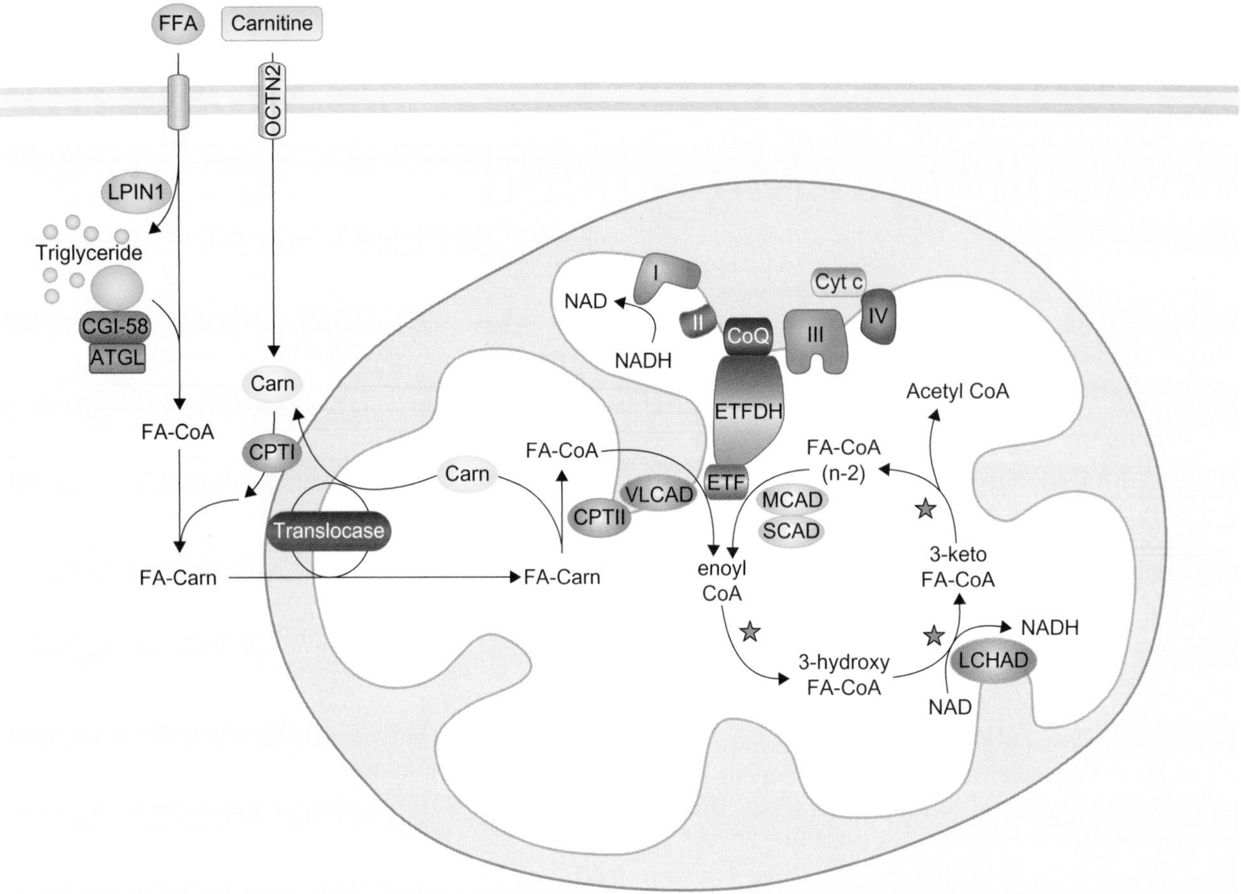

FIGURE 75.1 Overview of fat utilization in skeletal muscle indicating sites of genetic defects that impair fat metabolism. OCTN2 = carnitine transporter; FFA = free fatty acid; LPIN1 = protein involved in triglyceride synthesis; ATGL = adipose triglyceride lipase; GCI-58 = protein involved in activation of ATGL; Carn = carnitine; CPTI = carnitine palmitoyl transferase 1; Translocase = the carnitine, fatty acylCo-A transferase; CPTII = carnitine palmitoyl transferase 2; VLCAD = very long chain acyl Co-A dehydrogenase; MCAD and SCAD = medium and short chain acylCo-A dehydrogenase; ETF = electron transfer flavoprotein (receives electrons from the dehydrogenase reaction catalyzed by VLCAD, MCAD and SCAD); ETFDH = electron transfer flavoprotein dehydrogenase (receives electrons from ETF, transfers them to coenzyme Q10 for oxidation via respiratory chain complexes III and IV); enolyl CoA, 3-hydroxy FA-CoA, 3 keto FA-CoA are intermediates in beta oxidation ultimately yielding acetyl-CoA (for oxidation by the TCA cycle and a fatty acylCoA (FA-CoA) shortened by two carbons for further beta oxidation. LCHAD = long chain hydroxy-acylCo-A dehydrogenase, one of the three enzymatic reactions (indicated by stars) catalyzed by mitochondrial trifunctional protein. NADH produced in the reaction catalyzed by LCHAD is oxidized via complex I of the respiratory chain.

and yields acetyl-CoA and an acyl-CoA shortened by two carbons, which becomes the substrate of a new β-oxidation cycle. TP mutations affecting all enzyme activities or predominantly LCHAD produce severe, infantile or adult forms. In the adult forms, recurrent rhabdomyolysis triggered by exercise, fasting or infections is a leading symptom, often associated with respiratory failure. In contrast to adult CPT2 and VLCAD deficiencies, affected patients also have an axonal sensorimotor peripheral neuropathy and, often, pigmentary retinopathy. Most patients have mutations in the LCHAD domain of trifunctional protein and the Glu510Gln missense mutation accounts for nearly 90% mutant alleles in the adult form of the disease (4).

While exercise, especially exercise undertaken while fasting, is the most common trigger of rhabdomyolysis in CPT2, VLCAD, and TP/LCHAD deficiencies, infection/fever or fasting alone are also important causes of muscle injury in these FAO defects. Recently mutations in LPIN-1, a protein highly expressed in skeletal muscle and adipose tissue, have been implicated as a common cause of fever/fasting-induced rhabdomyolysis in childhood (8). LPIN-1 is important for normal lipid metabolism since it acts both as a phosphatidate phosphatase, converting phosphatidic acid to diacylglycerol during triglyceride and phospholipid biosynthesis, and as a regulator of fatty acid oxidation and mitochondrial biogenesis through an association with PPAR activators/coactivators.

Fatty Acid Defects Causing Muscle Weakness and Lipid Accumulation

Excess deposition of lipid in skeletal muscle is not characteristic of CPT2, VLCAD, or TP/LCHAD disorders and, between episodes of muscle injury, patients have normal muscle strength. In contrast, some disorders of muscle lipid metabolism typically produce a "lipid storage myopathy" with muscle weakness and increased numbers and size of lipid droplets within muscle fibers. These include primary carnitine deficiency, neutral lipid storage disease (NLSD), and multiple acyl CoA dehydrogenase deficiency.

Primary Carnitine Deficiency

Primary carnitine deficiency is due to mutations in the gene encoding the high affinity, sodium-dependent plasma membrane carnitine transporter OCTN2, causing impaired muscle carnitine transport across the plasma membrane of cells and impaired reabsorption of filtered carnitine by the kidney (9). Affected patients develop generalized muscle weakness and often cardiomyopathy along with massive lipid accumulation in skeletal muscle, heart and liver (10). Diagnosis is suggested by severe deficiency ($<10\%$ of normal) of free carnitine and acylcarnitines in plasma, muscle and other tissues, and may be confirmed by impaired carnitine uptake in patient lymphocytes or fibroblasts (4). Timely supplementation of L-carnitine usually reverses symptoms (1).

Neutral Lipid Storage Disease (NLSD)

Neutral lipid storage disease (NLSD) is due to mutations in neutral lipases necessary for the liberation of fatty acids from TG stores in skeletal muscle, adipocytes, and other tissues. Adipocyte triglyceride lipase (ATGL), activated by the protein CGI-58, catalyzes the first step in triglyceride hydrolysis. Mutations in the gene encoding CGI-58 (ABHD5) cause NLSD with icthyosis (NLSDI) or Chanarin–Dorfman syndrome (10). Patients typically have mild weakness associated with marked lipid accumulation in skeletal muscle and other tissues in conjunction with the characteristic dermatological feature of icthyosis (11). A signal laboratory feature is the accumulation of lipid droplets within leukocytes termed Jordan's anomaly.

NLSD with myopathy (NLSDM) is caused by mutations in the gene encoding ATGL (PNPLA2) (12). Affected patients develop muscle weakness usually in the second or third decade, sometimes associated with dilated cardiomyopathy. Jordan's anomaly and massive lipid accumulation in skeletal muscle, heart and, to a lesser extent, liver may precede overt symptoms of muscle weakness or cardiac disease (13).

Multiple Acyl CoA Dehydrogenase Deficiency (MADD)

MADD is due to mutations in electron transfer flavoprotein A or B or to mutations in electron transfer flavoprotein dehydrogenase (ETFDH, ETF:ubiquinone oxidoreductase) (4). The clinical spectrum ranges from a fatal multisystem disease of infancy to a less severe disorder in which symptoms emerge in adolescence or adult life. Late onset MADD may cause a severe lipid storage myopathy with proximal limb and axial muscle weakness sometimes associated with dysphagia. Elevated serum creatine kinase is typical, but myoglobinuria is rare (14). Patients with myopathic MADD may dramatically improve when treated with riboflavin. Recent studies indicate that riboflavin-responsive MADD is attributable primarily to mutations in ETFDH (14). Furthermore, myopathic MADD often is associated with deficiency of coenzyme Q_{10} and may respond to treatment with CoQ_{10} alone, riboflavin alone, or a combination of the two (15). The diagnosis is suggested by the accumulation of long, medium and short chain acylcarnitines in plasma or in cultured fibroblasts incubated with long chain acylcarnitine. Organic aciduria with excretion of hydroxyglutaric, ethylmalonic, and various dicarboxylic acids also is characteristic (14).

MUSCLE CARBOHYDRATE METABOLISM AND DISORDERS (FIGURE 75.2)

Carbohydrate Disorders Causing Muscle Weakness

Pompe Disease (Glycogen Storage Disease (GSD) II)

Pompe disease causes lysosomal glycogen storage due to loss of function mutations in the enzyme acid alpha glucosidase (GAA), also termed acid maltase. The fatal infantile variant is characterized by generalized weakness and hypotonia and cardiomyopathy with massive cardiomegaly, resulting in death from cardiorespiratory failure in the first months of life (16). "Late-onset" variants with isolated myopathic weakness manifest in childhood or adult life. There is both axial and proximal limb weakness, and diaphragmatic involvement explains why respiratory insufficiency may be the presenting symptom in adult-onset disease. Typical features include: serum creatine kinase elevation, myopathic motor unit potentials with pseudomyotonic discharges in some (especially paraspinal) muscles on EMG, and vacuolar myopathy with membrane-bound glycogen. The diagnosis is achieved by enzyme analysis in skeletal muscle, fibroblasts or dried blood spots. Virtually complete enzyme deficiency is found in infantile Pompe disease whereas residual enzyme

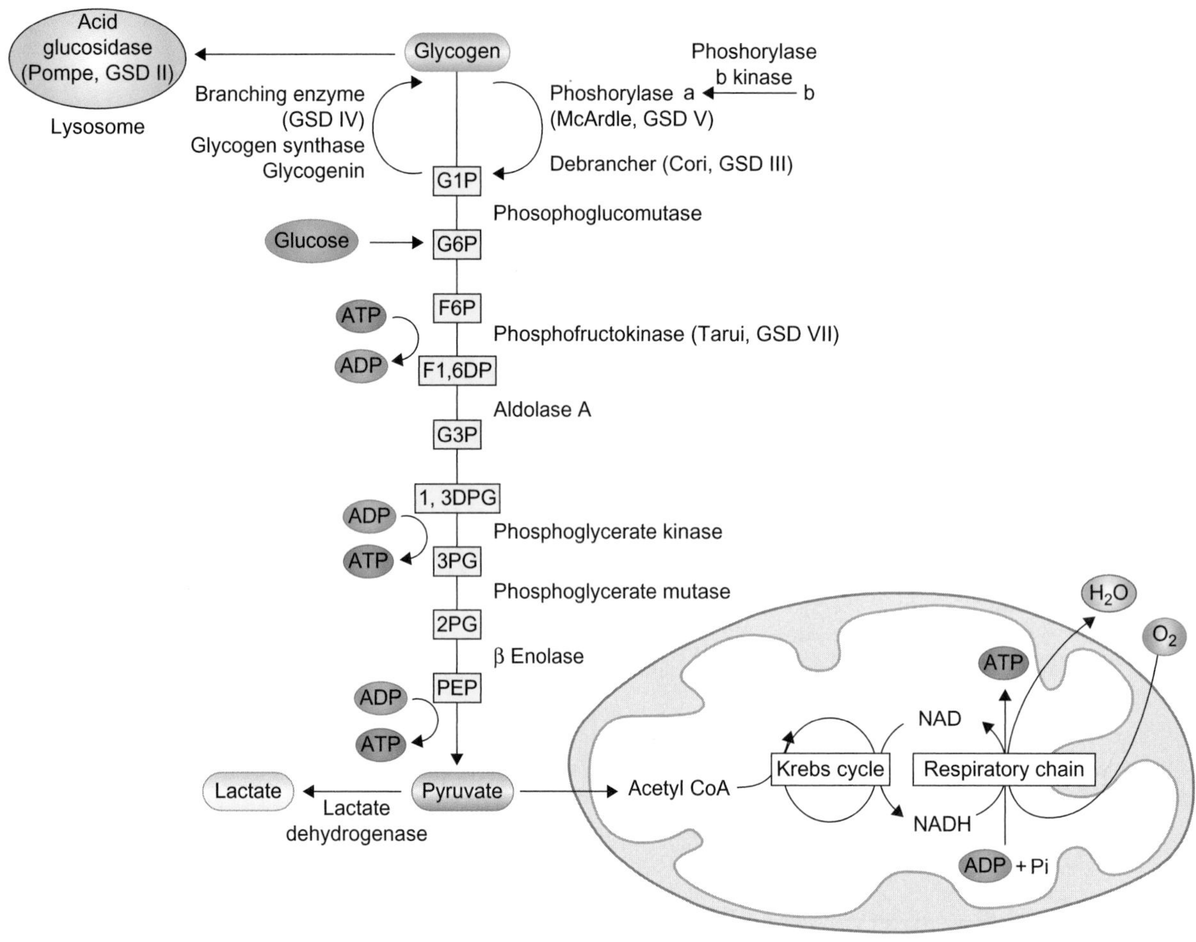

FIGURE 75.2 Outline of muscle glycogen/glucose metabolism indicating defects that impair glycogen/glucose breakdown and glycogen synthesis. For the most common muscle glycogen storage diseases, GSD designations (GSD II, III, IV, V, and VII) and eponyms are provided. Note that glycogen and glucose are metabolized anaerobically (with ATP generated by substrate level phosphorylation and pyruvate reduced to lactate) as well as aerobically with pyruvate metabolized to acetylCo-A with ATP produced via oxidative phosphorylation.

activity varying between 2% and 40% of normal may be found in juvenile and adult-onset forms (16). More than 100 pathogenic mutations have been identified with the IVS1(-13T>G) mutation accounting for approximately 50% of late-onset cases (16). Biweekly, intravenous enzyme replacement therapy (ERT) significantly ameliorates the infantile disease, especially when started very early, but the long-term outcome remains uncertain. In late-onset cases, ERT has achieved modest benefit (17).

Debrancher Deficiency (GSD III)

Debrancher is a single protein with two separate enzymatic domains: one is an oligo-1,4-1,4-glucantransferase; the other is an amylo-1,6-glucosidase. Once the peripheral chains of glycogen have been shortened by phosphorylase to four glucosyl units, these "stubs" are removed by debrancher in two steps. First, a maltotriosyl unit is transferred from a donor to an acceptor chain (transferase activity) leaving behind a single glucosyl unit. Second, the remaining glucosyl unit is hydrolyzed by the amylo-1,6-glucosidase, liberating a molecule of glucose. Debrancher is coded by a single gene, so multi-organ involvement is typical. In the common form of the disease, GSD IIIa, patients have liver, muscle, and sometimes cardiac involvement; approximately 15% of patients have selective hepatic involvement (GSD IIIb) (18). While myopathy in GSD IIIa is common, clinical manifestations are heterogeneous. In childhood, features of hepatic involvement (hepatomegaly, hypoglycemia, ketosis) predominate and muscle symptoms are usually absent or mild, consisting of hypotonia or mild weakness that is non-progressive and may mimic a congenital myopathy (19). Such weakness may resolve around puberty.

Significant weakness attributable to debrancher deficiency most often presents in the third or fourth decade of life with a course that generally is slowly progressive and not debilitating (20). Patients may have symmetrical, predominantly proximal or more generalized weakness. Another manifestation is distal weakness and atrophy, suggesting the diagnosis of Charcot–Marie Tooth or motor neuron disease (19). Although muscle glycogen is crucial for normal muscle energy metabolism, dynamic symptoms of exercise intolerance are not commonly recognized in GSD III even when ischemic forearm exercise reveals markedly blunted lactate production. Creatine kinase levels are routinely elevated but exertional muscle contractures or recurrent rhabdomyolysis are not typical of this disorder and pigmenturia has not been described (19).

Clinical heterogeneity is paralleled by genetic heterogeneity. Approximately 100 mutations have been described, but no clear genotype–phenotype correlation has emerged to account for the various neuromuscular manifestations of GSD III (19). Even among patients with the same mutation, the range of muscle symptoms has been shown to vary from minimal to severe. The responsible variables have yet to be identified.

Brancher Deficiency (GSDIV)

Glycogen branching enzyme (G BE) is a single polypeptide encoded by one gene. GBE deficiency (GSD IV) results in the deposit of an amylopectin-like polysaccharide that has fewer branching points and longer outer chains than normal glycogen and is known as polyglucosan. Polyglucosan is periodate/Schiff (PAS)-positive and only partially digested by diastase, which makes it easily recognizable in various tissues and offers an important clue to the correct diagnosis. GSD IV is a heterogeneous disease that may include hepatic, central nervous system, and cardiac as well as neuromuscular manifestations. Fatal perinatal (fetal akinesia with multiple deformities including arthrogryposis, craniofacial abnormalities, and pulmonary hypoplasia) and congenital (neonatal hypotonia, muscle wasting, neuronal involvement, and inconsistent cardiomyopathy) forms of GSD IV have been described (21). Rarely GSD IV may cause myopathy and cardiomyopathy in childhood or myopathy and CNS involvement or isolated myopathy in adult life.

Carbohydrate Disorders Causing Dynamic (Exercise-Induced) Muscle Symptoms

Phosphorylase b Kinase Deficiency (PhK, GSD IX)

Phosphorylase b kinase is a complex enzyme with four separate subunits, which, in turn, have tissue-specific isoforms: two alpha isozymes, A1 for muscle, A2 for liver; two gamma isozymes, G1 for muscle/testes, G2 for liver; one beta isozyme, and three delta isozymes bound to calmodulin. PhK activates glycogen phosphorylase by phosphorylating a specific serine residue in response to hormonal or neuronal activation, converting phosphorylase b to a. The clinical spectrum of PhK deficiency is broad and includes liver, muscle, or muscle and liver involvement. Cardiac phenotypes associated with glycogen accumulation and severe deficiency of PhK enzymatic activity have been shown to be associated with mutations in the gene encoding AMP-activated protein kinase (AMPK) (22). AMPK is not believed to directly regulate PhK, so the mechanism of PhK deficiency is unknown (23). Selective skeletal muscle involvement is due to mutations in the muscle-specific alpha (A1) subunit on the X chromosome; liver manifestations predominate in autosomal recessive beta subunit mutations with minor or asymptomatic muscle involvement. Muscle symptoms most commonly linked to muscle PhK deficiency are exercise intolerance, cramps, and, in some cases, pigmenturia. Serum creatine kinase and muscle glycogen levels are often, but not invariably, elevated. While muscle PhK deficiency has been considered to result in clinically significant muscle phosphorylase deficiency, ischemic forearm testing has been reported as normal or only blunted, raising the question whether energy production from glycogenolysis is significantly limited. Physiological investigation of one patient with PhK deficiency due to an A1 subunit mutation revealed normal lactate production with ischemic forearm testing but no lactate increase during submaximal cycle exercise (corresponding to 60% of maximal oxygen uptake) implying deficient phosphorylase with aerobic but not anaerobic exercise (24). The severity of PhK deficiency varies substantially, and the relationship between mutations, enzymatic activity, and muscle glycogenolysis under varying conditions remains to be clarified.

Muscle Phosphorylase Deficiency (McArdle Disease, GSD V)

The key manifestations of the disease that bears his name were described by Brian McArdle in 1951. The enzyme deficiency was defined separately by Larner and Villar-Palasi, Mommaerts et al., and Schmidt and Mahler eight years later. Pathogenic mutations in the muscle-specific isoform of glycogen phosphorylase on chromosome 11 were first identified in the early 1990s and have now increased to more than 100, with the R50X predominating in Northern Europe and North America (25). McArdle disease is the most common muscle GSD with an estimated prevalence of 1:100,000, and is one of the two metabolic myopathies (along with CPT2 deficiency) most commonly causing exertional myoglobinuria. Virtually all mutations result in a complete loss of enzyme function and thus a complete block in muscle glycogen breakdown (25). Both oxidative and anaerobic metabolism are severely impaired. Anaerobic glycogenolysis is needed to support maximal effort muscle contraction, hence activities such as lifting or pushing heavy objects, performing sit-ups, or running the bases in softball or baseball rapidly cause muscle fatigue. If patients push further, they develop the cardinal features of the disease, namely muscle stiffness and contractures, muscle pain, and rhabdomyolysis that may result in myoglobinuria (25). These symptoms are readily reproduced by ischemic exercise used to demonstrate the characteristic block in lactate production, indicating these symptoms are due to blocked anaerobic glycogenolysis. A less recognized feature of the disorder is low oxidative capacity that fluctuates with the availability of extramuscular fuels. Patients experience fatigue, tachycardia, and sometimes shortness of breath during sustained activity such as walking, especially uphill, and routinely must slow their pace or stop to rest after a few minutes. On resuming activity, patients may experience a "second wind" with enhanced exercise capacity. Formal exercise testing indicates the second wind reliably occurs after 6–8 minutes of exercise and is associated with a dramatic decrease in exercise heart rate that is proportional to an increase in muscle oxidative capacity, which, in turn is attributable to increased uptake of glucose and combustion of fatty acids (26).

Most patients experience muscle contractures, which are distinct from ordinary cramps. The affected muscle is locked in a condition similar to *rigor mortis* and may remain in that situation for a half hour or more. Unlike common neural cramps that may occur during prolonged exercise in athletes, a contracture cannot be relieved by stretching, and attempting to do so causes severe pain. About 50% of patients report episodes of pigmenturia, which typically occurs the first time they urinate after exertional muscle injury (25). About 25% of these patients experience renal failure. Creatine kinase is virtually always elevated between overt episodes of rhabdomyolysis, often 5–10 times the upper limit of normal or more. Muscle weakness has been reported in approximately 20% of patients (27). When present in younger patients, through the fourth to fifth decade, weakness is generally mild, affecting primarily proximal muscles and or neck flexors. In older patients, weakness is more frequent and may be severe.

Despite symptoms of exercise intolerance from early childhood, the diagnosis is almost never made in the first decade of life; about 25% of patients are diagnosed in each of the second, third, and fourth decade, with about 20% first diagnosed in the fifth decade or later. Generally, diagnostic testing is undertaken only after a sentinel event, such as an episode of rhabdomyolysis and myoglobinuria or the discovery of otherwise unexplained elevated creatine kinase. The characteristic history of exercise intolerance is often missed, because patients are not directly quizzed about their ability to run all four bases in baseball/softball or to run 100 meters with maximal effort. These activities invariably trigger muscle symptoms. Although the high prevalence of some mutations facilitates diagnosis by genetic testing, muscle enzyme analysis, preferably achieved with a needle muscle biopsy, is the gold standard. It is important to note that many patients in whom the diagnosis was not specifically considered prior to muscle biopsy are diagnosed by muscle phosphorylase histochemistry. Accordingly, it is important that muscle pathology laboratories include this test as a routine procedure.

Management includes counseling patients to: (i) avoid maximal effort muscle contractions (weight lifting, maximal effort running) that trigger muscle injury; and (ii) engage in regular moderate, aerobic exercise at an exercise intensity that elicits a heart rate of no more than 60–70% of maximal to optimize alternate fuel delivery and utilization (28). Adequate dietary protein is important to support muscle repair and regeneration but is not an important alternative source of energy. Adequate dietary carbohydrate is recommended to maintain hepatic glycogen stores and hepatic glucose production since blood glucose is a critical alternative fuel when glycogenolysis is blocked. Simple sugars ingested shortly before exercise increase exercise capacity, but must be used sparingly to avoid weight gain (29).

Muscle Phosphofructokinase (PFK) Deficiency (GSD VII)

In 1965, Tarui et al. described exercise intolerance mimicking McArdle disease and documented complete deficiency of PFK in muscle and a partial deficiency in erythrocytes (30). There are three isoforms of PFK, muscle (M), liver (L) and platelet (P), and PFK is a tetramer. In skeletal muscle, only the M isoform is expressed (M4) whereas red cells contain both M and L isoforms (M4, M3L1, M2L2. M1L3, L4) resulting in partial red cell enzyme deficiency in GSD VII. Clinical manifestations are virtually identical to McArdle disease with lifelong exercise intolerance and exercise-induced muscle contractures, rhabdomyolysis and myoglobinuria (31). However, in contrast to McArdle disease, patients also have compensated hemolytic anemia. Exertional nausea and vomiting are common. Because oxidative capacity is as low as in McArdle disease, modest aerobic exercise causes fatigue, but patients do not experience a second wind/improved oxidative capacity when exercise is sustained or resumed after rest (32). This is because the metabolic block prevents glucose metabolism, which is critical for the McArdle second wind. Furthermore, rather than improving exercise capacity as in McArdle patients, carbohydrate ingestion lowers oxidative capacity in PFK deficiency by lowering blood levels of fatty acids, on which muscle oxidative metabolism depends (31). Muscle weakness is common in later life and may be severe. Clinical variants have been described, including fatal infantile PFK deficiency.

PFK deficiency has been described in multiple racial and ethnic groups, but is prevalent in Ashkenazi Jews. Approximately 20 PFK-M mutations have been described. The most common in Ashkenazi Jewish patients, present in approximately 60% of alleles, is a splice site mutation resulting in the deletion of 78 bp of exon 5 (33).

The diagnosis is suggested by a compatible history and by the presence of compensated hemolytic anemia with reticulocytosis and increased serum bilirubin. Exercise monitored by ^{31}phosphorus magnetic spectroscopy reveals a characteristic phosphomonoester peak reflecting the accumulation of sugar phosphates behind the metabolic block (31). Diagnostic confirmation depends upon PFK histochemistry or enzyme assay of skeletal muscle. However, it is important to note that this enzyme is labile and enzyme activity is lost if tissue is not promptly frozen and properly maintained prior to analysis, and misdiagnosis due to artifactual PFK deficiency is common. In fact, in our experience, most patients referred based upon enzyme analysis by commercial laboratories have proven *not* to have PFK deficiency. Patient management involves education to avoid exercise-induced muscle injury, avoidance of carbohydrate prior to physical activity, and regular moderate aerobic exercise.

Distal Glycolytic Defects: Phosphoglycerate Kinase (PGK) Deficiency

PGK is encoded by a single gene on Xq13 for all tissues except testes. PGK deficiency can affect multiple tissues causing – in isolation or in various combinations – hemolytic anemia, central nervous system dysfunction, and myopathy (34). In isolated PGK myopathy, patients experience muscle contractures, rhabdomyolysis, and myoglobinuria triggered by brief, maximal effort exercise. Aerobic exercise capacity is preserved, presumably because of some residual enzyme activity. Forearm exercise testing results in a blunted increase in lactate. Patients in whom myopathy is associated with CNS or CNS and hematological features typically have more severe exercise intolerance with reduced aerobic capacity and greater susceptibility to exercise-induced muscle contractures and rhabdomyolysis. Diagnosis is achieved by enzyme analysis in skeletal muscle or red cell hemolysates. Management involves patient education to avoid severe episodes of muscle injury.

Muscle Phosphoglycerate Mutase (PGAM) Deficiency

PGAM is a dimeric enzyme containing muscle (M), brain (B) or both subunits in different tissues. About 95% of PGAM enzymatic activity in skeletal muscle is attributable to the MM homodimer. PGAM deficiency reduces muscle enzyme activity to about 5% of normal and causes premature fatigue, contractures, and rhabdomyolysis with myoglobinuria triggered by maximal effort exercise. Residual glycolysis is sufficient to support normal aerobic capacity so there is no evidence of substrate-limited oxidative metabolism. Nine of the 13 patients described with this disorder have been African Americans. Of the eight genetically characterized African American patients, seven were homozygous for a W78X nonsense mutation in exon 1, and one was compound heterozygous for this mutation and a novel missense mutation, suggesting a founder effect (35). Patients of different ethnic origins (Italian, Pakistani) harbored different mutations. Many affected patients also have tubular aggregates in the muscle biopsy.

Muscle Lactate Dehydrogenase (LDH) Deficiency

Lactate dehydrogenase is a tetrameric enzyme containing muscle (LDH-A), heart (LDH-B) or both subunits. LDH-A deficiency was first described in Japan and subsequently identified in two families from North America. Similar to PGAM and myopathic PGK deficiency, muscle LDH-deficient patients develop muscle contractures, rhabdomyolysis and myoglobinuria with maximal effort exercise (31). The disorder is purely a defect in anaerobic glycolysis. NADH formed via glyceraldehyde phosphate dehydrogenase (GADPH), and normally oxidized by LDH, builds up with levels of exercise that normally would result in accelerated lactate formation and ultimately blocks glycolysis at the level of GADPH. Some patients have an associated dermatitis related to the fact that LDH-A is the dominant subunit expressed in skin. Multiple mutations have been identified in both North American and Japanese patients (31).

Other Rare Defects

Two patients have been reported with *aldolase A deficiency*, the isoform that is dominant in skeletal muscle and red cells. Patients have hemolytic anemia and are subject to rhabdomyolysis during febrile illnesses related to the thermolability of the mutant enzyme (36). *Beta-enolase deficiency* has been described in a single patient with exercise-induced muscle pain and fatigability but no pigmenturia (37). Enolase is a dimeric enzyme composed potentially of three isoforms coded by separate genes, alpha (ubiquitous), beta (muscle), and gamma (brain). The beta isoform is found exclusively in muscle. The affected patient had 5% of normal enolase in muscle and a blunted lactate response to ischemic forearm exercise. A single patient with muscle *phosphoglucomutase deficiency* (1% residual enzymatic activity) was ascribed to a compound heterozygous mutation (38). The patient had a history of exertional cramps and exercise-induced pigmenturia. Muscle glycogen levels were not elevated and forearm exercise resulted in a normal rise in lactate. Two families have been described with defects in muscle glycogen synthesis (these disorders are labeled "GSD type 0"). In one family, three siblings had *glycogen synthase (GS) 1 deficiency* due to a homozygous nonsense mutation in the gene encoding the muscle form of GS (*GYS1*). They had low exercise capacity and a hypertrophic cardiomyopathy (39). Glycogen was absent in skeletal muscle and heart, and skeletal muscle showed marked type 1 fiber predominance and mitochondrial proliferation. A second report identified a patient with a missense mutation in the gene encoding the muscle primer glycogenin-1 (GYG1), resulting in failure of glycogenin to autoglycosylate, a crucial step for the initiation of glycogen synthesis (40). The clinical phenotype was similar to GS1 deficiency with exercise intolerance and cardiomyopathy. Muscle biopsy showed absent glycogen with marked type 1 fiber predominance and mitochondrial proliferation.

MITOCHONDRIAL MYOPATHIES

Mitochondrial myopathies are conventionally attributed to genetic defects that disrupt the mitochondrial respiratory chain. The clinical hallmark of muscle impairment in these defects is exercise intolerance and lactic acidosis at low levels of physical activity. Mitochondrial defects may also result in severe weakness. These muscle symptoms may occur in isolation or in association with multisystemic mitochondrial dysfunction. A great variety of mitochondrial or nuclear genetic defects may be responsible.

Myopathies Due to Mitochondrial DNA (mtDNA) Mutations

The first class of mitochondrial DNA mutations recognized to cause mitochondrial myopathy were heteroplasmic, *single large-scale deletions*. Affected patients characteristically have chronic progressive external ophthalmoplegia (CPEO) with or without a more generalized myopathy, or a multisystemic syndrome (Kearns–Sayre syndrome, KSS) with CPEO, pigmentary retinopathy, cardiac conduction defects, and CNS dysfunction (41). Muscle fibers with high levels of mutant mtDNA and sub-sarcolemmal mitochondrial proliferation appear "ragged-red" (ragged-red fibers, RRF) with the modified Gomori trichrome stain and lack cytochrome *c* oxidase (COX) histochemical activity (COX-negative fibers) whereas they stain intensely with succinate dehydrogenase (SDH) ("ragged blue" fibers). This muscle histology profile is typical of most mitochondrial DNA mutations and reflects deficiency of respiratory chain complexes that contain mitochondrial DNA-encoded subunits (complexes I, III, IV and V) while preserving complex II (SDH), which is exclusively nuclear encoded (Figure 75.3). More than 200 pathogenic maternally inherited or sporadic *mtDNA point mutations* in tRNA or coding region genes have been described (42). Muscle weakness or fatigability commonly accompanies multisystem mitochondrial disease, including classical maternally inherited mitochondrial encephalomyopathies due to the m.3243A>G mutation in tRNA$^{leu(UUR)}$, the most common cause of MELAS (mitochondrial encephalomyopathy, lactic acidosis and stroke like episodes), and the m.8344A>G mutation in tRNA^{lys}, the typical cause of MERRF (myoclonus epilepsy with ragged red fibers). Pure myopathy, often characterized by marked exercise intolerance, has been associated with heteroplasmic mutations in tRNA or protein-coding genes, especially the cytochrome *b* gene (43). Most mutations in protein-coding genes are sporadic and apparently de novo. While pathogenic mtDNA mutations that cause mitochondrial myopathy are typically heteroplasmic, homoplasmic mutations are receiving renewed attention. Notably, the reversible cytochrome c oxidase deficiency of infancy is due to a maternally inherited homoplasmic m.14674T>C mutation in tRNA^{glu} (44).

Mitochondrial Myopathy Due to Nuclear Mutations Causing Multiple mtDNA Deletions or mtDNA Depletion

Mutations in nuclear genes necessary for mtDNA replication and maintenance generally result in adult-onset CPEO, usually dominantly inherited (45). Most of these mutations are in the catalytic subunit of the mtDNA polymerase, polymerase gamma (POLG). However, mutations in other nuclear genes can cause CPEO and myopathy, including the mtDNA helicase, Twinkle, the muscle–heart isoform of the mitochondrial adenine nucleotide translocase (ANT1), and in the ribonucleotide reductase, p53-R2 subunit (RRM2B). Phenotypes include not only CPEO and weakness, but also CPEO with peripheral or central nervous system disorders and other symptoms. CPEO and multiple mtDNA deletions also may be seen in MNGIE syndrome, mitochondrial neurogastrointestinal encephalomyopathy, attributable to mutations in thymidine phosphorylase (TYMP) (46). POLG1, Twinkle, and TYMP mutations may also be associated with mitochondrial DNA depletion (47). Among other

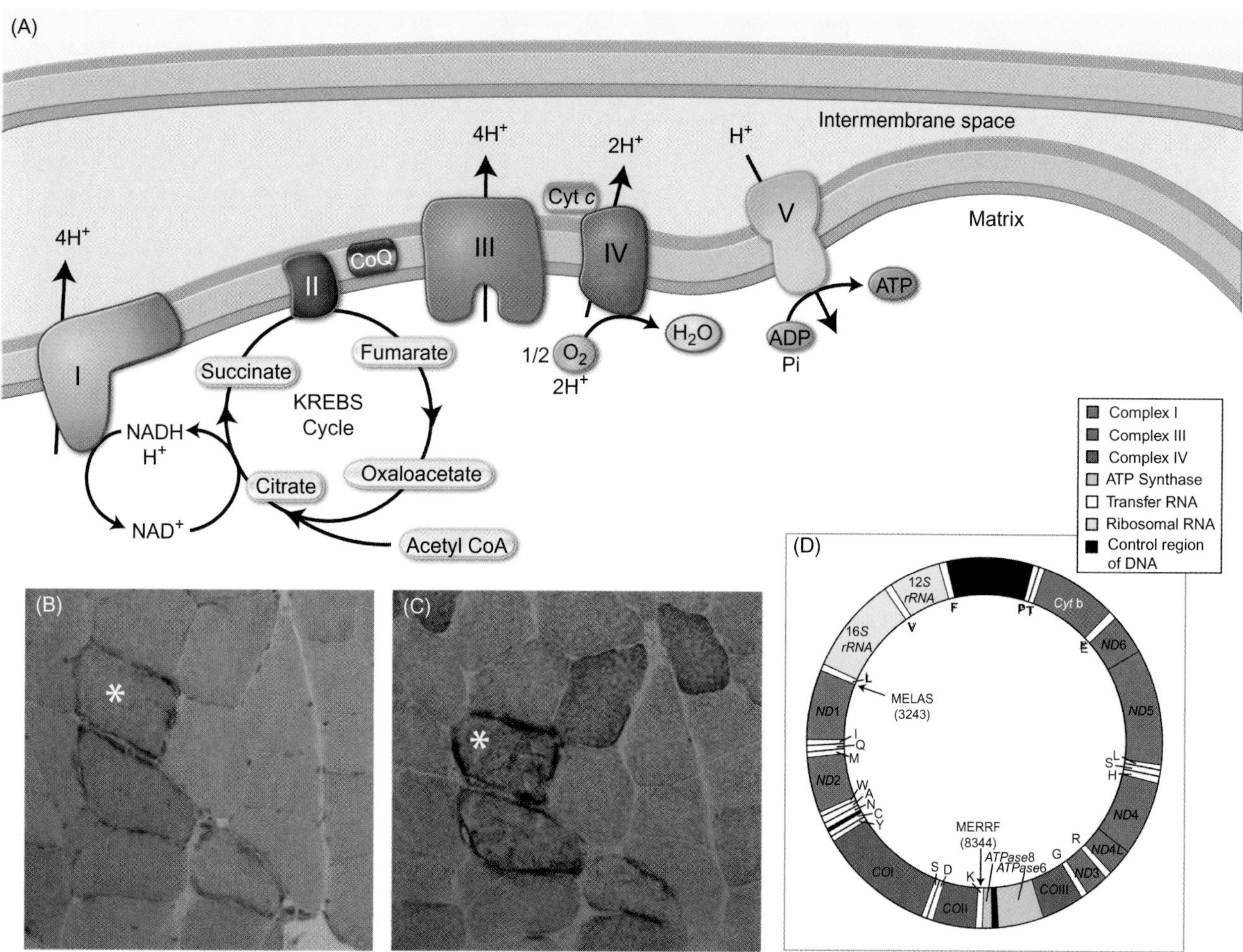

FIGURE 75.3 Cartoon illustrating mitochondrial respiratory chain complexes (A) and mitochondrial DNA (B) indicating tRNA genes (letters) and coding subunits that are components of complexes I, III, IV and V. Note that subunits of complex II are exclusively nuclear encoded so expression of complex II (succinate dehydrogenase, SDH) is preserved and typically enhanced in proportion to mitochondrial proliferation with mitochondrial DNA mutations. (C) and (D) are serial sections of muscle from a patient with a heteroplasmic mitochondrial DNA mutation. Muscle fibers with a high abundance of mutant mtDNA show subsarcolemmal mitochondrial proliferation resulting in "ragged red" fibers (*) with Gomori trichrome (C); the same fibers stain blue with combined cytochdrome c oxidase (COX, complex IV) and succinate dehydrogenase (SDH, complex II) stain.

defects responsible for mtDNA depletion, thymidine kinase 2 (TK2) defects are noteworthy. TK2 mutations cause a rapidly progressive myopathy of infancy or early childhood associated with elevated creatine kinase and muscle histology resembling muscular dystrophy or spinal muscular atrophy (47).

Mitochondrial Myopathy Due to Nuclear DNA Mutations

It is estimated that 70–80% of mitochondrial disease in children and a substantial percentage in adults is due to mutations in nuclear genes, but most remain unknown (42). Most of the nuclear gene defects that have been identified to date affect subunits or assembly factors that result in deficiency of complexes I or IV and cause childhood encephalopathy. However, a number of mitochondrial myopathies attributable to nuclear defects have been described. Myopathy with coenzyme Q deficiency has multiple causes. Some cases of weakness and exercise intolerance with CK elevation and muscle lipid accumulation have been shown to be attributable to riboflavin-responsive mutations in ETFDH. Another form of myopathic CoQ deficiency is associated with a mutation in CABC1, the human homologue of a gene necessary for ubiquinone synthesis in yeast (48). Additional genetic mechanisms of myopathic CoQ deficiency remain to be discovered. Acyl-CoA dehydrogenase 9 (ACAD9) which closely resembles VLCAD has been shown to be important for complex I assembly. Mutations in ACAD9 result in childhood onset, severe exercise intolerance and riboflavin-responsive complex I deficiency (49); other mutations in this gene may cause cardiomyopathy and encephalopathy (50). Another interesting mitochondrial myopathy is attributable to a splice site mutation in the iron-sulfur (Fe-S) cluster scaffold (ISCU) gene resulting in ISCU deficiency and reduced levels of Fe-S cluster containing proteins including the tricarboxylic acid cycle enzymes aconitase and succinate dehydrogenase and Fe-S subunits of respiratory chain complexes I and III (51). Symptoms are life-long severe exercise intolerance in which modest exercise causes fatigue, tachycardia and shortness of breath with episodes of myoglobinuria. Detailed physiological investigations performed in affected patients more than forty years ago represent the first description of exercise pathophysiology in a severe mitochondrial myopathy showing dramatically impaired extraction of oxygen from blood and a hyperkinetic circulation in exercise with a marked mismatch between O_2 delivery and O_2 utilization (52). Subsequent study has revealed that this exercise response is a consistent feature of all severe muscle oxidative defects (53).

REFERENCES

1. Bruno C, Dimauro S. Lipid storage myopathies. *Curr Opin Neurol* 2008;**21**:601–6.
2. Bonnefont JP, Djouadi F, Prip-Buus C, Gobin S, Munnich A, Bastin J. Carnitine palmitoyltransferases 1 and 2: biochemical, molecular and medical aspects. *Mol Aspects Med* 2004;**25**:495–520.
3. Orngreen MC, Duno M, Ejstrup R, Christensen E, Schwartz M, Sacchetti M, et al. Fuel utilization in subjects with carnitine palmitoyltransferase 2 gene mutations. *Ann Neurol* 2005;**57**:60–6.
4. Laforet P, Vianey-Saban C. Disorders of muscle lipid metabolism: diagnostic and therapeutic challenges. *Neuromuscul Disord* 2010;**20**:693–700.
5. Bonnefont JP, Bastin J, Laforet P, Aubey F, Mogenet A, Romano S, et al. Long-term follow-up of bezafibrate treatment in patients with the myopathic form of carnitine palmitoyltransferase 2 deficiency. *Clin Pharmacol Ther* 2010;**88**:101–8.
6. Laforet P, Acquaviva-Bourdain C, Rigal O, Brivet M, Penisson-Besnier I, Chabrol B, et al. Diagnostic assessment and long-term follow-up of 13 patients with Very Long-Chain Acyl-Coenzyme A dehydrogenase (VLCAD) deficiency. *Neuromuscul Disord* 2009;**19**:324–9.
7. Spiekerkoetter U, Bastin J, Gillingham M, Morris A, Wijburg F, Wilcken B. Current issues regarding treatment of mitochondrial fatty acid oxidation disorders. *J Inherit Metab Dis* 2010;**33**:555–61.
8. Michot C, Hubert L, Brivet M, De Meirleir L, Valayannopoulos V, Muller-Felber W, et al. LPIN1 gene mutations: a major cause of severe rhabdomyolysis in early childhood. *Hum Mutat* 2010;**31**: E1564–1573.
9. Nezu J, Tamai I, Oku A, Ohashi R, Yabuuchi H, Hashimoto N, et al. Primary systemic carnitine deficiency is caused by mutations in a gene encoding sodium ion-dependent carnitine transporter. *Nat Genet* 1999;**21**:91–4.
10. Lefevre C, Jobard F, Caux F, Bouadjar B, Karaduman A, Heilig R, et al. Mutations in CGI-58, the gene encoding a new protein of the esterase/lipase/thioesterase subfamily, in Chanarin–Dorfman syndrome. *Am J Hum Genet* 2001;**69**:1002–12.
11. Bruno C, Bertini E, Di Rocco M, Cassandrini D, Ruffa G, De Toni T, et al. Clinical and genetic characterization of Chanarin–Dorfman syndrome. *Biochem Biophys Res Commun* 2008;**369**:1125–8.
12. Fischer J, Lefevre C, Morava E, Mussini JM, Laforet P, Negre-Salvayre A, et al. The gene encoding adipose triglyceride lipase (PNPLA2) is mutated in neutral lipid storage disease with myopathy. *Nat Genet* 2007;**39**:28–30.
13. Akman HO, Davidzon G, Tanji K, Macdermott EJ, Larsen L, Davidson MM, et al. Neutral lipid storage disease with subclinical myopathy due to a retrotransposal insertion in the PNPLA2 gene. *Neuromuscul Disord* 2011;**20**:397–402.
14. Olsen RK, Olpin SE, Andresen BS, Miedzybrodzka ZH, Pourfarzam M, Merinero B, et al. ETFDH mutations as a major cause of riboflavin-responsive multiple acyl-CoA dehydrogenation deficiency. *Brain* 2007;**130**:2045–54.
15. Gempel K, Topaloglu H, Talim B, Schneiderat P, Schoser BG, Hans VH, et al. The myopathic form of coenzyme Q10 deficiency is caused by mutations in the electron-transferring-flavoprotein dehydrogenase (ETFDH) gene. *Brain* 2007;**130**:2037–44.
16. Kishnani PS, Steiner RD, Bali D, Berger K, Byrne BJ, Case LE, et al. Pompe disease diagnosis and management guideline. *Genet Med* 2006;**8**:267–88.
17. van der Ploeg AT, Clemens PR, Corzo D, Escolar DM, Florence J, Groeneveld GJ, et al. A randomized study of alglucosidase alfa in late-onset Pompe's disease. *N Engl J Med* 2010;**362**:1396–406.
18. Kishnani PS, Austin SL, Arn P, Bali DS, Boney A, Case LE, et al. Glycogen storage disease type III diagnosis and management guidelines. *Genet Med* 2010;**12**:446–63.
19. Moses SW, Gadoth N, Bashan N, Ben-David E, Slonim A, Wanderman KL. Neuromuscular involvement in glycogen storage disease type III. *Acta Paediatr Scand* 1986;**75**:289–96.
20. Cornelio F, Bresolin N, Singer PA, DiMauro S, Rowland LP. Clinical varieties of neuromuscular disease in debrancher deficiency. *Arch Neurol* 1984;**41**:1027–32.
21. Bruno C, van Diggelen OP, Cassandrini D, Gimpelev M, Giuffre B, Donati MA, et al. Clinical and genetic heterogeneity of branching enzyme deficiency (glycogenosis type IV). *Neurology* 2004;**63**:1053–8.
22. Burwinkel B, Scott JW, Buhrer C, van Landeghem FK, Cox GF, Wilson CJ, et al. Fatal congenital heart glycogenosis caused by a recurrent activating R531Q mutation in the gamma 2-subunit of AMP-activated protein kinase (PRKAG2), not by phosphorylase kinase deficiency. *Am J Hum Genet* 2005;**76**:1034–49.
23. Akman HO, Sampayo JN, Ross FA, Scott JW, Wilson G, Benson L, et al. Fatal infantile cardiac glycogenosis with phosphorylase kinase deficiency and a mutation in the gamma2-subunit of AMP-activated protein kinase. *Pediatr Res* 2007;**62**:499–504.
24. Orngreen MC, Schelhaas HJ, Jeppesen TD, Akman HO, Wevers RA, Andersen ST, et al. Is muscle glycogenolysis impaired in X-linked phosphorylase b kinase deficiency? *Neurology* 2008;**70**:1876–82.
25. Lucia A, Nogales-Gadea G, Perez M, Martin MA, Andreu AL, Arenas J. McArdle disease: what do neurologists need to know? *Nat Clin Pract Neurol* 2008;**4**:568–77.

26. Haller RG, Vissing J. Spontaneous "second wind" and glucose-induced second "second wind" in McArdle disease: oxidative mechanisms. *Arch Neurol* 2002;**59**:1395–402.
27. Quinlivan R, Buckley J, James M, Twist A, Ball S, Duno M, et al. McArdle disease: a clinical review. *J Neurol Neurosurg Psychiatry* 2010;**81**:1182–8.
28. Haller RG, Wyrick P, Taivassalo T, Vissing J. Aerobic conditioning: an effective therapy in McArdle's disease. *Ann Neurol* 2006;**59**:922–8.
29. Vissing J, Haller RG. The effect of oral sucrose on exercise tolerance in patients with McArdle's disease. *N Engl J Med* 2003;**349**:2503–9.
30. Tarui S, Okuno G, Ikura Y, Tanaka T, Suda M, Nishikawa M. Phosphofructokinase deficiency in skeletal muscle. A new type of glycogenosis. *Biochem Biophys Res Commun* 1965;**19**:517–23.
31. DiMauro S, Lamperti C. Muscle glycogenoses. *Muscle Nerve* 2001;**24**:984–99.
32. Haller RG, Vissing J. No spontaneous second wind in muscle phosphofructokinase deficiency. *Neurology* 2004;**62**:82–6.
33. Nakajima H, Raben N, Hamaguchi T, Yamasaki T. Phosphofructokinase deficiency; past, present and future. *Curr Mol Med* 2002;**2**:197–212.
34. Spiegel R, Gomez EA, Akman HO, Krishna S, Horovitz Y, DiMauro S. Myopathic form of phosphoglycerate kinase (PGK) deficiency: a new case and pathogenic considerations. *Neuromuscul Disord* 2009;**19**:207–11.
35. Naini A, Toscano A, Musumeci O, Vissing J, Akman HO, DiMauro S. Muscle phosphoglycerate mutase deficiency revisited. *Arch Neurol* 2009;**66**:394–8.
36. Yao DC, Tolan DR, Murray MF, Harris DJ, Darras BT, Geva A, et al. Hemolytic anemia and severe rhabdomyolysis caused by compound heterozygous mutations of the gene for erythrocyte/muscle isozyme of aldolase, ALDOA(Arg303X/Cys338Tyr). *Blood* 2004;**103**:2401–3.
37. Comi GP, Fortunato F, Lucchiari S, Bordoni A, Prelle A, Jann S, et al. Beta-enolase deficiency, a new metabolic myopathy of distal glycolysis. *Ann Neurol* 2001;**50**:202–7.
38. Stojkovic T, Vissing J, Petit F, Piraud M, Orngreen MC, Andersen G, et al. Muscle glycogenosis due to phosphoglucomutase 1 deficiency. *N Engl J Med* 2009;**361**:425–7.
39. Kollberg G, Tulinius M, Gilljam T, Ostman-Smith I, Forsander G, Jotorp P, et al. Cardiomyopathy and exercise intolerance in muscle glycogen storage disease. *N Engl J Med* 2007;**357**:1507–14.
40. Moslemi AR, Lindberg C, Nilsson J, Tajsharghi H, Andersson B, Oldfors A. Glycogenin-1 deficiency and inactivated priming of glycogen synthesis. *N Engl J Med* 2010;**362**:1203–10.
41. Moraes CT, DiMauro S, Zeviani M, Lombes A, Shanske S, Miranda AF, et al. Mitochondrial DNA deletions in progressive external ophthalmoplegia and Kearns–Sayre syndrome. *N Engl J Med* 1989;**320**:1293–9.
42. Tucker EJ, Compton AG, Thorburn DR. Recent advances in the genetics of mitochondrial encephalopathies. *Curr Neurol Neurosci Rep* 2010;**10**:277–85.
43. Andreu AL, Hanna MG, Reichmann H, Bruno C, Penn AS, Tanji K, et al. Exercise intolerance due to mutations in the cytochrome b gene of mitochondrial DNA. *N Engl J Med* 1999;**341**:1037–44.
44. Horvath R, Kemp JP, Tuppen HA, Hudson G, Oldfors A, Marie SK, et al. Molecular basis of infantile reversible cytochrome c oxidase deficiency myopathy. *Brain* 2009;**132**:3165–74.
45. Spinazzola A, Zeviani M. Disorders of nuclear-mitochondrial intergenomic communication. *Biosci Rep* 2007;**27**:39–51.
46. Lara MC, Valentino ML, Torres-Torronteras J, Hirano M, Marti R. Mitochondrial neurogastrointestinal encephalomyopathy (MNGIE): biochemical features and therapeutic approaches. *Biosci Rep* 2007;**27**:151–63.
47. Suomalainen A, Isohanni P. Mitochondrial DNA depletion syndromes – many genes, common mechanisms. *Neuromuscul Disord* 2010;**20**:429–37.
48. Mollet J, Delahodde A, Serre V, Chretien D, Schlemmer D, Lombes A, et al. CABC1 gene mutations cause ubiquinone deficiency with cerebellar ataxia and seizures. *Am J Hum Genet* 2008;**82**:623–30.
49. Gerards M, van den Bosch BJ, Danhauser K, Serre V, van Weeghel M, Wanders RJ, et al. Riboflavin-responsive oxidative phosphorylation complex I deficiency caused by defective ACAD9: new function for an old gene. *Brain* 2011;**134**:210–9.
50. Nouws J, Nijtmans L, Houten SM, van den Brand M, Huynen M, Venselaar H, et al. Acyl-CoA dehydrogenase 9 is required for the biogenesis of oxidative phosphorylation complex I. *Cell Metab* 2010;**12**:283–94.
51. Mochel F, Knight MA, Tong WH, Hernandez D, Ayyad K, Taivassalo T, et al. Splice mutation in the iron-sulfur cluster scaffold protein ISCU causes myopathy with exercise intolerance. *Am J Hum Genet* 2008;**82**:652–60.
52. Linderholm H, Muller R, Ringqvist R, Sornas R. Hereditary abnormal muscle metabolism with hyperkinetic circulation during exercise. *Acta Med Scand* 1969;**185**:153–66.
53. Taivassalo T, Jensen TD, Kennaway N, DiMauro S, Vissing J, Haller RG. The spectrum of exercise tolerance in mitochondrial myopathies: a study of 40 patients. *Brain* 2003;**126**:413–23.

Section D

Therapeutics

Chapter 76

Gene Therapy of Skeletal Muscle Disorders Using Viral Vectors

Andrea L.H. Arnett[1,2,3], Julian N. Ramos[1,3] and Jeffrey S. Chamberlain[1,3,4,5]

[1]Department of Neurology, [2]Medical Scientist Training Program, [3]Program in Molecular and Cellular Biology, [4]Department of Biochemistry, [5]Department of Medicine, University of Washington, Seattle, WA

INTRODUCTION

A large number of genetic disorders manifest in skeletal muscle, many of which have devastating consequences in affected individuals. Consequently, skeletal muscle is an important target for gene therapies, but one that presents numerous challenges. The significant volume and widespread distribution of striated muscle presents an imposing obstacle to the delivery of gene constructs, but recent studies show that delivery vectors derived from viruses can facilitate systemic gene transfer. In addition, the regenerative aspects of skeletal muscle pose unique challenges to the persistence of corrective transgenes. Nevertheless, several viral vector-mediated treatment strategies targeting skeletal muscle have progressed to preclinical and clinical trials, raising optimism that they may lead to a treatment for multiple muscle disorders.

GENE THERAPY VECTORS AND SKELETAL MUSCLE TRANSDUCTION

Several types of viral vectors have shown at least some potential for *in vivo* or *ex vivo* gene delivery to treat muscle disorders (Figure 76.1). These include host genome-integrating vectors, such as those derived from lentiviruses, as well as vectors with a low potential for integration, such as recombinant adenoviral (Ad) and adeno-associated viral (rAAV) vectors. Each vector system presents advantages and obstacles relating to immunogenicity, production and purification, and risk of mutagenesis, all of which influence and limit their use in gene therapy strategies. A brief summary of the major vector systems used for muscle gene therapy is outlined below.

Adenoviral Vectors

The initial attempts at developing gene therapies for skeletal muscle disease focused on vectors derived from adenovirus (Ad). Ad is a non-enveloped double-stranded DNA virus with a genome size of approximately 36 kb (1). Over 50 human serotypes have been identified, but the majority of recombinant Ad vectors are based on serotypes 2 and 5 (2). Adenoviruses transduce a wide array of cell types, but have a strong tropism for respiratory, ocular, and gastrointestinal epithelium. In addition, the liver is heavily targeted following intravascular administration, and this has been harnessed to treat canine and murine models of hemophilia A and B (3,4). Unfortunately, the tropism of Ad for mature skeletal muscle is limited. The composition and structure of the extracellular matrix and basal lamina surrounding muscle fibers serves as an impediment to the diffusion of large viral vectors (5). In addition, Ad transduction of skeletal muscle is hampered by reduced expression of the primary cell surface receptor used for entry (CAR) into mature muscle fibers (6). Despite these barriers, the host immune response remains the greatest impediment to Ad-mediated gene therapies. First-generation adenoviruses lack the E1a and b genes, rendering them markedly defective in replication. However, residual replication in mammalian cells enabled low expression of viral genes, resulting in an enhanced immune response that limited the duration of transgene expression (7). This situation was improved upon by the development of "gutted" Ad vectors that retained only the viral inverted terminal repeats (ITRs) and packaging signal (8,9). However, gutted Ad vectors are generated via co-infection of a helper virus that provides viral proteins in *trans*. Residual contamination of vector with helper-virus represents an obstacle to the use of large-scale Ad preps in a clinical setting (10). The use of muscle-specific promoters has been observed to significantly restrict transgene expression to muscle, and can prevent an immune response against Ad-transduced cells by preventing transduction of immune effector cells (11,12).

Muscle. DOI: http://dx.doi.org/10.1016/B978-0-12-381510-1.00076-4

Viral vectors

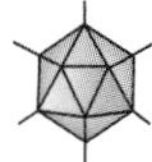

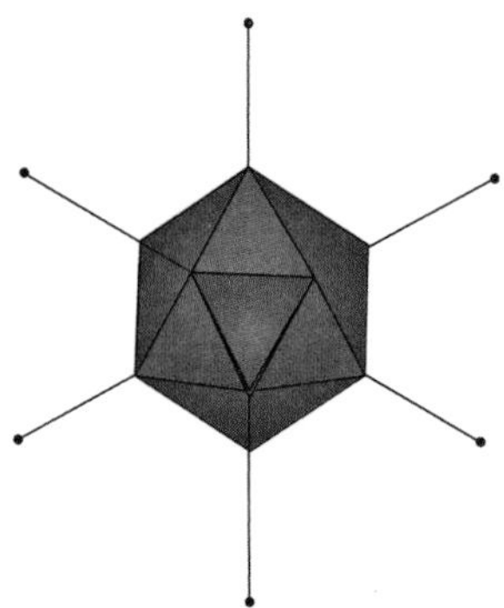

Adeno-associated virus	Lentivirus	Adenovirus
+ High tropism for striated muscle + Effective systemic delivery + Low immunogenicity – Low capacity	+ Permanent transduction + Works well for *ex vivo* modification of cells – Risk of insertional mutagenesis	+ High capacity – Highly immunogenic – Low tropism for skeletal muscle

FIGURE 76.1 **Characteristics of common viral vectors used for gene transfer studies.** Adeno-associated virus *(left)* has low immunogenicity and a high tropism for striated muscle, but the genome carrying capacity is low compared to other vectors. Lentivirus *(middle)* can achieve permanent transduction of targeted cells, but this characteristic is associated with an increased risk of insertional mutagenesis. Adenovirus *(right)* has a high carrying capacity, but is limited by a low tropism for muscle and high immunogenicity.

Lentiviral Vectors

Integrating lentiviruses from the *Retroviridae* family have also been used in gene therapy strategies. Lentiviruses are enveloped, ssRNA viruses, approximately 100 nm in diameter (13,14). Engineered lentiviral vectors retain minimal signals for packaging and integration, and are otherwise devoid of viral genes that could lead to the production of replication-competent virus (13). Unfortunately, only low to moderate levels of adult skeletal muscle transduction have been obtained via IM or systemic injection (15,16). However, neonatal skeletal muscle is more efficiently transduced, and *in utero* injection has demonstrated widespread transgene expression in both mature fibers and satellite cells (17–19). As integrating vectors, lentiviruses are incorporated into the host genome preferentially at sites of high transcriptional activity (20). Integration poses a risk of insertional mutagenesis (21) but also has the potential to provide a permanently corrected pool of stem cells that can replenish muscle fibers lost during normal muscle turnover. In this regard, lentiviruses have been shown to efficiently transduce muscle progenitor cells with a modified dystrophin construct prior to transplantation in a murine model of Duchenne muscular dystrophy (DMD) (15,22). Thus, *ex vivo* modification of stem cells remains an important aspect of lentiviral mediated therapies.

Adeno-Associated Viral (AAV) Vectors

AAV vectors are a very promising tool for use in gene therapy strategies for muscle disorders. The wild type virus has an ssDNA genome of 4.7 kb, and is a member of the parvovirus family. AAV was first identified as a contaminant in adenovirus preparations, and is unable to replicate *in vivo* without the assistance of a replication-competent helper virus (e.g. adenovirus or herpesvirus) (23). An attractive safety feature for AAV vectors is that the wild-type virus has no known pathogenicity. AAV can transduce a wide array of tissues and is significantly less able to elicit a host T-cell immune response than are adenoviral vectors (24). Widespread interest in using rAAV vectors for muscle gene therapy comes from observations that these vectors are expressed for years in transduced striated muscles (25), and the discovery that they can be systemically delivered to muscles body-wide via the vasculature (26). The major limitation of rAAV vectors is the limited cloning capacity of ~5 kb, precluding delivery of large gene cassettes. Unfortunately, attempts to modify the AAV capsid through mutations and chimeras of serotypes have not significantly expanded the packaging capacity (27).

Many AAV serotypes display a unique profile of tropism for different tissues (27). rAAV serotypes 6, 8, and 9 have demonstrated widespread transduction of striated muscle in mice upon systemic delivery (26,28–31). The most encompassing serotype comparison of striated muscle transduction to date lies within two studies by the Rabinowitz group (31,32). rAAV serotypes 1, 6, 7, 8, and 9 were found to efficiently transduce both cardiac and skeletal muscle when administered by tail vein injection. The most ubiquitous transduction among muscle and non-muscle tissues was observed in rAAV8 and rAAV9. Additionally, rAAV7 and rAAV9 exhibited the fastest transduction kinetics and were the first serotypes to plateau in expression levels. In cardiac gene delivery experiments, rAAV6 consistently displayed the highest levels of expression of all the serotypes compared, and was less prone to non-muscle transduction than rAAV8 and 9.

Although rAAV vectors are capable of integrating into the host genome, the frequency of this occurrence is very low (33,34). Instead, rAAV genomes predominately exist in cells as episomal DNA. However, systemic or vascular delivery of rAAV can result in transduction of a wide range of tissues, and appropriate tissue-specific regulatory elements will need to be incorporated into the vector design. In addition, immunity to wild-type AAV in humans presents an important obstacle to rAAV-mediated therapies. A significant percentage of the adult human population has pre-existing immunity to various AAV serotypes (35). These factors must be carefully considered and may complicate the design of therapies that require re-administration of vector.

GENE THERAPY OF THE MUSCULAR DYSTROPHIES

The muscular dystrophies are a diverse group of genetic disorders characterized by impaired function and wasting of skeletal and often cardiac muscle. Of these, DMD is the most common, and it arises almost exclusively from null allele mutations in the dystrophin gene (36). Becker muscular dystrophy (BMD) is a milder form of DMD caused by mutations that allow expression of reduced amounts of, or a partially functional, dystrophin protein (36). DMD has been a major target for gene therapies, and significant effort has been focused on the development of safe and effective methods for vector delivery.

The large size of the dystrophin cDNA (~13.9 kb) presents unique challenges to gene delivery strategies, as it is larger than the carrying capacity of both rAAV and lentiviral vectors. However, some truncated dystrophins can retain a high degree of functionality. In the case of the milder disorder BMD, deletion mutations in the dystrophin gene can result in the expression of truncated, yet partially functional, dystrophin (37). This observation led researchers to develop mini- and micro-dystrophins for therapeutic use, which have been used to achieve body-wide amelioration of the dystrophic phenotype in mice via rAAV-mediated gene delivery (28,38,39). Engineered micro-dystrophin constructs retain domains that are critical for the function of dystrophin, yet are small enough to be packaged within the rAAV capsid (Figure 76.2).

Creating a novel truncated dystrophin gene that can be packaged into a rAAV genome requires careful selection of the domains and sub-domains to be included within the engineered construct. To retain mechanical function and protein stability, a micro-dystrophin must simultaneously bind to both γ-actin filaments and β-dystroglycan (38) (Figure 76.3). The dystrophin-deficient *mdx* mouse is a well-established rodent model for DMD and has been utilized to evaluate the functionality of multiple truncated dystrophin constructs (see Figure 76.2). Assays to gauge the quality of a construct typically include quantification of the percentage of centrally nucleated fibers, a hallmark of myofibers having undergone regeneration, sarcolemmal integrity, protection against myofiber necrosis and relevant mechanical properties compared to wild-type and *mdx* mice. Transgenic *mdx* mice expressing a micro-dystrophin possessing a C-terminal domain deletion and hinge 2 linked directly to spectrin-like repeat 24 (ΔR4-23,ΔCT) showed no signs of dystrophic histopathology and a near-normal frequency of centrally nucleated fibers. Specific force generation was increased in comparison to untreated controls, but was still lower than wild-type levels (38). While greater muscle function is attained by expressing larger mini-dystrophins, those larger clones can only be delivered with rAAV by either splitting the gene into two overlapping rAAV vectors that will allow recombination *in vivo* (42) or utilizing a virus with a larger carrying capacity (i.e. adenovirus or lentivirus) (19).

rAAV-Mediated Transduction of Striated Muscle in Large Animal Models

Encouraging results using rAAV vectors to delivery genes systemically to striated muscles of mice have prompted a series of feasibility studies in larger animal models. Initial gene transfer studies in canines using rAAV2 resulted in strong expression that persisted for more than three years following intravascular delivery into an isolated hindlimb (43). However, subsequent studies using AAV serotypes 2, 6, 8, and 9 have had difficulty achieving similar success due to a cellular immune response against the vectors. Both transgene products and rAAV capsid proteins have been suggested to cause inflammation and clearance of transduced cells in canine muscle (44–47). However, it was also found that transient immunosuppression could circumvent the cellular immune response and permit long-term transgene expression in canine skeletal muscles (45). rAAV6 gene delivery in immune-suppressed canines

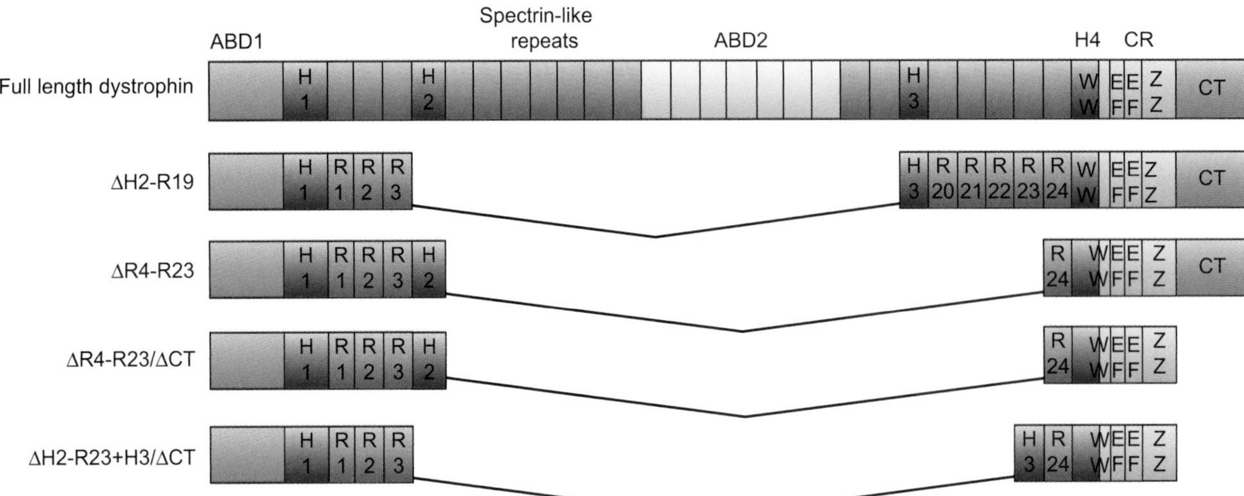

FIGURE 76.2 Schematic representation of domains of dystrophin and truncated dystrophin constructs. Full length dystrophin consists of an actin-binding domain (ABD1), four hinges (H1–4), 24 spectrin-like repeats (R1–R24) within which lies a second ABD (ABD2), a cysteine rich domain (CR), and the carboxy-terminal domain (CT). The CR contains 2 EF-hand regions and a zinc finger domain (ZZ) that together with a WW-domain in hinge 4 form the dystroglycan-binding site. Dystrophin also binds to α1, β1, and β2-syntrophin at the CT domain. A mini-dystrophin (ΔR4-R23) lacking 16 spectrin-like repeats was able to correct 95% of the morphological abnormalities in transgenic *mdx* mice and support near normal force development in skeletal muscles. A smaller construct (micro-dystrophin, ΔR4-R23) lacking an additional 4 spectrin-like repeats was able to prevent dystrophy in transgenic *mdx* mice but did not bring back as much strength as the larger mini-dystrophin (38). Further truncation of dystrophin by deletion of the CT domain (ΔR4-R23/ΔCT) did not further impair function (40). Recent work has shown that replacing hinge 2 with hinge 3 i (ΔH2-R23 + H3/ΔCT) significantly improves the functional capacity of truncated dystrophins (41). The full-length cDNA only fits into gutted or high-capacity adenoviral vectors, the larger mini-dystrophins can be delivered with lentiviral vectors, while the smallest micro-dystrophins can be systemically delivered using rAAV.

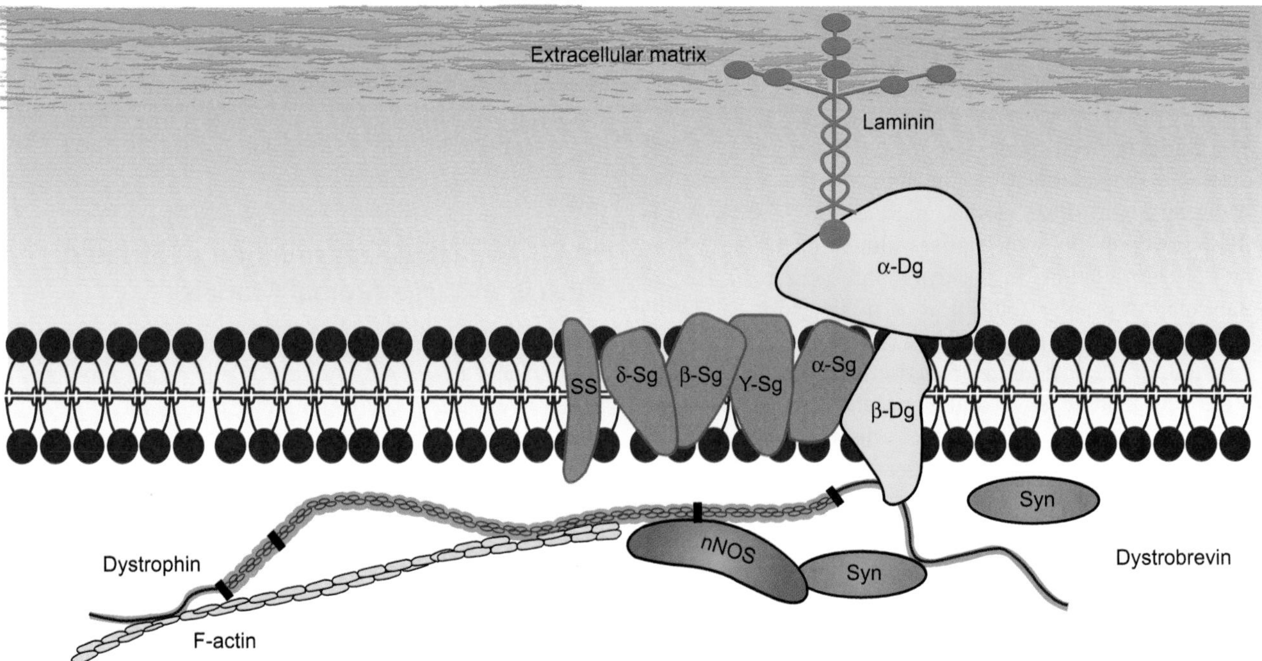

FIGURE 76.3 Model of dystrophin and the dystrophin–glycoprotein complex (DGC) in skeletal muscle. Dystrophin directs stable assembly of the DGC on the sarcolemma and mediates a strong, mechanical connection between the extracellular matrix and the subsarcolemmal actin cytoskeleton. nNOS, neuronal nitric oxide synthase; Syn, syntrophin; F-actin, filamentous γ-actin; SS, sarcospan; Sg, sarcoglycan; Dg, dystroglycan.

has led to successful and widespread transduction of striated muscle when administered at 2 months of age (48).

Intramuscular injection of rAAV1-CMV-erythropoietin into rhesus macaques resulted in more than 6 years of robust transgene expression (25). It is still unclear whether immunosuppression will be a necessary component of rAAV-mediated gene therapy, and there is no consensus for an immunosuppressive regimen that will result in optimal transduction. One group found that tolerance of the transgene product delivered to macaques by rAAV2 may be influenced by immunosuppressive drugs (49). In another study, the safety of delivering rAAV1 versus rAAV8 vectors was compared in macaques, where intramuscular and intravascular injections did not elicit a cellular immune response (50). In agreement with these findings, another group reported successful transduction of rAAV8-CMV-eGFP without immunomodulation (51). Differences between various studies may reflect differing doses and vector production methods, and further study will be necessary to clarify the nature of the rAAV-directed immune response in large animals and humans.

Regulating Muscle-specific Expression

Expression of full-length or truncated dystrophin at supraphysiological levels in transgenic mice has not been associated with detrimental effects. However, transgenic mouse models expressing these proteins were primarily generated using non-ubiquitously active promoters that restricted transgene expression to striated muscle (e.g., references 38,52). Conversely, viral-mediated dystrophin replacement studies typically utilized vectors with strong, ubiquitous viral promoters (e.g. Rous sarcoma virus and cytomegalovirus promoters and enhancers) (38,39,53). This raises concerns regarding off-target effects of exogenous expression following vector delivery to non-muscle tissues. The most implemented mechanism for achieving tissue-specific transgene expression has been through the use of muscle-specific promoters and enhancers. Regulatory elements derived from the muscle creatine kinase (MCK) gene are only active in differentiated myogenic cells and have demonstrated restricted expression within skeletal and cardiac muscle when delivered by adenovirus and multiple rAAV serotypes (26,54–56). Hybrid promoters incorporating enhancer and promoter regions of the α-myosin heavy chain and M-creatine kinase genes exhibit similar expression patterns and have gone through several generations of refinement (56,57). The synthetic promoter C5-12 has also demonstrated tissue-specific expression in both AAV1 and lentiviral vectors (58,59). These findings indicate the feasibility of utilizing tissue-specific regulatory elements to reduce the risk of off-target effects following vector delivery to non-muscle tissues.

rAAV Vectors for DMD in Clinical Trials

Plans are currently under way in several laboratories to test rAAV vectors in human clinical trials for treatment of DMD. These initial trials have been designed to determine safety and efficacy with relatively low doses. One study has already been completed, in which six DMD boys were intramuscularly injected with rAAV2.5-CMV-microdystrophin without immunosuppression. No expression of the transgene product was observed in any of the patients. However, vector genomes were detected in some of the muscle biopsies. The factors contributing to this failure to achieve expression are unclear, but the authors detected a T-cell mediated immune response against dystrophin in two of the six patients (60). If this T-cell mediated immune response contributed to a loss of dystrophin expression, then gene therapy approaches for DMD would need to be modified to prevent immune rejection of treated muscles. It should be noted that it remains unclear whether dystrophin immunity contributed to loss of expression, as most patients display revertant fiber expression of dystrophin without deleterious consequences, and one of the six treated patients in the rAAV trial had T-cell reactivity against revertant dystrophin even before initiation of the clinical trial. Still, if dystrophin immunogenicity does prove to be a limitation of gene therapy strategies then at least three approaches can be envisioned to prevent loss of expression. First, dystrophin gene delivery could be performed with the use of long-term immune suppression. Second, gene therapy vectors could incorporate a muscle-specific promoter to prevent antigen presentation in immune effector cells. Finally, one could perform gene therapy be delivering a non-immunogenic surrogate transgene, such as micro-utrophin (61).

CONCLUSIONS

Efforts to develop gene therapy for muscle disorders have utilized a wide array of different vector systems, gene regulatory elements, and transgenes. Currently, the only viral vector system showing significant potential for whole body gene delivery to skeletal and cardiac muscles are vectors derived from AAV. These vectors can achieve systemic gene transfer to striated muscles, and have been used in animal models to treat a variety of disorders caused by many recessively inherited mutations. Current efforts to deliver gene constructs expressing inhibitory RNAs may also allow this system to be applied to dominantly inherited disorders of muscle (62). The primary remaining obstacles to treatment of muscle disorders remain challenges related to the route of administration, dose, the use of immune suppressive strategies, and overall safety. Nonetheless, with the great progress witnessed over the past decade in treating mouse and canine models of muscle disorders, the clinical use of viral gene therapy for skeletal muscle appears to be within reach.

ACKNOWLEDGMENTS

We thank Lindsey Muir, Jane Seto, and Evan Thomas Schroeder for help with the figures.

REFERENCES

1. Doerfler W. In: Doerfler W, Becker Y, Hadar J, editors. *Adenovirus DNA, the viral genome and its expression*. Boston, MA: Martinus Nijhoff Publishing;1986.
2. Wilson JM. Adenoviruses as gene-delivery vehicles. *N Engl J Med* 1996;**334**:1185–7.
3. Brown BD, Shi CX, Powell S, Hurlbut D, Graham FL, Lillicrap D. Helper-dependent adenoviral vectors mediate therapeutic Factor VIII expression for several months with minimal accompanying toxicity in a canine model of severe hemophilia A. *Blood* 2004;**103**:804–10.
4. Ehrhardt A, Xu H, Dillow AM, Bellinger DA, Nichols TC, Kay MA. A gene-deleted adenoviral vector results in phenotypic correction of canine hemophilia b without liver toxicity or thrombocytopenia. *Blood* 2003;**102**:2403–11.
5. Huard J, Feero WG, Watkins SC, Hoffman EP, Rosenblatt DJ, Glorioso JC. The basal lamina is a physical barrier to herpes simplex virus-mediated gene delivery to mature muscle fibers. *J Virol* 1996;**70**:8117–23.
6. Nalbantoglu J, Pari G, Karpati G, Holland PC. Expression of the primary coxsackie and adenovirus receptor is downregulated during skeletal muscle maturation and limits the efficacy of adenovirus-mediated gene delivery to muscle cells. *Hum Gene Ther* 1999;**10**:1009–19.
7. Yang Y, Jooss KU, Su Q, Ertl HC, Wilson JM. Immune responses to viral antigens versus transgene product in the elimination of recombinant adenovirus-infected hepatocytes in vivo. *Gene Ther* 1996;**3**:137–44.
8. Alba R, Bosch A, Chillon M. Gutless adenovirus: last-generation adenovirus for gene therapy. *Gene Ther* 2005;**12**(Suppl. 1): S18–27.
9. DelloRusso C, Scott JM, Hartigan-O'Connor D, Salvatori G, Barjot C, Robinson AS, et al. Functional correction of adult *mdx* mouse muscle using gutted adenoviral vectors expressing full-length dystrophin. *Proc Natl Acad Sci USA* 2002;**99**:12979–84.
10. Hartigan-O'Connor D, Barjot C, Salvatori G, Chamberlain JS. Generation and growth of gutted adenoviral vectors. *Methods Enzymol.* 2002;**346**:224–46.
11. Hartigan-O'Connor D, Kirk CJ, Crawford R, Mule JJ, Chamberlain JS. Immune evasion by muscle-specific gene expression in dystrophic muscle. *Mol Ther* 2001;**4**:525–33.
12. Hauser MA, Robinson A, Hartigan-O'Connor D, Williams-Gregory DA, Buskin JN, Apone S, et al. Analysis of muscle creatine kinase regulatory elements in recombinant adenoviral vectors. *Mol Ther* 2000;**2**:16–25.
13. Escors D, Breckpot K. Lentiviral vectors in gene therapy: their current status and future potential. *Arch Immunol Ther Exp (Warsz)* 2010;**58**:107–19.
14. Vogt VM, Simon MN. Mass determination of rous sarcoma virus virions by scanning transmission electron microscopy. *J Virol* 1999;**73**:7050–5.
15. Li S, Kimura E, Fall BM, Reyes M, Angello JC, Welikson R, et al. Stable transduction of myogenic cells with lentiviral vectors expressing a minidystrophin. *Gene Ther* 2005;**12**:1099–108.
16. Peng KW, Pham L, Ye H, Zufferey R, Trono D, Cosset FL, et al. Organ distribution of gene expression after intravenous infusion of targeted and untargeted lentiviral vectors. *Gene Ther* 2001;**8**:1456–63.
17. MacKenzie TC, Kobinger GP, Louboutin JP, Radu A, Javazon EH, Sena-Esteves M, et al. Transduction of satellite cells after prenatal intramuscular administration of lentiviral vectors. *J Gene Med* 2005;**7**:50–8.
18. Talbot GE, Waddington SN, Bales O, Tchen RC, Antoniou MN. Desmin-regulated lentiviral vectors for skeletal muscle gene transfer. *Mol Ther* 2010;**18**:601–8.
19. Kimura E, Li S, Gregorevic P, Fall BM, Chamberlain JS. Dystrophin delivery to muscles of *mdx* mice using lentiviral vectors leads to myogenic progenitor targeting and stable gene expression. *Mol Ther* 2010;**18**:206–13.
20. Baum C. Insertional mutagenesis in gene therapy and stem cell biology. *Curr Opin Hematol* 2007;**14**:337–42.
21. Cavazzana-Calvo M, Fischer A. Gene therapy for severe combined immunodeficiency: are we there yet? *J Clin Invest* 2007;**117**:1456–65.
22. Kobinger GP, Louboutin JP, Barton ER, Sweeney HL, Wilson JM. Correction of the dystrophic phenotype by in vivo targeting of muscle progenitor cells. *Hum Gene Ther* 2003;**14**:1441–9.
23. Atchison RW, Casto BC, Hammon WM. Adenovirus-associated defective virus particles. *Science* 1965;**149**:754–6.
24. Nayak S, Herzog RW. Progress and prospects: immune responses to viral vectors. *Gene Ther* 2010;**17**:295–304.
25. Rivera VM, Gao GP, Grant RL, Schnell MA, Zoltick PW, Rozamus LW, et al. Long-term pharmacologically regulated expression of erythropoietin in primates following aav-mediated gene transfer. *Blood* 2005;**105**:1424–30.
26. Gregorevic P, Blankinship MJ, Allen JM, Crawford RW, Meuse L, Miller DG, et al. Systemic delivery of genes to striated muscles using adeno-associated viral vectors. *Nat Med* 2004;**10**:828–34.
27. Schultz BR, Chamberlain JS. Recombinant adeno-associated virus transduction and integration. *Mol Ther* 2008;**16**:1189–99.
28. Gregorevic P, Allen JM, Minami E, Blankinship MJ, Haraguchi M, Meuse L, et al. rAAV6-microdystrophin preserves muscle function and extends lifespan in severely dystrophic mice. *Nat Med* 2006;**12**:787–9.
29. Wang Z, Zhu T, Qiao C, Zhou L, Wang B, Zhang J, et al. Adeno-associated virus serotype 8 efficiently delivers genes to muscle and heart. *Nat Biotechnol* 2005;**23**:321–8.
30. Pacak CA, Mah CS, Thattaliyath BD, Conlon TJ, Lewis MA, Cloutier DE, et al. Recombinant adeno-associated virus serotype 9 leads to preferential cardiac transduction in vivo. *Circ Res* 2006;**99**:e3–9.
31. Zincarelli C, Soltys S, Rengo G, Rabinowitz JE. Analysis of AAV serotypes 1-9 mediated gene expression and tropism in mice after systemic injection. *Mol Ther* 2008;**16**:1073–80.
32. Zincarelli C, Soltys S, Rengo G, Koch WJ, Rabinowitz JE. Comparative cardiac gene delivery of adeno-associated virus

serotypes 1-9 reveals that AAV6 mediates the most efficient transduction in mouse heart. *Clin Transl Sci* 2011;**3**:81–9.
33. Nakai H, Montini E, Fuess S, Storm TA, Grompe M, Kay MA. AAV serotype 2 vectors preferentially integrate into active genes in mice. *Nat Genet* 2003;**34**:297–302.
34. Inagaki K, Lewis SM, Wu X, Ma C, Munroe DJ, Fuess S, et al. DNA palindromes with a modest arm length of greater, similar 20 base pairs are a significant target for recombinant adeno-associated virus vector integration in the liver, muscles, and heart in mice. *J Virol* 2007;**81**:11290–303.
35. Halbert CL, Miller AD, McNamara S, Emerson J, Gibson RL, Ramsey B, et al. Prevalence of neutralizing antibodies against adeno-associated virus (AAV) types 2, 5, and 6 in cystic fibrosis and normal populations: implications for gene therapy using AAV vectors. *Hum Gene Ther* 2006;**17**:440–7.
36. Emery AE, Muntoni F. *Duchenne muscular dystrophy*. Oxford: Oxford University Press;2003.
37. Koenig M, Beggs AH, Moyer M, Scherpf S, Heindrich K, Bettecken T, et al. The molecular basis for Duchenne versus Becker muscular dystrophy: correlation of severity with type of deletion. *Am J Hum Genet* 1989;**45**:498–506.
38. Harper SQ, Hauser MA, DelloRusso C, Duan D, Crawford RW, Phelps SF, et al. Modular flexibility of dystrophin: implications for gene therapy of Duchenne muscular dystrophy. *Nat Med* 2002;**8**:253–61.
39. Sakamoto M, Yuasa K, Yoshimura M, Yokota T, Ikemoto T, Suzuki M, et al. Micro-dystrophin cDNA ameliorates dystrophic phenotypes when introduced into *mdx* mice as a transgene. *Biochem Biophys Res Commun* 2002;**293**:1265–72.
40. Gregorevic P, Blankinship MJ, Allen JM, Chamberlain JS. Systemic microdystrophin gene delivery improves skeletal muscle structure and function in old dystrophic *mdx* mice. *Mol Ther* 2008;**16**:657–64.
41. Banks GB, Judge LM, Allen JM, Chamberlain JS. The polyproline site in hinge 2 influences the functional capacity of truncated dystrophins. *PLoS Genet* 2010;**6**:e1000958.
42. Odom GL, Gregorevic P, Allen JM, Chamberlain JS. Gene therapy of mdx mice with large truncated dystrophins generated by recombination using rAAV6. *Mol Ther* 2011;**19**:36–45.
43. Arruda VR, Stedman HH, Nichols TC, Haskins ME, Nicholson M, Herzog RW, et al. Regional intravascular delivery of AAV-2-FIX to skeletal muscle achieves long-term correction of hemophilia b in a large animal model. *Blood* 2005;**105**:3458–64.
44. Wang Z, Allen JM, Riddell SR, Gregorevic P, Storb R, Tapscott SJ, et al. Immunity to adeno-associated virus-mediated gene transfer in a random-bred canine model of Duchenne muscular dystrophy. *Hum Gene Ther* 2007;**18**:18–26.
45. Wang Z, Kuhr CS, Allen JM, Blankinship M, Gregorevic P, Chamberlain JS, et al. Sustained AAV-mediated dystrophin expression in a canine model of Duchenne muscular dystrophy with a brief course of immunosuppression. *Mol Ther* 2007;**15**:1160–6.
46. Yuasa K, Yoshimura M, Urasawa N, Ohshima S, Howell JM, Nakamura A, et al. Injection of a recombinant AAV serotype 2 into canine skeletal muscles evokes strong immune responses against transgene products. *Gene Ther* 2007;**14**:1249–60.
47. Yuasa K, Sakamoto M, Miyagoe-Suzuki Y, Tanouchi A, Yamamoto H, Li J, et al. Adeno-associated virus vector-mediated gene transfer into dystrophin-deficient skeletal muscles evokes enhanced immune response against the transgene product. *Gene Ther* 2002;**9**:1576–88.
48. Gregorevic P, Schultz BR, Allen JM, Halldorson JB, Blankinship MJ, Meznarich NA, et al. Evaluation of vascular delivery methodologies to enhance rAAV6-mediated gene transfer to canine striated musculature. *Mol Ther* 2009;**17**:1427–33.
49. Mingozzi F, Hasbrouck NC, Basner-Tschakarjan E, Edmonson SA, Hui DJ, Sabatino DE, et al. Modulation of tolerance to the transgene product in a nonhuman primate model of AAV-mediated gene transfer to liver. *Blood* 2007;**110**:2334–41.
50. Toromanoff A, Cherel Y, Guilbaud M, Penaud-Budloo M, Snyder RO, Haskins ME, et al. Safety and efficacy of regional intravenous (R.I.) versus intramuscular (I.M.) delivery of rAAV1 and rAAV8 to nonhuman primate skeletal muscle. *Mol Ther* 2008;**16**:1291–9.
51. Rodino-Klapac LR, Janssen PM, Montgomery CL, Coley BD, Chicoine LG, Clark KR, et al. A translational approach for limb vascular delivery of the micro-dystrophin gene without high volume or high pressure for treatment of Duchenne muscular dystrophy. *J Transl Med* 2007;**5**:45.
52. Cox GA, Cole NM, Matsumura K, Phelps SF, Hauschka SD, Campbell KP, et al. Overexpression of dystrophin in transgenic *mdx* mice eliminates dystrophic symptoms without toxicity. *Nature* 1993;**364**:725–9.
53. Wang B, Li J, Xiao X. Adeno-associated virus vector carrying human minidystrophin genes effectively ameliorates muscular dystrophy in *mdx* mouse model. *Proc Natl Acad Sci USA* 2000;**97**:13714–9.
54. Hauser MA, Robinson A, Hartigan-O'Connor D, Williams-Gregory DA, Buskin JN, Apone S, et al. Analysis of muscle creatine kinase regulatory elements in recombinant adenoviral vectors. *Mol Ther* 2000;**2**:16–25.
55. Donoviel DB, Shield MA, Buskin JN, Haugen HS, Clegg CH, Hauschka SD. Analysis of muscle creatine kinase gene regulatory elements in skeletal and cardiac muscles of transgenic mice. *Mol Cell Biol* 1996;**16**:1649–58.
56. Salva MZ, Himeda CL, Tai PW, Nishiuchi E, Gregorevic P, Allen JM, et al. Design of tissue-specific regulatory cassettes for high-level rAAV-mediated expression in skeletal and cardiac muscle. *Mol Ther* 2007;**15**:320–9.
57. Sun B, Young SP, Li P, Di C, Brown T, Salva MZ, et al. Correction of multiple striated muscles in murine pompe disease through adeno-associated virus-mediated gene therapy. *Mol Ther* 2008;**16**:1366–71.
58. Liu YL, Mingozzi F, Rodriguez-Colon SM, Joseph S, Dobrzynski E, Suzuki T, et al. Therapeutic levels of factor IX expression using a muscle-specific promoter and adeno-associated virus serotype 1 vector. *Hum Gene Ther* 2004;**15**:783–92.
59. Richard E, Douillard-Guilloux G, Batista L, Caillaud C. Correction of glycogenosis type 2 by muscle-specific lentiviral vector. *In Vitro Cell Dev Biol Anim* 2008;**44**:397–406.
60. Mendell JR, Campbell K, Rodino-Klapac L, Sahenk Z, Shilling C, Lewis S, et al. Dystrophin immunity in Duchenne's muscular dystrophy. *N Engl J Med* 2010;**363**:1429–37.
61. Odom GL, Gregorevic P, Allen JM, Finn E, Chamberlain JS. Microutrophin delivery through rAAV6 increases lifespan and improves muscle function in dystrophic dystrophin/utrophin-deficient mice. *Mol Ther* 2008;**16**:1539–45.
62. Arnett AL, Chamberlain JR, Chamberlain JS. Therapy for neuromuscular disorders. *Curr Opin Genet Dev* 2009;**19**:290–7.

Chapter 77

Cell-Based Therapies in Skeletal Muscle Disease

Denis Vallese, Erica Yada, Gillian Butler-Browne and Vincent Mouly
Université Pierre et Marie Curie-Paris 6, UM76, INSERM U974, and CNRS UMR 7215, Institut de Myologie, Paris, France

THERAPEUTIC STRATEGIES FOR MUSCULAR DYSTROPHIES

Muscular dystrophies are clinically and molecularly heterogeneous diseases characterized by muscle weakness, muscle wasting, and degeneration, affecting both children and adults (1). The majority of muscular dystrophies are caused by mutations in genes coding for proteins either associated with the muscle cell membrane, such as the dystrophin–glycoprotein complex (DGC) (2) or the extracellular matrix, such as laminin 2 and collagen VI (3), or the nuclear membrane such as lamin A/C or emerin (4); see www.musclegenetable.org/ for an updated table of genetic neuromuscular disorders.

Duchenne muscular dystrophy (DMD) has been an early target for cell therapy. DMD is the most common form of muscular dystrophy, since it occurs at a rate of approximately 1 in 3500 male births, and also one of the most severe, with onset in early childhood and progressive muscle wasting and weakness that leads to death in the third decade of life (1). So far, the only clinical treatments for DMD patients are limited to supportive care, such as surgery, corticosteroid administration for muscle weakness, ventilation for respiratory failure, and physiotherapy. These treatments result in amelioration of symptoms and improved quality of life (5). However, these corrective therapies show many side effects, such as weight gain and osteoporosis with the risk of bone fractures (6). Consequently, new pharmacological, gene-based and cell-based therapeutic strategies have been developed (7–9).

The major goals of many of the pharmacological therapies are either to delay the onset of pathological features, counteracting the consequences of the dystrophic process, or to ameliorate the muscle function by means of anti-inflammatory molecules or other drugs, such as protease inhibitors, calcium blockers or drugs that act on protein and lipid metabolism (10). For example, the upregulation of utrophin, an autosomal homologue of dystrophin, could be an alternative strategy to treat DMD patients, since its increased expression in *mdx* mice has been shown to prevent/reduce the dystrophic phenotype (11).

Anti-inflammatory drugs, such as glucocorticoids, have been shown to be effective in slowing the progression of the disease in DMD patients (6,12). Although steroid-induced side effects can be serious (e.g. weight gain, bone fractures, etc.), the treatment with anti-inflammatory drugs has been shown to prolong ambulation considerably and reduce the incidence of severe scoliosis (7).

Another promising pharmacological approach is based on the read-through of stop codons. Nonsense mutations (deletion or substitution of a single DNA base that leads to the formation of a premature stop codon) will cause the premature termination of the protein translation. Over 10 years ago, Barton-Davis et al. showed that administration of the aminoglycoside antibiotic gentamicin led to the read-through of the stop mutation in the *mdx* mouse and the production of significant quantities of dystrophin (13). A similar approach is now used in clinical trials by PTC pharmaceutics/Genzyme with PTC124 (14).

Gene therapy, in contrast, directly targets the genetic defects, attempting to overcome pathological mutations by providing the muscle with the correct form of the gene or by correcting the protein by using a gene splicing approach to restore the reading frame using exon-skipping vectors (8,15). While exon skipping strategy is now being tested in clinical trials following the first proofs of concept using oligonucleotides (16) and morpholinos (17), recent years have seen the development of other vectors, such as U7-based viral vectors (18), as well as a number of other strategies and tools for effective gene replacement therapies. Although this is in theory the simplest approach for the treatment of genetic diseases such as muscular dystrophies, its application to muscle diseases has faced problems common to other genetic diseases, such as ectopic gene expression, immune modulation

Muscle. DOI: http://dx.doi.org/10.1016/B978-0-12-381510-1.00077-6

against the vector and the transgene expression product itself, vector design and production, and also problems specific to muscular dystrophy, such as gene delivery to the majority of muscle fibers (19,20).

Cell therapy is based on stem cell-driven muscle regeneration, by local or systemic injections of precursor cells. Transplanted cells must be able to fuse with existing myofibers or form new muscle fibers, and transplanted cell nuclei, which are incorporated into the myofibers, will express the missing gene product. In addition to regeneration of myofibers, a major goal of stem cell therapies is the reconstitution of the satellite cell niche, which promotes future functional regeneration of the muscle.

Cell transplantation therapy was first explored in the mouse as early as 1978 by T. Partridge and colleagues (21). The positive results obtained in animal models led to several clinical trials in the early 1990s that demonstrated the safety of the technique but did not show functional benefits in the injected muscles. Failure was mainly due to the poor survival and migration of injected myoblasts and, in some cases, also to the host's immune response against transplanted cells (9). Among all myopathies, DMD has been the major target of myogenic cell transplantation, due to the existence of an animal model, the *mdx* mouse, lacking dystrophin (22). Two strategies are possible: (i) *heterologous* transplantation (also termed allotransplantation), when cells from a healthy donor are used; or (ii) *autologous* transplantation, when healthy cells from the patient himself are used. Both strategies are associated with distinct benefits and risks that should be taken into account when deciding which treatment a patient should undergo. In the case of heterologous transplantation the main hurdle is to find a suitable immunocompatible donor, with the potential risk of immune rejection if HLA (human leukocyte antigens, also known as MHC, major histocompatibility complex) matching is not achieved closely enough (for a review see 23).

In the case of an autologous transplantation the donor cells isolated from the patient must be derived from healthy or non-affected muscles. While this is applicable to some diseases such as oculo-pharyngeal muscular dystrophy (OPMD) where very few muscles are targeted by the disease (24), in most muscular dystrophies the cells would have to be genetically corrected, in order to restore the expression of the mutated protein.

CELL CANDIDATES

The ideal cell candidate for cell transplantation therapy should fulfill several criteria: (i) be easily expandable *in vitro* without losing their "stem-cell" and myogenic properties, in order to both replenish the satellite cell niche and repair/replace damaged fibers once injected *in situ*; (ii) for whole body treatment they should be able to be deliverable systemically, in order to reach all affected muscles; (iii) be able to survive, proliferate and migrate throughout the entire host muscle.

Over the past years several different types of precursor cells have been identified, characterized, and are now being considered for cell therapy approaches (25,26), these are summarized in Table 77.1 and will be discussed in detail below.

Satellite Cells

The most obvious candidates for cell therapy of muscular dystrophies are the **satellite cells**, which are called myoblasts when expanded *in vitro*. These cells were first identified over 40 years ago (27) and since then they have been clearly established to be the adult skeletal muscle stem cell (28). Located between the basal lamina and the sarcolemma of the muscle fiber, they are ideally positioned to repair degenerating muscle fibers. In mature skeletal muscle they are in quiescent state but are activated in response to muscle damage (Figure 77.1) or increased muscle load (29). The activation and proliferation of satellite cells during muscle regeneration is mainly controlled by two transcription factors, Myf5 and MyoD (30,31), and is followed by differentiation to form new myotubes. A small number of cells do not undergo terminal differentiation but restore the reserve pool of quiescent muscle stem cells available to mediate further cycles of muscle regeneration (32).

In mice, satellite cells are most abundant at birth (20%) (33) and their frequency declines to stabilize to between 1% and 5% of skeletal muscle nuclei in adult mice (34). In humans, the proportion of satellite cells in skeletal muscles also decreases with age, which could explain the decreased efficiency of muscle regeneration in older subjects, when the satellite cells will represent only 1–0.5% of the muscle nuclei (35). An essential parameter for cell therapy is their identification/purification. For years the characterization of satellite cells was made on the basis of electron microscopy. The discovery of numerous molecular markers, which can be used either to identify satellite cells on sections or to purify them using surface markers, has radically changed the field. Currently the most widely used markers in the mouse are Pax7, M-cadherin, caveolin-1, CD34, $\alpha7\beta1$ integrin, SM/C 2.6 (36) and syndecan 3 and 4 (32,37), whereas CD56/NCAM, a surface marker which, although not entirely satellite cell specific, has been used to purify these cells from mouse and humans muscles, and Pax7, a nuclear transcription factor, have been used in humans (38). The combination of these two latter markers with laminin

TABLE 77.1 Cell Candidates for Cell Therapy Strategies

Cell Type	Source	Molecular Markers	Proliferation	Myogenic Differentiation	Alternative Lineage Potential	Systemic Delivery
Myoblasts	Skeletal muscle	CD56, M-cadherin, MyoD caveolin-1, Pax7, Desmin, SM/C 2.6	+++	Spontaneous	Osteogenic and adipogenic differentiation	No
Perivascular cells (mesoangioblast-like cells/ pericytes)	Skeletal muscle (fetal/adult), pancreas (fetal/adult), placenta, white adipose tissue, fetal heart, fetal skin, lungs, brain, eyes, gut, bone marrow, umbilical cord	ALP, PDGF-Rβ, CD146, α-SMA, NG2, CD44	+++	Spontaneous (skeletal muscle, placenta, white adipose tissue, pancreas). Not described for other origins	Chondrogenic, osteogenic and adipogenic differentiation	Yes
Myo-endothelial cells	Skeletal muscle	CD56, CD34, CD144	+++	Spontaneous	Chondrogenic, osteogenic differentiation	Not tested
CD133$^+$	Pheripheral blood	CD133, CD34, CD90, CD45, CD44, LFA-1$^+$ PSGL-1, VLA-4, L selectin, CXCR4	–	Induced by C2C12 co-culture	Myeloid and endothelial differentiation	Yes
	Skeletal muscle	CD133, CD34 (d), CXCR4	+++	Spontaneous, but limited	Endothelial differentiation	Yes
SMALD (ALDH$^+$ CD34$^-$)	Skeletal muscle	ALDH br, SSClow	+++	Spontaneous	Osteogenic differentiation	Not tested
PICs (PW1 interstitial cells)	Skeletal muscle	PW1$^+$, Pax7$^-$	+++	Spontaneous (skeletal and smooth muscle)	Not tested	Not tested
hMADs (MSCs from adipose tissue)	Adipose tissue	CD44, CD105, CD90, CD13, CD49b, HLADR$^-$	+++	myoD, myogenin and desmin expression. No myotube formation	Osteoegnic and adipogenic differentiation	Not tested
MSCs (from synovial membrane)	Synovial membranes	CD71 CD90 CD29 CD44 CD49b CD49d CD49e CD54 CD106 CXCR4, CD14$^-$ CD45$^-$	+++	Sporadic myogenic differentiation	Osteogenic, chondrogenic and adipogenic differentiation	Yes

+++ = good proliferation rate,– = low proliferation rate; (d) = dystrophic sample; ALDH = aldehyde dehydrogenase 1A1; hMAD = human mesenchymal stem cell from adipose tissue; MSC = mesenchymal stem cell.

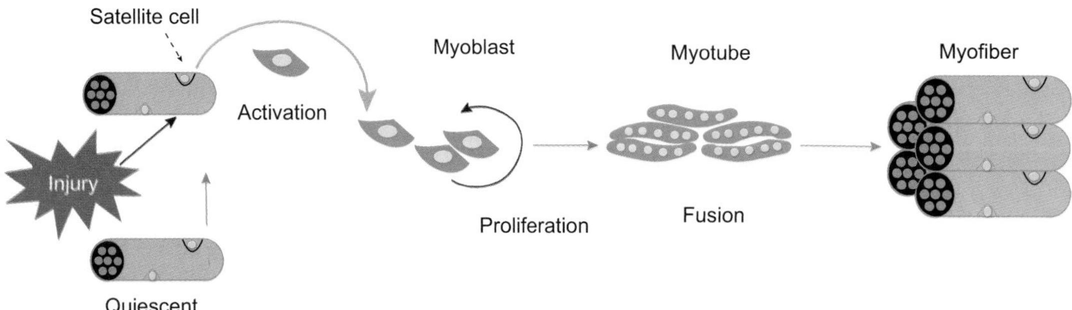

FIGURE 77.1 Satellite cells. Satellite cells are located beneath the basal lamina of muscle fibers and are normally in a quiescent state. They can become activated following mechanical stimulus or injury and then start to proliferate. Some of them differentiate to form multinucleated myofibers, whereas some others do not undergo terminal differentiation but restore the reserve pool of quiescent cells available to mediate further cycles of muscle regeneration.

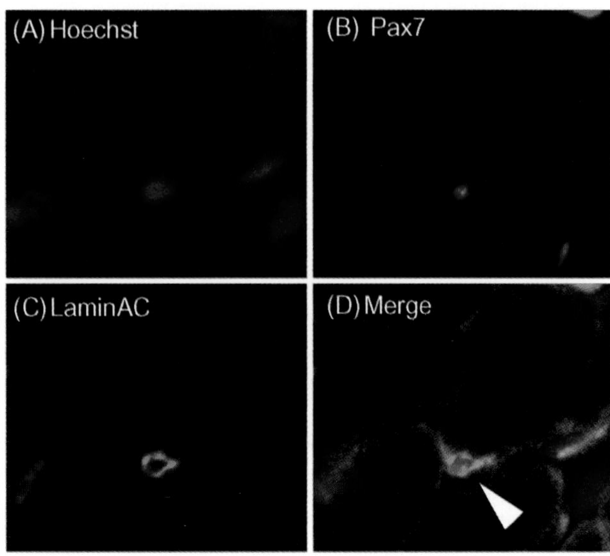

FIGURE 77.2 Satellite cell localization and identification by Pax7 expression. Human myoblasts injected into an immunodeficient mouse muscle are found in satellite cell position, located between the sarcolemma and the basal lamina (laminin staining in grey, D), one month after transplantation. Human cells are stained with laminAC (green, C and D), satellite cells (white arrow, D) are identified with a staining for Pax7 (red, B and D).

staining (for basal membrane identification) is the most valid method to identify human satellite cells in their *in vivo* niche (37,38) (Table 77.1, Figure 77.2).

Numerous trials aiming at reconstituting skeletal muscle in human muscle diseases (mainly DMD) using myoblast transfer therapy have been carried out over the past 20 years, and have provided many lessons concerning the hurdles that still remain to be faced in order to optimize cell therapy strategies. Isolation and expansion of myoblasts is feasible *in vitro*, and they were thus chosen as the first candidate cell to be tested for cell therapy. Myoblast transplantation was first explored in the mouse in 1978 by T. Partridge and colleagues (21), who showed that injecting normal healthy myoblasts into the tibialis muscle of an *mdx* mouse resulted in the restoration of dystrophin expression to the entire muscle. Many subsequent studies confirmed these results using myoblasts from newborn (39) or adult mice (40,41) as well as human myoblasts (42). These very promising preliminary results led to several clinical trials in the 1990s that, overall, failed to provide to the patients any relevant clinical benefit. The most commonly encountered difficulties were the poor survival of cells, the limited dispersion from the injection site, immunorejection of allogenic cells, and inefficient myogenic contribution (9). When applied in mice, muscle damage or irradiation (39,43) can improve the migration of myoblasts, but owing to obvious ethical reasons such a protocol is not clinically relevant. In a more clinical context, Skuk and colleagues were able to improve cell dispersion by performing multiple injections 1 mm apart (44). Although this was shown to greatly improve muscle reconstitution, this protocol remains more pertinent in the case of muscle dystrophies where only a limited number of small muscles are involved and would consequently only require a localized tissue repair, e.g. OPMD or facioscapulohumeral dystrophy (FSHD), for which cell therapy clinical trials are ongoing.

To further improve dispersion of transplanted cells, systemic injection could be a possible solution, but this strategy has been excluded for myoblasts following a study that demonstrated that they were unable to cross the endothelial wall (45).

More recent experimental studies on muscle satellite cells have used new powerful approaches, e.g. single fiber isolation, purification of satellite cells or subpopulations by FACS sorting followed by direct *in vivo* injection in the absence of *in vitro* amplification (46–48). Although these approaches showed better efficiency compared to those obtained using *in vitro* expanded myoblasts, their clinical application is not trivial.

At present, although myoblast transplantation can be applied to limited targets, such as pharyngeal muscles in OPMD patients, we are still a long way from a wide clinical application of myoblast transfer therapy. However, newly discovered myogenic stem cells, which are described in more details in the following sections, raise new hopes for cell therapy in muscular dystrophies.

Mesoangioblasts

So far, the most promising cells that can be delivered systemically to skeletal muscle are mesoangioblasts (or pericytes) (45,49) (for a review see 50) and cells derived from muscle that express the stem cell marker CD/AC133 (51) (next section).

Mesoangioblasts were initially isolated from the dorsal aorta of mouse embryos (52) but more recently this class of vessel-associated stem cells have also been characterized in dogs (53) and humans (45). The behavior of these cells in humans has been well characterized both *in vitro* and *in vivo*: adult cells do not express endothelial markers, but instead express markers of pericytes, such as NG2 proteoglycan and alkaline phosphatase (ALP), and can be easily isolated from freshly dissociated ALP^+ cells. These pericyte-derived cells readily proliferate *in vitro* and spontaneously differentiate into myosin heavy chain (MyHC)-expressing myotubes. Their ability to contribute to muscle regeneration has been tested in both mice and dogs. Arterial injections of *wild-type* mouse-derived mesoangioblasts into female α-sarcoglycan null dystrophic mice restored the expression of α-sarcoglycan and the dystrophin–glycoprotein complex (49). Interestingly, similar results were obtained in GRMD dystrophin-deficient dogs (53). Human-derived cells also showed good myogenic regeneration *in vivo*, when injected into the femoral artery of *scid/mdx* female mice, and were able to colonize the host muscle, either fuse to muscle fibers and express dystrophin, or localize to the satellite cell position and express typical satellite cell markers (45). Similarly, mesoangioblasts derived from DMD patients, transduced with a lentiviral vector expressing human mini-dystrophin (45), were able to reach the skeletal muscle tissue and participate to host muscle regeneration after intra-arterial injection in *scid/mdx* mice (45). Based on the positive results obtained with the above-mentioned studies, a phase I clinical trial using mesoangioblasts allotransplantation in DMD patients has been initiated in 2011 (26).

$CD133^+$ Cells

The glycosylated epitope CD133, normally expressed on circulating human hematopoietic/endothelial progenitors, has been recently used to identify a new cell subpopulation with myogenic capacities in the peripheral blood (54). These cells, called $CD133^+$ (or $AC133^+$), when co-cultured with mouse myoblasts or with Wnt-expressing cells, were able to form MyHC-expressing myotubes *in vitro*, and to participate to muscle regeneration and replenish the satellite cell compartment *in vivo*, when injected into dystrophic muscles of *scid/mdx* mice (54).

Recently, the *in vivo* regenerative potential of human skeletal muscle-derived $CD133^+$ cells has been quantified and compared with that of human myoblasts. After intramuscular injection into the cryo-damaged muscles of $Rag2^-\ \gamma C^-\ C5^-$ immunodeficient mice, $CD133^+$ cells showed a greater regenerative capacity in terms of number of fibers expressing human proteins and number of human cells in a satellite cell position, than *bona fide* satellite cell-derived myoblasts (51). Due to the promising results obtained in mice, a phase I clinical trial has been performed to confirm the safety of autologous transplantation of muscle-derived $CD133^+$ stem cells in DMD patients (55) and neither local nor systemic side effects were observed (55).

Side Population (SP) Cells

Side population (SP) cells are defined as the cell fraction that efficiently excludes Hoechst 33342 dye (DNA binding dye), and therefore shows a unique pattern on fluorescence-activated cell sorting (FACS) analysis (56). This cell population was initially described in bone marrow cultures, but has been identified consequently in several other tissues, such as liver, lung, kidney, brain, heart, and skeletal muscle. SP cells can differentiate into several lineages *in vitro*, e.g. adipocyte and osteocyte (57), but they do not differentiate into myotubes unless they are co-cultured with myoblasts (57,58), although they can be directed towards myogenic differentiation in response to the muscle environment, and have been shown to be also capable of giving rise to skeletal muscle and satellite cells *in vivo* (58). It has been established that SP cells are not derived from satellite cells because of the specific surface marker that they express (59).

The SP cell fraction is a heterogeneous cell population: more than half of the muscle-derived SP cells are $CD34^+$, and almost the entire fraction (90%) is also Sca-1^+ (57). The majority of muscle SP cells are positive for CD31, a marker of endothelial cells, and the $CD31^-CD45^-$ subfraction, whose number and ratio increase during muscle regeneration (57), can differentiate into myogenic, adipogenic, and osteogenic lineages *in vitro*, although it has a limited myogenic potential *in vivo* compared to satellite cells. In addition, it has been recently shown that this SP cell subfraction can support muscle regeneration by promoting proliferation and migration of myoblasts (60).

ES and iPS Cells

Embryonic stem (ES) cells are totipotent stem cells, able to differentiate into all types of somatic and germ-line tissues *in vitro* (61). ES cells have a high potential of proliferation and differentiation, therefore the differentiation process must be carefully controlled, in order to specifically guide the cells into the myogenic lineage and avoid the formation of teratomas, one of the major hurdles faced during ES cell-based therapies. The teratoma formation results from the presence of residual undifferentiated ES cells (62) and depends on the stages of embryogenesis or fetal development (63).

Several reports have indicated that mouse ES cells can be induced to differentiate into muscle fibers if myogenic genes, such as MyoD or IGF-II, are transfected into the cells (64,65). Recently, Chang and colleagues have described a new method to induce the differentiation of mouse ES cells into the skeletal muscle lineage (66): briefly, they modified the ES cell culture conditions in order to obtain more Pax7 positive cells, which were then FACS sorted using the SM/C 2.6 antibody. These sorted cells were able to generate muscle fibers both *in vitro* and *in vivo*, even after long-term engraftment (up to 24 weeks) (66).

Human ES cells were first established by Thomson et al. in 1998 (67); however, the ethical issues linked to their use are still a matter of debate. Barberi et al. described the derivation of multipotent mesenchymal precursors from human ES cells (68), however their study was limited to the qualitative detection of donor-derived differentiated cells in mouse recipient muscle upon injection of hESCs (human embryonic stem cells).

In 2006, Yamanaka and his colleagues established a new stem cell population, named induced pluripotent stem (iPS) cells, by reprogramming mouse fibroblasts with four transcription factors, Oct3/4, Sox2, KLF4 and c-Myc using retroviral vectors (69). iPS cells have been shown to be functionally equivalent to ES cells, as they express ES cell markers, have similar gene expression profiles, form teratomas when injected into immunodeficient mouse, and contribute to the cell types of chimeric animals, including the germ line. Moreover, Park et al. showed that it is also possible to generate iPS cells from DMD and BMD patient fibroblasts (70), thus increasing the hopes for possible future applications in cell therapy for DMD. In addition, it has been demonstrated that iPS cells, derived either from *mdx* mice or DMD patients, can be genetically corrected using a human artificial chromosome (HAC) containing the genomic dystrophin sequence (71). As mentioned above, the generation of iPS cell was initially obtained using 4 growth factors, which included an oncogene, c-Myc. Many studies have tried to reduce or replace the use of these genes (72–74), although, at present, no chemical compound can entirely replace the function of these transduced transcription factors.

This iPS approach avoids the ethical issues related to the use of ES cells, and allows the generation of autologous pluripotent stem cells, although the control of their differentiation is as critical as for ES cells.

Mesenchymal Stem Cells (MSCs)

Mesenchymal stem cells or multipotent stromal cells (MSCs) represent a heterogeneous subset of non-hematopoietic cells that can be identified in many tissues, including umbilical cord blood, placenta, adipose tissue, liver, muscle, synovial membrane and bone marrow (75,76). They can differentiate into mesodermal lineages, including adipose tissue, cartilage and muscle (77–79) and can form contractile myotubes *in vitro* (80).

MSCs can be identified by several markers (CD73, CD90 and CD105) – although none of these is MSC-specific – and by the lack of expression of hematopoietic antigens (CD45, CD34 and CD14 or CD11b, CD19 and HLA-DR) (81). MSCs have also been proposed to evade or modulate the immunological responses, which may be important for the induction of immunotolerance or to minimize the rejection of allogenic transplantation following cell therapy (82), although they may become targets of the immune system when they engage into a differentiation pathway.

Numerous papers have described the use of MSCs in cell therapies for DMD. MSCs have been shown to have myogenic potential in the *mdx* mouse (83), and Ferrari et al. showed that adherent MSCs derived from bone marrow could migrate into the regenerating muscle and participate to the regeneration giving rise to differentiated myofibers, although with a very low efficiency (84). More recently, adherent MSCs derived from human bone marrow were engrafted into *mdx*-nude mice and human dystrophin positive fibers could be detected two weeks after injection (85). The therapeutic potential of MSCs in skeletal muscle still needs to be confirmed, since their efficiency is very low, although their immunomodulating potential is promising.

Skeletal Muscle Aldehyde Dehydrogenase-Positive Cells (SMALD)

Recently, a new cell population has been identified in human skeletal muscle on the basis of aldehyde dehydrogenase 1A1 (ALDH) enzymatic activity. This enzymatic activity is known to be a characteristic feature of human bone marrow, umbilical cord/peripheral blood progenitors and was also found within the skeletal muscle, as shown by Vauchez and colleagues (86). This newly discovered ALDH$^+$ cell population can be divided into two sub-populations, according to the expression of the marker CD34, and only the CD34$^-$ fraction could develop CD56$^+$ myoblast *in vitro* that were able to form multinucleated myotubes.

Moreover, only the ALDH$^+$/CD34$^-$ population showed a strong myogenic potential *in vivo* after injection into irradiated and notexin-treated muscles of *scid* mice. The grafted cells were able to efficiently participate to muscle regeneration and localize in a satellite cell position (86). Although further studies are required for a more complete characterization, especially concerning their *in vivo* behavior, these new muscle progenitors demonstrate a good potential for cell therapy.

PW1$^+$/Pax7$^-$ Interstitial Cells (PICs)

Recently, the group of D. Sassoon has discovered a new population of muscle-resident stem cells in the mouse, called PW1$^+$/Pax7$^-$ interstitial cells (PICs), located within the interstitial space of skeletal muscle (87). These PICs show bipotential behavior *in vitro*, being able to differentiate towards the myogenic lineage and to generate both smooth and skeletal muscle. These cells were shown to be able to participate to myogenesis *in vivo* and contribute to skeletal muscle regeneration, at levels comparable to those obtained with freshly isolated satellite cells, when injected into cryo-damaged muscles of immunodeficient mice (87), although it is not yet clear whether these cells can be delivered *via* the system circulation and whether they represent in humans a population distinct from the CD133$^+$ and SMALD myogenic precursors.

GENETIC MANIPULATION FOR AUTOLOGOUS CELL THERAPY

Correction of the genetic defect in the transplanted cells would permit the use of autologous instead of heterologous donor-derived cells, thus avoiding concomitant immunosuppressive treatments. The majority of recent studies have addressed DMD, since it is the most common form of muscular dystrophy, and many synthetic quasi-, mini- and micro- dystrophin genes have been developed, in order to fit DNA packaging limitations given by viral vectors capacity. These are truncated versions of the dystrophin cDNA, which however retain only a partial functionality, thus providing a possible molecular rescue. However, the site of insertion of these constructs would have to be carefully monitored to avoid tumorigenicity.

As mentioned above in the iPS section, Kazuki et al. have recently validated the use of a human artificial chromosome (HAC) to restore full-length dystrophin in mouse and human iPS cells (71), and this would therefore avoid the use of truncated dystrophin isoforms, which have lost part of their functionality.

CLINICAL TRIALS

Attempts to reconstitute skeletal muscle in muscular dystrophy patients through myoblast transplantation started more than twenty years ago and it has mainly involved patients suffering from DMD. A number of clinical trials have been made (Table 77.2), all being encouraged by the promising results obtained in animal models. Different parameters have changed, single vs. multiple injections, the number of injected cells, the bolus volume, and the injection technique (88). The positive aspect of these clinical trials is that no severe side effects have ever been described in the literature, but on the other hand the results obtained have been, in the best-case scenario, short-lasting dystrophin expression and a slight improvement of muscle strength in a few cases (9).

The mostly common hurdles have been limited migration and proliferation of donor cells in dystrophic muscle, problems with poor donor-cell survival, immunorejection and inefficient myogenic contribution (89). Since difficulties in delivering myoblasts to a wide range of muscle tissue still has to be overcome, cell therapy using resident satellite cells can only be considered for diseases where a few muscle groups are affected, such as in OPMD or FSHD. In these cases the healthy muscles represent a source of myoblasts for autologous transplantation that can be used without any immunosuppression. According to this therapeutic strategy, two clinical trials are presently ongoing in France for OPMD and FSHD, supervised by Dr Lacau-Saint Guily and Dr Desnuelle respectively.

Recent discoveries have shown that many other cell types might be promising candidates for cell-therapy strategies, e.g. mesoangioblasts or CD133$^+$ cells, which already went through a safety and feasibility test recently (55). For other candidates, such as SMALD$^+$ cells or PICs, there is still a long way to go before a clinical application can be envisioned. For more updated information regarding currently ongoing clinical trials see http://clinicaltrials.org.

TABLE 77.2 Clinical Trials of Heterologous Cell Therapy for Duchenne Muscular Dystrophy

Author	Year	No. of Patients	Age	Immuno-suppression	No. of Myoblasts ($\times 10^6$)	Outcomes
Law	1990–1	3	9–10	+	8	All patients Dys$^+$ (IHC and WB) ↑ strength at 3 months
Huard	1992	9	5–20	−	77–845	7 patients Dys$^+$ (IHC/WB) 4 patients showed ↑ strength at 4 months
Law	1992	21	6–14	+	5000	↑ strength in 43% of muscles analyzed at 3 months
Gussoni	1992	8	6–10	−	100	3 patients Dys$^+$ (PCR) at 1 months
Karpati	1993	8	6–10	+	55	No Dys$^+$ at 1 year follow-up 3 patients showed ↑ strength
Tremblay	1993	1†	14	−	704	↑ strength (12–31%) at 6 months; very slight increase in Dys expression
Tremblay	1993	5	4–10	−	102–240	3 patients Dys$^+$ (IHC and WB)
Morandi	1995	3	6–9	+	55	No Dys$^+$
Mendell	1995	12	5–9	6 patients +	110	1 patients Dys$^+$ (IHC)
				6 patients −		
Miller	1997	10	5–10	+	80–100	3 patients Dys$^+$ (PCR) at 1 month; 1 out of 6 at 6 months
Neumeyer	1998	6#	>21	+	73–100	No patients Dys$^+$ (IHC) at 6 months
Skuk	2004–6	9	8–17	+	30	8 patients Dys$^+$ (IHC)
Skuk	2007	1	26	+	25–67.5	Some treated muscles were Dys$^+$ at 14 months (PCR) and 18 months (PCR and IHC)
Torrente	2007	8	8–12	−	0.02*	Safety test: no adverse effects were reported. ↑ vascularization in 4/5 treated muscles

*IHC = immunohistochemistry; WB = Western blot; ↑ = increase/improvement; † = donor was the monozygotic twin of symptomatic carrier; # = patients were affected by Becker muscular dystrophy; * = autologous transplantation of CD133$^+$ cells.*

CONCLUSION

At present, using myoblasts amplified *in vitro*, only small amounts of skeletal muscle tissue have been obtained at the injected sites in various clinical trials centered on DMD. Alternative myogenic cell types recently described have only been used in phase I clinical trials for skeletal muscle, while other gene-based therapies, such as exon skipping, are currently being tested in phase I and II clinical trials. Autologous myoblast (or any myogenic cell type) transplantation may be suited for localized forms of muscular dystrophy with a limited target, such as OPMD, or extended to FSHD if results are encouraging enough. We need to improve the conditions for isolation, expansion (which should be as limited as possible since it hampers the regenerative capacity *in vivo*) and implantation of cells to limit cell death and improve homing and migration within the tissue, with or without the help of cytokines, matrix or hydrogels. Reducing fibrosis or controlling inflammation may also improve the success of transplantation in recipient tissue. The ideal candidate should be easily isolated, amplified, and injected systemically while targeting the desired site, and more years of clinically oriented research will most probably be required. Collaborative efforts of both stem cell and gene therapy researchers should in the future enable safe and efficient dedicated clinical trials, most probably designed specifically for each muscular dystrophy, or even for each type of mutation.

AKNOWLEDGMENTS

The laboratory of the authors is supported by grants from the European Commission MYOAGE Network (contract FP7-LSHG-2007-B-223576), AFM, PPMD-nl, AFLD, ANR In-A-Fib, Région Ile-de-France, INSERM, CNRS and Université Pierre et Marie Curie. The authors wish to thank all members of the group, as well as the MSG, for fruitful discussions.

REFERENCES

1. Emery AE. The muscular dystrophies. *Lancet* 2002;**359**:687–95.
2. Blake DJ, Weir A, Newey SE, Davies KE. Function and genetics of dystrophin and dystrophin-related proteins in muscle. *Physiol Rev* 2002;**82**:291–329.
3. Zou Y, Zhang RZ, Sabatelli P, Chu ML, Bonnemann CG. Muscle interstitial fibroblasts are the main source of collagen VI synthesis in skeletal muscle: implications for congenital muscular dystrophy types Ullrich and Bethlem. *J Neuropathol Exp Neurol* 2008;**67**:144–54.
4. Wolff N, Gilquin B, Courchay K, Callebaut I, Worman HJ, Zinn-Justin S. Structural analysis of emerin, an inner nuclear membrane protein mutated in X-linked Emery–Dreifuss muscular dystrophy. *FEBS Lett* 2001;**501**:171–6.
5. Daftary AS, Crisanti M, Kalra M, Wong B, Amin R. Effect of long-term steroids on cough efficiency and respiratory muscle strength in patients with Duchenne muscular dystrophy. *Pediatrics* 2007;**119**:e320–4.
6. Manzur AY, Kuntzer T, Pike M, Swan A. Glucocorticoid corticosteroids for Duchenne muscular dystrophy. *Cochrane Database Syst Rev* 2008; CD003725.
7. Bushby K, Lochmuller H, Lynn S, Straub V. Interventions for muscular dystrophy: molecular medicines entering the clinic. *Lancet* 2009;**374**:1849–56.
8. Trollet C, Athanasopoulos T, Popplewell L, Malerba A, Dickson G. Gene therapy for muscular dystrophy: current progress and future prospects. *Expert Opin Biol Ther* 2009;**9**:849–66.
9. Negroni E, Vallese D, Vilquin JT, Butler-Browne G, Mouly V, Trollet C. Current advances in cell therapy strategies for muscular dystrophies. *Expert Opin Biol Ther* 2011;**11**:157–76.
10. Cossu G, Sampaolesi M. New therapies for Duchenne muscular dystrophy: challenges, prospects and clinical trials. *Trends Mol Med* 2007;**13**:520–6.
11. Deconinck AE, Rafael JA, Skinner JA, Brown SC, Potter AC, Metzinger L, et al. Utrophin-dystrophin-deficient mice as a model for Duchenne muscular dystrophy. *Cell* 1997;**90**:717–27.
12. Mendell JR, Moxley RT, Griggs RC, Brooke MH, Fenichel GM, Miller JP, et al. Randomized, double-blind six-month trial of prednisone in Duchenne's muscular dystrophy. *N Engl J Med* 1989;**320**:1592–7.
13. Barton-Davis ER, Cordier L, Shoturma DI, Leland SE, Sweeney HL. Aminoglycoside antibiotics restore dystrophin function to skeletal muscles of mdx mice. *J Clin Invest* 1999;**104**:375–81.
14. Welch EM, Barton ER, Zhuo J, Tomizawa Y, Friesen WJ, Trifillis P, et al. PTC124 targets genetic disorders caused by nonsense mutations. *Nature* 2007;**447**:87–91.
15. Lu QL, Morris GE, Wilton SD, Ly T, Artem'yeva OV, Strong P, et al. Massive idiosyncratic exon skipping corrects the nonsense mutation in dystrophic mouse muscle and produces functional revertant fibers by clonal expansion. *J Cell Biol* 2000;**148**:985–96.
16. Goemans NM, Tulinius M, van den Akker JT, Burm BE, Ekhart PF, Heuvelmans N, et al. Systemic administration of PRO051 in Duchenne's muscular dystrophy. *N Engl J Med* 2011;**364**:1513–22.
17. Kinali M, Arechavala-Gomeza V, Feng L, Cirak S, Hunt D, Adkin C, et al. Local restoration of dystrophin expression with the morpholino oligomer AVI-4658 in Duchenne muscular dystrophy: a single-blind, placebo-controlled, dose-escalation, proof-of-concept study. *Lancet Neurol* 2009;**8**:918–28.
18. Goyenvalle A, Babbs A, van Ommen GJ, Garcia L, Davies KE. Enhanced exon-skipping induced by U7 snRNA carrying a splicing silencer sequence: Promising tool for DMD therapy. *Mol Ther* 2009;**17**:1234–40.
19. Nayak S, Herzog RW. Progress and prospects: immune responses to viral vectors. *Gene Ther* 2010;**17**:295–304.
20. Odom GL, Gregorevic P, Chamberlain JS. Viral-mediated gene therapy for the muscular dystrophies: successes, limitations and recent advances. *Biochim Biophys Acta* 2007;**1772**:243–62.
21. Partridge TA, Grounds M, Sloper JC. Evidence of fusion between host and donor myoblasts in skeletal muscle grafts. *Nature* 1978;**273**:306–8.
22. Bulfield G, Siller WG, Wight PA, Moore KJ. X chromosome-linked muscular dystrophy (mdx) in the mouse. *Proc Natl Acad Sci USA* 1984;**81**:1189–92.
23. Palmieri B, Tremblay JP, Daniele L. Past, present and future of myoblast transplantation in the treatment of Duchenne muscular dystrophy. *Pediatr Transplant* 2010;**14**:813–9.
24. Perie S, Mamchaoui K, Mouly V, Blot S, Bouazza B, Thornell LE, et al. Premature proliferative arrest of cricopharyngeal myoblasts in oculo-pharyngeal muscular dystrophy: therapeutic perspectives of autologous myoblast transplantation. *Neuromuscul Disord* 2006;**16**:770–81.
25. Price FD, Kuroda K, Rudnicki MA. Stem cell based therapies to treat muscular dystrophy. *Biochim Biophys Acta* 2007;**1772**:272–83.
26. Tedesco FS, Dellavalle A, Diaz-Manera J, Messina G, Cossu G. Repairing skeletal muscle: regenerative potential of skeletal muscle stem cells. *J Clin Invest* 2010;**120**:11–9.
27. Mauro A. Satellite cell of skeletal muscle fibers. *J Biophys Biochem Cytol* 1961;**9**:493–5.
28. Partridge T. Reenthronement of the muscle satellite cell. *Cell* 2004;**119**:447–8.
29. Morgan JE, Partridge TA. Muscle satellite cells. *Int J Biochem Cell Biol* 2003;**35**:1151–6.
30. Tajbakhsh S, Bober E, Babinet C, Pournin S, Arnold H, Buckingham M. Gene targeting the myf-5 locus with nlacZ reveals expression of this myogenic factor in mature skeletal muscle fibres as well as early embryonic muscle. *Dev Dyn* 1996;**206**:291–300.
31. Cooper RN, Tajbakhsh S, Mouly V, Cossu G, Buckingham M, Butler-Browne GS. In vivo satellite cell activation via Myf5 and MyoD in regenerating mouse skeletal muscle. *J Cell Sci* 1999;**112** (Pt 17):2895–901.
32. Zammit PS, Partridge TA, Yablonka-Reuveni Z. The skeletal muscle satellite cell: the stem cell that came in from the cold. *J Histochem Cytochem* 2006;**54**:1177–91.
33. Cardasis CA, Cooper GW. An analysis of nuclear numbers in individual muscle fibers during differentiation and growth: a satellite cell-muscle fiber growth unit. *J Exp Zool* 1975;**191**: 347–58.
34. Bischoff R. The satellite cell and muscle regeneration. In: Engel A, Franzini-Armstrong C, editors. *Myology*. 2nd ed. New York: McGraw-Hill;1994.
35. Renault V, Thornell LE, Eriksson PO, Butler-Browne G, Mouly V. Regenerative potential of human skeletal muscle during aging. *Aging Cell* 2002;**1**:132–9.
36. Fukada S, Higuchi S, Segawa M, Koda K, Yamamoto Y, Tsujikawa K, et al. Purification and cell-surface marker characterization of quiescent satellite cells from murine skeletal muscle by a novel monoclonal antibody. *Exp Cell Res* 2004;**296**:245–55.

37. Boldrin L, Muntoni F, Morgan JE. Are human and mouse satellite cells really the same? *J Histochem Cytochem* 2010;**58**:941–55.
38. Lindstrom M, Thornell LE. New multiple labelling method for improved satellite cell identification in human muscle: application to a cohort of power-lifters and sedentary men. *Histochem Cell Biol* 2009;**132**:141–57.
39. Morgan JE, Hoffman EP, Partridge TA. Normal myogenic cells from newborn mice restore normal histology to degenerating muscles of the mdx mouse. *J Cell Biol* 1990;**111**:2437–49.
40. Kinoshita I, Huard J, Tremblay JP. Utilization of myoblasts from transgenic mice to evaluate the efficacy of myoblast transplantation. *Muscle Nerve* 1994;**17**:975–80.
41. Kinoshita I, Vilquin JT, Guerette B, Asselin I, Roy R, Tremblay JP. Very efficient myoblast allotransplantation in mice under FK506 immunosuppression. *Muscle Nerve* 1994;**17**:1407–15.
42. Huard J, Verreault S, Roy R, Tremblay M, Tremblay JP. High efficiency of muscle regeneration after human myoblast clone transplantation in SCID mice. *J Clin Invest* 1994;**93**:586–99.
43. Morgan JE, Pagel CN, Sherratt T, Partridge TA. Long-term persistence and migration of myogenic cells injected into pre-irradiated muscles of mdx mice. *J Neurol Sci* 1993;**115**:191–200.
44. Skuk D, Goulet M, Roy B, Chapdelaine P, Bouchard JP, Roy R, et al. Dystrophin expression in muscles of Duchenne muscular dystrophy patients after high-density injections of normal myogenic cells. *J Neuropathol Exp Neurol* 2006;**65**:371–86.
45. Dellavalle A, Sampaolesi M, Tonlorenzi R, Tagliafico E, Sacchetti B, Perani L, et al. Pericytes of human skeletal muscle are myogenic precursors distinct from satellite cells. *Nat Cell Biol* 2007;**9**:255–67.
46. Cerletti M, Jurga S, Witczak CA, Hirshman MF, Shadrach JL, Goodyear LJ, et al. Highly efficient, functional engraftment of skeletal muscle stem cells in dystrophic muscles. *Cell* 2008;**134**:37–47.
47. Montarras D, Morgan J, Collins C, Relaix F, Zaffran S, Cumano A, et al. Direct isolation of satellite cells for skeletal muscle regeneration. *Science* 2005;**309**:2064–7.
48. Sacco A, Doyonnas R, Kraft P, Vitorovic S, Blau HM. Self-renewal and expansion of single transplanted muscle stem cells. *Nature* 2008;**456**:502–6.
49. Sampaolesi M, Torrente Y, Innocenzi A, Tonlorenzi R, D'Antona G, Pellegrino MA, et al. Cell therapy of alpha-sarcoglycan null dystrophic mice through intra-arterial delivery of mesoangioblasts. *Science* 2003;**301**:487–92.
50. Peault B, Rudnicki M, Torrente Y, Cossu G, Tremblay JP, Partridge T, et al. Stem and progenitor cells in skeletal muscle development, maintenance, and therapy. *Mol Ther* 2007;**15**:867–77.
51. Negroni E, Riederer I, Chaouch S, Belicchi M, Razini P, Di Santo J, et al. In vivo myogenic potential of human CD133$^+$ muscle-derived stem cells: a quantitative study. *Mol Ther* 2009;**17**:1771–8.
52. De Angelis L, Berghella L, Coletta M, Lattanzi L, Zanchi M, Cusella-De Angelis MG, et al. Skeletal myogenic progenitors originating from embryonic dorsal aorta coexpress endothelial and myogenic markers and contribute to postnatal muscle growth and regeneration. *J Cell Biol* 1999;**147**:869–78.
53. Sampaolesi M, Blot S, D'Antona G, Granger N, Tonlorenzi R, Innocenzi A, et al. Mesoangioblast stem cells ameliorate muscle function in dystrophic dogs. *Nature* 2006;**444**:574–9.
54. Torrente Y, Belicchi M, Sampaolesi M, Pisati F, Meregalli M, D'Antona G, et al. Human circulating AC133(+) stem cells restore dystrophin expression and ameliorate function in dystrophic skeletal muscle. *J Clin Invest* 2004;**114**:182–95.
55. Torrente Y, Belicchi M, Marchesi C, Dantona G, Cogiamanian F, Pisati F, et al. Autologous transplantation of muscle-derived CD133$^+$ stem cells in Duchenne muscle patients. *Cell Transplant* 2007;**16**:563–77.
56. Goodell MA, Brose K, Paradis G, Conner AS, Mulligan RC. Isolation and functional properties of murine hematopoietic stem cells that are replicating in vivo. *J Exp Med* 1996;**183**:1797–806.
57. Uezumi A, Ojima K, Fukada S, Ikemoto M, Masuda S, Miyagoe-Suzuki Y, et al. Functional heterogeneity of side population cells in skeletal muscle. *Biochem Biophys Res Commun* 2006;**341**:864–73.
58. Asakura A, Seale P, Girgis-Gabardo A, Rudnicki MA. Myogenic specification of side population cells in skeletal muscle. *J Cell Biol* 2002;**159**:123–34.
59. Asakura A, Rudnicki MA. Side population cells from diverse adult tissues are capable of *in vitro* hematopoietic differentiation. *Exp Hematol* 2002;**30**:1339–45.
60. Motohashi N, Uezumi A, Yada E, Fukada S, Fukushima K, Imaizumi K, et al. Muscle CD31(-) CD45(-) side population cells promote muscle regeneration by stimulating proliferation and migration of myoblasts. *Am J Pathol* 2008;**173**:781–91.
61. Evans MJ, Kaufman MH. Establishment in culture of pluripotential cells from mouse embryos. *Nature* 1981;**292**:154–6.
62. Fujikawa T, Oh SH, Pi L, Hatch HM, Shupe T, Petersen BE. Teratoma formation leads to failure of treatment for type I diabetes using embryonic stem cell-derived insulin-producing cells. *Am J Pathol* 2005;**166**:1781–91.
63. Eventov-Friedman S, Katchman H, Shezen E, Aronovich A, Tchorsh D, Dekel B, et al. Embryonic pig liver, pancreas, and lung as a source for transplantation: optimal organogenesis without teratoma depends on distinct time windows. *Proc Natl Acad Sci USA* 2005;**102**:2928–33.
64. Dekel I, Magal Y, Pearson-White S, Emerson CP, Shani M. Conditional conversion of ES cells to skeletal muscle by an exogenous MyoD1 gene. *New Biol* 1992;**4**:217–24.
65. Prelle K, Wobus AM, Krebs O, Blum WF, Wolf E. Overexpression of insulin-like growth factor-II in mouse embryonic stem cells promotes myogenic differentiation. *Biochem Biophys Res Commun* 2000;**277**:631–8.
66. Chang H, Yoshimoto M, Umeda K, Iwasa T, Mizuno Y, Fukada S, et al. Generation of transplantable, functional satellite-like cells from mouse embryonic stem cells. *FASEB J* 2009;**23**:1907–19.
67. Thomson JA, Itskovitz-Eldor J, Shapiro SS, Waknitz MA, Swiergiel JJ, Marshall VS, et al. Embryonic stem cell lines derived from human blastocysts. *Science* 1998;**282**:1145–7.
68. Barberi T, Bradbury M, Dincer Z, Panagiotakos G, Socci ND, Studer L. Derivation of engraftable skeletal myoblasts from human embryonic stem cells. *Nat Med* 2007;**13**:642–8.
69. Takahashi K, Yamanaka S. Induction of pluripotent stem cells from mouse embryonic and adult fibroblast cultures by defined factors. *Cell* 2006;**126**:663–76.
70. Park IH, Arora N, Huo H, Maherali N, Ahfeldt T, Shimamura A, et al. Disease-specific induced pluripotent stem cells. *Cell* 2008;**134**:877–86.

71. Kazuki Y, Hiratsuka M, Takiguchi M, Osaki M, Kajitani N, Hoshiya H, et al. Complete genetic correction of ips cells from Duchenne muscular dystrophy. *Mol Ther* 2010;**18**:386–93.
72. Nakagawa M, Koyanagi M, Tanabe K, Takahashi K, Ichisaka T, Aoi T, et al. Generation of induced pluripotent stem cells without Myc from mouse and human fibroblasts. *Nat Biotechnol* 2008;**26**:101–6.
73. Wernig M, Meissner A, Cassady JP, Jaenisch R. c-Myc is dispensable for direct reprogramming of mouse fibroblasts. *Cell Stem Cell* 2008;**2**:10–2.
74. Zhu S, Li W, Zhou H, Wei W, Ambasudhan R, Lin T, et al. Reprogramming of human primary somatic cells by OCT4 and chemical compounds. *Cell Stem Cell* 2010;**7**:651–5.
75. Bianco P, Robey PG, Saggio I, Riminucci M. "Mesenchymal" stem cells in human bone marrow (skeletal stem cells): a critical discussion of their nature, identity, and significance in incurable skeletal disease. *Hum Gene Ther* 2010;**21**:1057–66.
76. Chamberlain G, Fox J, Ashton B, Middleton J. Concise review: mesenchymal stem cells: their phenotype, differentiation capacity, immunological features, and potential for homing. *Stem Cells* 2007;**25**:2739–49.
77. Pittenger MF, Mackay AM, Beck SC, Jaiswal RK, Douglas R, Mosca JD, et al. Multilineage potential of adult human mesenchymal stem cells. *Science* 1999;**284**:143–7.
78. Piersma AH, Brockbank KG, Ploemacher RE, van Vliet E, Brakel-van Peer KM, Visser PJ. Characterization of fibroblastic stromal cells from murine bone marrow. *Exp Hematol* 1985;**13**:237–43.
79. Prockop DJ. Marrow stromal cells as stem cells for nonhematopoietic tissues. *Science* 1997;**276**:71–4.
80. Wakitani S, Saito T, Caplan AI. Myogenic cells derived from rat bone marrow mesenchymal stem cells exposed to 5-azacytidine. *Muscle Nerve* 1995;**18**:1417–26.
81. Dominici M, Le Blanc K, Mueller I, Slaper-Cortenbach I, Marini F, Krause D, et al. Minimal criteria for defining multipotent mesenchymal stromal cells. The International Society for Cellular Therapy position statement. *Cytotherapy* 2006;**8**:315–7.
82. Kode JA, Mukherjee S, Joglekar MV, Hardikar AA. Mesenchymal stem cells: immunobiology and role in immunomodulation and tissue regeneration. *Cytotherapy* 2009;**11**:377–91.
83. Saito T, Dennis JE, Lennon DP, Young RG, Caplan AI. Myogenic expression of mesenchymal stem cells within myotubes of mdx mice *in vitro* and *in vivo*. *Tissue Eng* 1995;**1**:327–43.
84. Ferrari G, Stornaiuolo A, Mavilio F. Failure to correct murine muscular dystrophy. *Nature* 2001;**411**:1014–5.
85. Dezawa M, Ishikawa H, Itokazu Y, Yoshihara T, Hoshino M, Takeda S, et al. Bone marrow stromal cells generate muscle cells and repair muscle degeneration. *Science* 2005;**309**:314–7.
86. Vauchez K, Marolleau JP, Schmid M, Khattar P, Chapel A, Catelain C, et al. Aldehyde dehydrogenase activity identifies a population of human skeletal muscle cells with high myogenic capacities. *Mol Ther* 2009;**17**:1948–58.
87. Mitchell KJ, Pannerec A, Cadot B, Parlakian A, Besson V, Gomes ER, et al. Identification and characterization of a non-satellite cell muscle resident progenitor during postnatal development. *Nat Cell Biol* 2010;**12**:257–66.
88. Skuk D, Tremblay JP. Intramuscular cell transplantation as a potential treatment of myopathies: clinical and preclinical relevant data. *Expert Opin Biol Ther* 2011;**11**:359–74.
89. Negroni E, Butler-Browne GS, Mouly V. Myogenic stem cells: regeneration and cell therapy in human skeletal muscle. *Pathol Biol (Paris)* 2006;**54**:100–8.

Chapter 78

Immunological Components of Genetically Inherited Muscular Dystrophies: Duchenne Muscular Dystrophy and Limb-Girdle Muscular Dystrophy Type 2B

Melissa J. Spencer[1,3], Irina Kramerova[1,3], M. Carrie Miceli[2,3] and Kanneboyina Nagaraju[4]

[1]*Departments of Neurology,* [2]*Microbiology, Immunology and Molecular Genetics, David Geffen School of Medicine at UCLA,* [3]*Center for Duchenne Muscular Dystrophy at UCLA, Los Angeles, CA,* [4]*Research Center for Genetic Medicine, Children's National Medical Center, Washington, DC*

INTRODUCTION

Genetically inherited muscle diseases (the "muscular dystrophies") are not strictly autoimmune diseases, nor do they precisely replicate conditions of acute muscle injury; however, a large number of the genetically inherited dystrophies possess some level of intramuscular inflammation. Most of these dystrophies (DMD and LGMD2B in particular) share the common feature of membrane damage followed by satellite cell-mediated muscle repair; thus they more accurately represent a persistently healing wound. In the context of normal wound healing, inflammatory mediators released from the wound site induce expression of adhesion molecules that recruit immune cells to extravasate to the tissue. TGF-β, secreted by immune cells, stimulates fibroblast activation and secretion of extracellular matrix proteins that stabilize the wound until the damage resolves. Myeloid cells phagocytose the debris, secrete growth factors and the wound is repaired. In contrast, in the inherited muscular dystrophies, damage to the muscle cell membrane is persistent due to the genetic defect, thus creating a chronic inflammatory environment. Both "pro-inflammatory" (e.g. TNF, IL-1β, and interferon gamma) and "anti-inflammatory/pro-fibrotic" (e.g. TGF-β, IL-13, IL-10) mediators are present in the inflamed tissue. A delicate balance between these various factors is necessary to stabilize the wound, repair the injury, and resolve the inflammation; however, perturbation of this balance could have unwelcome consequences. In addition, the local environment of the muscle can slant the responding immune effectors towards inflammation, necrosis or fibrosis respectively. The inflammatory milieu of dystrophic muscle changes over time, but eventually becomes skewed to a more pro-fibrotic environment, evidenced by the abundant scar tissue in mouse and patients' muscles (Figure 78.1). At the present time, the role of the immune system has been investigated in only two muscular dystrophies; Duchenne muscular dystrophy due to mutations in dystrophin and limb-girdle muscular dystrophy type 2B due to mutations in dysferlin. The emphasis of this chapter will therefore be on DMD and LGMD2B dystrophies, which are the best studied. A lack of discussion of other dystrophies should not be interpreted to mean that other dystrophies do not involve inflammation and fibrosis, but only that there is a paucity of information on these other dystrophies at this time.

DUCHENNE MUSCULAR DYSTROPHY

The Immune Milieu of Dystrophin-Deficient Muscle

Dystrophic muscles contain representation of most immune cell types and chemical messengers. Early descriptions of infiltrating cell types reported a predominance of macrophages and T cells in DMD biopsies (1). The availability of the mouse model of DMD (the "mdx" mouse) has allowed for a more thorough investigation of the immune response to dystrophin deficiency. Dystrophic lesions in mdx muscles contain both myeloid and lymphoid cells that include $CD4^+$ T cells (2), $CD8^+$

Muscle. DOI: http://dx.doi.org/10.1016/B978-0-12-381510-1.00078-8

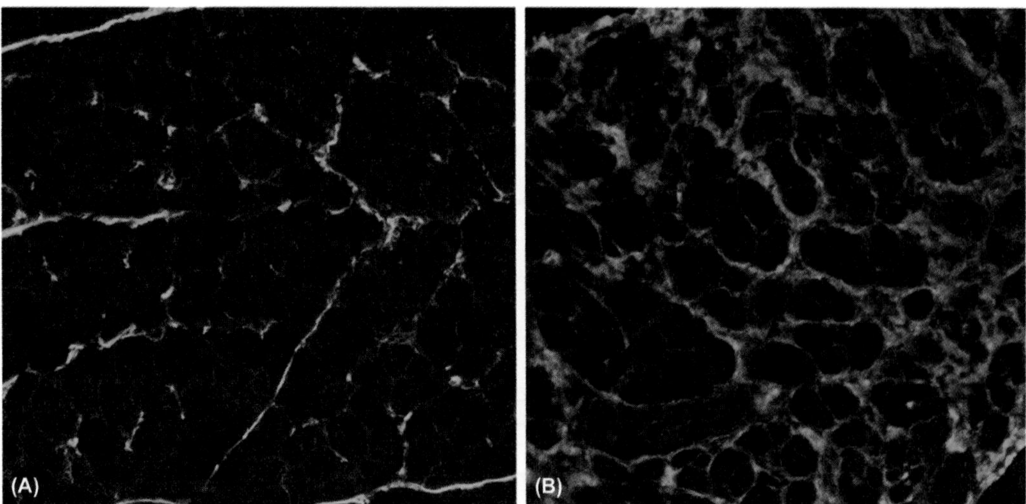

FIGURE 78.1 Fibrosis in mdx diaphragm muscle. Shown are cross-sections of diaphragm muscles from 8-month-old mice, stained with type I collagen (bright green). Note the increase in connective tissue deposition, between muscle fibers, in the mdx muscle section. (A) C57 BL/6 and (B) mdx.

T cells (2,3), double-negative (DN) (4) and double positive (DP) (4) T cells (2–4), NK cells (4), NKT cells (4), B cells (4), macrophages (5–7), mast cells (8), neutrophils (4), and eosinophils (9,10). Microarrays of mdx (11) and DMD (12,13) biopsies show a predominant signature of inflammatory mediators. In addition, many chemokines and chemokine receptors are elevated and likely perpetuate the inflammation (14). In this chapter we discuss the role of these cell types in the pathogenesis of DMD and present the research done on the known inflammatory mediators that show promise as therapeutic targets in this disease.

Macrophages

Macrophages represent the major cell type infiltrating both human and mouse dystrophic muscle. At the earliest stages of muscle necrosis, macrophages can be seen gravitating to and surrounding dying muscle fibers (1). Bone marrow-derived monocytes enter inflamed tissue and differentiate to macrophages. Like T cells that can be broadly phenotyped as either Th1 or Th2 subtypes (depending on their cytokine secretion profile), macrophages can polarize into M1 (i.e. pro-inflammatory, secreting TNF, IL-6, and IL-12,) or M2 (i.e. anti-inflammatory, pro-repair, pro-fibrotic secreting TGF-β, IFN-γ, IL-4, IL-10) phenotypes). In the case of acute muscle injury, it has been shown that M1 macrophages kill muscle cells through a nitric oxide-dependent mechanism (15) and that M2 macrophages contribute factors that support muscle repair (16), particularly through secretion of insulin-like growth factor-1 (IGF-1) (17). Several cytokines have been identified that polarize macrophages into these subtypes, including interferon gamma (which polarizes to the M1 type) or IL-4 (which polarizes to the M2 type) (6).

A series of papers have elucidated the macrophage-mediated mechanisms that take place during chronic inflammation that occurs in muscles of the mdx mouse model (5,6,18,19). In the early stages of the disease (3–4 weeks of age), M1 macrophages predominate (6). M1 macrophages express tumor necrosis factor and IL-6, which promote the chemotaxis of other cell types to muscle. Macrophage cytokines are activated through NF-κB (20) and fibrinogen binding to the Mac1 integrin (7). In addition, M1 macrophages express high levels of iNOS that generates cytotoxic concentrations of nitric oxide (NO) (6) which damages phospholipid membranes, affects signaling through S-nitrosylation, and/or induces protein denaturation. iNOS can also nitrosylate the ryanodine receptor and contribute to the calcium leak from the sarcoplasmic reticulum and calpain activation leading to worsened disease (21). While M1 macrophages seem to be more highly represented in early stages (4-week-old mdx mice), M2 macrophages become the predominant macrophage type in later stages (12 weeks old). M2 macrophages express the cytokine IL-10, which is inhibitory for M1 macrophages and promotes an environment conducive for muscle repair (19). While boosting IL-10 and other M2 cytokines in dystrophic muscle might benefit disease phenotype in the short term, the potential for its promotion of fibrosis with long-term overexpression is high, so long-term studies are needed to determine it effect on fibrotic processes. M2 macrophages can contribute to skeletal and cardiac muscle fibrosis through arginase-mediated metabolism of arginine (18). These macrophages express high levels of arginase, an enzyme that generates ornithine and

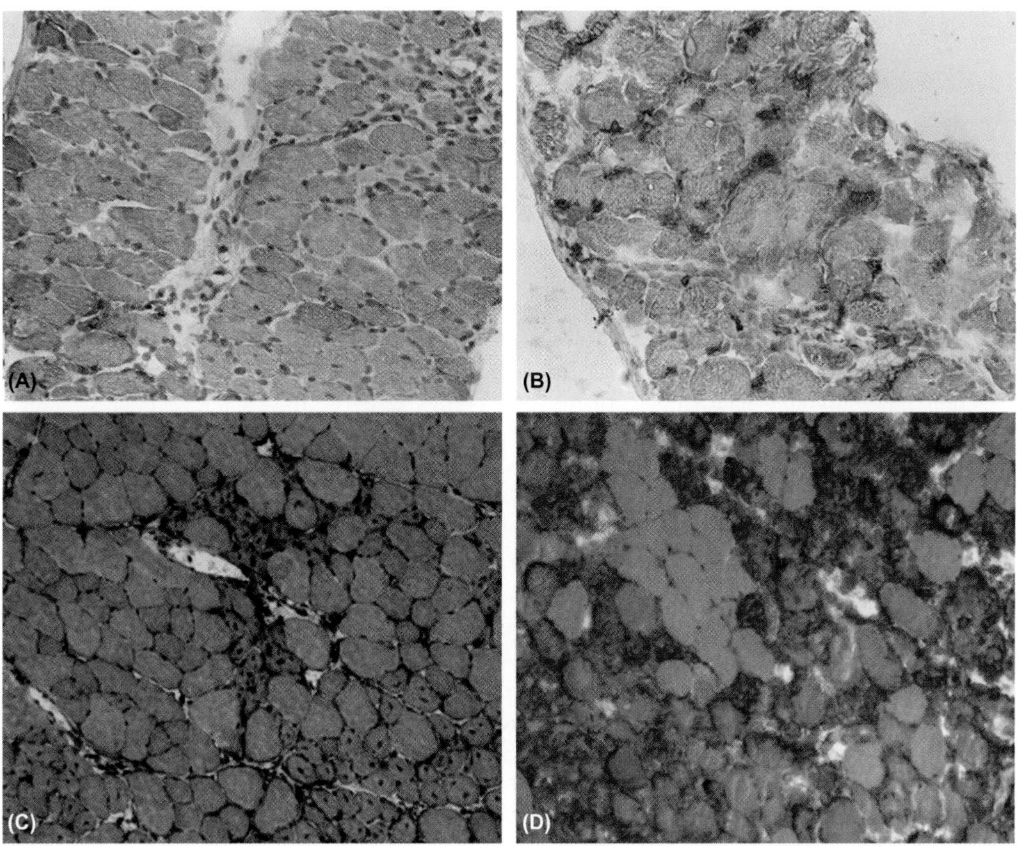

FIGURE 78.2 **Ablation of immunomodulators can suppress inflammation in mdx dystrophy.** Shown are cross-sections of 4-week-old, mdx muscles, stained with Gr-1 antibody (recognizes both neutrophils and macrophages) and CD68 (recognizes M1 macrophages). Staining is visualized as a red color. Sections are counterstained with hematoxylin (blue), which stains nuclei dark blue and cytoplasm light blue. Ablation of osteopontin (OPN) or matrix metalloproteinase 9 (MMP9) reduces the infiltration of both of these cell types. (A) $OPN^{-/-}$, mdx diaphragm, (B) mdx diaphragm, (C) $MMP9^{-/-}$, mdx quadriceps and (D) mdx quadriceps.

proline, byproducts which stimulate collagen synthesis in fibroblasts (18). Thus, the early stages of the mouse disease replicate conditions of acute muscle injury, but as the muscle never fully heals, a more M2-like, pro-repair but also pro-fibrotic environment is established over the remaining disease course (6). Thus, therapeutics aimed at immune modulation of macrophages must strive for a delicate balance between pro- and anti-inflammatory mediators, so as not to tip the balance further toward necrosis or fibrosis, both detrimental in their own right.

Neutrophils

Neutrophils are the second most abundant cell type in dystrophic muscle. Together with macrophages, they make up about 70% of all the infiltrating cell types. Interference with their presence in dystrophic muscle, either through antibody (22) or ablation of osteopontin (4) results in a greatly improved dystrophic phenotype (Figure 78.2). The mechanisms for how they might be impacting disease is unknown, but the muscle injury literature suggests that neutrophils harm muscle through free radical-mediated damage to membranes, primarily through superoxide dismutase generation of hydrogen peroxide, which is then converted to hypochlorous acid by neutrophil myeloloperoxidase (23). Free radicals are not only damaging to normal plasma membranes, but dystrophic membranes are even more susceptible to free-radical-mediated damage (24), so interference with neutrophil extravasation to muscle or activation will likely be beneficial for DMD.

T Cells

T cells represent a pivotal arm of adaptive immunity that regulates immune tolerance and activation. In response to exposure to specific antigen, T cells can be activated to differentiate into effector lineages including CTL, Th1, Th2, Th17, $\gamma\delta$ or Treg effector or memory T cells with different capacities to: migrate and reside within central lymphoid or peripheral tissues; mediate T cell effector functions; and influence processes of tissue destruction, repair, and fibrosis. In some circumstances, exposure to antigen selectively induces one or more T effector functions (such as cytotoxicity, TNF or γ-IFN production), whereas in other circumstances it can lead to T cell inactivation and tolerance through the induction of apoptosis, anergy (a state of non-responsiveness), or exhaustion (involving loss of activating and upregulation of inactivating surface receptors). Several factors aid in determining tolerance versus activation, including the maturational stage of the T cell, the type of cell involved in presenting the antigen, and cytokines and other immune mediators present in the local T cell microenvironment (25).

Self-antigens expressed sufficiently in the thymus microenvironment lead to deletion of autoreactive T cell precursors through negative selection and/or the development of nTregs (natural Tregs) that serve to monitor and dampen immune responses directed against these self-antigens. T cells that escape these modes of central tolerance induction are poised to respond to antigenic stimulation by professional antigen presenting cells (APC) or can be rendered tolerant through one of several peripheral tolerance mechanisms. The local cytokine environment and mode of antigen presentation help program these cells toward effectors with appropriate activating or tolerizing activity. While T effector differentiation was originally thought to represent a commitment to terminal differentiation of a T effector with defined activities, recent findings make clear that this process is more plastic, with some effector T cells retaining the capacity to be reprogrammed to alternate T lineages or to intermediate subset phenotypes capable of "mixed" effector functions. A striking example of this is the ability of auto-aggressive Th1 cells to be reprogrammed to immunosuppressive iTregs (induced Tregs) upon the induction of foxp3 and/or in the context of local exposure to TGF-β and retinoic acid; some iTregs retain the ability to produce pro-inflammatory γ-IFN in addition to mediating suppressor functions (26).

Both $CD4^+$ and $CD8^+$ T cells appear in dystrophic muscle at the onset of necrosis, and short-term depletion of each subtype is beneficial to disease features (2–4). Mdx mice crossed onto the nude mouse background lacking T cells have reduced diaphragm fibrosis, implicating T cells in this process (27). Many of the T cells in the mdx infiltrate represent $CD4^+CD8\alpha^+$ double-positive or $CD4^-CD8^-$ double negative subsets (4), known to arise within memory and exhausted T cell subpopulations. In addition T regulatory cells and NKT cells are also present in low numbers in mdx and human (4;and unpublished data). It is unclear which self-antigens these T cells are directed against. It is likely that loss of muscle integrity, inflammation and ensuing upregulation of MHC class I expression on myofibers in mdx and DMD muscle promotes the presentation of autoantigens above threshold levels and in the context of APC and costimulation not typically expressed in non-dystrophic muscle. Expansions of T cells with limited and conserved TCR Vα and Vβ element usage have been observed in both DMD and mdx (4,28) muscles, suggesting antigen-driven expansion or the development of NKT-like regulatory populations with limited TCR repertoires.

Of particular interest is the potential activation of dystrophin-reactive T cells stimulated by revertant fibers. Indeed, in most cases, dystrophic muscles contain revertant fibers expressing rescued dystrophin produced either through a compensatory mutation or exon skipping. While they are too rare to rescue muscle function, these revertants might stimulate or tolerize local dystrophin-reactive T cells. Several studies make clear that dystrophin-reactive T cells are not all deleted during negative selection. Indeed, functional dystrophin-reactive and CD8 CTL can readily be activated, stimulated to different effectors or tolerized in response to dystrophin in a number of experimental settings (29–31), depending on the context in which the dystrophin is presented as well as the species analyzed. rAAV vectors have emerged as front-runners for dystrophin gene therapy because they are less immunostimulatory and can be tolerogenic under some circumstances; inducing Tregs cells or T cells that are anergized, targeted for apoptosis, only express a subset of needed effector functions, or are otherwise incapacitated. Using rAAV vectors, mini-dystrophin can be stably expressed in mice to rescue the dystrophic phenotype; whereas these same rAAV DMD vectors are immunostimulatory in dogs, leading to T cells that prevent sustained dystrophin transgene expression (32,33). Transient immunosuppression appears sufficient to prevent response to capsid and dystrophin rejection in dogs, since stable expression of dystrophin positive fibers has been sustained under these circumstances (33).

Recent gene therapy studies in DMD boys have begun to characterize dystrophin reactive T cells in humans and provide a compelling need to better understand the regulation and contributions of dystrophin-reactive T cells in the context of dystrophic muscle (34,35). In DMD patients receiving intramuscular rAAV vector-mediated delivery of mini-dystrophin, 4/6 subjects generated dystrophin-reactive CD4 and/or CD8 IFN-γ-producing T cells in their peripheral blood lymphocytes (PBL) (34). As might be expected, some of these T cells were directed against novel sequences unique to mini-dystrophin or present in the mini-gene but deleted in the DMD patient. Others were directed against epitopes also found expressed in the subject's revertant fibers; in one case these cells were present prior to vector delivery and expanded quickly after gene therapy, consistent with the possibility that T cells were primed by endogenous revertants and could play a role in eliminating rescued revertant fibers throughout DMD pathogenesis. It is possible that IFN-γ produced by Th1 cells could promote antigen presentation and lysosomal activity of macrophages, promote lymphocyte migration or activate iNos; each of which could promote clearance of dystrophin-positive cells. However, it remains to be seen if the dystrophin-reactive T cells found in PBL can traffic to the muscle, survive and damage dystrophin-positive fibers. Once T cells traffic to the muscle they could be reprogrammed in the presence of high TGF-β levels and/or other factors to effect tolerance to dystrophin through conversion to iTregs or induced apoptosis. Alternatively, local TGF-β could aid in development of auto-aggressive Th17 cells, which have yet to be considered in dystrophic settings (25). While T cell targeting of dystrophin-positive cells may explain lack of robust and sustained dystrophin expression in this DMD gene therapy trial, low expression levels may also reflect non-optimal levels of vector/transgene delivery and expression.

Identification of dystrophin-reactive T cells in DMD PBL in response to dystrophin delivery by AAV prompted a similar analysis in the final cohort of DMD subjects in which gentamycin (36) was used to restore dystrophin by inducing readthrough of a premature stop codon. One patient treated with gentamycin expressed $CD4^+$ IFN-γ^+ T cells specific for a dystrophin epitope expressed on revertant fibers and which expanded in response to mini-dystrophin (35). These findings led the authors to speculate that aggressive Th1 type memory T cell responses to dystrophin might limit the frequency of naturally occurring revertants and pose a barrier to dystrophin replacement therapies in the absence of immunosuppression. In this instance, $CD4^+$ IFN-γ^+ dystrophin-reactive T cells were also cultured from a muscle biopsy. It remains unclear how they function *in vivo* and whether they played a role in limiting the stability of dystrophin-positive fibers. However, in the three patients tested, only the muscle biopsy with dystrophin-reactive T cells was entirely dystrophin-free.

In the context of proposed DMD exon-skipping strategies for dystrophin replacement, it is interesting to consider a report that 2-O-methyl modified RNA can act as a TLR7 antagonist (37). These findings raise the possibility that 2-O-methyl antisense oligonucleotide (AON)-based exon-skipping strategies might dampen inflammation and autoimmunity induced by TLR7, which is dramatically upregulated on infiltrating mononuclear cells and myofibers in human dystrophic muscle (13), and may explain the apparent lack of a limiting immune response to 2-O-methyl AON-directed DMD exon skipping. However, T cell reactivity to dystrophin has yet to be experimentally considered in recent exon skipping and readthrough clinical trials. As stem cell transfer, exon skipping, readthrough, gene correction, and dystrophin vector-based gene therapies move forward, more sophisticated analyses of dystrophin-specific T cell responses, assessing additional T cell surface markers and intracellular cytokine staining using multicolor flow cytometry and emerging technologies on a larger cohort of subjects, will be important in understanding their role in pathogenesis and disease progression and determining the need for immunosuppression for their long-term success as potential therapeutics.

The Relationship Between Inflammation and Fibrosis in DMD

Fibrosis is a prominent and progressive feature of DMD muscle that eventually induces significant functional impairment in both skeletal and cardiac muscle. An association between inflammation and fibrosis has been demonstrated in many studies using the mdx mouse. One key candidate immunomodulator involved in the fibrotic process in dystrophic muscles is TGF-β. This molecule is elevated in mdx (38) and DMD muscles (13,39) and high expression of TGF-β and its receptors correlates with more fibrotic stages of disease (13). The concentration of TGF-β is not perfectly correlated to the level of fibrosis in a given model or muscle (40), but in general, reduced TGF-β seems to accompany/result in reduced fibrosis (41–43). The lack of a perfectly tight correlation suggests that other fibrosis-promoting processes are occurring simultaneously, for example through regulation of TGF-β availability by binding proteins or alteration of arginase metabolism. The source of TGF-β in dystrophic muscles is still not known, but leukocytes are likely to be an important source of the cytokine (27,44). TGF-β can affect tissue fibrogenesis by increasing collagen secretion by fibroblasts or by converting myoblasts to fibroblasts (45), suggesting that it plays both direct and indirect roles in the fibrotic process. TGFβ's promotion of fibrosis is not the only manner in which it negatively impacts disease. It can also block terminal myogenic differentiation and therefore impair muscle repair. Thus, targeting TGFβ in DMD is likely to have more than a single beneficial effect.

Strong support for the important role of TGF-β in promotion of fibrosis derives from a recent study by McNally and colleagues in which they demonstrated that latent TGF-β binding protein 4 (LTPBP4) is an important modifier of the dystrophic phenotype (46). LTBP4 binds TGF-β and keeps it in a latent state. Proteolytic cleavage of LTPB4 by an unknown protease releases TGF-β and allows it to bind to its receptor and activate downstream signaling. The activity of LTBP4 is modified by the presence of a 12 amino acid insertion within its sequence, which prevents its cleavage, resulting in less available TGF-β. Dystrophic mouse strains that contained the 12 amino acid insertion in LTBP4 (e.g. 129 background) had less membrane damage and fibrosis than those on a background (D2) that omitted the insertion sequence. These studies showed for the first time, in an unbiased screen, that TGF-β is a potent modifier of the dystrophic phenotype.

Inflammatory Mediators that Impact DMD

Several previous studies have demonstrated that experimental interventions that reduce subsets of immune cells *in vivo* can reduce muscle pathology in the mdx mouse, including depletion of $CD8^+$ T cells (2), $CD4^+$ T cells (3), macrophages (5), TNF (38,47–50) and eosinophils (10). These studies lend support for the involvement of the immune system in DMD progression. More recently, immune mediators that regulate the extravasation, migration, activity, and survival of these various cell types have begun to be elucidated. In the next section, the role that each of these cell types or mediators has in these processes will be discussed.

Osteopontin

Osteopontin (OPN) is an acidic phosphoprotein that is highly expressed in DMD biopsies and mdx muscles (4). The primary source of OPN in dystrophic muscle is immune cells, although myogenic cells also express it (4; and unpublished data). OPN can be secreted, or it can be retained intracellularly where it is associated with the CD44 complex (51). Secreted OPN binds to integrins and CD44 as well as to several extracellular matrix molecules including fibronectin and collagen (52,53). OPN has also been shown to regulate the extravasation, phenotype, activation, and survival of multiple immune cell types (54). Recently it was demonstrated that ablation of OPN on the mdx background resulted in an abated dystrophic phenotype of increased strength and reduced fibrosis (4). Consistent with its role in other systems, OPN proved to be an immunomodulator, that when targeted, resulted in reduced neutrophils and NKT cells and reductions in TGF-β. Thus, in the mdx mouse, OPN promotes dystrophy and fibrosis, at least in part through its effect on inflammation.

There is preliminary evidence in humans that OPN also promotes progression of DMD. Researchers studied two cohorts of patients in the United States and Italy and identified a single nucleotide polymorphism (SNP) in the promoter of the OPN gene (*spp1*) that correlated with a more severe progression (55). Patients with a "GG" or "GT" in position -66 progressed to full wheelchair use at an earlier age than patients with a "TT" in position -66. Coinciding with the earlier loss of ambulation was a 2.7-fold increase in expression of OPN (55). Thus, this SNP in OPN appears to be the first genetic modifier of the DMD phenotype and lends strong support for OPN as a therapeutic target.

OPN can modulate different aspects of inflammation, including immune cell migration, where its effects can be direct through CD44 integrin binding or indirect, via modulation of matrix metalloproteinases (MMPs). OPN stimulates MMP expression (56) and there is reciprocal regulation of OPN by MMPs via proteolytic cleavage. OPN fragments derived from MMP9 cleavage can affect cell migration through binding to CD44 or integrin (57). On the other hand, OPN regulates MMP9 expression via NF-κB (58,59). Both MMP2 and MMP9 are greatly upregulated in mdx muscles (59,60) and ablation of MMP9 or broad inhibition of MMPs in mdx results in improved disease (59,60). Taking into account the reciprocal relationship between OPN and MMP9, it is feasible that pharmacological inhibition of both could be synergistic and therapeutically beneficial.

NF-κB

Nuclear factor-kappa B (NF-κB) signaling is comprised of a family of transcription factors that are widely associated with regulation of inflammation. They also respond to certain inflammatory mediators, especially TNF, or reactive oxygen species (ROS). The canonical pathway includes P65/p50 dimerization, which is activated after the inhibitor I-κB is targeted for degradation. In biopsies from DMD patients (13,61) and mdx mice (20,62), the canonical NF-κB pathway is greatly elevated and its elevation correlates with the onset of disease symptoms. Inhibitors of NF-κB, such as pyrrolidine dithiocarbamate (PDTC) (63,64) and NEMO-binding peptide (20), attenuate symptoms of dystrophy in the mdx mouse. It is not clear if the high expression of NF-κB is a master driver of muscle inflammation in dystrophic muscles or if the inflammatory environment (e.g. high TNF and IL-1) drives NF-κB activation; however, it is clear that both muscle-derived and immune cell-derived NF-κB contribute to promotion of disease in the mdx mouse (20). Interestingly, high expression of NF-κB signaling can trigger muscle atrophy in the absence of any type of dystrophy (65), likely due to its ability to maintain satellite cells in the proliferative state, which prevents fusion necessary for muscle repair (66). Thus, the beneficial effects of targeting NF-κB relate to both its promotion of inflammation and its inhibition of muscle repair. Long-term studies are needed to adequately assess its affect on muscle fibrosis and function with age.

LIMB-GIRDLE MUSCULAR DYSTROPHY TYPE 2B

Immunopathogenesis of Dysferlinopathy

Genetic defects in the dysferlin gene result in limb-girdle muscular dystrophy (LGMD2B) and distal muscular dystrophy of the Miyoshi type. The muscle weakness is slowly progressive, with loss of ambulation generally occurring in the fourth decade (67,68). Dysferlin is a C2 domain containing 230 kDa transmembrane protein, which primarily resides at the intracellular face of the plasma membrane and which plays a role in membrane vesicle trafficking and membrane repair. Muscle samples from patients with dysferlin deficiency show numerous extra-structural membrane defects when analyzed by electron microscopy, including tears in the plasma membrane and accumulation of subsarcolemmal vesicles and vacuoles (69).

Inflammation in Dysferlin Deficiency

The inflammatory infiltrate in dysferlin-deficient muscle has been well described (70–72). Prominent mononuclear cell infiltrates in muscle biopsies of dysferlin-deficient patients has often led to a misdiagnosis of polymyositis; however, there are several differences between the muscle inflammation in dysferlin deficiency and that which occurs in other inflammatory muscle diseases. In general, dysferlin-deficient muscle biopsies show more macrophages and fewer $CD8^+$ T cells than biopsies from polymyositis patients. The endomysial and perivascular infiltrates in dysferlin-deficient muscle consist of $CD4^+$ T cells, macrophages, and $CD8^+$ T cells whereas non-necrotic dysferlin-deficient fibers appear free of all types of infiltrates (70). Thus the nature of the infiltrate seems to differ from that of other inflammatory myopathies such as polymyositis, in which the predominant T-cell subset is $CD8^+$ T cells infiltrating otherwise normal myofibers. Muscle inflammation in dysferlin deficiency also differs from DMD, in which macrophages and T cells are found mainly in necrotic fibers.

Skeletal muscle inflammation is also prominent in a spontaneous mouse model of dysferlinopathy (*SJL/J (SJL-Dysf)*). Staining of frozen sections of dysferlin-deficient and control muscle biopsies showed that infiltrating mononuclear and dendritic cells, but not muscle fibers, expressed high levels of HLA-A, -B, -C, HLA-DR, and CD86 antigens (Figure 78.3). Low levels of HLA-A, -B, -C and HLA-DR antigen expression were also noted on capillary endothelial cells as well as in association with fiber phagocytosis and regeneration; their occasional expression in non-necrotic fibers might represent a marker of ongoing necrosis (70–73). Thus HLA-A, -B, -C staining pattern of dysferlin muscle biopsies is distinct from inflammatory myopathies, where muscle fibers express high levels of MHC class I antigen. Similarly, staining of frozen muscle sections of SJL/J mice for macrophage activation and dendritic cell markers showed that infiltrating mononuclear cells expressed the macrophage mononuclear cell marker (MoMa-2) and activation markers CD11c and ICAM-1. These data suggest that macrophages and monocytes present in the muscle tissues of dysferlin-deficient patients and SJL/J mice have an activated phenotype. Dysferlin is normally expressed in $CD14^+$ monocytes, and $CD14^+$ cells show dysferlin deficiency in LGMD2B and Miyoshi myopathy (74). Recent studies indicate that dysferlin-deficient monocytes showed increased phagocytic activity and siRNA-mediated inhibition of dysferlin expression in the J774 macrophage cell line was associated with significantly enhanced phagocytosis (72). These data indicate that mild myofiber damage in dysferlin-deficient muscle stimulates an inflammatory cascade that may initiate, exacerbate, and possibly perpetuate the underlying myofiber-specific dystrophic process (72).

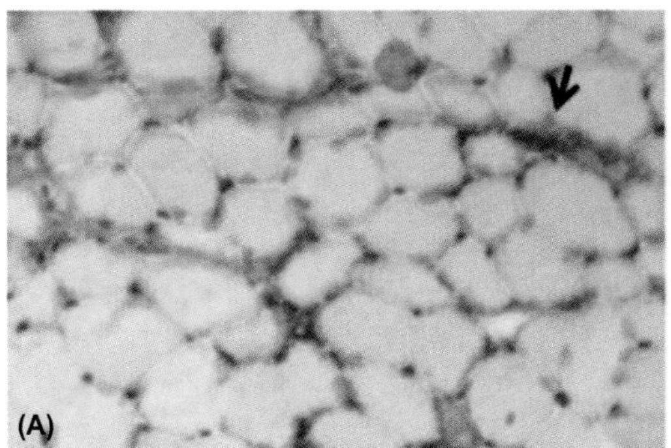

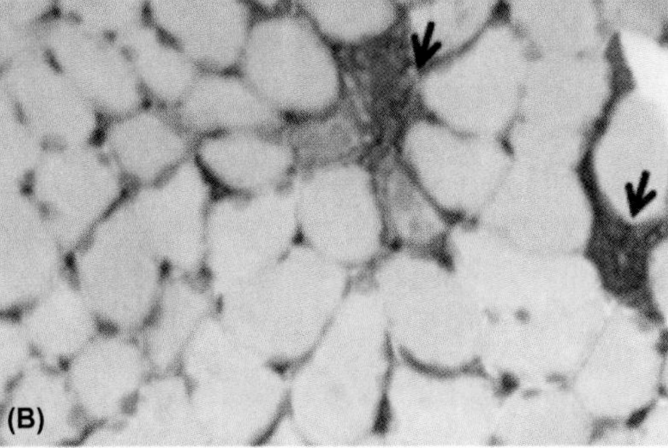

FIGURE 78.3 **Macrophage/monocyte activation markers in LGMD2B muscle biopsies.** Staining of muscle biopsies for HLA-ABC (A) and HLA-DR (B) showed most of the staining is localized to infiltrating mononuclear cells (arrow), capillaries, and some degenerating muscle fibers. Positive stain is brown. Nuclei are counterstained in blue.

Exocytosis and Secretion of Proinflammatory Molecules

Plasma membrane repair is initiated by an influx of calcium through a wound, resulting in an increase in calcium levels at the site of injury. This influx, in turn, triggers the accumulation of vesicles, which fuse with one another and then with the plasma membrane through soluble *N*-ethylmaleimide-sensitive factor attachment protein receptor (SNARE) complexes (SNARE) and synaptosome-associated protein (SNAP) family proteins at the site of injury; which reseal the wounded membrane. In LGMD2B biopsies, more than 50% of healthy-looking muscle fibers show small subsarcolemmal vacuoles, some of which are undergoing exocytosis. Query of inflammatory pathways in LGMD2B muscle biopsies showed increased expression of proinflammatory molecules such as versican and tenascin along with an increase in vesicular trafficking pathway proteins not normally observed in muscle (synaptotagmin-like protein Slp2a/SYTL2 and the small GTPase Rab27A) (75).

Recent studies suggest that thrombospondin 1 is significantly increased in dysferlin deficient muscle fibers and macrophages, suggesting that endogenous chemotactic triggers like TSP-1 have a role in sustaining muscle inflammation (76). It is known that inflammasome components (pro-IL-1β and pro-caspase-1) co-localize to lysosomes until they receive an exocytosis-inducing stimulus; in the absence of such a stimulus, these precursor molecules may undergo lysosomal degradation. The colocalization of pro-IL-1β and pro-caspase-1 and the secretion of mature IL-1β after ATP stimulation in lysosomes suggest that active caspase-1 cleaves pro-IL-1β and facilitates the secretion of mature IL-1β. The binding of extracellular ATP to P2X7 receptors facilitates lysosome exocytosis and IL-1β secretion. Indeed recent experiments demonstrate that normal primary skeletal muscle cells are capable of secreting IL-1β in response to combined treatment with lipopolysaccharide and the P2X7 receptor agonist, benzylated ATP (77). These data indicate that skeletal muscle is an active contributor of inflammatory proteins and strategies that interfere with muscle- and macrophage-derived pro-inflammatory molecules may be therapeutically useful for patients with LGMD2B.

There are very few studies that have addressed the relationship between accumulation of mutant dysferlin and inflammation in dysferlinopathy. A recent study showed that mutant but not wild-type dysferlin spontaneously aggregated in the endoplasmic reticulum (ER) and induced unfolded protein response and conversion of LC3, a marker of autophagosome formation (78). These data, coupled with recent data that overexpression of dysferlin in mouse skeletal muscle leads to accumulation of tubular aggregates and ER stress response, suggests that mutant dysferlin aggregates likely activate the endoplasmic reticulum overload response (EOR) (79). It is well known that EOR triggers NF-κB activation and inflammation, especially in multiple inflammatory muscle diseases (80). In addition, the presence of sarcolemmal and interstitial amyloid deposits in muscle fibers of patients with dysferlin mutations suggests that LGMD2B is associated with secondary amyloidosis and dysferlin protein is a constituent of these amyloid deposits and pro-inflammatory mediators such as IL-1 induce beta-amyloid associated muscle degeneration (81,82).

Role of Complement in Disease Pathogenesis

Initial electron microscopy studies showed the presence of the membrane attack complex (MAC) on the surface of isolated non-necrotic muscle fibers, indicating a role for complement activation in the disease progression (69,83). The susceptibility to complement-mediated damage is partly due to lack of the complement inhibitory factor CD55/DAF on dysferlin-deficient muscle fibers (84). Recent genetic experiments in mice that lack both dysferlin and central complement component C3 demonstrated that indeed the absence of complement activation resulted in amelioration of muscle disease in the mouse model (85).

A Model for Muscle Fiber Damage and Inflammation in Dysferlin Deficiency

Although they are born with a genetic defect in the dysferlin gene, LGMD2B patients are apparently normal until their late 'teens. As of now, the factors that initiate and perpetuate the disease are not well understood. Since dysferlin is expressed both in skeletal muscle and macrophages, it is likely that the phenotype is due to abnormalities in both cell types. We postulate that in LGMD2B, an increase in vesicular trafficking and plasma membrane repair defects result in the release of ATP and other endogenous danger/alarm signals (e.g. HMGB1 and S100 proteins). These, in turn, bind to their cellular receptors (toll-like receptors, P2X7 receptors) and activate the inflamasome and NF-κB pathways. Extracellular ATP and complement components, which are also activated, are known to induce additional pores in the plasma membrane, leading to an influx of calcium, which may potentially activate calcium-dependent proteases. Further, activation of NF-κB in this disease may induce not only muscle fiber wasting but also inhibition of myogenesis. All these downstream processes cause significant muscle fiber damage and dysfunction in addition to inflammation and fibrosis (77).

Although very little has been done to assess the contribution of inflammation to the pathogenesis of the genetically inherited muscular dystrophies, it is clear from the work in DMD and LGMD2B that mechanisms of muscle inflammation in each of these muscle diseases differs dramatically. Thus, each dystrophy must be investigated using suitable genetic models and appropriate human biopsies. Furthermore, since delivery of genes by viral vectors, or restoration of reading frame by exon skipping and stop-codon readthrough are becoming therapeutic realities, much work is necessary to evaluate the role of T cells in rejection of epitopes that are new to the immune system. Thus, even in the age of successful gene therapies, immunotherapies will need to be developed to both reduce scar tissue formation and other disease features, and to insure successful restoration of newly delivered genes.

REFERENCES

1. Arahata K, Engel AG. Monoclonal antibody analysis of mononuclear cells in myopathies. I: Quantitation of subsets according to diagnosis and sites of accumulation and demonstration and counts of muscle fibers invaded by T cells. *Ann Neurol* 1984;**16**:193–208.
2. Spencer MJ, Walsh CM, Dorshkind KA, Rodriguez EM, Tidball JG. Myonuclear apoptosis in dystrophic mdx muscle occurs by perforin-mediated cytotoxicity. *J Clin Invest* 1997;**99**:2745–51.
3. Spencer MJ, Montecino-Rodriguez E, Dorshkind K, Tidball JG. Helper (CD4(+)) and cytotoxic (CD8(+)) T cells promote the pathology of dystrophin-deficient muscle. *Clin Immunol* 2001;**98**:235–43.
4. Vetrone SA, Montecino-Rodriguez E, Kudryashova E, Kramerova I, Hoffman EP, Liu SD, et al. Osteopontin promotes fibrosis in dystrophic mouse muscle by modulating immune cell subsets and intramuscular TGF-beta. *J Clin Invest* 2009;**119**:1583–94.
5. Wehling M, Spencer MJ, Tidball JG. A nitric oxide synthase transgene ameliorates muscular dystrophy in mdx mice. *J Cell Biol* 2001;**155**:123–31.
6. Villalta SA, Nguyen HX, Deng B, Gotoh T, Tidball JG. Shifts in macrophage phenotypes and macrophage competition for arginine metabolism affect the severity of muscle pathology in muscular dystrophy. *Hum Mol Genet* 2009;**18**:482–96.
7. Vidal B, Serrano AL, Tjwa M, Suelves M, Ardite E, De Mori R, et al. Fibrinogen drives dystrophic muscle fibrosis via a TGFbeta/alternative macrophage activation pathway. *Genes Dev* 2008;**22**:1747–52.
8. Gorospe JR, Tharp MD, Hinckley J, Kornegay JN, Hoffman EP. A role for mast cells in the progression of Duchenne muscular dystrophy? Correlations in dystrophin-deficient humans, dogs, and mice. *J Neurol Sci* 1994;**122**:44–56.
9. Cai B, Spencer MJ, Nakamura G, Tseng-Ong L, Tidball JG. Eosinophilia of dystrophin-deficient muscle is promoted by perforin-mediated cytotoxicity by T cell effectors. *Am J Pathol* 2000;**156**:1789–96.
10. Wehling-Henricks M, Sokolow S, Lee JJ, Myung KH, Villalta A, Tidball JG. Major basic protein-1 promotes fibrosis of dystrophic muscle and attenuates the cellular immune response in muscular dystrophy. *Hum Mol Genet* 2008;**17**:2280–92.
11. Porter JD, Khanna S, Kaminski HJ, Rao JS, Merriam AP, Richmonds CR, et al. A chronic inflammatory response dominates the skeletal muscle molecular signature in dystrophin-deficient mdx mice. *Hum Mol Genet* 2002;**11**:263–72.
12. Chen YW, Zhao P, Borup R, Hoffman EP. Expression profiling in the muscular dystrophies: identification of novel aspects of molecular pathophysiology. *J Cell Biol* 2000;**151**:1321–36.
13. Chen YW, Nagaraju K, Bakay M, McIntyre O, Rawat R, Shi R, et al. Early onset of inflammation and later involvement of TGFbeta in Duchenne muscular dystrophy. *Neurology* 2005;**65**:826–34.
14. Demoule A, Divangahi M, Danialou G, Gvozdic D, Larkin G, Bao W, et al. Expression and regulation of CC class chemokines in the dystrophic (mdx) diaphragm. *Am J Respir Cell Mol Biol* 2005;**33**:178–85.
15. Nguyen HX, Tidball JG. Interactions between neutrophils and macrophages promote macrophage killing of rat muscle cells in vitro. *J Physiol* 2003;**547**:125–32.
16. Arnold L, Henry A, Poron F, Baba-Amer Y, van Rooijen N, Plonquet A, et al. Inflammatory monocytes recruited after skeletal muscle injury switch into antiinflammatory macrophages to support myogenesis. *J Exp Med* 2007;**204**:1057–69.
17. Lu H, Huang D, Saederup N, Charo IF, Ransohoff RM, Zhou L. Macrophages recruited via CCR2 produce insulin-like growth factor-1 to repair acute skeletal muscle injury. *FASEB J* 2011;**25**:358–69.
18. Wehling-Henricks M, Jordan MC, Gotoh T, Grody WW, Roos KP, Tidball JG. Arginine metabolism by macrophages promotes cardiac and muscle fibrosis in mdx muscular dystrophy. *PLoS One* 2010;**5**:e10763.
19. Villalta SA, Rinaldi C, Deng B, Liu G, Fedor B, Tidball JG. Interleukin-10 reduces the pathology of mdx muscular dystrophy by deactivating M1 macrophages and modulating macrophage phenotype. *Hum Mol Genet* 2010; [ePub ahead of print November 30, 2010. doi: 101093/hmg/ddq523]
20. Acharyya S, Villalta SA, Bakkar N, Bupha-Intr T, Janssen PM, Carathers M, et al. Interplay of IKK/NF-kappaB signaling in macrophages and myofibers promotes muscle degeneration in Duchenne muscular dystrophy. *J Clin Invest* 2007;**117**:889–901.
21. Bellinger AM, Reiken S, Carlson C, Mongillo M, Liu X, Rothman L, et al. Hypernitrosylated ryanodine receptor calcium release channels are leaky in dystrophic muscle. *Nat Med* 2009;**15**:325–30.
22. Hodgetts S, Radley H, Davies M, Grounds MD. Reduced necrosis of dystrophic muscle by depletion of host neutrophils, or blocking TNFalpha function with Etanercept in mdx mice. *Neuromuscul Disord* 2006;**16**:591–602.
23. Nguyen HX, Lusis AJ, Tidball JG. Null mutation of myeloperoxidase in mice prevents mechanical activation of neutrophil lysis of muscle cell membranes in vitro and in vivo. *J Physiol* 2005;**565**:403–13.
24. Rando TA, Disatnik MH, Yu Y, Franco A. Muscle cells from mdx mice have an increased susceptibility to oxidative stress. *Neuromuscul Disord* 1998;**8**:14–21.
25. Mays LE, Wilson JM. The complex and evolving story of T cell activation to AAV vector-encoded transgene products. *Mol Ther* 2011;**19**:16–27.
26. Hatton RD. TGF-beta in Th17 cell development: the truth is out there. *Immunity* 2011;**34**:288–90.

27. Morrison J, Lu QL, Pastoret C, Partridge T, Bou-Gharios G. T-cell-dependent fibrosis in the mdx dystrophic mouse. *Lab Invest* 2000;**80**:881–91.
28. Gussoni E, Pavlath GK, Miller RG, Panzara MA, Powell M, Blau HM, Steinman L. Specific T cell receptor gene rearrangements at the site of muscle degeneration in Duchenne muscular dystrophy. *J Immunol* 1994;**153**:4798–805.
29. Wilson JM. Autoimmunity, recessive diseases, and gene replacement therapy. *Mol Ther* 2010;**18**:2045–7.
30. Ohtsuka Y, Udaka K, Yamashiro Y, Yagita H, Okumura K. Dystrophin acts as a transplantation rejection antigen in dystrophin-deficient mice: implication for gene therapy. *J Immunol* 1998;**160**:4635–40.
31. Yuasa K, Sakamoto M, Miyagoe-Suzuki Y, Tanouchi A, Yamamoto H, Li J, et al. Adeno-associated virus vector-mediated gene transfer into dystrophin-deficient skeletal muscles evokes enhanced immune response against the transgene product. *Gene Ther* 2002;**9**:1576–88.
32. Gregorevic P, Allen JM, Minami E, Blankinship MJ, Haraguchi M, Meuse L, et al. rAAV6-microdystrophin preserves muscle function and extends lifespan in severely dystrophic mice. *Nat Med* 2006;**12**:787–9.
33. Odom GL, Banks GB, Schultz BR, Gregorevic P, Chamberlain JS. Preclinical studies for gene therapy of Duchenne muscular dystrophy. *J Child Neurol* 2010;**25**:1149–57.
34. Mendell JR, Campbell K, Rodino-Klapac L, Sahenk Z, Shilling C, Lewis S, et al. Dystrophin immunity in Duchenne's muscular dystrophy. *N Engl J Med* 2010;**363**:1429–37.
35. Malik V, Rodino-Klapac LR, Viollet L, Wall C, King W, Al-Dahhak R, et al. Gentamicin-induced readthrough of stop codons in Duchenne muscular dystrophy. *Ann Neurol* 2010;**67**:771–80.
36. Malik V, Rodino-Klapac LR, Viollet L, Mendell JR. Aminoglycoside-induced mutation suppression (stop codon readthrough) as a therapeutic strategy for Duchenne muscular dystrophy. *Ther Adv Neurol Disord* 2010;**3**:379–89.
37. Robbins M, Judge A, Liang L, McClintock K, Yaworski E, MacLachlan I. 2'-O-methyl-modified RNAs act as TLR7 antagonists. *Mol Ther* 2007;**15**:1663–9.
38. Gosselin LE, Barkley JE, Spencer MJ, McCormick KM, Farkas GA. Ventilatory dysfunction in mdx mice: impact of tumor necrosis factor-alpha deletion. *Muscle Nerve* 2003;**28**:336–43.
39. Bernasconi P, Di Blasi C, Mora M, Morandi L, Galbiati S, Confalonieri P, et al. Transforming growth factor-beta1 and fibrosis in congenital muscular dystrophies. *Neuromuscul Disord* 1999;**9**:28–33.
40. Zhou L, Porter JD, Cheng G, Gong B, Hatala DA, Merriam AP, et al. Temporal and spatial mRNA expression patterns of TGF-beta1, 2, 3 and TbetaRI, II, III in skeletal muscles of mdx mice. *Neuromuscul Disord* 2006;**16**:32–8.
41. Yamazaki M, Minota S, Sakurai H, Miyazono K, Yamada A, Kanazawa I, et al. Expression of transforming growth factor-beta 1 and its relation to endomysial fibrosis in progressive muscular dystrophy. *Am J Pathol* 1994;**144**:221–6.
42. Cohn RD, van Erp C, Habashi JP, Soleimani AA, Klein EC, Lisi MT, et al. Angiotensin II type 1 receptor blockade attenuates TGF-beta-induced failure of muscle regeneration in multiple myopathic states. *Nat Med* 2007;**13**:204–10.
43. Andreetta F, Bernasconi P, Baggi F, Ferro P, Oliva L, Arnoldi E, et al. Immunomodulation of TGF-beta 1 in mdx mouse inhibits connective tissue proliferation in diaphragm but increases inflammatory response: implications for antifibrotic therapy. *J Neuroimmunol* 2006;**175**:77–86.
44. Farini A, Meregalli M, Belicchi M, Battistelli M, Parolini D, D'Antona G, et al. T and B lymphocyte depletion has a marked effect on the fibrosis of dystrophic skeletal muscles in the scid/mdx mouse. *J Pathol* 2007;**213**:229–38.
45. Alexakis C, Partridge T, Bou-Gharios G. Implication of the satellite cell in dystrophic muscle fibrosis: a self-perpetuating mechanism of collagen overproduction. *Am J Physiol Cell Physiol* 2007;**293**:C661–9.
46. Heydemann A, Ceco E, Lim JE, Hadhazy M, Ryder P, Moran JL, et al. Latent TGF-beta-binding protein 4 modifies muscular dystrophy in mice. *J Clin Invest* 2009;**119**:3703–12.
47. Gosselin LE, Martinez DA. Impact of TNF-alpha blockade on TGF-beta1 and type I collagen mRNA expression in dystrophic muscle. *Muscle Nerve* 2004;**30**:244–6.
48. Radley HG, Davies MJ, Grounds MD. Reduced muscle necrosis and long-term benefits in dystrophic mdx mice after cV1q (blockade of TNF) treatment. *Neuromuscul Disord* 2008;**18**:227–38.
49. De Luca A, Nico B, Liantonio A, Didonna MP, Fraysse B, Pierno S, et al. A multidisciplinary evaluation of the effectiveness of cyclosporine a in dystrophic mdx mice. *Am J Pathol* 2005;**166**:477–89.
50. Pierno S, Nico B, Burdi R, Liantonio A, Didonna MP, Cippone V, et al. Role of tumour necrosis factor alpha, but not of cyclo-oxygenase-2-derived eicosanoids, on functional and morphological indices of dystrophic progression in mdx mice: a pharmacological approach. *Neuropathol Appl Neurobiol* 2007;**33**:344–59.
51. Suzuki K, Zhu B, Rittling SR, Denhardt DT, Goldberg HA, McCulloch CA, et al. Colocalization of intracellular osteopontin with CD44 is associated with migration, cell fusion, and resorption in osteoclasts. *J Bone Miner Res* 2002;**17**:1486–97.
52. Bayless KJ, Meininger GA, Scholtz JM, Davis GE. Osteopontin is a ligand for the alpha4beta1 integrin. *J Cell Sci* 1998;**111** (Pt 9):1165–74.
53. Mukherjee BB, Nemir M, Beninati S, Cordella-Miele E, Singh K, Chackalaparampil I, et al. Interaction of osteopontin with fibronectin and other extracellular matrix molecules. *Ann NY Acad Sci* 1995;**760**:201–12.
54. Wang KX, Denhardt DT. Osteopontin: role in immune regulation and stress responses. *Cytokine Growth Factor Rev* 2008;**19**:333–45.
55. Pegoraro E, Hoffman EP, Piva L, Gavassini BF, Cagnin S, Ermani M, et al. SPP1 genotype is a determinant of disease severity in Duchenne muscular dystrophy. *Neurology* 2011;**76**:219–26.
56. Rangaswami H, Bulbule A, Kundu GC. Nuclear factor-inducing kinase plays a crucial role in osteopontin-induced MAPK/IkappaBalpha kinase-dependent nuclear factor kappaB-mediated promatrix metalloproteinase-9 activation. *J Biol Chem* 2004;**279**:38921–35.
57. Takafuji V, Forgues M, Unsworth E, Goldsmith P, Wang XW. An osteopontin fragment is essential for tumor cell invasion in hepatocellular carcinoma. *Oncogene* 2007;**26**:6361–71.
58. Chen YJ, Wei YY, Chen HT, Fong YC, Hsu CJ, Tsai CH, Hsu HC, Liu SH, Tang CH. Osteopontin increases migration and MMP-9 up-regulation via alphavbeta3 integrin, FAK, ERK,

and NF-kappaB-dependent pathway in human chondrosarcoma cells. *J Cell Physiol* 2009;**221**:98–108.

59. Kumar A, Bhatnagar S. Matrix metalloproteinase inhibitor batimastat alleviates pathology and improves skeletal muscle function in dystrophin-deficient mdx mice. *Am J Pathol* 2010;**177**:248–60.
60. Li H, Mittal A, Makonchuk DY, Bhatnagar S, Kumar A. Matrix metalloproteinase-9 inhibition ameliorates pathogenesis and improves skeletal muscle regeneration in muscular dystrophy. *Hum Mol Genet* 2009;**18**:2584–98.
61. Monici MC, Aguennouz M, Mazzeo A, Messina C, Vita G. Activation of nuclear factor-kappaB in inflammatory myopathies and Duchenne muscular dystrophy. *Neurology* 2003;**60**:993–7.
62. Kumar A, Boriek AM. Mechanical stress activates the nuclear factor-kappaB pathway in skeletal muscle fibers: a possible role in Duchenne muscular dystrophy. *FASEB J* 2003;**17**:386–96.
63. Messina S, Altavilla D, Aguennouz M, Seminara P, Minutoli L, Monici MC, et al. Lipid peroxidation inhibition blunts nuclear factor-kappaB activation, reduces skeletal muscle degeneration, and enhances muscle function in mdx mice. *Am J Pathol* 2006;**168**:918–26.
64. Siegel AL, Bledsoe C, Lavin J, Gatti F, Berge J, Millman G, et al. Treatment with inhibitors of the NF-kappaB pathway improves whole body tension development in the mdx mouse. *Neuromuscul Disord* 2009;**19**:131–9.
65. Van Gammeren D, Damrauer JS, Jackman RW, Kandarian SC. The IkappaB kinases IKKalpha and IKKbeta are necessary and sufficient for skeletal muscle atrophy. *FASEB J* 2009;**23**:362–70.
66. Guttridge DC, Mayo MW, Madrid LV, Wang CY, Baldwin Jr AS. NF-kappaB-induced loss of MyoD messenger RNA: possible role in muscle decay and cachexia. *Science* 2000;**289**:2363–6.
67. Liu J, Aoki M, Illa I, Wu C, Fardeau M, Angelini C, et al. Dysferlin, a novel skeletal muscle gene, is mutated in Miyoshi myopathy and limb girdle muscular dystrophy. *Nat Genet* 1998;**20**:31–6.
68. Bashir R, Britton S, Strachan T, Keers S, Vafiadaki E, Lako M, et al. A gene related to Caenorhabditis elegans spermatogenesis factor fer-1 is mutated in limb-girdle muscular dystrophy type 2B. *Nat Genet* 1998;**20**:37–42.
69. Selcen D, Stilling G, Engel AG. The earliest pathologic alterations in dysferlinopathy. *Neurology* 2001;**56**:1472–81.
70. Gallardo E, Rojas-Garcia R, de Luna N, Pou A, Brown Jr RH, Illa I. Inflammation in dysferlin myopathy: immunohistochemical characterization of 13 patients. *Neurology* 2001;**57**:2136–8.
71. Confalonieri P, Oliva L, Andreetta F, Lorenzoni R, Dassi P, Mariani E, et al. Muscle inflammation and MHC class I up-regulation in muscular dystrophy with lack of dysferlin: an immunopathological study. *J Neuroimmunol* 2003;**142**:130–6.
72. Nagaraju K, Rawat R, Veszelovszky E, Thapliyal R, Kesari A, Sparks S, et al. Dysferlin deficiency enhances monocyte phagocytosis: a model for the inflammatory onset of limb-girdle muscular dystrophy 2B. *Am J Pathol* 2008;**172**:774–85.
73. Fanin M, Angelini C. Muscle pathology in dysferlin deficiency. *Neuropathol Appl Neurobiol* 2002;**28**:461–70.
74. Ho M, Gallardo E, McKenna-Yasek D, De Luna N, Illa I, Brown Jr RH. A novel, blood-based diagnostic assay for limb girdle muscular dystrophy 2B and Miyoshi myopathy. *Ann Neurol* 2002;**51**:129–33.
75. Kesari A, Fukuda M, Knoblach S, Bashir R, Nader GA, Rao D, et al. Dysferlin deficiency shows compensatory induction of Rab27A/Slp2a that may contribute to inflammatory onset. *Am J Pathol* 2008;**173**:1476–87.
76. De Luna N, Gallardo E, Sonnet C, Chazaud B, Dominguez-Perles R, Suarez-Calvet X, et al. Role of thrombospondin 1 in macrophage inflammation in dysferlin myopathy. *J Neuropathol Exp Neurol* **69**:643–53.
77. Rawat R, Cohen TV, Ampong B, Francia D, Henriques-Pons A, Hoffman EP, et al. Inflammasome up-regulation and activation in dysferlin-deficient skeletal muscle. *Am J Pathol* 2010;**176**:2891–900.
78. Fujita E, Kouroku Y, Isoai A, Kumagai H, Misutani A, Matsuda C, et al. Two endoplasmic reticulum-associated degradation (ERAD) systems for the novel variant of the mutant dysferlin: ubiquitin/proteasome ERAD(I) and autophagy/lysosome ERAD(II). *Hum Mol Genet* 2007;**16**:618–29.
79. Glover LE, Newton K, Krishnan G, Bronson R, Boyle A, Krivickas LS, et al. Dysferlin overexpression in skeletal muscle produces a progressive myopathy. *Ann Neurol* 2010;**67**:384–93.
80. Nagaraju K, Casciola-Rosen L, Lundberg I, Rawat R, Cutting S, Thapliyal R, et al. Activation of the endoplasmic reticulum stress response in autoimmune myositis: potential role in muscle fiber damage and dysfunction. *Arthritis Rheum* 2005;**52**:1824–35.
81. Spuler S, Carl M, Zabojszcza J, Straub V, Bushby K, Moore SA, et al. Dysferlin-deficient muscular dystrophy features amyloidosis. *Ann Neurol* 2008;**63**:323–8.
82. Schmidt J, Barthel K, Wrede A, Salajegheh M, Bahr M, Dalakas MC. Interrelation of inflammation and APP in sIBM: IL-1 beta induces accumulation of beta-amyloid in skeletal muscle. *Brain* 2008;**131**:1228–40.
83. Spuler S, Engel AG. Unexpected sarcolemmal complement membrane attack complex deposits on nonnecrotic muscle fibers in muscular dystrophies. *Neurology* 1998;**50**:41–6.
84. Wenzel K, Zabojszcza J, Carl M, Taubert S, Lass A, Harris CL, et al. Increased susceptibility to complement attack due to down-regulation of decay-accelerating factor/CD55 in dysferlin-deficient muscular dystrophy. *J Immunol* 2005;**175**:6219–25.
85. Han R, Frett EM, Levy JR, Rader EP, Lueck JD, Bansal D, et al. Genetic ablation of complement C3 attenuates muscle pathology in dysferlin-deficient mice. *J Clin Invest* 2010;**120**:4366–74.

Chapter 79

Myostatin: Regulation, Function, and Therapeutic Applications

Se-Jin Lee
Johns Hopkins University School of Medicine, Department of Molecular Biology and Genetics, Baltimore, MD

DISCOVERY OF MYOSTATIN AND ITS BIOLOGICAL FUNCTION AS A NEGATIVE REGULATOR OF MUSCLE MASS

Myostatin (MSTN; also called growth/differentiation factor-8 or GDF-8) was originally identified in a screen for new members of the transforming growth factor (TGF-ß) superfamily of signaling molecules (1). A possible role for MSTN in regulating skeletal muscle development and function was suggested by its expression pattern, as *Mstn* mRNA was detected almost exclusively in the skeletal muscle lineage both during embryogenesis and in adult tissues. The biological function of MSTN was elucidated through gene targeting studies in mice, which revealed that loss of MSTN led to dramatic increases in skeletal muscle mass throughout the body, with individual muscles growing to about twice the normal size. The fact that both fiber numbers and fiber sizes were increased in *Mstn* null mice suggested that MSTN normally plays two roles to limit muscle mass, a developmental role to regulate the number of muscle fibers that are formed and a postnatal role to regulate muscle fiber growth.

The discovery of MSTN immediately suggested the possibility that inhibitors of MSTN signaling might have applications for increasing muscle growth both for enhancing livestock production and for treating human muscle-wasting conditions. Indeed, a large number of subsequent studies have provided compelling impetus for pursuing these types of applications. In particular, although the initial studies identifying MSTN and its biological function were carried out in mice, it is now clear that both the amino acid sequence of MSTN and its function as a negative regulator of muscle mass have been highly conserved across species. The predicted amino acid sequence of the active MSTN molecule is identical, for example, between chickens and humans (2), and naturally-occurring mutations in the *MSTN* gene leading to increased muscling have now been identified in cattle (2–5), sheep (6), dogs (7), and humans (8). Furthermore, the identification of regulatory and signaling components of the MSTN pathway (Figure 79.1) has led to the development of a variety of pharmacological agents capable of blocking MSTN activity *in vivo* (9–14), and a number of these agents have been shown to be capable of causing significant muscle growth when administered systemically to normal adult mice, demonstrating conclusively that this regulatory system plays an important role in suppressing muscle growth postnatally.

REGULATION OF MSTN EXTRACELLULARLY BY BINDING PROTEINS

MSTN is synthesized as a precursor protein that undergoes proteolytic processing to generate the active species (1). Following removal of the signal peptide, pro-MSTN is cleaved by furin proteases to generate a C-terminal fragment of 109 amino acids, a disulfide-linked dimer of which is the biologically-active molecule. There is some evidence to suggest that processing of the precursor protein may be one step at which the levels of active MSTN may be regulated (15). Following processing, the C-terminal dimer remains non-covalently bound to the N-terminal propeptide, which maintains the C-terminal dimer in an inactive or latent state (16,17). This latent complex of C-terminal dimer and N-terminal propeptide appears to represent the major circulating form of MSTN in the blood (18,19).

The C-terminal dimer in the latent complex can be activated *in vitro* by causing dissociation of the propeptide, such as by acid or heat treatment (11,18). A major question has been how the latent complex is activated *in vivo*, and there is now considerable evidence that this occurs predominantly by proteolytic cleavage of the propeptide by members of the BMP-1/TLD family of metalloproteases (11,20). Purified forms of each of the four known members of this protease family (BMP-1, TLD,

Muscle. DOI: http://dx.doi.org/10.1016/B978-0-12-381510-1.00079-X

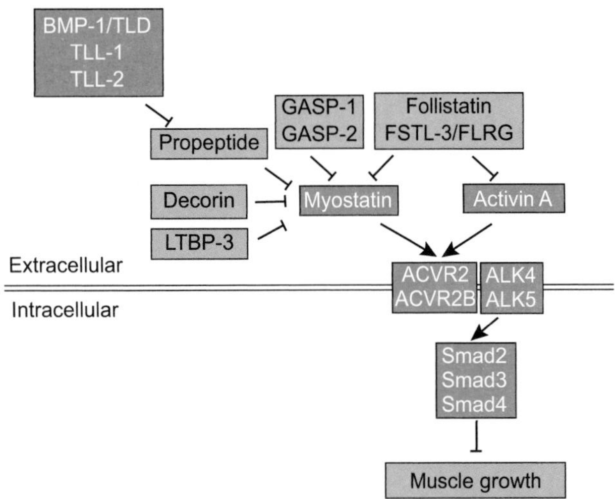

FIGURE 79.1 Regulatory and signaling components. Components shown in red promote signaling through this pathway and thereby suppress muscle growth. Components shown in green block signaling through this pathway and thereby stimulate muscle growth.

TLL-1, and TLL-2) are capable of cleaving and activating the purified MSTN latent complex *in vitro* (11). Moreover, targeted mutations either in the *Mstn* gene rendering the propeptide resistant to cleavage or in at least one member of this protease gene family (*Tll2*) have been shown to partially phenocopy the *Mstn* deletion mutation in terms of increased muscle mass, consistent with an inability to activate fully the latent complex in these mutant mice (20).

In addition to the propeptide, a number of other proteins have been shown to bind MSTN and inhibit its activity. One of these is follistatin (FST), which is a protein originally identified for its ability to inhibit FSH secretion by pituitary cells (21,22). Follistatin was shown to exert its activity by binding to activins (23), which like MSTN, are members of the TGF-ß family of secreted proteins. Subsequent studies demonstrated that follistatin is also capable of binding other TGF-ß family members, most notably the bone morphogenetic proteins (BMPs) and GDF-11, which is highly related to MSTN (1,24). The latter finding raised the possibility that follistatin may also be capable of binding and inhibiting MSTN, and this has been borne out both by *in vitro* studies using purified proteins and by *in vivo* studies in which follistatin was overexpressed as a transgene in skeletal muscle (16). In support of a normal role for endogenous follistatin as an antagonist of MSTN signaling *in vivo* is the finding that mice heterozygous for an *Fst* loss-of-function mutation (homozygous *Fst* mutants are not viable) exhibit decreased muscle mass (25), which is the opposite of what is observed in mice lacking MSTN. Although these findings are consistent with increased MSTN signaling in *Fst* mutant mice, genetic studies analyzing compound *Fst/Mstn* mutant mice have demonstrated that follistatin appears to be regulating muscle mass by blocking not only MSTN but also an additional ligand with similar biological activity. The existence of additional ligands that seem to cooperate with MSTN to limit muscle mass was also uncovered in transgenic studies in which overexpression of follistatin in muscle was found to cause another doubling of muscle mass (i.e. an overall quadrupling) in mice completely lacking MSTN (26) (Figure 79.2). Although the identity of the ligand or ligands that cooperate with MSTN is still being investigated, a variety of studies have implicated activin A as the most likely candidate.

Besides follistatin, a number of other MSTN inhibitory proteins have also been identified. One of these is FSTL-3 (also called FLRG), which is another member of the follistatin family. FSTL-3 is capable of binding MSTN and inhibiting its activity *in vitro* (19), and overexpression of FSTL-3 in mice was shown to cause increased muscle mass (26), consistent with inhibition of MSTN activity *in vivo*. Although mice lacking FSTL-3 appear to have relatively normal muscle mass (25,27), FSTL-3 has been detected in a complex with MSTN in serum (19), suggesting that it may play some role in regulating MSTN activity *in vivo*. Two other proteins containing follistatin domains, namely GASP-1 and GASP-2, have also been shown to be capable of functioning as MSTN inhibitors (28,29). Although the ability of GASP-1 and GASP-2 to bind and inhibit MSTN *in vitro* has been well documented, what role these molecules play *in vivo* is not yet clear, as the phenotype of mice carrying mutations in these genes has not yet been reported; however, as in the case of FSTL-3, an *in vivo* role for GASP-1 in regulating MSTN activity has been suggested by the finding that GASP-1 appears to be complexed to MSTN in the blood (28). The role of GASP-1 and GASP-2 in regulating MSTN activity is likely to be complex, as these proteins contain multiple distinct protease inhibitory domains and are capable of binding both the mature C-terminal portion of MSTN as well as its propeptide. Finally, two other extracellular proteins, LTBP-3 (latent TGF-ß binding protein-3) (15) and decorin (30), have also been shown to bind MSTN and have been proposed to regulate the processing of pro-MSTN and to maintain MSTN bound to the extracellular matrix, respectively.

When not bound to inhibitory proteins, the mature MSTN molecule appears to signal through a two component receptor system that is typical of members of the TGF-ß superfamily. MSTN binds initially to the activin type II receptors (ACVR2 and ACVR2B; also called ActRII and ActRIIB) (16), exhibiting a higher affinity for ACVR2B than for ACVR2. Based on the analysis of mice carrying mutations in each of these receptor genes, the two receptors appear to be functionally redundant

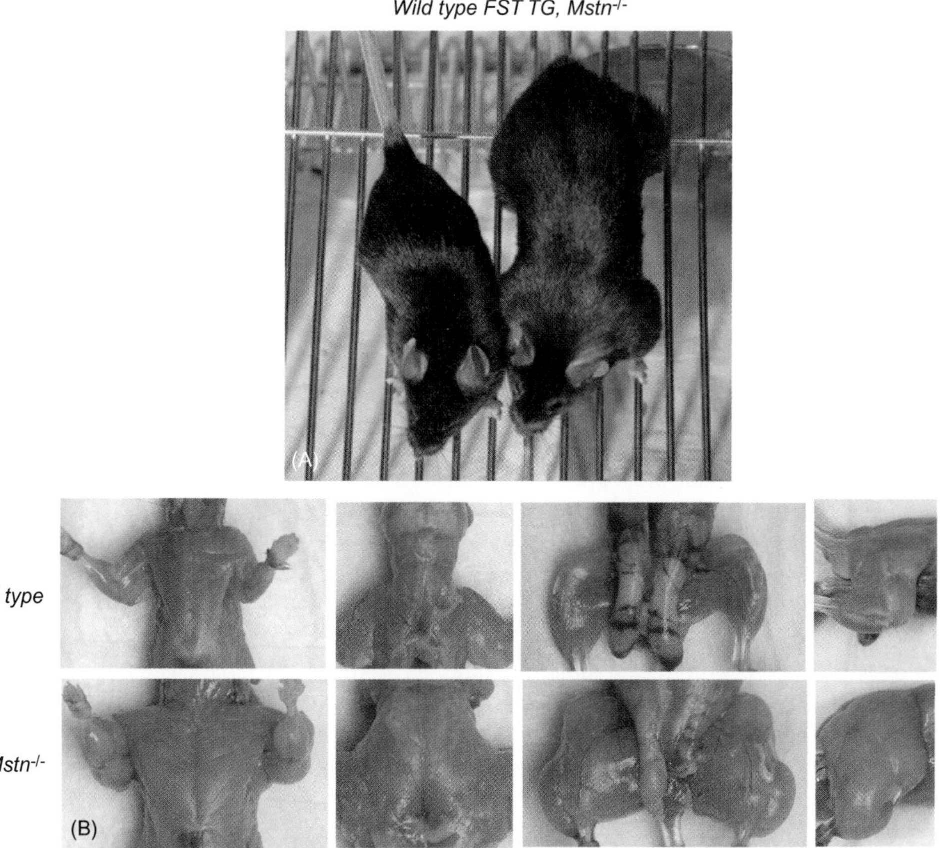

FIGURE 79.2 Effect of overexpressing follistatin in mice lacking myostatin. (a) *Wild-type* mouse (left) next to a quadruple-muscled *Mstn* null, *Fst* transgenic (TG) mouse (right). (b) Comparison of muscles of a *wild-type* mouse (top panels) with those of a quadruple-muscled *Mstn* null, *Fst* TG mouse (bottom panels). *(Images reproduced from Lee, 2007 (26), with permission from the author.)*

with respect to the control of muscle mass, and it seems likely that MSTN utilizes both receptors *in vivo* (12). Binding of MSTN to the activin type II receptors then leads to binding and phosphorylation of type I receptors. *In vitro* studies have suggested that either of two type I receptors, ALK4 or ALK5, seems to mediate MSTN signaling (31), but genetic studies targeting these receptors in muscle *in vivo* have not yet been reported. The activated type I receptors then almost certainly propagate the intracellular signal via phosphorylation of Smad2 and/or Smad3. Although some of the gene expression changes resulting from activation and inhibition of this pathway have been identified, which of these are essential for the physiological effects seen upon manipulation of this pathway are not known.

DEVELOPMENT OF MSTN INHIBITORS AS POTENTIAL THERAPEUTIC AGENTS

Based on the biological function of MSTN, an enormous amount of effort has been directed at developing agents capable of blocking this signaling pathway *in vivo*. The fact that MSTN is a secreted signaling protein immediately raised the possibility that neutralizing monoclonal antibodies directed against MSTN might be effective as therapeutic agents. Several pharmaceutical and biotechnology companies have reported the development of either monoclonal antibodies or peptibodies that are highly specific for MSTN (10,13,14). In general, these molecules have been reported to be capable of causing muscle growth by about 25–30% when administered systemically to adult mice. At least several such molecules have progressed to human testing, although the results of only one such clinical trial have been reported in the literature to date (see below).

In addition to monoclonal antibodies, a number of other pharmacologic agents have been developed that are capable of blocking MSTN activity. All of these have exploited the known regulatory and signaling mechanisms that have been elucidated to date, and most of these agents have been biologics that have been engineered as Fc fusion proteins in order to enhance their stability *in vivo*. One such agent is a form of the MSTN propeptide, which as discussed above, is capable of binding the mature MSTN molecule and preventing it from signaling. The most active form of the propeptide *in vivo* is a fusion of an Fc domain to a mutant version of the propeptide carrying a single amino acid change (D76A) that renders it resistant to cleavage by members of the BMP-1/TLD family of proteases (11). This molecule, which is capable of binding both MSTN and the highly related protein, GDF-11, can induce muscle growth in mice to a similar extent as the MSTN monoclonal antibodies.

The most potent pharmacological agent that has been reported to date is a soluble form of the activin type IIB receptor (ACVR2B/Fc or ActRIIB/Fc) (12). This soluble receptor is capable of inducing much more substantial muscle growth than either the D76A mutant propeptide/Fc fusion protein or monoclonal antibodies directed against MSTN. Just two intraperitoneal injections of the soluble receptor have been shown to be sufficient to induce a 40–60% increase in skeletal muscle mass throughout the body over a two-week period. A major reason for the enhanced effect seen with the soluble receptor compared to other MSTN inhibitors is that the soluble receptor, like follistatin, is capable of inhibiting other TGF-ß family members besides MSTN that also appear to function to limit muscle growth. The clearest demonstration of this expanded range of the soluble receptor compared to other MSTN inhibitors is that the soluble receptor can induce muscle growth even in *Mstn* null mice. At least one biotechnology company, namely Acceleron Pharma, has tested this soluble receptor in human trials, and this company is currently conducting a phase II clinical trial with their version of this molecule in patients with muscular dystrophy.

Although considerable progress has been made in terms of developing biologic agents capable of targeting this pathway *in vivo*, much less progress has been made in terms of developing small molecule inhibitors of MSTN signaling. Small molecule inhibitors of the type I receptors, ALK4 and ALK5, have been developed for other applications, and these have been shown to be capable of blocking MSTN signaling *in vitro* (32); however, there has not yet been a report demonstrating that these inhibitors can induce muscle growth *in vivo*. The only other obvious potential targets for small molecule drug discovery based on what is known currently about the regulatory and signaling components of this pathway would be the type II receptors, ACVR2 and ACVR2B, and the metalloproteases in the BMP-1/TLD family. Finally, there have been reports suggesting that certain HDAC inhibitors can induce expression of the MSTN antagonist, follistatin (33), and some studies have reported beneficial effects of HDAC inhibitors in the setting of muscle degeneration, which have been attributed to their ability to upregulate follistatin expression (34). Clearly, the development of small molecule inhibitors of this pathway is still in its infancy, and a major challenge for this effort will be either to limit effects of targeting the known components to muscle or to identify additional components that may be more specific for muscle.

PHYSIOLOGICAL EFFECTS OF TARGETING MSTN SIGNALING IN NORMAL AND DISEASE SETTINGS

The availability of both genetic and pharmacological tools to manipulate levels of signaling *in vivo* has led to an explosion of studies investigating the effects of manipulating this pathway in both normal and disease settings. What is clear is that inhibition of this signaling pathway in normal mice can lead to dramatic and widespread increases in skeletal muscle mass. Genetic manipulations that result in inhibition of this pathway during development lead to increased muscle fiber numbers, and several studies have shown that the increases in fiber numbers seen in *Mstn* null mice are restricted just to type II fibers (mostly IIx and IIb) (35–38). In contrast, either genetic or pharmacological manipulations that result in postnatal inhibition of this pathway lead to muscle fiber hypertrophy, and in this case, both type I and type II fibers seem to be affected (39–41). There is also general agreement that these increases in muscle mass are accompanied by increases in muscle strength and contractile force, with perhaps the most striking illustration being the enhanced racing performance of whippets that are heterozygous for a *MSTN* loss-of-function mutation (7); however, some studies reported a reduction in specific force when the pathway is downregulated, suggesting that the effects on muscle function may not be commensurate with the overall effects on muscle mass (36). Finally, it is clear that the range of effects that can be generated by manipulating this signaling pathway is enormous and that within this range, the regulatory system operates much like a rheostat, with mutations in many of the regulatory components exhibiting haploinsufficiency (for review see reference 42); hence, effects on muscle mass and growth can be finely tuned by subtly manipulating the homeostatic regulatory balance among the various components.

These properties of the MSTN regulatory system and the availability of tools and methods to manipulate levels of signaling have made this pathway an area of intensive investigation with respect to identifying human disease states in which targeting MSTN signaling may provide therapeutic benefit. A large part of this effort has been directed at investigating the potential benefit of targeting this pathway in primary muscle degenerative diseases, such as muscular dystrophy. The rationale has been that although this strategy would not address the underlying cause of muscle degeneration, targeting MSTN signaling in this disease setting might allow for additional muscle growth and/or regeneration and thereby perhaps compensate for the loss of muscle function resulting from mutations in genes such as *dystrophin*. A large number of studies have reported the effects of either crossing in the *Mstn* loss-of-function mutation or administering MSTN inhibitors directly to a wide range of genetic models of muscular dystrophy, including models of Duchenne muscular dystrophy, congenital muscular dystrophy type 1A, and various subtypes of limb girdle muscular dystrophy (for review see reference 43). Although the results of these studies were somewhat variable depending on the specific models that were examined, the specific interventions that were employed, and the stage of disease that was investigated, the positive finding was that loss or inhibition of signaling could generally increase muscle mass and strength in many of these models. Moreover, in several cases, beneficial effects on reducing muscle fibrosis were also observed. The results of these preclinical studies were sufficiently encouraging for two clinical trials to move forward in patients with muscular dystrophy, one using a monoclonal antibody directed against MSTN (MYO-029) in a heterogenous group of adult patients (44) and the other using a soluble ACVR2B receptor in children with Duchenne muscular dystrophy.

Several preclinical studies have also tested the efficacy of MSTN inhibition in models of other neuromuscular diseases in addition to muscular dystrophy (for review see reference 43). Specifically, both genetic and pharmacological approaches have been used to inhibit the MSTN pathway in mouse models of amyotrophic lateral sclerosis (ALS) and spinal muscular atrophy (SMA). The results of these studies have been somewhat mixed in that although increases in muscle mass were observed in some of these studies, the interventions did not lead to significant improvement in terms of overall survival.

Although much of the focus of MSTN inhibition as a therapeutic strategy has been on genetic models of muscle degenerative diseases, there is considerable interest in the possibility that this therapeutic strategy may be effective in settings of more acute muscle loss. A major area of investigation in this regard is in the setting of cachexia, which can accompany a variety of disease states, including cancer, AIDS, sepsis, burns, kidney failure, and congestive heart failure. Although the etiology of cachexia is not well understood, the finding that overexpression of MSTN could itself induce a cachexia-like syndrome in mice raised the possibility that overactivity of this pathway might play a causative role in inducing muscle wasting in cachectic patients (18). Indeed, several studies have found components of this regulatory system to be misregulated in experimental models of cachexia, and a recent study found that a number of human tumors produce high levels of activin A, raising the possibility that activin A may be the culprit that activates this signaling pathway at least in some patients with cancer cachexia (45). Several studies have reported that blocking the MSTN pathway pharmacologically in experimental models of cachexia in mice can be effective in preserving muscle mass or reversing muscle loss (14,45,46). Moreover, in one of these studies, blocking this pathway with the soluble ACVR2B receptor was shown to increase survival in mice bearing cachexia-inducing tumors even though actual tumor growth was not affected, suggesting that preservation of muscle mass in itself might prolong survival in cancer patients (45).

Although these studies provide compelling support for further evaluating this therapeutic strategy in humans with cachexia, the question of whether activation of this pathway plays a causative role in inducing wasting is still not completely answered, at least with respect to cancer cachexia. A causative role for MSTN in cachexia has been more firmly established in the case of cardiac cachexia. Although the predominant source of MSTN in the body under normal conditions is skeletal muscle, *MSTN* expression in cardiac muscle has been found to be upregulated during heart failure both in humans and in experimental models in animals (47–50). Moreover, a heart-specific knockout of the *Mstn* gene in mice was shown to prevent the increase in circulating MSTN protein levels following transverse aortic constriction and to render the mice resistant to the skeletal muscle atrophy that is normally induced in this injury paradigm (51). Assuming that this same mechanism is responsible for the induction of cardiac cachexia in humans, this is perhaps the most clear-cut example to date of a disease setting in which MSTN overactivity plays a direct role in the pathogenesis of muscle wasting. It will be important to determine the extent to which MSTN plays a causative role in cachexia induced by other disease states.

Besides muscle degenerative diseases and cachexia, a third area being actively explored for potential therapeutic applications for MSTN inhibition is the muscle loss that occurs during aging, or age-related sarcopenia. It is well known that humans lose muscle mass as a function of age, and although a variety of hypotheses have been put forth to explain the molecular and physiological basis for this phenomenon, the cause of age-related muscle loss is not fully understood. A variety of studies have investigated the possibility that changes in levels of MSTN signaling as a function of age might play a role in the etiology of age-related sarcopenia (for review see reference 52). These have included studies measuring levels of MSTN and some of the known signaling components in young versus old mice and humans, analyzing the pattern of muscle loss in aged *Mstn* knockout mice, and attempting to correlate polymorphisms in human genes encoding signaling components with muscle function in the elderly. Although these studies have identified some tantalizing associations, additional studies will be required to establish more conclusively whether MSTN does play a role in the etiology of sarcopenia. What is clear, at least in animal studies, is that aged muscle is responsive to pathway inhibition. Several studies have shown that the anabolic effects of pharmacological agents targeting this pathway in young mice can also be seen in old mice (13). It is simply too early to know whether the same will turn out to be case in humans.

Finally, it is well established that targeting the MSTN pathway can have profound effects not only in terms of enhancing muscle mass and function but also in terms of improving metabolic function. Indeed, an early study showed that mice lacking MSTN have reduced fat stores and that loss of MSTN could partially suppress fat accumulation and the development of insulin resistance in mouse models of obesity and type II diabetes (53). Whether these metabolic effects result from loss of MSTN signaling directly to adipose tissue or are an indirect result of the anabolic effects of MSTN loss on skeletal muscle has not been definitively established. The former possibility has been supported by both *in vitro* and *in vivo* studies showing that MSTN can signal directly to adipocytes (for review see reference 54) as well as by the observation that MSTN expression in adipose tissue is dramatically elevated in obese mice (55); however, based on the fact that similar metabolic effects have been observed in a variety of different mouse lines with increased muscling, it seems more likely that the metabolic effects seen in mice in which this pathway has been targeted are an indirect result of the loss of signaling to skeletal muscle. Whatever the underlying basis for these metabolic effects may be, numerous follow up studies have demonstrated the potential benefits of targeting this pathway in experimental models of metabolic disease, including studies in which MSTN inhibitors have been administered systemically to mice (13,56). As a result, there is considerable interest in the possibility that agents targeting this pathway may have applications not only for muscle degenerative and wasting conditions but perhaps also for diseases like obesity and type II diabetes.

CONCLUSIONS AND SPECULATION

Since the initial discovery of myostatin in 1997 as a negative regulator of muscle mass, an enormous amount of progress has been made in terms of understanding the regulation of myostatin, identifying key components of this signaling system, and assessing the effects of manipulating the MSTN pathway *in vivo*. Numerous pharmacological agents have been developed that have been demonstrated to be effective in blocking this pathway *in vivo*. Many of these have been tested in a wide range of experimental models of muscle and metabolic diseases, and based on these preclinical studies, several such agents have progressed to the stage of human testing. Despite this progress, however, a number of important questions remain regarding the biology of MSTN. Perhaps the most basic questions relate to the evolution of this regulatory system. Why, for example, has this system evolved to encompass such a complex network of regulatory components? Moreover, given that it would seem to make the most sense to be able to control the growth of individual muscles locally, why develop a system in which such a key mediator like MSTN circulates in the blood? Perhaps most fundamentally, why has this regulatory system been so strongly maintained through evolutionary selection?

In attempting to answer such basic questions, it is critical to keep in mind that loss of MSTN not only leads to dramatic increases in skeletal muscle mass but also has significant effects on fat accumulation and glucose metabolism. In this regard, I speculated previously (42,57) that perhaps the fundamental physiological role of MSTN may be to regulate the homeostatic balance between muscle and fat and that perhaps levels of MSTN signaling may be modulated in response to various physiological stimuli in order to shift the metabolic balance either toward muscle growth or toward fat storage. An appealing aspect of this model is that it provides a rationale for explaining not only the complexity of this regulatory system but also one of the conundrums of MSTN biology, namely, the fact that MSTN circulates in the blood. According to this model, levels of circulating MSTN protein might be regulated in order to set overall limits on the amount of skeletal muscle mass maintained throughout the body, but because this circulating MSTN protein is bound to inhibitory proteins and therefore biologically latent, the growth of individual muscles could be controlled locally by regulating the extent to which the latent MSTN complex is activated at the target site. In this manner, MSTN could function as a systemic regulator of the overall metabolic balance between muscle and fat while at the same time acting locally to control the growth of individual muscles.

If this hypothesis is correct, the implication would be that although MSTN plays a critical role for animals in the wild, this entire regulatory system may be largely dispensable for humans; that is, given that we are no longer subject to environmental stressors such as threats from predators, lack of food availability, and extended exposure to extremes in temperatures, our survival may be less dependent on exactly where we maintain our homeostatic set point in balancing muscle versus fat. In this respect, for humans, the MSTN regulatory system may essentially be an evolutionary vestige, which would make MSTN an ideal target for pharmacologic intervention. Certainly, based on the extensive efforts by both the academic and pharmaceutical communities to date, it is clear that agents capable of modulating MSTN activity can result in profound effects *in vivo*. The challenges moving forward will be to define more precisely those disease settings in which pharmacological manipulation of this pathway will lead to therapeutic benefit and to match those clinical indications with specific MSTN inhibitors.

REFERENCES

1. McPherron AC, Lawler AM, Lee S-J. Regulation of skeletal muscle mass in mice by a new TGF-ß superfamily member. *Nature* 1997;**387**:83–90.
2. McPherron AC, Lee S-J. Double muscling in cattle due to mutations in the myostatin gene. *Proc Natl Acad Sci USA* 1997;**94**:12457–61.
3. Grobet L, Martin LJR, Poncelet D, Pirottin D, Brouwers B, Riquet J, et al. A deletion in the bovine myostatin gene causes the double-muscled phenotype in cattle. *Nature Genet* 1997;**17**:71–4.
4. Kambadur R, Sharma M, Smith TL, Bass JJ. Mutations in myostatin (GDF8) in double-muscled Belgian Blue and Piedmontese cattle. *Genome Res* 1997;**7**:910–5.
5. Grobet L, Poncelet D, Royo LJ, Brouwers B, Pirottin D, Michaux C, et al. Molecular definition of an allelic series of mutations disrupting the myostatin function and causing double-muscling in cattle. *Mamm Genome* 1998;**9**:210–3.
6. Clop A, Marcq F, Takeda H, Pirottin D, Tordoir X, Bibe B, et al. A mutation creating a potential illegitimate microRNA target site in the myostatin gene affects muscularity in sheep. *Nature Genet.* 2006;**38**:813–8.
7. Mosher DS, Quignon P, Bustamante CD, Sutter NB, Mellersh CS, Parker HG, et al. A mutation in the myostatin gene increases muscle mass and enhances racing performance in heterozygote dogs. *PLoS Genetics* 2007;**3**:779–86.
8. Schuelke M, Wagner KR, Stolz LE, Hübner C, Riebel T, Kömen W, et al. Myostatin mutation associated with gross muscle hypertrophy in a child. *N Engl J Med* 2004;**350**:2682–8.
9. Bogdanovich S, Krag TOB, Barton ER, Morris LD, Whittemore L-A, Ahima RS, et al. Functional improvement of dystrophic muscle by myostatin blockade. *Nature* 2002;**420**:418–21.
10. Whittemore L-A, Song K, Li X, Aghajanian J, Davies MV, Girgenrath S, et al. Inhibition of myostatin in adult mice increases skeletal muscle mass and strength. *BBRC* 2003;**300**:965–71.
11. Wolfman NM, McPherron AC, Pappano WN, Davies MV, Song K, Tomkinson KN, et al. Activation of latent myostatin by the BMP-1/tolloid family of metalloproteinases. *Proc Natl Acad Sci USA* 2003;**100**:15842–6.
12. Lee S-J, Reed A, Davies M, Girgenrath S, Goad M, Tomkinson K, et al. Regulation of muscle growth by multiple ligands signaling through activin type II receptors. *Proc Natl Acad Sci USA* 2005;**102**:18117–22.
13. LeBrasseur NK, Schelhorn TM, Bernardo BL, Cosgrove PG, Loria PM, Brown TA. Myostatin inhibition enhances the effects of exercise on performance and metabolic outcomes in aged mice. *J Gerontol A Biol Sci Med Sci* 2009;**64**:940–8.
14. Zhang L, Rajan V, Lin E, Hu Z, Han HQ, Zhou X, et al. Pharmacological inhibition of myostatin suppresses systemic inflammation and muscle atrophy in mice with chronic kidney disease. *FASEB J* 2011;**25**:1653–63.
15. Anderson SB, Goldberg AL, Whitman M. Identification of a novel pool of extracellular pro-myostatin in skeletal muscle. *J Biol Chem* 2008;**283**:7027–35.
16. Lee S-J, McPherron AC. Regulation of myostatin activity and muscle growth. *Proc Natl Acad Sci USA* 2001;**98**:9306–11.
17. Thies RS, Chen T, Davies MV, Tomkinson KN, Pearson AA, Shakey QA, et al. GDF-8 propeptide binds to GDF-8 and antagonizes biological activity by inhibiting GDF-8 receptor binding. *Growth Factors* 2001;**18**:251–9.
18. Zimmers TA, Davies MV, Koniaris LG, Haynes P, Esquela AF, Tomkinson KN, et al. Induction of cachexia in mice by systemically administered myostatin. *Science* 2002;**296**:1486–8.
19. Hill JJ, Davies MV, Pearson AA, Wang JH, Hewick RM, Wolfman NM, et al. The myostatin propeptide and the follistatin-related gene are inhibitory binding proteins of myostatin in normal serum. *J Biol Chem* 2002;**277**:40735–41.
20. Lee S-J. Genetic analysis of the role of proteolysis in the activation of latent myostatin. *PLoS One* 2008;**3**:e1628.
21. Robertson DM, Klein R, de Vos FL, McLachlan RI, Wettenhall RE, Hearn MT, et al. The isolation of polypeptides with FSH suppressing activity from bovine follicular fluid which are structurally different to inhibin. *Biochem Biophys Res Commun* 1987;**149**:744–9.
22. Ueno N, Ling N, Ying SY, Esch F, Shimasaki S, Guillemin R. Isolation and partial characterization of follistatin: a single-chain Mr 35,000 monomeric protein that inhibits the release of follicle-stimulating hormone. *Proc Natl Acad Sci USA* 1987;**84**:8282–6.
23. Nakamura T, Takio K, Eto Y, Shibai H, Titani K, Sugino H. Activin-binding protein from rat ovary is follistatin. *Science* 1990;**247**:836–8.
24. Gamer LW, Wolfman NM, Celeste AJ, Hattersley G, Hewick R, Rosen V. A novel BMP expressed in developing mouse limb, spinal cord, and tail bud is a potent mesoderm inducer in Xenopus embryos. *Dev Biol* 1999;**208**:222–32.
25. Lee S-J, Lee Y-S, Zimmers T, Soleimani A, Matzuk MM, Tsuchida K, et al. Regulation of muscle mass by follistatin and activins. *Mol Endocrinol* 2010;**24**:1998–2008.
26. Lee S-J. Quadrupling muscle mass in mice by targeting TGF-ß signaling pathways. *PLoS One* 2007;**2**:e789.
27. Mukherjee A, Sidis Y, Mahan A, Raher MJ, Xia Y, Rosen ED, et al. FSTL3 deletion reveals roles for TGF-ß family ligands in glucose and fat homeostasis in adults. *Proc Natl Acad Sci USA* 2007;**104**:1348–53.
28. Hill JJ, Qiu Y, Hewick RM, Wolfman NM. Regulation of myostatin in vivo by growth and differentiation factor-associated serum protein-1: a novel protein with protease inhibitor and follistatin domains. *Mol Endocrinol* 2003;**17**:1144–54.
29. Kondás K, Szláma G, Trexler M, Patthy L. Both WFIKKN1 and WFIKKN2 have high affinity for growth and differentiation factors 8 and 11. *J Biol Chem* 2008;**283**:23677–84.
30. Li Y, Li J, Zhu J, Sun B, Branca M, Tang Y, et al. Decorin gene transfer promotes muscle cell differentiation and muscle regeneration. *Mol Ther* 2007;**15**:1616–22.
31. Rebbapragada A, Benchabane H, Wrana J, Celeste AJ, Attisano L. Myostatin signals through a transforming growth factor ß-like

signaling pathway to block adipogenesis. *Mol Cell Biol* 2003;**23**:7230–42.

32. Trendelenburg AU, Meyer A, Rohner D, Boyle J, Hatakeyama S, Glass DJ. Myostatin reduces Akt/TORC1/p70S6K signaling, inhibiting myoblast differentiation and myotube size. *Am J Physiol Cell Physiol* 2009;**296**:C1258–70.
33. Iezzi S, Di Padova M, Serra C, Caretti G, Simone C, Maklan E, et al. Deacetylase inhibitors increase muscle cell size by promoting myoblast recruitment and fusion through induction of follistatin. *Dev Cell* 2004;**6**:673–84.
34. Minetti GC, Colussi C, Adami R, Serra C, Mozetta C, Parente V, et al. Functional and morphological recovery of dystrophic muscles in mice treated with deacetylase inhibitors. *Nat Med* 2006;**12**:1147–50.
35. Girgenrath S, Song K, Whittemore L-A. Loss of myostatin expression alters fiber-type distribution and expression of myosin heavy chain isoforms in slow- and fast-type skeletal muscle. *Muscle Nerve* 2005;**31**:34–40.
36. Amthor H, Macharia R, Navarrete R, Schuelke M, Brown SC, Otto A, et al. Lack of myostatin results in excessive muscle growth but impaired force generation. *Proc Natl Acad Sci USA* 2007;**104**:1835–40.
37. Elashry MI, Otto A, Matsakas A, El-Morsy SE, Patel K. Morphology and myofiber compostion of skeletal musculature of the forelimb in young and aged wild type and myostatin null mice. *Rejuvenation Res* 2009;**12**:269–81.
38. McPherron AC, Huynh TV, Lee S-J. Redundancy of myostatin and growth/differentiation factor 11. *BMC Dev Biol* 2009;**9**:24–32.
39. Foster K, Graham IR, Otto A, Foster H, Trollet C, Yaworsky PJ, et al. Adeno-associated virus-8-mediated intravenous transfer of myostatin propeptide leads to systemic functional improvements of slow but not fast muscle. *Rejuvenation Res* 2009;**12**:85–94.
40. Matsakas A, Foster K, Otto A, Macharia R, Elashry MI, Feist S, et al. Molecular, cellular and physiological investigation of myostatin propeptide-mediated muscle growth in adult mice. *Neuromuscul Disord* 2009;**19**:489–99.
41. Cadena SM, Tomkinson KN, Monnell TE, Spaits ME, Kumar R, Underwood KW, et al. Administration of a soluble activin tpe IIB receptor promotes skeletal muscle growth independent of fiber type. *J Appl Physiol* 2010;**109**:635–42.
42. Lee S-J. Extracellular regulation of myostatin: a molecular rheostat for muscle mass. *Immunol Endocr Metabol Agents Med Chem* 2010;**10**:183–94.
43. Wagner KR. Clinical applications of myostatin inhibitors for neuromuscular diseases. *Immunol Endocr Metabol Agents Med Chem* 2010;**10**:204–10.
44. Wagner KR, Fleckenstein JL, Amato AA, Barohn RJ, Bushby K, Escolar DM, et al. A Phase I/II trial of MYO-029 in adult subjects with muscular dystrophy. *Ann Neurol* 2008;**63**:561–71.
45. Zhou X, Wang JL, Lu J, Song Y, Kwak KS, Jiao Q, et al. Reversal of cancer cachexia and muscle wasting by ActRIIB antagonism leads to prolonged survival. *Cell* 2010;**142**:531–43.
46. Benny Klimek ME, Aydogdu T, Link MJ, Pons M, Koniaris LG, Zimmers TA. Acute inhibition of myostatin-family proteins preserves skeletal muscle in mouse models of cancer cachexia. *Biochem Biophys Res Commun* 2010;**391**:1548–54.
47. Sharma M, Kambadur R, Matthews KG, Somers WG, Devlin GP, Conaglen JV, et al. Myostatin, a transforming growth factor-beta superfamily member, is expressed in heart muscle and is upregulated in cardiomyocytes after infarct. *J Cell Physiol* 1999;**180**:1–9.
48. Shyu KG, Lu MJ, Wang BW, Sun HY, Chang H. Myostatin expression in ventricular myocardium in a rat model of volume-overload heart failure. *Eur J Clin Invest* 2006;**36**:713–9.
49. Lenk K, Schur R, Linke A, Erbs S, Matsumoto Y, Adams V, et al. Impact of exercise training on myostatin expression in the myocardium and skeletal muscle in a chronic heart failure model. *Eur J Heart Fail* 2009;**11**:342–8.
50. Bish LT, Morine KJ, Sleeper MM, Sweeney HL. Myostatin is upregulated following stress in an Erk-dependent manner and negatively regulates cardiomyocyte growth in culture and in a mouse model. *PLoS One* 2010;**5**:e10230.
51. Heineke J, Auger-Messier M, Xu J, Sargent M, York A, Welle S, et al. Genetic deletion of myostatin from the heart prevents skeletal muscle atrophy in heart failure. *Circulation* 2010;**121**:419–25.
52. Wilkinson HA. Role of myostatin signaling in aging: applications for age related sarcopenia. *Immunol Endocr Metabol Agents Med Chem* 2010;**10**:211–6.
53. McPherron AC, Lee S-J. Suppression of body fat accumulation in myostatin-deficient mice. *J Clin Invest* 2002;**109**:595–601.
54. LeBrasseur NK. Building muscle, browning fat and preventing obesity by inhibiting myostatin. *Diabetologia* 2012;**55**:13–7.
55. Allen DL, Cleary AS, Speaker KJ, Lindsay SF, Uyenishi J, Reed JM, et al. Myostatin, activin receptor IIb, and follistatin-like-3 gene expression are altered in adipose tissue and skeletal muscle of obese mice. *Am J Physiol Endocrinol Metab* 2008;**294**:E918–27.
56. Akpan I, Goncalves MD, Dhir R, Yin X, Pistilli EE, Bogdanovich S, et al. The effects of a soluble activin type IIB receptor on obesity and insulin sensitivity. *Int J Obes (Lond)* 2009;**33**: 1265–73.
57. Lee S-J. Regulation of muscle mass by myostatin. *Ann Rev Cell Dev Biol* 2004;**20**:61–86.

Chapter 80

Insulin-Like Growth Factor I Regulation and Its Actions in Skeletal Muscle Growth and Repair

Elisabeth R. Barton

School of Dental Medicine, Department of Anatomy and Cell Biology, University of Pennsylvania, Philadelphia, PA

INTRODUCTION

Skeletal muscle development, growth, and repair are orchestrated by many growth factors, which are proteins produced locally or delivered systemically. Because the muscle tissue consists not only of contractile muscle fibers, but also vasculature, innervating neurons, and extracellular matrix (ECM), there is a requirement for coordinated actions of the growth factors to ensure that each system is optimally regulated to result in a functioning organ. This chapter focuses on insulin-like growth factor I (IGF-I), but several additional growth factors are also involved in skeletal muscle growth in addition to IGF-I and myostatin. For example, hepatocyte growth factor (HGF) is one of the primary activators of quiescent satellite cells (1). Upon HGF binding to its receptor (c-met), satellite cells enter into the cell cycle and contribute to formation or repair of muscle fibers. Many members of the fibroblast growth factors (FGF) family have been implicated in myoblast proliferation and differentiation, as well as ECM remodeling (2). Vascular endothelial growth factor (VEGF) acts through tyrosine kinase receptors found predominantly on endothelial cells to promote both physiological and pathological angiogenesis (3). However, in regenerating muscle there is transient upregulation of both VEGF and its receptors in fibers, potentially coordinating the vascularization process during repair, and simultaneously acting directly on fibers (4). The growth factor cocktail that bathes skeletal muscle and directs the regeneration process is well tuned in normal healthy tissue. However, in disease and aging, the mixture may become disregulated, and so the goals of therapies to repair muscle are to re-tune and re-optimize the components to efficiently resolve damage and regain functional muscle.

IGF-I ACTIVITY AND ITS REGULATION

Insulin, IGF-I, and IGF-II are related in protein structure and their ability to bind to their specific receptors. Mature IGF-I and IGF-II consist of A, B, C, and D-domains. The A- and B-domains of IGFs are homologous to those of insulin. Unlike insulin, the C-domain is not cleaved off in mature IGFs. IGFs contain an additional D-domain, which is absent in insulin. IGF-I and IGF-II mediate effects predominantly via the IGF-I receptor (IGF-IR). IGF-I and its activation of the IGF-IR can promote growth in virtually all tissues. A second receptor, the mannose-6-phosphate receptor, binds IGF-II, although its role in skeletal muscle has not been clarified. The IGF-IR is encoded by a single gene producing an α and β subunit (for review see 5, 6). During processing, these subunits form a disulphide-linked heterodimer. Formation of the receptor requires a second dimerization between two $\alpha\beta$ heterodimers connected by disulfide bonds between the α subunits to result in a 300 kD hetero-tetrameric glycoprotein. The extracelullar α subunits contain the ligand-binding site. The transmembrane β subunits contain the inherent tyrosine kinase activity of the receptor, which mediates multiple signaling processes and lead to changes in gene expression and protein synthesis after ligand binding (Figure 80.1A).

Upon ligand binding, activation of the inherent tyrosine kinase occurs, and then receptors mediate their actions via phosphorylation of insulin receptor substrate (IRS) proteins, Shc, and Gab-1 (Figure 80.1B). Activated IRS and Shc complexes can bind src homology 2 (SH2) domains on adapter molecules such as grb2 and the p85 subunit of PI-3K, among others, leading to the downstream signaling events associated with these proteins. Divergence in signaling begins, in part, at adaptor molecule association to IRS proteins. Grb2 couples to the

Muscle. DOI: http://dx.doi.org/10.1016/B978-0-12-381510-1.00080-6

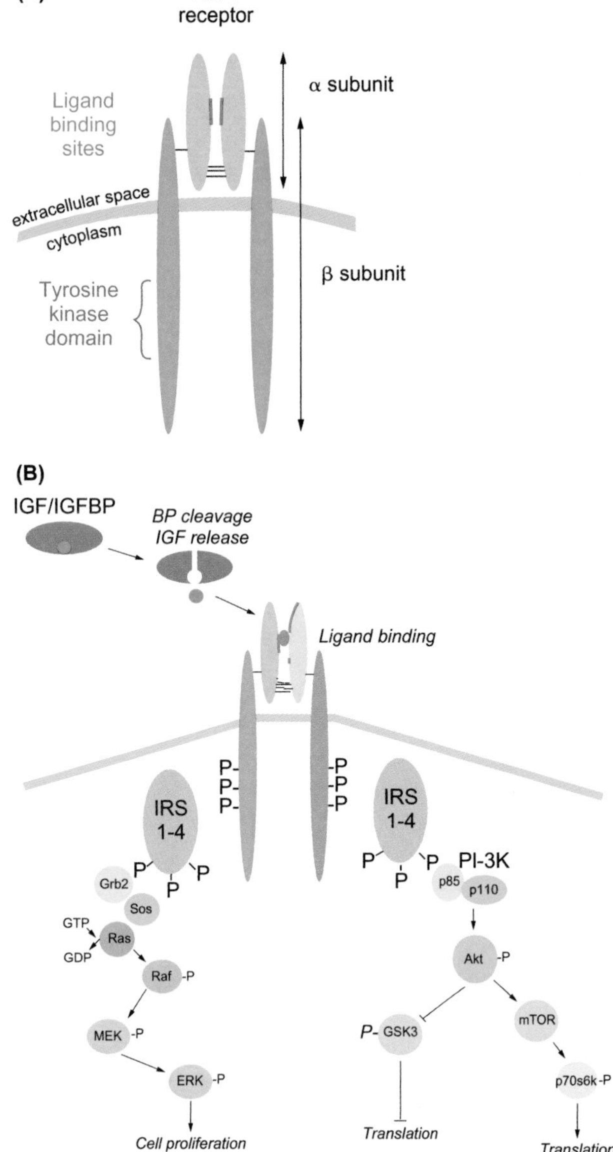

FIGURE 80.1 Domains and signaling pathways of the IGF-I receptor. (A) The IGF-IR is a hetero-tetrameric glycoprotein formed from two heterodimers. The extracellular alpha subunit contains the ligand-binding site, and the inherent tyrosine kinase activity is on the intracellular portion of the transmembrane beta subunit. (B) IGF-I is bound to IGF binding proteins. Protease cleavage of the binding proteins release IGF-I and enable it to bind to IGF-IR. Ligand-binding activates the receptor tyrosine kinase activity, and instigates a signaling cascade via phosphorylation of a number of proteins, including IRS, Shc, and Gab-1. These complexes bind to SH2 domains on adaptor proteins. Association with Grb2 couples to the ras-raf1-MEK-ERK (MAPK) pathway, which promotes cell proliferation. Association with p85 subunit of phosphoinositol-3 kinase (PI-3K) ultimately activates Akt, which is central to promoting muscle hypertrophy and cell survival. Signaling activity is turned off following internalization of the receptor.

ras-raf1-MEK-Erk (MAPK) pathway, whereas p85 is part of the PI-3K/Akt pathway (7,8). Signaling activity is turned off following internalization of the ligand-receptor complex, after which receptors are degraded through both the ubiquitin and lysosomal pathways (9) or recycled back to the membrane.

The insulin receptor (IR) and IGF-IR have a high level of homology, and this enables interchangeable ligand binding. However, the ligand-binding pocket confers preferential binding: IGF-I can bind to IGF-IR at 1000-fold lower concentration than insulin, whereas IGF-I levels must be three-fold higher than insulin concentrations for equivalent binding to IR. Thus, although insulin is the preferred ligand for IR and is the primary mediator for GLUT4 translocation and glucose clearance in muscle, IGF-I can also bind and activate IR as well. This is a significant consideration for IGF-I therapies, because of the potential impact on glucose homeostasis. In addition to IGF-IR and IR, the high homology affords the formation of hybrid receptors through association of hemireceptors of each type. In muscle, hybrid receptors comprise at least half of the IR, IGF-IR population (10,11). Ligand-binding studies have shown that hybrid receptors preferentially bind IGF-I with equivalent affinity as IGF-IR (12,13), yet how downstream actions of the hybrid receptor differ from IGF-IR is not understood.

IGF-I is a potent mitogen, enhancing cell proliferation via the MAPK arm of the signaling pathway (14). Because muscle fibers are post-mitotic, the proliferative actions are observed in satellite cells, which express the IGF-IR following activation by HGF. Satellite cells divide, and then can undergo differentiation, fusing either to damaged sites on muscle fibers, or forming new fibers. High levels of IGF-I can enhance satellite cell division, which increases the pool of cells available for repair and growth. In addition to mitogenic actions, IGF-I also enhances the formation of muscle through regulation of differentiation and stimulation of protein synthesis. IGF-I promotes increased gene expression of the myogenic transcription factors, such as myogenin, in myoblasts. Activation of IGF-IR on the post-mitotic muscle fibers leads to hypertrophy of the fibers. Signaling via the PI-3K/Akt pathway is the primary regulator of the hypertrophic response, such that pharmacologic blockade of Akt actions prevents hypertrophy and constitutively active Akt is sufficient to drive hypertrophy (15). IGF-I actions on both satellite cells and the muscle fibers contribute to muscle growth (16), but the proportion is dependent on the initial state of the muscle. For instance, in aging muscle, where satellite cells are less active, then the muscle fibers are the primary source for increases in mass. However, in regenerating tissue, the activated satellite pool may not only fuse to existing fibers, but upon IGF-I stimulation, there is an increased appearance of new fibers, or hyperplasia, that leads to increases in mass (17). Complementary to these actions, IGF-I can also protect against cell death, or apoptosis, through the PI-3K/Akt signaling arm, which drives Bcl-2 expression (reviewed in 18). Thus, there is a multi-pronged mechanism by which IGF-I promotes muscle survival, growth, and regenerative capacity.

REGULATION OF IGF-I PRODUCTION AND ACTIVITY

There are at least six proteins that have extremely high binding affinity for IGF-I and IGF-II, such that they are the preferable binding partners for IGFs compared to the receptors. These proteins are called the IGF-binding proteins (IGFBPs), and stably associate with IGFs in the circulation and in tissues to modulate IGF availability for receptor activation, and to stabilize the pool of IGFs produced (reviewed in 19). The IGFBPs have conserved N- and C-termini that coordinate binding to the IGFs, and the divergent central domains have site for wide range of proteolytic enzymes. The central domains also have different N-glycosylation and phosphorylation sites, as well as regions for heparin binding. These regions of the IGFBPs afford association to the extracellular matrix, providing docking sites for the IGFBP-IGF complexes in tissues. Upon IGFBP cleavage, IGF-I is released, and is then able to bind to nearby receptors. Further, it is now becoming clear that the IGFBPs have independent activity, adding complexity to the regulation of growth.

IGFBP3 is the major binding partner in the circulation, and together with acid-labile-subunit (ALS), for a very stable ternary complex that comprises the predominant pool of circulating IGF. As such, only ~1% of the total IGF-I in the circulation is free, or "unbound" IGF. In skeletal muscle, modulation of IGFBP4 and IGFBP5 expression occurs depending upon the loading state of the muscle and the availability of ligand (see, for example, reference 20).

The regulation of somatic growth was a central question more than 50 years ago, and resulted in the somatomedin hypothesis (21), which proposed that growth hormone (GH) secreted from the pituitary controlled growth by stimulating the liver to produce circulating substances, or somatomedins (later identified as IGF-I and IGF-II). In line with the original hypothesis, the liver is the major source for circulating, or endocrine, pool of IGF-I. However, other tissues, including the brain, kidney, and muscle, can produce their own paracrine/autocrine source of IGF-I. A large body of work has examined the impact of these separate sources of IGF-I on organismal and tissue-specific growth using animal models with tissue-targeted ablation of IGF-I expression. As a result, the original somatomedin hypothesis has been modified and refined in the past several decades. The general consensus is that limiting liver IGF-I does not control the growth of many of the tissues that make their own IGF-I, such as skeletal muscle or brain, but that such limitations can reduce bone density, and also drive compensatory GH release (reviewed in 22). However, if local production of IGF-I is blocked, then the growth of those specific tissues is impaired. To complicate things further, boosting circulating levels of IGF-I, either through injections of recombinant growth factor or by enhancing liver production, can rescue the local needs of those tissues. These observations have raised the question: is there a special property of the paracrine IGF-I sources that provides unique control of tissue growth? Or are all IGF-I molecules equivalent? Potential mechanisms for generating different forms of IGF-I occur during transcription and after translation, and these will be described in the following sections.

ALTERNATIVE SPLICING

While the predominant focus of research and therapies has been on the physiological impact and benefit of IGF-I, the existence of additional potentially active peptides produced by the *igf1* gene is being considered. Alternative splicing of the gene results in multiple isoforms that retain the identical sequence for mature IGF-I, but also produces divergent C-terminal peptides, called the E-peptides. Proposed functions for the peptides include modulation of the actions, stability, or bioavailability of IGF-I, as well as activity unique to the E-peptides (23–28). These possibilities have gained the attention of the skeletal muscle field, where novel actions of IGF-I and the E-peptides could have significant impact on muscle mass, strength and repair.

The prepropeptide expressed by the *igf1* gene is >90% identical in mammals (reviewed in 29,30). There are six exons in the *igf1* gene (Figure 80.2A) (31,32). Exons 1 and 2 are used interchangeably, and constitute Class I and II, respectively, of the IGFI isoforms. These encode the 5′ untranslated region (UTR), and a portion of the signal peptide. Utilization of Exon 1 or 2 seems dependent on two different promoters that are regulated in a tissue-specific manner (29). Exons 3 and 4 are invariant, and encode the remaining portion of the signal peptide, the mature IGF-I peptide, and a portion of the E peptide. The rest of the E peptide is encoded by Exons 5 or 6. Most IGF-I transcripts skip Exon 5 and splice Exon 4 directly to Exon 6, and are defined as *class A*. The inclusion of all of rodent Exon 5 or a portion of human Exon 5, causes a frame shift in the open reading frame of the subsequent exon and gives rise to a premature stop within Exon 6. This splice form (*class B*

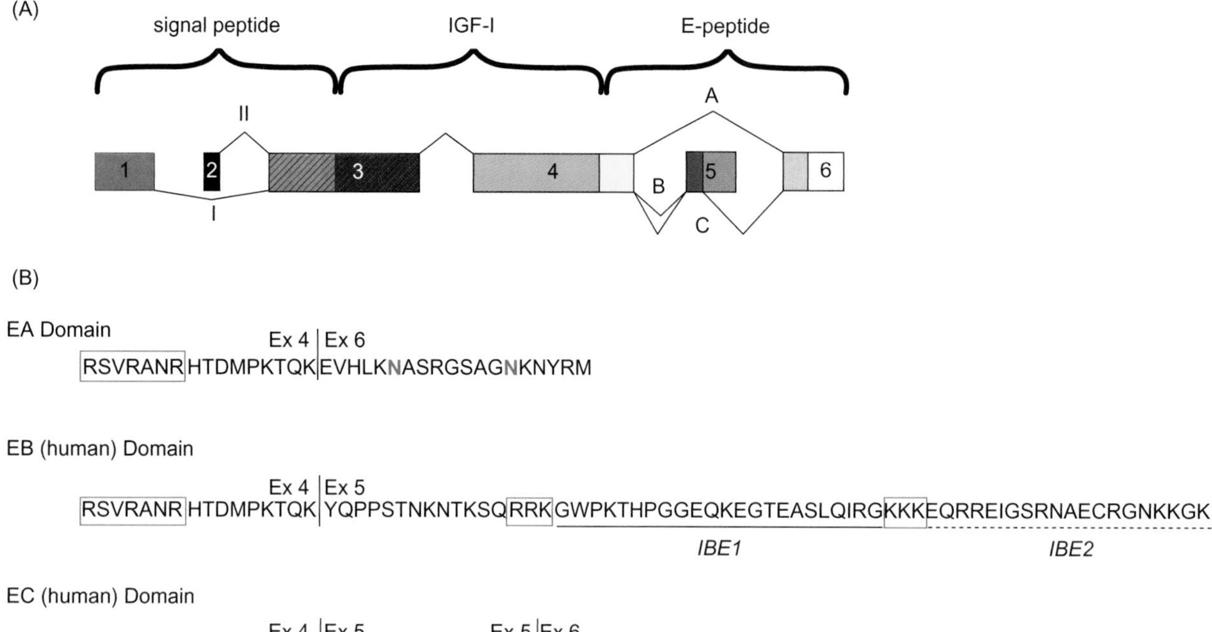

FIGURE 80.2 Alternative splicing and modifications in the *Igf1* gene. (A) The human *Igf1* gene has six exons. Class 1 and 2 arise from the utilization of either Exon 1 or 2, respectively, by alternative splicing at the 5′ end. Class A transcripts skip Exon 5. Class B utilizes only Exon 5, and appears to be unique to human IGF-I. Class C is produced by an internal splice site within Exon 5 that causes a frame shift and premature termination in Exon 6, and the resultant peptide bears high homology to rodent class B IGF-I. (B) The C-terminal sequences of these isoforms bear only ~50% homology. The common region encoded by Exon 4 contains a series of protease cleavage sites (green boxes) that can release the E peptides from mature IGF-I. EB and EC have additional potential cleavage sites. The EA domain contains putative N-glycosylation sites (in bold red). The IBE1 and IBE2 peptides underlined in the EB peptide are produced by protease cleavage sites; IBE1 has been shown to have mitogenic activity (28). The peptide utilized for MGF studies *in vitro* is underlined in the EC peptide (35).

in rodents and *class C* in humans) only occurs in up to 10% of the *igf1* transcripts. A third form (human class B) contains only Exon 5 (significantly longer in humans (515nucleotides)) (31), resulting in a unique E peptide extension which, to date, has not been observed in other species. The E-peptides share only 50% sequence homology at the amino acid level.

POTENTIAL FUNCTIONS OF IGF-I E-PEPTIDES

Bioactivity of the E-peptides was demonstrated twenty years ago (28). A predicted amidated peptide found only in human IGF-IB (IBE1) caused concentration-dependent stimulation of cell growth in human bronchial epithelial cells (sequence shown in Figure 80.2B). Further studies demonstrated that the specific binding activity of the peptide in cells was not affected by the presence of insulin or IGF-I, nor was its activity prevented by presence of a neutralizing antibody to the IGF-I receptor. This study was the first to report that IGF-I, similar to other prohormones, such as proglucagon (33) could contain multiple bioactive peptides. The third human isoform (hIGF-IC) was identified later in liver tissue (34), and the authors speculated that the alternative splicing mechanism found in IGF-IC (and by extension, rodent IGF-IB) was one way a cell could reduce proliferative effects caused by IBE1 production. This scheme was challenged in later studies reporting that the C isoform could induce cell proliferation and migration (27,35). Splice forms inclusive of Exon 5 were called mechano-growth factor (MGF) to indicate the increased expression of this isoform in response to stretch or damage. The ability to express MGF in response to damage or overload diminished with age in skeletal muscle from both humans and rats (36,37), suggesting that the aging-related loss in the ability to repair after damage might be correlated to diminished MGF expression. Recently, the comparison of IGF-I precursor sequences from non-human primates, human, and dog reveals that the EA domain is strongly conserved across species, whereas the human EC and EB domains are highly variable (38). While this does not preclude the general biological importance of these variable regions, the function is apt to be species specific.

IGF-I PROCESSING

Once translated, IGF-I prepropeptides require multiple processing steps prior to producing a mature IGF-I peptide that is 70 amino acids long and identical for all isoforms. Post-translational processing has been examined in 293 Chinese hamster ovary cell lines, and occurs via a constitutive secretory pathway, similarly directed by Class 1 and 2 signal peptides (reviewed in 39). The peptide precursor (proIGF-I) contains the E-peptide in addition to the domains in the mature peptide. A pentabasic motif near the end of the D-domain (Lys65-X-X-Lys68-x-x-Arg71-x-x-Arg74-x-x-Arg77) contains two putative cleavage sites, Arg71, and Arg77. This motif is included in all classes of IGF-I. Cleavage at Arg71 is mediated by serine proteases from the subtilisin-related proprotein convertase family (SPC). SPCs are expressed in many tissues, and have also been shown to cleave precursors of the insulin receptor and nerve growth factor. The final removal of Arg71 is possibly accomplished by a carboxypeptidase. While efficient cleavage of the E-peptide has been shown to occur by furin and other SPCs in culture, not all E-peptides seem to be cleaved prior to IGF-I secretion. Several reports have detected the secretion of proIGF-IA and rodent proIGF-IB from fibroblasts and myoblasts (40–42). Whether cleavage of EA–peptide occurs extracellularly, or if proIGF-IA possesses bioactivity has not been determined.

The IGF-IA E-peptides contains potential N-glycosylation sites (Figure 80.2, shown in bold red). Due to the frame shift caused by the insertion of Exon 5, these sites are non-existent in other splice forms. Glycosylation is detected *in vitro* and *in vivo* (42,43), but the significance to IGF-I function has yet to be determined.

As summarized above, the expression and processing of the gene encoding IGF-I has been well characterized *in vitro*. It is generally accepted that the mature IGF-I peptide is the main mediator of IGF-I actions via the IGF-IR, and the fact that IGF-I can drive cell proliferation and differentiation in multiple cell types and tissues has been repeatedly demonstrated. However, it as not been confirmed that this is the only activity associated with the entire IGF-I propeptide. Specifically, it is not known if IGF-I mediated effects are also due, in part, to the presence of a particular E-peptide, or if there are completely novel cellular responses to E peptide expression.

TARGETS FOR THERAPY

IGF-I has long been recognized as one of the critical factors for coordinating muscle growth, enhancing muscle repair, and increasing muscle mass and strength. As stated above, IGF-I can help in two main ways. First, IGF-I acts directly on the muscle fibers to increase protein synthesis and muscle mass. It also drives activated satellite cells to fuse to existing muscle fibers, helping to repair damaged regions of the fibers, and to promote muscle growth (44). IGF-I coordinates efficient muscle repair, enhanced muscle growth, and motor neuron survival. These actions can result in improved muscle function, which have been demonstrated in several animal models with many different modes of delivery. While IGF-I may not prevent the initial loss of muscle mass associated with disuse, its pro-growth actions can accelerate the process of recovery of both muscle size and function. In addition, there is a growing awareness that the additional products of the *igf1* gene, the E-peptides, may also contribute to recovery and to prevention of atrophy, although a systematic evaluation of their therapeutic potential has not been performed.

More than 30 genetic disorders of muscle have been identified and arise from mutations in a wide range of genes including those that encode proteins of the dystrophin glycoprotein complex, the nuclear membrane, and extracellular matrix. While each disease is unique in onset, severity and pattern, there is a common set of shared pathologies. The hallmarks of the muscular dystrophies include muscle weakness, fragility, and degeneration. Significant progress has been made to understand the mechanisms underlying each of the muscular dystrophies, yet even more will be required to design therapies specific to each genetic disorder. In the meantime, agents that counter the common pathologies can be utilized to promote muscle regeneration, maintain mass and strength, and prolong quality of life. IGF-I is a strong candidate for use as a therapeutic in muscle disease because it aids in the repair and maintenance of tissue health.

In addition to genetic muscle disease, IGF-I could be utilized to enhance recovery after acute atrophy or injuries in the healthy population. Muscle atrophy is a common clinical phenomenon observed in multiple rehabilitation settings, and is characterized by reductions in several morphological and physiological parameters, including decreases in muscle fiber size and number, protein content, and protein/DNA ratios, as well as losses in muscle strength and shifts in contractile properties toward those of fast fiber types. Disuse atrophy is often a secondary consequence of disease or injury, such as in systemic diseases that require bed rest or orthopedic injuries that demand cast immobilization or a change in weight-bearing status. Because apoptosis may contribute to the loss of mass, or atrophy, when muscle is unloaded, IGF-I activity could protect against muscle atrophy in unloading by multiple ways. However, animal studies have showed that the IGF-I signaling axis appears to be blocked in unweighting (45). Still, it is clear that once re-loading occurs, the IGF-I pathway is clearly part of the therapeutic strategies that can boost recovery.

Finally, boosting muscle regenerative capacity to counter sarcopenia has been considered, particularly as the aging population increases (46). With aging there is a decrease in the production and activity of the growth hormone/IGF-I axis which lead to an increase in catabolic processes and is exhibited by the age-related loss of muscle mass and strength. Animal studies have demonstrated that muscle specific overexpression of IGF-I improved regenerative capacity and maintained muscle mass and function, and ultimately blocked age-related muscle atrophy in mice (47,48). In human studies, normalizing circulating IGF-I levels in aging men or women either through administration of IGF-I, GH, or GH releasing hormone shows some benefit, with improvements in strength and bone density reported (49). While aging skeletal muscle exhibits functional benefits from increased IGF-I, it is not clear that the rest of the body is in agreement. Counter to the muscle, low circulating IGF-I as well as depressed IGF-I signaling is associated with increased lifespan, presumably due to improved metabolic status and the reduction of tumorigenesis. IGF-I based therapeutics for sarcopenia may need to increase IGF-I exclusively in the muscle to avoid the significant risks to longevity.

RISKS OF IGF-I FOR THERAPY

Virtually every cell in the body expresses IGF-IR, and so they are responsive to IGF-I. The pro-growth actions of IGF-I may be beneficial for muscle, but they have devastating consequences for other tissues. The risk of cancer arising from increased IGF-I is a very real concern, where IGF-I has been implicated in breast, prostate, and colorectal tumor formation. In fact, the research efforts to *combat* IGF-I actions likely outweigh those looking to boost its activity. As such, any therapeutic strategy for increasing IGF-I for muscle growth must consider carcinogenic side effects. A second side effect of increasing IGF-I involves glucose homeostasis. Recalling that IGF-I can also bind to and activate IR, rapid spikes in circulating IGF-I can cause increased glucose clearance and hypoglycemia. Prolonged elevation of IGF-I has more significant metabolic consequences. Finally, increased circulating IGF-I can disrupt the feedback to GH regulation of endogenous IGF-I production. Because GH not only regulates the expression of IGF-I and its binding proteins, but also has direct anabolic actions, considerations for maintaining the GH/IGF axis are important.

CURRENT AND EMERGING STRATEGIES FOR THERAPY

To boost IGF-I levels for promoting increased muscle growth and regenerative capacity, the most straightforward approach is to deliver IGF-I systemically. Several clinical trials have assessed the efficacy of systemic delivery of recombinant IGF-I in patients who could benefit from strength gains. These include the aging population, patients with growth hormone deficiency, and those who suffer from amyotrophic lateral sclerosis and myotonic dystrophy (50–58). In addition, recombinant GH has also been utilized in a subset of these patient groups to allow for both direct actions of GH as well as those mediated through IGF-I to provide benefit. Because IGF-I is a potent growth factor in many tissues of the body and poses a potential carcinogenic risk, investigators have introduced IGF-I in limiting amounts. Thus, these trials have produced mixed results because the ability for IGF-I to provide any benefit to skeletal muscle is constrained by both the low level of protein administered as well as the limited distribution of IGF-I to the muscle by the circulation (e.g., 51–53). Therefore, new strategies are needed to allow for heightened levels of IGF-I where it is needed, while avoiding the systemic risks.

Two strategies have been considered that could reduce the risks of systemic effects. First, one can "mask" the IGF-I by chelating it to an agent that reduces its bioavailability until it is needed. Mecasermin rinfabate, which is a complex of recombinant IGF-I and IGF binding protein 3 (IGFBP3) called IPLEX™ (59), was developed recently. Because the free IGF-I pool is what is sensed for GH regulation of IGF-I production, this strategy boosts the pool associated with the major circulating binding protein (IGFBP3) (19). Patients could receive higher effective doses of IGF-I via IPLEX™ compared to recombinant IGF-I to patients with less systemic risk due to the longer half-life of the complex. This drug targeted patients suffering from GH-insensitive Short Stature, bypassing the loss of GH actions of IGF-I expression. Here it has been successful in increasing height in pre-pubertal children. Because trials using recombinant IGF-I in myotonic dystrophy (DM1) patients showed some promise, and because IPLEX™ could provide a more stable source of IGF-I for these patients, a clinical trial was performed in DM1 patients (60). While there was some metabolic benefit for the patients, there was no significant improvement in the functional outcome measures associated with skeletal muscle. This does not eliminate IPLEX™ or other stabilized forms for IGF-I from the clinical horizon for all dystrophies, but suggests that each genetic muscle disease may derive differential benefit from IGF-I therapies dependent on the primary cause.

An emerging strategy for IGF-I therapy chemically modifies the mature peptide to dramatically increase stability. Rather than a complex with a second protein, a single polyethylene glycol (PEG) residue was added to Lys68, near the C-terminus of the mature IGF-I protein (61). PEG-IGF-I has a half-life of more than 30 hours in mice *in vivo*, providing almost 100-fold increase in

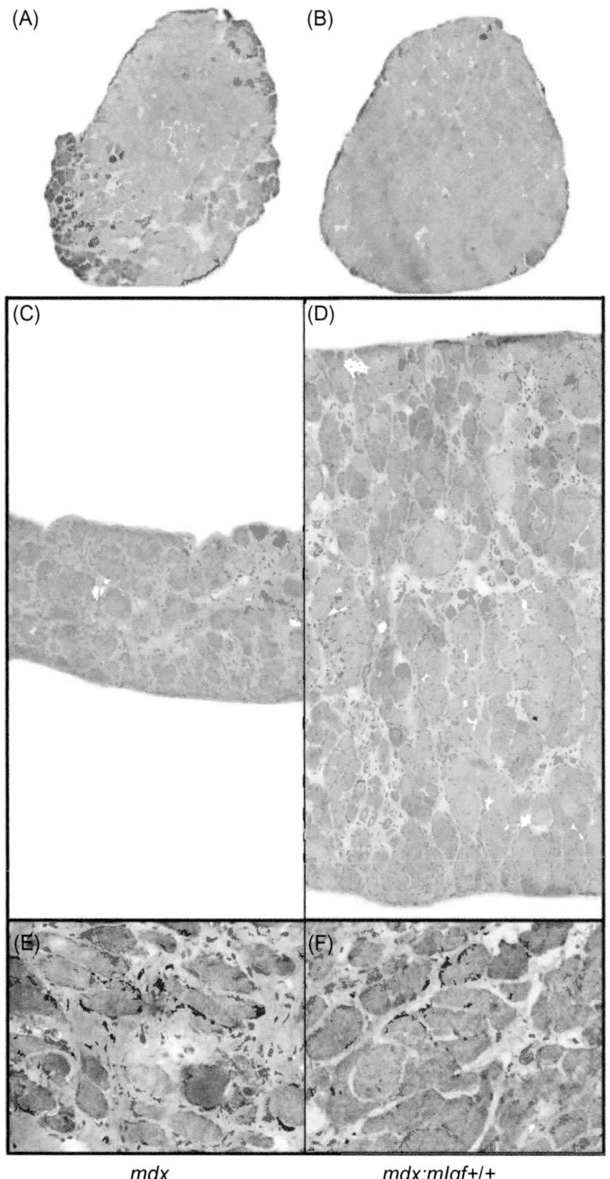

FIGURE 80.3 **Effect of muscle-specific IGF-IA overexpression on the morphology of dystrophic muscle.** Cross-sections of extensor digitorum muscles from mdx mice aged 14 months show that in muscles from mdx mice (A), there is widespread fiber necrosis indicated by the rounded, darkly stained fibers, focal regions of degeneration, and a high variability in fiber size. Transgenic expression of IGF-IA (B) significantly reduces all of these hallmarks of dystrophic pathology. Sagittal cross-sections of diaphragms from the same 14-month-old mdx mice reveal the fibrotic replacement of muscle fibers (C,E) from mdx mice. Transgenic expression of IGF-IA in the diaphragm caused a tripling of muscle thickness, primarily by hyperplasia (D), and a reduction in the extent of fibrosis (E) shown in sections stained by Gomori's trichrome. Scale bars = 50 μm. *(From Barton et al., 2002 (17).)*

stability over the native protein. Although this modification appears to interfere with IGFBP binding, PEG-IGF-I retains high specificity for the IGF-IR, and reduced activation of the IR. In myoblast cultures, PEG-IGF-I enhanced proliferation and differentiation to the same extent as recombinant IGF-I, and in the mdx mouse model for Duchenne muscular dystrophy (DMD), PEG-IGF-I improved the susceptibility to contraction-induced injury similar to recombinant IGF-I. However, the changes in serum glucose that are caused by recombinant IGF-I were distinctly absent with administration of PEG-IGF-I. This suggests that PEG modification of IGF-I may avoid one of the side effects of recombinant IGF-I therapies: namely, hypoglycemia.

The above strategies are geared toward modulating the systemic levels of IGF-I, and may be optimal for acute treatments. However, if muscle IGF-I were to increase without changing circulating levels, then the carcinogenic risks, and possibly the GH disregulation could be avoided. Further, increasing the local muscle production of IGF-I could provide an effective therapy for enhancing functional and repair capacity. Multipronged benefits of IGF-I were demonstrated in *mdx* mice crossbred to transgenic animals with muscle specific expression of IGF-I, resulting in increased functional muscle mass, decreased fibrotic replacement of muscle, and no apparent effects on non-expressing tissues (17) (Figure 80.3). Obviously, germ line transmission of any gene is not a rational approach for people. However, viral administration of the cDNA encoding for IGF-I into target tissues is a viable option, and could provide therapeutic benefits to muscle. Viral gene delivery of IGF-I into mouse and rat muscle boosts muscle mass in young animals, maintains muscle mass and strength in old animals, accelerates rehabilitation after disuse atrophy, and enhances and prolongs the hypertrophic effects of resistance training (16,23,47). Thus, tailoring the delivery of IGF-I to the tissues that benefit from its actions may ultimately be the way forward when long term treatments are necessary.

REFERENCES

1. Allen RE, Sheehan SM, Taylor RG, Kendall TL, Rice GM. Hepatocyte growth factor activates quiescent skeletal muscle satellite cells in vitro. *J Cell Physiol* 1995;**165**:307–12.
2. Yun YR, Won JE, Jeon E, Lee S, Kang W, Jo H, et al. Fibroblast growth factors: biology, function, and application for tissue regeneration. *J Tissue Eng* 2010;**2010**:218142.
3. Cross MJ, Dixelius J, Matsumoto T, Claesson-Welsh L. VEGF-receptor signal transduction. *Trends Biochem Sci* 2003;**28**:488–94.
4. Wagatsuma A, Tamaki H, Ogita F. Sequential expression of vascular endothelial growth factor, Flt-1, and KDR/Flk-1 in regenerating mouse skeletal muscle. *Physiol Res* 2006;**55**:633–40.
5. Adams TE, Epa VC, Garrett TP, Ward CW. Structure and function of the type 1 insulin-like growth factor receptor. *Cell Mol Life Sci* 2000;**57**:1050–93.
6. De Meyts P, Whittaker J. Structural biology of insulin and IGF1 receptors: implications for drug design. *Nat Rev Drug Discov* 2002;**1**:769–83.

7. Urso B, Cope DL, Kalloo-Hosein HE, Hayward AC, Whitehead JP, O'Rahilly S, et al. Differences in signaling properties of the cytoplasmic domains of the insulin receptor and insulin-like growth factor receptor in 3T3-L1 adipocytes. *J Biol Chem* 1999;**274**:30864–73.
8. Dupont J, Dunn SE, Barrett JC, LeRoith D. Microarray analysis and identification of novel molecules involved in insulin-like growth factor-1 receptor signaling and gene expression. *Recent Prog Horm Res* 2003;**58**:325–42.
9. Vecchione A, Marchese A, Henry P, Rotin D, Morrione A. The Grb10/Nedd4 complex regulates ligand-induced ubiquitination and stability of the insulin-like growth factor I receptor. *Mol Cell Biol* 2003;**23**:3363–72.
10. Federici M, Porzio O, Zucaro L, Fusco A, Borboni P, Lauro D, et al. Distribution of insulin/insulin-like growth factor-I hybrid receptors in human tissues. *Mol Cell Endocrinol* 1997;**129**:121–6.
11. Bailyes EM, Nave BT, Soos MA, Orr SR, Hayward AC, Siddle K. Insulin receptor/IGF-I receptor hybrids are widely distributed in mammalian tissues: quantification of individual receptor species by selective immunoprecipitation and immunoblotting. *Biochem J* 1997;**327**(Pt 1):209–15.
12. Kristensen C, Wiberg FC, Andersen AS. Specificity of insulin and insulin-like growth factor I receptors investigated using chimeric mini-receptors. Role of C-terminal of receptor alpha subunit. *J Biol Chem* 1999;**274**:37351–6.
13. Entingh-Pearsall A, Kahn CR. Differential roles of the insulin and insulin-like growth factor-I (IGF-I) receptors in response to insulin and IGF-I. *J Biol Chem* 2004;**279**:38016–24.
14. Coolican SA, Samuel DS, Ewton DZ, McWade FJ, Florini JR. The mitogenic and myogenic actions of insulin-like growth factors utilize distinct signaling pathways. *J Biol Chem* 1997;**272**:6653–62.
15. Bodine SC, Stitt TN, Gonzalez M, Kline WO, Stover GL, Bauerlein R, et al. Akt/mTOR pathway is a crucial regulator of skeletal muscle hypertrophy and can prevent muscle atrophy in vivo. *Nat Cell Biol* 2001;**3**:1014–9.
16. Barton-Davis ER, Shoturma DI, Sweeney HL. Contribution of satellite cells to IGF-I induced hypertrophy of skeletal muscle. *Acta Physiol Scand* 1999;**167**:301–5.
17. Barton ER, Morris L, Musaro A, Rosenthal N, Sweeney HL. Muscle-specific expression of insulin-like growth factor I counters muscle decline in mdx mice. *J Cell Biol* 2002;**157**:137–48.
18. Kooijman R. Regulation of apoptosis by insulin-like growth factor (IGF)-I. *Cytokine Growth Factor Rev* 2006;**17**:305–23.
19. Firth SM, Baxter RC. Cellular actions of the insulin-like growth factor binding proteins. *Endocr Rev* 2002;**23**:824–54.
20. Stevens-Lapsley JE, Ye F, Liu M, Borst SE, Conover C, Yarasheski KE, et al. Impact of viral-mediated IGF-I gene transfer on skeletal muscle following cast immobilization. *Am J Physiol Endocrinol Metabol* 2010;**299**:E730–40.
21. Salmon Jr WD, Daughaday WH. A hormonally controlled serum factor which stimulates sulfate incorporation by cartilage in vitro. *J Lab Clin Med* 1957;**49**:825–36.
22. Butler AA, LeRoith D. Minireview: tissue-specific versus generalized gene targeting of the igf1 and igf1r genes and their roles in insulin-like growth factor physiology. *Endocrinology* 2001;**142**:1685–8.
23. Barton ER. Viral expression of insulin-like growth factor-I isoforms promotes different responses in skeletal muscle. *J Appl Physiol* 2006;**100**:1778–84.
24. Goldspink G. Cloning of local growth factors involved in the determination of muscle mass. *Br J Sports Med* 2000;**34**:159–60.
25. Hepler JE, Van Wyk JJ, Lund PK. Different half-lives of insulin-like growth factor I mRNAs that differ in length of 3' untranslated sequence. *Endocrinology* 1990;**127**:1550–2.
26. Kuo YH, Chen TT. Novel activities of pro-IGF-I E peptides: regulation of morphological differentiation and anchorage-independent growth in human neuroblastoma cells. *Exp Cell Res* 2002;**280**:75–89.
27. Mills P, Lafreniere JF, Benabdallah BF, El Fahime el M, Tremblay JP. A new pro-migratory activity on human myogenic precursor cells for a synthetic peptide within the E domain of the mechano growth factor. *Exp Cell Res* 2007;**313**:527–37.
28. Siegfried JM, Kasprzyk PG, Treston AM, Mulshine JL, Quinn KA, Cuttitta F. A mitogenic peptide amide encoded within the E peptide domain of the insulin-like growth factor IB prohormone. *Proc Natl Acad Sci USA* 1992;**89**:8107–11.
29. Adamo ML, Neuenschwander S, LeRoith D, Roberts Jr CT. Structure, expression, and regulation of the IGF-I gene. *Adv Exp Med Biol* 1993;**343**:1–11.
30. Barton ER. The ABCs of IGF-I isoforms: impact on muscle hypertrophy and implications for repair. *Appl Physiol Nutr Metab* 2006;**31**:791–7.
31. Rotwein P, Pollock KM, Didier DK, Krivi GG. Organization and sequence of the human insulin-like growth factor I gene. Alternative RNA processing produces two insulin-like growth factor I precursor peptides. *J Biol Chem* 1986;**261**:4828–32.
32. Shimatsu A, Rotwein P. Mosaic evolution of the insulin-like growth factors. Organization, sequence, and expression of the rat insulin-like growth factor I gene. *J Biol Chem* 1987;**262**:7894–900.
33. Bell GI, Sanchez-Pescador R, Laybourn PJ, Najarian RC. Exon duplication and divergence in the human preproglucagon gene. *Nature* 1983;**304**:368–71.
34. Chew SL, Lavender P, Clark AJ, Ross RJ. An alternatively spliced human insulin-like growth factor-I transcript with hepatic tissue expression that diverts away from the mitogenic IBE1 peptide. *Endocrinology* 1995;**136**:1939–44.
35. Yang SY, Goldspink G. Different roles of the IGF-I Ec peptide (MGF) and mature IGF-I in myoblast proliferation and differentiation. *FEBS Lett* 2002;**522**:156–60.
36. Hameed M, Orrell RW, Cobbold M, Goldspink G, Harridge SD. Expression of IGF-I splice variants in young and old human skeletal muscle after high resistance exercise. *J Physiol* 2003;**547**:247–54.
37. Owino V, Yang SY, Goldspink G. Age-related loss of skeletal muscle function and the inability to express the autocrine form of insulin-like growth factor-1 (MGF) in response to mechanical overload. *FEBS Lett* 2001;**505**:259–63.
38. Wallis M. New insulin-like growth factor (IGF)-precursor sequences from mammalian genomes: the molecular evolution of IGFs and associated peptides in primates. *Growth Horm IGF Res* 2009;**19**:12–23.
39. Duguay SJ. Post-translational processing of insulin-like growth factors. *Horm Metab Res* 1999;**31**:43–9.
40. Conover CA, Baker BK, Hintz RL. Cultured human fibroblasts secrete insulin-like growth factor IA prohormone. *J Clin Endocrinol Metab* 1989;**69**:25–30.

41. Pfeffer LA, Brisson BK, Lei H, Barton ER. The insulin-like growth factor (IGF)-I E-peptides modulate cell entry of the mature IGF-I protein. *Mol Biol Cell* 2009;**20**:3810–7.
42. Wilson HE, Westwood M, White A, Clayton PE. Monoclonal antibodies to the carboxy-terminal Ea sequence of pro-insulin-like growth factor-IA (proIGF-IA) recognize proIGF-IA secreted by IM9 B-lymphocytes. *Growth Horm IGF Res* 2001;**11**:10–7.
43. Bach MA, Roberts Jr CT, Smith EP, LeRoith D. Alternative splicing produces messenger RNAs encoding insulin-like growth factor-I prohormones that are differentially glycosylated in vitro. *Mol Endocrinol* 1990;**4**:899–904.
44. Florini JR, Ewton DZ, Coolican SA. Growth hormone and the insulin-like growth factor system in myogenesis. *Endocr Rev* 1996;**17**:481–517.
45. Criswell DS, Booth FW, DeMayo F, Schwartz RJ, Gordon SE, Fiorotto ML. Overexpression of IGF-I in skeletal muscle of transgenic mice does not prevent unloading-induced atrophy. *Am J Physiol* 1998;**275**:E373–9.
46. Berger MJ, Doherty TJ. Sarcopenia: prevalence, mechanisms, and functional consequences. *Interdisciplin Topics Gerontol* 2010;**37**:94–114.
47. Barton-Davis ER, Shoturma DI, Musaro A, Rosenthal N, Sweeney HL. Viral mediated expression of insulin-like growth factor I blocks the aging-related loss of skeletal muscle function. *Proc Natl Acad Sci USA* 1998;**95**:15603–7.
48. Musaro A, McCullagh K, Paul A, Houghton L, Dobrowolny G, Molinaro M, et al. Localized Igf-1 transgene expression sustains hypertrophy and regeneration in senescent skeletal muscle. *Nat Genet* 2001;**27**:195–200.
49. Borst SE. Interventions for sarcopenia and muscle weakness in older people. *Age Ageing* 2004;**33**:548–55.
50. Cusi K, DeFronzo R. Recombinant human insulin-like growth factor I treatment for 1 week improves metabolic control in type 2 diabetes by ameliorating hepatic and muscle insulin resistance. *J Clin Endocrinol Metab* 2000;**85**:3077–84.
51. Lai EC, Felice KJ, Festoff BW, Gawel MJ, Gelinas DF, Kratz R, et al. Effect of recombinant human insulin-like growth factor-I on progression of ALS. A placebo-controlled study. The North America ALS/IGF-I Study Group. *Neurology* 1997;**49**:1621–30.
52. Borasio GD, Robberecht W, Leigh PN, Emile J, Guiloff RJ, Jerusalem F, et al. A placebo-controlled trial of insulin-like growth factor-I in amyotrophic lateral sclerosis. European ALS/IGF-I Study Group. *Neurology* 1998;**51**:583–6.
53. Friedlander AL, Butterfield GE, Moynihan S, Grillo J, Pollack M, Holloway L, et al. One year of insulin-like growth factor I treatment does not affect bone density, body composition, or psychological measures in postmenopausal women. *J Clin Endocrinol Metab* 2001;**86**:1496–503.
54. Mauras N, O'Brien KO, Welch S, Rini A, Helgeson K, Vieira NE, et al. Insulin-like growth factor I and growth hormone (GH) treatment in GH-deficient humans: differential effects on protein, glucose, lipid, and calcium metabolism. *J Clin Endocrinol Metab* 2000;**85**:1686–94.
55. Waters D, Danska J, Hardy K, Koster F, Qualls C, Nickell D, et al. Recombinant human growth hormone, insulin-like growth factor 1, and combination therapy in AIDS-associated wasting. A randomized, double-blind, placebo-controlled trial. *Ann Intern Med* 1996;**125**:865–72.
56. Moxley 3rd RT. Potential for growth factor treatment of muscle disease. *Curr Opin Neurol* 1994;**7**:427–34.
57. Thompson JL, Butterfield GE, Gylfadottir UK, Yesavage J, Marcus R, Hintz RL, et al. Effects of human growth hormone, insulin-like growth factor I, and diet and exercise on body composition of obese postmenopausal women. *J Clin Endocrinol Metab* 1998;**83**:1477–84.
58. Butterfield GE, Thompson J, Rennie MJ, Marcus R, Hintz RL, Hoffman AR. Effect of rhGH and rhIGF-I treatment on protein utilization in elderly women. *Am J Physiol* 1997;**272**:E94–9.
59. Kemp SF, Fowlkes JL, Thrailkill KM. Efficacy and safety of mecasermin rinfabate. *Expert Opin Biol Ther* 2006;**6**:533–8.
60. Heatwole CR, Eichinger KJ, Friedman DI, Hilbert JE, Jackson CE, Logigian EL, et al. Open-label trial of recombinant human insulin-like growth factor 1/recombinant human insulin-like growth factor binding protein 3 in myotonic dystrophy type 1. *Arch Neurol* 2011;**68**:37–44.
61. Metzger F, Staudenmaier C, Sänger S, Sajid W, van der Poel C, Sobottka B, et al. Separation of fast from slow anabolism by site-specific pegylation of insulin-like growth factor I. *J Biol Chem* 2011;**286**:19501–10.

Chapter 81

Novel Targets and Approaches to Treating Skeletal Muscle Disease

Elizabeth McNally

Department of Medicine, Section of Cardiology, Department of Human Genetics, University of Chicago, Chicago, IL

INTRODUCTION

In many forms of muscle disease, multiple muscle groups are weakened and are the targets for therapy. Limb muscle weakness reduces voluntary movement such as ambulation, and weakness of involuntary muscles renders difficulty for posture maintenance and breathing. Many inherited diseases of skeletal muscle are caused by recessive mutations that result in a loss of protein function. In this sense, gene replacement strategies that restore gene products and function are logical but significantly challenged by the large mass of tissue to be targeted. Viral gene replacement, while conceptually a simple approach, is complicated by the need to deliver virus to many muscle groups to achieve efficacy and improve strength and function of multiple muscle groups. This led investigators to contemplate alternative novel approaches using both biological agents and small compounds as therapy. Small molecules offer the advantage of ready delivery to the wide target of many muscle groups. At this same time, these compounds must have an acceptable therapeutic window since they will be systemically delivered for the lifetime of the recipient. Currently there are no cures for the muscular dystrophies and myopathies. The purpose of this chapter is to highlight future areas for therapy development. Use of these novel strategies is likely to complement existing pharmacological agents and may also augment gene replacement/correction strategies since each of these methods on its own may prove insufficient.

DISEASE TARGETS

In the past two decades remarkable progress has been made in defining the precise genes and mutations that cause inherited muscle weakness. In the muscular dystrophies the most common mechanisms leading to disease are typified by what occurs in Duchenne muscular dystrophy (DMD) and in its milder form, Becker muscular dystrophy (BMD). Namely, there is progressive breakdown and ongoing destruction of existing myofibers (Figure 81.1). There is a variable inflammatory response in degenerating skeletal muscle depending on the cause of disease. Skeletal muscle damage, unlike cardiac muscle, is associated with robust regeneration due to muscle stem cells called satellite cells. Cell-based therapy is aggressively being pursued for muscle treatment and is described in Chapters 62 and 77. Viral gene replacement is addressed in Chapter 76. In developing new approaches to treating muscle disease, each of these steps in muscle disease – the primary molecular defect, the signaling cascades triggered by damage, the breakdown of myofibers and the regenerative response, including both the cell intrinsic and cell extrinsic mechanisms – is in itself a target for therapy.

RESEALING MUSCLE MEMBRANE DISRUPTION

Synthetic Surfactants – P188

In DMD, the absence of dystrophin leads to an unusually fragile plasma membrane. Seminal work by Rybakova and colleagues demonstrated that dystrophin participates in a mechanically strong link between the cytoskeleton, the plasma membrane and the membrane itself (1). When the sarcolemma is peeled from the underlying cytoskeleton, the actin cytoskeletal remains intact on the inner surface of the plasma membrane. In the absence of dystrophin, cytoplasmic γ-actin no longer links to the sarcolemma. The absence of dystrophin or the dystrophin-associated proteins, the sarcoglycans, leads to microdisruptions manifested as abnormal membrane permeability (Figure 81.2). In the case of dystrophin, muscle contraction enhances membrane breakdown, and this can be visualized through the use of the vital tracer Evans blue dye.

Resealants have been tested to subvert the fragile properties of the dystrophin-deficient membrane.

Muscle. DOI: http://dx.doi.org/10.1016/B978-0-12-381510-1.00081-8

Poloxamer 188 (P188) is a nonionic synthetic surfactant of small molecular mass 8.4 kDa that reseals the plasma membrane in dystrophin-deficient cardiomyocytes and skeletal myofibers. P188 is a triblock copolymer of the form poly(ethylene oxide) − poly(propylene oxide) − poly(ethylene oxide) (PEO − PPO − PEO) and can serve as an effective membrane sealant in muscle in response to trauma such as that induced by electrical shock, burns or irradiation. P188 was shown to prevent mechanical-stretch induced damage in isolated dystrophin-deficient cardiomyocytes (2), and further to prevent dobutamine-induced cardiac dysfunction in the *mdx* mouse model. More recently, this use of P188 was tested in chronic infusion and also in a larger model of cardiomyopathy, more akin to what occurs in humans (3).

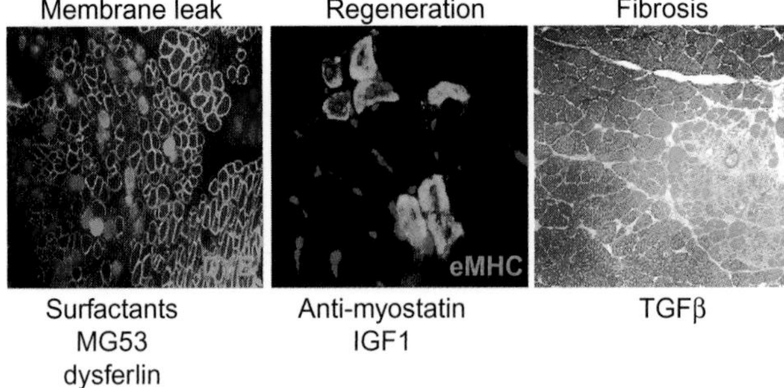

FIGURE 81.1 **Pathological progression in muscular dystrophy.** The sarcolemma is fragile in DMD and becomes disrupted in many different forms of muscle disease. This can be visualized by injecting vital tracers such as Evans blue dye (DYE, red), which is visible as red fluorescence. Note the red opacified myofibers in this mouse model of muscular dystrophy. Normal muscle has no opacified fibers. In the middle panel, dystrophic muscle has been stained with an antibody to embryonic myosin heavy chain (eMHC, green). Normal muscle does not express eMHC unless it has been injured. Dystrophic muscle has myofibers that express eMHC marking the attempted regeneration. In muscular dystrophy, regeneration does not keep pace with degeneration. IGF1 and anti-myostatin compounds are being tested for therapy. The right panel shows fibrosis in muscular dystrophy. Anti-fibrotic agents that target TGF-β or its intracellular signaling pathways are being tested for utility in muscular dystrophy.

The use of P188 has also been suggested to be of benefit for skeletal muscle where it has been shown to protect against contraction-induced force deficits in *mdx* skeletal muscle. In the absence of dystrophin, repeated contraction, particularly lengthening contractions also known as eccentric contraction, reduces force production. In a series of rapidly repeated contractions, dystrophin-deficient muscle becomes highly disrupted and can exhibit as much as a 50% reduction in force. Contractile properties were partially improved by P188 administration in the lumbrical muscles of the *mdx* mouse (4). The side-effect profile for P188 delivery is thought to be reasonable, even in the face of chronic administration. The challenge with delivery of P188 centers on the need to provide intravenous or intramuscular dosing. This delivery method is not insurmountable given the availability of pumps, both extracorporeal and subcutaneous.

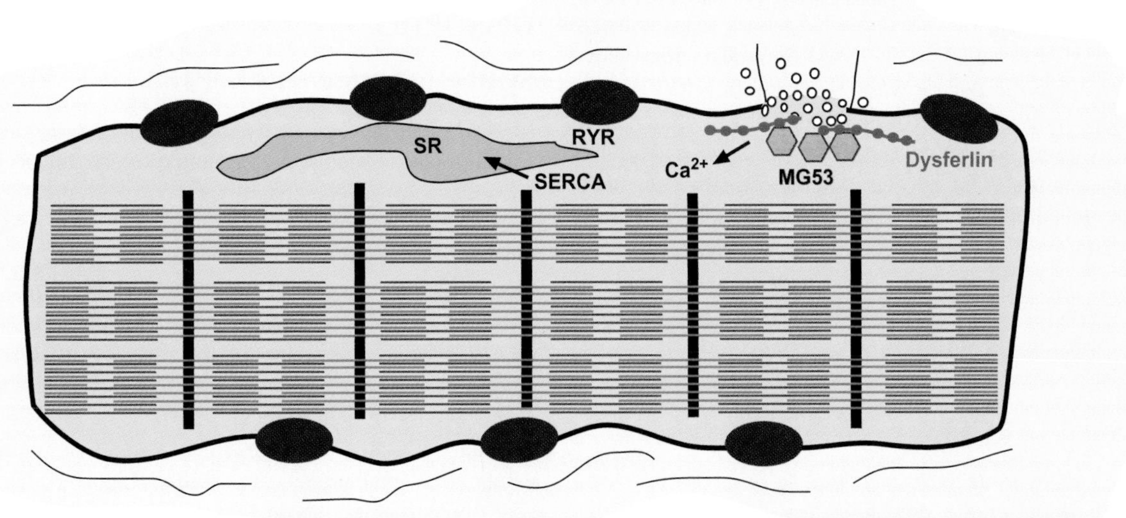

FIGURE 81.2 **Membrane disruption in muscle.** With membrane disruption, vesicles accumulate to promote resealing. MG53 (green) and dysferlin (blue) have been implicated in resealing. Disruption of the plasma membrane leads to increased intracellular calcium. Increased SERCA expression or decreased ryanodine receptor (RYR) leak can be used to offset the detrimental effects of increased intracellular calcium.

MG53

Mitsugumin 53 (MG53) also contributes to membrane repair. MG53, also known as TRIM72, is a member of the tripartite motif protein family in that it contains a RING finger, B box, and coiled coil domain. MG53 is highly enriched in skeletal and cardiac muscle, although is broadly expressed. MG53 interacts with caveolin-3 and is involved in exocytosis and muscle growth and myoblast fusion. Mice lacking MG53 develop a mild myopathy and display exercise intolerance and exercise-induced damage (5). Notably, MG53 is a protein that is rapidly recruited to sites of muscle membrane disruption where it is thought to nucleate a repair complex that includes caveolin-3 and dysferlin (see below). It has also been observed that MG53's cysteine sulphydryl groups are redox-sensitive and that under conditions of increased oxidative damage, a conformational change in MG53 is triggered that promotes muscle repair (5). In a reduced environment MG53 is largely monomeric, whereas in an oxidized state MG53 is observed to oligomerize. In the presence of the reducing agent dithiothreitol, MG53 recruitment to sites of muscle membrane disruption was diminished. It was also observed using lipid profiling that MG53 has a preference for binding the negatively charged phosphotidylserine, and this negatively charged phospholipid is usually enriched on the inner surface or cytoplasmic face of the plasma membrane.

It has been proposed that MG53 could be useful to reseal membrane disruptions in muscle disease (6). It remains to be shown that MG53 is effective in a chronic disease setting such as that seen in genetically mediated forms of myopathy or muscular dystrophy. Delivering MG53 to muscle or heart may require a tissue-specific approach; it is unclear whether the protein must be delivered from an intracellular vantage or whether extracellular application is viable. It is possible that MG53-dependent repair is most effective in the acute injury setting since chronic and acute injury may employ some distinct molecular mechanisms. Of note, it has been suggested that MG53/TRIM72 is a negative regulator of myoblast fusion and that loss of MG53 is associated with enhanced muscle growth (7). Therefore, additional studies on the primary mechanisms of MG53 are required prior to this moving into the therapeutic setting.

Dysferlin

Mutations in dysferlin lead to a recessive form of muscular dystrophy, limb girdle muscular dystrophy type 2B. Dysferlin is a membrane-associated protein that is highly expressed in multinucleated myofibers and it is implicated in muscle repair. Dysferlin, like the other ferlin proteins, is defined by multi-C2 domain composition. The ferlin proteins, including dysferlin, typically contain at least six C2 domains; C2 domains are independently folding domains that bind calcium, phospholipids or other proteins. They are found in more than 100 membrane-associated proteins, but most C2 domain-containing proteins contain only one or two C2 domains. The C2 domains in dysferlin are similar to those found in synaptotagmins, proteins implicated in fast exocytosis at nerve terminals. The first C2 domain of dysferlin called C2A is positioned at the amino terminus and directly binds negatively charged phospholipids (8). A mutation within C2A that is associated with inherited muscular dystrophy was shown to have disrupted calcium-sensitive phospholipid binding.

Experimental evidence supports dysferlin's role in membrane resealing. Specifically, when dysferlin null myofibers are subjected to wounding with a laser, the membrane reseals more slowly. Notably, membrane resealing after laser wounding occurs equally slowly in normal cells when calcium is absent (9). Laser wounding experiments were conducted in the presence of FM1-43, a membrane-associated but impermeant dye. FM1-43 is applied to the myofiber prior to wounding where it inserts into the sarcolemma. Upon injury, there is an accumulation of dye at the site of wounding, and because this dye is embedded in the membrane, this dye accumulation represents vesicles. The origin of these submembranous vesicles is not clear, but the fluorescence of FM1-43 increases when lipophilic content increases. The protein components that regulate vesicle trafficking at the sites of wounding are not clear but dysferlin interacting proteins include caveolin, MG-53, AHNAK, and annexins (5,10,11). The biological *in vivo* significance of laser-induced wounding is unclear since the nature of the membrane disruption may be much larger than what occurs *in vivo* from contraction-induced damage. The elevation of serum creatine kinase in LGMD 2B patients is even higher than in other forms of muscular dystrophy, and this substantial elevation may be useful in identifying dysferlin mutant patients. Elevated serum muscle proteins reflect significant leak and defective membrane repair.

Membrane wounding and repair has also been studied with other assays, including a bead wounding assay where 40–70 μm acid-washed beads are rolled over myotubes in culture to induce sarcolemmal injury (12). Like the laser injury model, the bead-wounding assay is also conducted in the presence of fluorescent dextran to visualize membrane disruption. Response to osmotic shock assay can also be used (13). Normal myotubes form blebs along the surface of the sarcolemma within seconds of being placed in 25–50% hypotonic solution. Like the resealing assays the formation of blebs is calcium-dependent since it does not occur in the presence of EGTA. Interestingly, dysferlin null myotubes failed to form membrane blebbing in hypotonic solution. It was suggested that the formation of blebs requires vesicle fusion to provide additional membrane. It is also possible that the absence of membrane blebs also reflects an abnormal underlying subsarcolemmal network since the membrane remains intact in this assay. These assays document that repair after injury is abnormal in the absence of dysferlin, however the *in vivo* relevance is not clear. Replacement of dysferlin either through viral or pharmacologic approaches was sufficient to correct laser injury or blebbing, but how these findings translate to *in vivo* correction of pathology is not clear.

Dysferlin is also linked more broadly to membrane trafficking. Dysferlin, and other ferlin family members, mediate the endocytic recycling. Endocytic recycling is the process where internalized vesicles are recycled to plasma membrane. Endocyctic recycling is not only important for the recycling of the lipid components of vesicles, but also for their protein content, such as specific receptors. The loss of ferlin proteins, including dysferlin, impairs the recycling and activity of the insulin-like growth factor (IGF) receptor (14). IGF receptors are critical for muscle growth and repair both in the prenatal and postnatal state. In the absence of dysferlin, IGF receptor is redirected to lysosomes rather than back to the plasma membrane. These data imply that ferlin protein, including dysferlin, are important for vesicle trafficking beyond resealing. Therefore, upregulation of ferlin proteins or dysferlin itself as a means of augmenting muscle repair may be complicated by more finely tuned regulation. Interestingly, it has been shown that a mini-dysferlin that contains only the carboxy-terminal two C2 domains and the transmembrane domain is effective to regulate membrane resealing (15). With further dissection of the functional elements within dysferlin, it may be possible to target more effectively regions of the protein essential for the resealing process.

Dysferlin is highly expressed in myofibers. Dysferlin is expressed at lower levels in myoblasts and is also found in immune cells leading to the hypothesis that dysferlin's role in non-myofiber cells contributes to pathology. Restoring dysferlin expression in using a muscle-specific transgene in the A/J mouse that lacks dysferlin was found to correct the histological findings of muscular dystrophy, suggesting that the muscle-specific role of dysferlin is essential for pathogenesis (16). In this study, mice were examined at 8 months of age, a time point where pathological changes were evident.

LGMD 2B patients are often normal, or even athletic in early life and typically show progressive decline. This course has been hypothesized to reflect progressive damage over time owing to the inability to repair damage. A nonmutually exclusive hypothesis is that the regeneration capacity of dysferlin null muscle is deficient. Several lines of evidence support impaired regeneration and a role for the ferlin family members in mediating repair. Since vesicle transport and membrane fusion are important features of myoblast fusion to myofibers as they are to membrane resealing, it could be expected that dysferlin-deficient muscle would show regenerative defects. In support of this, when injured by notexin injection, dysferlin-deficient muscle fails to regain its normal architecture in the expected time frame. Dysferlin null myoblasts fuse less well to form large myofibers in culture (14). Additionally, human dysferlin null myoblast cultures have a decreased fusion potential, suggestive of a fusion defect in dysferlinopathy patients (17). These data provide evidence that dysferlin has a role in myoblasts, in addition to mature skeletal muscle, that may effect the capacity for muscle regeneration. Therapy for dysferlin is focused on replacing dysferlin since its myriad functions in vesicle trafficking may be difficult to target with small molecules.

Utrophin

Utrophin is highly related to dystrophin and can substitute for dystrophin's function. Normally, utrophin is expressed highly in developing muscle, and in mature muscle is enriched at the neuromuscular junction. As the myofiber matures, utrophin levels are decreased and dystrophin is the protein expressed in the mature myofiber. Like dystrophin, utrophin interacts with the dystrophin-associated protein complex to complete a link from the cytoskeleton through the membrane and to the extracellular matrix. Since utrophin is a naturally occurring protein that can largely substitute for dystrophin, several approaches have been taken to stimulate utrophin's expression (18) (Figure 81.3). Upregulation of utrophin can be achieved by protein delivery or by upregulating the native endogenous utrophin promoter. Increasing native utrophin levels by 2–3-fold may be sufficient to improve muscle degeneration in DMD since muscles showing this modest level of overexpression are protected. The utrophin promoter has been dissected and compounds that are thought to stimulate the utrophin promoter have been characterized. Notably heregulin, a member of the neuregulin family, has been shown to induce utrophin expression and ameliorate muscular dystrophy in the *mdx* mouse (19).

Peptide translocation domains, or PTDS, are small positively charged units that when coupled to proteins or other molecules permit transport across membranes. PTD-coupled utrophin was translocated into muscle cells where it was effective in improving muscle pathology and muscle function in the *mdx* mouse (20). The PTD was able to deliver both full utrophin and a miniutrophin effectively. This approach may prove more generally useful to deliver proteins to muscle after intraperitoneal delivery. However, to treat larger mammals will require adequate protein production and purification. One advantage to

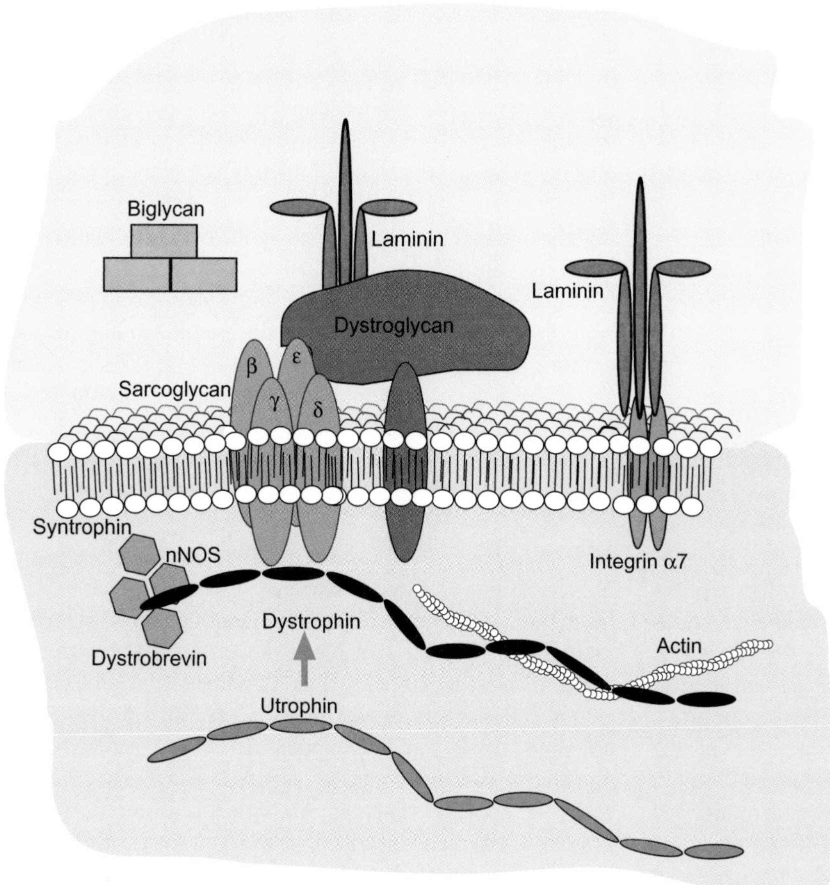

FIGURE 81.3 **Membrane stabilizing therapy in muscular dystrophy.** The dystrophin complex is found at the plasma membrane of muscle. Extracellular components such as biglycan and laminin 111 have been shown to be effective in mouse models of muscular dystrophy. Upregulation of alternative transmembrane linkages such as integrin α7 has also been shown to be useful. Dystrophin replacement with utrophin is also being pursued using compounds that stimulate utrophin expression.

delivering utrophin is that it is less likely to elicit an immune response. Viral gene delivery of dystrophin into DMD patients has been associated with an immune response that limits expression of dystrophin (21). It remains to be seen whether the immune system can be overwhelmed to effectively deliver dystrophin. A protein such as utrophin, which is normally expressed in DMD patients, should not be associated with a similar immune response.

Utrophin, while highly similar to dystrophin, does not share all of dystrophin's exact binding domains, and therefore may not fully substitute for dystrophin. Specifically, utrophin's actin binding domain properties differ from those found in dystrophin (22). Also, it is not clear that nitric oxide synthase will adhere to the utrophin protein complex with the same affinity and function as a dystrophin protein complex (23). These biochemical observations may limit the ability for utrophin to fully substitute for dystrophin or for smaller dystrophin products to fully correct all aspects of dystrophin deficiency.

Biglycan

Biglycan is an extracellular matrix protein that is also being pursued for the treatment of DMD. Biglycan is a small molecular mass leucine-rich proteoglycan that interacts with multiple components of the dystrophin complex including dystroglycan and sarcoglycan components. Intraperitoneal or intramuscular delivery of purified biglycan was associated with upregulation of utrophin (24). Upregulation of utrophin in the *mdx* background was associated with improved phenotype in the *mdx* mouse. Interestingly, biglycan and the related protein proteoglycan decorin may also regulate transforming growth factor-β family members. These extracellular matrix proteins may also regulate myostatin, a negative inhibitor of muscle growth. Therefore, there may be additional mechanisms by which biglycan exerts its effect. Current efforts on biglycan are focused on upscale purification and optimization of delivery methods. The finding that biglycan exerts its effect through utrophin upregulation supports that biglycan delivery may be most appropriate for DMD therapy.

Integrin α7

Integrin α7 is a major laminin-binding integrin that can stabilize the muscle plasma membrane. Integrin α7 couples with β1 integrin in mature muscle fibers. Mutation in the gene encoding integrin α7 can also lead to muscular dystrophy in humans and mice. Transgenic overexpression of integrin α7 was shown to improve the phenotype in mice lacking dystrophin and utrophin (25). While it may prove complicated to try to deliver a transmembrane protein as a therapy, approaches to stimulate the integrin α7 promoter are being pursued. The mechanism by which integrin α7 functions to improve outcome in muscular dystrophy may rely on multiple mechanisms including providing an alternative compensatory transmembrane linkage to the sarcoglycan complex (26).

Laminin 111 and Glycosylating Enzymes

Laminin 111 is an extracellular matrix protein that has also been promoted for its ability to improve muscle regeneration and stabilize the plasma membrane in multiple forms of muscular dystrophy. Laminin 111 is composed of α1-β1-γ1 chains of laminin, a prominent extracellular matrix component. When delivered intramuscularly to mice lacking integrin α7 it was found to improve muscle regeneration. Interestingly, intraperitoneal delivery of laminin 111 was also shown to improve pathology in the *mdx* mouse (27). While some of the improvement of *mdx* pathology in response to laminin 111 delivery is likely due to improved regeneration, the effect likely extends beyond regeneration. It was observed that laminin 111 delivery was associated with increased expression of integrin α7 and it is thought that increased expression of integrin α7 in part explains some improvement in membrane stability. Most notable was that after systemic, intraperitoneal delivery that there was improvement in cardiac and diaphragm muscles in the *mdx* mouse.

The complexity of molecular attachments for the muscle membrane has focused attention on the specific carbohydrate moieties that participate in this linkage with an emphasis on potential therapy. Dystroglycan, provides a major link between the extracellular matrix and the sarcolemma (28). Dystroglycan undergoes O-linked glycosylation and the congenital muscular dystrophies that arise from mutations in the genes that help modify these proteins underscores the importance of these post-translational modifications (covered in Chapters 67 and 70). Upregulation of the glycosylating enzymes is also being tested in mouse models of muscular dystrophy. Given that these are enzymes, it may be possible to stimulate enzymatic activity as a therapeutic target.

STIMULATING MUSCLE GROWTH

Growth stimulators for muscle disease are a rational tactic for the atrophic muscle disorders such as disuse atrophy and sarcopenia. For the muscle degenerative disorders, such as the muscular dystrophies, it remains a theoretical question whether larger muscles may be more susceptible to damage. However, because muscle weakness and wasting are the major clinical concern from patients, muscle stimulators are actively being pursued. It is clear that muscle growth stimulants hold interest well beyond the muscle disease population. Therefore, when contemplating the underlying mechanism of growth stimulants, the effect on normal muscle must be considered separately from the effect on diseased muscle, since it remains possible that these effects may be different. Among considerations for muscle growth stimulants are their tissue specificity since growth stimulants may promote other unwanted growth, such as carcinogenesis.

Myostatin Inhibitors

Myostatin is a TGF-β family member that negatively regulates of muscle mass. Several approaches have been tried for therapeutically manipulating this pathway including antibodies that block the activin IIB receptor or using myostatin pro-peptide as a competitor for the receptor (29). Follistatin overexpression may also prove useful although these methods appear to lack specificity for myostatin and also bind to activins. However, in some cases it appears that the activity to promote muscle growth is independent of myostatin and therefore binding other family members like activins may be therapeutically useful. Antibodies that block myostatin were tested in patients with muscle disease including limb girdle muscular dystrophy (30). The trial did not show improvement of muscle mass but was stopped because of side effects deriving from repeated exposure to the antibodies.

Insulin-Like Growth Factor (IGF)-1

IGF-1 promotes muscle growth and is being actively pursued for muscle disease (31). IGF-1 acts downstream from growth hormone and is related to insulin. Processing differs between IGF-1 and insulin in that the former retains the C domain and has a longer A and additional D domain. IGF-1 is multiply spliced to produce distinct products, and the presence of the E peptide is thought to be important for some aspects of muscle growth. IGF-1 is stabilized in the serum by binding to IGF binding proteins (IGFBPs) and acts though the IGF-1-receptor. IGF-1s bind the type 1 IGF receptor, a receptor serine threonine kinase that, in turn, stimulates a cascade of signaling responses. In response to ligand binding, the IGF-1 receptor is phosphorylated and activates the MAP kinase-dependent signaling (MAPK) and the PI3K/AKT pathways. Overexpression of IGF-1 results in larger mice with an increase in muscle fiber number and larger cross sectional area (32). Treatment with IGF-1 improves muscle size in the *mdx* mouse (33,34). Because of its effects on growth of muscle, IGF-1 is being investigated for its use to treat muscle disorders. The utility of IGF-1 may extend to sarcopenia and muscle wasting associated with chronic disorders such as liver disease and heart failure. Inhibiting IGF-1 is being pursued in early phase oncology trials. Whether IGF-1 will promote untoward tissue growth such as malignancy will be closely followed in clinical trials.

INFLAMMATION AND FIBROSIS

Inhibiting TGF-β

Muscular dystrophy, especially DMD, is accompanied by excessive inflammation and fibrosis. One of the major mediators of fibrosis is transforming growth factor (TGF)-β. TGF-β is increased in the muscle of DMD patients (35) paralleling what has been observed in fibrotic diseases of the lung and kidney. A number of approaches have been used to reduce TGF-β signaling including halofuginone (36) and pirfenidone (37). Osteopontin is an extracellular matrix protein that is regulated by TGF-β and ablation of the osteopontin locus improves the phenotype in the mdx mouse (38). Intriguingly in a study of DMD patients, the osteopontin gene was identified as a modifier of severity of disease (39). A promoter mutation associated with increased expression of *SPP1* gene encoding osteopontin was associated with earlier loss of ambulation and reduced grip strength. This finding may be paradoxical given that loss of osteopontin reduced disease in the *mdx* mouse, but many interacting proteins may regulate TGF-β. A genome-wide scan for modifier genes of fibrosis and membrane leak in a mouse model of limb girdle muscular dystrophy identified latent TGF-β binding protein 4 (*LTBP4*) as a significant modifier of skeletal muscle (40). Using this same approach, additional genomic loci were identified as modifiers of cardiac and diaphragm muscle (41). The identification of these modifier genes may reveal pathways useful for modulating in therapy.

Treating the *mdx* mouse with the angiotensin receptor blocker (ARB) losartan reduced TGF-β signaling and improved outcome in the *mdx* mouse by reducing fibrosis (42). It has been shown in DMD patients that pretreatment prior to the development of cardiomyopathy with angiotensin-converting enzyme inhibitors (ACEI) delays the onset of cardiomyopathy and improves mortality (43). It is not clear whether ACEI or ARBs or both should be used in DMD patients, and ongoing clinical trials will test this question. These agents are thought to target the TGF-β pathway including the canonical TGF-β signaling pathway involving the SMADs. It was recently shown using a *Drosophila* model of muscle disease that reduction of SMADs improved walking and heart function (44). Whether inhibiting the non-canonical pathways will also be useful in treating muscle disease remains to be shown. With all these approaches, it is also believed that reducing fibrosis will also improve regeneration since the fibrotic matrix is thought to be less favorable for efficient myoblast differentiation and engraftment.

CALCIUM AND MITOCHONDRIAL DYSREGULATION IN MUSCLE DISEASE

Elevated intracellular calcium is a feature of muscle disease where the sarcolemma has been disrupted such as in DMD. Increased calcium may interfere with normal excitation–contraction coupling and also triggers activation of calcium-sensitive proteases and contributes to muscle degeneration. Reduction of the transient receptor potential channels (TRPC) reduced calcium leak channels in dystrophic muscle (45). Genetic overexpression of TRPC3 alone mimics aspects of muscular dystrophy, and overexpression of a dominant negative TRPC6 abrogates histopathological changes in mouse models of muscular dystrophy (46).

The ryanodine receptor 1 (RyR1) is the major calcium release channel of the sarcoplasmic reticulum in muscle. RyR1 is abnormally nitrosylated in muscular dystrophy leading to leaky channels. S107 is a small molecule that binds to RyR1 and promotes its stable binding to calstabin/FKB12. S107 was shown to improve histopathology and cardiac arrhythmias in the *mdx* mouse model and underscores the link between abnormal intracellular calcium regulation and fibrosis (47,48). Similarly, virally mediated overexpression of SERCA, the sarcoplasmic reticulum calcium uptake channel, also improves histopathology in muscular dystrophy (49). These calcium-associated therapies are not thought to stabilize the plasma membrane but rather treat the intracellular consequences of membrane instability in muscle disease. It is possible that these therapies will prove most effective in those forms of muscle disease such as DMD that are typified by aggressive membrane instability and cellular degeneration. Intracellular calcium dysregulation is linked to mitochondrial dysfunction and compounds that limit abnormal mitochondrial function are also being examined (50). Coenzyme Q10 and idebenone are commonly used in clinical practice for muscle disease, although results from clinical trials have been limited.

GENE CORRECTION STRATEGIES

In addition to the pharmacological targets above, gene correction has evolved from viral gene replacement approaches to gene correction. Stop codon therapy developed from the observation that the aminoglycoside gentamicin promotes stop codon readthrough and restores dystrophin expression in the *mdx* mouse (51). This is an appealing avenue since even modest increases in dystrophin expression will likely lead to clinical improvement based on genotype-phenotype examination of DMD and BMD patients. Small molecules are currently in clinical trials in DMD patients using a nonaminoglycoside compound, PTC-124 (52). Stop codon suppression is not limited to DMD but should also prove useful in other forms of genetic disease. Exon skipping of mutant exons in the dystrophin gene bypasses the defect and can be used to generate internally truncated but functional dystrophin proteins (53). Exon skipping can be induced by viruses or small modified nucleotides and clinical trials are ongoing.

CONCLUSIONS

Gene correction tactics may only result in partial restoration of protein function, but even partial restoration is likely to be clinically meaningful. Combination therapy using gene correction, muscle growth promoters, and anti-fibrotics could be linked to calcium handling agents to result in even greater functional improvement. Combination therapy, where individual agents treat distinct aspects of pathogenesis, is the mainstay of anticancer therapy and even the treatment of simpler disorders such as hypertension. The future for muscle therapy will likely embrace combinatorial drug treatment with a better understanding of the precise pathways most responsible for unique diseases. In this sense, muscle disease will benefit from a personalized medicine in the full sense of its meaning.

REFERENCES

1. Rybakova IN, Patel JR, Ervasti JM. The dystrophin complex forms a mechanically strong link between the sarcolemma and costameric actin. *J Cell Biol* 2000;**150**:1209–14.
2. Yasuda S, Townsend D, Michele DE, Favre EG, Day SM, Metzger JM. Dystrophic heart failure blocked by membrane sealant poloxamer. *Nature* 2005;**436**:1025–9.
3. Townsend D, Turner I, Yasuda S, Martindale J, Davis J, Shillingford M, et al. Chronic administration of membrane sealant prevents severe cardiac injury and ventricular dilatation in dystrophic dogs. *J Clin Invest* 2010;**120**:1140–50.
4. Ng R, Metzger JM, Claflin DR, Faulkner JA. Poloxamer 188 reduces the contraction-induced force decline in lumbrical muscles from mdx mice. *Am J Physiol Cell Physiol* 2008;**295**:C146–50.
5. Cai C, Masumiya H, Weisleder N, Matsuda N, Nishi M, Hwang M, et al. MG53 nucleates assembly of cell membrane repair machinery. *Nat Cell Biol* 2009;**11**:56–64.
6. McNeil P. Membrane repair redux: redox of MG53. *Nat Cell Biol* 2009;**11**:7–9.
7. Lee CS, Yi JS, Jung SY, Kim BW, Lee NR, Choo HJ, et al. TRIM72 negatively regulates myogenesis via targeting insulin receptor substrate-1. *Cell Death Differ* 2010;**17**:1254–65.
8. Davis DB, Doherty KR, Delmonte AJ, McNally EM. Calcium-sensitive phospholipid binding properties of normal and mutant ferlin C2 domains. *J Biol Chem* 2002;**277**:22883–8.
9. Bansal D, Miyake K, Vogel SS, Groh S, Chen CC, Williamson R, et al. Defective membrane repair in dysferlin-deficient muscular dystrophy. *Nature* 2003;**423**:168–72.
10. Huang Y, Laval SH, van Remoortere A, Baudier J, Benaud C, Anderson LV, et al. AHNAK, a novel component of the dysferlin protein complex, redistributes to the cytoplasm with dysferlin during skeletal muscle regeneration. *FASEB J* 2007;**21**:732–42.
11. Lennon NJ, Kho A, Bacskai BJ, Perlmutter SL, Hyman BT, Brown Jr. RH. Dysferlin interacts with annexins A1 and A2 and mediates sarcolemmal wound-healing. *J Biol Chem* 2003;**278**:50466–73.
12. Klinge L, Laval S, Keers S, Haldane F, Straub V, Barresi R, et al. From T-tubule to sarcolemma: damage-induced dysferlin translocation in early myogenesis. *FASEB J* 2007;**21**:1768–76.
13. Wang B, Yang Z, Brisson BK, Feng H, Zhang Z, Welch EM, et al. Membrane blebbing as an assessment of functional rescue of dysferlin-deficient human myotubes via nonsense suppression. *J Appl Physiol* 2010;**109**:901–5.
14. Demonbreun AR, Fahrenbach JP, Deveaux K, Earley JU, Pytel P, McNally EM. Impaired muscle growth and response to insulin-like growth factor 1 in dysferlin-mediated muscular dystrophy. *Hum Mol Genet* 2011;**20**:779–89.
15. Krahn M, Wein N, Bartoli M, Lostal W, Courrier S, Bourg-Alibert N, et al. A naturally occurring human minidysferlin protein repairs sarcolemmal lesions in a mouse model of dysferlinopathy. *Sci Transl Med* 2010;**2**:50ra69.
16. Millay DP, Maillet M, Roche JA, Sargent MA, McNally EM, Bloch RJ, et al. Genetic manipulation of dysferlin expression in skeletal muscle: novel insights into muscular dystrophy. *Am J Pathol* 2009;**175**:1817–23.
17. de Luna N, Gallardo E, Soriano M, Dominguez-Perles R, de la Torre C, Rojas-Garcia R, et al. Absence of dysferlin alters myogenin expression and delays human muscle differentiation "in vitro". *J Biol Chem* 2006;**281**:17092–8.
18. Khurana TS, Davies KE. Pharmacological strategies for muscular dystrophy. *Nat Rev Drug Discov* 2003;**2**:379–90.
19. Krag TO, Bogdanovich S, Jensen CJ, Fischer MD, Hansen-Schwartz J, Javazon EH, et al. Heregulin ameliorates the dystrophic phenotype in mdx mice. *Proc Natl Acad Sci USA* 2004;**101**:13856–60.
20. Sonnemann KJ, Heun-Johnson H, Turner AJ, Baltgalvis KA, Lowe DA, Ervasti JM. Functional substitution by TAT-utrophin in dystrophin-deficient mice. *PLoS Med* 2009;**6**:e1000083.
21. Mendell JR, Campbell K, Rodino-Klapac L, Sahenk Z, Shilling C, Lewis S, et al. Dystrophin immunity in Duchenne's muscular dystrophy. *N Engl J Med* 2010;**363**:1429–37.
22. Rybakova IN, Humston JL, Sonnemann KJ, Ervasti JM. Dystrophin and utrophin bind actin through distinct modes of contact. *J Biol Chem* 2006;**281**:9996–10001.
23. Lai Y, Thomas GD, Yue Y, Yang HT, Li D, Long C, et al. Dystrophins carrying spectrin-like repeats 16 and 17 anchor nNOS to the sarcolemma and enhance exercise performance in a mouse model of muscular dystrophy. *J Clin Invest* 2009;**119**:624–35.
24. Amenta AR, Yilmaz A, Bogdanovich S, McKechnie BA, Abedi M, Khurana TS, et al. Biglycan recruits utrophin to the sarcolemma and counters dystrophic pathology in mdx mice. *Proc Natl Acad Sci USA* 2011;**108**:762–7.

25. Burkin DJ, Wallace GQ, Nicol KJ, Kaufman DJ, Kaufman SJ. Enhanced expression of the alpha 7 beta 1 integrin reduces muscular dystrophy and restores viability in dystrophic mice. *J Cell Biol* 2001;**152**:1207–18.
26. Allikian MJ, Hack AA, Mewborn S, Mayer U, McNally EM. Genetic compensation for sarcoglycan loss by integrin alpha7beta1 in muscle. *J Cell Sci* 2004;**117**:3821–30.
27. Rooney JE, Gurpur PB, Burkin DJ. Laminin-111 protein therapy prevents muscle disease in the mdx mouse model for Duchenne muscular dystrophy. *Proc Natl Acad Sci USA* 2009;**106**:7991–6.
28. Yoshida-Moriguchi T, Yu L, Stalnaker SH, Davis S, Kunz S, Madson M, et al. O-mannosyl phosphorylation of alpha-dystroglycan is required for laminin binding. *Science* 2010;**327**:88–92.
29. Bogdanovich S, Krag TO, Barton ER, Morris LD, Whittemore LA, Ahima RS, et al. Functional improvement of dystrophic muscle by myostatin blockade. *Nature* 2002;**420**:418–21.
30. Wagner KR, Fleckenstein JL, Amato AA, Barohn RJ, Bushby K, Escolar DM, et al. A phase I/IItrial of MYO-029 in adult subjects with muscular dystrophy. *Ann Neurol* 2008;**63**:561–71.
31. Barton ER, Morris L, Musaro A, Rosenthal N, Sweeney HL. Muscle-specific expression of insulin-like growth factor I counters muscle decline in mdx mice. *J Cell Biol* 2002;**157**:137–48.
32. Musaro A, McCullagh KJ, Naya FJ, Olson EN, Rosenthal N. IGF-1 induces skeletal myocyte hypertrophy through calcineurin in association with GATA-2 and NF-ATc1. *Nature* 1999;**400**:581–5.
33. Lynch GS, Cuffe SA, Plant DR, Gregorevic P. IGF-I treatment improves the functional properties of fast- and slow-twitch skeletal muscles from dystrophic mice. *Neuromuscul Disord* 2001;**11**:260–8.
34. Gregorevic P, Plant DR, Leeding KS, Bach LA, Lynch GS. Improved contractile function of the mdx dystrophic mouse diaphragm muscle after insulin-like growth factor-I administration. *Am J Pathol* 2002;**161**:2263–72.
35. Bernasconi P, Torchiana E, Confalonieri P, Brugnoni R, Barresi R, Mora M, et al. Expression of transforming growth factor-beta 1 in dystrophic patient muscles correlates with fibrosis. Pathogenetic role of a fibrogenic cytokine. *J Clin Invest* 1995;**96**:1137–44.
36. Huebner KD, Jassal DS, Halevy O, Pines M, Anderson JE. Functional resolution of fibrosis in mdx mouse dystrophic heart and skeletal muscle by halofuginone. *Am J Physiol Heart Circ Physiol* 2008;**294**:H1550–61.
37. Van Erp C, Irwin NG, Hoey AJ. Long-term administration of pirfenidone improves cardiac function in mdx mice. *Muscle Nerve* 2006;**34**:327–34.
38. Vetrone SA, Montecino-Rodriguez E, Kudryashova E, Kramerova I, Hoffman EP, Liu SD, et al. Osteopontin promotes fibrosis in dystrophic mouse muscle by modulating immune cell subsets and intramuscular TGF-beta. *J Clin Invest* 2009;**119**:1583–94.
39. Pegoraro E, Hoffman EP, Piva L, Gavassini BF, Cagnin S, Ermani M, et al. SPP1 genotype is a determinant of disease severity in Duchenne muscular dystrophy. *Neurology* 2011;**76**:219–26.
40. Heydemann A, Ceco E, Lim JE, Hadhazy M, Ryder P, Moran JL, et al. Latent TGF-beta-binding protein 4 modifies muscular dystrophy in mice. *J Clin Invest* 2009;**119**:3703–12.
41. Swaggart KA, Heydemann A, Palmer AA, McNally EM. Distinct genetic regions modify specific muscle groups in muscular dystrophy. *Physiol Genomics* 2011;**43**:24–31.
42. Cohn RD, van Erp C, Habashi JP, Soleimani AA, Klein EC, Lisi MT, et al. Angiotensin II type 1 receptor blockade attenuates TGF-beta-induced failure of muscle regeneration in multiple myopathic states. *Nat Med* 2007;**13**:204–10.
43. Duboc D, Meune C, Pierre B, Wahbi K, Eymard B, Toutain A, et al. Perindopril preventive treatment on mortality in Duchenne muscular dystrophy: 10 years' follow-up. *Am Heart J* 2007;**154**:596–602.
44. Goldstein JA, Kelly SM, LoPresti PP, Heydemann A, Earley JU, Ferguson EL, et al. SMAD signaling drives heart and muscle dysfunction in a Drosophila model of muscular dystrophy. *Hum Mol Genet* 2011;**20**:894–904.
45. Vandebrouck C, Martin D, Colson-Van Schoor M, Debaix H, Gailly P. Involvement of TRPC in the abnormal calcium influx observed in dystrophic (mdx) mouse skeletal muscle fibers. *J Cell Biol* 2002;**158**:1089–96.
46. Millay DP, Goonasekera SA, Sargent MA, Maillet M, Aronow BJ, Molkentin JD. Calcium influx is sufficient to induce muscular dystrophy through a TRPC-dependent mechanism. *Proc Natl Acad Sci USA* 2009;**106**:19023–8.
47. Bellinger AM, Reiken S, Carlson C, Mongillo M, Liu X, Rothman L, et al. Hypernitrosylated ryanodine receptor calcium release channels are leaky in dystrophic muscle. *Nat Med* 2009;**15**:325–30.
48. Fauconnier J, Thireau J, Reiken S, Cassan C, Richard S, Matecki S, et al. Leaky RyR2 trigger ventricular arrhythmias in Duchenne muscular dystrophy. *Proc Natl Acad Sci USA* 2010;**107**:1559–64.
49. Goonasekera SA, Lam CK, Millay DP, Sargent MA, Hajjar RJ, Kranias EG, et al. Mitigation of muscular dystrophy in mice by SERCA overexpression in skeletal muscle. *J Clin Invest* 2011;**121**:1044–52.
50. Millay DP, Sargent MA, Osinska H, Baines CP, Barton ER, Vuagniaux G, et al. Genetic and pharmacologic inhibition of mitochondrial-dependent necrosis attenuates muscular dystrophy. *Nat Med* 2008;**14**:442–7.
51. Barton-Davis ER, Cordier L, Shoturma DI, Leland SE, Sweeney HL. Aminoglycoside antibiotics restore dystrophin function to skeletal muscles of mdx mice. *J Clin Invest* 1999;**104**:375–81.
52. Welch EM, Barton ER, Zhuo J, Tomizawa Y, Friesen WJ, Trifillis P, et al. PTC124 targets genetic disorders caused by nonsense mutations. *Nature* 2007;**447**:87–91.
53. Wilton SD, Fletcher S. Splice modification to restore functional dystrophin synthesis in Duchenne muscular dystrophy. *Curr Pharm Des* 2010;**16**:988–1001.

Part IV

Smooth Muscle

Section A

Basic Physiology

Chapter 82

Development of the Smooth Muscle Cell Lineage

Nina Bowens[1] and Michael S. Parmacek[2]

[1]*Department of Surgery and* [2]*Department of Medicine, and* [1,2]*University of Pennsylvania Cardiovascular Institute, Philadelphia, PA*

DIVERSITY OF THE SMOOTH MUSCLE CELL LINEAGE(S)

Smooth muscle cells (SMCs) play important roles throughout the body, subserving diverse functions including the modulation of arterial tone and blood flow distribution, control of gastrointestinal and genitourinary tract motility, and the regulation of bronchial and airway resistance. The diverse functions of SMCs are ultimately dependent upon the contractile properties of this muscle cell lineage which in turn are dependent upon the expression of a unique repertoire of lineage-restricted contractile proteins, cell surface receptors, and signaling molecules (for review see 1, 2, 3). The lineage relationships that define and distinguish functionally distinct subsets of vascular and visceral SMCs remain poorly defined. The embryological origins of the smooth muscle cell lineage are remarkably diverse, raising fundamental questions about the relationship and developmental programs that underlie SMC diversity and heterogeneity. Better understanding of the molecular programs that regulate SMC development and differentiation will undoubtedly provide important new insights into the unique physiology of tissue-restricted and morphologically-distinct subsets of SMCs.

The SMC lineage is characterized by its remarkable plasticity and ability to respond and adapt (or mal-adapt) to environmental cues (for review see 3, 4). In the postnatal vasculature and in most visceral organs, SMCs are maintained in a "contractile state", in the G_0/G_1 phase of the cell cycle, where they express high levels of SMC lineage-restricted contractile proteins which are required for homeostatic regulation of organismal function. However, during development and in response to specific growth factors and cytokines, SMCs assume a "synthetic" phenotype resembling a fibroblast. This is accompanied by the coordinate downregulation of genes encoding SMC contractile proteins and the upregulation of genes promoting synthetic functions and extracellular matrix (ECM). In contrast to terminally differentiated cardiac and skeletal muscle cells, SMCs possess the capacity to re-enter the cell cycle, proliferate, and to migrate. It is important to recognize that the nomenclature defining SMCs as either "contractile" or "synthetic" generally reflects the behavior of primary SMC cultures *in vitro* and fails to account for the spectrum of phenotypes observed *in vivo* (4). For example, in the embryo and in some pathological circumstances, SMCs express abundant contractile proteins, while at the same time proliferating and secreting high levels of extracellular matrix (for review see 3).

Differentiation Markers of the SMC Lineage

The unique physiological properties of SMCs are ultimately attributable to the expression of a discrete subset of SMC lineage-restricted contractile proteins, signaling molecules and cytoskeletal elements including smooth muscle (SM)-α-actin (*Acta2*), SM-myosin heavy chain (*Myh11*), SM22α (*Tagln*), SM-calponin (*Cnn1*), telokin (*Mylk*), and smoothelin (*Smtn*) (for review see 2). Multiple studies have shown that the muscle-restricted transcriptional co-activator myocardin plays a critical role in regulating the "contractile SMC gene program" acting via its capacity to physically associate with the transcription factor, SRF, which in turn binds to CArG box-containing regulatory elements controlling the transcription of these SMC lineage-restricted genes (for review see 5). Recent studies have shown that alternatively spliced isoforms of myocardin regulate transcription in smooth and cardiac muscle cells, respectively (6). Myocardin sits at a nodal point regulating SMC phenotype which is influenced by multiple signaling pathways that converge upon the myocardin-SRF complex in the nucleus of SMCs influencing its activity (for review see 5).

There is ongoing debate over whether a true SMC lineage-specific marker exists. Most SMC-restricted proteins are expressed at least transiently in other muscle cell

Muscle. DOI: http://dx.doi.org/10.1016/B978-0-12-381510-1.00082-X

lineages. Smooth muscle myosin heavy chain (SM-MyHC) is considered the most definitive marker of the SMC lineage (7). In situ hybridization studies performed in the developing mouse have revealed SM-MyHC is restricted to vascular and visceral SMCs (7). Cell fate-mapping studies utilizing the SM-MyHC promoter/enhancer demonstrated restricted expression of the *LacZ* reporter gene in vascular and visceral SMCs with the exception of a small population of cells within the right atrium of the heart (8). However, the failure to detect SM-MyHC gene or protein expression does not preclude a cell from belonging to the SMC lineage. In the mouse embryo, there is at least a 48-hour temporal delay between the expression of early SMC markers, such as SMA and SM22α, and the expression of SM-MyHC in the embryonic aorta (7). Similarly, SM-MyHC is frequently not observed in synthetic SMCs following vascular injury or in other pathological circumstances (9).

Smooth muscle α-actin (SMA) is one of the earliest markers and it is the most abundant protein expressed in SMCs (for review see 3). However, SMA is transiently expressed in embryonic cardiomyocytes and skeletal muscle and in transforming growth factor-beta (TGF-β)-stimulated endothelial cells and myofibroblasts (10,11). Like SMA, the cytoskeletal SMC-restricted protein SM22α is an early marker of the SMC lineage which is transiently expressed in the embryonic heart and skeletal muscle (12). Smoothelin-A and -B are also cytoskeletal proteins that are expressed selectively in visceral and vascular SMCs, respectively (13,14). Smoothelin isoforms have also been detected in other tissues and tumor cells (13,14). SM-calponin, a SMC lineage-restricted calcium-regulatory protein involved in SMC contraction, is also expressed transiently in cardiomyocytes and myofibroblasts (15). Telokin, the 17 kDa non-catalytic myosin light chain kinase isoform, is expressed at high levels in visceral SMCs and at lower levels in vascular SMCs (16).

Pericytes

Pericytes share some common origins with SMCs and subserve an overlapping set of functions in the vasculature (for review see 17). Pericytes include a population of cells surrounding capillaries that signal directly to the underlying endothelial cells and form a permeability barrier. Pericytes also play critical roles in hemostasis, maintenance of the blood–brain barrier, angiogenesis, and neovascularization. Several studies have suggested that pericytes and vascular mural cells may overlap with, or represent a unique population of, differentiated mesenchymal stem cells (18). However, the precise derivation and embryological origins of pericytes remains poorly defined. Given their anatomic relationships to endothelial cells and overlapping set of functions, it is not surprising that pericyte and SMC markers overlap. Pericyte markers include SM-α-actin, platelet-derived growth factor receptor-β, angiopoietin 1 (Ang-1), regulator of G protein signaling 5 (RGS-5), desmin and chondroitin sulfate proteoglycan (for review see 17). Each of these markers is also expressed in other vascular cells.

Myofibroblasts and Myoepithelial Cells

The myofibroblast also shares common functions and overlapping markers with the SMC (for review see 19). In the heart, kidney, intestine, and other tissues, in response to mechanical and stress-related signals, a subset of fibroblasts modulate their phenotype and become myofibroblasts. Myofibroblasts are distinguished by their spindle-like morphology, high concentration of SMC-restricted markers including SMA, SM22α, SM-calponin and enhanced secretion of ECM (for review see 20). Recently it has been shown that the transcriptional coactivator myocardin-related transcription factor-A (MRTF-A) plays a critical role in promoting the conversion of cardiac fibroblasts to myofibroblasts activating a fibrotic gene program (21). MRTF-A is a member of the MRTF family of transcriptional coactivators, which also includes myocardin and myocardin-related transcription factor-B (MRTF-B) (for review see 5). MRTF-A differs from myocardin as it is expressed in multiple cell lineages including undifferentiated embryonic stem (ES) cells and fibroblasts. However, like myocardin, MRTF-A is a remarkably potent transcriptional coactivator that physically associates with SRF to synergistically activate transcription of a subset of CArG box-containing genes (22). Both myocardin and MRTF-A are influenced by biomechanical signals transduced via the actin cytoskeleton to the nucleus (for review see 5).

Mammary myoepithelial cells are ectodermally-derived cells that possess characteristics of both epithelial cells and SMCs (for review see 23). As true epithelial cells they express cytokeratins as the major component of the intermediate filament and they form desmosomes and cadherin-mediated junctions. However, like SMCs, they express myofilaments and express a subset of SMC-restricted contractile proteins including SMA, SM22α and SM-calponin (24). Myoepithelial cell muscle filaments are required for oxytocin-stimulated contraction and release of milk (24). In this regard it is noteworthy that *Mrtf-a*$^{-/-}$ null mutant dams cannot effectively nurse their pups due to a failure to maintain the differentiated state of mammary myoepithelial cells which is accompanied by decreased expression of genes encoding SMC contractile proteins including SMA, SM22α, and SM-MyHC (25). From an evolutionary standpoint, it is tempting to speculate that MRTF-A (and MRTF-B) has evolved to promote the expression of genes encoding SMC contractile proteins required to enhance cell contractility and motility *in non-muscle cell lineages* including the cardiac myofibroblast and myoepithelial cell.

SMC PROGENITORS AND STEM CELLS

Embryonic Stem Cells

An understanding of the processes whereby SMCs are specified and differentiate from embryonic stem (ES) cells and/or progenitor cells is required in order to elucidate and distinguish lineage relationships underlying the function(s) of SMCs during embryonic and postnatal development. ES cells are pluripotent cells derived from the inner cell mass of the blastocyst possessing the capacity for self-renewal and the ability to differentiate into all cell types. Multiple laboratories have shown that under specific cell culture conditions, embryonic stem cells may be induced to differentiate into a population of cells enriched for definitive SMCs. Exposure to TGF-β or collagen promotes ES cells to differentiate toward the SMC fate suggesting that differentiation of SMCs is dependent, at least in part, upon signals transduced from the extracellular matrix (26,27). At a transcriptional level, the forced expression of the SMC lineage-restricted transcriptional co-activator myocardin activates most, but not all, SMC lineage-restricted genes in undifferentiated embryonic stem cells (28,29). However, myocardin is not required for differentiation of vascular SMCs from ES cells, as myocardin null (*Myocd*$^{-/-}$) ES cells differentiate into SMCs *in vitro* and contribute to the vasculature of chimeric mice (30). As such, dependent upon the specific developmental context myocardin-dependent and -independent SMC differentiation programs may be activated.

Cardiovascular Progenitor Cells

Cardiovascular progenitor cells are multipotent cells possessing the capacity to differentiate into cardiomyocytes, endothelial cells, and vascular SMCs (31,32). In the presence of specific growth factors including BMP4, Activin A, VEGF, DKK, and FGF, ES cells differentiate to form cardiovascular progenitor cells. These cells express the mesodermal primitive streak marker, *brachyury*, as well as vascular endothelial growth factor receptor 2 (VEGFR2, Flk-1) and PDGFRα. Under different cell culture conditions, ES cells give rise to a subset of vascular progenitor cells which differentiate into enriched populations of endothelial cells and SMCs, but not cardiomyocytes (33). Vascular progenitor cells express the endothelial/hematopoietic cell surface marker CD34, and are induced by exposure to platelet-derived growth factor ($PDGF_{BB}$) (33). Both cardiovascular progenitors and vascular progenitors may be distinguished from the hemangioblast, which gives rise to endothelial cells as well as hematopoietic cell lineages (34).

EMBRYOLOGIC ORIGINS OF SMOOTH MUSCLE CELL LINEAGE

Origin(s) of Vascular Smooth Muscle Cells

Vascular and visceral SMCs arise from multiple distinct locations and origins in the embryo in a precise spatially- and temporally-restricted manner. In the mouse, vascular SMCs are first observed on the ventral surface of the dorsal aorta at embryonic day (E) 9.0–9.5 (35). For many years it was believed that aortic SMCs were derived primarily from the splanchnic lateral plate mesoderm (36). Cell fate-mapping studies have confirmed that the first aortic SMCs in posterior regions of the embryo are derived from the lateral plate mesoderm (35). However, it is now recognized that these cells are subsequently replaced by somite-derived cells and that SMCs populating the adult aorta beyond the insertion site of the ligamentum arteriosum are derived from the paraxial mesoderm (35,37). Similarly, SMCs populating the renal and intercostal arteries are derived from the paraxial mesoderm (35). These somite-derived SMCs are believed to arise from progenitor cells in the sclerotome (37).

Cell fate-mapping studies have also revealed that SMCs populating the vasculature of the mesentery and gut are derived from a subset of Wilm's tumor protein (Wt1)-expressing serosal mesothelial cells (38). As such, this represents a conserved mechanism recapitulating some aspects of the differentiation of epicardial vascular cells from the proepicardium which is also of mesothelial origin. It is also noteworthy that the renal and intercostal arteries arise via angiogenic sprouting from the aorta, while the mesenteric and celiac vessels are formed by remodeling of the vitelline artery (39). It has been postulated that the mesothelium may serve as a reservoir of SMC precursors in other tissues and in adult tissues following stress or injury (1).

Cardiac Neural Crest-Derived Vascular SMCs

A subpopulation of cephalic neural crest cells located between the mid-otic placode and the caudal boundary of the third somite, designated as the "cardiac neural crest", migrate ventrally through pharyngeal arches 3–6, where they invest and subsequently differentiate into vascular SMCs forming the tunica media of the great arteries and aorticopulmonary septum (for review see 40). As shown in Figure 82.1, cardiac neural crest cells delaminate from the neural tube and migrate to populate the 3rd, 4th and

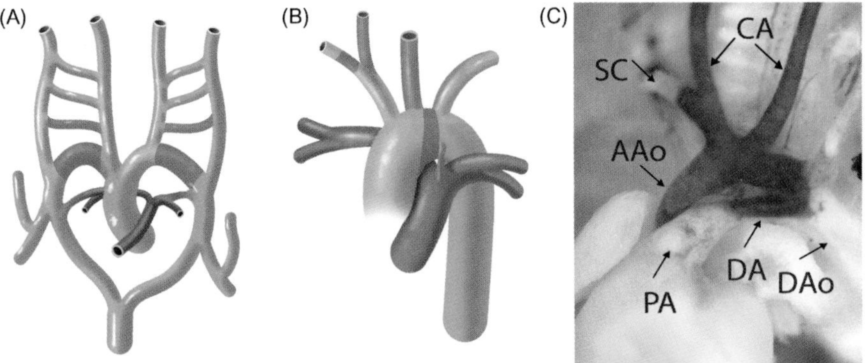

FIGURE 82.1 Neural crest-derived SMCs populate the cardiac outflow tract and great arteries. (A) A schematic representation of the embryonic vascular system at E10.5 in the mouse. Cardiac neural crest cells migrate from their origin in the neural tube to populate the 3rd, 4th, and 6th pharyngeal arch arteries and the cardiac outflow tract where they differentiate into vascular SMCs. Arterial segments contributing to the great arteries (see panel B) are color coded in blue, purple, and green. (B) Patterning of the postnatal circulation illustrating the origin (color coded from panel A) of the great arteries. (C) *Wnt1-Cre* transgenic mice were interbred with *R26R* indicator mice to define the pattern of Cre-mediated gene excision and the origin of neural crest-derived vascular SMCs. This panel shows a postnatal day (P)2 *Wnt1-Cre*$^+$/*R26R*$^+$ mouse demonstrating β-galactosidase expression (blue stain) in arteries populated by neural crest-derived SMCs including the ductus arteriosus (DA), ascending aorta (AAo), carotid arteries (CA), but not in the pulmonary artery (PA) or descending aorta (DAo) beyond the insertion site of the DA.

6th pharyngeal arch arteries. Subsequently, a subpopulation of cells invades the cardiac outflow tract where they condense and contribute to the aortico-pulmonary septum (41). Neural crest cells populating the pharyngeal arch arteries differentiate into vascular SMCs expressing abundant levels of SMC-restricted contractile proteins (Figure 82.1A). Subsequently, in response to the local release of growth factors, the pharyngeal arch arteries undergo a complex remodeling process ultimately establishing the cardiac outflow tract and discrete pulmonary and systemic circulations (Figure 82.1B).

Cell fate-mapping studies have shown that neural crest-derived SMCs contribute to the ascending aorta (AAo), aortic arch to the level of the ductus arteriosus (DA), ductus arteriosus, and common carotid arteries (CA) (Figure 82.1C) (42). Interestingly, myocardin is not expressed in the pre-migratory, or migratory, cardiac neural crest demonstrating neural crest-derived SMC differentiation is not dependent upon myocardin (43). However, myocardin-related transcription factor (MRTF)-B is expressed abundantly in the cardiac neural crest and MRTF-B null and loss-of-function mutant mice exhibit a cell autonomous block in vascular SMC differentiation from cardiac neural crest cells (43,44).

The local expression of growth factors and signaling molecules plays a critical role in regulating cardiac neural crest-derived SMC differentiation and formation of the cardiac outflow tract and great arteries (for review see 45,46). Disruption of several components of the bone morphogenetic protein (BMP)/TGF-β signaling complex leads to defective remodeling of the branchial arch arteries and cardiac outflow tract. Tissue-specific inactivation of Alk2 (type I BMP receptor) in neural crest cells causes defective aorticopulmonary septation attributable, at least in part, to a block in SMC differentiation (47). TGF-β_2 is expressed abundantly in the cardiac outflow tract and great arteries and TGF-β_2 null embryos display a spectrum of aortic arch malformations, double outlet right ventricle (DORV) and endocardial cushion defects (48,49). The observed pathology in BMP/TGF-β mutant mice is also attributable to alterations in extracellular matrix components which bind to TGF-β ligands and signal to endothelial cells and medial SMCs. Mice lacking the long form of latent TGF-β binding protein 1 exhibit improper aorticopulmonary septation and a spectrum of pharyngeal arch remodeling defects (50).

Notch signaling also influences neural crest-derived SMC differentiation and cardiac outflow tract formation (for review see 51). Notch is a highly conserved cell−cell signaling pathway that plays a critical role in cell fate decisions, development and disease (for review see 52). Mice expressing a dominant-negative inhibitor of Notch signaling in the cardiac neural crest exhibit pulmonary artery stenosis and pharyngeal arch patterning defects that are associated with a block in smooth muscle cell differentiation (53). This is attributable, at least in part, to a block in Notch2 signaling as neural crest-restricted inactivation of Notch2 produces hypoplasia of the aorta and pulmonary arteries accompanied by defects in vascular SMC differentiation (54). Human mutations in both JAGGED1 and NOTCH2 are associated with Alagille syndrome, demonstrating a conserved role for Notch signaling in formation of the cardiac outflow tract and great arteries (55).

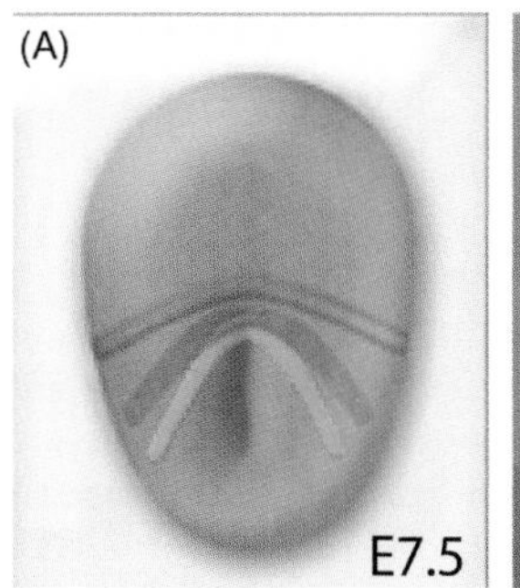

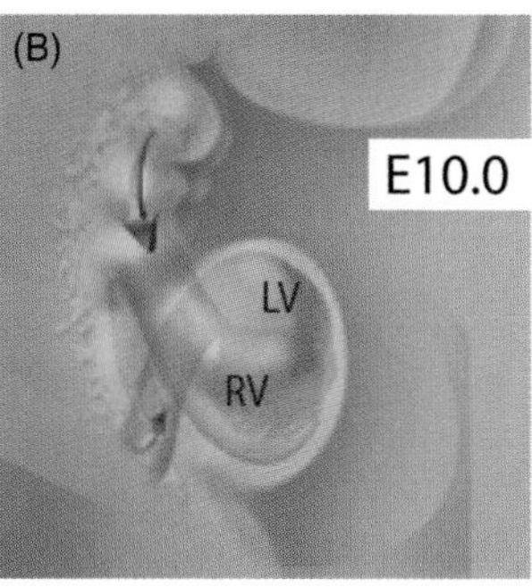

FIGURE 82.2 The second heart field contributes to SMCs at the arterial pole of the heart. (A) A schematic representation of the E7.5 mouse embryo showing the locations of cardiomyocyte progenitors in the first heart field (red) and cardiomyocyte and vascular SMC progenitors in the second heart field (green). (B) A schematic representation of the mouse embryo at E10.0 illustrating the migration of cells (green) from the second heart field into the embryonic heart where they contribute to cardiomyocytes in the right ventricle (RV) and atrial and to vascular SMCs at the arterial pole of the heart.

Second Heart Field-Derived Vascular SMCs

As shown in Figure 82.2, the second heart field is a population of progenitor cells lying beneath the floor of the foregut that gives rise to cardiomyocytes and SMCs at the arterial pole of the heart (for review see 56). In the cardiac crescent stage (E7.5 in the mouse), the second heart field (green color) lies anterior to the first heart field (red color) (Figure 82.2A). SMCs at the arterial pole of the heart in the aortic root and pulmonary trunk arise from the second heart field. Two temporally distinct migrations of precursor cells from the second heart field are observed in the embryo. First, cells from the second heart field migrate to the cardiac outflow tract and differentiate into cardiac myocytes (Figure 82.2B). Subsequently, a sub-population of cells from the second heart field migrates to the aortic sac and differentiates into SMCs that form the origin of the aorta and pulmonary artery (Figure 82.2B). Although, species variation in the spatial relationships between second heart field- and neural crest-derived SMCs is observed at the arterial pole of the heart, both populations play roles in patterning of the cardiac outflow tract and these progenitor cell populations have been implicated in the pathogenesis of common forms of congenital heart disease (56).

Proepicardium and Coronary Vessels

In mammals, the proepicardial organ is a primordial structure that arises from the septum transversum near the venous pole of the heart in the area of the sinoatrial junction (57). The proepicardial organ is a source of epicardial epithelium which gives rise to the coronary endothelial cells, SMCs, and cardiac fibroblasts (57). Early in development, the proepicardium does not express markers of differentiated endothelial cells or their precursors (CD34, PECAM-1, VEGFR1, VEGFR2), fibroblast, hematopoietic (CD45, CD34) or SMC (SM-α-actin) lineages (58). In mammals, formation of the epicardium from the proepicardium occurs via release of vesicles from the tips of the proepicardium into the pericardial cavity. These vesicles attach to the dorsal surface of the heart, proliferate, and migrate in a precise temporal and spatial pattern to form the epicardium. The proepicardial organ disappears by the end of the 5th week of human gestation.

In response to Friend of GATA (FOG)-2-dependent signals from the myocardium (59,60), a sub-population of epicardially-derived cells lose their epithelial character, undergo epithelial-to-mesenchymal transformation (EMT) and invaginate into the myocardium (61). It is not known whether there are separate populations of epicardially-derived mesothelial cells that differentiate into endothelial, smooth muscle or fibroblast sub-populations. In the embryonic heart, the coronary vessels develop from the blood islands which are aggregates of endothelial cells and erythrocytes that are not connected to the systemic circulation (58). Blood islands coalesce to form capillaries which grow within the subepicardium. Subsequently, coronary SMCs arise from the epicardial mesothelium via EMT and undergo SMC differentiation (62). These cells approach the vascular wall before the connection with the aorta is established (58). The coronary arterial circulation is established by directional capillary growth toward the sinuses of Valsalva ultimately establishing luminal patency via apoptosis of the aortic wall. Connection between the coronary arteries and aorta is established at day 44–49 in the human embryo (63). Further differentiation of mesenchymal cells into vascular SMCs occurs after blood flows within the patent coronary vasculature. Formation of the tunica media of larger coronary vessels starts at the proximal end of the coronary artery by building up a layer of mesenchymal cells.

Visceral Mesoderm and Visceral SMCs

In contrast to vascular SMCs, the derivation and molecular programs regulating visceral SMC development and differentiation remain poorly characterized. Visceral smooth muscle is derived from the splanchnic layer of the lateral plate mesoderm which forms an outer coat around the primary epithelial lining of hollow organs. In the gastrointestinal tract, it involves formation of the primitive gut tube from the endoderm and apposition of the inner leaflet of the lateral plate mesoderm against the endoderm. The inner leaflet encircles the gut to become the visceral mesoderm. The visceral mesoderm is a complex tissue that gives rise to smooth muscle, mesenchyme, and other cells. The visceral mesoderm and its components confer instructive and permissive signals that regulate development of the mesoderm and underlying endodermal derivatives (for review see 64).

The molecular programs that govern lateral plate mesoderm development are dependent upon signals from the underlying endoderm (64). Interactions between sonic hedgehog (Shh), BMP4, and Foxf1 participate in visceral mesoderm morphogenesis and are conserved across species. Foxf1 expression localizes to the interfaces between mesenchyme and epithelium. The earliest known function of Foxf1 is to specify visceral mesoderm (splanchnic) from somatic mesoderm. In the gastrointestinal tract, early muscle progenitors called "smooth muscle myoblasts" differentiate from loose mesenchyme surrounding the primitive gut (65). The smooth muscle myoblast expresses SMA, while mature enteric SMCs express both SMA and SM-γ-actin. Appropriate SMC development requires precise regulation of ligand concentration with either excessive or deficient quantities inhibiting SMC development. BMP transcription in the visceral mesoderm is initiated in response to endodermal Hh signals (66). In the gut, BMP2 and BMP4 play critical roles during development signaling via the BMP receptor-1a. BMP-4 in the visceral mesoderm controls smooth muscle proliferation and differentiation throughout most of the developing vertebrate GI tract (67). Expression of BMP-4 during development is tightly regulated as insufficient expression of BMP-4 in the mesenchyme of the small intestine causes inadequate formation of the muscularis propria, while overexpression of BMP-4 in the mesenchyme of the embryonic gut retards smooth muscle differentiation (68).

CONCLUSIONS AND FUTURE DIRECTIONS

For decades the diverse embryological origins and remarkable phenotypic plasticity of the SMC lineage has challenged investigators examining the molecular and genetic programs regulating SMC development and differentiation. However, the application of modern molecular tools, including most notably cell fate-mapping and the generation of mice harboring conditional gene mutations, has provided exciting new insights into the molecular programs underlying SMC heterogeneity and function. In particular the discovery of the transcriptional coactivator myocardin and myocardin-related transcription factors, stands as a singular achievement which has illuminated a central pathway underlying the contractile smooth muscle cell gene program.

REFERENCES

1. Majesky MW. Developmental basis of vascular smooth muscle diversity. *Arterioscler Thromb Vasc Biol* 2007;**27**:1248–58.
2. Owens GK. Molecular control of vascular smooth muscle cell differentiation. *Acta Physiol Scand* 1998;**164**:623–35.
3. Owens GK, Kumar MS, Wamhoff BR. Molecular regulation of vascular smooth muscle cell differentiation in development and disease. *Physiol Rev* 2004;**84**:767–801.
4. Parmacek MS. Transcriptional programs regulating vascular smooth muscle cell development and differentiation. *Curr Top Dev Biol* 2001;**51**:69–89.
5. Parmacek MS. Myocardin-related transcription factors: critical coactivators regulating cardiovascular development and adaptation. *Circ Res* 2007;**100**:633–44.
6. Creemers EE, Sutherland LB, McAnally J, Richardson JA, Olson EN. Myocardin is a direct transcriptional target of Mef2, Tead and Foxo proteins during cardiovascular development. *Development* 2006;**133**:4245–56.
7. Miano JM, Cserjesi P, Ligon KL, Periasamy M, Olson EN. Smooth muscle myosin heavy chain exclusively marks the smooth muscle lineage during mouse embryogenesis. *Circ Res* 1994;**75**:803–12.
8. Madsen CS, Regan CP, Hungerford JE, White SL, Manabe I, Owens GK. Smooth muscle-specific expression of the smooth muscle myosin heavy chain gene in transgenic mice requires 5'-flanking and first intronic DNA sequence. *Circ Res* 1998;**82**:908–17.
9. Sartore S, Scatena M, Chiavegato A, Faggin E, Giuriato L, Pauletto P. Myosin isoform expression in smooth muscle cells during physiological and pathological vascular remodeling. *J Vasc Res* 1994;**31**:61–81.
10. Arciniegas E, Sutton AB, Allen TD, Schor AM. Transforming growth factor beta 1 promotes the differentiation of endothelial cells into smooth muscle-like cells in vitro. *J Cell Sci* 1992;**103**:521–9.
11. Tomasek JJ, McRae J, Owens GK, Haaksma CJ. Regulation of alpha-smooth muscle actin expression in granulation tissue myofibroblasts is dependent on the intronic CArG element and the transforming growth factor-beta1 control element. *Am J Pathol* 2005;**166**:1343–51.
12. Li L, Miano JM, Cserjesi P, Olson EN. SM22 alpha, a marker of adult smooth muscle, is expressed in multiple myogenic lineages during embryogenesis. *Circ Res* 1996;**78**:188–95.
13. Rensen SS, Thijssen VL, De Vries CJ, Doevendans PA, Detera-Wadleigh SD, Van Eys GJ. Expression of the smoothelin gene is mediated by alternative promoters. *Cardiovasc Res* 2002;**55**:850–63.
14. van der Loop FT, Gabbiani G, Kohnen G, Ramaekers FC, van Eys GJ. Differentiation of smooth muscle cells in human blood vessels as defined by smoothelin, a novel marker for the contractile phenotype. *Arterioscler Thromb Vasc Biol* 1997;**17**:665–71.
15. Samaha FF, Ip HS, Morrisey EE, Seltzer J, Tang Z, Solway J, et al. Developmental pattern of expression and genomic organization of the calponin-h1 gene. A contractile smooth muscle cell marker. *J Biol Chem* 1996;**271**:395–403.
16. Herring BP, Smith AF. Telokin expression is mediated by a smooth muscle cell-specific promoter. *Am J Physiol* 1996;**270**: C1656–65.
17. Kutcher ME, Herman IM. The pericyte: cellular regulator of microvascular blood flow. *Microvasc Res* 2009;**77**:235–46.

18. Corselli M, Chen CW, Crisan M, Lazzari L, Peault B. Perivascular ancestors of adult multipotent stem cells. *Arterioscler Thromb Vasc Biol* 2010;**30**:1104–9.
19. Tomasek JJ, Gabbiani G, Hinz B, Chaponnier C, Brown RA. Myofibroblasts and mechano-regulation of connective tissue remodelling. *Nat Rev Mol Cell Biol* 2002;**3**:349–63.
20. Souders CA, Bowers SL, Baudino TA. Cardiac fibroblast: the renaissance cell. *Circ Res* 2009;**105**:1164–76.
21. Small EM, Thatcher JE, Sutherland LB, Kinoshita H, Gerard RD, Richardson JA, et al. Myocardin-related transcription factor-A controls myofibroblast activation and fibrosis in response to myocardial infarction. *Circ Res* 2010;**107**:294–304.
22. Miralles F, Posern G, Zaromytidou AI, Treisman R. Actin dynamics control SRF activity by regulation of its coactivator MAL. *Cell* 2003;**113**:329–42.
23. Jolicoeur F. Intrauterine breast development and the mammary myoepithelial lineage. *J Mammary Gland Biol Neoplasia* 2005;**10**:199–210.
24. Deugnier MA, Moiseyeva EP, Thiery JP, Glukhova M. Myoepithelial cell differentiation in the developing mammary gland: progressive acquisition of smooth muscle phenotype. *Dev Dyn* 1995;**204**:107–17.
25. Li S, Chang S, Qi X, Richardson JA, Olson EN. Requirement of a myocardin-related transcription factor for development of mammary myoepithelial cells. *Mol Cell Biol* 2006;**26**:5797–808.
26. Han Y, Li N, Tian X, Kang J, Yan C, Qi Y. Endogenous transforming growth factor (TGF) beta1 promotes differentiation of smooth muscle cells from embryonic stem cells: stable plasmid-based siRNA silencing of TGF beta1 gene expression. *J Physiol Sci* 2010;**60**:35–41.
27. Sinha S, Hoofnagle MH, Kingston PA, McCanna ME, Owens GK. Transforming growth factor-beta1 signaling contributes to development of smooth muscle cells from embryonic stem cells. *Am J Physiol Cell Physiol* 2004;**287**:C1560–8.
28. Du KL, Ip HS, Li J, Chen M, Dandre F, Yu W, et al. Myocardin is a critical serum response factor cofactor in the transcriptional program regulating smooth muscle cell differentiation. *Mol Cell Biol* 2003;**23**:2425–37.
29. Yoshida T, Kawai-Kowase K, Owens GK. Forced expression of myocardin is not sufficient for induction of smooth muscle differentiation in multipotential embryonic cells. *Arterioscler Thromb Vasc Biol* 2004;**24**:1596–601.
30. Pipes GC, Sinha S, Qi X, Zhu CH, Gallardo TD, Shelton J, et al. Stem cells and their derivatives can bypass the requirement of myocardin for smooth muscle gene expression. *Dev Biol* 2005;**288**:502–13.
31. Kattman SJ, Witty AD, Gagliardi M, Dubois NC, Niapour M, Hotta A, et al. Stage-specific optimization of activin/nodal and BMP signaling promotes cardiac differentiation of mouse and human pluripotent stem cell lines. *Cell Stem Cell* 2011;**8**:228–40.
32. Yamashita J, Itoh H, Hirashima M, Ogawa M, Nishikawa S, Yurugi T, et al. Flk1-positive cells derived from embryonic stem cells serve as vascular progenitors. *Nature* 2000;**408**:92–6.
33. Levenberg S, Ferreira LS, Chen-Konak L, Kraehenbuehl TP, Langer R. Isolation, differentiation and characterization of vascular cells derived from human embryonic stem cells. *Nat Protoc* 2010;**5**:1115–26.
34. Yokomizo T, Takahashi S, Mochizuki N, Kuroha T, Ema M, Wakamatsu A, et al. Characterization of GATA-1(+) hemangioblastic cells in the mouse embryo. *EMBO J* 2007;**26**:184–96.
35. Wasteson P, Johansson BR, Jukkola T, Breuer S, Akyurek LM, Partanen J, et al. Developmental origin of smooth muscle cells in the descending aorta in mice. *Development* 2008;**135**:1823–32.
36. Hungerford JE, Owens GK, Argraves WS, Little CD. Development of the aortic vessel wall as defined by vascular smooth muscle and extracellular matrix markers. *Dev Biol* 1996;**178**:375–92.
37. Pouget C, Pottin K, Jaffredo T. Sclerotomal origin of vascular smooth muscle cells and pericytes in the embryo. *Dev Biol* 2008;**315**:437–47.
38. Wilm B, Ipenberg A, Hastie ND, Burch JB, Bader DM. The serosal mesothelium is a major source of smooth muscle cells of the gut vasculature. *Development* 2005;**132**:5317–28.
39. Gest TR, Carron MA. Embryonic origin of the caudal mesenteric artery in the mouse. *Anat Rec A Discov Mol Cell Evol Biol* 2003;**271**:192–201.
40. Stoller JZ, Epstein JA. Cardiac neural crest. *Semin Cell Dev Biol* 2005;**16**:704–15.
41. Jiang Y, Prosper F, Verfaillie CM. Opposing effects of engagement of integrins and stimulation of cytokine receptors on cell cycle progression of normal human hematopoietic progenitors. *Blood* 2000;**95**:846–54.
42. Huang J, Cheng L, Li J, Chen M, Zhou D, Lu MM, et al. Myocardin regulates expression of contractile genes in smooth muscle cells and is required for closure of the ductus arteriosus in mice. *J Clin Invest* 2008;**118**:515–25.
43. Li J, Zhu X, Chen M, Cheng L, Zhou D, Lu MM, et al. Myocardin-related transcription factor B is required in cardiac neural crest for smooth muscle differentiation and cardiovascular development. *Proc Natl Acad Sci USA* 2005;**102**:8916–21.
44. Oh J, Richardson JA, Olson EN. Requirement of myocardin-related transcription factor-B for remodeling of branchial arch arteries and smooth muscle differentiation. *Proc Natl Acad Sci USA* 2005;**102**:15122–7.
45. Scholl AM, Kirby ML. Signals controlling neural crest contributions to the heart. *Wiley Interdiscip Rev Syst Biol Med* 2009;**1**:220–7.
46. Gittenberger-de Groot AC, Azhar M, Molin DG. Transforming growth factor beta-SMAD2 signaling and aortic arch development. *Trends Cardiovasc Med* 2006;**16**:1–6.
47. Kaartinen V, Dudas M, Nagy A, Sridurongrit S, Lu MM, Epstein JA. Cardiac outflow tract defects in mice lacking ALK2 in neural crest cells. *Development* 2004;**131**:3481–90.
48. Bartram U, Molin DG, Wisse LJ, Mohamad A, Sanford LP, Doetschman T, et al. Double-outlet right ventricle and overriding tricuspid valve reflect disturbances of looping, myocardialization, endocardial cushion differentiation, and apoptosis in TGF-beta(2)-knockout mice. *Circulation* 2001;**103**:2745–52.
49. Molin DG, Poelmann RE, DeRuiter MC, Azhar M, Doetschman T, Gittenberger-de Groot AC. Transforming growth factor beta-SMAD2 signaling regulates aortic arch innervation and development. *Circ Res* 2004;**95**:1109–17.
50. Todorovic V, Frendewey D, Gutstein DE, Chen Y, Freyer L, Finnegan E, et al. Long form of latent TGF-beta binding protein 1 (Ltbp1L) is essential for cardiac outflow tract septation and remodeling. *Development* 2007;**134**:3723–32.

51. Jain R, Rentschler S, Epstein JA. Notch and cardiac outflow tract development. *Ann NY Acad Sci* 2010;**1188**:184–90.
52. Artavanis-Tsakonas S, Rand MD, Lake RJ. Notch signaling: cell fate control and signal integration in development. *Science* 1999;**284**:770–6.
53. High FA, Epstein JA. The multifaceted role of Notch in cardiac development and disease. *Nat Rev Genet* 2008;**9**:49–61.
54. High FA, Lu MM, Pear WS, Loomes KM, Kaestner KH, Epstein JA. Endothelial expression of the Notch ligand Jagged1 is required for vascular smooth muscle development. *Proc Natl Acad Sci USA* 2008;**105**:1955–9.
55. Oda T, Elkahloun AG, Pike BL, Okajima K, Krantz ID, Genin A, et al. Mutations in the human Jagged1 gene are responsible for Alagille syndrome. *Nat Genet* 1997;**16**:235–42.
56. Vincent SD, Buckingham ME. How to make a heart: the origin and regulation of cardiac progenitor cells. *Curr Top Dev Biol* 2010;**90**:1–41.
57. Mikawa T, Gourdie RG. Pericardial mesoderm generates a population of coronary smooth muscle cells migrating into the heart along with ingrowth of the epicardial organ. *Dev Biol* 1996;**174**:221–32.
58. Ratajska A, Czarnowska E, Ciszek B. Embryonic development of the proepicardium and coronary vessels. *Int J Dev Biol* 2008;**52**:229–36.
59. Svensson EC, Huggins GS, Lin H, Clendenin C, Jiang F, Tufts R, et al. A syndrome of tricuspid atresia in mice with a targeted mutation of the gene encoding Fog-2. *Nat Genet* 2000;**25**:353–6.
60. Tevosian SG, Deconinck AE, Tanaka M, Schinke M, Litovsky SH, Izumo S, et al. FOG-2, a cofactor for GATA transcription factors, is essential for heart morphogenesis and development of coronary vessels from epicardium. *Cell* 2000;**101**:729–39.
61. Dettman RW, Denetclaw Jr W, Ordahl CP, Bristow J. Common epicardial origin of coronary vascular smooth muscle, perivascular fibroblasts, and intermyocardial fibroblasts in the avian heart. *Dev Biol* 1998;**193**:169–81.
62. Gittenberger-de Groot AC, Vrancken Peeters MP, Mentink MM, Gourdie RG, Poelmann RE. Epicardium-derived cells contribute a novel population to the myocardial wall and the atrioventricular cushions. *Circ Res* 1998;**82**:1043–52.
63. Conte G, Pellegrini A. On the development of the coronary arteries in human embryos, stages 14-19. *Anat Embryol (Berl)* 1984;**169**:209–18.
64. McLin VA, Henning SJ, Jamrich M. The role of the visceral mesoderm in the development of the gastrointestinal tract. *Gastroenterology* 2009;**136**:2074–91.
65. McHugh KM. Molecular analysis of smooth muscle development in the mouse. *Dev Dyn* 1995;**204**:278–90.
66. Roberts DJ, Johnson RL, Burke AC, Nelson CE, Morgan BA, Tabin C. Sonic hedgehog is an endodermal signal inducing Bmp-4 and Hox genes during induction and regionalization of the chick hindgut. *Development* 1995;**121**:3163–74.
67. Batts LE, Polk DB, Dubois RN, Kulessa H. Bmp signaling is required for intestinal growth and morphogenesis. *Dev Dyn* 2006;**235**:1563–70.
68. De Santa Barbara P, Williams J, Goldstein AM, Doyle AM, Nielsen C, Winfield S, et al. Bone morphogenetic protein signaling pathway plays multiple roles during gastrointestinal tract development. *Dev Dyn* 2005;**234**:312–22.

Chapter 83

Smooth Muscle Myocyte Ultrastructure and Contractility

Avril V. Somlyo[1] and Marion J. Siegman[2]

[1]*Department of Molecular Physiology and Biological Physics, University of Virginia, Charlottesville, VA,* [2]*Department of Molecular Physiology and Biophysics, Thomas Jefferson University, Philadelphia, PA*

INTRODUCTION

Smooth muscle (SM) comprising the walls of many hollow organs is structurally and functionally diverse, reflecting the specialized contractile needs of the blood vessel, airway, uterus, bladder or gut. This chapter is intended as an overview of the general basic characteristics of SM ultrastructural features and of the contractile proteins with their implications for specialized functions. SM will be compared to skeletal and cardiac muscle illustrating the similarities but emphasizing the differences that account for the unique SM phenotype. Many of these features are also relevant to migrating non-muscle cells.

THE CONTRACTILE APPARATUS

The rise of intracellular Ca^{2+} serves as the initial switch to turn on the contractile apparatus in smooth, cardiac, and skeletal muscle. The pathways subsequently diverge with Ca^{2+} binding to the actin filament-associated protein, troponin in striated muscles, whereas in SM Ca^{2+} binds to calmodulin (CaM) forming an active complex with myosin light chain kinase (MLCK). MLCK/CaM/Ca_4 phosphorylates Ser19 of the 20 kDa myosin regulatory light chain (RLC_{20}) permitting actin activation of the actomyosin ATPase, cross-bridge cycling and contraction (1). A myosin light chain phosphatase (MLCP) dephosphorylates RLC_{20}. The magnitude of force output depends on the balance of MLCK and MLCP activities. Stimulus specific secondary levels of Ca^{2+}-independent regulation occur through multiple signaling pathways that modify MLCK and MLCP activities (2). Ultimately, all of these processes converge on the contractile cytoskeleton responsible for the mechanical contractile event. Thus, an appreciation of the players involved and the organization of the contractile apparatus is necessary to understand the unique mechanical properties of SM cells needed to carry out their specialized functions in the body.

General Organization and Relationship to Mechanical Properties

The thin actin filaments, thick myosin filaments and dense bodies constitute a contractile unit in SM (3,4). In cross-sections of portal vein SM cells myosin filaments form a 60–80 nm lattice (Figure 83.1), with each myosin surrounded by an orbit of actin filaments. The measured actin to myosin filament ratio is 15:1 (5) in agreement with ratios determined biochemically (6). At higher magnification, cross-bridges project from the myosin filaments (Figure 83.1, lower left panel). Stereoscopic imaging of longitudinal sections revealed a longitudinal order of 3–5 neighboring myosin filaments 2.2 μm in length (3) that are considered to be the A-band of a mini-sarcomere (Figure 83.2). As the maximal force developed by muscle is proportional to the sarcomere length or to the number of cross-bridges acting in parallel, the greater length of SM compared with skeletal myosin filaments (2.2 vs. 1.5 μm) contributes to the ability of SM to develop nearly the same amount of force as striated muscle, in spite of the lower concentration of myosin (3). Actin filaments emanating from plasma membrane and cytosolic dense bodies can be followed to the myosin filaments and make up the equivalent of the I-bands and Z-bands of striated muscles (4) (Figure 83.2). Importantly, the polarity of the actin filaments determined by decoration with subfragment 1 of myosin, point away from the dense bodies just as observed at Z-bands and are thus correctly positioned for a sliding filament mechanism of contraction (4). In cultured SM cells, membrane-dense bodies become focal adhesion sites consisting of large dynamic protein complexes where the cytoskeleton connects to the extracellular matrix. The actin cross-linking protein, α-actinin, also found at striated muscle Z-bands, and vimentin localize to dense bodies and focal adhesions. It is now apparent that like focal adhesions, dense bodies and Z-bands are not only anchoring sites for the cytoskeleton but also serve as scaffolds

Muscle. DOI: http://dx.doi.org/10.1016/B978-0-12-381510-1.00083-1

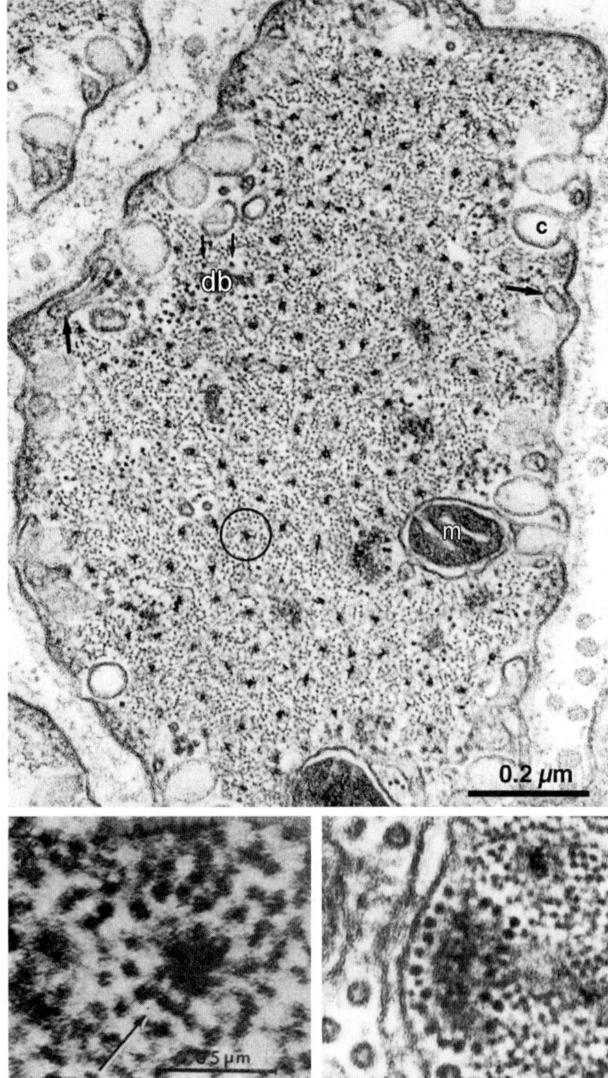

FIGURE 83.1 Electron micrograph from rabbit vas deferens SM cell showing transversely sectioned thick (myosin) filaments surrounded by actin filaments (encircled region) and dense bodies (db) with associated 10 nm filaments (small arrows). Surface couplings, where the sarcoplasmic reticulum is apposed to the plasma membrane, are also present (large arrows). Caveolae (c), and mitochondria (m) are indicated. (Lower left panel) High magnification view (320,000×) of a transverse section showing a 14.6 nm diameter myosin filament surrounded by 16 actin filaments. Three cross-bridges (arrow) at different levels can be seen in stereo views (pair not included) as well as a suggestion of other cross-bridges lying close to the myosin filament. (Lower right panel) High magnification view (210,000×) of a transversely sectioned dense body where some substructure and amorphous material is surrounded by 10 nm filaments. Profiles with the diameter of actin filaments are visible within the dense body. *(From Ashton et al., 1975 (3), with permission.)*

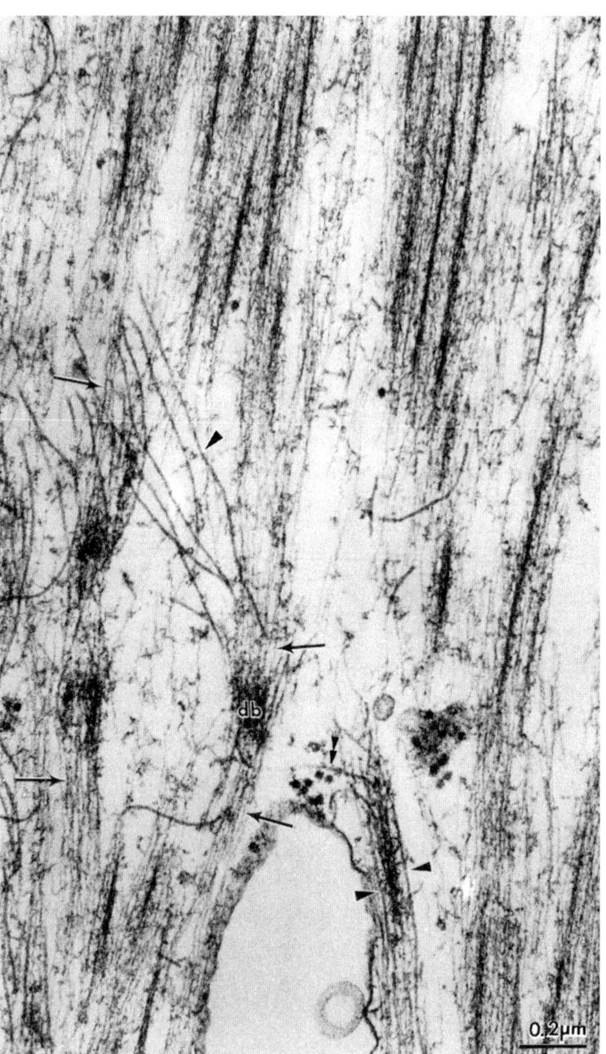

FIGURE 83.2 Mini-sarcomeres in a longitudinal section of a saponin-skinned portal vein SM cell. Filaments are spread out, revealing relationships of dense bodies with associated actin to neighboring myosin filaments. Thin filaments *(arrows)* that emerge from cytoplasmic dense bodies (db) can be traced to where they are adjacent to (overlap) myosin filaments. The 10 nm filaments (arrowheads) do not run parallel to the mini-sarcomere-like units, but appear to interconnect dense bodies (double arrowhead). *(From Bond and Somlyo, 1982 (4), with permission.)*

for many signaling molecules influencing myofibrillogenesis, cell migration, actin dynamics, mechanosensing, hypertrophy and atrophy (7,8; see Chapter 87). Intermediate or 10 nm filaments make up a third filament type found surrounding dense bodies (Figure 83.1, lower right panel). They do not run parallel to the mini-sarcomeres but are obliquely oriented linking up to dense bodies of different sarcomeres forming a non-contractile cytoskeleton. SM 10 nm filaments consist of two proteins, desmin and vimentin, which can be expressed individually or together in the same cell. They can massively increase in hypertrophied vascular SM (9).

THE MYOSIN MOTOR

Smooth, cardiac, skeletal, and non-muscle myosins constitute class II of the myosin superfamily that form filaments through self-association of their long α-helical coiled-coil tails forming the filament backbone. The motor domain hydrolyzes ATP and its rigid lever arm or neck project from the backbone. During the working stroke of the cross-bridge, the motor domain is bound to actin and the lever arm swings from a converter domain or fulcrum point at the base of the motor domain, translating the actin filament by 10 nm (10). The lever arm binds two light chains, the essential light chain (ECL_{17}) and the regulatory light chain (RLC_{20}), both members of the calmodulin superfamily. ELC_{17} wraps around the long α-helical segment of the lever arm adjacent to the converter region at the fulcrum of the head-lever arm and with RLC_{20} stabilize the lever arm. There are two isoforms, acidic (ELC_{17a}) and basic (ELC_{17b}), that differ in five of the nine COOH-terminal amino acid residues and are products of a single gene (11). ELC_{17a} is associated with fast phasic and ELC_{17b} with slow tonic type SMs. The role of the two isoforms on contractile kinetics is not clear, although ELC_{17a} isoform exchange for the slow ELC_{17b} in SM lead to an increase in velocity of shortening and rate of force development by non-phosphorylated cross-bridges (12). Regulation of SM myosin through RLC_{20} is discussed below.

There is a single myosin heavy chain (MHC) gene. Alternative splicing of two sites gives rise to four isoforms: SMB and SMA with or without a 7 amino acid insert near the ATP-binding pocket which modifies the rate of ATP hydrolysis and ADP release; SM1 and SM2 with 9 or 34 amino acids respectively in the non-helical C-terminal tail thought to contribute to filament stability and possibly filament formation (13). No differences were found in the ability of SM1 and SM2 myosins to propel actin filaments, reviewed in (13). Homodimer and heterodimer pairing of all four MHCs may occur and individual SM cells may express one or more of the isoforms. The 7 amino acid insert confers functional differences being absent in the tonic aorta but present in phasic SM such as intestine reviewed in (13).

MYOSIN FILAMENTS

Myosin is organized into filaments in relaxed and contracted SM and does not depend on phosphorylation of RLC_{20} for assembly (5,14,15). Furthermore, most of the myosin in mature SM is filamentous in view of the close agreement between SDS gels and quantitative electron microscopy of relaxed SM (3). Therefore, recently proposed pools of non-assembled myosin that polymerizes when trachealis muscle is activated at short muscle lengths and that contributes to force development must be very small (16). The difficulty in these studies may arise from the technically challenging counting of filament profiles where cell length cannot be easily controlled in tissues. However, in cultured cells undergoing mitosis and migration smooth and non-muscle myosin II filaments must assemble and disassemble as stress fibers turn over and the leading edges and tails project and retract. Furthermore, as in striated muscles, the regular cytoskeletal structure in SM is not static and myofibrillar proteins likely turnover continually to maintain or rebuild damaged proteins (17) contributing to a small pool of non-assembled myosin in mature SM.

Whether SM myosin filaments are bipolar or side polar is controversial and stems from *in vitro* studies where the length, diameter, and polarity of the filaments are influenced by ionic strength, pH, cations, myosin concentration, and the rapidity of dilution (18). SM myosin readily assembles into side polar filaments *in vitro* (19). However, isolated filaments do not necessarily recapitulate the *in vivo* structure. In striated muscle antiparallel myosin tail interactions give rise to bipolar filaments with a central bare zone lacking myosin heads. This is easily seen in the A-band with multiple precisely aligned filaments but cannot be seen in SM either due to its absence or the lack of alignment. Side polar filaments are non-helical with the orientation of the myosin molecules reversed on opposite sides of the filament giving rise to a square profile in cross-section, with cross-bridges on two faces only (20). Electron microscopy has shown both square and round profiles using intact, permeabilized, chemically fixed or rapidly frozen muscles, methods that are all open to artifacts. Thus, this has been a difficult issue to resolve. A further complication is that if a round bipolar filament is obliquely oriented it appears as a rectangle (3). Thus new approaches are needed to resolve this issue, for example by showing the polarity of the actin filaments on either side of myosin filaments. Both bipolar and side polar filaments are compatible with the ability of SM to undergo extreme shortening to 25% of initial length (21). Actin filaments of opposite polarity from opposing dense bodies could be pulled along the side polar filament whereas in the case of bipolar filaments, the high actin to myosin ratio of 13:1 (21) could also bring into play additional correctly oriented actin filaments as the muscle shortens.

CONTRACTILE REGULATION

The contractile regulation in SM is distinctly different than in striated muscles where Ca^{2+} binding to troponin on the actin filament acts as a derepressor removing the inhibitory effect of troponin. In SM, Ca^{2+} is a true activator increasing the low ATPase activity of the dormant myosin motor (1). This activation is through phosphorylation of the RLC_{20} by the Ca_4CaM-dependent MLCK upon an increase in cytosolic Ca^{2+}. Double-headed myosin is needed for regulation (22). Phosphorylation of both heads increases the actomyosin ATPase activity >1000-fold (23). The two heads of myosin each bind actin, hydrolyze ATP, and work cooperatively (23). Both heads are needed for the "off state" as removal of one head results in the "on state" even in the absence of phosphorylation (24). Two big questions in the field are: how does phosphorylation of Ser19 on the RLC_{20} turn on the active site of the myosin head at a >10 nm distance and how do non-phosphorylated $RLCs_{20}$ maintain the "off state"? Based on structural analysis of two-dimensional crystalline arrays of a two-headed fragment of myosin (HMM) in the unphosphorylated and phosphorylated states a mechanism for inhibition was suggested (25). An asymmetric head–head interaction was found in the inactive state where the ATPase activity of one head is "blocked" through its actin-binding interface abutting the converter domain of its partner head preventing hydrolysis. Upon phosphorylation the heads straighten. This conformation resembles the much-studied folded 10S myosin molecules, distinctive of smooth and non-muscle myosins, that upon phosphorylation assume an extended 6S active conformation (reviewed in 26). It remains to be determined whether this asymmetric head–head interaction occurs in myosin filaments either isolated or *in vivo*. Interestingly, cooperatively cycling non-phosphorylated cross-bridges can develop up to 40% of maximal force indicating that under some circumstance unphosphorylated heads are not "blocked" (27). Using cryoelectron microscopy and fitting of the SM HMM atomic structure, this asymmetric interaction of the heads has also been visualized on isolated non-phosphorylated cardiac and tarantula myosin filaments, which are stable in contrast to SM. This is surprising as the major "on" switch in cardiac muscle is regulated through Ca^{2+} binding to troponin with light chain phosphorylation only playing a modulatory role under some conditions. Thus, this asymmetric head state may be a general relaxed state of the heads on the filament applicable to myosins in general and being more stable in SM (26). The detailed interactions of the off state are not yet established and await an atomic structure. A recent model, based on single ATP turnover data and on the functional dependence of the two SM myosin heads with one strongly and one weakly bound at any point in time, proposes a phosphorylation-dependent equilibrium between the compact inhibited state and the active state (28). In this model non-phosphorylated, singly or doubly phosphorylated SM myosin may form the inhibited state but phosphorylation makes it more difficult. It is also worth noting that phosphorylation significantly increases the stiffness of SM cross-bridges in rigor (29) expected to give a mechanical advantage to the lever arm. Ultimately, recent advances in live time biophysical measurements of the SM myosin motor *in situ*, in the context of mechanical performance and the atomic structure are needed to reveal the essence of the "on" and "off" states in relation to SM contractility.

Regulatory Molecules Trafficking at the Myosin Head

The myosin lever arm and its RLC_{20} is a major intersection for the trafficking of molecules that regulate contractility with MLCK and MLCP serving as traffic lights to regulate phosphorylation of Ser19 of RLC_{20}. These in turn can be regulated, reviewed in (2). Regulation of MLCK and MLCP will be reviewed in Chapter 87. Multiple kinases including ROCK, Zip-kinase associated with MLCP and integrin-linked kinase can phosphorylate MYPT1 and inhibit MLCP activity as does the phosphorylated inhibitory protein CPI-17 (30). On the other hand cyclic nucleotides can activate MLCP through phosphorylation of telokin (31) or binding to the C-termini leucine zipper of MYPT1, reviewed in (2). Ultimately interaction domains and high-resolution structures are needed for insight into the molecular mechanisms underlying these processes.

ACTIN

Thin filaments are two-stranded helical polymers of actin with the two strands crossing at ~36 nm encompassing seven actin monomers. Asymmetric actin monomers (G-actin) polymerize to form actin filaments (F-actin) 5–8 nm in diameter. Based on weight, the ratio of actin to myosin is strikingly different in SM compared with rabbit skeletal muscle, 3:1 vs. 1:3 respectively. The ratio of actin to myosin filaments is ~13:1 in SM (Figure 83.1) in contrast to 2:1 in striated muscle. Arterial has a somewhat higher ratio than venous SM. The total myosin content in SM is ~5 times less than in skeletal muscle yet it can develop equivalent maximal force/myocyte cross section (6). In motility assays the rate of movement of smooth and skeletal actin over phosphorylated or non-phosphorylated myosins, with and without a load was not different (32) in keeping with their similar biochemical properties. Thus, SM actin is not making a major contribution to the different contractile properties of smooth and striated muscle.

Actin Isoforms

Actin is a highly conserved protein with the six mammalian isoforms encoded by six different genes, α-skeletal, α-cardiac, α-smooth, γ-smooth, and two ubiquitously expressed cytoplasmic (non-muscle) isoforms, β-cytoplasmic and γ-cytoplasmic (33). The isoforms can be separated by isoelectric focusing even though any two isoforms have >93% sequence homology differing in only a few

N-terminal amino acids. In SM, the expression of actin isoforms is tissue- rather than species-specific, with isoform expression changing during development (1). The α-smooth or γ-smooth actin isoforms may be expressed exclusively or in combination with the α-isoform more prevalent in tonic type and γ-isoform in phasic type SMs (34). Alpha-smooth actin is highest in vascular with the γ-smooth and non-muscle isoforms most prevalent in visceral SM (34). However, the functional significance is unclear as RLC_{20} phosphorylation is the dominant regulator of contractility (1). In addition, isolated native actin filaments have been shown to consist of randomly copolymerized isoactins in each filament in the same proportions as found in the tissue (35). Therefore, although different SM tissues express different isoform ratios, these isoforms are not segregated into different cells or domains within cells, also suggesting that isoform diversity does not translate into diversity of contractile function. Differential localizations of the non-muscle-actin isoforms have been reported in striated muscle, stereocilia, and cultured cells but are subject to the vagaries of antibody specificity and fixation and await other technologies to reveal specific isoform functions (36). Actin isoforms could play distinctive roles in cultured cells where actin dynamics drive migration at the leading edge and the cytoskeleton is rapidly turning over. In experimental rat aortic intimal thickening and atherosclerotic plaques as well as in cultured aortic cells the predominance of α-smooth actin switches to β-smooth actin with an increase in the γ-smooth isoform (37). Thus, the pattern of actin expression can be used as a marker of atheromatous SMCs. In smooth α-actin null mice, surprisingly, the formation of the cardiovascular system is not impaired even though SM α-actin is normally the most prevalent isoform in blood vessels and is expressed in early stages of heart development (38). A minor upregulation of skeletal α-actin did not prevent the disorganization and reduction of myofilaments with fewer myosin filaments resulting in a compromised vascular contractility in these mice supporting an important role for the smooth α-actin isoform. Support for special functions of some of the actin isoforms derives from the inability of overexpressed alternate actin isoforms to rescue a given actin isoform knockout (for review see (36)). While intriguing the necessity for specific actin isoforms for specific functions remains to be explored further.

Actin Associated Proteins

Tropomyosin (TM), a long fibrous protein lies along the long pitch double-helical thin filament spanning seven actin monomers and through end-to-end contacts continuously covers the actin filament in all muscles. The troponin complex discovered by Ebashi (39) binds TM with a 38 nm periodicity along the actin filament. Ca^{2+} binding to troponin results in a shift in the position of TM allowing interaction of actin and myosin, known as the "steric blocking model". Troponin is absent in SM yet the shift in the actin layer lines of the X-ray pattern considered to reflect the movement of TM occurs when SM is activated (40). If this interpretation is correct other Ca-binding proteins such as caldesmon (CD) may play a role to control TM (41). Nevertheless, while there is evidence for Ca^{2+} regulation of the thin filament, albeit largely *in vitro*, Ca/CaM/MLCK phosphorylation of myosin RLC_{20} is the dominant regulator for activation of force in SM while striated muscles are Ca^{2+}-regulated through the troponin switch on the actin filament. On the other hand CD regulation of thin filaments has been proposed to explain relaxation that under some conditions can occur at high levels of RLC_{20} phosphorylation (reviewed in 42) and in the presence of significant basal RLC_{20} phosphorylation (reviewed in 42). Conditional knock down of CD isoforms targeted to SM has yet to be achieved. Caldesmon first identified as a CaM binding protein, is a widely expressed 75 nm long molecule bound to the thin filament in a ratio of 1 CD:2 TM:14 actin in SM (reviewed in 41). Of the two isoforms the heavy isoform h-CD is restricted to SM. At low [Ca^{2+}.CaM] or when unphosphorylated, CD inhibits the actomyosin ATPase. In a steric blocking model, upon increased Ca^{2+} or phosphorylation, CD working allosterically through TM switches actin "on". However, it is still not clear whether CD functions like troponin. In another model CD competes with myosin for a common actin-binding site. The concentration of CD may be too low to displace myosin unless CD is concentrated in regions in the cell. While the *in vitro* studies are compelling, the contribution of CD to the contractility of SM awaits studies in transgenic animals. In non-muscle cells, cultured or dedifferentiated SM cells, CD may play additional roles related to enhanced actin dynamics in these cells, for example in inhibition of the Arp2/3 mediated actin nucleation and in cell migration (43).

Calponin (CaP), a CaM-binding protein, also binds to actin filaments and inhibits the actomyosin ATPase activity but unlike CD, independently of TM (44). CD and CaP do not interact and have been found on different populations of thin filaments (45). CP was first isolated by Takahashi (46) and of the three isoforms identified the more basic, h1-CaP, is most prevalent in differentiated SM, with other isoforms dominant during development (47). CaP expression is downregulated in cultured SM cells. Although widely studied, the physiological or pathophysiological function of CaP *in vivo* in SM tissues remains to be resolved. Knock out of h1-CaP in mice did not abolish force, Ca^{2+}sensitivity, Ca^{2+}sensitization, delays in onset and half-times of force development nor Ca^{2+}sensitized force initiated by photolysis of caged

GTPγS (48). However, unloaded shortening velocity (V_{us}) of thiophosphorylated fibers was significantly faster in the h1-CaP null SM consistent with the possibility that CaP exerts a regulatory influence on the cross-bridge cycle. However the findings are not unequivocal as actin content was decreased by 25–50% and the electrophoretic mobility of h-CaD changed. Thus, the loss of actin filaments could alter the number of contractile units in series as well as the cross-bridge detachment rate accounting for the decrease in V_{us} (48). While the role of CaP in contractility remains unclear, its main function may lie elsewhere. CaP isoforms are expressed in non-muscle cells and are thought to play a regulatory role in cell motility and proliferation in for example, developing and remodeling of SM cells, fibroblasts, endothelial cells and keratinocytes (reviewed in 49). It is worth noting that many proteins have a CaP homology domain (CH) which serves to bind actin and signaling molecules and this has led to the suggestion that CaP could play a role in signaling (see Chapter 87).

Actin Dynamics Regulate Gene Transcription

Stimuli that alter the equilibrium between monomeric G- and filamentous F-actin leading to a decrease in G-actin feed forward to increase the expression of actin in SM in a RhoA-dependent manner (50,51). In cultured smooth and non-muscle cells RhoGTPases control the cytoskeletal dynamics thus regulating cell adhesion and migration, both relevant to SM during development and disease states. RhoA regulates the potent myocardin-related transcription factors, MRTFs. These are known to be co-activators of serum response factor that binds to CArG boxes in the promoter region of SM marker genes such as actin and myosin (52). MRTF activity is inhibited, by binding through its RPEL domain, to G-actin and preventing translocation of MRTF to the nuclei to activate transcription (51,53,54). Thus actin dynamics can regulate its own expression and that of other SM specific proteins. This mechanism could also be responsive to the continual turnover of the actin cytoskeleton during normal maintenance and repair and following injury.

MECHANICS AND ENERGETICS OF CONTRACTION

Length-Tension Relationships of Smooth Muscle

As described above, contractile proteins are arranged in filaments and may be organized as contractile units. The relationships between muscle length and force production have been studied in a variety of vertebrate and invertebrate smooth muscles and, qualitatively, these have proved to be similar to striated muscle (55,56), indicating that contraction in smooth muscle also operates by means of a sliding filament mechanism (57). The relationship between active force and muscle length (or sarcomere length) is approximately bell shaped, with peak force (*Po*) occurring at an optimum length designated *Lo* (Figure 83.3). The sliding filament hypothesis relies primarily on the finding of a proportional relationship between active force production and contractile filament overlap at muscle lengths exceeding the optimum length for force development, *Lo*, and this is traced to the number of myosin cross-bridges interacting with actin (57). Like striated muscles, all smooth muscles studied exhibit an optimum length (*Lo*) for force development. In most smooth muscles, there is considerable passive force at short muscle lengths, with slack length, *Ls*, occurring

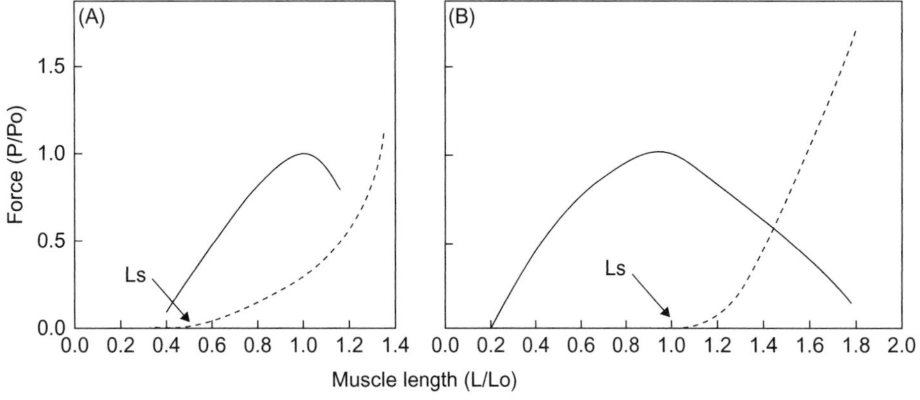

FIGURE 83.3 Typical length–force relationships for SMs. Passive force, resulting from extension of resting muscles (dashed lines) and active force, resulting from maximal stimulation of the muscles at each length (solid) lines, are shown. In panel (A), *Ls*, the length at which passive force is just detectable, occurs at ~0.5 *Lo*, the length at which active force is maximal (Po = 1). Muscle can shorten to about 0.3 *Lo*. In panel (B), *Ls* coincides with *Lo*. The muscle can shorten to ~0.2 *Lo*. The muscle is readily extensible to long lengths where there is a linear relationship between active force and muscle length.

at ~0.4–0.5 *Lo* (Figure 83.3A). In such muscles, passive force rises steeply upon extension of the muscle so that there is a large component of passive force at *Lo*, which has two major consequences. First, as the muscle shortens, these elements become compressed and provide a resistance to and possible limit to shortening. Also, their presence makes it difficult to measure active force production at longer lengths without irreversible damage to the muscle (56,58). In certain vascular and intestinal preparations (mesenteric vein and artery, *anococcygeus m.*), in which the steep rise in the passive force curve occurs at slightly *longer* lengths than in other preparations (58), force decreased linearly with increasing length, which extrapolated to zero force at ~1.9 *Lo*, providing strong evidence for a sliding filament mechanism in smooth muscle (Figure 83.3B). These muscles can shorten to 0.2–0.5 *Lo*, so that the relationship of active force production to length is asymmetric, as in skeletal muscle, in that active force production declines gradually at lengths exceeding *Lo* but declines sharply at lengths shorter than *Lo*.

A well-known characteristic of intact smooth muscle is its ability to contract to very short lengths, yet little is known about the basis of the decline in active force production at short lengths in smooth muscle. There is a disparity among measured force and parameters that are accepted indices of actin–myosin interaction, such as dynamic stiffness and energy usage; in general the latter exceeds force to varying degrees at short muscle lengths in different muscles (59,60). In contrast, at lengths exceeding slack length, *Ls*, cells and filaments are aligned parallel to the longitudinal axis of the tissue, and measured force is consistent with indices of events at the cross-bridge. In intact tissue, passive structural elements such as cell–cell connections and linkages through the extracellular matrix that are in series with the contractile apparatus limit mechanotransmission as they become increasingly slack and floppy at short lengths, with cells and filaments becoming misaligned (60). In isolated cells where these constraints are absent, stimulation leads to evaginations of the plasma membrane (blebs) between dense bodies and the contractile apparatus becomes helically oriented (61). *In situ* there is a tendency towards such extreme changes only at short muscle lengths, and then only to the extent that the floppy extracellular matrix permits. The appearance of blebs is a fingerprint for cell shortening (60) as is an increase in density of myosin filaments per cross-sectional area although myosin content is unchanged. Without adequate control of cell length, conclusions about remodeling of contractile filaments based on filament count must be made with caution. These structural factors become important functionally particularly in reservoir organs, where emptying or propulsion of contents relies on the ability of the muscle to generate force and shorten. This is complicated further in disease, since smooth muscles readily adapt to changes in functional demand by remodeling, with structural changes in contractile and passive elastic elements that modify the length-dependences of active and passive force production, resting compliance and the ability to shorten (62–64).

F–V Relationship

The hyperbolic relationship between shortening velocity and force first described by Hill (65) for skeletal muscle also applies to smooth muscle tissues and single cells (56,66). This similarity in shape of the relationship in the two muscle types was taken as strong evidence for the operation of qualitatively similar cross-bridge mechanisms. Although maximum force production is the same or greater in smooth muscle, the maximum velocities of shortening reported for smooth muscle are much slower than skeletal muscle.

There seems to be an invariant relationship among mechanical parameters such as Vmax for shortening, time to maximum force development, and the rates of energy usage (67), and all are consistent with the overall actomyosin ATPase of the two muscle types (68). The differences between skeletal and smooth muscles become apparent when comparing the time courses of total high energy phosphate utilization (ΔATP + ΔPCr − ΔAMP) and force production during isometric tetani in the two muscles. At the temperatures shown, the frog sartorius muscle (Figure 83.4) developed force about 45 times faster and had a rate of chemical energy usage about 45 times higher than the taenia coli (67). This shows that there is an inverse relationship between the time required to develop maximum force and the rate of energy utilization.

In smooth and striated muscles, measurements of the force–velocity (F–V) relationship are typically made at the plateau of a tetanic contraction, either by imposing isovelocity shortenings under isometric conditions (69) or during after loaded isotonic contractions (70). When only a measure of (V_{us}) is sought, unloaded shortening velocity is measured (71) at the time of interest. However, the interpretation of the F–V relations and Vmax in particular in smooth muscle must be made with caution, in light of the fact that in smooth muscle the velocity of cross-bridge cycling is regulated, and varies with time during the course of a contraction (discussed below).

Energy Usage During Force Development and Force Maintenance

A unique property that smooth muscles share is the ability to regulate the energy cost of force production and force maintenance. Direct measurements of high energy phosphate utilization in the rabbit taenia coli smooth muscle showed that during the initial development of force the chemical energy requirement is some four times greater than that for subsequent force maintenance. The higher average rate of energy utilization during force development was not due to the cost of work done against the series elasticity, but was, rather, consistent with a faster rate of cross-bridge cycling (72). Estimates of energy usage, based on steady-state oxygen consumption and lactate production (58) are in good agreement with the direct measurements of high-energy phosphate usage during force maintenance in vascular smooth muscles in the taenia coli. If the major calcium regulatory system in smooth muscle was simply a calcium-dependent MLCK, then it would be expected that the degree of light chain phosphorylation would directly reflect the number of cycling cross-bridges and the average rate of chemical energy usage. However, the relative degrees of light chain phosphorylation during development and subsequent isometric force maintenance were not proportional to the relative rates of ATP utilization during those times. Indeed, a four-fold decrease in energy usage occurred with only a ~4% decrease in the degree of myosin light chain phosphorylation (72). Such a small change in the degree of light chain phosphorylation might give rise to a large change in cross-bridge cycling rate if some cooperative regulatory process operated (27,73–75) (discussed below).

Economy

It has long been recognized that there are a variety of energy requirements for isometric force maintenance in different muscle types (76), and these have been compared on the basis of their "economy". Economy is calculated as the force per cross-sectional area divided by the rate of energy utilization per gram tissue. The economy of the rabbit taenia coli obtained from direct measurements of high-energy phosphate utilization, 700 (N/cm^2)/($\mu mol\ g^{-1} s^{-1}$) is similar to that in other smooth muscles estimated from measurement of oxygen consumption or heat production (72). The economy of the taenia coli is 100-fold higher than the frog sartorius (Figure 83.4), and this can be traced in part to a slower cross-bridge cycle and the 40% longer myosin filament, which puts more cross-bridges in parallel in smooth muscle (3). In contrast, the economy of the invertebrate smooth muscle (anterior byssus retractor muscle, ABRM) of *Mytilus edulis* during the catch state (78) is an order of magnitude greater than the taenia coli. However, when the 30-fold longer myosin filament length of the ABRM is accounted for, the economy of force maintenance in this muscle would be similar to the taenia coli.

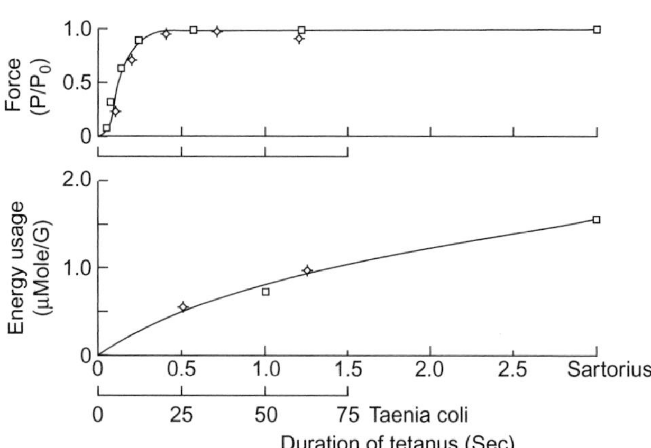

FIGURE 83.4 Comparison of relative rates of force development and associated energy usage under isometric conditions in frog sartorius at 0 °C and rabbit taenia coli at 18 °C. Note 50-fold difference in time scales for the two muscles: The frog develops tension 50 times faster, and its rate of chemical usage is 50 times greater. □, data for frog sartorius; ○, data for taenia coli. *(From Butler and Davies 1980 (77), with permission.)*

Latch

Certain invertebrate smooth muscles, such as the anterior byssus retractor muscle (ABRM) of *Mytilus edulis*, show the catch state, which is similar in many ways to vertebrate smooth muscles. Catch is a condition that ensues following force development and the cessation of stimulation, characterized by a prolonged period (minutes to hours) of high force maintenance, high resistance to stretch, no force recovery on quick-release and extremely low energy cost when intracellular calcium concentrations have returned to just supra-basal concentrations. This is in contrast to the initial period of stimulation, when there is a high intracellular calcium concentration and force development, high rate of energy usage and the muscle shows force redevelopment following quick release. Unlike vertebrate smooth muscles, where the economy is based on cross-bridge kinetics, we now know that the high economy in catch derives from the fact that the mini-titin twitchin acts as a force-maintaining tether between actin and myosin filaments (see review in 79). Nevertheless, catch-like mechanical behavior, expressed as the absence of force redevelopment following quick release during force maintenance, was noted during tonic contractions in vertebrate vascular smooth muscle by the Somlyos (80). It is not yet known whether there is a counterpart to twitchin in vertebrate smooth muscles that show catch-like behavior. It is interesting that there are many structural and functional similarities between twitchin and MyC-protein of cardiac muscle (79).

Dillon and colleagues (81) measured shortening velocity at a low fixed afterload in arterial smooth muscle and found a time-dependent slowing of velocity during the course of a contraction. The similarity in the time course of changes in shortening velocity to the time course phosphorylation of the 20 kD light chains of myosin together with energetic evidence (72) led to the development of a model for what is known as the "latch" state of mammalian smooth muscle. The mechanical and energetic similarities to the catch state inspired the term "latch." The latch-bridge hypothesis has evolved into one in which the unique properties of smooth muscle result from the dephosphorylation of an attached cross-bridge. The idea that high force output with low levels of myosin light chain phosphorylation could be explained on the basis of phosphatase activity was independently proposed by Driska (82) and Hai and Murphy (83). They suggested that myosin light chain phosphorylation is required for the transition of the cross-bridge into the force-producing state, and that phosphorylated myosin goes through the normal cross-bridge cycle in which there is attachment and detachment of the cross-bridge with concomitant splitting of ATP. A cross-bridge that is dephosphorylated while attached to actin and generating force, a latch-bridge, has a detachment rate that is very slow and would alter the kinetics of the completion of the cross-bridge cycle. The dephosphorylated cross-bridges would act as an internal load on the remaining phosphorylated cross-bridges, producing a decrease in velocity. Under steady-state conditions, there is high force production from dephosphorylated cross-bridges so that high forces can be maintained when only a small fraction of myosin is phosphorylated at any time. The decline in phosphorylation and in cycling rates with maintained numbers of cross-bridges would account for the high economy of force maintenance. This is a very attractive model and has led to a large experimental effort that has tested its applicability.

Relaxation is a specific condition where there is strong evidence for dephosphorylation of myosin resulting in the formation of force-bearing cross-bridges with very slow detachment rates. In the rabbit taenia coli and permeabilized portal vein, force declines very slowly at a time when the ability to redevelop force following a quick-release, myosin light chain phosphorylation and ATPase activity have all decreased to near-resting values (84–86). Moreover, no significant suprabasal energy usage could be detected during relaxation from an isometric tetanus (72). The energy used to maintain an equivalent impulse ($\int Pdt/\Delta \sim P$) was higher during stimulation than during relaxation. That is, force was maintained with less energy usage during relaxation than during stimulation. This suggested that the extra force per unit of energy used during relaxation might be due to the presence of attached but non-cycling cross-bridges in the relaxing muscle, a state that had been proposed to exist in resting smooth muscles (87). These events in smooth muscle stand in contrast to those of skeletal muscle, where the energy usage during relaxation is very low, and correlates with the dissipation of force generated by the slowing of cross-bridge cycling (88).

There are certain critical features that are not supported by the latch-bridge model. The rate of energy usage and maximum velocity of shortening are often correlated to the degree of light chain phosphorylation (89). However, certain inconsistencies in the relationships occur, including large changes in ATPase activity and maximum shortening can occur in some muscles with disproportionately small changes in the degree of myosin light chain phosphorylation (90,91) maximum force production with very low degrees of phosphorylation (92,93) or no increase in phosphorylation (94). These inconsistencies raised the question of the quantitative relationship between the degree of myosin light chain phosphorylation and the number of molecules that increase their ATPase activity under activated conditions. Single turnover techniques (in which the rate at which ADP bound to myosin is replaced with a new ADP derived from ATP splitting) showed that a small degree of myosin light chain phosphorylation cooperatively turns on the maximum number of myosin molecules. Cooperatively activated myosin would have a slower ATPase than that directly activated by light chain phosphorylation, but higher degrees of phosphorylation increased the rate of cross-bridge cycling (74,75). Further evidence for cooperative attachment of cross-bridges and its potential magnitude is based on studies where the release of micromolar ATP from caged ATP in smooth muscle depleted of ATP caused force development up to 40% of maximal tension in the absence of Ca^{2+} and RLC_{20} phosphorylation (27). Thus, cooperativity can directly account for high force output and low rates of energy usage with low levels of light chain phosphorylation.

Energy Usage During Shortening and Work Production and the Question of Internal Loads

Fenn (95) showed that energy output from skeletal muscle could be varied by changes in the mechanical constraints placed upon the muscle. When skeletal muscle shortened and performed work, a quantity of energy was liberated above that seen during an isometric contraction; this is part of what is known as the Fenn effect. In smooth muscle, a Fenn effect is observed when an isovelocity shortening is initiated during maximum force maintenance, but not at the onset of stimulation when isometric force would ordinarily be developed (84). Recall that the average rate of energy usage during isometric force development is four-fold greater than during force maintenance. Thus, at a time when energy usage under isometric conditions is low, the average rate of energy usage during shortening increases some 2.5-fold. A possible cause for a high chemical energy cost of external work production could be the existence of attached but non-cycling cross-bridges (81,87).

A prediction of the latch hypothesis is that dephosphorylated cross-bridges would provide an internal load on phosphorylated, cycling cross-bridges. This was tested under conditions in which the "latch" state was induced (high force with decreased maximum velocity of shortening, chemical energy usage, and myosin light chain phosphorylation), yet there was no evidence of an increase in the chemical energy cost of active external work production (92). That is, there was no energetic evidence for the dissipation of work against an internal load under conditions during which most of the force would be expected to be generated by latch-bridges. It has been shown under rather simple conditions of the *in vitro* motility assay that a population of unphosphorylated cross-bridges can act as a load on a population of cycling (thiophosphorylated) cross-bridges (96). These results were not consistent with the latch-bridge model in that the latter required the dephosphorylation of myosin cross-bridges while attached to actin. Once detached, the dephosphorylated bridges could not reattach unless phosphorylated again. Thus, detached unphosphorylated cross-bridges would presumably not interact with actin. However, recent single myosin force assays in the laser trap suggest that monomeric smooth muscle myosin is in a dynamic equilibrium between an inhibited/folded and an active/extended conformation, whereby RLC_{20} phosphorylation shifts the equilibrium to the active, force-generating state (28,97). Interestingly, for myosin molecules that have only one of their two RLC_{20} phosphorylated, a situation that most likely occurs during dephosphorylation within tissue, these singly phosphorylated myosin molecules are still capable of generating significant force (97) and thus potential contributors to the latch state.

The observation that velocity of actin filament movement in the *in vitro* motility assay depended on the ratio of phosphorylated to unphosphorylated myosin suggests that the two cross-bridge populations can interact mechanically. The experiments were also interesting in that they showed that unphosphorylated smooth muscle myosin could impede skeletal muscle myosin to a greater extent than it does phosphorylated smooth muscle myosin, strongly suggesting that smooth muscle cross-bridges spend a greater fraction of their cycle time in the strongly bound, high-force producing state than skeletal muscle cross-bridges, which was directly confirmed at the molecular level using single molecule force assays (98,99). This, together with a longer myosin filament (3), would explain the ability of smooth muscles to generate as much force as striated muscles.

ARCHITECTURE AND FUNCTION OF THE SARCOPLASMIC RETICULUM

General Properties

The sources and sinks of activator Ca^{2+} are both extracellular and intracellular and mediated by a variety of Ca^{2+} channels and pumps localized on the plasma membrane and sarcoplasmic reticulum (SR). The SR and rough ER form a continuous network (Figure 83.1) that also connects to the nuclear envelope. This continuity implies that Ca^{2+} can diffuse throughout the system. The SR/ER volume and distribution of the tubules, fenestrated sheets, and surface couplings differ in phasic and tonic SMs. The fenestrated sheets of SR (Figure 83.5) are reminiscent of the longitudinal SR encircling the A-band in striated muscles. The SR volume is 5% in large arteries and is distributed as a network throughout the cells (Figure 83.5), while phasic portal vein and taenia coli have a scanty 2% distributed around the cell periphery (101). The more extensive arterial central SR/ER is likely associated with a role in the synthesis of elastin, collagen, and glycosaminoglycans. However, even the scanty 2% volume is sufficient to maintain full size agonist-induced contractions repetitively over a 15 min period in the absence of extracellular Ca^{2+}. This provides functional evidence for an intracellular compartment capable of releasing and sequestering Ca^{2+} in SM (102). The first evidence of divalent cation transport into the SR of SM was the direct electron microscopic visualization of strontium, used as

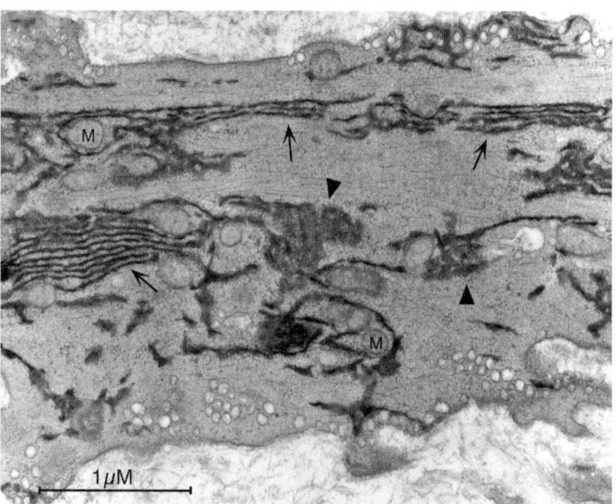

FIGURE 83.5 Sarcoplasmic reticulum network in a portion of a main pulmonary artery SM cell highlighted by staining with osmium ferricyanide. Stacks of sarcoplasmic reticulum can be easily recognized (arrows) in the central region of the cell. Arrowheads denote possible fenestrated stacks or tubules of SR viewed *en face*. SR tubules can also be seen in close apposition to mitochondria (m) and close to the plasma membrane. Note SR fenestrations surrounding caveolae. *(From Nixon et al., 1994 (100), with permission.)*

an electron opaque marker of Ca, in the lumen of the SR (103). Subsequently, using X-ray microprobe analysis to directly detect Ca, agonists were shown to release Ca from both the peripheral and central SR (102,104). Localized Ca storage, in the range of 48 mmol/kg SR dry wt in the SR/ER, is enhanced largely by Ca^{2+}-binding proteins; a cardiac-like form of calsequestrin and calreticulin with other less studied Ca^{2+}-binding proteins playing a minor role in storage (105). Calsequestrin is the major SR Ca^{2+}-binding protein in striated muscles and found in most but not all SMs (106). In the phasic vas deferens, calsequestrin is largely localized to the peripheral SR (100), suggesting accessibility of this Ca-store to excitatory signals from the plasma membrane. Ca^{2+} flow into the SR is mediated by isoforms of the ATP-driven SR/ER Ca^{2+}ATPase that pumps Ca^{2+} into the SR and contributes to the restoration and maintenance of basal sub-micromolar $[Ca^{2+}]_i$. These isoforms are also found in slow skeletal, cardiac and non-muscle cells (for review see 107). Many but not all SMs also express the SR membrane-associated protein, phospholamban (108), a cAMP-dependent target that regulates the SR Ca^{2+} pump contributing to the β-adrenergic response in the heart and thought to function in a similar fashion promoting relaxation in some SMs.

Surface Couplings: Role in Excitation–Contraction Coupling

Electromechanical coupling through changes in the membrane potential and pharmacomechanical coupling through mechanisms independent of the membrane potential (109) are the two major forms of excitation–contraction coupling in SM. Electromechanical coupling may use both Ca^{2+}-influx and Ca^{2+}-release as sources of activator Ca^{2+} and is initiated at surface couplings where SR tubules approach the plasma membrane. The narrow 12–18 nm gap between the two membrane systems is traversed by bridging structures (Figure 83.6) (101,113). The lumen of the junctional SR of SM and striated muscle contains amorphous material consisting largely of calsequestrin (100). These surface couplings are sites for excitation–contraction coupling analogous to the triad and dyad structures in skeletal and cardiac muscle as well as the surface couplings in cardiac myocytes, albeit that the bridging structures have a different periodicity in SM (114). In striated muscles the "feet" bridging the junctional gap consist of ryanodine receptors serving as Ca^{2+} release channels in the SR junctional membrane and dihydropyridine receptors in the transverse tubules or plasma membrane (see Chapter 86). In SM the identity of the bridging structures is unknown. Immunoelectron microscopy has demonstrated that both inositol 1,4,5-trisphosphate (InsP3) and ryanodine receptors (RyRs) are localized both on the peripheral and central SR (100,115) in keeping with the finding of Ca^{2+} storage and release sites in both locations. Thus, InsP3 receptors likely constitute some of the bridging structures at surface couplings. The localized sites of InsP3, RyRs and Ca^{2+} stores in the SM central SR resemble the striated muscle corbular SR (116) although a role for agonist-induced Ca^{2+}-induced Ca^{2+}-release in intact SM is not well established. Corbular SR containing Ca^{2+}, calsequestrin and RyRs consists of outpocketings of SR not associated with the cell membrane and considered to function as Ca^{2+}-induced Ca^{2+}-release sites (116). Surface couplings and central Ca^{2+}-induced Ca^{2+}-release sites with InsP3 and RyRs are good candidates for the sites of origin of Ca^{2+} sparks and Ca^{2+} waves recorded in SM cells (see Chapter 87). Store operated channels (SOCS) are also likely localized at surface couplings. High $[Ca^{2+}]$ sparks are thought to occur in the restricted junctional space between the SR and plasma membrane resulting in activation of BK_{ca} channels and hyperpolarization to modify constriction (117). The localized Ca^{2+} release at a spark may be high enough to trigger Ca^{2+}-induced Ca^{2+}-release. Caffeine releases Ca^{2+} through RyRs in SM just as in striated muscles although the role of RyRs in SM is less well established. Ca^{2+} influx can also induce Ca^{2+}-induced Ca^{2+} release consistent with this being one of the mechanisms of electromechanical coupling in SM as in cardiac muscle, reviewed in (107). On the other hand, InsP3 production can induce Ca^{2+} release independently of a change in membrane potential and this is a major mechanism of pharmacomechanical coupling induced by many physiological agonists. The generation of InsP3 from caged InsP3 was shown to precede force development unlike in skeletal muscle fibers, supporting its physiological role in SM but not skeletal muscle (118). A large fraction (1.2 ec) of the lag between agonist activation and force onset lies in the time required for InsP3 production (0.5–1.0 sec) (Figure 83.7), whereas InsP3-induced Ca^{2+} release is rapid ~30 ms (reviewed in 107). The remaining time reflects the reactions needed for RLC_{20} phosphorylation. The long lag for InsP3 generation rules it out as a messenger for electromechanical coupling where depolarization-induced rise in cytosolic Ca^{2+} occurs within a few milliseconds. Another major mechanism of pharmacomechanical coupling is through modulation of the sensitivity of the contractile apparatus through signaling pathways that alter the activities of MLCK or MLCP (reviewed in 107 and in Chapter 87). For example, agonist activation of the small GTPase RhoA and its target Rho kinase (ROCK) lead to inhibitory phosphorylation of MLCP resulting in an increase in phosphorylated RLC_{20} and an increase in force without a concomitant increase in Ca^{2+}, reviewed in (2,107). The lag phase for this Ca^{2+} sensitization pathway is several seconds occurring after Ca^{2+} has crested and

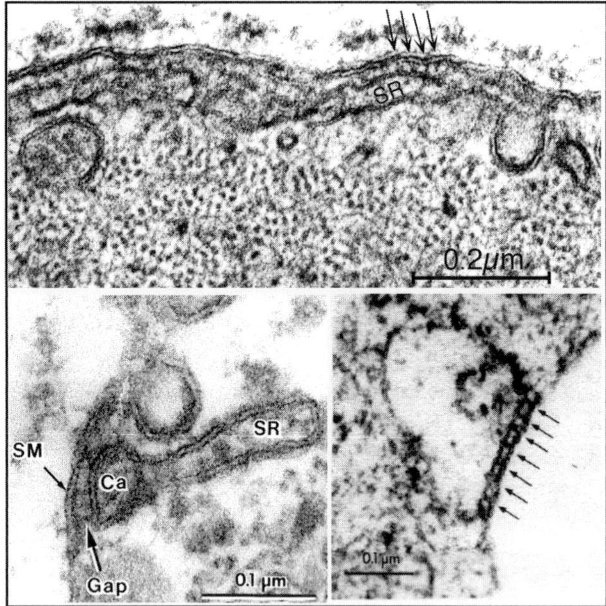

FIGURE 83.6 Typical surface coupling of sarcoplasmic reticulum (SR) in SM. Dense periodic structures (arrows) are present across the 15–20 nm junctional gap between SR and plasma membrane. Upper and lower left panels from rabbit portal vein and lower right from chicken amnion. *(From Somlyo and Somlyo, 2002 (110); Somlyo, 1985 (111); Somlyo et al., 1980 (112), respectively, with permission.)*

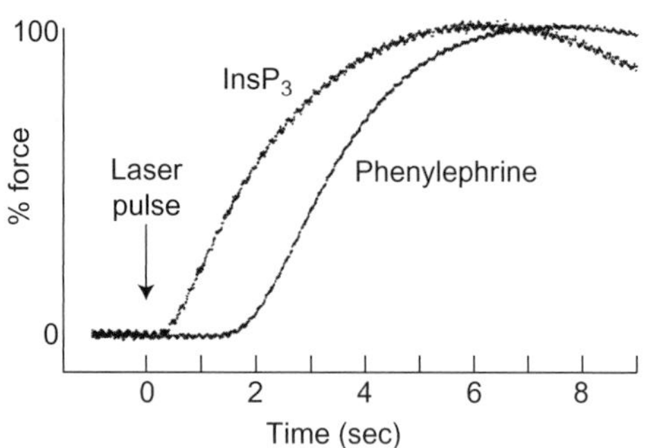

FIGURE 83.7 Force transients recorded after photolysis of caged Ins[1,4,5]P_3 in a permeabilized muscle strip and caged phenylephrine in an intact muscle strip of guinea pig portal vein at 20 °C. A 50 nsec laser pulse at 347 nm is indicated by the arrow. Lag phase preceding force development was 0.4 sec for Ins(1,4,5)P_3 and 1.8 sec for phenylephrine. The intact strip used for the caged phenylephrine experiment had been treated with 6-hydroxydopamine for 20 min to produce adrenergic denervation. This experiment was done in presence of 143 mmol/l K to depolarize the cell membrane and 50 μmol/l caged phenylephrine. Ins(1,4,5) P_3 response was obtained in a muscle strip permeabilized with 50 μg/ml saponin for 15 min, calcium loaded for 5 min, at pCa 6.6 with 10 μm caged Ins(1,4,5)P_3. Approximately 10% Ins[I,4,5]P_3 and phenylephrine were released from the caged precursors. *(From Somlyo et al., 1988 (119); Somlyo and Somlyo, 1992 (120), with permission.)*

fallen, thus, contributing to the tonic component of the contractile response evoked by agonists (121). Likewise ROCK or PKC can phosphorylate and activate CPI-17 to inhibit the catalytic subunit of MLCP (reviewed in 30). Cyclic nucleotides can activate MLCP through phosphorylation of telokin (31,122,123) or can inhibit MLCK (124) but this MLCK inhibition is not likely to occur in SM *in situ* (125). Overall, it is likely that electromechanical coupling and pharmacomechanical coupling are both important for excitation–contraction coupling and operate simultaneously with the relative contribution of each varying with different agonists and tissues. While the SR serves as an important source and sink for the control of cytosolic Ca^{2+} with contributions from plasma membrane Ca^{2+} channels, the Ca^{2+} ATPase, and the Na/Ca exchanger, other mechanisms are overlaid on this basic grid providing secondary modulation to tune the contractile response for the particular SM function.

MITOCHONDRIA

Mitochondria are mostly encircled by and in close proximity to SR/ER in SM (105) (Figure 83.5) where in some cases a gap of only 20 nm exists between the membranes of the two organelles (110). There are two views, one that high local Ca^{2+} release into this space is taken up by the low-affinity mitochondrial uniporter or the other that the high affinity SR protects the mitochondria from Ca^{2+} influx. While massive pathophysiological Ca uptake into mitochondria occurs in all types of muscle with Ca overload upon cell damage, whether mitochondria accumulate significant amounts of Ca^{2+} under physiological conditions to buffer cytosolic $[Ca^{2+}]_i$ remains debatable. It is generally agreed that in resting cells free mitochondrial Ca^{2+} $[Ca^{2+}]_{mt}$ is ~100 nM and total mitochondrial Ca is 0.4-1.0 mmol/kg mitochondrial dry wt (110) resulting in a total/free mitochondrial Ca of at least 4000:1. Published $[Ca^{2+}]_{mt}$ (measured by fluorescent indicators) of 10 μM would lead to an estimate of ~40 mmol/kg mitochondrial dry wt. This is highly unlikely considering the partial mitochondrial volume and total Ca content of SM cells and never found in normal cells. Enzymatic isolation of cells and the uncertainty of calibration of luminescent and fluorescent Ca^{2+} indicators within the mitochondrial matrix may contribute to the reported values and remain to be resolved.

SURFACE VESICLES

Surface vesicles or caveolae are flask-shaped invaginations of the plasma membrane (50–80 nm diameter) (Figure 83.6) increasing the surface area by 25–70% in SM. They are organized in longitudinal rows along the surface of the cell surrounded by a fenestration of SR tubules with dense bodies in the intervening vesicle free space (reviewed in 112). Caveolae composed of specialized protein lipid raft domains house a very large number of molecules involved in signal transduction and transport as well as the protein caveolin with its isoforms (reviewed in 126). These molecules in turn are temporarily and spatially regulated by cyclic nucleotides, Ca^{2+}, kinases, and phosphatases. Caveolin-1 has been shown to be necessary for functional InsP3R coupling to the plasma membrane and canonical transient receptor potential (TRPC3) channels necessary for cerebral arterial SMC contractility (127). Caveolin-1 knockout mice display pulmonary arterial hypertension that can be idiopathic (IPAH) or secondary to other disorders (reviewed in 126).

CONCLUSION

Overall, structure informs the function of smooth muscles and together they provide insight into the fundamental mechanisms of SM contractility opening possibilities for treatment of diseases of SM, which are a major cause of death, and for improved public health.

ACKNOWLEDGMENTS

We thank Dr David Warshaw for comments on the discussion of latch. Supported by R01GM086457-02 and R01DK088905-01 to AVS.

REFERENCES

1. Hartshorne DJ. Biochemistry of the contractile process in smooth muscle. In: Johnson LR, editor. *Physiology of the gastrointestinal tract*. 2nd ed. New York: Raven Press;1987. p. 423–82.
2. Somlyo AP, Somlyo AV. Ca^{2+} sensitivity of smooth muscle and nonmuscle myosin II: modulated by G proteins, kinases, and myosin phosphatase. *Physiol Rev* 2003;**83**:1325–58.
3. Ashton FT, Somlyo AV, Somlyo AP. The contractile apparatus of vascular smooth muscle: intermediate high voltage stereo electron microscopy. *J Mol Biol* 1975;**98**:17–29.
4. Bond M, Somlyo AV. Dense bodies and actin polarity in vertebrate smooth muscle. *J Cell Biol* 1982;**95**:403–13.
5. Devine CE, Somlyo AP. Thick filaments in vascular smooth muscle. *J Cell Biol* 1971;**49**:636–49.
6. Murphy RA, Herlihy JT, Megerman J. Force-generating capacity and contractile protein content of arterial smooth muscle. *J Gen Physiol* 1974;**64**:691–705.
7. Linke WA, Kruger M. The giant protein titin as an integrator of myocyte signaling pathways. *Physiology (Bethesda)* 2010;**25**:186–98.
8. Sanger JM, Sanger JW. The dynamic Z bands of striated muscle cells. *Sci Signal* 2008;**1**:pe37.
9. Berner PF, Somlyo AV, Somlyo AP. Hypertrophy-induced increase of intermediate filaments in vascular smooth muscle. *J Cell Biol* 1981;**88**:96–100.
10. Holmes KC, Geeves MA. The structural basis of muscle contraction. *Philos Trans R Soc Lond B Biol Sci* 2000;**355**:419–31.
11. Nabeshima Y, Nonomura Y, Fujii-Kuriyama Y. Nonmuscle and smooth muscle myosin light chain mRNAs are generated from a single gene by the tissue-specific alternative RNA splicing. *J Biol Chem* 1987;**262**:10608–12.
12. Matthew JD, Khromov AS, Trybus KM, Somlyo AP, Somlyo AV. Myosin essential light chain isoforms modulate the velocity of shortening propelled by nonphosphorylated cross-bridges. *J Biol Chem* 1998;**273**:31289–96.
13. Eddinger TJ, Meer DP. Myosin II isoforms in smooth muscle: heterogeneity and function. *Am J Physiol Cell Physiol* 2007;**293**: C493–508.
14. Somlyo AP, Devine CE, Somlyo AV. Thick filaments in unstretched mammalian smooth muscle. *Nature* 1971;**233**:218–9.
15. Somlyo AV, Butler TM, Bond M, Somlyo AP. Myosin filaments have non-phosphorylated light chains in relaxed smooth muscle. *Nature* 1981;**294**:567–9.
16. Kuo KH, Wang L, Pare PD, Ford LE, Seow CY. Myosin thick filament lability induced by mechanical strain in airway smooth muscle. *J Appl Physiol* 2001;**90**:1811–6.
17. Gautel M, Ehler E. Cell biology. Gett'N-WASP stripes. *Science* 2010;**330**:1491–2.
18. Sanger JW. Formation of synthetic myosin filaments: influence of pH, ionic strength, cation substitution, dielectric constant and method of preparation. *Cytobiologie* 1971;**4**:450–66.
19. Craig R, Megerman J. Assembly of smooth muscle myosin into side-polar filaments. *J Cell Biol* 1977;**75**:990–6.
20. Xu JQ, Harder BA, Uman P, Craig R. Myosin filament structure in vertebrate smooth muscle. *J Cell Biol* 1996;**134**:53–66.
21. Somlyo AP, Devine CE, Somlyo AV, Rice RV. Filament organization in vertebrate smooth muscle. *Philos Trans R Soc Lond B Biol Sci* 1973;**265**:223–9.
22. Trybus KM. Role of myosin light chains. *J Muscle Res Cell Motil* 1994;**15**:587–94.
23. Adelstein RS, Sellers JR. Myosin structure and function. In: Barany M, editor. *Biochemistry of smooth muscle contraction*. London: Academic Press;1996. p. 3–19.
24. Cremo CR, Sellers JR, Facemyer KC. Two heads are required for phosphorylation-dependent regulation of smooth muscle myosin. *J Biol Chem* 1995;**270**:2171–5.
25. Wendt T, Taylor D, Messier T, Trybus KM, Taylor KA. Visualization of head–head interactions in the inhibited state of smooth muscle myosin. *J Cell Biol* 1999;**147**:1385–90.
26. Lowey S, Trybus KM. Common structural motifs for the regulation of divergent class II myosins. *J Biol Chem* 2010;**285**:16403–7.
27. Somlyo AV, Goldman YE, Fujimori T, Bond M, Trentham DR, Somlyo AP. Cross-bridge kinetics, cooperativity, and negatively strained cross-bridges in vertebrate smooth muscle. A laser-flash photolysis study. *J Gen Physiol* 1988;**91**:165–92.
28. Walcott S, Warshaw DM. Modeling smooth muscle myosin's two heads: long-lived enzymatic roles and phosphorylation-dependent equilibria. *Biophys J* 2010;**99**:1129–38.
29. Khromov AS, Somlyo AV, Somlyo AP. Thiophosphorylation of myosin light chain increases rigor stiffness of rabbit smooth muscle. *J Physiol* 1998;**512**(Pt 2):345–50.
30. Eto M. Regulation of cellular protein phosphatase-1 (PP1) by phosphorylation of the CPI-17 family, C-kinase-activated PP1 inhibitors. *J Biol Chem* 2009;**284**:35273–7.

31. Khromov AS, Wang H, Choudhury N, McDuffie M, Herring BP, Nakamoto R, Owens GK, et al. Smooth muscle of telokin-deficient mice exhibits increased sensitivity to Ca^{2+} and decreased cGMP-induced relaxation. *Proc Natl Acad Sci USA* 2006;**103**:2440–5.
32. Harris DE, Warshaw DM. Smooth and skeletal muscle actin are mechanically indistinguishable in the in vitro motility assay. *Circ Res* 1993;**72**:219–24.
33. Vandekerckhove J, Weber K. Mammalian cytoplasmic actins are the products of at least two genes and differ in primary structure in at least 25 identified positions from skeletal muscle actins. *Proc Natl Acad Sci USA* 1978;**75**:1106–10.
34. Fatigati V, Murphy RA. Actin and tropomyosin variants in smooth muscles. Dependence on tissue type. *J Biol Chem* 1984;**259**:14383–8.
35. Drew JS, Murphy RA. Actin isoform expression, cellular heterogeneity, and contractile function in smooth muscle. *Can J Physiol Pharmacol* 1997;**75**:869–77.
36. Perrin BJ, Ervasti JM. The actin gene family: function follows isoform. *Cytoskeleton (Hoboken)* 2010;**67**:630–4.
37. Gabbiani G, Kocher O, Bloom WS, Vandekerckhove J, Weber K. Actin expression in smooth muscle cells of rat aortic intimal thickening, human atheromatous plaque, and cultured rat aortic media. *J Clin Invest* 1984;**73**:148–52.
38. Schildmeyer LA, Braun R, Taffet G, Debiasi M, Burns AE, Bradley A, et al. Impaired vascular contractility and blood pressure homeostasis in the smooth muscle alpha-actin null mouse. *FASEB J* 2000;**14**:2213–20.
39. Ebashi S. Third component participating in the superprecipitation of 'natural actomyosin'. *Nature* 1963;**200**:1010.
40. Vibert PJ, Haselgrove JC, Lowy J, Poulsen FR. Structural changes in actin-containing filaments of muscle. *J Mol Biol* 1972;**71**:757–67.
41. Marston S, El-Mezgueldi M. Role of tropomyosin in the regulation of contraction in smooth muscle. *Adv Exp Med Biol* 2008;**644**:110–23.
42. Pfitzer G, Schroeter M, Hasse V, Ma J, Rosgen KH, Rosgen S, et al. Is myosin phosphorylation sufficient to regulate smooth muscle contraction? *Adv Exp Med Biol* 2005;**565**:319–28; discussion **328**:405–15.
43. Yamakita Y, Oosawa F, Yamashiro S, Matsumura F. Caldesmon inhibits Arp2/3-mediated actin nucleation. *J Biol Chem* 2003;**278**:17937–44.
44. Winder SJ, Walsh MP. Smooth muscle calponin. Inhibition of actomyosin MgATPase and regulation by phosphorylation. *J Biol Chem* 1990;**265**:10148–55.
45. Makuch R, Birukov K, Shirinsky V, Dabrowska R. Functional interrelationship between calponin and caldesmon. *Biochem J* 1991;**280**(Pt 1):33–8.
46. Takahashi K, Abe M, Hiwada K, Kokubu T. A novel troponin T-like protein (calponin) in vascular smooth muscle: interaction with tropomyosin paracrystals. *J Hypertens Suppl* 1988;**6**:S40–3.
47. Jin JP, Walsh MP, Resek ME, McMartin GA. Expression and epitopic conservation of calponin in different smooth muscles and during development. *Biochem Cell Biol* 1996;**74**:187–96.
48. Matthew JD, Khromov AS, McDuffie MJ, Somlyo AV, Somlyo AP, Taniguchi S, et al. Contractile properties and proteins of smooth muscles of a calponin knockout mouse. *J Physiol* 2000;**529**(Pt 3):811–24.
49. Wu KC, Jin JP. Calponin in non-muscle cells. *Cell Biochem Biophys* 2008;**52**:139–48.
50. Mack CP, Somlyo AV, Hautmann M, Somlyo AP, Owens GK. Smooth muscle differentiation marker gene expression is regulated by RhoA-mediated actin polymerization. *J Biol Chem* 2001;**276**:341–7.
51. Miralles F, Posern G, Zaromytidou AI, Treisman R. Actin dynamics control SRF activity by regulation of its coactivator MAL. *Cell* 2003;**113**:329–42.
52. Wang Z, Wang DZ, Hockemeyer D, McAnally J, Nordheim A, Olson EN. Myocardin and ternary complex factors compete for SRF to control smooth muscle gene expression. *Nature* 2004;**428**:185–9.
53. Jin L, Gan Q, Zieba BJ, Goicoechea SM, Owens GK, Otey CA, et al. The actin associated protein palladin is important for the early smooth muscle cell differentiation. *PLoS One* 2010;**5**: e12823.
54. Vartiainen MK, Guettler S, Larijani B, Treisman R. Nuclear actin regulates dynamic subcellular localization and activity of the SRF cofactor MAL. *Science* 2007;**316**:1749–52.
55. Cornelius F, Lowy J. Tension-length behaviour of a molluscan smooth muscle related to filament organisation. *Acta Physiol Scand* 1978;**102**:167–80.
56. Gordon AR, Siegman MJ. Mechanical properties of smooth muscle. I. Length-tension and force-velocity relations. *Am J Physiol* 1971;**221**:1243–9.
57. Gordon AM, Huxley AF, Julian FJ. The variation in isometric tension with sarcomere length in vertebrate muscle fibres. *J Physiol* 1966;**184**:170–92.
58. Paul RJ. Chemical energetics of vascular smooth muscle. In: Bohr DF, Somlyo AP, Sparks HV, editors. *Handbook of physiology: The cardiovascular system*, Vol. II. Bethesda, MD: American Physiological Society;1980. p. 201–35.
59. Meiss RA. Dynamic stiffness of rabbit mesotubarium smooth muscle: effect of isometric length. *Am J Physiol* 1978;**234**: C14–26.
60. Siegman MJ, Butler TM, Mooers SU. Energetic, mechanical and ultrastructural correlates of the length-tension relationship in smooth muscle. In: Stephens NL, editor. *Smooth muscle contraction*. New York: Marcel Dekker;1984. p. 189–98.
61. Fay FS, Delise CM. Contraction of isolated smooth muscle cells – structural changes. *Proc Natl Acad Sci USA* 1973;**70**:641–5.
62. Katsuda S, Okada Y, Minamoto T, Oda Y, Matsui Y, Nakanishi I. Collagens in human atherosclerosis. Immunohistochemical analysis using collagen type-specific antibodies. *Arterioscler Thromb* 1992;**12**:494–502.
63. Siegman MJ, Butler TM, Mooers SU, Trinkle-Mulcahy L, Narayan S, Adam L, et al. Hypertrophy of colonic smooth muscle: contractile proteins, shortening velocity, and regulation. *Am J Physiol* 1997;**272**:G1571–80.
64. Siegman MJ, Butler TM, Mooers SU, Trinkle-Mulcahy L, Narayan S, Stirewalt WS, et al. Hypertrophy of colonic smooth muscle: structural remodeling, chemical composition, and force output. *Am J Physiol* 1997;**272**:G1560–70.
65. Hill AV. The heat of shortening and the dynamic constants of muscle. *Proc. R. Soc. Lond. B* 1938;**126**:136–95.
66. Warshaw DM. Force: velocity relationship in single isolated toad stomach smooth muscle cells. *J Gen Physiol* 1987;**89**:771–89.

67. Butler TM, Siegman MJ, Mooers SU, Davies RE. Chemical energetics of single isometric tetani in mammalian smooth muscle. *Am J Physiol* 1978;**235**:C1–7.
68. Barany M. ATPase activity of myosin correlated with speed of muscle shortening. *J Gen Physiol* 1967;**Suppl:197-218**:50.
69. Kushmerick MJ, Davies RE. The chemical energetics of muscle contraction. II. The chemistry, efficiency and power of maximally working sartorius muscles. Free energy and enthalpy of ATP hydrolysis in the sarcoplasm. *Proc R Soc Lond B Biol Sci* 1969;**174**:315–53.
70. Wilkie DR. The mechanical properties of muscle. *Br Med Bull* 1956;**12**:177–82.
71. Edman KA. The velocity of unloaded shortening and its relation to sarcomere length and isometric force in vertebrate muscle fibres. *J Physiol* 1979;**291**:143–59.
72. Siegman MJ, Butler TM, Mooers SU, Davies RE. Chemical energetics of force development, force maintenance, and relaxation in mammalian smooth muscle. *J Gen Physiol* 1980;**76**:609–29.
73. Persechini A, Hartshorne DJ. Phosphorylation of smooth muscle myosin: evidence for cooperativity between the myosin heads. *Science* 1981;**213**:1383–5.
74. Vyas TB, Mooers SU, Narayan SR, Siegman MJ, Butler TM. Cross-bridge cycling at rest and during activation. Turnover of myosin-bound ADP in permeabilized smooth muscle. *J Biol Chem* 1994;**269**:7316–22.
75. Vyas TB, Mooers SU, Narayan SR, Witherell JC, Siegman MJ, Butler TM. Cooperative activation of myosin by light chain phosphorylation in permeabilized smooth muscle. *Am J Physiol* 1992;**263**:C210–9.
76. Ruegg JC. Smooth muscle tone. *Physiol Rev* 1971;**51**:201–48.
77. Butler TM, Davies RE. High-energy phosphates in smooth muscle. In: Bohr DF, Somlyo AP, Sparks HV, editors. *Handbook of physiology: The cardiovascular system*, Vol. II. Bethesda, MD: American Physiological Society;1980. p. 237–52.
78. Baguet F, Gillis JM. Energy cost of tonic contraction in a lamellibranch catch muscle. *J Physiol* 1968;**198**:127–43.
79. Butler TM, Siegman MJ. Mechanism of catch force: tethering of thick and thin filaments by twitchin. *J Biomed Biotechnol* 2010;**2010**:725207.
80. Somlyo AP, Somlyo AV. Active state and catch-like state in rabbit main pulmonary artery. *J Gen Physiol* 1967;**50**:168–9.
81. Dillon PF, Aksoy MO, Driska SP, Murphy RA. Myosin phosphorylation and the cross-bridge cycle in arterial smooth muscle. *Science* 1981;**211**:495–7.
82. Driska SP. High myosin light chain phosphatase activity in arterial smooth muscle: Can it explain the latch phenomenon? In: Siegman MJ, Somlyo AP, Stephens NL, editors. *Regulation and contraction of smooth muscle*. New York: Alan R. Liss;1987. p. 387–99.
83. Hai CM, Murphy RA. Cross-bridge phosphorylation and regulation of latch state in smooth muscle. *Am J Physiol* 1988;**254**: C99–106.
84. Butler TM, Siegman MJ, Mooers SU. Chemical energy usage during shortening and work production in mammalian smooth muscle. *Am J Physiol* 1983;**244**:C234–42.
85. Butler TM, Siegman MJ, Mooers SU, Narayan SR. Myosin-product complex in the resting state and during relaxation of smooth muscle. *Am J Physiol* 1990;**258**:C1092–9.
86. Siegman MJ, Butler TM, Mooers SU, Davies RE. Mechanical and energetic correlates of isometric relaxation. In: Casteels R, Godfraind T, Ruegg JC, editors. *Excitation–contraction coupling in smooth muscle*. Amsterdam: Elsevier/North-Holland;1977. p. 449–53.
87. Siegman MJ, Butler TM, Mooers SU, Davies RE. Crossbridge attachment, resistance to stretch, and viscoelasticity in resting mammalian smooth muscle. *Science* 1976;**191**:383–5.
88. Curtin NA, Woledge RC. Energetics of relaxation in frog muscle. *J Physiol* 1974;**238**:437–46.
89. Hai CM, Murphy RA. Ca^{2+}, crossbridge phosphorylation, and contraction. *Annu Rev Physiol* 1989;**51**:285–98.
90. Haeberle JR, Hott JW, Hathaway DR. Regulation of isometric force and isotonic shortening velocity by phosphorylation of the 20,000 dalton myosin light chain of rat uterine smooth muscle. *Pflugers Arch* 1985;**403**:215–9.
91. Siegman MJ, Butler TM, Mooers SU, Michalek A. Ca^{2+} can affect Vmax without changes in myosin light chain phosphorylation in smooth muscle. *Pflugers Arch* 1984;**401**:385–90.
92. Butler TM, Siegman MJ, Mooers SU. Slowing of cross-bridge cycling in smooth muscle without evidence of an internal load. *Am J Physiol* 1986;**251**:C945–50.
93. Moreland S, Moreland RS. Effects of dihydropyridines on stress, myosin phosphorylation, and V0 in smooth muscle. *Am J Physiol* 1987;**252**:H1049–58.
94. Jiang MJ, Morgan KG. Agonist-specific myosin phosphorylation and intracellular calcium during isometric contractions of arterial smooth muscle. *Pflugers Arch* 1989;**413**:637–43.
95. Fenn WO. A quantitative comparison between the energy liberated and the work performed by the isolated sartorius muscle of the frog. *J Physiol* 1923;**58**:175–203.
96. Warshaw DM, Desrosiers JM, Work SS, Trybus KM. Smooth muscle myosin cross-bridge interactions modulate actin filament sliding velocity in vitro. *J Cell Biol* 1990;**111**:453–63.
97. Walcott S, Fagnant PM, Trybus KM, Warshaw DM. Smooth muscle heavy meromyosin phosphorylated on one of its two heads supports force and motion. *J Biol Chem* 2009;**284**:18244–51.
98. Guilford WH, Dupuis DE, Kennedy G, Wu J, Patlak JB, Warshaw DM. Smooth muscle and skeletal muscle myosins produce similar unitary forces and displacements in the laser trap. *Biophys J* 1997;**72**:1006–21.
99. VanBuren P, Work SS, Warshaw DM. Enhanced force generation by smooth muscle myosin in vitro. *Proc Natl Acad Sci USA* 1994;**91**:202–5.
100. Nixon GF, Mignery GA, Somlyo AV. Immunogold localization of inositol 1,4,5-trisphosphate receptors and characterization of ultrastructural features of the sarcoplasmic reticulum in phasic and tonic smooth muscle. *J Muscle Res Cell Motil* 1994;**15**:682–700.
101. Devine CE, Somlyo AV, Somlyo AP. Sarcoplasmic reticulum and excitation-contraction coupling in mammalian smooth muscles. *J Cell Biol* 1972;**52**:690–718.
102. Bond M, Kitazawa T, Somlyo AP, Somlyo AV. Release and recycling of calcium by the sarcoplasmic reticulum in guinea-pig portal vein smooth muscle. *J Physiol* 1984;**355**:677–95.
103. Somlyo AV, Somlyo AP. Strontium accumulation by sarcoplasmic reticulum and mitochondria in vascular smooth muscle. *Science* 1971;**174**:955–8.

104. Kowarski D, Shuman H, Somlyo AP, Somlyo AV. Calcium release by noradrenaline from central sarcoplasmic reticulum in rabbit main pulmonary artery smooth muscle. *J Physiol* 1985;**366**:153–75.
105. Milner RE, Famulski KS, Michalak M. Calcium binding proteins in the sarcoplasmic/endoplasmic reticulum of muscle and non-muscle cells. *Mol Cell Biochem* 1992;**112**:1–13.
106. Raeymaekers L, Verbist J, Wuytack F, Plessers L, Casteels R. Expression of Ca^{2+} binding proteins of the sarcoplasmic reticulum of striated muscle in the endoplasmic reticulum of pig smooth muscles. *Cell Calcium* 1993;**14**:581–9.
107. Somlyo AP, Somlyo AV. Signal transduction and regulation in smooth muscle. *Nature* 1994;**372**:231–6.
108. Raeymaekers L, Jones LR. Evidence for the presence of phospholamban in the endoplasmic reticulum of smooth muscle. *Biochim Biophys Acta* 1986;**882**:258–65.
109. Somlyo AV, Somlyo AP. Electromechanical and pharmacomechanical coupling in vascular smooth muscle. *J Pharmacol Exp Ther* 1968;**159**:129–45.
110. Somlyo AP, Somlyo AV. The sarcoplasmic reticulum: then and now. *Novartis Found Symp* 2002;**246**:258–71.
111. Somlyo AP. The messenger across the gap. *Nature* 1985;**316**:298–9.
112. Somlyo AV. Ultrastructure of vascular smooth muscle. In: Bohr DF, Somlyo AP, Sparks HV, editors. *Handbook of physiology: The cardiovascular system*, Vol. II. Bethesda, MD: American Physiological Society;1980. p. 33–67.
113. Somlyo AV. Bridging structures spanning the junctioning gap at the triad of skeletal muscle. *J Cell Biol* 1979;**80**:743–50.
114. Somlyo AV, Franzini-Armstrong C. New views of smooth muscle structure using freezing, deep-etching and rotary shadowing. *Experientia* 1985;**41**:841–56.
115. Lesh RE, Nixon GF, Fleischer S, Airey JA, Somlyo AP, Somlyo AV. Localization of ryanodine receptors in smooth muscle. *Circ Res* 1998;**82**:175–85.
116. Jorgensen AO, Shen AC, Arnold W, McPherson PS, Campbell KP. The Ca^{2+}-release channel/ryanodine receptor is localized in junctional and corbular sarcoplasmic reticulum in cardiac muscle. *J Cell Biol* 1993;**120**:969–80.
117. Nelson MT, Cheng H, Rubart M, Santana LF, Bonev AD, Knot HJ, et al. Relaxation of arterial smooth muscle by calcium sparks. *Science* 1995;**270**:633–7.
118. Walker JW, Somlyo AV, Goldman YE, Somlyo AP, Trentham DR. Kinetics of smooth and skeletal muscle activation by laser pulse photolysis of caged inositol 1,4,5-trisphosphate. *Nature* 1987;**327**:249–52.
119. Somlyo AP, Walker JW, Goldman YE, Trentham DR, Kobayashi S, Kitazawa T, et al. Inositol trisphosphate, calcium and muscle contraction. *Philos Trans R Soc Lond B Biol Sci* 1988;**320**:399–414.
120. Somlyo AP, Somlyo AV. Smooth muscle structure and function. In: Fozzard HA, editor. *The heart and cardiovascular system*. 2nd ed. New York: Raven Press;1992. p. 1295–324.
121. Fujihara H, Walker LA, Gong MC, Lemichez E, Boquet P, Somlyo AV, et al. Inhibition of RhoA translocation and calcium sensitization by in vivo ADP-ribosylation with the chimeric toxin DC3B. *Mol Biol Cell* 1997;**8**:2437–47.
122. Wu X, Haystead TA, Nakamoto RK, Somlyo AV, Somlyo AP. Acceleration of myosin light chain dephosphorylation and relaxation of smooth muscle by telokin. Synergism with cyclic nucleotide-activated kinase. *J Biol Chem* 1998;**273**:11362–9.
123. Wu X, Somlyo AV, Somlyo AP. Cyclic GMP-dependent stimulation reverses G-protein-coupled inhibition of smooth muscle myosin light chain phosphate. *Biochem Biophys Res Commun* 1996;**220**:658–63.
124. Conti MA, Adelstein RS. The relationship between calmodulin binding and phosphorylation of smooth muscle myosin kinase by the catalytic subunit of 3':5' cAMP-dependent protein kinase. *J Biol Chem* 1981;**256**:3178–81.
125. Stull JT, Hsu LC, Tansey MG, Kamm KE. Myosin light chain kinase phosphorylation in tracheal smooth muscle. *J Biol Chem* 1990;**265**:16683–90.
126. Insel PA, Patel HH. Membrane rafts and caveolae in cardiovascular signaling. *Curr Opin Nephrol Hypertens* 2009;**18**:50–6.
127. Adebiyi A, Narayanan D, Jaggar JH. Caveolin-1 assembles type 1 inositol 1,4,5-trisphosphate receptors and canonical transient receptor potential 3 channels into a functional signaling complex in arterial smooth muscle cells. *J Biol Chem* 2011;**286**:4341–8.

Chapter 84

Potassium, Sodium, and Chloride Channels in Smooth Muscle Cells

Keshari M. Thakali, Asif R. Pathan, Sujay V. Kharade and Nancy J. Rusch
Department of Pharmacology and Toxicology, College of Medicine, University of Arkansas for Medical Sciences, Little Rock, AR

INTRODUCTION

The plasma membrane of a vascular smooth muscle cell (SMC) expresses unique populations of K^+ channels, and the K^+ currents generated by these channels regulate electromechanical coupling and contraction of the blood vessel wall. The opening of K^+ channels in the SMCs results in K^+ efflux, and this hyperpolarizing current contributes to the resting membrane potential (E_m) of the SMC and promotes vasodilation. Multiple types of K^+ channels often work in concert to regulate the level of resting E_m and to establish excitation patterns in a single SMC. Additionally, the vascular SMCs can form electrical syncytia with adjacent endothelial cells to establish an optimal level of tone in the blood vessel wall that, under normal circumstances, will permit tissues to be perfused commensurate with their needs.

This chapter primarily focuses on the structure and physiological role of K^+ channels in vascular SMCs. Two other types of ion channels, the voltage-gated Na^+ channel and the Cl^- channels, also are considered since there is growing evidence for their role in regulating vascular tone. Finally, a short mention of these ion channels in the respiratory and gastrointestinal (GI) tracts is included to extend the discussion to non-vascular SMCs. Notably, the ion channel families discussed here (Figure 84.1) interact extensively with the Ca^{2+}-permeable channels discussed elsewhere in this book. In particular, the intracellular Ca^{2+} contributed by Ca^{2+}-permeable channels can bind to K^+ and Cl^- channels to dramatically alter their activity. Ultimately, a complex interaction between hundreds of ion channel subunits and signaling molecules will help to finely tune the level of excitability and contraction in SMC-containing organs.

POTASSIUM CHANNELS

Under resting conditions, K^+ efflux across the plasma membrane is the primary driving force that confers a negative level of membrane potential (E_m) to the SMCs of the blood vessel wall. There are several unique characteristics that distinguish the electrical properties of vascular SMCs from those of striated muscle cells. First, the range of resting E_m in vascular SMCs is generally between −60 mV and −35 mV, which is considerably more depolarized than the E_m range between −90 mV and −70 mV generally observed in cardiac and skeletal muscle cells. Importantly, the more positive resting E_m of the SMCs is near or even resides within the lower E_m range for opening of voltage-gated Ca^{2+} channels. Thus, the level of E_m in SMCs is regarded as the primary determinant of contraction because even small reductions in E_m corresponding to SMC depolarization will result in the opening of voltage-gated Ca^{2+} channels, Ca^{2+} influx, and SMC activation. Second, vascular SMCs rely more predominantly than striated muscle on the inhibition of resting K^+ efflux for depolarization, because the plasma membrane of SMCs often lacks the dense expression of fast Na^+ channels that mediate the initial excitatory inward current in cardiac and skeletal myocytes. Finally, SMCs appear to be electrically coupled to adjacent endothelial cells that line the blood vessel lumen by gap junction proteins, permitting ionic crosstalk between these two cell types to coordinate electrical events and the level of excitability within the blood vessel wall. In healthy individuals, the endothelial cells exert a hyperpolarizing effect on the vascular SMCs that promotes vasodilation and blood flow to distal tissues.

Voltage-Gated K^+ Channels

The voltage-gated K^+ (K_v) channels are multi-protein complexes that share the common properties of K^+ selectivity and voltage-dependent activation. More than 40 mammalian genes encode the pore-forming α subunits of K_v channels, which are the transmembrane proteins that mediate conduction of K^+ across the plasma membrane (1). Structurally, these α-subunits contain six transmembrane

Muscle. DOI: http://dx.doi.org/10.1016/B978-0-12-381510-1.00084-3

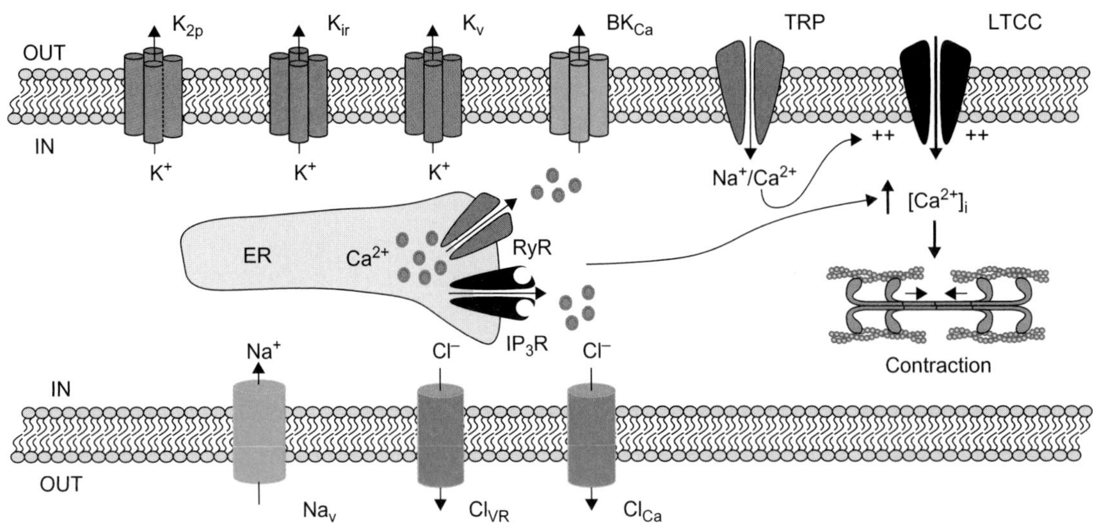

FIGURE 84.1 Ion channels in vascular SMCs. The K^+ channels include the two pore domain (K_{2P}), inwardly rectifying (K_{ir}), voltage-gated (K_v) and high-conductance, Ca^{2+}-sensitive (BK_{Ca}) K^+ channels. Voltage-gated Na^+ (Na_v) channels, volume-regulated Cl^- (Cl_{VR}) channels and Ca^{2+}-sensitive Cl^- (Cl_{Ca}) channels also are expressed. These K^+ channels interact with the ryanodine receptors (RyR), inositol triphosphate receptors (IP_3R), transient receptor potential (TRP) channels and L-type Ca^{2+} channels (LTCC) to modulate SMC excitability.

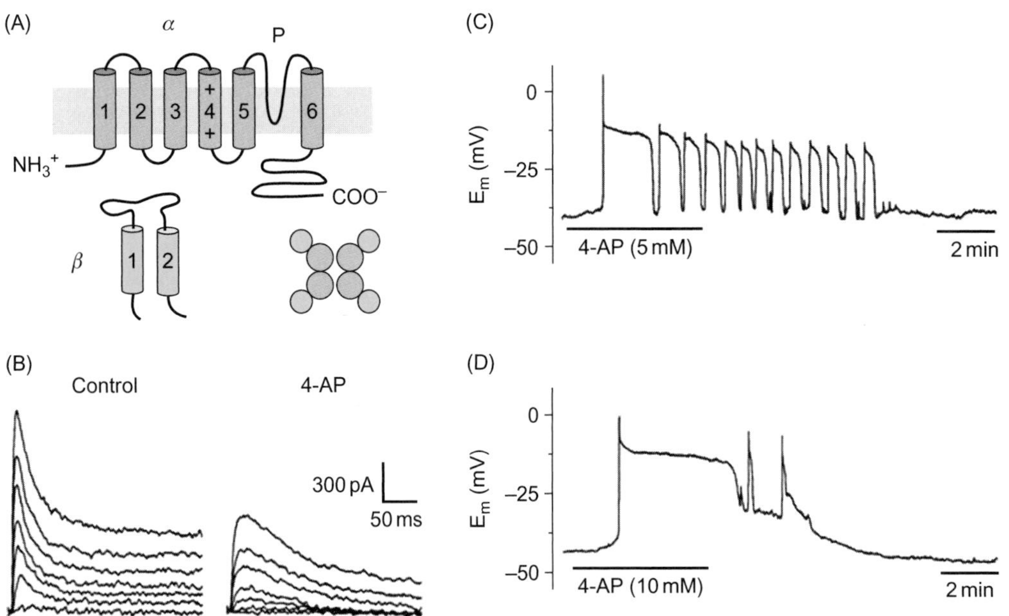

FIGURE 84.2 Voltage-gated (K_v) channels. (A) Topology of the K_v channel. Four α- and β-subunits compose the multi-protein channel (inset). The β-subunit is assumed to be intracellular. (B) 4-Aminopyridine (4-AP, 10 mM) exerts a blocking effect on whole-cell K_v channel currents. (C,D) Effect of 4-AP on the resting E_m of current-clamped rat pulmonary SMCs. Bath application of 5 mM 4-AP in (C) resulted in depolarizing spikes; addition of 10 mM 4-AP in (D) caused a profound steady-state depolarization. *(Panels B, C, and D reproduced from Yuan, 1995 (2), with permission.)*

segments (S1–S6) flanked by amino- and carboxyl-termini located in the cell interior (Figure 84.2A). Domains S1 to S4 form the voltage sensor that confers "voltage sensitivity" to the K_v channel and enables its opening in response to membrane depolarization; the S5 and S6 domains form the channel pore. Four α-subunits emanating from the same or different isoforms of the same gene family form the tetrameric pore complex. The "mixing and matching" of α-subunits creates diverse populations of K_v channels with different biophysical properties and responses to intracellular signaling molecules and pharmacological modulators. Some degree of channel inhibition is usually conferred by 4-aminopyridine (4-AP), and this drug is often used as a screening tool to detect functional K_v channels in SMCs (Figure 84.2B) (1,2). An additional level of complexity is introduced by the ability of the α-subunits to bind regulatory β-subunits (Figure 84.2A), which can interact with the cytoplasmic domains of the α-subunit to modify cell surface expression and alter channel gating (3). Several β-subunit genes have been detected in vascular SMCs, but their role in regulating the expression and behavior of K_v channels is poorly understood.

The complex structure of the K_v channels has thwarted efforts to identify their molecular composition. Tens of transcripts encoding the α-subunits have been detected in different vascular beds, but the number of functional proteins appears much lower. For example, only several α isoforms arising from the *Shaker*-related (K_v1) gene have been confirmed to form functional K_v channels in rat cerebral, pulmonary, and renal arteries, and in rabbit portal vein, despite the detection of many K_v1 transcripts in SMCs (4–7). In the SMCs of the rat cerebral and pulmonary circulation, α-subunits from the *Shab*-related (K_v2) gene family also may form functional channels (7,8). These α-subunits may co-assemble with K_v5 to K_v9 family members, that cannot alone form K_v channel pores, to provide unique populations of oxygen-sensitive K^+ channels in pulmonary SMCs. Regardless of their molecular composition, it is well established that K_v channels contribute importantly to the resting E_m and diameter of SMCs in the small arteries and arterioles of many vascular beds. During excitation of the SMCs, the voltage-dependent opening of the K_v channels mediates a compensatory hyperpolarizing current that closes voltage-gated Ca^{2+} channels to buffer vasoconstriction. For example, pharmacological block of the K_v channels in the SMCs of the rat pulmonary circulation by 4-AP (5 mM) results in a profound loss of resting E_m and the induction of an abnormal oscillating E_m pattern (Figure 84.2C). A higher concentration of 4-AP (10 mM) establishes a sustained and profound depolarization of the SMCs (Figure 84.2D) (2). Similar excitatory responses occur in response to block of K_v channels in the SMCs of many other vascular preparations. Not surprisingly considering their important dilator function, a loss of K_v channels has been observed in pathologies of elevated vascular tone (9–11). Thus, the K_v channels broadly mediate vasodilation in many vascular beds and may play a critical role in buffering abnormal vascular tone.

High-Conductance, Calcium-Sensitive K^+ (BK_{Ca}) Channels

The high-conductance, Ca^{2+}-sensitive K^+ channels are often referred to as "Maxi-K" or "Big K" (BK_{Ca}) channels to recognize their high single-channel conductance (200–300 pS), which may be 10-fold higher than the current amplitudes generated by K_v channels. Thus, the opening of BK_{Ca} channels unleashes a powerful hyperpolarizing force in vascular SMCs. As reviewed elsewhere in detail (12), the pore-forming α-subunit shows partial homology with the K_v channels in six (S1–S6) of its seven (S0–S6) transmembrane domains that confer voltage-sensitivity and pore-formation (Figure 84.3A). However, the additional property of Ca^{2+}-sensitivity (Figure 84.3B) is conferred by four intracellular domains (S7–S10) and by the interaction of a unique extracellular N-terminus with a β_1-subunit. Unlike the α-subunits of K_v channels that originate from multiple gene families, BK_{Ca} channels appear to arise from a single *hSlo* gene, although phenotypic diversity is generated by a high level of alternative splicing. Iberiotoxin, a scorpion toxin, selectively blocks BK_{Ca} channels when applied to the external membrane surface.

The BK_{Ca} channels are densely expressed in vascular SMCs, and are particularly evident in the small arteries and arterioles of the cerebral, coronary, and renal circulations. These vessels show a high level of pressure-induced depolarization and constriction ("myogenic" tone). The depolarizing response to pressure in these SMCs coupled to rises in intracellular Ca^{2+} act synergistically to activate the BK_{Ca} channels, which in turn, act as a biological brake to buffer further depolarization and SMC activation. The BK_{Ca} channels in some SMCs appear to be in close proximity to the IP_3Rs and RyRs in the sarcoplasmic reticulum, and the Ca^{2+} released by the RyRs is a powerful stimulus for the opening of BK_{Ca} channels (Figure 84.3C) (13). Accordingly, deletion of the *hSlo* gene that encodes the pore-forming α-subunit of the BK_{Ca} channel results in a loss of membrane hyperpolarizing spontaneous K^+ outward currents (Figure 84.3D) and a significant blood pressure elevation associated with increased vascular tone and endocrine abnormalities (14). Similarly, disruption of the BK_{Ca} channel β_1 subunit gene in mice that compromises the Ca^{2+}-sensitivity of the BK_{Ca} channel is associated with arterial activation and blood pressure elevation (15). Conversely, genetic epidemiological studies suggest that a gain-of-function BK_{Ca} channel β_1-subunit variant in humans that promotes BK_{Ca} channel activity appears to protect against diastolic hypertension (16). Thus, the BK_{Ca} channel appears to be a powerful dilator influence that regulates organ blood flow, peripheral vascular resistance, and systemic blood pressure.

Inwardly Rectifying K^+ (K_{ir}) Channels

The inwardly rectifying K^+ (K_{ir}) channels share the property of "inward rectification", indicating that they conduct inward K^+ current more readily than outward K^+ current.

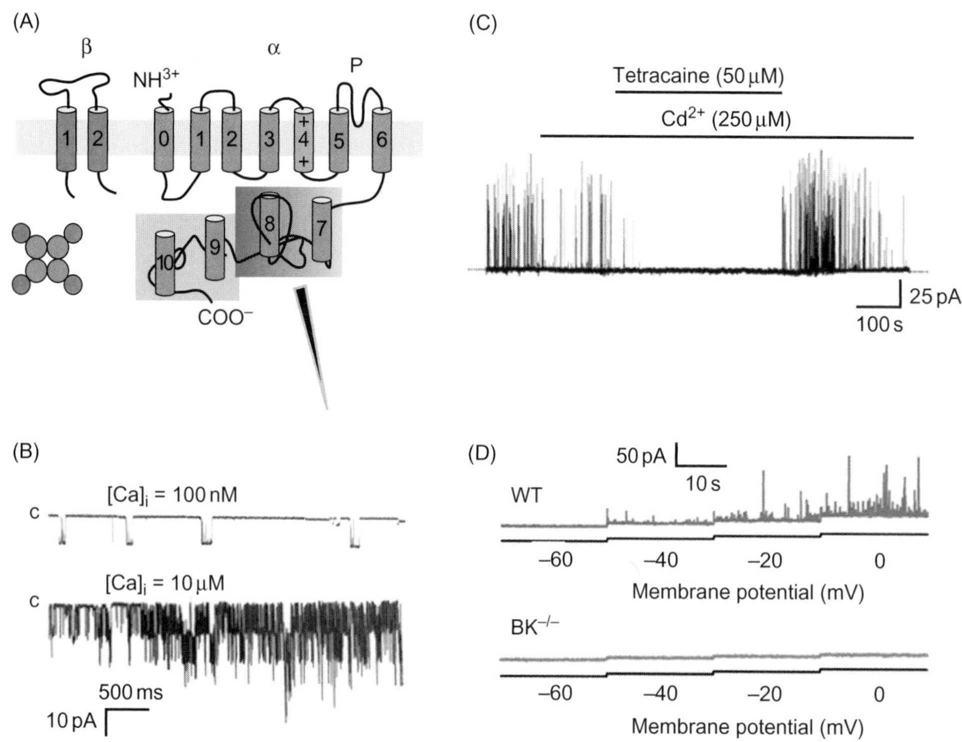

FIGURE 84.3 **High-conductance, Ca^{2+}-activated K^+ (BK_{Ca}) channels.** (A) The BK_{Ca} channel topology. The α-subunit assembles as a tetramer (inset) associated with β-subunits that may be membrane delineated. (B) Increasing the Ca^{2+} concentration from 100 nM to 10 μM at the cytosolic surface of an inside-out patch of rat cerebral SMC results in profound activation of BK_{Ca} channels. Patch potential was −40 mV; c = channel closed state. (C) Spontaneous outward currents mediated by BKCa channels in a patch-clamped rat cerebral SMC. BK_{Ca} currents persisted in the presence of cadmium (Cd^{2+}), an inorganic blocker of voltage-gated Ca^{2+} channels. The currents were inhibited when ryanodine receptors were blocked by tetracaine. (D) BK_{Ca} channel currents in cerebral SMCs of wild-type (WT) mice increase in response to depolarization. The currents were absent in SMCs of $BK^{-/-}$ mice. *(Panel C reproduced from Cheranov and Jaggar, 2002 (13), with permission; panel D reproduced from Sausbier et al., 2005 (14), with permission.)*

Another key property is that their single-channel conductance rises in response to elevations of extracellular K^+. As reviewed by others (17), the pore-forming α-subunit of the K_{ir} channel has a unique membrane topology of only two transmembrane regions (M1 and M2) linked by a pore-forming loop (Figure 84.4A). Similar to the K_v and BK_{Ca} channels, four α-subunits from the same gene family ($K_{ir}2$) assemble to form the channel pore. Inward rectification is at least partially conferred by channel block from intracellular Mg^{2+} and polyamines at specific residues located in the M2 domain and carboxyl-terminal regions of the channel. Another gene family of K_{ir} channels, $K_{ir}6$, can associate with membrane-delineated sulphonylurea receptors (SUR) that contain binding sites for adenosine triphosphate (ATP) (Figure 84.4B) (18). The resulting "ATP-sensitive K^+ (K_{ATP}) channels" close as intracellular ATP rises, resulting in the depolarization of energy-replete SMCs that can enact vasoconstriction. Currents attributed to K_{ATP} channels have been detected in the SMCs of skeletal muscle arterioles and other resistance arteries using pharmacological approaches, and appear to contribute importantly to resting E_m and diameter of these microvessels (19).

In contrast, the absence of selective pharmacological blockers for the prototypical K_{ir} channels has hampered efforts to define their role in regulating vascular tone. Although the K_{ir} channels are blocked by micromolar concentrations of barium (Ba^{2+}), this inorganic cation also can interfere with other ionic processes. With this caveat in mind, K_{ir} channels have been described in SMCs from a number of arterial sites and may be active under some conditions. For example, channel block by Ba^{2+} has been demonstrated to depolarize rat cerebral SMCs with the biggest effect at more negative resting E_m levels (Figure 84.4C) (20). A corresponding vasoconstriction ensues that is proportional to the loss of resting E_m (Figure 84.4D). Additionally, the K_{ir} channels may act as metabolic sensors, because their single-channel conductance increases as a function of the extracellular K^+ concentration ($[K_o]$). Thus, small elevations of $[K_o]$ may enhance K^+ efflux through K_{ir} channels resulting in a Ba^{2+}-sensitive hyperpolarization and relaxation. Indeed,

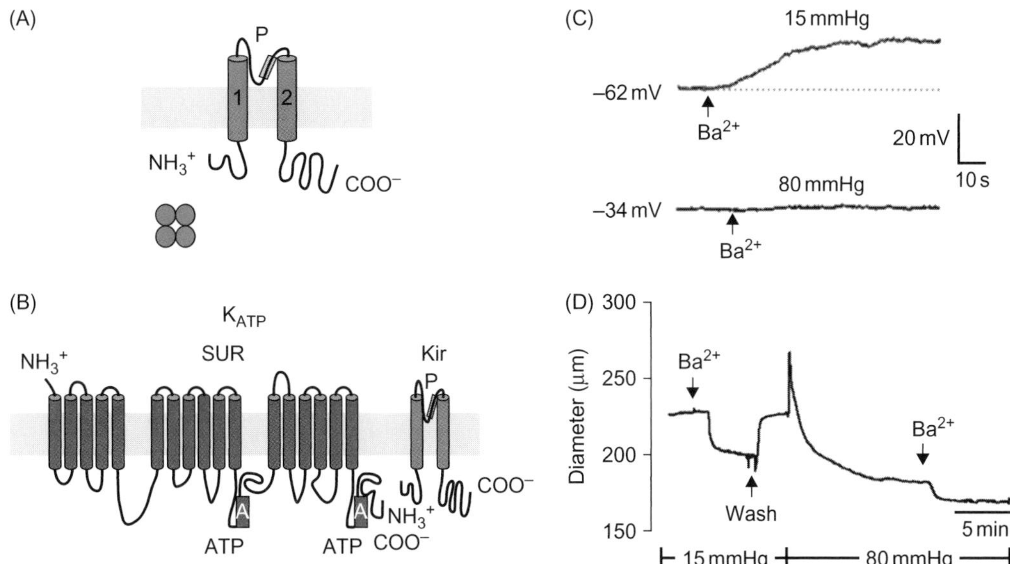

FIGURE 84.4 Inwardly rectifying K^+ (K_{ir}) channels. (A) Topology of the K_{ir} channel. Four α-subunits co-assemble to form a functional tetramer (inset). (B) ATP-sensitive (K_{ATP}) channels are composed of a K_{ir} channel associated with a sulphonylurea receptor (SUR). (C) Rat cerebral arteries were cannulated and pressurized at 15 mmHg (top) or 80 mmHg (lower). Pressurizing the artery from 15 mmHg to 80 mmHg depolarized the SMCs from −62 mV to −34 mV, respectively. Subsequently, block of K_{ir} channels by barium (Ba^{2+}) caused a depolarization that was more predominant at the more negative resting E_m. (D) Diameter measurements corresponding to the E_m responses in (C). Block of K_{ir} channels by Ba^{2+} induces vasoconstriction that predominates at the more negative E_m. *(Panels C and D reproduced from Wu et al., 2007 (20), with permission.)*

the cerebral arteries of Kir2.1$^{-/-}$ mice lacking the α-subunit to encode vascular K_{ir} channels show an inability to dilate in response to elevated [K_o]. Thus, the capability to respond to local metabolic challenges by increasing arterial diameter and blood flow may rely in part on the K_{ir} channels (21).

Two Pore Domain K^+ (K_{2P}) Channels

The two pore domain K^+ (K_{2P}) channels are structurally unique K^+ channels with two pore (P) domains (rather than the standard single pore) in each α- subunit, which also contains four transmembrane domains (Figure 84.5A). Two α-subunits co-assemble to form the channel pore. The first K_{2P} channel to be cloned in the 1990s was given the name TWIK-1 (Tandem of P domains in a Weak Inward rectifying K^+ channel) (22). Since the cloning of TWIK-1, many genes coding for K_{2P} channels have been identified and assigned to the *KCNK* gene family and then further subdivided into six classes according to their biophysical and biological properties (for review see 23).

The K_{2P} channels are typically open at negative E_m levels and, therefore, are often referred to as "leak", "background", or "baseline" K^+ channels. They are postulated to contribute to the resting E_m in vascular SMCs and also mediate hyperpolarizing currents in response to vasoactive stimuli. For example, one prominent *KCNK* channel in vascular SMCs appears to be TASK-1, which may contribute to the resting E_m of the SMCs of rabbit pulmonary artery. The TASK-1 protein has been detected in the pulmonary SMCs (Figure 84.5B), and appears to be sensitive to changes in pH, hypoxia and other metabolic stimuli that regulate pulmonary vascular tone (24). For example, the E_m responses triggered by changes in pH in pulmonary SMCs have been attributed to the opening and closing of TASK-1 channels (Figure 84.5C) (24). Another type of K_{2P} channel, TREK-1, is thought to be activated by arachidonic acid and other polyunsaturated fatty acids (PUFAs) in addition to membrane stretch, pH, temperature, signaling molecules and anesthetic agents (23). Initially the dilator response to PUFAs was reported to be abolished in isolated basilar arteries of TREK-1$^{-/-}$ mice (25), but new observations in similar animals suggest that PUFA-induced dilations do not rely on K_{2P} channels (26). Currently, the characterization of these channels is confounded by the lack of specific pharmacological blockers and the need to design and characterize K_{2P} channel-specific null mice. Regardless, there is sufficient evidence to regard these newly discovered K^+ channels as potentially important regulators of vascular tone.

K^+ Channels in Non-Vascular Smooth Muscles

Direct comparisons of K^+ channels between vascular and non-vascular SMCs have been rare, but the SMCs of

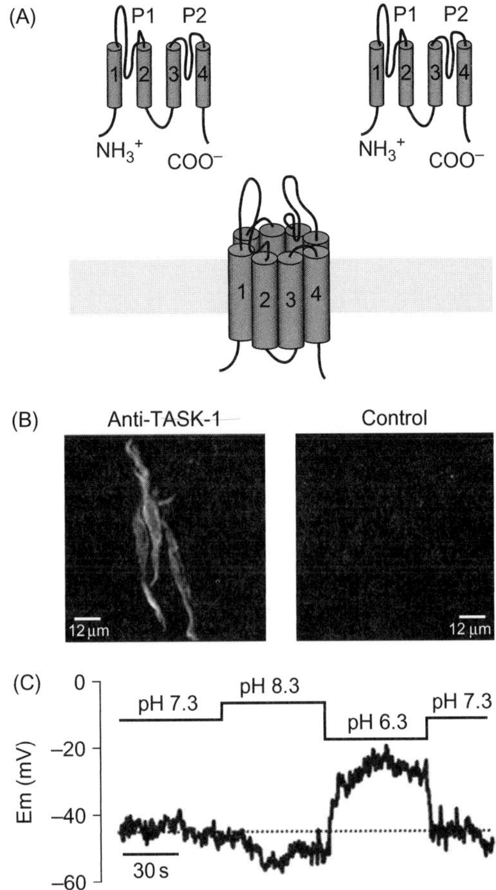

FIGURE 84.5 Two pore domain K^+ (K_{2P}) channels. (A) The α-subunit contains two P domains and four transmembrane domains. Two α-subunits form a functional channel. (B) Immunofluorescence associated with the K_{2P} channel, TASK-1, in isolated rat pulmonary SMCs. The negative control lacked primary antibody. (C) The resting Em of rat pulmonary SMCs is regulated by pH. The underlying change in K^+ conductance was attributed to TASK-1 channels. *(Panels C and D reproduced from Gurney et al., 2003 (24), with permission.)*

non-vascular tissues, such as the SMCs in the respiratory and GI tracts, appear to express a diverse assortment of K^+ channels similar to vascular SMCs (27,28). However, the expression levels and signaling pathways that determine K^+ channel activity clearly differ between and within SMC-containing organs. For example, the range of resting E_m values from −70 mV to −30 mV in airway SMCs is wider than the voltage range of −60 mV to −35 mV reported for vascular SMCs (29). These highly variable E_m values presumably partially reflect regional changes in the types and activity of K^+ channels between the SMCs in different segments of the respiratory tract. Not surprisingly, K^+ channel profiles appear to be tailored to local airway SMC function. For example, more depolarized resting E_m values have been reported for the SMCs of bronchi compared to trachea, which may position the bronchiolar SMCs to contract more readily to perform their critical role of regulating airflow (30,31). Similar to their role in other types of SMCs, the K^+ channels in airway SMCs also exert an important dilator influence in the respiratory tract. The airway SMCs are uniquely exposed to a broad spectrum of environmental factors and local autocoids that influence airway diameter. Many of these substances activate G-protein-coupled receptors to generate spontaneous Ca^{2+} oscillations caused by Ca^{2+} release from inositol triphosphate receptors (IP_3R) in the sarcoplasmic reticulum of airway SMCs (28,32). This characteristic pattern of oscillating Ca^{2+} mobilization and airway constriction appears to occur without major changes in E_m or voltage-gated Ca^{2+} influx. Thus, unlike vascular SMCs that rely heavily on K^+ channels to buffer voltage-gated Ca^{2+} influx and thereby attenuate contraction, airway SMCs rely primarily on intracellular Ca^{2+} stores for SMC activation and K^+ channels may play a less dominant role in regulating SMC excitability (28). This is not to infer, however, that K^+ channels fail to contribute to resting E_m levels and promote airway SMC relaxation, but that their primary role in the respiratory tract may be to buffer abnormal SMC excitation rather than modulate physiological responses. The BK_{Ca} channels and numerous gene families of K_v channels are densely expressed in the SMCs of the respiratory tract (28). Also the airway SMCs of mice in which the BK_{Ca} channel gene is deleted show membrane depolarization and excessive voltage-gated Ca^{2+} influx, indicating functional K^+ channels (33). Additionally, all of the recognized K^+ channel types, including the K_{ir} and K_{ATP} channels, have been identified as targets of bronchodilator substances including endogenous autocoids and oxidative metabolites (34,35). Hence, pharmacological openers of the K^+ channels are being designed to treat pathologies involving airway hyper-reactivity (36).

Potassium channels in the SMCs of the GI tract are fundamentally important for the function of this organ system. Highly coordinated movements of circular and longitudinal smooth muscle are required to enable the mixing and propulsion of gastric contents, and a complex scheme of electrical profiles is required to accomplish the diverse functions of the GI tract. For example, the stomach and small intestine enable digestion and absorption, whereas the large intestine enables drying and compaction of waste. The main classes of K^+ channels in the SMCs of the GI tract resemble those in other SMCs, but regional differences in K^+ channel expression and regulation have evolved to confer site-specific functions. Thus, the resting E_m that reflects the basal level of K^+ efflux in SMCs varies between −85 mV and −40 mV along the GI tract with the cells of the small intestine more depolarized (~ −55 mV) compared to stomach or colon (~ −75 mV) (37,38). In the GI tract, this level of resting E_m is vital since it determines the ability of the SMCs to respond to endogenous substances and depolarizing stimuli from the interstitial cells of Cajal (ICC) that coordinate SMC contraction. The ICC network generates the pacemaker activity that initiates and propagates "slow waves" down the GI tract, which subsequently opens voltage-dependent Ca^{2+} channels to cause contraction (37,38). As reviewed by Vogalis (39), the K^+ channel types that regulate these phasic contractions include the BK_{Ca} channels, which repolarize the SMC membrane after a slow wave or an action potential occurs. Additionally, diverse populations of K_v channels are widely expressed in GI SMCs that can dampen the rate of SMC depolarization, increase the threshold for action potential firing, and contribute to the resting E_m in some cell types (39). Hyperpolarizing K^+ currents also may be mediated by the opening of K_{ir} channels and the recently characterized K_{2P} channels in the SMCs of the GI tract (39,40). For example, mechanosensitive TREK-1 channels belonging to the K_{2P} gene family have been described in murine colonic SMCs (40). In this tissue, they apparently open in response to stretch, thereby providing a repolarizing influence to facilitate SMC relaxation during distension of the GI lumen (40). Similar to other types of smooth muscle, the diverse populations of K^+ channels in the SMCs of the GI tract can coordinately open to regulate cell excitability and patterns of contraction. In some cases, release of a single signaling molecule may activate several types of K^+ channels to elicit a powerful repolarizing current. Thus, nitric oxide can activate both BK_{Ca} and K_v channels in GI SMCs (39). Other agonists may elicit more subtle hyperpolarizing responses and rely on a single type of K^+ channel type to buffer SMC depolarization and contraction.

VOLTAGE-SENSITIVE SODIUM CHANNELS

Although K^+ and Ca^{2+}-permeable channels are thought to predominate in vascular SMCs, other types of ion channels also appear more sparsely, or alternatively, have not been targeted for intense study. One of these is the voltage-gated, "fast" Na^+ (Na_v) channel that mediates action potential initiation and propagation in cardiac and skeletal muscle. Historically, vascular SMCs were viewed as lacking these channels. Additionally, it was assumed that Na_v channels would be mostly inactivated at the more positive levels of resting E_m found in vascular SMCs. However, recent reports have confirmed the presence of Na^+ currents in freshly isolated vascular SMCs, raising the possibility that they contribute to vascular SMC excitability.

The molecular biology of the Na_v channels is reviewed elsewhere (41), and we will focus on evidence for the functional expression of these channels in vascular SMCs. The initial reports of vascular Na^+ currents often relied on findings in cultured SMCs, which are known to phenotypically drift and express ion channels not necessarily detected in freshly isolated cells. Thus, Cox et al. (42) reported that primary cultures of human aortic SMCs showed abundant tetrodotoxin-sensitive Na^+ currents, whereas freshly isolated SMCs from the same artery were devoid of Na^+ currents. Additionally, Meguro and colleagues (43) demonstrated that transcripts and currents attributed to Na_v channels were absent in normal SMCs but were abundant in the SMCs of balloon-injured aortae. These reports and similar observations documenting the induction of Na^+ channels in vascular SMCs in short-term culture and other conditions favoring SMC proliferation generated skepticism regarding a physiological role for Na_v channels in vascular SMCs *in situ*.

More recently, however, a number of investigators have directly recorded currents attributable to Na_v channels in freshly isolated arterial SMCs, and have suggested that the enzymes used for cell isolation may minimize Na^+ currents under some conditions. For example, tetrodotoxin-sensitive Na^+ currents were measured in mouse and rat mesenteric arterial SMCs enzymatically dissociated with collagenase and elastase (Figure 84.6A), but could not be detected in similar SMCs dissociated with papain and collagenase (44). When steady-state activation and inactivation curves for the Na^+ current were plotted, a window current between −40 mV and −20 mV was revealed (Figure 84.6B), suggesting that Na_v channels may be active in the range of resting E_m found in vascular SMCs (43). The functional role of Na_v channels in regulating vascular reactivity has been explored using the Na_v channel opener veratridine, an alkaloid that slows channel inactivation. In endothelium-denuded rings of rat aorta, veratridine potentiated constrictions to low concentrations (6–8 mmol/l) of the depolarizing agent KCl, and tetrodotoxin prevented this constriction as did pharmacological block of the Na^+/Ca^{2+} exchanger (45). These results imply that Na^+ influx through Na_v channels in vascular SMCs may cause the Na^+/Ca^{2+} exchanger to function in the reverse mode, i.e., extruding Na^+ in exchange for extracellular Ca^{2+}, with the resulting rise in $[Ca]_i$ contributing to SMC contraction. A similar coupling of Na_v channel activation to the Na^+/Ca^{2+} exchanger has been associated with vascular activation in the rat femoral artery and mouse portal vein (46,47).

There are several reports of Na_v channels in the SMCs of other hollow organs, such as those found in the respiratory and GI tracts. For example, Na_v channel transcript and corresponding Na^+ current were detected in cultured human bronchial SMCs, but this finding was not confirmed in freshly isolated SMCs from the same preparation (48,49). Additionally, currents attributed to Na_v channels have been recorded from freshly isolated human jejunum circular but not longitudinal SMCs (50,51),

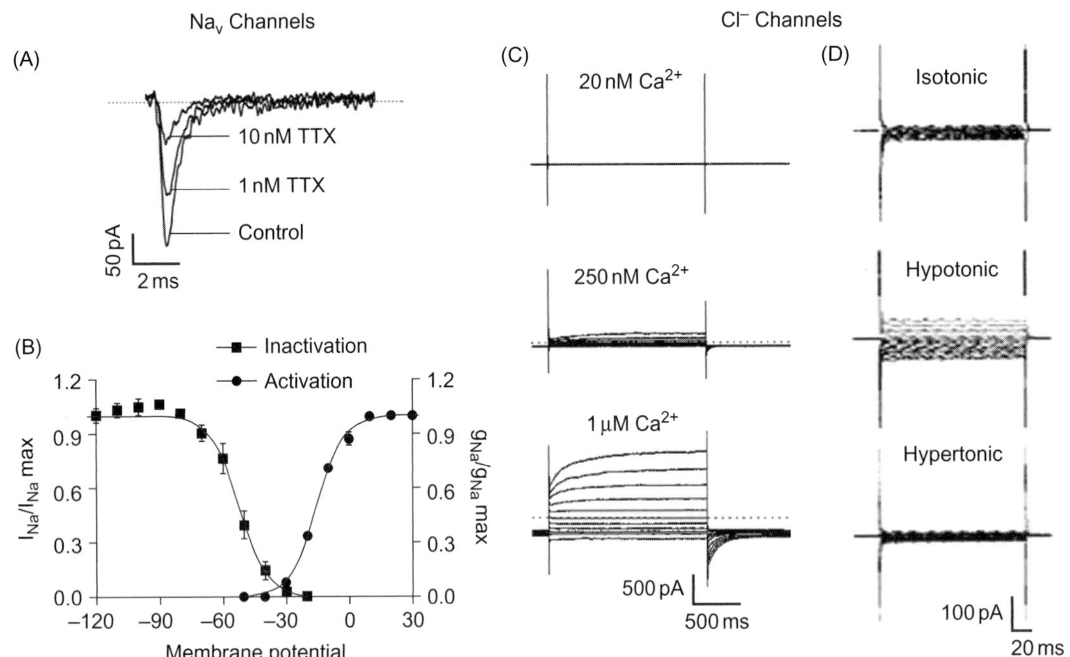

FIGURE 84.6 Voltage-gated Na$^+$ (Na$_v$) channels and two types of Cl$^-$ channels in vascular SMCs. (A) Na$^+$ currents elicited in mouse mesenteric SMCs are blocked by tetrodotoxin (TTX). (B) Steady-state activation and inactivation plots reveal a "window current" between −40 mV and −20 mV, suggesting that Na$_v$ channels may be active at physiological E$_m$. (C) Calcium-activated Cl$^-$ currents elicited in mouse portal vein SMCs are activated by increasing concentrations of Ca^{2+} in the pipette solution dialyzing the cell. (D) Currents attributed to volume-regulated Cl$^-$ currents in canine pulmonary SMCs are evoked by hypotonic but not isotonic or hypertonic solutions. *(Panel B reproduced from Berra-Romani, 2004 (44), with permission; panel C reproduced from Saleh, 2007 (54), with permission; panel D reproduced from Yamazaki, 1998 (58), with permission.)*

human and rat colonic SMCs (52), and human esophageal SMCs (53). Although the Na$_v$ channels in these hollow organs purportedly are important mediators of SMC depolarization, further studies to confirm their physiological roles are needed.

CHLORIDE CHANNELS

The Cl$^-$ channels in vascular SMCs appear to represent a diverse population of Cl$^-$-permeable channels with subtypes involved in responses to vasoactive agonists, intracellular pH, and changes in [Ca]$_i$ and cell volume. However, a lack of specific pharmacological blockers has hampered efforts to identify the role of Cl$^-$ channels in regulating vascular tone. It also has been difficult to identify the precise gene families that encode Cl$^-$ channels in vascular SMCs. Thus, whereas it is unclear if Cl$^-$ channels modulate the resting E$_m$ in vascular SMCs, recent findings infer that they may be under-appreciated players in this process.

Calcium-activated Cl$^-$ (Cl$_{Ca}$) channels have been detected in coronary, mesenteric, pulmonary, and other small arteries of several mammalian species. For example, increasing the Ca^{2+} concentration in the pipette solution dialyzing mouse portal vein myocytes reveals a prominent Cl$^-$ current (Figure 84.6C) (54). Agonist-induced Ca^{2+} entry also may trigger the opening of Cl$_{Ca}$ channels, resulting in Cl$^-$ efflux, SMC depolarization, and vasoconstriction (for review see 55). Recently, a candidate gene, transmembrane protein 16A (TMEM16A), has been suggested to encode the Cl$_{Ca}$ channel in vascular SMCs based on its biophysical properties and detection in different vascular beds (56). Indeed, the siRNA-mediated knockdown of TMEM16A in rat pulmonary SMCs results in a loss of Cl$_{Ca}$ channel-mediated current that otherwise is a prominent feature of these cells (57). With a candidate gene identified, the role of the Cl$_{Ca}$ channels in regulating vascular SMC excitability may be an emerging story.

Volume-regulated Cl$^-$ (Cl$_{VR}$) channels also can be activated in vascular SMCs by decreasing the osmotic pressure to enact membrane deformation. For example, canine pulmonary SMCs bathed in isotonic solution (300 mosmol) revealed Cl$_{VR}$ channel currents in response to hypotonic solution (230 mosmol). Superfusing the SMC with hypertonic solution (370 mosmol) abolished the Cl$^-$ current (Figure 84.6D) (58). There is some evidence that Cl$_{VR}$ also may be activated in SMCs *in situ*. For example, pharmacological block of Cl$^-$ channels relaxes pressurized rat cerebral arteries, and this response appears to rely on the Cl$_{VR}$ channels (59). Thus, Cl$^-$ efflux through Cl$_{VR}$ channels may provide a depolarizing influence in some SMCs that contributes to vascular activation under some conditions. It is proposed that the Cl_{VR} channels in vascular SMCs belong to the ClC gene family with ClC-3 as the predominant isoform (60). Indeed, the Cl_{VR} channel currents elicited by hypotonic cell swelling in canine pulmonary SMCs can be abolished by intracellular dialysis with anti-C1C-3 antibodies that appear to interact specifically with C1C-3 (61). Other types of Cl^- channels including a cAMP-dependent Cl^- channel have been detected in vascular SMCs, but the molecular identities and physiological functions of these channels have not been established.

Some non-vascular SMCs also express Cl_{Ca} channels. In the GI tract, rat intestinal and colonic SMCs (62–64), opossum esophageal circular SMCs (65), guinea pig ileal circular SMCs (65), and guinea pig tracheal SMCs (66) exhibit Cl_{Ca} channel current. More recently, Huang et al. (67) localized the Cl_{Ca} channel candidate gene TMEM16A to airway SMCs to provide a molecular candidate for the Cl_{Ca} currents. There are fewer reports of Cl_{VR} channels in non-vascular SMCs, although Dick et al. (68) detected ClC-3 mRNA in canine colonic SMCs and recorded Cl_{VR} currents in response to hypotonic solution in the freshly isolated cells. Thus, while there is some evidence of Cl^- channels in non-vascular SMCs, the expression patterns and functional roles of these Cl^- channels are not clearly defined.

PERSPECTIVES

There is an extensive network of ion channels in the plasma membrane of SMCs that regulates cell excitability. With the development of more sophisticated molecular biology tools and new pharmacological channel blockers, the functional impact of various ion channels in normal and pathophysiological conditions is being pinpointed and the channels targeted for the development of new therapeutics. For example, new classes of K^+ channels including the voltage-gated KCNQ (K_V7) channels are being recognized as important repolarizing influences in SMCs. Initially reported in murine portal vein myocytes (69), KCNQ channels have since been identified in aorta (70), pulmonary (71), tibial (70), cerebral (72,73) and mesenteric arteries (74,75) from rats, mice, and humans. In rat cerebral arteries, the KCNQ channels buffer the development of myogenic tone (73) suggesting that KCNQ channel openers may effectively treat cerebral vasospasm (72). Similarly, new gene families that encode the K_{2P} channels were recently discovered (76). Exciting roles for these unique K^+ channels that open in response to stretch, pH fluctuations. and other important physiological stimuli that regulate SMC tone are only starting to be realized. Finally, the molecular identity and role of the Cl^- channels expressed in SMCs is an evolving story with the recent discovery of TMEM16A as a candidate gene (56). Thus, whereas much is known about ion channel expression and function in SMCs, there surely are ion channels yet to be discovered and unanswered questions about how these ion channels act in concert to regulate SMC contraction in health and disease.

REFERENCES

1. Coetzee WA, Amarillo Y, Chiu J, Chow A, Lau D, McCormack T, et al. Molecular diversity of K^+ channels. *Ann. NY Acad. Sci* 1999;**868**:233–85.
2. Yuan XJ. Voltage-gated K^+ currents regulate resting membrane potential and $[Ca^{2+}]_i$ in pulmonary arterial myocytes. *Circ Res* 1995;**77**:370–8.
3. Pongs O, Schwarz JR. Beta subunit ancillary subunits associated with voltage-dependent K^+ channels. *Physiol Rev* 2010;**90**:755–96.
4. Albarwani S, Nemetz LT, Madden JA, Tobin AA, England SK, Pratt PF, et al. Voltage-gated K^+ channels in rat small cerebral arteries: molecular identity of the functional channels. *J. Physiol* 2003;**551**:751–63.
5. Chen TT, Luykenaar KD, Walsh EJ, Walsh MP, Cole WC. Key role of Kv1 channels in vasoregulation. *Circ. Res* 2006;**99**:53–60.
6. Fergus DJ, Martens JR, England SK. Kv channel subunits that contribute to voltage-gated K^+ current in renal vascular smooth muscle. *Eur J Physiol* 2003;**445**:697–704.
7. Archer SL, Souil E, Dinh-Xuan AT, Schremmer B, Mercier JC, El Yaagoubi A, et al. Molecular identification of the role of voltage-gated K^+ channels, Kv1.5 and Kv2.1, in hypoxic pulmonary vasoconstriction and control of resting membrane potential in rat pulmonary artery myocytes. *J Clin Inv* 1998;**101**:2319–30.
8. Amberg GC, Santana LF. Kv2 channels oppose myogenic constriction of rat cerebral arteries. *Am. J. Physiol* 2006;**291**:C348–56.
9. Yuan XJ, Wang J, Juhaszova M, Gaine SP, Rubin LJ. Attenuated K^+ channel gene transcription in primary pulmonary hypertension. *Lancet* 1998;**351**:726–7.
10. Li H, Gutterman DD, Rusch NJ, Bubolz A, Liu Y. Nitration and functional loss of voltage-gated K^+ channels in rat coronary microvessels exposed to high glucose. *Diabetes* 2004;**53**:2436–42.
11. Tobin AA, Joseph BK, Al-Kindi HN, Albarwani S, Madden JA, Nemetz LT, et al. Loss of cerebrovascular Shaker-type K^+ channels: a shared vasodilator defect of genetic and renal hypertensive rats. *Am J Physiol* 2009;**297**:H293–303.
12. Cui J, Yang H, Lee US. Molecular mechanisms of BK channel activation. *Cell. Mol. Life Sci* 2009;**66**:852–75.
13. Cheranov SY, Jaggar JH. Sarcoplasmic reticulum calcium load regulates rat arterial smooth muscle calcium sparks and transient K_{Ca} currents. *J. Physiol* 2002;**544**:71–84.
14. Sausbier M, Arntz C, Bucurenciu I, Zhao H, Zhou XB, Sausbier U, et al. Elevated blood pressure linked to primary hyperaldosteronism and impaired vasodilation in BK channel-deficient mice. *Circulation* 2005;**112**:60–8.
15. Brenner R, Perez GJ, Bonev AD, Eckman DM, Kosek JC, Wiler SW, et al. Vasoregulation by the β1 subunit of the calcium-activated potassium channel. *Nature* 2000;**407**:870–6.
16. Fernandez-Fernandez JM, Tomas M, Vazquez E, Orio P, Latorre R, Senti M, et al. Gain-of-function mutation in the KCNMB1

potassium channel subunit is associated with low prevalence of diastolic hypertension. *J Clin Inv* 2004;**113**:1032–9.

17. Hibino H, Inanobe A, Furutani K, Murakami S, Findlay I, Kurachi Y. Inwardly rectifying potassium channels: their structure, function, and physiological roles. *Physiol Rev* 2010;**90**:291–366.
18. Yamada M, Isomoto S, Matsumoto S, Kondo C, Shindo T, Horio Y, et al. Sulphonylurea receptor 2B and $K_{ir}6.1$ form a sulphonylurea-sensitive but ATP-insensitive K^+ channel. *J Physiol* 1997;**499**:715–20.
19. Jackson WF, Huebner JM, Rusch NJ. Enzymatic isolation and characterization of single vascular smooth muscle cells from cremasteric arterioles. *Microcirculation* 1997;**4**:35–50.
20. Wu B-N, Luykenaar KD, Brayden JE, Giles WR, Corteling RL, Wiehler WB, et al. Hyposmotic challenge inhibits inward rectifying K^+ channels in cerebral arterial smooth muscle cells. *Am J Physiol Heart Circ Physiol* 2007;**292**:H1085–94.
21. Zaritsky JJ, Eckman DM, Wellman GC, Nelson MT, Schwarz TL. Targeted disruption of the Kir2.1 and Kir2.2 genes reveals the essential role of the inwardly rectifying K^+ current in K^+-mediated vasodilation. *Circ Res* 2000;**87**:160–6.
22. Lesage F, Guillemare E, Fink M, Duprat F, Lazdunski M, Romey G, et al. TWIK-1, a ubiquitous human weakly inward rectifying K^+ channel with a novel structure. *EMBO J* 1996;**15**:1004–11.
23. Enyedi P, Czirjak G. Molecular background of leak K^+ currents: two-pore domain potassium channels. *Physiol Rev* 2010;**90**:559–605.
24. Gurney AM, Osipenko ON, MacMillan D, McFarlane KM, Tate RJ, Kempsill FEJ. Two-pore domain K channel, TASK-1, in pulmonary artery smooth muscle cells. *Circ Res* 2003;**93**:957–64.
25. Blondeau N, Pétrault O, Manta S, Giordanengo V, Gounon P, Bordet R, et al. Polyunsaturated fatty acids are cerebral vasodilators via the TREK-1 potassium channel. *Circ Res* 2007;**101**:176–84.
26. Namiranian K, Lloyd EE, Crossland RF, Marrelli SP, Taffet GE, Reddy AK, et al. Cerebrovascular responses in mice deficient in the potassium channel, TREK-1. *Am J Physiol* 2010;**299**:R461–9.
27. Bardou O, Trinh NT, Brochiero E. Molecular diversity and function of K^+ channels in the airway and alveolar epithelial cells. *Am J Physiol* 2009;**296**:L145–55.
28. Hirota S, Helli P, Janssen LJ. Ionic mechanisms and Ca^{2+} handling in airway smooth muscle. *Eur Respir J* 2007;**30**:114–33.
29. Honda K, Tomita T. Electrical activity in isolated human tracheal muscle. *Jap Physiol* 1987;**37**:333–6.
30. Oonuma H, Nakajima T, Nagata T, Iwasawa K, Wang Y, Hazama H, et al. Endothelin-1 is a potent activator of non-selective cation currents in human bronchial smooth muscle cells. *Am J Respir Cell Mol Biol* 2000;**23**:213–21.
31. Bai Y, Sanderson MJ. Airway smooth muscle relaxation results from a reduction in the frequency of Ca^{2+} oscillations induced by a cAMP-mediated inhibition of the IP3 receptor. *Respir. Res* 2006;**7**:34–53.
32. Perez-Zoghbi JF, Karner C, Ito S, Shepherd M, Alrashdan Y, Sanderson MJ. Ion channel regulation of intracellular calcium and airway smooth muscle function. *Pulm Pharmacol Ther* 2009;**22**:388–97.
33. Sausbier M, Zhou X-B, Beier C, Sausbier U, Wolpers D, Maget S, et al. Reduced rather than enhanced cholinergic airway constriction in mice with ablation of the large conductance Ca^{2+}-activated K^+ channel. *FASEB J* 2007;**21**:812–22.
34. Gupta JB, Prasad K. Mechanism of H^2O^2-induced modulation of airway smooth muscle. *Am J Physiol* 1992;**263**:L714–22.
35. Morin C, Sirois M, Echave V, Rizcallah E, Rousseau E. Relaxing effects of 17(18)-EpETE on arterial and airway smooth muscles in human lung. *Am J Physiol* 2009;**296**:L130–9.
36. Fozard JR, Manley PW. Potassium channel openers: agents for the treatment of airway hyperreactivity. In: Hansel TT, Barnes PJ, editors. *New Drugs for Asthma, Allergy and COPD*. Basel: Karger;2001*Prog Respir Res* **31**:77–80.
37. Sanders KM, Koh SD, Ward SM. Interstitial cells of cajal as pacemakers in the gastrointestinal tract. *Annu Rev Physiol* 2006;**68**:307–43.
38. Sanders KM. Regulation of smooth muscle excitation and contraction. *Neurogastroen Motil* 2008;**20**:S39–53.
39. Vogalis F. Potassium channels in gastrointestinal smooth muscle. *J Auton Pharmacol* 2001;**20**:207–19.
40. Sanders KM, Koh SD. Two-pore-domain potassium channels in smooth muscles: new components of myogenic regulation. *J Physiol* 2006;**570**:37–43.
41. Catterall WA, Goldin AL, Waxman SG. International Union of Pharmacology. XLVII. Nomenclature and structure-function relationships of voltage-gated sodium channels. *Pharmacol Rev* 2005;**57**:397–409.
42. Cox RH, Zhou Z, Tulenko TN. Voltage-gated sodium channels in human aortic smooth muscle cells. *J Vasc Res* 1998;**35**:310–7.
43. Meguro K, Iida H, Takano H, Morita T, Sata M, Nagai R, et al. Function and role of voltage-gated sodium channel $Na^v1.7$ expressed in aortic smooth muscle cells. *Am J Physiol Heart Circ Physiol* 2009;**296**:H211–9.
44. Berra-Romani R, Blaustein MP, Matteson DR. TTX-sensitive voltage-gated Na^+ channels are expressed in mesenteric artery smooth muscle cells. *Am J Physiol Heart Circ Physiol* 2005;**289**:H137–45.
45. Fort A, Cordaillat M, Thollon C, Salazar G, Mechaly I, Villeneuve N, et al. New insights in the contribution of voltage-gated Na^v channels to rat aorta contraction. *PLoS One* 2009;**4**:e7360.
46. Bocquet A, Sablayrolles S, Vacher B, Le Grand B. F 15845, a new blocker of persistent sodium current prevents consequences of hypoxia in rat femoral artery. *Br J Pharmacol* 2010;**161**:405–15.
47. Saleh S, Yeung SYM, Prestwich S, Pucovsky V, Greenwood I. Electrophysiological and molecular identification of voltage-gated sodium channels in murine vascular myocytes. *J Physiol* 2005;**568**:155–69.
48. Snetkov VA, Hirst SJ, Ward JP. Ion channels in freshly isolated and cultured human bronchial smooth muscle cells. *Exp Physiol* 1996;**81**:791–804.
49. Jo T, Nagata T, Iida H, Imuta H, Iwasawa K, Ma J, et al. Voltage-gated sodium channel expressed in cultured human smooth muscle cells: involvement of SCN9A. *FEBS Lett* 2004;**567**:339–43.
50. Ou Y, Gibbons SJ, Miller SM, Strege PR, Rich A, Distad MA, et al. SCN5A is expressed in human jejunal circular smooth muscle cells. *Neurogastroenterol Motil* 2002;**14**:477–86.
51. Holm AN, Rich A, Miller SM, Strege P, Ou Y, Gibbons S, et al. Sodium current in human jejunal circular smooth muscle cells. *Gastroenterology* 2002;**122**:178–87.
52. Xiong Z, Sperelakis N, Noffsinger A, Fenoglio-Preiser C. Fast Na^+ current in circular smooth muscle cells of the large intestine. *Pflugers Arch* 1993;**423**:485–91.
53. Deshpande MA, Wang J, Preiksaitis HG, Laurier LG, Sims SM. Characterization of a voltage-dependent Na^+ current in human esophageal smooth muscle. *Am J Physiol Cell Physiol* 2002;**283**:C1045–55.

54. Saleh SN, Angermann JE, Sones WR, Leblanc N, Greenwood IA. Stimulation of Ca^{2+}-gated Cl^- currents by the calcium-dependent K^+ channel modulators NS1619 [1,3-dihydro-1-[2-hydroxy-5-(trifluoromethyl)phenyl]-5-(trifluoromethyl)-2H-benzimidazol-2-one] and isopimaric acid. *J Pharmacol Exp Ther* 2007;**321**:1075–84.
55. Leblanc N, Ledoux J, Saleh S, Sanguinetti A, Angermann J, O'Driscoll K, et al. Regulation of calcium-activated chloride channels in smooth muscle cells: a complex picture is emerging. *Can J Physiol Pharmacol* 2005;**83**:541–56.
56. Davis AJ, Forrest AS, Jepps TA, Valencik ML, Wiwchar M, Singer CA, et al. Expression profile and protein translation of TMEM16A in murine smooth muscle. *Am J Physiol Cell Physiol* 2010;**299**: C948–59.
57. Manoury B, Tamuleviciute A, Tammaro P. TMEM16A/anoctamin 1 protein mediates calcium-activated chloride currents in pulmonary arterial smooth muscle cells. *J Physiol* 2010;**588**:2305–14.
58. Yamazaki J, Duan D, Janiak R, Kuenzli K, Horowitz B, Hume JR. Functional and molecular expression of volume-regulated chloride channels in canine vascular smooth muscle cells. *J Physiol* 1998;**507**:729–36.
59. Nelson MT, Conway MA, Knot HJ, Brayden JE. Chloride channels inhibit myogenic tone in rat cerebral arteries. *J Physiol* 1997;**502**:259–64.
60. Duan D, Winter C, Cowley S, Hume JR, Horowitz B. Molecular identification of a volume-regulated chloride channel. *Nature* 1997;**390**:417–21.
61. Wang G-X, Hatton WJ, Wang GL, Zhong J, Yamboliev I, Duan D, et al. Functional effects of novel anti-ClC-3 antibodies on native volume-sensitive osmolyte and anion channels in cardiac and smooth muscle cells. *Am J Physiol* 2003;**285**:H1453–63.
62. Ohta T, Ito S, Nakazato Y. Chloride currents activated by caffeine in rat intestinal smooth muscle cells. *J Physiol* 1993;**465**:149–62.
63. Matchkov VV, Aalkjaer C, Nilsson H. Distribution of cGMP-dependent and cGMP-independent Ca^{2+}-activated Cl^- conductances in smooth muscle cells from different vascular beds and colon. *Pflugers Arch* 2005;**451**:371–9.
64. Xu L, Ting-Lou Lv N, Zhu X, Chen Y, Yang J. Emodin augments calcium activated chloride channel in colonic smooth muscle cells by G_i/G_o protein. *Eur J Pharmacol* 2009;**615**:171–6.
65. Zhang Y, Paterson WG. Role of Ca^{2+}-activated Cl^- channels and MLCK in slow IJP in opossum esophageal smooth muscle. *Am J Physiol Gastrointest Liver Physiol* 2002;**283**:G104–14.
66. Janssen LJ, Sims SM. Histamine activates Cl^- and K^+ currents in guinea-pig tracheal myocytes: convergence with muscarinic signalling pathway. *J. Physiol* 1993;**465**:661–77.
67. Huang F, Rock JR, Harfe BD, Cheng T, Huang X, Jan YN, et al. Studies on expression and function of the TMEM16A calcium-activated chloride channel. *Proc Natl Acad Sci USA* 2009;**106**:21413–8.
68. Dick GM, Bradley KK, Horowitz B, Hume JR, Sanders KM. Functional and molecular identification of a novel chloride conductance in canine colonic smooth muscle. *Am J Physiol* 1998;**275**: C940–50.
69. Ohya S, Sergeant GP, Greenwood IA, Horowitz B. Molecular variants of KCNQ channels expressed in murine portal vein myocytes: a role in delayed rectifier current. *Circ Res* 2003;**92**:1016–23.
70. Schleifenbaum J, Köhn C, Voblova N, Dubrovska G, Zavarirskaya O, Gloe T, et al. Systemic peripheral artery relaxation by KCNQ channel openers and hydrogen sulfide. *J. Hypertens* 2010;**28**:1875–82.
71. Joshi S, Sedivy V, Hodyc D, Herget J, Gurney AM. KCNQ modulators reveal a key role for KCNQ potassium channels in regulating the tone of rat pulmonary artery smooth muscle. *J Pharmacol Exp Ther* 2009;**329**:368–76.
72. Mani BK, Brueggemann LI, Cribbs LL, Byron KL. Activation of vascular KCNQ (K^v7) potassium channels reverses spasmogen-induced constrictor responses in rat basilar artery. *Br J Pharmacol* 2011; ePub ahead of print 22 August, 2011, doi: 10.1111/j.1476-5381.2011.01273.x.
73. Zhong XZ, Harhun MI, Olesen SP, Ohya S, Moffatt JD, Cole WC, et al. Participation of KCNQ (K^v7) potassium channels in myogenic control of cerebral arterial diameter. *J Physiol* 2010;**588**:3277–93.
74. Mackie AR, Brueggemann LI, Henderson KK, Shiels AJ, Cribbs LL, Scrogin KE, et al. Vascular KCNQ potassium channels as novel targets for the control of mesenteric artery constriction by vasopressin, based on studies in single cells, pressurized arteries, and in vivo measurements of mesenteric vascular resistance. *J Pharmacol Exp Ther* 2008;**325**:475–83.
75. Ng FL, Davis AJ, Jepps TA, Harhun MI, Yeung SY, Wan A, et al. Expression and function of the K^+ channel KCNQ genes in human arteries. *Br J Pharmacol* 2011;**162**:42–53.
76. Ketchum KA, Joiner WJ, Sellers AJ, Kaczmarek LK, Goldstein SA. A new family of outwardly rectifying potassium channel proteins with two pore domains in tandem. *Nature* 1995;**376**:690–5.

Chapter 85

G-Protein-Coupled Receptors in Smooth Muscle

Angela Wirth[1,2] and Stefan Offermanns[1]

[1]*Department of Pharmacology, Max-Planck-Institute for Heart and Lung Research, Bad Nauheim, Germany,* [2]*Institute of Pharmacology, University of Heidelberg, Heidelberg, Germany*

INTRODUCTION

Smooth muscles are widely distributed in the body and show a high degree of functional specialization. Smooth muscle cells regulate the tone and movement of the wall of most hollow organs like the vascular, gastrointestinal, bronchial system or the urogenital system and uterus. However, smooth muscle cells are also found in many other places where they serve very specific functions, ranging from the control of the pupillary diameter to the movement of body hairs. In contrast to the more uniform function of heart or skeletal muscle, the wide variety of smooth muscle functions requires their regulation by many different mediators. Most of these mediators act locally or systemically as hormones or are released as transmitters from nerve endings innervating smooth muscle tissue. Most of the mediators regulating smooth muscle contractility act through G-protein-coupled receptors (GPCRs), the largest and most versatile receptor system in higher organisms. In this chapter, we will give an overview on GPCRs involved in the regulation of smooth muscle function, and we will describe basic signal transduction mechanisms employed by GPCRs to regulate the tone of smooth muscle cells.

G-PROTEIN-COUPLED RECEPTORS

The mammalian genome encodes about 400 non-olfactory G-protein-coupled receptors that are activated by particular hormones, neurotransmitters or other mediators. Once a GPCR has been activated by a ligand, it couples to a heterotrimeric G-protein, which in turn then regulates one or several effectors like second messenger-producing enzymes or ion channels (1,2). This modular structure of the G-protein-mediated signaling system is the basis of the large functional versatility of the GPCR system. There are at least four basic families of G-proteins which are defined by particular G-protein α-subunits, G_s, G_i/G_o, G_q/G_{11}, and G_{12}/G_{13} (3). Each of the G-protein families regulates particular effectors after activation through a GPCR, and an activated receptor couples to a subset of individual G-protein subtypes. Also the G-protein $\beta\gamma$-complex takes part in the regulation of downstream signaling processes by regulating a variety of effector proteins (4). In smooth muscle cells, the coupling of receptors to particular G-protein subfamilies determines whether the receptor agonist induces an increase or a decrease in the smooth muscle tone. Typical smooth muscle-relaxing agonists acting through GPCRs will activate receptors coupled to the G-protein G_s which in turn stimulates the activity of adenylyl cyclases and thereby mediates an increase in the intracellular cAMP concentration (5). In contrast, GPCRs mediating contraction of smooth muscle cells typically couple to G-proteins of the G_q/G_{11} family which couple receptors to β-isoforms of phospholipase C resulting in the formation of diacylglycerol, an activator of protein kinase C, as well as in the formation of inositol-1,4,5-trisphosphate which releases Ca^{2+} from intracellular stores (6). Many of the contraction-inducing receptors also couple to G-proteins of the G_{12}/G_{13} family, which link these receptors via Rho guanine nucleotide exchange factors (RhoGEF) to the activation of the small GTPase RhoA (7). Some of the receptors mediating smooth muscle contraction also couple to G_i/G_o-type G-proteins which mediate an inhibition of adenylyl cyclase and thereby antagonize the activity of active receptors coupling to G_s.

G-Protein-Mediated Signaling Pathways Mediating Smooth Muscle Contraction

The regulation of the phosphorylation of myosin light chain (MLC) is a central process in the control of smooth muscle cell contraction (8,9). The Ca^{2+}-calmodulin-activated MLC kinase (MLCK) phosphorylates MLC,

Muscle. DOI: http://dx.doi.org/10.1016/B978-0-12-381510-1.00085-5

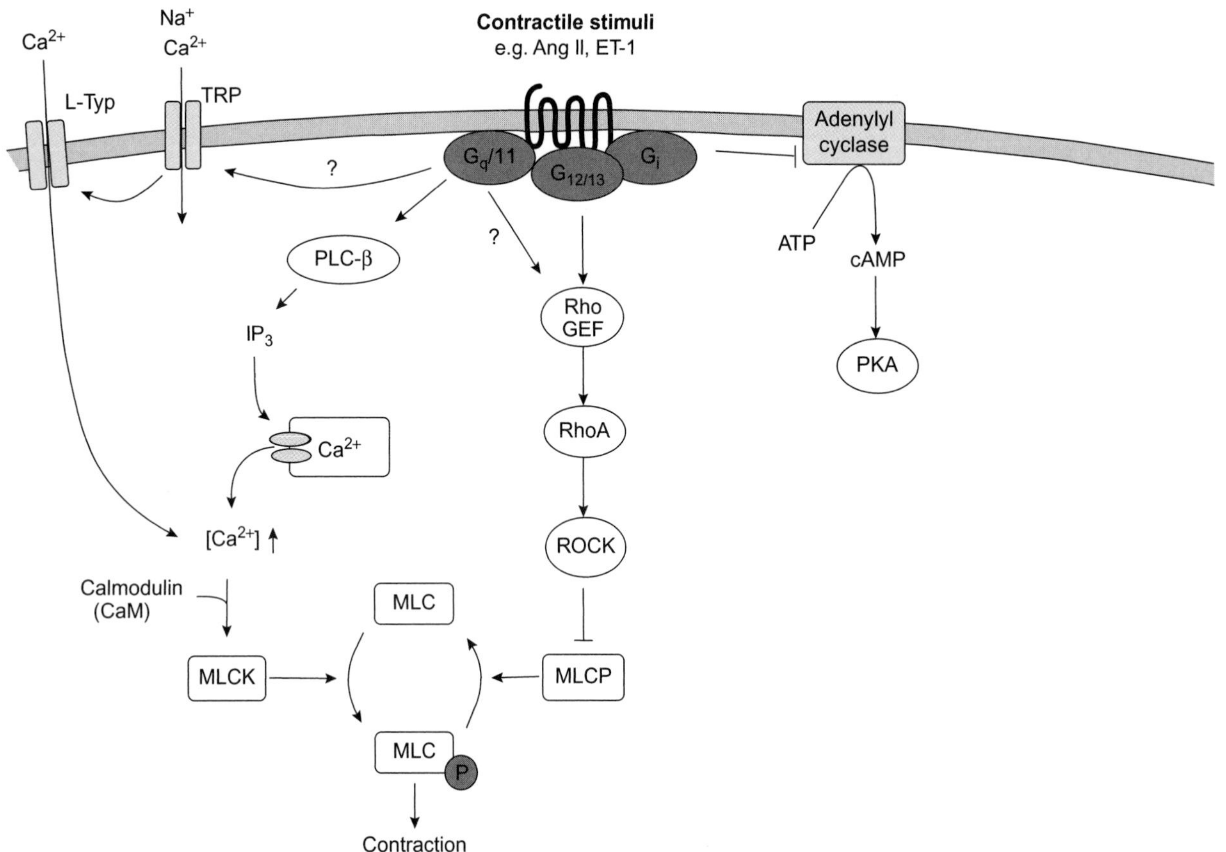

FIGURE 85.1 Mechanisms of GPCR-mediated smooth muscle contraction. GPCRs mediating contraction of smooth muscle cells typically couple to G-proteins of the G_q/G_{11} family; in some cases also of the G_{12}/G_{13} and G_i family. Activation of β-isoforms of phospholipase C (PLC-β) by G_q/G_{11} results in inositol-1,4,5,-trisphosphate (IP_3) formation and release of intracellularly stored Ca^{2+}. Ca^{2+} together with calmodulin activates the myosin light chain kinase (MLCK) resulting in phosphorylation of the myosin light chain (MLC). In addition, G_q/G_{11} may activate cation channels resulting in depolarization and opening of voltage-dependent Ca^{2+} channels. Activation of G_{12}/G_{13} stimulates the activity of particular Rho guanine nucleotide exchange factors (Rho-GEFs). The activated small GTPase RhoA via stimulation of Rho-kinase (ROCK) activity then inhibits the myosin light chain phosphatase (MLCP). G_i type G-proteins release relatively high amounts of βγ-subunits which may result in activation of particular PLC-β isoforms. In addition, α-subunits of G_i type G-proteins inhibit adenylyl cyclase resulting in decreased activity of protein kinase A (PKA) (see Figure 85.2). TRP, transient receptor potential channel. For details: see text.

whereas its dephosphorylation is catalyzed by the MLC phosphatase (MLCP). While Ca^{2+} appears to be the major regulator of the activity of MLCK, regulation of MLCP occurs in a Ca^{2+}-independent manner. The classic pathway through which GPCRs increase smooth muscle contraction is initiated by coupling of the receptors to G-proteins of the G_q/G_{11} family. Activation of G_q/G_{11} results in an increase in the activity of β-isoforms of phospholipase C leading to the formation of inositol-1,4,5-trisphosphate and the release of intracellularly stored Ca^{2+} (see Figure 85.1). Ca^{2+} then together with calmodulin activates MLCK resulting in the phosphorylation of MLC and an increase in smooth muscle tone. In various smooth muscle types, evidence has been provided that the Ca^{2+} leading to MLCK activation is not solely derived from intracellular stores but can also be supplied through a transmembrane influx via particular cation channels (10,11). This is strongly suggested by the fact that the GPCR-mediated contraction of various smooth muscle cell types can be inhibited by the blockade of L-type Ca^{2+} channels or by genetic inactivation of the genes encoding the pore-forming subunit of L-type calcium channels (12). Opening of L-type Ca^{2+} channels results from depolarization of smooth muscle cells which may be induced through the GPCR-dependent activation of cation channels like transient receptor potential channels (TRP channels) (13,14) (see section Calcium Homeostasis below).

Besides this classic Ca^{2+}-dependent signaling pathway resulting in MLCK activation, a parallel Ca^{2+}-independent pathway is operating in smooth muscle cells, which links GPCRs to the regulation of the myosin phosphatase. This pathway involves the small GTP-binding protein RhoA which, after activation, stimulates activity of Rho kinase which then phosphorylates and inhibits myosin phosphatase (15). The G-proteins G_{12}/G_{13} have been shown to link receptors to the Rho/Rho-kinase pathway in smooth muscle cells (8,16,17). The α-subunits of G_{12} and G_{13} are able to bind to particular RhoGEF proteins and thereby stimulate the formation of active RhoA able to stimulate Rho-kinase activity (18). In particular, the RhoGEF protein LARG has been shown to couple G_{12}/G_{13} to the Rho/Rho-kinase pathway in vascular smooth muscle cells *in vivo* (17). In several cases, evidence has also been provided that activated G_q/G_{11} can induce activation of RhoA. There are probably different mechanisms by which G_q/G_{11} mediate activation of the Rho/Rho-kinase pathway. The α-subunits of G_q/G_{11} can directly regulate the activity of RhoGEF proteins like p63 RhoGEF (19) or LARG (20). However, there are also indirect mechanisms linking G_q/G_{11} to RhoA activation, like the recently described Ca^{2+}- and Jak2-dependent stimulation of the RhoGEF protein p115 RhoGEF in vascular smooth muscle cells initiated via the angiotensin II (AT_1) receptor (21).

Several GPCRs that mediate smooth muscle contraction also couple to G-proteins of the G_i/G_o family. The exact mechanism how activation of G_i type proteins contributes to the contractile response to agonists of G_i-coupled receptors is not completely clear. In some smooth muscle systems, activation of G_i may lead to the release of considerable amounts of free G-protein $\beta\gamma$-subunits which are then able to activate phospholipase C β-isoforms and result in increases in intracellular Ca^{2+} concentrations similar to the events following the activation of G_q/G_{11}. Activated G_i/G_o type proteins directly inhibit adenylyl cyclases resulting in a decrease in the intracellular cAMP levels, which would promote an increase in smooth muscle tone.

G-Protein-Mediated Signaling Pathways Mediating Smooth Muscle Relaxation

The relaxation of smooth muscle cells is mediated by increases in the concentration of the cyclic nucleotides cAMP and cGMP (22). While the formation of cGMP by guanylyl cyclases is not under the control of GPCRs, formation of cAMP results from activation of G_s-coupled receptors that stimulate the activity of membranous adenylyl cyclases. Multiple mechanisms have been described for cAMP-induced smooth muscle relaxation. Major mediators of this process are protein kinase A (PKA) as well as protein kinase G (PKG), which are both activated by cAMP (23). Both PKA and PKG inhibit GPCR-mediated smooth muscle contraction via various mechanisms affecting the G_q/G_{11}-mediated Ca^{2+}-dependent pathway as well as the Ca^{2+}-independent, Rho/Rho-kinase-mediated signaling pathway (see Figure 85.2).

Both PKA and PKG can inhibit GPCR-mediated IP_3 formation. A major mechanism by which cAMP/cGMP-dependent kinases reduce IP_3 formation in smooth muscle cells is the phosphorylation and activation of RGS4 (regulator of G-protein signaling 4) which results in a rapid inactivation of the G-proteins G_q/G_{11} and subsequent inhibition of both PLC-β activity and IP_3 formation (24,25). Furthermore, PKA reduces calcium influx by activation of K^+-channels, resulting in a hyperpolarization of the smooth muscle cell (26–28). PKG, but not PKA, can phosphorylate certain isoforms of the IP_3 receptor resulting in an inhibition of the IP_3 receptor-mediated Ca^{2+} release from intracellular stores (29,30).

PKA and PKG also interfere with the Rho/Rho-kinase pathway and with the subsequent inhibition of myosin phosphatase activity. PKA and PKG are capable of directly phosphorylating and inactivating RhoA thereby abolishing the activation of Rho-kinase (31). In addition, myosin phosphatase appears to be an important target for PKG and also PKA. Both kinases can phosphorylate myosin phosphatases thereby preventing the inhibition of the enzyme by Rho-kinase-dependent phosphorylation (32); however, it is not clear whether this mechanism operates *in vivo*. In addition, active PKG has been shown to interact with myosin phosphatase and to activate the enzyme (33,34). Both inhibition of Rho-kinase-mediated phosphorylation of myosin phosphatase as well as activation of myosin phosphatase result in an increased de-phosphorylation of MLC and relaxation of smooth muscle cells.

There is also evidence that activation of G_s-coupled receptors can induce smooth muscle relaxation via a cAMP-independent pathway (35–37). This pathway appears in some cases to involve the regulation of Ca^{2+}-activated K^+ channels. However, the exact mechanisms underlying this cAMP-independent effect are unknown.

Other Smooth Muscle Functions Regulated through G-Protein-Coupled Receptors (Migration, Differentiation, etc.)

GPCRs are not only involved in the regulation of smooth muscle tone but also play an important role in other cellular processes like the regulation of smooth muscle migration and differentiation.

Smooth muscle cells unlike most other differentiated cells retain the capacity to modulate their phenotype in response to certain stimuli. The contractile phenotype of smooth muscle cells is characterized by the coordinated expression of several genes encoding contractile and cytoskeletal proteins (38). Under certain conditions, e.g. after injury of blood vessels resulting in neointima formation

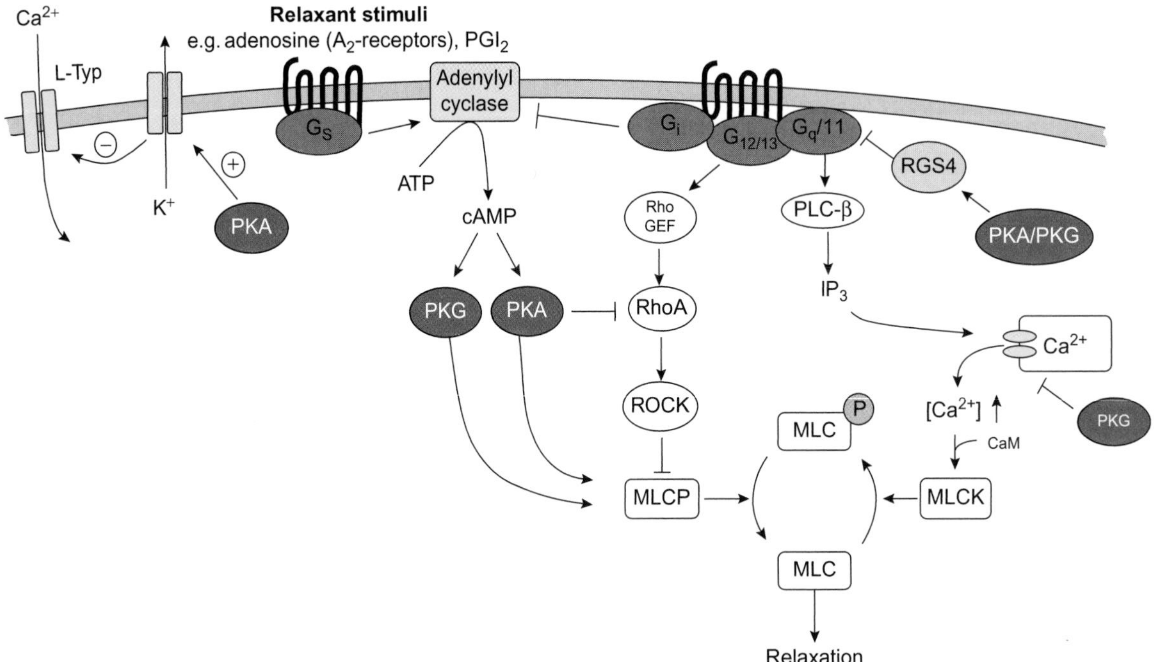

FIGURE 85.2 **Mechanisms of GPCR-mediated smooth muscle relaxation.** GPCR-mediated relaxation of smooth muscle cells involves receptors coupled to the G-protein G_s which by activation of adenylyl cyclase increases cAMP levels. Cyclic AMP, primarily via activation of the protein kinase A (PKA), and in part also of protein kinase G (PKG), induces relaxation. PKA inhibits the RhoA-mediated signaling pathway, activates myosin light chain phosphatase (MLCP) activity and can activate K^+-channels. In addition, PKA and PKG activate a regulator of G-protein signaling protein (RGS4) which inhibits G_q/G_{11}-mediated signalling. Finally, PKG has been shown to inhibit the release of intracellularly stored Ca^{2+}. For details: see text.

or during advanced atherosclerosis, this gene expression pattern is switched to an increased formation of extracellular matrix accompanied by the proliferation of smooth muscle cells (38). There is evidence that signaling pathways initiated by GPCRs are critically involved in the differentiation and dedifferentiation processes of smooth muscle cells. Activation of receptors that couple to the G-protein families G_q/G_{11} and G_{12}/G_{13} tend to promote the expression of contractile genes (39–41) and to stimulate smooth muscle cell differentiation (42,43). The underlying signaling events include the activation of different MAP-kinases, the generation of reactive oxygen species (44–46) or the stimulation of the RhoA/Rho-kinase pathway (47–49).

Migration of smooth muscle cells is a fundamental process during the development of hollow organs, like, for example, blood vessels, but can also be induced in the adult organism, for example after dedifferentiation. Migration of cells, including smooth muscle cells, depends on several orchestrated events that include reorganization of the actin filament network, de- and re-assembly of focal adhesions, and contraction of the actomyosin motor (50). Several GPCRs are involved in these processes. GPCRs like those for angiotensin II, thrombin or lysophospholipids, which couple to G-proteins of the G_q/G_{11}, G_{12}/G_{13}, and G_i/G_o families, are capable of stimulating smooth muscle cell migration by various intracellular signaling processes (50–56).

Thus, by activating different heterotrimeric G-proteins, GPCRs are capable of activating an intricate network of signaling events, mainly including MAPK cascades, the formation of reactive oxygen species and crosstalk to different tyrosine kinases to elicit various cellular effects in smooth muscle cells like migration, proliferation and differentiation.

G-PROTEIN-COUPLED RECEPTORS INVOLVED IN THE REGULATION OF SMOOTH MUSCLE CELL FUNCTION

A wide variety of GPCRs can be found to be involved in the regulation of smooth muscle (Tables 85.1 and 85.2). A particular smooth muscle type usually expresses a variety of different GPCRs that allows integration of multiple influences by neurotransmitters as well as local and systemic humoral factors. Well-studied examples are the vascular and airway smooth muscle organs, which are subject to multiple regulatory influences sensed by many different GPCRs (57,58).

TABLE 85.1 GPCRs Mediating Contraction of Smooth Muscle Cells

Ligand	Receptor(s)	G-Protein Coupling	SM Expression					
			Blood vessel	Airway	Uterus	GI tract	Urogenital	Ciliary
Acetylcholine	M_2	G_i/G_o	X	X		X	X	X
	M_3	G_q/G_{11}		X		X	X	X
Adenosine	A_1	G_i/G_o	X	X				
Angiotensin	AT_1	G_q/G_{11}, G_i/G_o, G_{12}/G_{13}	X					
Apelin	APJ	G_i/G_o	X			X		
ATP/UTP	$P2Y_1$	G_q/G_{11}	X					
	$P2Y_2$	G_q/G_{11}	X	X		X		
	$P2Y_6$	G_q/G_{11}	X	X				
Bradykinin	B_1	G_q/G_{11}, G_i/G_o	X					
	B_2	G_q/G_{11}, G_i/G_o	X	X				
Cholecystokinin	CCK_1	G_q/G_{11}				X		
Endothelin	ET_A	G_q/G_{11}, G_{12}/G_{13}	X	X	X	X		
	ET_B	G_q/G_{11}, G_i/G_o		X		X		
Epinephrine, norepinephrine	α_{1A}	G_q/G_{11}	X				X	
	α_{1B}	G_q/G_{11}	X					
	α_{1D}	G_q/G_{11}	X				X	
	α_{2A} and α_{2c}	G_i/G_o	X		X	X		
	α_{2B}	G_i/G_o	X		X			
Histamine	H_1	G_q/G_{11}	X	X		X	X	
Leukotriene B4	BLT_1	G_q/G_{11}, G_i/G_o	X					
Leukotriene C4/D4	$CysLT_2$	G_q/G_{11}		X				
LPA	LPA_1, LPA_2, LPA_3	G_q/G_{11}, G_{12}/G_{13}, G_i/G_o	X	X	X	X		
Melatonin	MT_1	G_q/G_{11}	X					
Motilin	MTLR	G_q/G_{11}, G_{12}/G_{13}				X		
Neurokinin A	NK_2	G_q/G_{11}, G_i/G_o	X	X		X		
Neurokinin B	NK_3	G_q/G_{11}				X		
Neuromedin U	NMU_1	G_q/G_{11}	X			X	X	
Neuropeptide S	NPS	G_q/G_{11}	?	X				
Neuropeptide Y	Y_1	G_i/G_o	X			X	X	
Neurotensin	NTS_1	G_q/G_{11}				X		
Oxytocin	OT	G_q/G_{11}			X			
Prostaglandin E_2	EP_1	G_q/G_{11}	X			X		X
	EP_3	G_i/G_o	X	X	X	X		
Prostaglandin $F_{2\alpha}$	FP	G_i/G_o	X		X			X
S1P	$S1P_2$, $S1P_3$	G_q/G_{11}, G_{12}/G_{13}	X	X	X	X		

(Continued)

TABLE 85.1 (Continued)

Ligand	Receptor(s)	G-Protein Coupling	SM Expression					
			Blood vessel	Airway	Uterus	GI tract	Urogenital	Ciliary
Serotonin	5-$HT_{1A/1B}$	G_i/G_o	X	X				
	5-HT_{1F}	G_i/G_o			X			
	5-$HT_{2A/2B}$	G_q/G_{11}	X	X		X		
Somatostatin	SST_2	G_i/G_o	X	X		X	X	X
Thromboxane A_2	TP	G_q/G_{11}, G_{12}/G_{13}	X	X	X			
Thrombin	PAR1,2,3	G_q/G_{11}, G_{12}/G_{13}	X	X	X	X	X	
Urotensin II	UT	G_q/G_{11}	X					
Vasopressin	V_{1a}	G_q/G_{11}	X		X			

TABLE 85.2 GPCRs Mediating Relaxation of Smooth Muscle Cells

Ligand	Receptor(s)	G-Protein-Coupling	SM Expression					
			Blood vessel	Airway	Uterus	GI tract	Urogenital	Ciliary
Adenosine	A_{2A}, A_{2B}	G_s	X	X		X		
Dopamine	$D_{1/5}$	G_s	X				X	
Epinephrine, norepinephrine	β_1	G_s				X		
	β_2	G_s	X	X	X	X		
Prostaglandin D_2	DP_1	G_s	X	X	X			
Prostaglandin E_2	EP_2	G_s	X	X	X			
	EP_4	G_s	X					
Prostacyclin	IP	G_s	X	X	X			
Relaxin	$RXFP_1$	G_s	X		X			
Vasopressin	V_2	G_s	X					
VIP, PACAP	$VPAC_2$	G_s		X	X	X		

The expression of many receptors is restricted to particular smooth muscle types in certain organ systems where they mediate organ-specific regulation of smooth muscle contraction by particular hormones or transmitters (Tables 85.1 and 85.2). However, there are also GPCRs that are found widely expressed in smooth muscle tissues of different organs. As most smooth muscle organs are under the control of the autonomic nervous system, most smooth muscle cells express adrenergic, and many also muscarinic, receptors. Also other biogenic amine receptors like those for serotonin and histamine are found on many smooth muscle cells. Most smooth muscle cells also have various receptors responding to classic local mediators like adenosine, nucleotides and prostanoids. There are quite a few peptide (57) and lipid mediators like lysophosphatidic acid and sphingosine-1 phosphate (59) which have only recently been identified, and which act through particular receptor subtypes to regulate various cell types including smooth muscle cells.

PHARMACOLOGICAL REGULATION OF SMOOTH MUSCLE FUNCTION THROUGH GPCRS

Dysregulations of smooth muscle tone are centrally involved in the pathology of various diseases. For instance, cardiovascular diseases like coronary heart disease or arterial hypertension are aggravated by increased vascular tone; gastrointestinal diseases like diarrhea or

TABLE 85.3 Pharmacological Regulation of Smooth Muscle Cells through GPCRs

Receptor	Drug (Example)	Wanted Effect (Disease)
Receptor agonists		
Acetylcholine (M_3)	Bethanechol	Contraction of *M. detrusor vesicae* → Emptying of urinary bladder
	Pilocarpin (local appl.)	Contraction of *M. sphincter pupillae* → Miosis
Vasopressin (V_1)	Terlipressin	Vasoconstriction
α_1 adrenergic	Phenylephrine	Vasoconstriction
Oxytocin (OT)	Oxytocin	Induction of labor
Prostaglandin E_2 (EP)	Misoprostol	Uterus contraction
β_2-adrenergic	Fenoterol (e.g.)	Bronchial relaxation (bronchial asthma), tocolysis
Prostacyclin (IP)	Iloprost	Vasodilation
Receptor antagonists		
α_1 adrenergic	Prazosin	Vasodilation (hypertension)
	Tamsulosin	Relaxation of lower urinary tract smooth muscle (benign prostatic hyperplasia)
Angiotensin II (AT_1)	Losartan	Vasodilation (arterial hypertension)
Acetylcholine (M_3)	Ipratropium	Bronchial relaxation (bronchial asthma)
	Tropicamide	Relaxation of *M. sphincter pupillae* → Mydriasis
	Solifenacin	Relaxation of *M. detrusor vesicae* (urge incontinence)
Endothelin (ET_A)	Sitaxentan	Relaxation of pulmonary vessels (pulmonary hypertension)
Prostaglandin D_2 (DP_1)	Laropiprant	Reduced prostaglandin D_2-dependent cutaneous vasodilation (flushing) under nicotinic acid therapy

obstipation are intimately linked to the regulation of peristalsis by the gastrointestinal smooth muscle. Similarly, obstructive pulmonary diseases, in particular bronchial asthma, result from an increased tone of bronchial smooth muscle cells. The wide variety of GPCRs expressed specifically in particular smooth muscle organs makes them ideal targets for drugs interfering with organ-specific smooth muscle functions. In fact, many drugs have been developed as agonists or antagonists of GPCRs expressed by smooth muscle cells in order to regulate their functions (see Table 85.3).

CONCLUSIONS

Smooth muscle cells are quite heterogeneous, depending on the organ system in which they serve their function. Their major role is to control the diameter, wall movement, and wall stiffness of hollow organs like the vascular, bronchial, gastrointestinal or urogenital system as well as the uterus. Besides a variety of myogenic regulatory mechanisms, the function of smooth muscle cells is under the control of external stimuli released from autonomous nerves, adjacent cells or distant sites. Many of these smooth muscle regulators act through GPCRs to modulate smooth muscle function. While the basal mechanisms of GPCR-mediated smooth muscle tone regulation are very similar between different organs, the sensitivity of organ-specific smooth muscle cells to smooth muscle regulators can vary profoundly depending on the receptor subtypes expressed by a particular organ-specific smooth muscle cell. More recent data also indicate that the response of smooth muscle cells to organ damage, which typically results in the dedifferentiation of smooth muscle cells and an increased tendency to migrate and proliferate, is also under the control of various locally produced mediators acting on specific GPCRs expressed by smooth muscle cells. In the future, it will be of interest to better understand the downstream signaling mechanisms used by GPCRs to regulate smooth muscle functions under physiological and pathophysiological conditions, to identify specific GPCRs playing critical roles in the regulation of smooth muscle functions under pathophysiological conditions and to finally exploit this knowledge to develop new pharmacological strategies in order to interfere with altered smooth muscle functions which are responsible for the initiation or progression of common diseases like bronchial hyperreactivity, arterial hypertension, or disorders of bowel motility.

REFERENCES

1. Lefkowitz RJ. Seven transmembrane receptors: something old, something new. *Acta Physiol (Oxf)* 2007;**190**:9–19.
2. Oldham WM, Hamm HE. How do receptors activate G proteins? *Adv Protein Chem* 2007;**74**:67–93.
3. Wettschureck N, Offermanns S. Mammalian G proteins and their cell type specific functions. *Physiol Rev* 2005;**85**:1159–204.
4. Dupre DJ, Robitaille M, Rebois RV, Hebert TE. The role of G-betagamma subunits in the organization, assembly, and function of GPCR signaling complexes. *Annu Rev Pharmacol Toxicol* 2009;**49**:31–56.
5. Simonds WF. G protein regulation of adenylate cyclase. *Trends Pharmacol Sci* 1999;**20**:66–73.
6. Mizuno N, Itoh H. Functions and regulatory mechanisms of Gq-signaling pathways. *Neurosignals* 2009;**17**:42–54.
7. Worzfeld T, Wettschureck N, Offermanns S. G(12)/G(13)-mediated signalling in mammalian physiology and disease. *Trends Pharmacol Sci* 2008;**29**:582–9.
8. Somlyo AP, Somlyo AV. Ca^{2+} sensitivity of smooth muscle and nonmuscle myosin II: modulated by G proteins, kinases, and myosin phosphatase. *Physiol Rev* 2003;**83**:1325–58.
9. Somlyo AP, Somlyo AV. Signal transduction and regulation in smooth muscle. *Nature* 1994;**372**:231–6.
10. Wang Y, Deng X, Hewavitharana T, Soboloff J, Gill DL. Stim, ORAI and TRPC channels in the control of calcium entry signals in smooth muscle. *Clin Exp Pharmacol Physiol* 2008;**35**:1127–33.
11. Albert AP, Saleh SN, Peppiatt-Wildman CM, Large WA. Multiple activation mechanisms of store-operated TRPC channels in smooth muscle cells. *J Physiol* 2007;**583**:25–36.
12. Moosmang S, Kleppisch T, Wegener J, Welling A, Hofmann F. Analysis of calcium channels by conditional mutagenesis. *Handb Exp Pharmacol* 2007;469–90.
13. Vennekens R. Emerging concepts for the role of TRP channels in the cardiovascular system. *J Physiol* 2010;**589**:1527–34.
14. Watanabe H, Murakami M, Ohba T, Takahashi Y, Ito H. TRP channel and cardiovascular disease. *Pharmacol Ther* 2008;**118**:337–51.
15. Puetz S, Lubomirov LT, Pfitzer G. Regulation of smooth muscle contraction by small GTPases. *Physiology (Bethesda)* 2009;**24**:342–56.
16. Gohla A, Schultz G, Offermanns S. Role for G(12)/G(13) in agonist-induced vascular smooth muscle cell contraction. *Circ Res* 2000;**87**:221–7.
17. Wirth A, Benyo Z, Lukasova M, Leutgeb B, Wettschureck N, Gorbey S, et al. G12-G13-LARG-mediated signaling in vascular smooth muscle is required for salt-induced hypertension. *Nat Med* 2008;**14**:64–8.
18. Fukuhara S, Chikumi H, Gutkind JS. RGS-containing RhoGEFs: the missing link between transforming G proteins and Rho? *Oncogene* 2001;**20**:1661–8.
19. Wuertz CM, Lorincz A, Vettel C, Thomas MA, Wieland T, Lutz S. p63RhoGEF – a key mediator of angiotensin II-dependent signaling and processes in vascular smooth muscle cells. *FASEB J* 2010;**24**:4865–76.
20. Booden MA, Siderovski DP, Der CJ. Leukemia-associated Rho guanine nucleotide exchange factor promotes G alpha q-coupled activation of RhoA. *Mol Cell Biol* 2002;**22**:4053–61.
21. Guilluy C, Bregeon J, Toumaniantz G, Rolli-Derkinderen M, Retailleau K, Loufrani L, et al. The Rho exchange factor Arhgef1 mediates the effects of angiotensin II on vascular tone and blood pressure. *Nat Med* 2010;**16**:183–90.
22. Hofmann F. Smooth muscle tone regulation. In: Offermanns S, Rosenthal W, editors. *Encyclopedic reference of molecular pharmacology*. Heidelberg: Springer-Verlag;2004. p. 870–5.
23. Murthy KS. Signaling for contraction and relaxation in smooth muscle of the gut. *Annu Rev Physiol* 2006;**68**:345–74.
24. Tang KM, Wang GR, Lu P, Karas RH, Aronovitz M, Heximer SP, et al. Regulator of G-protein signaling-2 mediates vascular smooth muscle relaxation and blood pressure. *Nat Med* 2003;**9**:1506–12.
25. Huang J, Zhou H, Mahavadi S, Sriwai W, Murthy KS. Inhibition of Galphaq-dependent PLC-beta1 activity by PKG and PKA is mediated by phosphorylation of RGS4 and GRK2. *Am J Physiol Cell Physiol* 2007;**292**:C200–8.
26. Standen NB, Quayle JM. K^+ channel modulation in arterial smooth muscle. *Acta Physiol Scand* 1998;**164**:549–57.
27. Schubert R, Nelson MT. Protein kinases: tuners of the BKCa channel in smooth muscle. *Trends Pharmacol Sci* 2001;**22**:505–12.
28. Johnson RP, El-Yazbi AF, Hughes MF, Schriemer DC, Walsh EJ, et al. Identification and functional characterization of protein kinase A-catalyzed phosphorylation of potassium channel Kv1.2 at serine 449. *J Biol Chem* 2009;**284**:16562–74.
29. Murthy KS, Zhou H. Selective phosphorylation of the IP3R-I in vivo by cGMP-dependent protein kinase in smooth muscle. *Am J Physiol Gastrointest Liver Physiol* 2003;**284**:G221–30.
30. Komalavilas P, Lincoln TM. Phosphorylation of the inositol 1,4,5-trisphosphate receptor. Cyclic GMP-dependent protein kinase mediates cAMP and cGMP dependent phosphorylation in the intact rat aorta. *J Biol Chem* 1996;**271**:21933–8.
31. Loirand G, Guilluy C, Pacaud P. Regulation of Rho proteins by phosphorylation in the cardiovascular system. *Trends Cardiovasc Med* 2006;**16**:199–204.
32. Wooldridge AA, MacDonald JA, Erdodi F, Ma C, Borman MA, Hartshorne DJ, et al. Smooth muscle phosphatase is regulated in vivo by exclusion of phosphorylation of threonine 696 of MYPT1 by phosphorylation of Serine 695 in response to cyclic nucleotides. *J Biol Chem* 2004;**279**:34496–504.
33. Surks HK, Mochizuki N, Kasai Y, Georgescu SP, Tang KM, Ito M, et al. Regulation of myosin phosphatase by a specific interaction with cGMP- dependent protein kinase Ialpha. *Science* 1999;**286**:1583–7.
34. Surks HK. cGMP-dependent protein kinase I and smooth muscle relaxation: a tale of two isoforms. *Circ Res* 2007;**101**:1078–80.
35. Matsushita M, Tanaka Y, Koike K. Studies on the mechanisms underlying beta-adrenoceptor-mediated relaxation of rat abdominal aorta. *J Smooth Muscle Res* 2006;**42**:217–25.
36. Kume H, Hall IP, Washabau RJ, Takagi K, Kotlikoff MI. Beta-adrenergic agonists regulate KCa channels in airway smooth muscle by cAMP-dependent and -independent mechanisms. *J Clin Invest* 1994;**93**:371–9.
37. Tanaka Y, Yamashita Y, Yamaki F, Horinouchi T, Shigenobu K, Koike K. Evidence for a significant role of a Gs-triggered mechanism unrelated to the activation of adenylyl cyclase in

the cyclic AMP-independent relaxant response of guinea-pig tracheal smooth muscle. *Naunyn Schmiedebergs Arch Pharmacol* 2003;**368**:437–41.

38. Owens GK, Kumar MS, Wamhoff BR. Molecular regulation of vascular smooth muscle cell differentiation in development and disease. *Physiol Rev* 2004;**84**:767–801.
39. Dulin NO, Orlov SN, Kitchen CM, Voyno-Yasenetskaya TA, Miano JM. G-protein-coupled-receptor activation of the smooth muscle calponin gene. *Biochem J* 2001;**357**:587–92.
40. Hautmann MB, Thompson MM, Swartz EA, Olson EN, Owens GK. Angiotensin II-induced stimulation of smooth muscle alpha-actin expression by serum response factor and the homeodomain transcription factor MHox. *Circ Res* 1997;**81**:600–10.
41. di Gioia CR, van de Greef WM, Sperti G, Castoldi G, Todaro N, Ierardi C, et al. Angiotensin II increases calponin expression in cultured rat vascular smooth muscle cells. *Biochem Biophys Res Commun* 2000;**279**:965–9.
42. Martin K, Weiss S, Metharom P, Schmeckpeper J, Hynes B, O'Sullivan J, et al. Thrombin stimulates smooth muscle cell differentiation from peripheral blood mononuclear cells via protease-activated receptor-1, RhoA, and myocardin. *Circ Res* 2009;**105**:214–8.
43. Saeed AE, Parmentier JH, Malik KU. Activation of alpha1A-adrenergic receptor promotes differentiation of rat-1 fibroblasts to a smooth muscle-like phenotype. *BMC Cell Biol* 2004;**5**:47.
44. Viedt C, Soto U, Krieger-Brauer HI, Fei J, Elsing C, Kubler W, et al. Differential activation of mitogen-activated protein kinases in smooth muscle cells by angiotensin II: involvement of p22phox and reactive oxygen species. *Arterioscler Thromb Vasc Biol* 2000;**20**:940–8.
45. Su B, Mitra S, Gregg H, Flavahan S, Chotani MA, Clark KR, et al. Redox regulation of vascular smooth muscle cell differentiation. *Circ Res* 2001;**89**:39–46.
46. Schauwienold D, Plum C, Helbing T, Voigt P, Bobbert T, Hoffmann D, et al. ERK1/2-dependent contractile protein expression in vascular smooth muscle cells. *Hypertension* 2003;**41**:546–52.
47. Lockman K, Hinson JS, Medlin MD, Morris D, Taylor JM, Mack CP. Sphingosine 1-phosphate stimulates smooth muscle cell differentiation and proliferation by activating separate serum response factor co-factors. *J Biol Chem* 2004;**279**:42422–30.
48. Grabski AD, Shimizu T, Deou J, Mahoney Jr WM, Reidy MA, Daum G. Sphingosine-1-phosphate receptor-2 regulates expression of smooth muscle alpha-actin after arterial injury. *Arterioscler Thromb Vasc Biol* 2009;**29**:1644–50.
49. Medlin MD, Staus DP, Dubash AD, Taylor JM, Mack CP. Sphingosine 1-phosphate receptor 2 signals through leukemia-associated RhoGEF (LARG), to promote smooth muscle cell differentiation. *Arterioscler Thromb Vasc Biol* 2010;**30**:1779–86.
50. Gerthoffer WT. Mechanisms of vascular smooth muscle cell migration. *Circ Res* 2007;**100**:607–21.
51. Touyz RM, Schiffrin EL. Signal transduction mechanisms mediating the physiological and pathophysiological actions of angiotensin II in vascular smooth muscle cells. *Pharmacol Rev* 2000;**52**:639–72.
52. Clempus RE, Griendling KK. Reactive oxygen species signaling in vascular smooth muscle cells. *Cardiovasc Res* 2006;**71**:216–25.
53. Nishio E, Watanabe Y. Role of the lipoxygenase pathway in phenylephrine-induced vascular smooth muscle cell proliferation and migration. *Eur J Pharmacol* 1997;**336**:267–73.
54. Wang Z, Castresana MR, Newman WH. Reactive oxygen species-sensitive p38 MAPK controls thrombin-induced migration of vascular smooth muscle cells. *J Mol Cell Cardiol* 2004;**36**:49–56.
55. Kyotani Y, Zhao J, Tomita S, Nakayama H, Isosaki M, Uno M, et al. Olmesartan inhibits angiotensin II-Induced migration of vascular smooth muscle cells through Src and mitogen-activated protein kinase pathways. *J Pharmacol Sci* 2010;**113**:161–8.
56. Mugabe BE, Yaghini FA, Song CY, Buharalioglu CK, Waters CM, Malik KU. Angiotensin II-induced migration of vascular smooth muscle cells is mediated by p38 mitogen-activated protein kinase-activated c-Src through spleen tyrosine kinase and epidermal growth factor receptor transactivation. *J Pharmacol Exp Ther* 2010;**332**:116–24.
57. Maguire JJ, Davenport AP. Regulation of vascular reactivity by established and emerging GPCRs. *Trends Pharmacol Sci* 2005;**26**:448–54.
58. Billington CK, Penn RB. Signaling and regulation of G protein-coupled receptors in airway smooth muscle. *Respir Res* 2003;**4**:2.
59. Igarashi J, Michel T. Sphingosine-1-phosphate and modulation of vascular tone. *Cardiovasc Res* 2009;**82**:212–20.

Chapter 86

Calcium Homeostasis and Signaling in Smooth Muscle

Theodor Burdyga[1] and Richard J. Paul[2]

[1]Department of Cellular and Molecular Physiology, Institute of Translational Medicine, University of Liverpool, Liverpool, UK, [2]Department of Molecular and Cellular Physiology, University of Cincinnati College of Medicine, Cincinnati, OH

INTRODUCTION

Intracellular Ca^{2+} is a universal second messenger that regulates a large number of cellular functions, such as contraction, metabolism, excitability, secretion, transcription, immune responses, fertilization, and development. Ca^{2+} signaling ultimately rests on the control of $[Ca^{2+}]_i$, both in a local as well as a global sense, which depends not only on Ca^{2+} influx and release from intracellular stores, but also the mechanisms of Ca^{2+} clearance. Complex spatiotemporal patterns of Ca^{2+} signaling are believed to be responsible for this diversity of functions performed by one signaling molecule. Smooth muscle is not a uniform tissue throughout the body and its type and function vary not only among different organs but also depend on its location. Smooth muscles range from myogenic where Ca^{2+} transients are controlled by the action potentials or waves of slow depolarizations to neurogenic, where Ca^{2+} signaling is largely controlled by nervous activity. Each SMC type has a Ca^{2+} signaling system that is uniquely adapted to control its particular function. Apart from contraction other Ca^{2+} signaling-related functions have been recognized in the smooth muscles and it is likely that there are many others that remain to be discovered. In smooth muscles, Ca^{2+} entry into the cytosol is regulated by the influx of Ca^{2+} *via* the plasma membrane and/or release of Ca^{2+} from intracellular Ca^{2+} stores, predominantly the sarcoplasmic reticulum (SR). A population of channels which includes voltage-, receptor-, and store-operated channels of the plasma membrane (PM) are involved in control of Ca^{2+} influx and two types of Ca^{2+}-release channels, the ryanodine receptor (RyR) and the inositol 1,4,5-trisphosphate receptor (IP_3R), are involved in intracellular Ca^{2+} mobilization in smooth muscles. The major cytosolic Ca^{2+} clearance systems are the sarcoplasmic/endoplasmic reticulum Ca^{2+} ATPase (SERCA), Na^+/Ca^{2+}-exchanger (NCX) powered by the Na^+-K^+ ATPase (NKA), and the plasma membrane Ca^{2+} ATPase (PMCA), with potential mitochondrial participation and coordination.

In the past 15 years significant progress has been made in the area of Ca^{2+} signaling in smooth muscles using Ca^{2+}-sensitive fluorescent indicators combined with advances in a new technology allowing Ca^{2+} imaging, particularly with the confocal microscope. Combined with electrophysiological techniques and new biochemical and molecular biology methods, these studies have revealed a spectrum of Ca^{2+} signals characterized by a high degree of spatial and temporal complexity ranging from elemental events such as Ca^{2+} sparks and puffs to intra- and intercellular Ca^{2+} waves and oscillations. This complex Ca^{2+} signaling results from the interactions of ion transport and pump proteins located in the PM, the SR, and mitochondria. The aim of this chapter is to review the Ca^{2+} entry and clearance mechanisms identified in smooth muscle cells and relate them to the hierarchy of Ca^{2+} signaling.

SOURCES OF Ca^{2+} IN SMOOTH MUSCLE CELLS

In smooth muscles Ca^{2+} entry into the cytosol is regulated by the influx of Ca^{2+} via the plasma membrane channels and the Na^+/Ca^{2+}-exchanger in reverse mode (i.e., Ca^{2+} in, Na^+ out of the cell), and/or release of Ca^{2+} from intracellular Ca^{2+} stores. Ca^{2+} entry channels include voltage, receptor- and store-operated Ca^{2+} channels.

Voltage Operated Ca^{2+} Channels

The electrical potential across the SMC membrane plays a pivotal role in control of all phasic and some tonic smooth muscle contraction, through its depolarization and the subsequent influx of Ca^{2+} through voltage-gated

Muscle. DOI: http://dx.doi.org/10.1016/B978-0-12-381510-1.00086-7

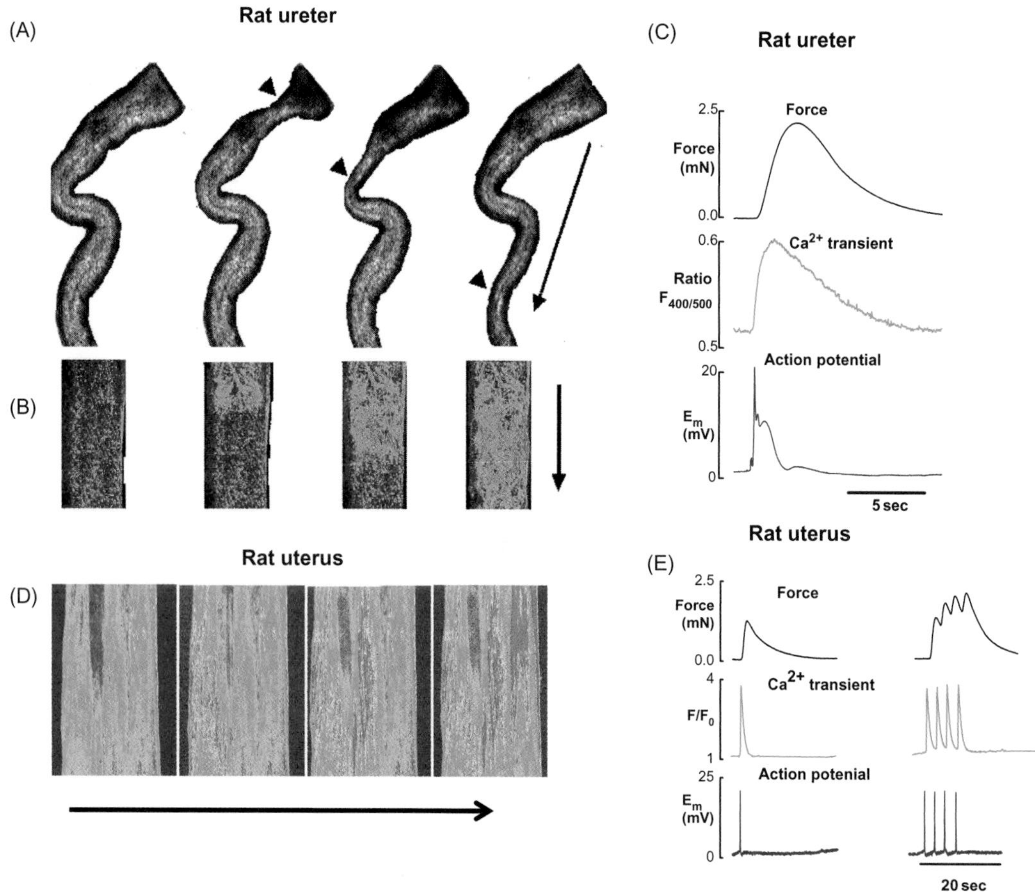

FIGURE 86.1 **Propagating intercellular action potential-mediated Ca^{2+} wave recorded with digital confocal imaging in intact ureter and uterine smooth muscles loaded with Ca-sensitive indicator fluo-4.** (A) Transmitted light images showing axial propagation of mechanical wave (arrow head) from proximal to distal ends (arrow) of rat ureter. (B) Pseudo-color images of segment of rat uterus loaded with fluo-4 showing axial propagation of the intercellular Ca^{2+} wave associated with the action potential underlying phasic contraction. (C) Graph showing temporal relationship between action potential (bottom trace), Ca^{2+} wave (middle trace), and phasic contraction (top trace) recorded from segment of ureter shown in (B). (D) Pseudo-color images of strip of fluo-4 loaded longitudinal smooth muscles of pregnant rat uterus showing transverse propagation of the intercellular Ca^{2+} wave associated with the action potentials underlying single or fused phasic contractions. (E) Graph showing temporal relationship between action potential (bottom trace), Ca^{2+} wave (middle trace), and phasic contractions (top trace) recorded from segment of uterus shown in (D).

Ca^{2+} channels (1,2). The voltage-operated Ca^{2+} channel is an ion channel population that opens as the potential across the membrane is reduced and is responsible for the upstroke of the action potential (AP). Influx of Ca^{2+} into electrically excitable smooth muscle cells occurs mainly through activation of long-lasting (L-type) high voltage-activated Ca^{2+} channels which have large conductance (8–25 pS) and are sensitive to dihydropyridine (DHP) derivatives: antagonists (e.g., nifedipine) or agonist (BayK-8644) (1). For this reason these channels are termed as DHP-sensitive Ca^{2+} channels. These channels are present in all types of smooth muscle cells, although the level of expression and their contribution to Ca^{2+} signaling is tissue- and stimulus-dependent. In some types of smooth muscle low-voltage activated transient (T-type) voltage-gated Ca^{2+} channels have also been detected; however, the functional role of these channels is still not clear (1). Action potential (AP)-mediated Ca^{2+} transients result from direct influx of Ca^{2+} via DHP-sensitive channels and appear as a Ca^{2+} spike in smooth muscles controlled by spike-like APs, such as uterus, bladder, GI tract, portal vein (Figure 86.1e). In ureter smooth muscle, the Ca^{2+} transient has a plateau phase controlled by the plateau type AP (Figure 86.1c).

SMCs are interconnected as a three-dimensional electrical syncytium and not only possess mechanical but also electrical intercommunication, so that electrophysiological phenomena can be interpreted in relation to tissue structure and cell relationships. Collective behavior would seem to be common to all smooth muscles, though the extent of its spatial spread is variable. Low-resistance pathways between the interiors of adjacent cells allow electrotonic spread of current or, more extensively, propagation of APs through the smooth muscle tissue.

Confocal imaging of intact strips loaded with fluo-4 combined with recording of electrical activity and force showed that in ureter AP-mediated Ca^{2+} spike propagates mainly in the axial direction (Figures 86.1a,b), while in some other types of smooth muscles such as bladder, GI tract, and uterus (Figure 86.1d), it propagates in axial, and less effectively in the transverse direction. Maximal force is produced only when all muscle bundles are recruited and contribute to force generation. The functional connections between smooth muscle cells consist of gap junctions that control electrical coupling between smooth muscle cells. In tonic non-spiking smooth muscles, such as small resistance arteries and arterioles, smooth muscles can be partially depolarized by a variety of direct stimulants which open DHP-sensitive Ca^{2+} channels activating small but sustained Ca^{2+} influx, thus eliciting tonic contractions (3). The generation of the regenerative AP in these types of smooth muscle is impeded by rapid activation of a family of K^+ channels sensitive to TEA (3). DHP-sensitive Ca^{2+} channels are capable of opening at moderate depolarizations (−40, −20 mV) and generate the so called "window current", which causes a steady increase in intracellular Ca^{2+} associated with the development of tonic contraction (3). Unlike Ca^{2+} spikes elicited by all-or-none regenerative APs , which give rise to the stereotypic, constant amplitude Ca^{2+} spike, "window" Ca^{2+} current can be graded depending on the level of depolarization.

Ca^{2+} Entry Coupled to Receptor Activation

More than 30 years ago, it was suggested that receptor activation could lead to Ca^{2+} entry into smooth muscle cells by mechanisms independent of membrane depolarization, and the concept of receptor-operated Ca^{2+} channels (ROC) and pharmaco-mechanical coupling in smooth muscle was introduced (4,5). Therefore, at that time, ROCs represented any plasma membrane Ca^{2+}-permeable channels other than voltage-sensitive Ca^{2+} channels, which were opened as a result of the binding of an agonist to its receptor. Based on new evidence, agonists can activate voltage-independent Ca^{2+} entry in smooth muscle cells in three different ways that represent different aspects of pharmaco-mechanical coupling in smooth muscles.

The first type of ROC reported for smooth muscles is the model of capacitative Ca^{2+} entry (CCE) via store-operated Ca^{2+} channels (SOC) (6) (Figure 86.2). The

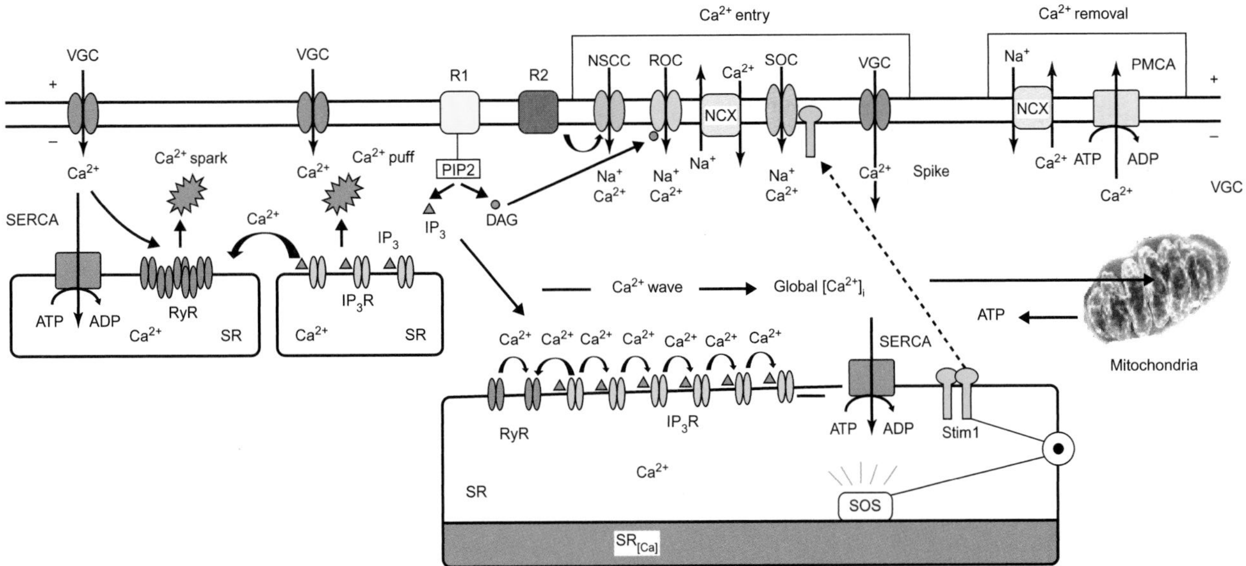

FIGURE 86.2 **Ca^{2+} mobilization and clearance pathways in smooth muscle cells.** Voltage-gated, L-type Ca channels (VGC) are opened by membrane depolarization and generate Ca^{2+} spikes underlying the upstroke of the propagating action potential in phasic and steady state graded Ca^{2+} influx in tonic smooth muscles. Ca^{2+} influx through VGC can trigger Ca^{2+} sparks directly (via CICR) or indirectly (via increasing the SR Ca^{2+} load). Agonist binding to G-protein-coupled receptors activates phospholipase C (PLC) generating diacylgycerol (DAG) and inositol trisphosphate (IP3). DAG activates receptor-operated channels (ROCs), eliciting Na^+ and Ca^{2+} entry, while IP_3 activates IP_3 receptors on the SR, causing local (Ca^{2+} puffs) or global (Ca^{2+} waves/oscillations) via activation of IP_3R. Ca^{2+} release through IP3R can additionally recruit adjacent RyRs. Store depletion is sensed by stromal interacting molecule 1 (STIM1) within the SR, which translocates to and activates store-operated channels (SOCs). The elevation in subplasmalemmal [Na^+] resulting from activation of non-selective cation channels (NSCC), non-selective receptor operated (ROCs) or SOCs may be sufficient to drive reverse-mode operation of Na^+/Ca^{2+} exchanger (NCX), leading to Ca^{2+} entry. Much of the Ca^{2+} entering the cell and released from stores may be sequestered by the superficial SR through SERCAs and mitochondria. Cycling between SR Ca^{2+} uptake and release mechanisms leads to Ca^{2+} oscillations. Ca^{2+} is removed from the cell by the plasma membrane Ca^{2+} ATPase (PMCA) and forward mode operation of the NCX.

idea of Ca^{2+} release/Ca^{2+} entry coupling in smooth muscles was originally proposed by Casteels and Droogmans (7). According to these authors refilling of the noradrenaline-sensitive Ca^{2+} store in vascular smooth muscle cells occurs via coupling between the Ca^{2+} store and the surface membrane which allows rapid inward movement of Ca ions into the cell that is resistant to voltage-gated Ca^{2+} channel blockers. SOCs are defined as plasma membrane Ca^{2+} channels that are opened in response to a decrease in the concentration of Ca^{2+} in the lumen of the sarcoplasmic reticulum ($[SR]_{[Ca]}$) (6). The key event that initiates the opening of SOCs is the decrease in $[SR]_{[Ca]}$, but not the Ca^{2+} released from ER. Experimentally, this can be demonstrated using cyclopiazonic acid (CPA) and thapsigargin, which act as selective inhibitors of the SERCA pump. These drugs cause depletion of SR Ca^{2+} stores by inhibiting sequestration of Ca^{2+} ions without activation of G proteins, and are used to provide an important distinction between Ca^{2+} entering through SOCs and other receptor operated channels. Ca^{2+} influx activated by SR Ca^{2+}-ATPase inhibitors is considered as a good functional marker for the Ca^{2+} entry via SOC. Numerous studies show that the SERCA pump inhibitors increase Ca^{2+} influx in various types of smooth muscles, which is resistant to L-type Ca^{2+} channel blockers (8,9). Members of the canonical transient receptor potential family (TRPC), particularly TRPC1, are involved in SOCE in vascular smooth muscles cells (8). Some studies suggest that the channels underlying SOC in smooth muscles are non-selective (10). More recently, a single membrane-spanning protein termed STIM1 (stromal-interacting molecule 1) was shown to play an essential role in the activation of SOCs. The STIM1 protein serves as a sensor of Ca^{2+} within the stores (9). Other studies provide convincing evidence showing that Orai1 (Orai, the keepers of the gates of Heaven in Greek mythology) is a pore subunit of the store-operated Ca^{2+} release-activated Ca^{2+} channels (6). The STIM1–Orai complex incorporating TRPC proteins is suggested to serve as a mechanism controlling activation of SOC in smooth muscles (9). A second type of ROC is the non-selective cationic channels (NSCC), which are opened by direct interaction with the receptor proteins (Figure 86.2). The NSCC are equally permeable to monovalent cations, such as Na^{+} and K^{+} in the extra- and intracellular compartments, but there is controversy over whether this conductance is a significant direct source for Ca^{2+} entry. NSCC current is voltage-dependent in many cells, and the current reverses near 0 mV, demonstrating its non-selectivity. The molecular mechanisms of NSCC activation are still not entirely clear. In ileal smooth muscles NSCC may be opened by ACh binding to M2 receptors working through Gi/Go, and facilitated via M3 receptors that are coupled to phospholipase C (PLC), IP_3 production, and Ca^{2+} release (3). The molecular entities responsible for non-selective cation conductances in smooth muscles have not yet been identified; however, Inoue and co-workers (11) showed that expression of a transient receptor potential protein (TRP6) in HEK293 cells resulted in a current with biophysical and pharmacological properties similar to the non-selective cation current activated by adrenergic stimuli in vascular smooth muscle cells.

The third mechanism is an activation of Ca^{2+} entry through receptor operated (ROC) channels independent of Ca^{2+} store(s) (Figure 86.2). This type of ROC is a non-selective cation channel, which is opened by receptor stimulation of GPCRs through the production of second messengers such as IP3 or DAG (10). The currents through ROCs have shown the properties of non-selective cation currents, with varying degrees of Ca^{2+} selectivity. Several members of the TRPC family are accepted to form ROC channels, including TRPC3, TRPC6, and TRPC7 (10).

Ca^{2+} Signals Associated with the SR Ca^{2+} Release

Ca^{2+} release from the SR in smooth muscle cells occurs through activation of two families of Ca^{2+} release channels, which have substantial homology and general structure called the ryanodine (RyRs) and inositol 1,4,5-trisphosphate receptors (IP_3R). Both types of receptors occur in three isoforms, RyR1, RyR 2, RyR3, and IP3R1, IP3R2, IP3R3, respectively. The RyR1 subtype is predominantly expressed in skeletal muscle, RyR2 in cardiac muscle, RyR3 seem to be expressed in many types of cells including smooth muscle. IP_3Rs are poorly expressed in skeletal and cardiac muscle but gene products have been identified in many types of excitable and non-excitable cells. Smooth muscle cells express multiple RyR and IP_3R isoforms in different proportions; depending on the type of smooth muscle or species, they can share the same store or be located on separate stores. These channels are involved in control of various functions in smooth muscle cells such as contraction, relaxation, proliferation, and differentiation (for recent review see 12). The functional role of RyRs and IP_3Rs channels in these processes critically depends on the molecular identity, level and proportion of expression, subcellular distribution, and types of functional units they form with other cellular structures, which is currently under investigation.

Ca^{2+} Sparks

Ca^{2+} sparks, mediated by activation of clusters of RyR channels, have been identified in skeletal, cardiac, and smooth muscles. In skeletal muscle, Ca^{2+} sparks are produced by direct mechanical interaction of the L-type channel ($Ca_v1.1$) with clusters of RyR1 channels to trigger the release of Ca^{2+} from the SR. In cardiac muscle Ca^{2+} sparks are produced by Ca^{2+} entering through the $Ca_v1.2$ channels during an action potential, stimulating the opening of the RyR2 channel via a Ca^{2+}-induced Ca^{2+} release mechanism. The Ca^{2+} sparks of smooth muscle are not quite the same as those in cardiac muscle, although in both tissues they arise from the opening of clusters of RyR channels, and reflect the activation of an elementary Ca^{2+}-release unit. In cardiac muscle, the Ca^{2+} sparks are recruited throughout the cell producing a global rise in $[Ca^{2+}]$ which amplifies the Ca^{2+} signal arising from the PM. In smooth muscles, Ca^{2+} sparks repeatedly arise from only a few discrete cytoplasmic microdomains adjacent to the superficially located SR within the myocytes termed frequent discharge sites (FDS) % (13) (Figure 86.3a). Despite the SR being a continuous network lining the internal side of the plasmalemma, in the majority of smooth muscle cells, there were only 1–4 FDS. This FDS invariably coincided with a prominent portion of the SR enriched with RyRs (14). The FDS-related SR element was a part of the superficial SR network and was within 1–2 μm of the nuclear envelope sites from which calcium is first released upon depolarization of the cell (15). However RyR channel opening is not always tightly linked to the gating of L-type Ca^{2+} channels. This led Kotlikoff and his group to postulate the concept of "loose coupling" (16). The most efficacious calcium spark trigger in the majority of smooth muscles appears to be the luminal SR Ca^{2+}, (SR $_{[Ca]}$), which is loaded via Ca^{2+} influx through voltage-gated Ca^{2+} channels. The $SR_{[Ca]}$ regulates Ca^{2+} release by stimulating RyRs on the luminal side. The mechanism of this facilitation is still poorly understood. In smooth muscle cells, ryanodine-sensitive Ca^{2+} release units are perfectly positioned to communicate with the plasma membrane ion channels (Figure 86.2). Nelson and colleagues (17) were the first to present strong evidence linking Ca^{2+} sparks and STOCs acting as a negative feedback mechanism to determine the degree of myogenic tone. Walsh and colleagues (18) in their elegant work directly demonstrated a

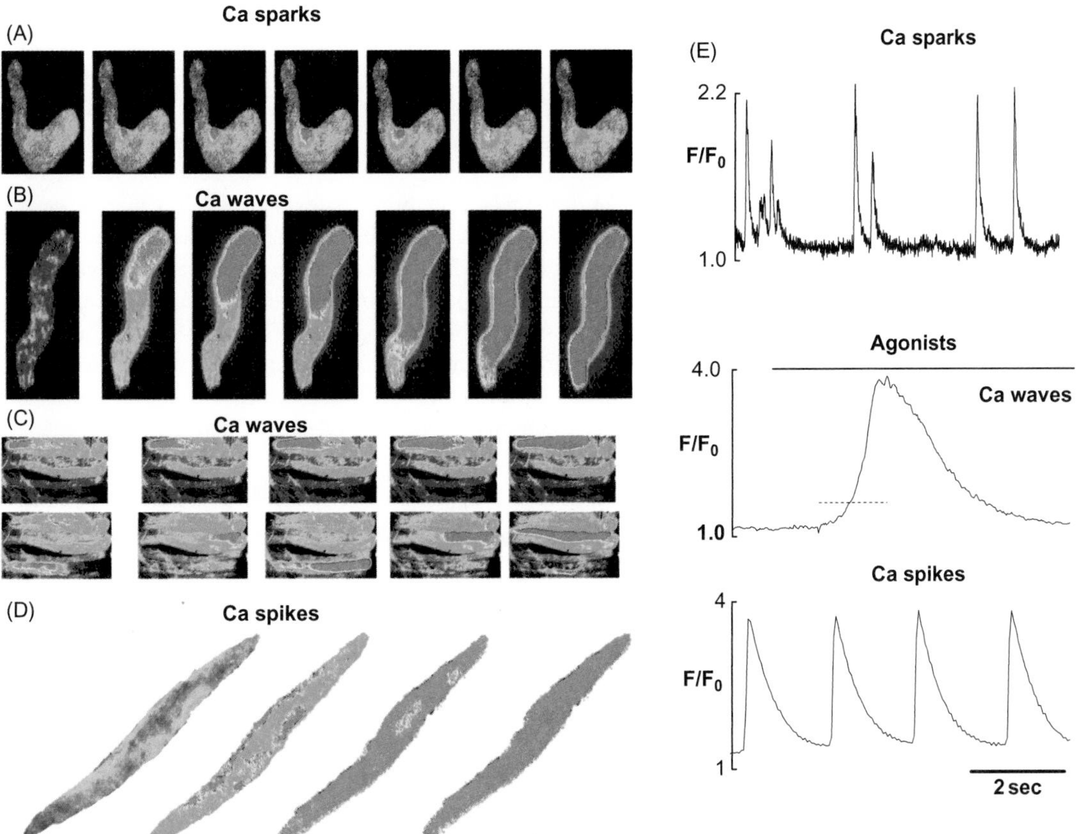

FIGURE 86.3 **Examples of different types of Ca^{2+} signaling identified in smooth muscles.** (A) Spontaneous Ca^{2+} sparks recorded from fluo-4-loaded guinea pig ureteric cell. (B,C) Propagating Ca^{2+} wave induced by carbachol (10 μM) or phenylephrine (10 μM) in rat ureteric myocytes and ureteric precapillary arteriole *in situ.* (D) Spontaneous Ca^{2+} spikes recorded from individual uterine myocyte in situ. (E) Temporal characteristics of Ca^{2+} sparks (top trace), Ca^{2+} wave (middle trace), and Ca^{2+} spike (bottom trace).

steep relationship between the level of luminal Ca^{2+} and the frequency of Ca^{2+} sparks and STOCs. It was suggested that the $SR_{[Ca]}$ provides a mechanism whereby agents could govern Ca^{2+}sparks and STOCs and hence the excitability of smooth muscle (19–21). By hyperpolarizing the cell membrane, the Ca^{2+} sparks/STOCs coupling mechanism can relax or oppose vasoconstriction in arteries (17), control excitability and the relative refractory period in ureter (22), and directly affect the duration of the action potentials in several types of phasic smooth muscles (11,12). Ca^{2+} sparks also appear to be involved in the important pacemaking potentials of gut and other smooth muscles (14,21). They also exert a depolarizing influence through Cl^-_{ca} channels in other smooth muscles such as pulmonary vascular myocytes (20).

Ca^{2+} Puffs

The term Ca^{2+} puffs refers to the small local increases in $[Ca^{2+}]$ that occur when IP_3Rs open spontaneously or in response to low concentrations of agonists. Polymorphisms of Ca^{2+} events mediated by opening of IP_3R channels, ranging from solitary Ca^{2+} puffs to propagating regenerative Ca^{2+} waves, have been well characterized and described in a number of non-excitable cells (23). Digital Ca^{2+} imaging techniques have revealed that in the majority of smooth muscle types, intracellular Ca^{2+} signals in response to IP_3 or IP_3-producing agents often present themselves as propagating Ca^{2+} waves or Ca^{2+} oscillations (Figure 86.3). In non-excitable cells an increase in $[Ca^{2+}]_i$ arising from the generation of IP_3 appears as localized transient increases of Ca^{2+}. So far, Ca^{2+} puffs have been detected in only two smooth muscles: rat ureter, in which agonist-induced Ca^{2+} release plays a dominant role in modulating contraction (24) and murine colonic myocytes (25). Unlike Ca^{2+} sparks, Ca^{2+} puffs showed large variability in amplitude, time course, and spatial spread, suggesting that IP_3R-gated channels in ureteric myocytes exist in clusters containing variable numbers of channels and that within these clusters a variable number of channels can be recruited (24). Ca^{2+} puffs in rat ureteric myocytes were blocked selectively by intracellular applications of heparin or an anti-IP_3R antibody, but were immune to ryanodine or an anti-ryanodine receptor antibody (24). When stimulated by higher concentrations of agonist, propagated, ryanodine-resistant Ca^{2+} waves appeared to result from the spatial recruitment of Ca^{2+} release sites by diffusion. This is consistent with data from multicellular preparations, where ryanodine-resistant agonist-induced Ca^{2+} release was reported (26). Localized Ca^{2+} transients and puffs, resistant to ryanodine and inhibited by xestospongin, U-73122 (an inhibitor of PLC), occurred spontaneously or during P2Y receptor stimulation in murine colonic myocytes (25). The puffs were coupled to the activation of both BK and small-conductance Ca^{2+}-activated K (SK) channels. Thus the release of Ca^{2+} by G protein-mediated activation of PLC can be linked to inhibitory responses via Ca^{2+} puffs targeting SK channels. This is in marked contrast to the usual finding that IP_3-dependent mechanisms are used by excitatory agonists in smooth muscles. Strong muscarinic stimulation can trigger an abrupt sub-plasmalemmal (sub-PM) $[Ca^{2+}]_i$ upstroke (SPCU), produced by an IP_3R-mediated Ca^{2+} release from sub-PM SR elements in guinea-pig ileum (where sub-PM SR elements are enriched with IP3Rs). These events were closely associated with action potentials and were strongly depended on Ca^{2+} entry through voltage-operated Ca^{2+} channels, suggesting that in this type of smooth muscle excitation–contraction involves an initial localized IP_3R-mediated Ca^{2+} release facilitated by voltage-gated Ca^{2+} entry (27).

Ca^{2+} Waves and Oscillations

Digital Ca^{2+} imaging of intact blood vessels loaded with Ca^{2+} sensitive dyes has shown that in many blood vessels, agonist-induced contractions are maintained by asynchronous wavelike Ca^{2+} oscillations in single smooth muscle cells (28–30) (Figure 86.3). Ca^{2+} oscillations appear as recurrent intracellular Ca^{2+} waves travelling through the longitudinal axis of the SMCs (Figure 86.3) and can be initiated by agonists, caffeine, or an increase in cytoplasmic or luminal level of Ca^{2+}. Calcium waves in smooth muscle cells are believed to be propagated along the SR. It is generally accepted that such waves are primarily propagated by regenerative calcium release, a process called calcium-induced calcium release or CICR. In the CICR mechanism, fast calcium waves are propagated by a reaction-diffusion cycle, whereby calcium ions diffuse along the outside of the ER and induce the release of more calcium stored inside the SR/ER. Waves are induced from the IP_3R on the SR by IP_3-generating agonists and proceed, at nearly constant amplitude, by sequential Ca^{2+} release from one release site or cluster (Figure 86.3). Each wave comprises a rising and a declining phase. The rising phase consists of a localized "initiation" component derived from the release of Ca^{2+} from the IP_3R followed by an "amplification" component during which this release feedback process thus amplifies the initiation (local) response to produce the rising phase of the wave. Examination of the propagation of Ca^{2+} waves suggests that the critical factor that determines propagation between domains is a time-dependent change in sensitivity of IP_3R and/or RyRs to Ca^{2+}, which can give rise to "loose coupling" between release sites and described by the "fire-diffuse-fire" model (31). The regenerative nature of Ca^{2+} waves depends on the positive feedback of increasing $[Ca^{2+}]_i$ on the IP_3R and recruitment of Ca^{2+}-sensitive RyRs. An alternative mechanism for the activation of RyRs in smooth muscles is an agonist-stimulated increase in cyclic ADP ribose (cADPR). cADPR, generated from NAD by ADP-ribosyl cyclase located as a cell surface receptor (CD38), is believed to facilitate the activation of RyRs via the FK506-binding protein 12.6 (FKBP12.6) (32,33). The cADPR/CD38 pathway of Ca^{2+} release is thought to be recruited by G-protein-coupled receptors (GPCRs), but the details are largely unknown. The relative involvement of IP_3R and RyR appears to vary between different types of smooth muscles. In smooth muscles displaying a higher density of IP_3Rs than that of RyRs (e.g. rat ureter or colonic smooth muscles), the Ca^{2+} responses to neurotransmitters will mainly depend on activation of IP_3 receptors alone. In smooth muscles displaying a higher density of RyRs than IP_3Rs (e.g. rat tail artery and rat portal vein), the Ca^{2+} waves and oscillations induced by neurotransmitters depend on activation of both IP_3Rs and RyRs. However, comparative functional experiments correlated with expression and distribution of IP_3R and RyR channels are needed to expand this conclusion to all types of smooth muscles. The delayed negative feedback on release, which is essential for oscillatory behavior, can be explained by inhibition of IP_3R type 1 isoform by high cytoplasmic and/or low luminal $[Ca^{2+}]$, time-dependent inactivation of IP_3R, or activation of SR Ca^{2+} uptake via SERCA. The observation that wave oscillations tend to originate from the same area within the cell can be explained by higher local density of SR Ca^{2+} release channels and/or SERCA pump units. FDS generating Ca^{2+} sparks could act as an initiation site in some types of smooth muscles (13). The frequency of Ca^{2+} oscillations depends on the type of agonist used and its concentration; the higher the concentration, the higher the frequency of Ca^{2+} oscillations. In precapillary arterioles that consist of a monolayer of smooth muscle cells, low concentrations of agonist induce low frequencies of asynchronous Ca^{2+} oscillations. Low frequency Ca^{2+} oscillation produce rhythmic phasic contractions seen as local vasomotion controlled by a single cell (29). An increase in concentration of agonist causes an increase in the number of oscillating cells and the frequency of Ca^{2+} oscillations, which result in summation of individual phasic contractions leading to generation of dynamic non-propagating vasoconstriction (30). In precapillary arterioles vasomotion will facilitate blood perfusion while vasoconstriction can decrease or fully block local blood flow, i.e., act as a local precapillary "sphincter". In macro vessels, the force of contraction will depend on the number of oscillating cells and the frequency of Ca^{2+} oscillations (30,34). In addition, Ca^{2+} waves also exert a depolarizing influence through activation of $Cl^-{}_{Ca}$ channels, which in phasic smooth muscles lead to generation of a burst of action potentials (14,35). In small resistance arteries, low-frequency (<0.05 Hz) asynchronous wavelike Ca^{2+} oscillations, which themselves are associated with only minimal development of tone, appear to be instrumental in the initiation of regional vasomotion (36). Ca^{2+} waves activate depolarizing current through activation of $Cl^-{}_{Ca}$ channels, which results in synchronized but intermittent activation of DHP sensitive, L-type Ca^{2+} channels that subsequently produce synchronized Ca^{2+} oscillations in a group of cells that underlie regional vasomotion (36). Since some of the released Ca^{2+} can be extruded to the extracellular space; recurrence of the Ca^{2+} waves will depend on reloading of the SR by Ca^{2+} influx. This can occur through several mechanisms: the store-operated non-selective cation channels, L-type voltage gated Ca^{2+} channels, and the reverse mode of NCX (30). More studies are required to identify the contributions of these or other mechanisms involved in replenishment of the SR. The relative contribution of RyRs and IP_3Rs to intracellular $[Ca^{2+}]_i$ mobilization and the role of these receptors in the genesis of localized Ca^{2+}-release events (sparks or puffs), propagating Ca^{2+} waves of $[Ca^{2+}]_i$ oscillations varies in different types of SMCs, and often depends on the strength and mechanism of SMC stimulation.

Ca^{2+} CLEARANCE SYSTEMS

Separately discussing Ca^{2+} sources and Ca^{2+} clearance is somewhat arbitrary, as either system may play dual roles; for example, the Na^+/Ca^{2+}-exchanger. The advantage is seeing each from a different view point. Even though ion fluxes through channels are several orders of magnitude greater than that of clearance by ion pumps, the time course of Ca^{2+} transients can be significantly underestimated without inhibition of Ca^{2+} clearance pathways (37). The speed of ions through channels may dominate initial Ca^{2+} transients, but the steady state brings Ca^{2+} clearance mechanisms into play, and they are a major factor in determining steady state $[Ca^{2+}]_i$. A Ca^{2+} influx under basal conditions estimated at 16 μmol/l per minute is more than 2 orders of magnitude greater than the resting $[Ca^{2+}]_i$. Thus, Ca^{2+} clearance from the cytosol is critical to the maintenance of a quiescent baseline.

The major Ca^{2+} clearance systems are sarco(endo) plasmic reticulum Ca^{2+} ATPase (SERCA), Na^+/Ca^{2+}-exchanger (NCX) powered by the Na^+-K^+ ATPase (NKA), and the plasma membrane Ca^{2+} ATPase (PMCA). NCX is generally considered to be a high-capacity exchanger with rapid turnover with but low affinity for Ca^{2+} ($K_d \approx 1$ μM), but high turnover. SERCA and PMCA, on the other hand, have a higher affinity for Ca^{2+} ($K_d \approx 0.1-0.3$ μM), but lower turnover than NCX (for review see 38). For smooth muscle, the relative contribution of each to Ca^{2+} clearance component is dependent on conditions and smooth muscle type. Estimates generally rely on inhibitors and often are linearly extrapolated from clearance rates so they must be viewed cautiously. There are also tissue, tissue preparation, and species differences.

In mouse bladder, NCX accounts for about 60% of calcium clearance, while PMCA and SERCA facilitate about 20–30% each (39). In uterine smooth muscle, 35% can be attributed to NCX and the remaining attributed to PMCA (40). In cells isolated from mouse aorta, NCX accounts for 90% of the Ca^{2+}-extrusion following inhibition of SERCA by cyclopiazonic acid (37). Mitochondrial Ca^{2+} uptake can also be a factor under certain conditions, but its apparent affinity is thought to be relatively low (~10–20 μM, (41)). Microdomains with relatively high $[Ca^{2+}]_i$ are posited to circumvent this relatively low affinity (42). Recent evidence, however, suggests mitochondria may play some role as both a buffer and/or regulator of Ca^{2+} clearance (discussed below).

The distribution, localization, and interactions of these Ca^{2+} clearance systems are a focus of recent interest in smooth muscle Ca^{2+} handling; in particular, the role of caveolae, and their corresponding subsarcolemmal compartments. Caveolae represent a Ca^{2+} pool that is partially sequestered from that of the general extracellular environment (for review see 43). These vesicular membrane structures are suggested to be a source of Ca^{2+} that can be recycled to and from the SR. Localization to this compartment has been firmly established in smooth muscle colocalization of PMCA and NCX with caveolae suggest a role for Ca^{2+} extrusion and regulation in this subsarcolemmal compartment (Figure 86.1). There is currently no direct evidence for its colocalization in the caveolae of smooth muscle. However, the colocalization of NCX and the α2-isoform of NKA in smooth muscle (44) (Figure 86.1), suggests that it may exist. In addition to this potential coupling, recent evidence suggests that the major players in Ca^{2+}-clearance may also be genetically regulated as a unit (45).

Sarcoplasmic Reticulum (SR) and Sarco (endo)plasmic Reticulum Ca^{2+} ATPase (SERCA)

In vascular smooth muscle cells, the sarcoplasmic reticulum Ca^{2+} store contributes significantly to the regulation of contraction as well as other cellular functions such as gene regulation both via Ca^{2+} release via IP_3 receptors (IP_3R) and ryanodine receptors (RyR) and by further modulation of $[Ca^{2+}]_i$ via Ca^{2+} uptake (for an excellent review see 12). The SR has been estimated at 5–7% of the volume of smooth muscle and there is evidence for an SR Ca^{2+} store which is a single luminally continuous entity that contains both IP_3R and RyR and within which Ca^{2+} is accessed freely by each receptor. One of the more interesting aspects of SERCA and the SR is that they are reported to be localized spatially and interact directly or indirectly with PMCA, NKA–NCX, and mitochondria, as well as with the plasma membrane and cell nucleus (46,47). This suggests a central role for SERCA and the SR in Ca^{2+} homeostasis.

SERCA Ca^{2+} pumps are transmembrane proteins of ~110 kDa and belong to a family of highly conserved proteins in the P-type superfamily of ion transport ATPases, which are encoded by three homologous genes, SERCA1-3. SERCA2b, one of two alternatively spliced transcripts, is a major SR Ca^{2+} pump of most smooth muscle tissue. A functional role for SERCA in the regulation of smooth muscle $[Ca^{2+}]_i$ and contractility, largely based on the use of the inhibitors thapsigargin and cyclopiazonic acid, has been long established. A SERCA2 gene-targeted mouse, in which one allele of both SERCA2a and SERCA2b are deleted, exhibited a 35% reduction in both SERCA2a protein levels and the maximal velocity of SR Ca^{2+} uptake (48). Somewhat surprisingly, neither aorta nor portal vein demonstrated altered mechanical characteristics after a 30–40% reduction in SERCA2 protein level, suggesting that SERCA2 has a large functional reserve in VSM.

A clearer picture of the role of SERCA in regulation of vascular $[Ca^{2+}]_i$ emerged from studies on an associated 52 amino acid protein, phospholamban (PLN), which acts as in inhibitor of SR Ca^{2+} pump activity (for reviews see 49). In its unphosphorylated form, the PLN monomer inhibits SERCA, while phosphorylation of PLN-Ser16 via PKA or PLN-Thr17 via CaMKII relieves such inhibition by increasing the apparent affinity of the pump for Ca^{2+}. PLN exists as both a monomer, which is a potent inhibitor of SERCA, and a less inhibitory pentameric form in the SR membrane. Phosphorylation of the PLN monomer acts to reduce the net charge of its cytoplasmic domain, which favors self-association into a less inhibitory pentameric structure. This modulation of the SERCA:PLN ratio is an important determinant of contractility in both cardiac and smooth muscle tissues (50).

Phospholamban is present in smooth muscle but the amount expressed varies both in a species-and tissue-specific way. Both cyclic AMP- and cyclic GMP-dependent protein kinase phosphorylate phospholamban, and this results in an increased Ca^{2+} accumulation by the smooth muscle endoplasmic reticulum. Unlike the other proteins that we have reviewed, PLN is a single copy gene with no known isoforms, which facilitated developing gene-targeted mice. Concentration-force responses to KCl or PE stimulation of aorta from the PLN-null mouse were less sensitive than wild-type tissues. SR Ca^{2+} pump inhibition with cyclopiazonic acid (CPA) abolished these differences, identifying the SR as the source of this rightward shift. The rate of rise of the rapid phase of PE-induced contraction was twice as great in PLN-KO aorta consistent with disinhibition of SERCA and concomitant with increased SR Ca^{2+} loading. Also of interest to regulation of the vasculature, the endothelium-dependent relaxation to ACh or to PKA activation with forskolin was blunted in aortae of PLN-KO mice (51).

Studies in the bladder extended contractility studies showing that $[Ca^{2+}]_i$ responses paralleled the force responses (52). CCh stimulation of PLN-deficient bladder exhibited significant attenuation of the maximal increases in $[Ca^{2+}]_i$ and force when compared to wild-type controls. Furthermore, the EC_{50} values for CCh-induced contraction of the PLN-KO bladder were increased in comparison to those for wild-type bladder. As was observed in the study of PLN-deficient aortae, the functional inhibition of SERCA with CPA eliminated these differences, again localizing the observed effects to the SR. Addition of function using mice (PLN-SMOE) carrying a transgene with PLN cDNA driven by the smooth muscle-specific SMP8 α-actin promoter showed that effects were specific to PLN, and not just SR. Intracellular Ca^{2+} and force vs. CCh relations in PLN-SMOE bladders were significantly shifted leftward, the opposite of that observed with PLN-KO bladders. CPA little effect on the PLN-SMOE tissues, suggesting that SERCA and the SR Ca^{2+} uptake in PLN-SMOE bladders was already substantially inhibited.

In phasic smooth muscle the rapid contraction/relaxation cycles demand a quicker rate of intracellular Ca^{2+} cycling. PLN might be expected to play a crucial role in contractility in such tissue and observed in portal vein (53) and antrum from PLB-KO mice (54). Associated with this increased phasic contractile activity were more rapid kinetics of contraction and decay.

Two major hypotheses have been proposed to explain the role of PLN and SERCA vascular smooth muscle contractility. As discussed in the section on Ca^{2+} sparks, one is dependent on activation of Ca^{2+}-activated potassium (K_{Ca}) channels, and the other on an increased rate of cytosolic Ca^{2+} sequestration into the SR. Nelson and colleagues (55) argue for a Ca^{2+} spark-driven mechanism of decreased contractility in smooth muscle. Ca^{2+} sparks are transient elevations in Ca^{2+} concentration in a small subsarcolemmal region of the cell elicited by the activation of a small number of ryanodine receptors. In smooth muscle, Ca^{2+} "sparks" are proposed to lead to an enhanced relaxation via activation of large-conductance K_{Ca} (BK) channels in the plasma membrane. The concomitant hyperpolarization closes voltage-dependent Ca^{2+} channels, leading to a lower $[Ca^{2+}]_i$ and relaxation. A second theory proposed for the altered contractility in PLN-deficient mice suggests a direct role for an increased rate of cytosolic Ca^{2+} sequestration into the SR. This enhanced removal of Ca^{2+} from the cytosol would effectively lower the $[Ca^{2+}]_i$, in turn leading to a lesser degree of contraction and greater Ca^{2+} loading of the SR. Such a role is supported by data from several independent studies. One compelling argument from the work of Paul and colleagues (38) is that the suppression of force was also observed upon depolarization with KCl. Under these conditions, Ca^{2+} sparks would not be anticipated to play a role. A seemingly logical objection to this would be that Ca^{2+} uptake by the SR could be saturated and suppression of force lost with prolonged contractions. However, there is evidence suggesting that the SR can be vectorially unloaded via a compartmented NCX and NKA (37), as originally suggested by van Breemen and colleagues (56). Ultimately, both an indirect role for augmented SR Ca^{2+} sequestration in the modulation of Ca^{2+} sparks, as well as a direct role for enhanced cytosolic Ca^{2+} removal in the reduction of $[Ca^{2+}]_i$, will likely underlie the modulatory effects of PLN and, of course, with the usual animal and tissue variability.

SERCA has been reported to be involved in NO-mediated relaxation by both cGMP and cGMP-independent pathways (57). NO has been reported to directly activate SERCA and reload Ca^{2+} stores, which inactivates store-operated Ca^{2+} channels, decreasing intracellular calcium and relaxes arteries. This mechanism is predominantly cGMP independent and is impaired in vascular diseases (58), however in PLN gene-ablated mice, cGMP relaxation of aorta was not affected (59). Another aspect of SERCA in Ca^{2+}-homeostasis is an increasing literature indicating the potential importance of redox regulation of SERCA (60). Finally, studies of PLN interactions with SERCA and its modulation by accessory proteins, HAX-1 (61), Hsp20 (62), junction, and HRC (63), have recently illustrated other potential sites for regulation of SERCA in cardiac muscle and will undoubtedly filter down in the near future to vascular smooth muscle.

Plasma Membrane Ca^{2+} ATPase

PMCA, a calmodulin-dependent calcium ATPase, is a ubiquitous transport protein that acts to extrude Ca^{2+} across the plasmalemma (for review see 38). It also has been reported to counter-transport a proton, which in turn might affect its activity. Four PMCA isoforms have been established, with further variability arising from alternative splicing (for review see 64). PMCA1 and PMCA4 are the only isoforms currently reported in smooth muscle. The lack of specific inhibitors has limited studies on the physiological significance of PMCA, and much of our knowledge comes from studies on gene-altered mice.

However, recently synthesized peptide inhibiters of PMCA have been reported (65).

PMCA can be a major regulator of contractility in vascular, bladder, and uterine smooth muscle. Neyses and co-workers, using transgenic mice overexpressing human PMCA4b (hPMCA4b) targeted to vascular smooth muscle, suggested that PMCA4b regulates vascular tone via inhibition of nitric oxide synthase I (neuronal (n)NOS) in a caveolar compartment. They reported an elevated blood pressure and an increased maximum contraction to KCl in de-endothelized aortic rings as well as enhanced sensitivity to phenylephrine and prostaglandin F2α of the transgenic mice compared to controls. PMCA4 and nNOS were reported to co-immunoprecipitate (66) suggesting that PMCA4 regulates vascular tone by decreasing localized $[Ca^{2+}]$ thus inhibiting nNOS. Utilizing $Pmca1^{+/-}$, $Pmca4^{-/-}$, and $Pmca1^{+/-} \times Pmca4^{-/-}$ mice, Paul and colleagues (39) observed a significant prolongation of the half-time for force development to potassium chloride (KCl) in suggesting that the ablation of the *Pmca4* allele (s) may limit depolarization-induced Ca^{2+} influx, as total PMCA was not affected in $Pmca1^{+/-}$ mice. Stimulation of NCX-mediated Ca^{2+} extrusion via an increased near membrane $[Ca^{2+}]$ in PMCA gene-ablated smooth muscles was proposed.

Isoform-specific roles for PMCA1 and PMCA4 in bladder smooth muscle were reported (67). $Pmca1^{+/-}$ bladders had higher $[Ca^{2+}]_i$ and force responses (Figure 86.2) to both KCl and carbachol (CCh) stimulation upon comparison to wild-type (WT) controls. In contrast, $Pmca4^{-/-}$ bladder responses to CCh were significantly suppressed (Figure 86.2), but not peak tension and $[Ca^{2+}]_i$ in response to KCl. These data plus the fact that $Pmca1^{-/-}$ genotype is embryonically lethal (68) support the house-keeping role for PMCA1, while modulation of receptor signaling appears to be the function of PMCA4. Potential mechanisms for the suppressed responses to CCh $Pmca4^{-/-}$ bladder include a high $[Ca^{2+}]$ in a sarcoplasmic reticulum (SR)-associated sub-sarcolemmal space which lead to a hyperloaded SR, suppressing store-operated Ca^{2+} entry and/or the activation of Ca^{2+}-activated K^+ channels via an increased $[Ca^{2+}]$ in PMCA4-associated sub-cellular compartments.

Ca^{2+} Clearance via Na^+/Ca^{2+} Exchanger Driven by NKA

Na^+/Ca^{2+}-exchanger utilizing the Na^+ gradient powered by the Na^+-K^+ ATPase can be a potent Ca^{2+} clearance system. The mammalian NCX family consists of at least three isoforms, NCX1–3, which, in turn, give rise to various splice variants (for reviews see 69, 70). NCX exchanges one Ca^{2+} ion across the plasma membrane for 2–3 Na^+ ions, thus can be electrogenic and modulated by membrane potential, as well as transmembrane gradients of Na^+ and Ca^{2+}. Since it is bidirectional, inhibition of the Na^+-K^+ ATPase can lead to a reversal of NCX, increasing $[Ca^{2+}]_i$ and contractility; a mechanism which is postulated to underlie salt-sensitive hypertension (71).

The Na^+-K^+ ATPase is the archetypal P-type ATPase, discovered by Shou in 1957 (72). NKA transports three Na^+ ions out of the cell and two K^+ ions into the cell per ATP hydrolyzed. It thus underlies the membrane potential and Na^+ and K^+ gradients. It is generally described as being an $\alpha\beta$ dimer, with four known α-isoforms and three β-isoforms currently identified (for reviews see 73). The β-subunit appears to be involved in localization of the ATPase to the plasma membrane and maturation of the enzyme. More recent evidence suggests an association with another protein now often considered a γ-subunit, which is a member of a larger class of proteins, called FXYD proteins, which add additional diversity as there are seven such proteins (74). Whether $Na^{+-}K^+$ ATPase is always associated with one member of the FXYD family of proteins is not known. Four known isoforms of the catalytic α-subunit exist, but only the α_1 and α_2 subunits are associated with adult murine aortic smooth (75). The α_1-isoform has a higher affinity for Na^+ ($K_{Na+} \approx 12$ mM) than α_2- ($K_{Na+} \approx 22$ mM). Unique to rodents and providing a useful experimental tool, the α_2-isoform has a much higher affinity ($IC_{50} = 58$ nM) for the inhibitor ouabain, than that ($IC_{50} = 48$ μM) of the α_1 subunit. In most other mammals, including humans, the sensitivity of the α-isoforms to ouabain is of similar magnitude.

Recent emphasis in research on NKA isoforms is their location and the colocalization with other Ca^{2+} clearance proteins. Colocalization of NCX, NKA, and the SR in smooth muscle has long been established (44). In cultured vascular smooth muscle (75) and astrocytes (76), the α_1-isoform is uniformly distributed across the plasmalemma; the α_2-isoform displays a punctate distribution. Blaustein and colleagues (77) reported that NKA α_2 (or α_3)-isoforms were localized in the same microdomains that included NCX and the SR (Figure 86.1), and proposed a model in which the α_2-isoform modulates $[Ca^{2+}]$ via NCX in a microdomain which, through communications with SERCA, regulates SR Ca^{2+} loading and contractility. Despite NCX's reported low affinity for Ca^{2+}, the close structural coupling of NCX with SR Ca^{2+} storage sites, where local $[Ca^{2+}]_i$ can be considerably higher than the cell global average, suggests that Na/Ca exchanger activity may have a significant role in filling of Ca^{2+} stores. Given the widespread distribution of the α_1-isoform, it was suggested to fulfill a "housekeeping" function. Again, gene-targeted and transgenic models have further advanced our understanding of the function of both the NCX and NKA enzymes.

In smooth muscle, the role of NCX in Ca^{2+} homeostasis shows a considerable variation between smooth muscle types and tissues and still remains controversial in many cases. Its role in smooth muscle has been either inferred or dismissed largely from indirect studies, often on complex multicellular preparations. Despite the difficulties introduced by multicellular preparations, in the intact sodium-loaded guinea-pig ureter, there is evidence for the NCX operating in reverse mode (78). Aaronson and Benham (79) using single cells isolated from the guinea-pig ureter under voltage clamp conditions, confirmed these observations and obtained evidence for NCX which, operating in reverse mode, elevated $[Ca^{2+}]_i$ but had little effect on $[Ca^{2+}]_i$ removal. In cells isolated from the guinea-pig bladder Ganitkevich and Isenberg (80) showed that NCX played little role in regulating $[Ca^{2+}]_i$. Similarly, in voltage-clamped guinea pig colonic myocytes, NCX did not appear to regulate bulk average $[Ca^{2+}]_i$ (81); however, in single cells isolated from *Bufo marinus*, there is evidence for a functional NCX that can operate in forward mode; i.e., Na^+ in, Ca^{2+} out of the cell (82).

NCX, on the other hand can play a major role in vascular smooth muscle accounting for 90% of Ca^{2+} clearance in mouse aorta cells (37). Kanaide and colleagues (83) expressed canine NCX1.3 in a mouse model utilizing the human smooth muscle α-actin promoter. In these mice expressing NCX1.3, forskolin activation of PKA induced decreases in $[Ca^{2+}]_i$ and tension that were greater in aortas compared with those from the wild-type controls (83). These changes were inhibited in the presence of NCX inhibition with low Na^+ PSS or SEA0400, implicating a role for the Na^+/Ca^{2+} exchanger in these forskolin-induced phenomena. Knockdown of NCX1, using a smooth muscle (SM)-specific promoter, attenuated vasoconstriction, L-type Ca^{2+} channel current and lowered blood pressure in mice (84). Vasoconstriction and myogenic tone in pressurized mesenteric arteries under conditions favoring reverse Ca^{2+} exchange, low extracellular Na^+ concentration, nanomolar ouabain, or treatment with an NCX inhibitor, SEA0400, was also attenuated. The reduced myogenic tone and BP was attributed to reduced Ca^{2+} entry via NCX1 1 leading to a lower cytosolic Ca^{2+} concentration.

Utilizing $\alpha_1^{+/-}$-, $\alpha_2^{-/-}$- and $\alpha_2^{+/-}$-mice, Paul and colleagues (75) found the $\alpha_2^{-/-}$-aortae to be more sensitive to receptor-mediated stimulation than wild-type aortae, while also exhibiting a faster rate of force development. The $\alpha_2^{-/-}$-aortae were also less sensitive to relaxation by either A- or G-kinase pathway activation. The contractility values for the $\alpha_1^{+/-}$-aortae, on the other hand, were identical to those of the wild-types. The $\alpha_2^{+/-}$-aortic contractility values generally fell between those of $\alpha_2^{-/-}$- and wild-type aortae. If the α_2-isoform does indeed modulate SR function via colocalization with NCX and SERCA, its absence in $\alpha_2^{-/-}$-aortae would lead to the inhibition or reversal of Na^+/Ca^{2+} exchange, ultimately causing an increase in Ca^{2+} content in the subsarcolemmal compartment. This could, in turn, result in greater SR loading, which might explain the increased sensitivity to receptor-mediated stimulation and the faster rate of force development. Such a "hyperloaded" SR might also explain the observed decreased sensitivity to agonist-stimulated relaxation, as it is long established that SERCA can be inhibited by elevated SR Ca^{2+}.

An alternative hypothesis based on a direct role for NKA in signaling (for further details, see below) has been proposed by Xie and colleagues (85). The increased contractility observed with low levels of ouabain, which, in the murine model, bind only to the α2-isoform, is proposed to be related not only to altered pumping, but also to the activation of Src kinase, ultimately leading to the generation of inositol triphosphate (IP_3), sensitization of the IP_3 receptor and SR Ca^{2+} release. Thus, ouabain inhibition of NKA could favor both SR Ca^{2+} store enhancement and depletion. Recent modeling in vascular smooth muscle cells comparing these alternatives (86) indicates that ouabain can lead to enhanced $[Ca^{2+}]_i$ transients when its predominant effect is inhibition of α2 NKA, leading to enhanced SR Ca^{2+} loading. Further complicating matters is a recent study on cultured aortic smooth muscle cells from 18-day fetal $\alpha_2^{-/-}$, mice indicating that the SR Ca^{2+} load is similar to the control, wild-type mice (37). Altered PMCA activity and capacitative Ca^{2+} entry were potential compensatory pathways affecting Ca^{2+} handling in these cultured cells.

Of particular interest to any discussion of smooth muscle Ca^{2+} signaling are sequelae to the regulation of blood pressure. Blaustein and colleagues (87) found that $\alpha_2^{+/-}$-mice to be hypertensive, while $\alpha_1^{+/-}$-mice were normotensive. Increased myogenic tone was observed in isolated, pressurized mesenteric arteries from $\alpha_2^{+/-}$-arteries but not in those from $\alpha^{\prime +/-}$-arteries. These investigators suggested that the hypertension observed in the $\alpha_2^{+/-}$-mice might result from this elevated myogenic tone. As NCX inhibitors SEA0400 and KB-R7943 blocked the augmentation of myogenic tone in $\alpha_2^{+/-}$ arteries, one might suspect that NCX is a major player. A decrease in the α_2-Na^+ pump activity could lead to an increase in $[Na^+]_i$ and myogenic tone via reverse NCX activity. Ultimately, the α_2-isoform of the arterial myocyte appears to be involved in long-term regulation of blood pressure.

Paul and colleagues (88) generated mice carrying the transgene for either the α_1- or α_2-isoform of NKA coupled with the smooth muscle-specific α-actin promoter, SMP8. Mice carrying the α_2-transgene (α_{2sm+}) were hypotensive, whereas the mice carrying the α_1-transgene (α_{1sm+}) were normotensive. A surprising observation was the coordinate expression of the α-isoforms. Regardless of which transgene was being expressed, both α-isoforms and total NKA were increased to a similar degree at both the protein and mRNA levels. These increases were greater in the α_{2sm+} line, suggesting that the observed decrease in blood pressure is dependent on the extent of the increase in α-isoform expression. No differences in contractility parameters were detected in α_{1sm+}-aortae, consistent with the lack of change in blood pressure. Complicating interpretation of the decreased blood pressure in the α_{2sm+}-aortae, it was found that not only was the α_2-isoform protein increased, but so also were the other Ca^{2+} clearance proteins, PMCA, NCX, and SERCA. Importantly, there was no generalized increase in proteins and specifically, contractile associated proteins, actin, myosin light chain, and calponin were unchanged. Ca^{2+} clearance may be so critical to Ca^{2+} homeostasis and signaling, that all its elements may be coordinately regulated as a single unit. Thus, an alternative explanation to the decreased blood pressure and contractile effects in the $\alpha 2_{sm+}$ aortae is related to the greater expression of Ca^{2+} clearance proteins. While NKA–NCX are clearly important in Ca^{2+} clearance, the effects of the α-isoforms in NKA's role in Ca^{2+} clearance appear to be distinct but mechanism(s) are yet to be fully resolved.

Na^+–K^+ ATPase and Signaling

A relatively new wrinkle in the role of NKA in Ca^{2+} homeostasis is its potential involvement in cell signaling. The NKA α1-isoform contains three distinct domains (89,90), whose binding motifs are reported to interact with signaling molecules, such as IP3R (91), PLC-γ (92), PI3K (93), ERK (94), and Src (95). Caveolae appear to be required for NKA receptor function (96), and specifically for vascular smooth muscle (97). These interactions, largely based on studies of inhibition of NKA with ouabain, indicate the potential for endogenous cardiotonic steroids to generate second messengers and modulate the activity of protein kinase cascades. A role for such cardiotonic steroids is not without skeptics (98). More recent studies, however, tend to be convincing; for reviews see (73,99). The most extensive literature on such signaling relates to activation of Src. Xie and colleagues propose a model in which the Src bound to NKA is located in caveolae. Ouabain binding activates Src, which then activates other downstream signaling pathways. Many downstream systems are reported to be involved (for review see 73), including early response genes and a number of metabolic pathways. One of the dilemmas in distinguishing between mechanisms is that even inhibition of NKA by nanomolar ouabain can lead to increased $[Ca^{2+}]_i$ and contractility which could also augment signaling pathways within several minutes in small mouse mesenteric arteries (87).

Mitochondria and Ca^{2+} Homeostasis

It has been long known that mitochondria can take up Ca^{2+} (100). The question here is the relevance to vascular smooth muscle Ca^{2+}-clearance, which of course, will depend on the particular vascular smooth muscle. Mitochondria have been proposed to be a major player in Ca^{2+} signaling (101), but their role as a major clearance component rather than as a modulator of the interacting systems of Ca^{2+}-clearance is less secure (102). Given their role in ATP synthesis, cellular redox potential, generation of reactive oxygen species (ROS), and ability to accumulate Ca^{2+}, it would be remarkable if mitochondria did not play any role in Ca^{2+} homeostasis.

Mitochondria develop negative membrane potentials by extrusion of protons via the electron transport chain. Ca^{2+} is accumulated via an electrogenic uniporter when $[Ca^{2+}]_i$ exceeds≈100 nM, using the potential, $\Delta\Psi_m$, generated across the inner mitochondrial membrane by the activity of the electron-transport chain (103). Mitochondria release Ca^{2+} more slowly back to the cytosol via a Na^+- or H^+-antiporter (104). In this way, mitochondria can act as Ca^{2+} buffer (105,106). Much of the current interest for smooth muscle focuses on the close apposition of mitochondria with the SR in a microdomain (107,108). In some cells, mitochondria are located close to sites of initiation of Ca^{2+} release units generating Ca^{2+} sparks. Mitochondria can possibly act as a "fire wall" in smooth muscles, buffering Ca^{2+} released by clusters of RyR generating Ca^{2+} spark protecting smooth muscles from generation of global rather than local Ca^{2+} signaling.

In smooth muscle, Van Breemen and colleagues have shown that mitochondria can modulate Ca^{2+} homeostasis in a variety of ways (109). Much of the knowledge reviewed in the studies above, relied on mitochondrial inhibitors. One might anticipate this to affect not only Ca^{2+} uptake, but also to alter ROS, redox potential, and ATP supply. The latter is worth considering, in that ATP powers Ca^{2+} clearance ion pumps. Tonic arteries have basal rates of ATP utilization in the range of 0.5 to 2 μmol ATP/min × gwt. Phasic arteries are generally higher and when maintaining active isometric force, this rate of usage can double. Total phosphagen (ATP + PCr) content of vascular smooth muscle is generally 3–6 μmol/gwt, so one needs an ongoing metabolic supply of phosphagen. Depending on the conditions, mitochondria inhibition limiting phosphagen production could blur straightforward interpretation of such data. Interestingly, in terms of supporting ion pump function, glycolytic enzymes associated with a plasma membrane microcompartment are known to preferentially fuel Na^+–K^+ ATPase under aerobic conditions (110). Glycolysis can easily double or more under hypoxia and large arteries can maintain significant force under hypoxia, where signaling, rather than ATP limitation appears to account for the loss of force from aerobic conditions (111). One can thus use hypoxia to investigate Ca^{2+} clearance without mitochondria ATP production and presumably Ca^{2+}-uptake; though ROS production could still be an issue.

Systemic vessels in general do not contract but modestly relax when exposed to hypoxia under non-stimulated conditions, suggesting that any potential mitochondrial Ca^{2+} release is not large or rapidly taken up by SR or extruded. Since baseline levels of force are maintained under hypoxia, Ca^{2+} clearance continues to occur against an appreciable Ca^{2+} leak. In stimulated arteries, such as porcine coronary arteries, hypoxia decreases both force and $[Ca^{2+}]_i$ (111), which is reversible upon reoxygenation. These arteries can reversibly contract and relax under anoxic conditions, indicating a significant Ca^{2+} clearance capacity in the absence of mitochondrial oxidative metabolism. Mitochondria are not required for Ca^{2+} clearance and their contribution under aerobic conditions can be compensated by other Ca^{2+} clearance mechanisms. This can in part be explained by a robust glycolytic capacity in VSM (112).

Despite the apparent low affinity of mitochondria for Ca^{2+}, mitochondrial $[Ca^{2+}]_m$ has been shown to mirror that of the cytosol $[Ca^{2+}]_i$ (113). The explanation is that local $[Ca^{2+}]$ can be significantly higher than that of the cytosol (for review see 114). The question is how large a factor is mitochondria in Ca^{2+} clearance, as compared to, for example the SR? Mitochondria have been estimated to occupy about 5% of the volume of vascular smooth muscle, similar to that for the SP, and thus require some Ca^{2+} buffer to avoid Ca^{2+} overload in order to clear cytosolic Ca^{2+}. This is generally thought to be PO_4. Mitochondria Ca^{2+} content is reported as high as 100 nmol/mg protein (115), would seem capable of exceeding its entire P content (116), which could be expected to limit ATP production. This would be one limit on mitochondria as a Ca^{2+} sink, and/or require a way to extrude Ca^{2+}, which has been postulated via the SR. Moreover, mitochondria are also suggested to participate in SR Ca^{2+} loading (109). This, however, is not favorable in terms of energy used per ion cycled compared to that of other Ca^{2+} sequestering organelles. The cost of Ca^{2+} entry into the inner mitochondrial matrix is about twice as high as a Ca^{2+} pump in terms of loss of ATP due to the reduction of the mitochondrial membrane potential (117). If would clearly be more efficient for the SR to load and unload Ca^{2+} directly from the cytosol. Perhaps coordination with mitochondrial oxidative phosphorylation by Ca^{2+} is worth the extra cost.

In terms of the role of mitochondria in Ca^{2+} clearance, measurements of $[Ca^{2+}]_i$ in cultured smooth muscle cells have been ambivalent. In addition to tissue and species differences, one must keep in mind the well-known changes in smooth muscle EC coupling associated with cell culture. In rat aorta (118) and pulmonary artery smooth muscle cells (119), moderate ($<1\ \mu M$) increases in $[Ca^{2+}]_i$ did not affect mitochondria $[Ca^{2+}]$. In voltage-clamped rat femoral artery cells, mitochondrial inhibition with CCCP altered Ca^{2+} release by caffeine and Ca^{2+} clearance (120). In cultured mouse aortic cells, $[Ca^{2+}]_i$ after store release with CPA, was moderately affected by CCCP or ruthenium red when NCX and PMCA were also inhibited (37), suggesting a role for mitochondria at high $[Ca^{2+}]_i$. Studies using permeabilized coronary artery suggested that mitochondria play a minor role (121). Based on studies using inhibitors of Ca^{2+} clearance, mitochondrial clearance does not appear to be a major factor compared to NCX, PMCA and SERCA (39,122). On the other hand, mitochondria appear to have a much clearer role in Ca^{2+} signaling and potential coordination of Ca^{2+} clearance systems (47,114,123).

Though we have treated the Ca^{2+} clearance systems, PMCA, NCX-NKA, and SERCA-PLN as separate entities, they are linked. For example, Ca^{2+} extrusion by PMCA leads to a counter transport of H^+, and thus coupling to NKA via the Na^+/H^+ exchanger. This is in addition to the coupling of NCX and NKA discussed earlier. SERCA is also interrelated, particularly as proposed to a subsarcolemmal compartmentalization with α2-NKA and NCX. Moreover as described in the section on capacitative Ca^{2+} entry (above) $SR_{[Ca]}$, modulated by SERCA is linked to Ca^{2+} influx via store-operated Ca^{2+} entry.

CONCLUSION

The differences between smooth muscle types themselves are often greater than those between smooth and skeletal muscle. So it is not surprising given the wide range of functionality that the mechanisms for modulating and maintaining Ca^{2+} homeostasis also differ widely. We now have a better understanding of the major players in Ca^{2+} entry and clearance. We have also made gains in, if not understanding, at least recognizing the interactions between the players are central to the regulation of $[Ca^{2+}]_i$. These complex interactions, given the importance of $[Ca^{2+}]_i$ homeostasis to cell signaling and function, will continue to be a major foci of smooth muscle research.

REFERENCES

1. Kuriyama H, Kitamura K, Nabata H. Pharmacological and physiological significance of ion channels and factors that modulate them in vascular tissues. *Pharmacol Rev* 1995;**47**:387–573.
2. Karaki H, Ozaki H, Hori M, Mitsui-Saito M, Amano K, Harada K, et al. Calcium movements, distribution, and functions in smooth muscle. *Pharmacol Rev* 1997;**49**:157–230.

3. Sanders KM. Invited review: mechanisms of calcium handling in smooth muscles. *J Appl Physiol* 2001;**91**:1438–49.
4. Somlyo AV, Somlyo AP. Electromechanical and pharmacomechanical coupling in vascular smooth muscle. *J Pharmacol Exp Ther* 1968;**159**:129–45.
5. Bolton TB. Mechanisms of action of transmitters and other substances on smooth muscle. *Physiol Rev* 1979;**59**:606–718.
6. Parekh AB, Putney Jr JW. Store-operated calcium channels. *Physiol Rev* 2005;**85**:757–810.
7. Casteels R, Droogmans G. Exchange characteristics of the noradrenaline-sensitive calcium store in vascular smooth muscle cells or rabbit ear artery. *J Physiol* 1981;**317**:263–79.
8. Leung FP, Yung LM, Yao X, Laher I, Huang Y. Store-operated calcium entry in vascular smooth muscle. *Br J Pharmacol* 2008;**153**:846–57.
9. Roos J, DiGregorio PJ, Yeromin AV, Ohlsen K, Lioudyno M, Zhang S, et al. STIM1, an essential and conserved component of store-operated Ca^{2+} channel function. *J Cell Biol* 2005;**169**:435–45.
10. Wynne BM, Chiao CW, Webb RC. Vascular smooth muscle cell signaling mechanisms for contraction to angiotensin II and endothelin-1. *J Am Soc Hypertens* 2009;**3**:84–95.
11. Inoue R, Okada T, Onoue H, Hara Y, Shimizu S, Naitoh S, et al. The transient receptor potential protein homologue TRP6 is the essential component of vascular alpha(1)-adrenoceptor-activated Ca(2 +)-permeable cation channel. *Circ Res* 2001;**88**:325–32.
12. Wray S, Burdyga T. Sarcoplasmic reticulum function in smooth muscle. *Physiol Rev* 2010;**90**:113–78.
13. Gordienko DV, Greenwood IA, Bolton TB. Direct visualization of sarcoplasmic reticulum regions discharging Ca(2+)sparks in vascular myocytes. *Cell Calcium* 2001;**29**:13–28.
14. Bolton TB. Calcium events in smooth muscles and their interstitial cells; physiological roles of sparks. *J Physiol* 2006;**570**:5–11.
15. Imaizumi Y, Torii Y, Ohi Y, Nagano N, Atsuki K, Yamamura H, et al. Ca^{2+} images and K^{+} current during depolarization in smooth muscle cells of the guinea-pig vas deferens and urinary bladder. *J Physiol* 1998;**510**(Pt 3):705–19.
16. Kotlikoff MI. Calcium-induced calcium release in smooth muscle: the case for loose coupling. *Prog Biophys Mol Biol* 2003;**83**:171–91.
17. Nelson MT, Cheng H, Rubart M, Santana LF, Bonev AD, Knot HJ, et al. Relaxation of arterial smooth muscle by calcium sparks [see comments]. *Science* 1995;**270**:633–7.
18. ZhuGe R, Tuft RA, Fogarty KE, Bellve K, Fay FS, Walsh Jr. JV. The influence of sarcoplasmic reticulum Ca^{2+} concentration on Ca^{2+} sparks and spontaneous transient outward currents in single smooth muscle cells. *J Gen Physiol* 1999;**113**:215–28.
19. Jaggar JH, Mawe GM, Nelson MT. Voltage-dependent K^{+} currents in smooth muscle cells from mouse gallbladder. *Am J Physiol* 1998;**274**:G687–93.
20. Remillard CV, Zhang WM, Shimoda LA, Sham JS. Physiological properties and functions of Ca(2 +) sparks in rat intrapulmonary arterial smooth muscle cells. *Am J Physiol Lung Cell Mol Physiol* 2002;**283**:L433–44.
21. Wellman GC, Nelson MT. Signaling between SR and plasmalemma in smooth muscle: sparks and the activation of Ca^{2+}-sensitive ion channels. *Cell Calcium* 2003;**34**:211–29.
22. Burdyga T, Wray S. Action potential refractory period in ureter smooth muscle is set by Ca sparks and BK channels. *Nature* 2005;**436**:559–62.
23. Berridge MJ, Bootman MD, Roderick HL. Calcium signalling: dynamics, homeostasis and remodelling. *Nat Rev Mol Cell Biol* 2003;**4**:517–29.
24. Boittin FX, Coussin F, Morel JL, Halet G, Macrez N, Mironneau J. Ca(2 +) signals mediated by Ins(1,4,5)P(3)-gated channels in rat ureteric myocytes. *Biochem J* 2000;**349**:323–32.
25. Bayguinov O, Hagen B, Bonev AD, Nelson MT, Sanders KM. Intracellular calcium events activated by ATP in murine colonic myocytes. *Am J Physiol Cell Physiol* 2000;**279**:C126–35.
26. Burdyga TV, Taggart MJ, Crichton C, Smith GL, Wray S. The mechanism of Ca^{2+} release from the SR of permeabilised guinea-pig and rat ureteric smooth muscle. *Biochim Biophys Acta* 1998;**1402**:109–14.
27. Gordienko DV, Harhun MI, Kustov MV, Pucovsky V, Bolton TB. Sub-plasmalemmal [Ca2 +]i upstroke in myocytes of the guinea-pig small intestine evoked by muscarinic stimulation: IP3R-mediated Ca^{2+} release induced by voltage-gated Ca^{2+} entry. *Cell Calcium* 2008;**43**:122–41.
28. Iino M, Kasai H, Yamazawa T. Visualization of neural control of intracellular Ca^{2+} concentration in single vascular smooth muscle cells in situ. *EMBO J* 1994;**13**:5026–31.
29. Borisova L, Wray S, Eisner DA, Burdyga T. How structure, Ca signals, and cellular communications underlie function in precapillary arterioles. *Circ Res* 2009;**105**:803–10.
30. Sanderson MJ, Bai Y, Perez-Zoghbi J. Ca(2 +) oscillations regulate contraction of intrapulmonary smooth muscle cells. *Adv Exp Med Biol* 2010;**661**:77–96.
31. Keizer J, Smith GD, Ponce-Dawson S, Pearson JE. Saltatory propagation of Ca^{2+} waves by Ca^{2+} sparks. *Biophys J* 1998;**75**:595–600.
32. Fritz N, Macrez N, Mironneau J, Jeyakumar LH, Fleischer S, Morel JL. Ryanodine receptor subtype 2 encodes Ca^{2+} oscillations activated by acetylcholine via the M2 muscarinic receptor/cADP-ribose signalling pathway in duodenum myocytes. *J Cell Sci* 2005;**118**:2261–70.
33. Prakash YS, Kannan MS, Walseth TF, Sieck GC. Role of cyclic ADP-ribose in the regulation of [Ca2 +]i in porcine tracheal smooth muscle. *Am J Physiol* 1998;**274**:C1653–60.
34. Kasai Y, Iino M, Tsutsumi O, Taketani Y, Endo M. Effects of cyclopiazonic acid on rhythmic contractions in uterine smooth muscle bundles of the rat. *Br J Pharmacol* 1994;**112**:1132–6.
35. Mironneau J, Arnaudeau S, Macrez-Lepretre N, Boittin FX. Ca^{2+} sparks and Ca^{2+} waves activate different Ca(2+)-dependent ion channels in single myocytes from rat portal vein. *Cell Calcium* 1996;**20**:153–60.
36. Peng H, Matchkov V, Ivarsen A, Aalkjaer C, Nilsson H. Hypothesis for the initiation of vasomotion. *Circ Res* 2001;**88**:810–5.
37. Lynch RM, Weber CS, Nullmeyer KD, Moore ED, Paul RJ. Clearance of store-released Ca^{2+} by the Na^{+}/Ca^{2+} exchanger is diminished in aortic smooth muscle from $Na^{+}-K^{+}$-ATPase alpha 2-isoform gene-ablated mice. *Am J Physiol Heart Circ Physiol* 2008;**294**:H1407–16.
38. Oloizia B, Paul RJ. Ca(2 +) clearance and contractility in vascular smooth muscle: evidence from gene-altered murine models. *J Mol Cell Cardiol* 2008;**45**:347–62.
39. Liu L, Ishida Y, Okunade G, Shull GE, Paul RJ. Role of plasma membrane Ca^{2+}-ATPase in contraction-relaxation processes of

the bladder: evidence from PMCA gene-ablated mice. *Am J Physiol Cell Physiol* 2006;**290**:C1239–47.

40. Floyd R, Wray S. Calcium transporters and signalling in smooth muscles. *Cell Calcium* 2007;**42**:467–76.
41. Broderick R, Somlyo AP. Calcium and magnesium transport by in situ mitochondria: electron probe analysis of vascular smooth muscle. *Circ Res* 1987;**61**:523–30.
42. Rizzuto R, Pozzan T. Microdomains of intracellular Ca^{2+}: molecular determinants and functional consequences. *Physiol Rev* 2006;**86**:369–408.
43. Daniel EE, El-Yazbi A, Cho WJ. Caveolae and calcium handling, a review and a hypothesis. *J Cell Mol Med* 2006;**10**:529–44.
44. Moore ED, Etter EF, Philipson KD, Carrington WA, Fogarty KE, Lifshitz LM, et al. Coupling of the Na^+/Ca^{2+} exchanger, Na^+/K^+ pump and sarcoplasmic reticulum in smooth muscle. *Nature* 1993;**365**:657–60.
45. Pritchard TJ, Bowman PS, Jefferson A, Tosun M, Lynch RM, Paul RJ. Na(+)-K(+)-ATPase and Ca(2+) clearance proteins in smooth muscle: a functional unit. *Am J Physiol Heart Circ Physiol* 2010;**299**:H548–56.
46. Tong WC, Sweeney M, Jones CJ, Zhang H, O'Neill SC, Prior I, et al. Three-dimensional electron microscopic reconstruction of intracellular organellar arrangements in vascular smooth muscle – further evidence of nanospaces and contacts. *J Cell Mol Med* 2009;**13**:995–8.
47. Poburko D, Lee CH, van Breemen C. Vascular smooth muscle mitochondria at the cross roads of Ca(2 +) regulation. *Cell Calcium* 2004;**35**:509–21.
48. Periasamy M, Huke S. SERCA pump level is a critical determinant of Ca(2+)homeostasis and cardiac contractility. *J Mol Cell Cardiol* 2001;**33**:1053–63.
49. Kiriazis H, Kranias EG. Genetically engineered models with alterations in cardiac membrane calcium-handling proteins. *Annu Rev Physiol* 2000;**62**:321–51.
50. Paul RJ, Shull GE, Kranias EG. The sarcoplasmic reticulum and smooth muscle function: evidence from transgenic mice. *Novartis Found Symp* 2002;**246**:228–38 [discussion 238–43, 272–76.]
51. Sutliff RL, Hoying JB, Kadambi VJ, Kranias EG, Paul RJ. Phospholamban is present in endothelial cells and modulates endothelium-dependent relaxation. Evidence from phospholamban gene-ablated mice. *Circ Res* 1999;**84**:360–4.
52. Nobe K, Sutliff RL, Kranias EG, Paul RJ. Phospholamban regulation of bladder contractility: evidence from gene-altered mouse models. *J Physiol* 2001;**535**:867–78.
53. Sutliff RL, Conforti L, Weber CS, Kranias EG, Paul RJ. Regulation of the spontaneous contractile activity of the portal vein by the sarcoplasmic reticulum: evidence from the phospholamban gene-ablated mouse. *Vascul Pharmacol* 2004;**41**:197–204.
54. Kim M, Hennig GW, Smith TK, Perrino BA. Phospholamban knockout increases CaM kinase II activity, intracellular Ca^{2+} wave activity, and alters contractile responses of murine gastric antrum. *Am J Physiol Cell Physiol* 2008;**294**:C432–41.
55. Nelson MT, Cheng H, Rubart M, Santana LF, Bonev AD, Knot HJ, et al. Relaxation of arterial smooth muscle by calcium sparks. *Science* 1995;**270**:633–7.
56. van Breemen C, Chen Q, Laher I. Superficial buffer barrier function of smooth muscle sarcoplasmic reticulum. *Trends Pharmacol Sci* 1995;**16**:98–105.
57. Adachi T. Modulation of vascular sarco/endoplasmic reticulum calcium ATPase in cardiovascular pathophysiology. *Adv Pharmacol* 2010;**59**:165–95.
58. Ying J, Tong X, Pimentel DR, Weisbrod RM, Trucillo MP, Adachi T, et al. Cysteine-674 of the sarco/endoplasmic reticulum calcium ATPase is required for the inhibition of cell migration by nitric oxide. *Arterioscler Thromb Vasc Biol* 2007;**27**:783–90.
59. Lalli MJ, Shimizu S, Sutliff RL, Kranias EG, Paul RJ. [Ca2 +]i homeostasis and cyclic nucleotide relaxation in aorta of phospholamban-deficient mice. *Am J Physiol Heart Circ Physiol* 1999;**277**:H963–70.
60. Trebak M, Ginnan R, Singer HA, Jourd'heuil D. Interplay between calcium and reactive oxygen/nitrogen species: an essential paradigm for vascular smooth muscle signaling. *Antioxid Redox Signal* 2010;**12**:657–74.
61. Zhao W, Waggoner JR, Zhang ZG, Lam CK, Han P, Qian J, et al. The anti-apoptotic protein HAX-1 is a regulator of cardiac function. *Proc Natl Acad Sci USA* 2009;**106**:20776–81.
62. Fan GC, Kranias EG. Small heat shock protein 20 (HspB6) in cardiac hypertrophy and failure. *J Mol Cell Cardiol* 2011;**51**:574–7.
63. Pritchard TJ, Kranias EG. Junctin and the histidine-rich Ca^{2+} binding protein: potential roles in heart failure and arrhythmogenesis. *J Physiol* 2009;**587**:3125–33.
64. Strehler EE, Zacharias DA. Role of alternative splicing in generating isoform diversity among plasma membrane calcium pumps. *Physiol Rev* 2001;**81**:21–50.
65. Szewczyk MM, Pande J, Akolkar G, Grover AK. Caloxin 1b3: a novel plasma membrane Ca(2 +)-pump isoform 1 selective inhibitor that increases cytosolic Ca(2 +) in endothelial cells. *Cell Calcium* 2010;**48**:352–7.
66. Schuh K, Quaschning T, Knauer S, Hu K, Kocak S, Roethlein N, et al. Regulation of vascular tone in animals overexpressing the sarcolemmal calcium pump. *J Biol Chem* 2003;**278**:41246–52.
67. Liu L, Ishida Y, Okunade G, Pyne-Geithman GJ, Shull GE, Paul RJ. Distinct roles of PMCA isoforms in Ca^{2+} homeostasis of bladder smooth muscle: evidence from PMCA gene-ablated mice. *Am J Physiol Cell Physiol* 2007;**292**:C423–31.
68. Okunade GW, Miller ML, Pyne GJ, Sutliff RL, O'Connor KT, Neumann JC, et al. Targeted ablation of plasma membrane Ca^{2+}-ATPase (PMCA) 1 and 4 indicates a major housekeeping function for PMCA1 and a critical role in hyperactivated sperm motility and male fertility for PMCA4. *J Biol Chem* 2004;**279**:33742–50.
69. Philipson KD, Nicoll DA. Sodium-calcium exchange: a molecular perspective. *Annu Rev Physiol* 2000;**62**:111–33.
70. Lytton J. Na^+/Ca^{2+} exchangers: three mammalian gene families control Ca^{2+} transport. *Biochem J* 2007;**406**:365–82.
71. Blaustein MP, Hamlyn JM. Signaling mechanisms that link salt retention to hypertension: endogenous ouabain, the Na(+) pump, the Na(+)/Ca(2 +) exchanger and TRPC proteins. *Biochim Biophys Acta* 2010;**1802**:1219–29.
72. Skou JC. The influence of some cations on an adenosine triphosphatase from peripheral nerves. *Biochim Biophys Acta* 1957;**23**:394–401.
73. Lingrel JB. The physiological significance of the cardiotonic steroid/ouabain-binding site of the Na,K-ATPase. *Annu Rev Physiol* 2010;**72**:395–412.
74. Garty H, Karlish SJ. Role of FXYD proteins in ion transport. *Annu Rev Physiol* 2006;**68**:431–59.

75. Shelly DA, He S, Moseley A, Weber C, Stegemeyer M, Lynch RM, et al. Na(+) pump alpha 2-isoform specifically couples to contractility in vascular smooth muscle: evidence from gene-targeted neonatal mice. *Am J Physiol Cell Physiol* 2004;**286**:C813–20.
76. Juhaszova M, Blaustein MP. Na^+ pump low and high ouabain affinity alpha subunit isoforms are differently distributed in cells. *Proc Natl Acad Sci USA* 1997;**94**:1800–5.
77. Blaustein MP, Lederer WJ. Sodium/calcium exchange: its physiological implications. *Physiol Rev* 1999;**79**:763–854.
78. Aickin CC, Brading AF, Burdyga TV. Evidence for sodium-calcium exchange in the guinea-pig ureter. *J Physiol* 1984;**347**:411–30.
79. Aaronson PI, Benham CD. Alterations in [Ca2 +]i mediated by sodium-calcium exchange in smooth muscle cells isolated from the guinea-pig ureter. *J Physiol* 1989;**416**:1–18.
80. Ganitkevich V, Isenberg G. Stimulation-induced potentiation of T-type Ca^{2+} channel currents in myocytes from guinea-pig coronary artery. *J Physiol* 1991;**443**:703–25.
81. Bradley KN, Flynn ER, Muir TC, McCarron JG. Ca(2+) regulation in guinea-pig colonic smooth muscle: the role of the Na (+)-Ca(2 +) exchanger and the sarcoplasmic reticulum. *J Physiol* 2002;**538**:465–82.
82. McCarron JG, Walsh Jr JV, Fay FS. Sodium/calcium exchange regulates cytoplasmic calcium in smooth muscle. *Pflugers Arch* 1994;**426**:199–205.
83. Karashima E, Nishimura J, Iwamoto T, Hirano K, Hirano M, Kita S, et al. Involvement of Na^+-Ca^{2+} exchanger in cAMP-mediated relaxation in mice aorta: evaluation using transgenic mice. *Br J Pharmacol* 2007;**150**:434–44.
84. Zhang J, Ren C, Chen L, Navedo MF, Antos LK, Kinsey SP, et al. Knockout of Na^+/Ca^{2+} exchanger in smooth muscle attenuates vasoconstriction and L-type Ca^{2+} channel current and lowers blood pressure. *Am J Physiol Heart Circ Physiol* 2010;**298**:H1472–83.
85. Xie Z, Cai T. Na^+-K^+–ATPase-mediated signal transduction: from protein interaction to cellular function. *Mol Interv* 2003;**3**:157–68.
86. Edwards A, Pallone TL. Ouabain modulation of cellular calcium stores and signaling. *Am J Physiol Renal Physiol* 2007;**293**:F1518–32.
87. Zhang J, Lee MY, Cavalli M, Chen L, Berra-Romani R, Balke CW, et al. Sodium pump alpha2 subunits control myogenic tone and blood pressure in mice. *J Physiol* 2005;**569**:243–56.
88. Pritchard TJ, Parvatiyar M, Bullard DP, Lynch RM, Lorenz JN, Paul RJ. Transgenic mice expressing Na^+-K^+-ATPase in smooth muscle decreases blood pressure. *Am J Physiol Heart Circ Physiol* 2007;**293**:H1172–82.
89. Sweadner KJ, Donnet C. Structural similarities of Na,K-ATPase and SERCA, the Ca(2+)-ATPase of the sarcoplasmic reticulum. *Biochem J* 2001;**356**:685–704.
90. Morth JP, Pedersen BP, Toustrup-Jensen MS, Sorensen TL, Petersen J, Andersen JP, et al. Crystal structure of the sodium-potassium pump. *Nature* 2007;**450**:1043–9.
91. Zhang S, Malmersjo S, Li J, Ando H, Aizman O, Uhlen P, et al. Distinct role of the N-terminal tail of the Na,K-ATPase catalytic subunit as a signal transducer. *J Biol Chem* 2006;**281**:21954–62.
92. Kim M, Jung J, Lee K. Roles of ERK, PI3 kinase, and PLC-gamma pathways induced by overexpression of translationally controlled tumor protein in HeLa cells. *Arch Biochem Biophys* 2009;**485**:82–7.
93. Yudowski GA, Efendiev R, Pedemonte CH, Katz AI, Berggren PO, Bertorello AM. Phosphoinositide-3 kinase binds to a proline-rich motif in the Na^+, K^+-ATPase alpha subunit and regulates its trafficking. *Proc Natl Acad Sci USA* 2000;**97**:6556–61.
94. Dmitrieva RI, Doris PA. Ouabain is a potent promoter of growth and activator of ERK1/2 in ouabain-resistant rat renal epithelial cells. *J Biol Chem* 2003;**278**:28160–6.
95. Tian J, Cai T, Yuan Z, Wang H, Liu L, Haas M, et al. Binding of Src to Na^+/K^+-ATPase forms a functional signaling complex. *Mol Biol Cell* 2006;**17**:317–26.
96. Liu L, Mohammadi K, Aynafshar B, Wang H, Li D, Liu J, et al. Role of caveolae in signal-transducing function of cardiac Na^+/K^+-ATPase. *Am J Physiol Cell Physiol* 2003;**284**:C1550–60.
97. Hardin CD, Vallejo J. Caveolins in vascular smooth muscle: form organizing function. *Cardiovasc Res* 2006;**69**:808–15.
98. Hansen O. No evidence for a role in signal-transduction of Na^+/K^+-ATPase interaction with putative endogenous ouabain. *Eur J Biochem* 2003;**270**:1916–9.
99. Liu J, Xie ZJ. The sodium pump and cardiotonic steroids-induced signal transduction protein kinases and calcium-signaling microdomain in regulation of transporter trafficking. *Biochim Biophys Acta* 2010;**1802**:1237–45.
100. Rossi CS, Lehninger AL. Stoichiometry of respiratory stimulation, accumulation of Ca^{++} and phosphate, and oxidative phosphorylation in rat liver mitochondria. *J Biol Chem* 1964;**239**:3971–80.
101. Duchen MR, Verkhratsky A, Muallem S. Mitochondria and calcium in health and disease. *Cell Calcium* 2008;**44**:1–5.
102. Franzini-Armstrong C. ER-mitochondria communication. How privileged? *Physiology (Bethesda)* 2007;**22**:261–8.
103. Becker GL, Fiskum G, Lehninger AL. Regulation of free Ca^{2+} by liver mitochondria and endoplasmic reticulum. *J Biol Chem* 1980;**255**:9009–12.
104. Crompton M, Heid I. The cycling of calcium, sodium, and protons across the inner membrane of cardiac mitochondria. *Eur J Biochem* 1978;**91**:599–608.
105. Collins TJ, Lipp P, Berridge MJ, Li W, Bootman MD. Inositol 1,4,5-trisphosphate-induced Ca^{2+} release is inhibited by mitochondrial depolarization. *Biochem J* 2000;**347**:593–600.
106. Chalmers S, McCarron JG. The mitochondrial membrane potential and Ca^{2+} oscillations in smooth muscle. *J Cell Sci* 2008;**121**:75–85.
107. Poburko D, Liao CH, van Breemen C, Demaurex N. Mitochondrial regulation of sarcoplasmic reticulum Ca^{2+} content in vascular smooth muscle cells. *Circ Res* 2009;**104**:104–12.
108. McCarron JG, Chalmers S, Bradley KN, MacMillan D, Muir TC. Ca^{2+} microdomains in smooth muscle. *Cell Calcium* 2006;**40**:461–93.
109. Poburko D, Kuo KH, Dai J, Lee CH, van Breemen C. Organellar junctions promote targeted Ca^{2+} signaling in smooth muscle: why two membranes are better than one. *Trends Pharmacol Sci* 2004;**25**:8–15.
110. Paul RJ, Bauer M, Pease W. Vascular smooth muscle: aerobic glycolysis linked to sodium and potassium transport processes. *Science* 1979;**206**:1414–6.

111. Shimizu S, Bowman PS, Thorne III G, Paul RJ. Effects of hypoxia on isometric force, intracellular Ca(2+), pH, and energetics in porcine coronary artery. *Circ Res* 2000;**86**:862–70.
112. Hardin CD, Allen TJ, Paul RJ, editors. *Metabolism and energetics of vascular smooth muscle*. San Diego, CA: Academic Press;2000.
113. Rizzuto R, Pinton P, Carrington W, Fay FS, Fogarty KE, Lifshitz LM, et al. Close contacts with the endoplasmic reticulum as determinants of mitochondrial Ca^{2+} responses. *Science* 1998;**280**:1763–6.
114. Carafoli E. The fateful encounter of mitochondria with calcium: how did it happen? *Biochim Biophys Acta* 2010;**1797**:595–606.
115. Gunter TE, Pfeiffer DR. Mechanisms by which mitochondria transport calcium. *Am J Physiol* 1990;**258**:C755–86.
116. Seguin A, Santos R, Pain D, Dancis A, Camadro JM, Lesuisse E. Co-precipitation of phosphate and iron limits mitochondrial phosphate availability in *Saccharomyces cerevisiae* lacking the yeast frataxin homologue (YFH1). *J Biol Chem* 2010; [ePub ahead of print December 28, 2010, doi: 10.1074/jbc.M110.163253.]
117. Lehninger AL, Reynafarje B, Vercesi A, Tew WP. Transport and accumulation of calcium in mitochondria. *Ann NY Acad Sci* 1978;**307**:160–76.
118. Monteith GR, Blaustein MP. Heterogeneity of mitochondrial matrix free Ca^{2+}: resolution of Ca^{2+} dynamics in individual mitochondria in situ. *Am J Physiol* 1999;**276**:C1193–204.
119. Drummond RM, Tuft RA. Release of Ca^{2+} from the sarcoplasmic reticulum increases mitochondrial [Ca2 +] in rat pulmonary artery smooth muscle cells. *J Physiol* 1999;**516**(Pt 1):139–47.
120. Kamishima T, Quayle JM. Mitochondrial Ca^{2+} uptake is important over low [Ca2 +]i range in arterial smooth muscle. *Am J Physiol Heart Circ Physiol* 2002;**283**:H2431–9.
121. Ueno H. Calcium mobilization in enzymically isolated single intact and skinned muscle cells of the porcine coronary artery. *J Physiol* 1985;**363**:103–17.
122. Shmygol A, Wray S. Functional architecture of the SR calcium store in uterine smooth muscle. *Cell Calcium* 2004;**35**:501–8.
123. Szabadkai G, Duchen MR. Mitochondria: the hub of cellular Ca^{2+} signaling. *Physiology (Bethesda)* 2008;**23**:84–94.

Chapter 87

Regulation of Smooth Muscle Contraction

Susanne Vetterkind and Kathleen G. Morgan
Health Sciences Department, Boston University, Boston, MA

TYPES OF CONTRACTILE STIMULATION

In smooth muscle there are three types of contractile stimulation to be considered: electrical, chemical, and mechanical (Figure 87.1). Some types of smooth muscle (e.g. phasically active muscles in the gut) display spontaneous electrical activity similar to cardiac pacemaker potentials that trigger action potentials (electrical stimulation or electromechanical coupling). However, other smooth muscles (e.g. tonically active smooth muscles of the large arteries) do not. Additionally, chemicals (e.g. hormones and neurotransmitters) binding to cell surface receptors (chemical stimulation or pharmacomechanical coupling) can activate signaling pathways that lead to contraction in the absence of depolarization. The release of autonomic neurotransmitters can modulate spontaneous electrical activity or cause graded depolarization of tonic smooth muscles. Mechanical forces like stretch or pressure can similarly trigger signaling pathways that regulate contractility (mechanical stimulation or mechanomechanical coupling).

Electrical Stimulation

Depolarization of the sarcolemma leads to opening of voltage-gated Ca^{2+} channels and influx of Ca^{2+} from the extracellular space. This Ca^{2+} pulse can also trigger the release of intracellular Ca^{2+} from the sarcoplasmic reticulum (Ca^{2+}-induced Ca^{2+} release, CICR). Contraction is then triggered by elevated intracellular Ca^{2+} levels.

In skeletal muscle, depolarization is mediated by impulses from motor nerves, which are under the control of the somatic nervous system. In smooth muscle, although it is innervated by the visceral (autonomous) nervous system (and therefore not under voluntary control), neural input is not always of the same central importance as in skeletal muscle. For example, uterine smooth muscle contractility is largely controlled by hormones and other biochemical factors, as well as by mechanical stimulation such as stretch, whereas neural input plays a minor modulating and organizing role (see Chapter 90). Yet, in many smooth muscles, including uterine smooth muscle, depolarization can occur spontaneously or be triggered by cytoskeletal activation.

Chemical Stimulation

A wide variety of biological effectors, including neurotransmitters, paracrine and endocrine factors, can induce contraction or relaxation of smooth muscle. Typically, these factors bind to specific receptors in the cell membrane, which then activate either receptor-operated channels to cause depolarization, or trigger a signaling cascade that ultimately leads to regulation of contractility. Since the majority of these factors, as well as their signaling pathways, are tissue-specific, they will not be covered here in detail (for examples, see chapters in the subsection Heterogeneities).

Common chemical signals in many types of smooth muscles are neurotransmitters released by nerve activity. The most important types of neurotransmission in smooth muscle are the adrenergic and cholinergic pathways. The responses to neurotransmitters, however, can vary significantly in a tissue-specific manner. For example, norepinephrine by primarily binding to α_1-adrenergic receptors triggers contraction in vascular smooth muscle, but by primarily binding to β-receptors causes relaxation of airway smooth muscle. Conversely, stimulation of M3 muscarinic receptors by acetylcholine leads to contraction of airway smooth muscle, but by releasing nitric oxide from the endothelium, causes relaxation of vascular smooth muscle.

Mechanical Stimulation

In 1902 the physiologist Sir William Bayliss published his findings on an autoregulatory mechanism that controls the muscle tone in the arterial wall by a nerve-independent, stretch-dependent contraction (1). This contraction in response to enhanced pressure on the arterial wall, known as the Bayliss effect or myogenic response, is a vital mechanism that keeps blood flow constant despite

Muscle. DOI: http://dx.doi.org/10.1016/B978-0-12-381510-1.00087-9

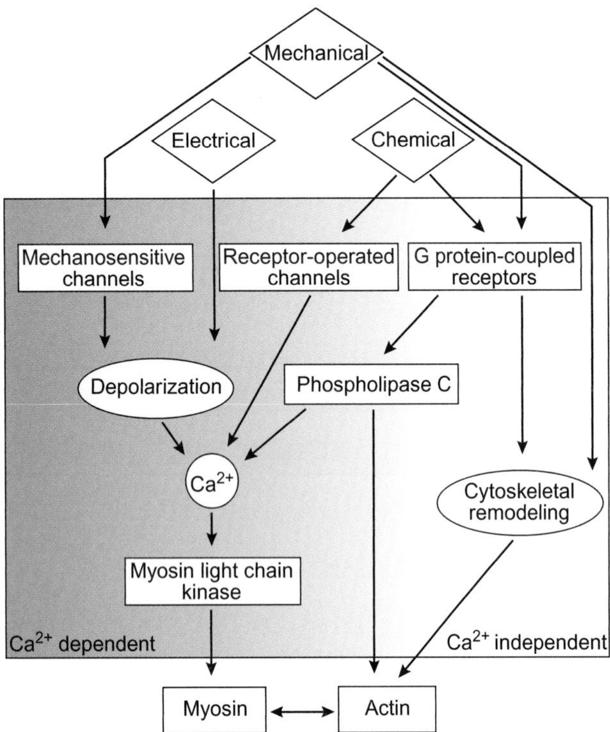

FIGURE 87.1 **Contractile signaling pathways in smooth muscle (simplified overview).** Three types of stimulation – mechanical, electrical, and chemical – target at myosin activation and/or actin–myosin interaction through pathways that show varying degrees of Ca^{2+} dependency (schematically indicated by blue gradient).

changes in arterial pressure. The myogenic response is mediated by two main factors: (i) depolarization of the smooth muscle cell membrane, accompanied by influx of extracellular Ca^{2+}; and (ii) post-translational changes in focal adhesion proteins connected to the cytoskeleton, a kind of "outside-in signaling".

Sensing of stretch by pressure-sensitive signaling proteins depends on cytoskeletal integrity of the cell. Stretch of the vascular wall and, with it, the plasma membrane and cytoskeleton of smooth muscle cells, leads to the opening of pressure-sensitive non-selective cation channels. The subsequent depolarization elicits activation of voltage-gated Ca^{2+} channels, and thereby contraction of the smooth muscle cell (see Chapter 84 on ion channels and Chapter 86 on calcium homeostasis). Also, focal adhesion proteins are post-translationally modified (e.g. phosphorylated) in response to stretch. This mechanism of stretch signaling includes trimeric G-protein-mediated activation of phospholipase C (PLC), which leads to release of Ca^{2+} from intracellular stores (see Chapter 85) and activation of non-receptor tyrosine kinases such as sarcoma kinase (Src) and focal adhesion kinase (FAK). Apart from these short-term regulatory mechanisms, altered protein expression of pressure sensitive channels or adhesion plaque proteins can be a part of long-term adaptations, e.g. to compensate for chronically elevated blood pressure.

Sensing of, and consequently, responding to stretch and pressure would not be possible without tension on the cell. Cellular tension, in turn, is produced by the opposing forces of contractile filaments and resisting structural elements, which can be either the extracellular matrix or rigid components of the cytoskeleton (intermediate filaments, cross-linked actin bundles), or both. This balance of forces generated by contractile and rigid elements can be described by the term "tensegrity" (2). Many of the proteins that provide cytoskeletal integrity and cell-matrix connectivity, including integrins and dystroglycans, have multiple functions as structural, signaling, and/or organizing (scaffold) proteins. Various actin-binding cytoskeletal proteins are also regulators of actin function. Equally important are cytoskeletal scaffolds as organizers of signaling pathways.

CONTRACTILE SIGNALING PATHWAYS BY TARGET

A variety of signaling pathways exists that trigger contraction. All of them ultimately regulate cross-bridge cycling between actin and myosin, and hence aim at only two targets: actin and myosin. While regulation of myosin is almost exclusively mediated by phosphorylation of the myosin regulatory light chain, regulation of actin occurs through a variety of actin-binding proteins.

Myosin

Just as in cardiac and skeletal muscle, the molecular mechanism for contraction of smooth muscle actin–myosin filaments is based on cross-bridge cycling. However, cross-bridge formation and myosin ATPase activity are regulated primarily by phosphorylation of the myosin regulatory light chain, as opposed to troponin/tropomyosin in skeletal muscle.

Myosin Light Chain Phosphorylation

Phosphorylation of myosin regulatory light chain (MLC) is an obligatory step in the activation of smooth muscle myosin and the initiation of smooth muscle contraction. This is in marked contrast to striated muscle myosin, which is enzymatically active in the absence of phosphorylation.

The regulatory light chains of myosin II bind to the neck region of the myosin heavy chain, which connects the rod-shaped alpha-helical coiled coil domain and the globular motor domains. Phosphorylation of MLC at the primary regulatory site, serine 19, induces a conformational change of the myosin molecule that activates the myosin ATPase function and hence, allows for cross-bridge cycling.

Myosin Light Chain Kinase

MLC phosphorylation is primarily mediated by myosin light chain kinase (MLCK). MLCK is a central enzyme in smooth muscle contraction, linking the increase in intracellular Ca^{2+}, as it occurs after contractile stimulation, to contraction of actin–myosin filaments: Ca^{2+} is released in response to contractile stimulation and binds to calmodulin. MLCK is then activated by binding of the Ca^{2+}/calmodulin complex. Once activated by Ca^{2+}/calmodulin binding, MLCK enzyme activity, or rather its sensitivity towards Ca^{2+}, can be modulated by phosphorylation, both in an inhibitory/desensitizing manner (protein kinase A, protein kinase C, Ca^{2+}/calmodulin dependent kinase II, and p21-activated kinase), and an activating/sensitizing manner (extracellular signal regulated kinase, ERK) (see Chapter 83).

MLCK is encoded by a very interesting gene, *mylk1* (3). It encodes two long, 220 kDa isoforms of MLCK, as well as a short, 130 kDa isoform and a small protein named telokin. Each of the four gene products is under the control of its own, independent promoter within the *mylk1* gene. The different MLCK isoforms, although showing distinct subcellular distribution and tissue-specific expression patterns, appear to have largely redundant functions. In smooth muscle, the 130 kDa isoform is the predominant form. Since the smooth muscle-specific protein telokin corresponds to the C-terminal, myosin-binding region of MLCK, but lacks the catalytic domain, it acts as a natural dominant-negative regulator and inhibits MLC phosphorylation. The relative expression levels of the MLCK isoforms and telokin therefore may have implications on tissue contractility and Ca^{2+} sensitivity.

The molecular evolution of MLC is noteworthy in that this molecule, like troponin-C, has emerged from the calmodulin family of Ca^{2+}-binding proteins by gene duplication (and indeed, some isoforms of MLC can bind and are activated by Ca^{2+}). The advantage of an indirect and tunable effector, MLCK, over direct activation of myosin by Ca^{2+}, is that it allows for a tighter and more precise regulation of contractility.

Myosin Light Chain Phosphatase

The activity of MLCK and other MLC kinases is opposed by the activity of a single myosin phosphatase. This enzyme is a trimeric complex consisting of a catalytic subunit (protein phosphatase 1, PP1), a regulatory subunit (myosin phosphatase targeting subunit, MYPT), and a third subunit of unknown function (M20). Myosin phosphatase was originally assumed to be unregulated and constitutively active, however, it has since become clear that myosin phosphatase is embedded in a network of regulatory pathways (see Figure 87.2).

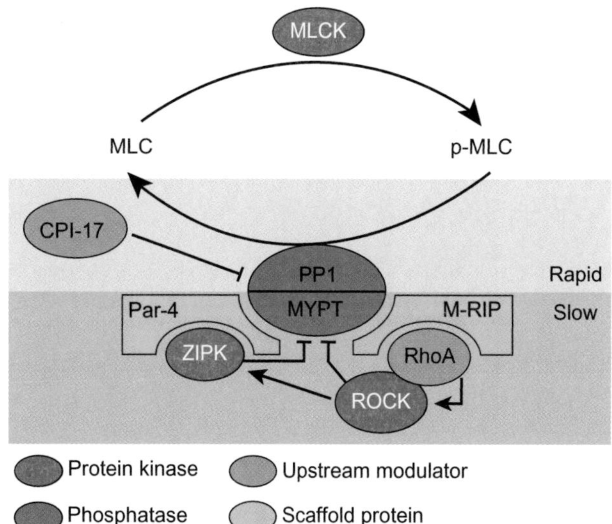

FIGURE 87.2 **Inhibition of myosin phosphatase.** Myosin phosphatase, a complex of the catalytic subunit PP1 and the regulatory subunit MYPT (M20 not shown), is regulated on different levels in space and time. The inhibitory mechanisms shown in the diagram can be categorized as "rapid" (CPI-17) and "slow" (phosphorylation of MYPT by ZIPK or ROCK). The kinases ZIPK and ROCK are directed to their substrate MYPT by their respective scaffold proteins, Par-4 and M-RIP. p-MLC = phosphorylated myosin light chain.

The most prominent regulator of myosin phosphatase is its regulatory subunit, MYPT, which acts like a scaffold to enhance enzymatic activity of the enzyme complex. It can also act as an inhibitor, since it harbors two inhibitory phosphorylation sites. These sites can be phosphorylated in response to activation of a RhoA pathway. The respective downstream kinases that phosphorylate the myosin phosphatase regulatory subunit and thus inhibit myosin phosphatase activity, are Rho kinase (ROCK) and zipper interacting kinase (ZIPK), as well as integrin-linked kinase. The small protein CPI-17 (protein kinase C potentiated inhibitor 17), a substrate of protein kinase C, acts as another myosin phosphatase inhibitor in its phosphorylated form.

The pathways that impede the phosphatase are counterbalanced by the nitric oxide pathway, which activates the phosphatase. The highly diffusible cellular messenger, nitric oxide, leads to elevation of intracellular cyclic guanosine monophosphate (cGMP), which then activates the type Ia protein kinase G (PKG). Among the substrates of PKG are the MYPT and RhoA. Phosphorylation of MYPT by PKG blocks subsequent inhibitory phosphorylation of MYPT and has therefore an activating effect on myosin phosphatase. Inhibition of RhoA signaling by

PKG also prevents MYPT inhibitory phosphorylation. Furthermore, PKG supports myosin phosphatase activity (and relaxation of the muscle) by activating protein phosphatase 2a (PP2a), which dephosphorylates and thus, deactivates the myosin phosphatase inhibitor CPI-17.

Ca^{2+} Sensitization

Apart from MLCK, which is clearly Ca^{2+}-dependent, other kinases exist that are capable of phosphorylating MLC in a Ca^{2+}-independent manner, among them ROCK, integrin-linked kinase, and ZIPK. The same set of kinases also inhibits myosin phosphatase by targeting MYPT at its inhibitory phosphorylation sites. Phosphorylation of MLC and simultaneous inhibition of myosin phosphatase can promote contraction through shifting the balance towards phosphorylation of MLC at constant Ca^{2+} levels, or it can sustain contraction at decreasing Ca^{2+} levels. Similarly, the actin regulatory pathway described below can regulate force in the absence of changes in Ca^{2+}. These modifications have been referred to as changes in the Ca^{2+} sensitivity of the muscle (4).

Actin

Actin is the most abundant protein in many cells and makes up approximately 20% of total protein content in smooth muscle. Reflecting its important role in many cellular processes, the actin sequence is highly conserved across species and through evolution.

Smooth muscle actin can exist in two forms: a monomeric globular G-actin and a filamentous polymeric F-actin. Classically, it has been assumed that the actin in differentiated, non-migrating, smooth muscle is rather static, performing primarily a structural role. However, recent work with both airway and vascular smooth muscles has now shown that an important part of the actin cytoskeleton is dynamic and remodels in the presence of agonists (5,6). This plasticity of the actin cytoskeleton is also consistent with the dramatic ability of unrestrained freshly dissociated vascular smooth muscle cells to shorten to 50–25% of their cell length when activated by vasoconstrictors (Figure 87.3). In contrast, striated muscle cells can only shorten to ~80% of their initial length because of the presence of Z-bands.

Actin Isoforms

There are six vertebrate isoforms of actin, all separate gene products, four of which are expressed in smooth muscle. Alpha smooth muscle actin is the major isoform in vascular smooth muscle but gamma smooth muscle actin predominates in gastrointestinal muscles. The alpha and gamma smooth muscle actins are primarily found in

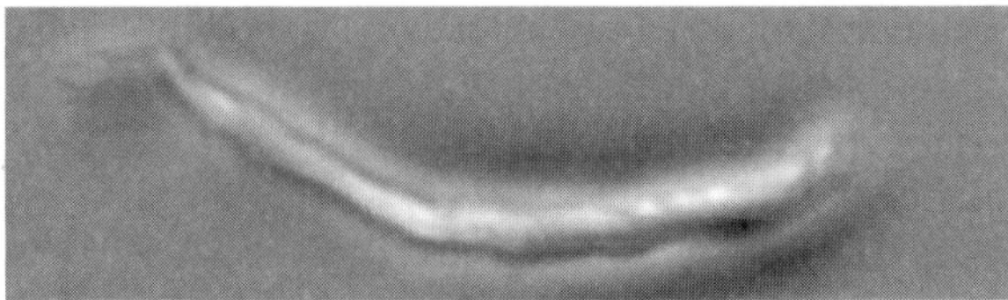

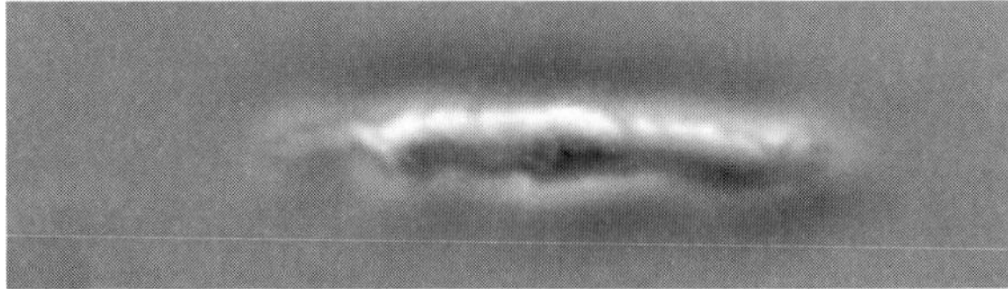

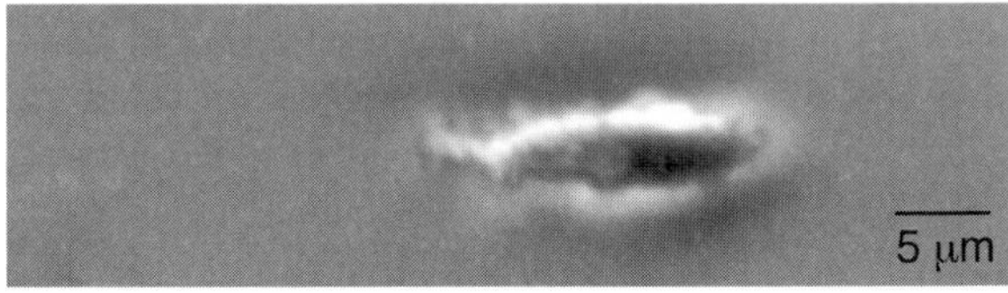

FIGURE 87.3 Shortening of a contractile smooth muscle cell. A single freshly enzymatically dissociated portal vein smooth muscle cell shows plasticity of its cytoskeleton by shortening dramatically in response to a depolarizing stimulus (KCl exchanged for NaCl in the physiological saline solution).

the myosin II-containing contractile filaments. All smooth muscles also contain nonmuscle beta and gamma actins in a nonmuscle actin cytoskeleton. Although the nonmuscle actins are of lesser abundance, it appears that they are the more dynamic forms of actin (5).

As is true for striated muscle actin, smooth muscle actin monomers (G actin) form filaments (F actin) that appear as two helically twisted chains. Smooth muscle actin filaments bind to a range of actin-binding proteins that regulate its straight, branched or cross-linked structure, its relative stability, and its interaction with other actin filaments and with myosin. The actin found in the contractile filaments of smooth muscle is associated with several actin-binding proteins. The best studied are tropomyosin, caldesmon, and calponin.

The contractile filaments insert directly or indirectly into alpha actinin-containing structures called dense bodies. The dense bodies function in a manner similar to that of the Z-lines of striated muscle. In a model developed for avian gizzard smooth muscle (7), it is proposed that the force generating elements between two dense bodies transmit force to adjacent mini-sarcomeres of contractile filaments in a diagonal manner across the cell until, eventually, a connection is made with adhesion plaques at the cell membrane. Recent studies suggest that the connection may be indirect via a connection with a cortical nonmuscle cytoskeleton (Figure 87.4).

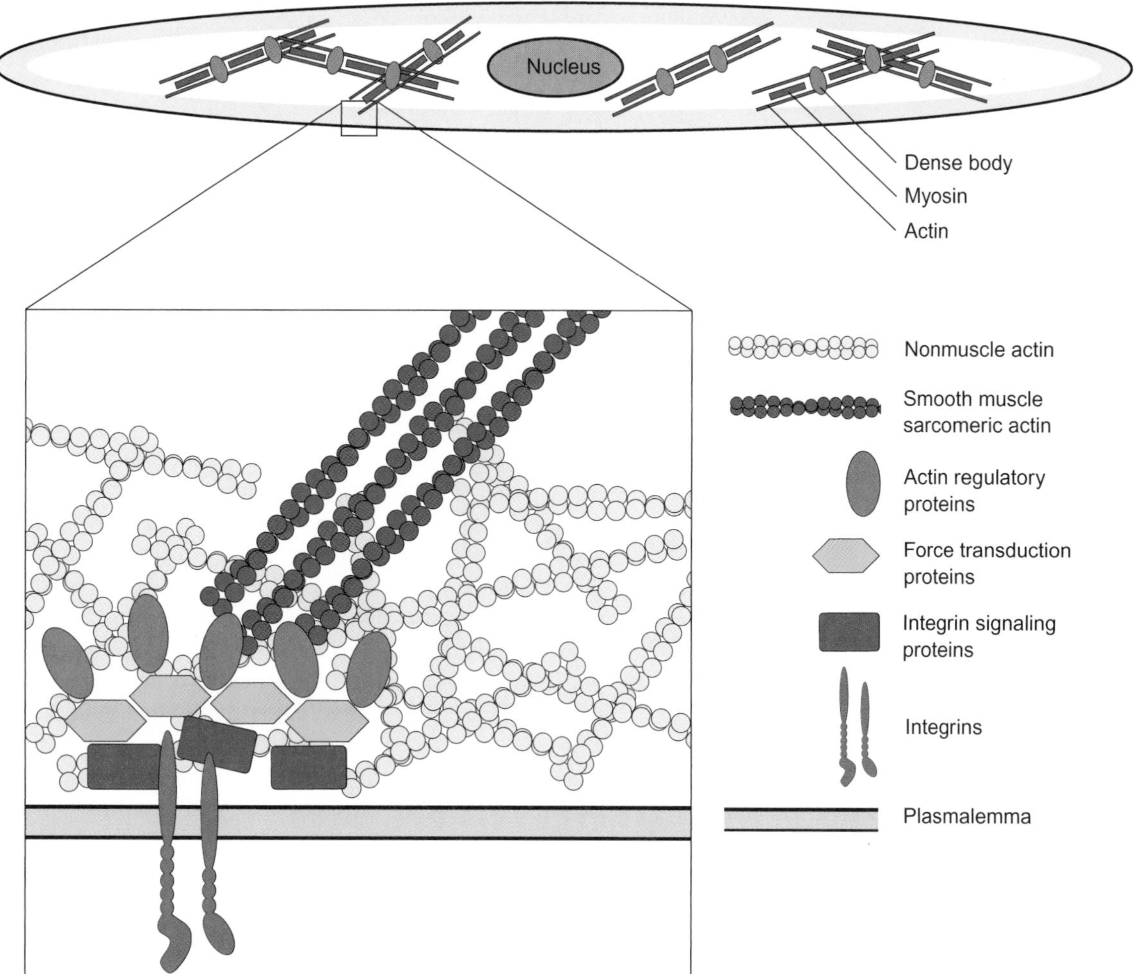

FIGURE 87.4 **Actin cytoskeleton and focal adhesions (schematic drawing).** Contractile actin–myosin filaments criss-cross the cell, anchored internally to dense bodies and externally to focal adhesions at the cell cortex. The inset illustrates the basic layered structure of a focal adhesion with integrin signaling proteins shown in red (e.g. FAK, paxillin, Src), force transduction proteins in yellow (e.g. vinculin, talin), and actin regulatory proteins in green (e.g. zyxin, VASP, N-WASP) (9). Focal adhesions and bundles of smooth muscle actin (dark blue) are embedded in a cortical network of nonmuscle actin (light blue). Please note that proteins are not drawn to scale.

Tropomyosin

Tropomyosin is a coiled coil dimeric protein that snakes along the major groove of actin filaments. By gating the binding of a host of actin-binding proteins, it acts as a major regulator of actin function. In smooth muscle myosin-containing contractile filaments, tropomyosin plays a major role in its interactions with the actin-binding protein caldesmon, which can be thought of as filling the role of the troponin complex in the regulation of actin–myosin interactions.

Caldesmon

Caldesmon is an actin- and myosin-binding protein that exists as two alternatively spliced isoforms. The heavy isoform is a marker of differentiated contractile smooth muscle cells but the light isoform exists in both contractile and proliferative smooth muscle cells. In contractile smooth muscle the heavy isoform is associated with the actin in the contractile filaments but the light isoform is thought to be associated with the nonmuscle actin cytoskeleton. Caldesmon, together with tropomyosin, regulate the access of myosin to actin. In relaxed smooth muscle the binding site on myosin is blocked by the caldesmon-tropomyosin complex. In response agonist stimulation such as alpha-agonist-mediated stimulation of vascular smooth muscle, a PKC- and possibly adhesion plaque-dependent signaling cascade is activated, resulting in an ERK-dependent phosphorylation of caldesmon and a consequent movement of the caldesmon-tropomyosin complex away from the myosin binding site on actin.

This allows the initiation of cross-bridge cycling and contraction.

Calponin

There are three calponin isoforms: the basic (CNN1), neutral (CNN), and acidic (CNN3) isoforms, all separate gene products. Basic calponin is a selective biomarker for differentiated smooth muscle whereas the neutral and acidic isoforms are more widely expressed. All are actin-binding proteins and *in vitro* calponin regulates myosin ATPase activity. Calponin's function in smooth muscle cells remains a matter of controversy. Several studies have implicated calponin in the direct regulation of actin–myosin interactions, but calponin is also known to be displaced from the contractile filaments during agonist activation and to undergo a cortical translocation. It has been suggested that it acts as an adaptor protein linking PKC and ERK signaling and in this way facilitates ERK-mediated pathways in the smooth muscle cell as well as nonmuscle cells (5).

Focal Adhesion/Actin Interactions

Over 150 proteins have been suggested to be contained in focal adhesions (8,9). Focal adhesions, via integrins, link the extracellular matrix to the actin cytoskeleton of smooth muscle cells. Interestingly, dystroglycans are also known to connect the extracellular matrix with the actin cytoskeleton through an organized set of proteins, the dystrophin–glycoprotein complex, and are known to be present in smooth muscle. However, the function and significance of the dystroglycan complex in smooth muscle are not yet fully understood.

Since smooth muscles, unlike skeletal muscles, do not possess tendons, force generated by the myosin-containing contractile filaments is funneled through the adhesion plaques to the rest of the smooth muscle tissue. In this way, the forces generated by individual "mini-sarcomeres" are added in parallel, producing a more effective force transmission than the addition of striated muscle sarcomeric forces in series at the tendon.

Focal adhesions also facilitate signaling pathways that control differentiation, apoptosis, and cell division. The "adhesome" includes actin regulatory proteins, integrin signaling proteins, and scaffolding proteins. Included in these diverse proteins are many kinases and phosphatases. Interestingly, many of the focal adhesion kinases are tyrosine kinases and in the contractile smooth muscle cell this is essentially the only major site of tyrosine phosphorylation. Other signaling pathways that directly regulate contractility (see Figure 87.1) involve primarily Ser/Thr kinases.

For nonmuscle cells it is known that focal adhesions are vertically separated into three strata going from the integrin signaling layer (including Src, FAK, and paxillin) to a force transduction or scaffolding layer (including talin and vinculin) to an actin-regulatory layer (including vasodilator-stimulated phosphoprotein (VASP), neural Wiskott–Aldrich syndrome protein (N-WASP) and zyxin) (9). Talin and vinculin in the force transduction layer connect the integrin signaling layer with the actin-regulatory layer in a controllable manner by tethering integrins to actin. A similar arrangement is expected for the focal adhesions (also called adhesion plaques or dense plaques) in the smooth muscle cell (Figure 87.4).

Focal adhesion signaling (in the form of tyrosine phosphorylation of focal adhesion proteins in response to vasoconstrictors and translocations of paxillin and talin) occurs in airway smooth muscle in response to agonists, suggesting ongoing agonist-induced focal adhesion remodeling. However, the relative degree of focal adhesion remodeling and the possible function of such remodeling are currently little understood for non-migrating, non-proliferating contractile smooth muscle cells. Furthermore, the significance of focal adhesion remodeling is not clear. However, much recent attention has been given to the fact that the stiffness of the aorta increases with age. This increased aortic stiffness is an early and independent predictor of negative cardiovascular outcomes such as hypertension, myocardial infarction, kidney disease, and cardiovascular-mediated dementia (10,11). Thus, it is possible that actin/focal adhesion/matrix connections play a role in such abnormal vascular stiffness.

ORGANIZATION OF SIGNALING PATHWAYS

To prevent disorganization, the large number of proteins that are involved in contractile signaling are ordered in space and time. In many cases, this is achieved by pathway-specific scaffold proteins. As mentioned above, the actin-binding protein calponin links protein kinase C signaling with ERK signaling. It is characteristic of scaffold proteins that they interact simultaneously with several components of a specific signaling pathway. Pre-assembly of signaling modules by scaffolds not only increases speed and efficiency of signaling. Specificity, too, is enhanced through the spatial and/or temporal separation of signaling pathways that have effectors in common. Smooth muscle Archvillin (SmAV), caveolin, paxillin, and calponin have all been described as scaffolds for the promiscuous kinase ERK and presumably help to target the kinase to specific substrates under specific conditions. Similarly, both myosin phosphatase-rho interacting protein (M-RIP) (12) and prostate apoptosis response-4

(Par-4) (13) have been described to have scaffolding functions related to myosin phosphatase (Figure 87.2). In this case it is assumed that the scaffolds regulate the input to the phosphatase from upstream signaling pathways.

Spatial Organization

The components of signaling pathways are usually not floating free in the cytoplasm, but are rather located at specific intracellular compartments, often in highly structured complexes. Examples for this sort of organization are the caveolae ("little caves"), small membrane invaginations decorated with the characteristic protein caveolin-1. Decades after their initial discovery, the function of caveolae, which are abundant in smooth muscle cell membranes, is still not well understood, and many controversies remain. It is widely agreed upon, though, that caveolae are scaffolds for various cell surface channels and receptors as well as many of their downstream effectors, and that caveolar function in signaling is important for regulation of smooth muscle tone (14,15).

Other examples for spatial organization of signaling pathways are focal adhesions, which serve not only as structural anchors of the cell on the substrate, but also organize the components of the integrin signaling pathway. The focal adhesion protein paxillin, for example, acts as a scaffold for the ERK cascade and also for focal adhesion kinase, FAK.

Specialized structures like focal adhesions and caveolae are not the only way signaling pathways are spatially separated within the cell. In some cases, apparently redundant protein isoforms show specific subcellular distributions and consequently direct upstream signals to distinct targets. Tropomyosin isoforms, for example, show distinct subcellular localization patterns, that reflect different actin filament subpopulations. Of note, different actin isoforms locate to specific filament types (16), suggesting that the isoform composition of actin fibers determines filament properties.

Temporal Organization

Some signaling pathways are organized in time. For example, Ca^{2+} sensitization through inhibition of myosin phosphatase can be achieved by two apparently redundant pathways: phosphorylation of the small inhibitor CPI-17 in response to protein kinase C activation, and phosphorylation of the regulatory subunit MYPT in response to Rho/ROCK activation. However, CPI-17 is more rapidly phosphorylated than MYPT (17), so that the two pathways complement each other in time and moreover, tissue-specific variations in their relative contribution to myosin phosphatase inhibition can modulate the time course of Ca^{2+} sensitization (Figure 87.2).

Also the Ca^{2+}/calmodulin dependent kinase II (CaMKII), known to regulate vascular tone through various mechanisms, is involved in the temporal organization of signaling. Binding of Ca^{2+}/calmodulin initially activates CaMKII. Once activated, the kinase autophosphorylates, which confers a "molecular memory" in form of autonomous activity even after Ca^{2+}/calmodulin has dissociated from the kinase.

CONCLUSIONS

Originally regarded as purely mechanical structures, actomyosin filaments have revealed more and more of their regulatable nature in the past decades. Since smooth muscle exerts very different functions in various organ systems of the body, it is not surprising that regulation of smooth muscle contraction is particularly complex, with regulatory mechanisms ranging from autoregulatory stretch sensing to modulation of gene expression.

As techniques evolve to allow not only for higher resolution, but also more comprehensive analysis of subcellular structures, we are beginning to understand how force is transmitted on the molecular level at focal adhesions. New perspectives on smooth muscle function have also come from the expanding collective of scaffold proteins as regulators of contraction.

Thus, although the basic control of smooth muscle contraction, centered around myosin light chain phosphorylation, is quite well understood, many aspects of its regulation are still in the process of unfolding.

REFERENCES

1. Bayliss WM. On the local reactions of the arterial wall to changes of internal pressure. *J Physiol* 1902;**28**:220–31.
2. Ingber DE. Tensegrity: the architectural basis of cellular mechanotransduction. *Annu Rev Physiol.* 1997;**59**:575–99.
3. Herring BP, El-Mounayri O, Gallagher PJ, Yin F, Zhou J. Regulation of myosin light chain kinase and telokin expression in smooth muscle tissues. *Am J Physiol Cell Physiol* 2006;**291**:C817–27.
4. Bradley AB, Morgan KG. Alteration in cytoplasmic calcium sensitivity during porcine coronary artery contractions as detected by aequorin. *J. Physiol. (Lond)* 1987;**385**:437–48.
5. Kim HR, Appel S, Vetterkind S, Gangopadhyay SS, Morgan KG. Smooth muscle signalling pathways in health and disease. *J Cell Mol Med.* 2008;**12**:2165–80.
6. Gunst SJ, Zhang W. Actin cytoskeletal dynamics in smooth muscle: a new paradigm for the regulation of smooth muscle contraction. *Am J Physiol Cell Physiol* 2008;**295**:C576–87.
7. North AJ, Gimona M, Lando Z, Small JV. Actin isoform compartments in chicken gizzard smooth muscle cells. *J. Cell Sci.* 1994;**107**:445–55.
8. Zaidel-Bar R, Itzkovitz S, Ma'ayan A, Iyengar R, Geiger B. Functional atlas of the integrin adhesome. *Nat Cell Biol* 2007;**9**:858–67.

9. Kanchanawong P, Shtengel G, Pasapera AM, Ramko EB, Davidson MW, Hess HF, et al. Nanoscale architecture of integrin-based cell adhesions. *Nature* 2010;**468**:580–4.
10. Dernellis J, Panaretou M. Aortic stiffness is an independent predictor of progression to hypertension in nonhypertensive subjects. *Hypertension* 2005;**45**:426–31.
11. Qiu H, Zhu Y, Sun Z, Trzeciakowski JP, Gansner M, Depre C, et al. Vascular smooth muscle cell stiffness as a mechanism for increased aortic stiffness with aging. *Circ Res* 2010;**107**:615–9.
12. Riddick N, Ohtani K, Surks HK. Targeting by myosin phosphatase-RhoA interacting protein mediates RhoA/ROCK regulation of myosin phosphatase. *J Cell Biochem* 2008;**103**:1158–70.
13. Vetterkind S, Lee E, Sundberg E, Poythress RH, Tao TC, Preuss U, et al. Par-4: a new activator of myosin phosphatase. *Mol Biol Cell* 2010;**21**:1214–24.
14. Bergdahl A, Sward K. Caveolae-associated signalling in smooth muscle. *Can J Physiol Pharmacol* 2004;**82**:289–99.
15. Je HD, Gallant C, Leavis PC, Morgan KG. Caveolin-1 regulates contractility in differentiated vascular smooth muscle. *Am J Physiol Heart Circ Physiol* 2004;**286**:H91–8.
16. Gallant C, Appel S, Graceffa P, Leavis PC, Lin JJ, Gunning PW, et al. Tropomyosin variants describe distinct functional subcellular domains in differentiated vascular smooth muscle cells. *Am J Physiol Cell Physiol* 2011;**300**:C1356–65.
17. Dimopoulos GJ, Semba S, Kitazawa K, Eto M, Kitazawa T. Ca^{2+}-dependent rapid Ca^{2+} sensitization of contraction in arterial smooth muscle. *Circ Res* 2007;**100**:121–9.

Section B

Heterogeneities

Chapter 88

Heterogeneity of Smooth Muscle

Richard Arnoldi[1], Christine Chaponnier[1], Giulio Gabbiani[1] and Boris Hinz[2]

[1]*Department of Pathology and Immunology, Faculty of Medicine, University of Geneva, Geneva, Switzerland,* [2]*Laboratory of Tissue Repair and Regeneration, Matrix Dynamics Group, Faculty of Dentistry, University of Toronto, Toronto, ON, Canada*

INTRODUCTION

Smooth muscle (SM) consists of mononucleated fusiform cells generally disposed as dense layers in the wall of vertebrate blood vessels and hollow organs (with the exception of the heart). Its contraction and relaxation is critical for the function of the vascular, digestive, respiratory, and urogenital systems. SMs are usually classified into enteric SM (ESM) and vascular SM (VSM), and occasionally into airways SM (ASM). In the walls of hollow organs, ESMs are present in several distinct layers: a thin layer just beneath the epithelium (muscularis mucosae), responsible for microcontractions affecting the epithelium, and two or three thick layers forming the muscularis propria, which is responsible for peristalsis. In blood vessels, VSM is restricted to the central layer (tunica media) where it is involved in maintaining tone and producing the contraction necessary for sustaining blood pressure. In addition to classic SMCs, other cell types display some SM-like features such as the ability to contract and the expression of typical SM proteins, namely actin isoforms, intermediate filaments and actin-binding proteins. These cells, which include myofibroblasts, myoepithelial cells, and myoid cells, will therefore also be discussed in this chapter.

SMOOTH MUSCLE

Heterogeneity

Although the primary function of SM is to mediate the contraction phenomena in the circulatory, respiratory, gastrointestinal, and urogenital systems, SMCs also have an important role in the organ resistance to compliance and regeneration, as well as significant properties of synthesis and secretion. The variety of physiological roles played by SMCs in the body explains the heterogeneity underlying their functional and anatomic specializations. Although SM heterogeneity has been established for a long time, the commonly accepted definition criteria have been refined over the past several decades in parallel with new techniques, taking into account function, morphology, organization, response to stimuli, type of innervations, and protein content. SMs have been first classified on the basis of their organization in the 1940s by Bozler into "multi-unit" and "unitary" (syncytial) (1). Multi-unit SM is found in ciliary muscle, iris muscle, piloerector muscles, but also in large airways and arteries. These types of SM are composed of separate fibers, which operate independently from one another and form few gap junctions. They are richly innervated with often one single nerve ending per fiber and are insulated by a thin basement membrane layer. Similar to skeletal muscle, multi-unit SMs are mainly controlled by nerve signals, and their stretching does not produce a contractile response. In contrast, unitary SMs are composed of bundles or sheets of fibers highly enriched with gap junctions, which allow synchronized response to stimuli. Their innervation is limited and their stimulation is controlled by factors such as hormones or mechanical factors. They respond to stretching and are found around all enteric organs and most vessels. This classification cannot, however, be regarded as rigid, since SMs in some organs, like bladder, and some blood vessels show features of both types.

With advances in electron microscopy and physiology techniques, additional criteria of heterogeneity have been proposed for SMs, largely based on their morphologic, neurologic, and mechanical properties. ESMCs are generally larger, more densely packed, and show a lower actin/myosin ratio than VSMCs (2,3). SMs have also been characterized according to their contraction features (Figure 88.1). Tonic SMs, which contract and relax slowly, can maintain tone for prolonged periods. The capacity to maintain a sustained contraction with little energy utilization is particularly important for blood vessels, bronchioles, and some sphincters. In contrast, phasic SMs contract and relax rapidly and, thus maintain tone poorly. The phasic response, for example, drives substances through the lumen of the gastrointestinal tract

Muscle. DOI: http://dx.doi.org/10.1016/B978-0-12-381510-1.00088-0

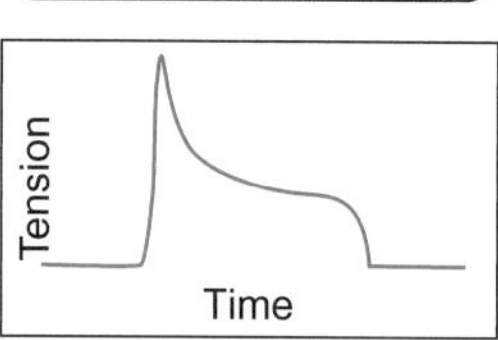

FIGURE 88.1 **Classification of SM-containing organs according to their contraction features.** SMs can be characterized by their phasic/tonic properties. Phasic SMs, which contract and relax rapidly, include most ESMs, whereas tonic SMs, which contract and relax slowly, correspond to VSMs and ASMs.

during peristalsis. The different mechanical properties of phasic and tonic SMs depend either on their signal transduction activity or on their contractile proteins composition. In tonic SMCs, initial contraction in response to acetylcholine is mediated through 1,4,5-IP_3-induced Ca^{2+} release from intracellular stores, and activation of the calmodulin-dependent pathway. In contrast, in phasic SMCs, acetylcholine-induced contraction is mediated by muscarinic M2 receptors linked to G proteins which activate HSP27-linked p38 kinase or ERK1/ERK2 pathways (4). Alternatively, high shortening velocity of phasic SMs has been associated with an increased proportion of γ-actin and β-tropomyosin, at the expense of α-actin and α-tropomyosin (5), but also with higher proportions of some SM-myosin heavy chains (MHCs) isoforms such as SM-MHC-1 (6) and SM-MHC-B (7). SM-myosin light chain (MLC) 17a (8) is highly expressed in phasic SMs such as the relatively fast muscles of porcine gastrointestinal tract, whereas the slow tracheal, aortic, pulmonary, and carotid arteries contain relatively high proportions of MLC_{17b} (9).

More recently, cultured SMCs from various tissues have been analyzed using DNA microarrays to profile their gene expression pattern. Although all SMCs display a relatively uniform spindle-shape, they can be clustered according to their gene expression pattern in a way that reflects their site of origin. Using genomic analysis, two SMCs groups emerge: (1) "vascular" including arterial, venous, and airway SMCs, and (2) "visceral" (i.e. enteric) including gastrointestinal, reproductive, and urinary SMCs (10). Very recently, the discovery of microRNAs (miRNAs), provided a palette of novel cell phenotypic regulators and markers. Single-stranded miRNAs are 20–24 nucleotides short and non-coding RNAs. miRNAs regulate post-transcriptionally the expression of at least 30% of genes in the cell by binding to 3′ untranslated regions (3′UTR) of target mRNAs, leading to either their degradation or their translational repression. Hundreds of miRNAs exist in eukaryotic cells with often cell-specific expression patterns. Among them, miR-145 is a phenotypic marker for mature VSMCs. miR-143 and miR-145 are enriched in VSMCs and their overexpression is sufficient to promote differentiation of VSMCs *in vitro* (11). In contrast, VSMCs of miR-143- and miR-145-deficient mice display a significant downregulation of SMC-specific differentiation markers (e.g. α-SM actin (SMA)), and do not respond to contractile stimuli (12). In other terms, deficiency of these two miRNAs leads to VSMC phenotypic switching from a contractile to a synthetic phenotype. PDGF-induced dedifferentiation of VSMCs causes indeed a rapid decrease of miR-145, whereas the expression of miR-221 is increased (13). miR-221/222 are regulators for VSMC proliferation and neointimal hyperplasia after vascular injury. Notably, in human ascending aortic aneurysms, the expression of miR-143 and miR-145 is significantly decreased (~0.5-fold) compared to control aortas (12). Deletion of Dicer, one of the two endonuclease processing miRNAs, in VSM results in late embryonic mice lethality due to an internal hemorrhage associated with dilated, thin-walled blood vessels caused by the reduction in cellular proliferation and an impaired contractility due to the loss of α-SMA filaments (14). A similar implication of miRNAs starts to emerge in ESMCs, with some pioneering studies, showing for instance that 45 miRNAs are aberrantly expressed in uterine leiomyomas (15,16).

With the development of immunoanalytical techniques in the 1980s, the expression of specific proteins ("markers") has become the instrument of choice for the phenotypic characterization of a given cell type. SMCs have been classified according to their proteomic profile signature, in particular the expression of cytoskeletal proteins. As of today, the expression of SMC-specific proteins and, in particular, the relative expression of α- and γ-SMAs remains the best criterion to appraise SMC heterogeneity. In the following section we will discuss various aspects of SMC heterogeneity in light of these two isoforms.

Actin Isoforms: Markers of Specific Tissues

Actin is highly conserved across species. Six highly homologous actin isoforms are expressed in higher vertebrates (17), each encoded by a distinct gene and displaying a unique temporal and spatial expression pattern (18). In addition to the two ubiquitous cytoplasmic actins, β-cytoplasmic (β-CYA) and γ-cytoplasmic (γ-CYA), mammalian SM contains two SM-dedicated isoforms differing in their sequence by only three amino acids, α-SMA and γ-SMA, which predominate in vascular and

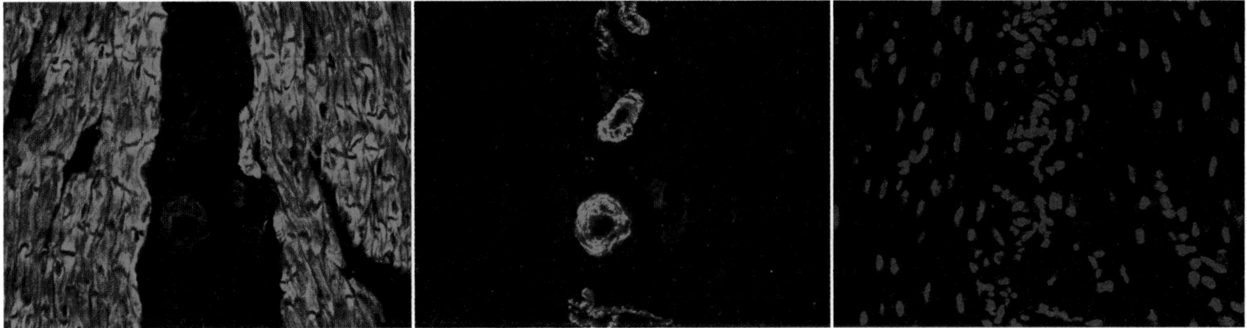

FIGURE 88.2 **Actin isoform expression is a valuable tool for investigating SM heterogeneity.** Nuclear staining with DAPI (blue) and immunofluorescence labeling with γ-SMA (green) and α-SMA (red) of chicken gizzard. In chicken gizzard, γ-SMA expression is confined to ESMCs, whereas α-SMA expression is limited to VSMCs.

enteric SM respectively (Figure 88.2). Isoactin differences lie predominantly in a cluster of acidic residues within their N-terminus (19). In different animals and organs, the relative isoactin composition varies between SMs. In particular, α-SMA and γ-SMAs contents display an inverse relationship, with α-SMA predominating in tonic vascular and airway SMs and γ-SMA predominating in phasic visceral SMs. Heterogeneous isoactin distribution has been amply demonstrated in early reports using either mRNA or protein analysis (18,20–25) (Figure 88.3), and more recently by DNA analysis (26). This heterogeneity seems to represent a general pattern of SM isoactin expression in vertebrates.

The different relative amounts of actin isoforms in SM and SM-like cells and their distinct subcellular compartmentalization and regulation suggest that they have, at least in part, different functions within a multifunctional SM tissue. We will now elaborate how changes in isoactin expression patterns correlate with SM organ development, adaptation to physiological challenges and pathologic conditions.

Actin Isoform Expression Varies During Development

The phenotypic diversity of SMCs may result from different embryonic origin and/or reflect a marked plasticity. In vertebrate embryos VSMCs originate from several distinct structures, such as somites, neural crest, or mesothelium (reviewed in 27). Different vessels, or even different segments of the same vessel, are thus composed of SMC populations that arise from distinct sources of progenitors, each with its own lineage and developmental history. This may be of particular importance since SMCs of different origins show little or no intermixing, and may respond differently to the same stimuli (28). SM differentiation is first apparent in developing vasculature at E9.0. This is followed by differentiation of SM tissues of the foregut and airways by E11.0 and then in the entire gastrointestinal tract by E13.0. Appearance of SM tissues in the urogenital tract starts in the bladder at E13.0 and continues in the ureter and genitals to E15.0 (29). Expression of α-SMA always precedes the expression of γ-SMA and becomes first visible in discrete cells lining the embryonic vasculature and around the dorsal aorta around E.9.5 (25,30). Many studies (31,32), showed that SMCs undergo a "developmental maturation" from a high proliferative, high biosynthetic, and non-contractile to a low proliferative, low biosynthetic, and contractile phenotype. This process implies, among others, an actin isoform switching. For instance, during the embryonic development of chicken gizzard muscle, the relative amount of γ-SMA rises at the expense of the cytoplasmic isoforms (33), and in adult, γ-actin is dominant (about 80%), β-actin is readily detected, and α-actin is almost absent (31).

In human early development, a multistep progressive modulation of cytoskeletal, contractile, and ECM proteins takes place in VSMCs. SM specific proteins such as α-SMA, γ-SMA, SM-MHCs, h-caldesmon, desmin, calponin, meta-vinculin, and SM α-tropomyosin (17,24,34,35) (Figure 88.4) increase at the expense of cytoplasmic actins (36) and nonmuscle MHCs. Although in the adult organism the majority of SMCs exhibits a differentiated phenotype, the specific distribution of actin isoforms remains regulated by factors affecting cell proliferation and adaptation. Thus, an uninterrupted expression of negative and positive regulators such as myogenin is probably essential for inducing and maintaining the SM differentiation program (37). This program can be further modulated by cell–cell and cell–ECM interactions, as well as by local soluble factors.

Changes in Actin Isoform Expression During Physiological Organ Adaptation

A number of different SMs can be structurally adapted according to physiological requirements, such as

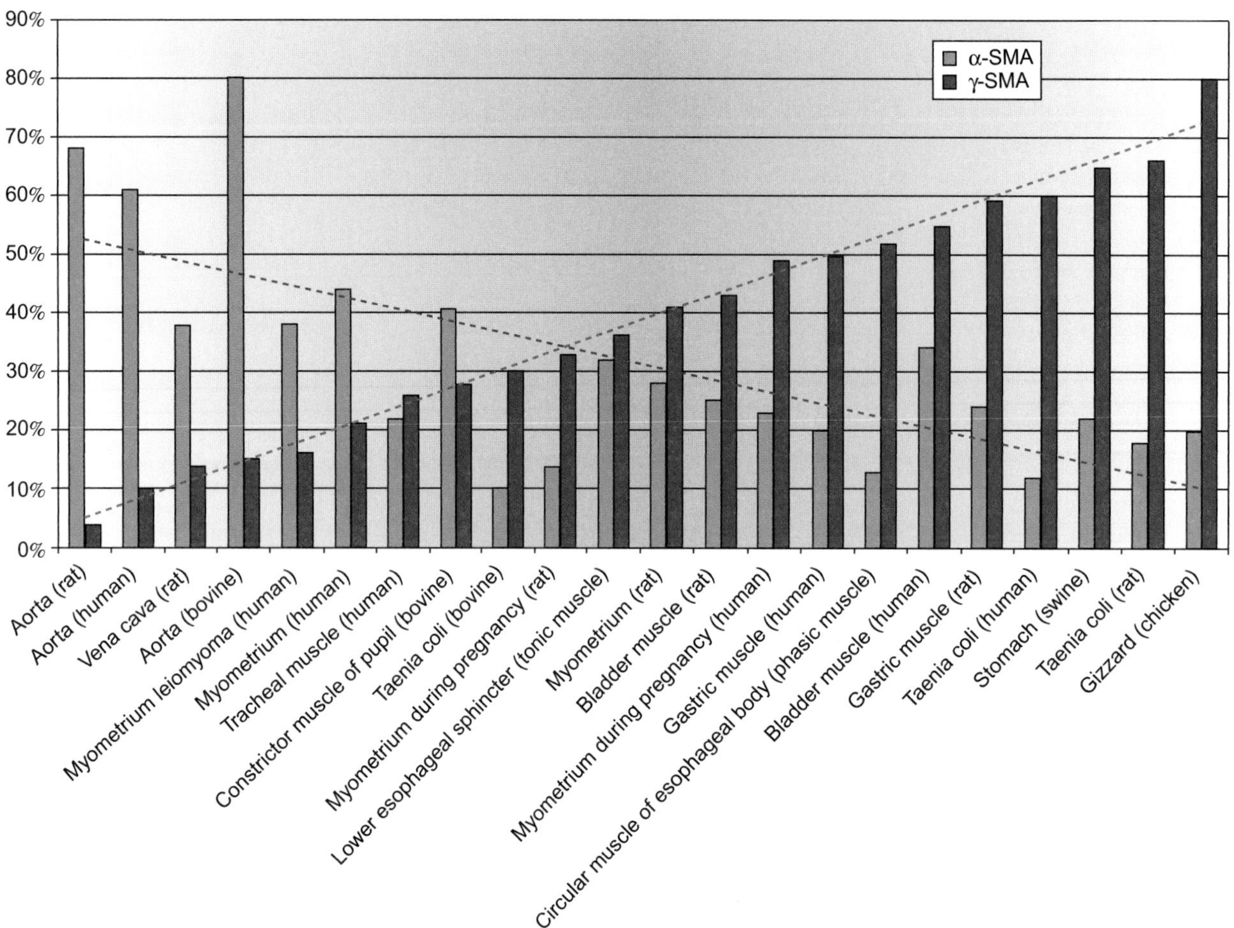

FIGURE 88.3 Summary of α-SMA (lilac) and γ-SMA (red) contents in various organs from several species. In many early reports using either mRNA or protein analysis, the two SM actin isoforms display an inverse relationship in a given SM, with α-SMA predominating in tonic VSMs and ASMs and γ-SMA predominating in phasic ESMs.

increased pressure or volume. Such adaptations can occur in ESM, such as bladder, and uterus or VSM, such as arteries and veins.

Bladder

One can consider the bladder musculature as a single unit. The bladder musculature is arranged in relatively coarse bundles, widely separated, with no sheet formation. Bundles have no definite orientation, except around the bladder neck, where three layers can be distinguished. The contractile properties of bladder SMCs are well suited for both urine storage and release. An experimental denervation of dog bladder indicates that while neural input is required for the rapid SM contraction that accompanies voiding, the intrinsic properties of cellular and extracellular components are responsible for bladder compliance (38).

Mechanical forces were shown to be essential to control bladder function and stimulate hypertrophy of vascular and urinary bladder SMCs. Rat urinary bladder exhibits both hyperplasia and hypertrophy of SMCs in response to urinary flow obstruction (39), and hypertrophy is associated with decreased force (40). SM hypertrophy is associated with alterations in the cellular cytoskeleton such as an overexpression of α-tropomyosin, h1-calponin, β- and γ-CYAs (41), and intermediate filaments (42).

Uterus

The uterus undergoes dramatic physiological adaptations during the course of pregnancy, resulting in major hypertrophy and remodelling of the SM wall (myometrium). Enlargement occurs in two distinct phases: (i) a "proliferative" phase with myocyte hyperplasia coupled with an increase in anti-apoptotic proteins in the first half of gestation, and (ii) a "synthetic" phase with an increase in SMC size in the second half of gestation (43). Postpartum uterus rapidly recovers original shape and size. Whereas activation of the IGF1/PI3K/mTOR signaling

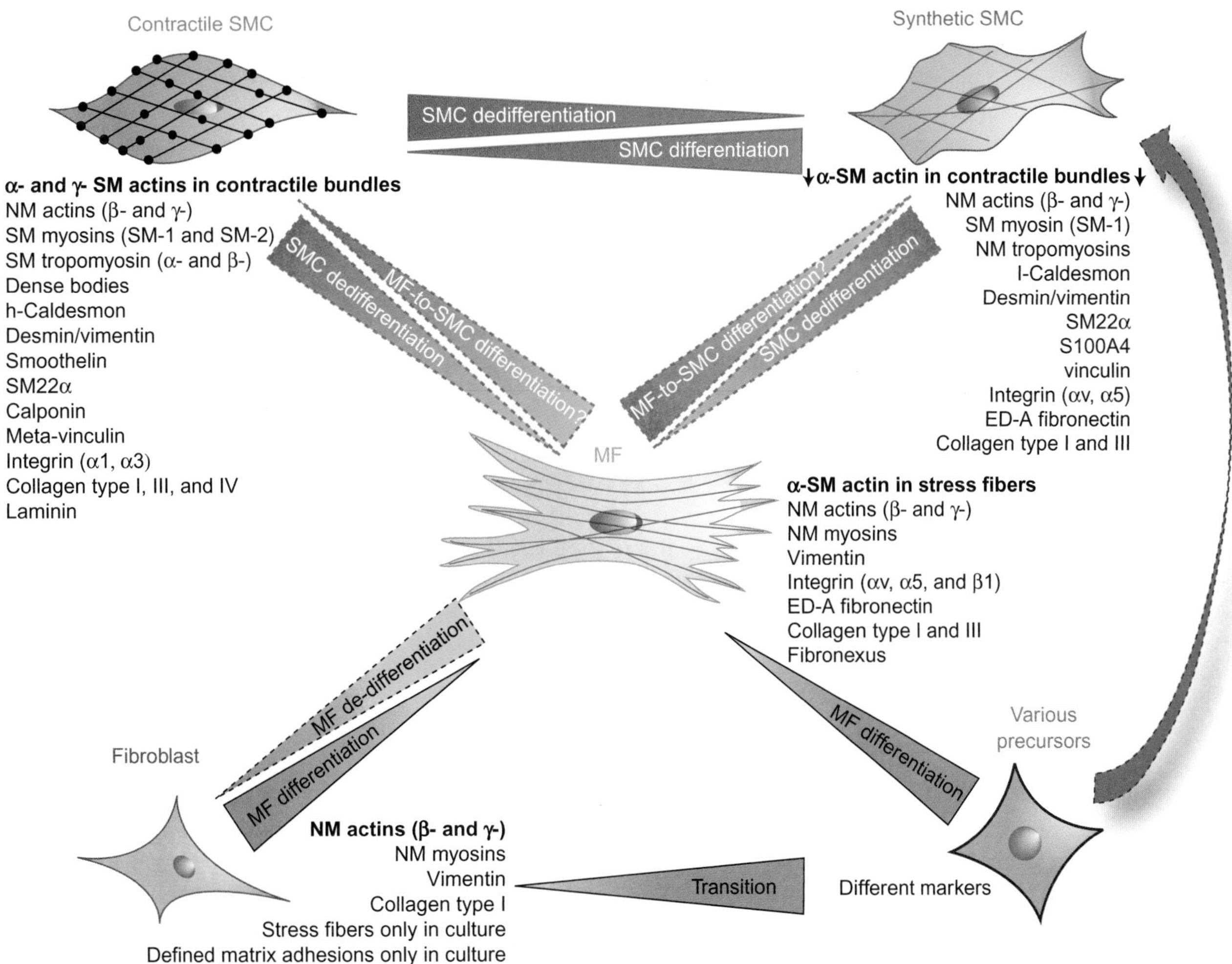

FIGURE 88.4 Differentiation spectra of SMCs and fibroblasts. SMCs display a remarkable level of plasticity that is reflected in changes of specific molecular markers in response to physiological or pathological conditions. Loss of late differentiation markers generates an SMC phenotype that resembles or may even coincide with the myofibroblast. Myofibroblasts generally differentiate from fibroblasts and other precursor cells by acquiring SMC functional and molcular characteristics.

pathway in uterine myocytes by estrogen could be responsible for the induction of myometrial hyperplasia during the proliferative phase of gestation (44), myometrial hypertrophy could be caused either by hormones (45) or by the stretching imposed on the uterine wall by the enlarging fetus (46). Mechanical stretch exerted by the growing fetus might be one of the main signals that cause the uterine myocytes to shift from a proliferative to a synthetic phenotype during pregnancy. This hypothesis is confirmed by the experimental use of unilaterally pregnant rats, in which the mean SMC volume increased three-fold with gestation in the gravid horn, while no change in cellular volume was observed in the non-gravid horn (47). The same two-steps mechanism has been reported for intestinal SM: immediately after induction of intestinal obstruction, SMCs enter a proliferative phase, while hypertrophy occurred later (48).

Although α-SMA and γ-SMA are both highly expressed in resting myometrium, rat and human pregnant myometria are characterized by a considerable increase in the amount of γ-SMA relative to α-SMA (24,49). The rat myometrium does not display significant changes in α-SMA gene expression, whereas γ-SM level increased by up to 32-fold at mRNA level, and 16-fold at the protein level, followed by a rapid return to non-pregnant levels in the postpartum period (50). This result strongly indicates a distinct mechanical function for the two isoforms in the SM.

Vascular Smooth Muscle

While arteries can be mechanically qualified as highly contractile and poorly compliant vessels, veins are the opposite, being poorly contractile but highly compliant.

Since systemic veins are eight-fold more distensible than arteries and have a three-fold greater volume, they are about 24-fold more compliant than their corresponding arteries. In a yet-unpublished study, we show that α-SMA is abundant and homogenous in the whole media of arteries, whereas γ-SMA is restricted to the outer layer (where cells are most stretched). Expression of γ-SMA is similar to that of α-SMA, in both vein adventitia and media (51).

Increased wall pressure initiates SM growth in arterial and venous vessels (52,53), similar to other hollow organs such as uterus, intestine, and urinary bladder (39,54,55). Experimental portal hypertension causes a hypertrophy of portal vein SMCs (56). Although the increase in muscle mass is usually accompanied by an increased force-generating ability, in rat portal vein, hypertrophy is associated with decreased force (57). In a rat model of portal vein hypertrophy induced by partial ligation, the cross-sectional area of wall doubled after 7 days, with a moderate decrease of α-SMA and increases of γ-actin, desmin and vimentin (58).

Actin Isoform Expression Changes in Pathological Conditions

Changes in the general pattern of SM isoactin expression in vertebrates can be set into relation with various human pathologies (see reviews 59,60). The type and the relative amounts of actin isoforms can vary in the same SMC. Recent data obtained from knockout and mutation experiments in mice indicate that isoactin ratio changes are not only indicative but could also be causal for pathologic developments (29,61). Although very similar, the different isoforms cannot perfectly compensate or substitute to one another. Homozygous α-SMA-deficient mice are viable, although they display defects in vascular contractility and basal blood pressure (62); this loss is partially compensated by α-skeletal actin (α-SKA) in defective vessels. No appreciable consequences are seen in the enteric system, probably due to γ-SMA compensation, or in skeletal and cardiac muscles, where α-SMA is abundantly expressed in normal animals, but only in early development. To date, no γ-SMA knockout has been described. Mutations in α-SMA gene lead to thoracic aneurysms and dissections (63).

Changes in the pattern of actin isoform expression occur in SMC in response to tissue challenge or insult and are often associated with changes in the cell differentiation state. Cellular differentiation has been defined as "the process by which multipotential cells ... acquire those cell-specific characteristics that distinguish them from other cell types" (64). However, differentiation of SMCs seems to remain highly dependent on environmental cues even in adult individuals. As a consequence, mature SMCs exposed to particular conditions can easily undergo a dedifferentiation process characterized by the downregulation of muscle-specific isoactins and the reexpression of developmental isoforms. The term "dedifferentiation" has been used to describe the process in which mature SMCs in culture rapidly evolve into modified SMCs, and then even into rapidly-proliferating fibroblast-like cells (65) (Figure 88.4). This phenomenon appears to be not a one-way process, hence Chamley-Campbell et al. have suggested the term "phenotypic modulation" from a "contractile" to a "synthetic" state (66).

Actin isoform switching parallels the modulation from a contractile to proliferative phenotype *in vivo* (67) and *in vitro* (23); namely, α-SMA content decreases/increases upon growth stimulation/arrest. This inverse relationship between the synthesis of α-SMA and cell proliferation suggests a correlation between specific muscle cell differentiation and accumulation of the muscle-type isoform (68). Hence, the pattern of actin isoform expression and, in particular, the expression of α-SMA in VSMCs, is related to the degree of SMC differentiation (69).

SM neoplasms, which range from benign leiomyomas to malignant leiomyosarcomas, differentially express α-SMA and γ-SMA (24). α-SMA expression is observed in all normal and neoplastic SM tissues, whereas γ-SMA expression seems to be limited to normal SM tissues and benign SM neoplasms. The latter has been therefore considered as a specific molecular marker for distinguishing leiomyomas versus leiomyosarcomas using a PCR-based diagnostic test (70).

Smooth Muscle Cell Phenotypic Heterogeneity

Associated with the heterogeneity of SM, it has been suggested that different SMC subpopulations exist, which promote different functions in the normal SM and that become differentially activated in pathophysiological conditions. To date, this concept has been verified for VSMCs as elaborated below.

Different Arterial Populations: Lessons Learned from Intimal Lesions

VSMCs are important players in the onset of the atheromatous plaque and of restenotic lesions (71). Upon migration from the media to the intima they switch phenotype from contractile to synthetic and contribute in various ways to plaque formation, including production of ECM components; they may also represent an efficient barrier to thrombus formation (72). However, it remains controversial whether any medial VSMC can contribute to intimal lesions or whether this task is restricted to a VSMC population of "atheroma prone cells". The latter possibility is based on the seminal observation by Benditt and

TABLE 88.1 Biological and Biochemical Features of Smooth Muscle Cell Subpopulations in Different Species

Species	Rat		Cow			Pig		Human	
Phenotype	Spindle	Epithelioid	Spindle	Rhomboid	Epithelioid	Spindle	Rhomboid	Spindle	Epithelioid
Autonomous growth	No	Yes	No	Yes	Yes	No	No	No	No
Migratory activity	Low	High	ND	ND	ND	Low	High	Low*	High*
Differentitation features									
α-SMA	++	+	++	+/−	+	+++	+	+++	++
Desmin	+/−	−	ND	ND	ND	+	+/−	ND	ND
SMMHC	+	+/−	++	−	−	++	+	+++	++
Smoothelin	ND	ND	ND	ND	ND	+	+/−	ND	ND
SM22α	++	ND	++	+/−	+	ND	ND	ND	ND
CRBP-1**	−	+++	ND	ND	ND	−	−	−	−
S100A4	−	−	ND	ND	ND	−	+++	−	+++

Adapted from Hao et al., 2003 (71), with permission from the American Heart Association.
**Under PDFG-BB stimulation.*
***Cellular retinol binding protein.*

Benditt that atheromatous plaque VSMCs have features of monoclonal or oligoclonal population and has now been confirmed by several other laboratories (73). The most used approach to verify VSMC heterogeneity is culturing distinct VSMC populations from arteries of several species; this has been successful in the rat, dog, cow, pig, and man (for review see 71). Among the isolated subpopulations in each species, at least one exhibits atheroma-prone cells features, such as high proliferative activity, dedifferentiated phenotype, and production of proteolytic enzymes (Table 88.1; for more details, see 71). The atheroma-prone cell subpopulation is called "epithelioid" in the rat and "rhomboid" in the pig. Moreover, rat clonal populations exhibiting epithelioid or spindle features have been isolated and characterized, thus confirming that a single SMC can give rise to a whole population with a given phenotype (71).

Biological and Biochemical Features of Different Vascular Populations

Using a variety of techniques, specific markers have been identified for many subpopulations of atheroma-prone cells and were successfully identified in the experimental thickening of at least rat and pig intima. Interestingly, the identified atheroma-prone cell markers vary in different species: in the adult rat, cellular retinol binding protein-1 (CRBP-1) is practically absent from the normal arterial media, but appears to be rapidly activated upon endothelial injury in a subset of VSMCs located toward the vascular lumen and to be expressed in the vast majority of intimal VSMCs. When the rat endothelium is repaired, CRBP-1 disappears from the intima mainly through VSMC apoptosis. However, when CRBP-1 expression was analyzed in pig and humans *in vitro* and *in vivo*, it did not appear as a marker of the atheroma-prone cell subpopulation. Hence, such markers seem to be species-specific and this complicates the experimental analysis (71). In the pig, atheroma-prone cells or rhomboid cells were isolated by collecting VSMCs from coronary artery explants very early after explantation, thus selecting cells that had migrated rapidly (74). One specific marker for these cells was identified by proteomic analysis to be S100A4, a member of the S100 protein family that had been previously associated with cancer invasion and metastasis (74). S100A4 was localized in coronary intimal VSMCs in a pig model of restenosis, confirming this marker property *in vivo*. Notably, it was also localized in VSMCs of human coronary and aortic plaques as well as in coronary restenotic lesions, but not in the normal media of the same vessels, indicating that, contrary to CRBP-1 in rat, this protein represents also a marker of the human situation. The observation that silencing S100A4 mRNA reduces mitotic activity of cultured porcine rhomboid VSMCs (74) suggests that interfering with the expression of this protein may represent a new promising strategy to interfere with atheroma or restenosis development.

The heterogeneity of VSMCs has been correlated with their multiple embryological origins according to the vessel type, such as mesoderm, neuroectoderm, epicardium (for coronary VSMCs), and more recently endothelium

(71,75). Endothelial cells have been shown to acquire VSMC features, such as the expression of α-SMA *in vitro* (76) and *in vivo* (75); moreover, the origin of intimal VSMCs from circulating bone marrow-derived cells has been suggested in transplant arteriopathy, after experimental endothelial lesion (77) or during hypercholesterolemia (78). Using differential cDNA screening it was shown that the pattern of gene expression in rat neointimal cells following endothelial lesion is similar to that expressed by cells during the neonatal period, suggesting that intimal VSMCs undergo dedifferentiation (79).

Cytokeratins 8 and 18, α-cardiac actin (α-CAA), as well as zonula occludens-2 protein, previously thought to be expressed exclusively in epithelial cells or cardiomyocytes, have been shown to be also present in epithelioid VSMCs in culture, in VSMCs of rat experimental intimal thickening, and human atheromatous plaque (80–82). Although neither the mechanisms nor the consequences of such expression are known, VSMCs appear to be more plastic than previously assumed.

Phenotypic analysis of VSMCs in different types of human coronary plaques revealed that, differently from medial VSMCs, VSMCs of all types of plaque lose their differentiation markers, such as SM myosin and smoothelin, and assume a myofibroblastic profile (Figure 88.4); this change is less developed in stable plaques and maximal in erosions (83). In view of recent findings indicating that the mechanisms regulating force production are different in myofibroblasts compared to classical VSMCs (84); and see following section on the myofibroblast), it is conceivable that the long-lasting tensile activity of the myofibroblast plays a role in facilitating plaque rupture, an event that characterizes erosions.

In conclusion, VSMCs appear to possess a high degree of plasticity. The existence of several VSMC populations has been convincingly described *in vitro* and is more and more evident *in vivo*. Further studies defining the biological activities of these populations will probably be important for the understanding of the pathogenesis of devastating vascular diseases, such as atheromatosis.

SMOOTH MUSCLE-LIKE CELLS

Myofibroblasts

Myofibroblasts share contractile features with SMCs and ECM-protein secreting activities with fibroblasts. Due to their phenotypic and functional similarity to SMC they are discussed in this chapter.

Myofibroblasts Prevalence and Origin

The controlled and transient appearance of myofibroblasts in healing processes is important for restoring the integrity of damaged tissues by forming a collagenous and mechanically resistant scar (84). Scars form in the heart after myocardial infarction, in skin after trauma, and in tendon, bone, and cartilage after fracture or rupture (for a review see 85). Excessive and detrimental myofibroblast activities turn beneficial tissue repair into devastating tissue deformations (86). A paradigm is fibrosis that can affect virtually all organs, such as skin, systemic sclerosis, palmar fascia in Dupuytren's disease, as well as heart, lung, liver, and kidney (reviewed in 85,86). Another condition relating to fibrosis is the stroma reaction to epithelial tumors, during which myofibroblasts generate a chemical and mechanical environment that promotes tumor progression (87). Myofibroblasts are *de novo* recruited from a multitude of different progenitor cells, mostly of mesenchymal origin (for elaborate listings see 85,87).

Myofibroblasts: Smooth Muscle or Fibroblast – or Both?

A defining feature of myofibroblasts is the neo-expression of α-SMA which is instrumental for generating the high contractile forces needed to remodel a collagen-rich ECM. Overexpression of α-SMA enhances the contraction of 3T3 fibroblasts significantly more than the similar overexpression of α-CAA, γ-CYA, and β-CYA isoforms (88). It is presently unclear how α-SMA produces this elevated contractile force without evident changes in the expression of other contractile proteins, such as non-muscle or SM myosins (88). General lack of SM myosin expression also provokes the question how similar myofibroblasts are to SMCs (Figure 88.4). Desmin, being the predominant intermediate filament protein of muscle, can often be used for a distinction although it is expressed by myofibroblasts under few specific conditions (88). Moreover, not all SMCs express desmin but the fibroblastic intermediate filament protein vimentin (22); both cytoskeletal proteins are therefore not unique markers. In normal adult tissue, SMCs express a number of late differentiation markers that are not part of the common myofibroblast repertoire, including SM myosin heavy chain, h-caldesmon, and smoothelin (85). However, in conditions of SM injury and in cell culture, SMCs lose these late differentiation markers and attain a myofibroblastic and collagen synthesizing phenotype (89) (Figure 88.4). Furthermore, gene expression profiling supported by protein biochemistry suggests that some of these late SMC markers can be induced in cultured fibroblasts by treatment with the pro-fibrotic cytokine TGF-β_1 (90). Hence, considering the expression profile of cytoskeletal proteins, differentiated myofibroblasts appears to exist in a continuum between fibroblasts and SMCs and no unique marker exist to date to attribute them to either side of the spectrum (Figure 88.4).

Regulation of Myofibroblast Contraction

Myofibroblast-containing tissues were shown to contract upon stimulation with SMC contraction agonists in seminal studies using tissue strips in organ baths (for a review see 91). This short-term behavior *in situ* is comparable to the reversible contraction of SM *in vivo* but different from the long-term contractile behavior of tissue myofibroblasts that cause irreversible contractures over days, months and years (84). It is generally accepted that the mechanical and architectural state of the ECM will have an effect on cell contractile behavior (84,92,93). Whereas SMCs under normal conditions reside in a defined and established tissue organization, myofibroblasts populate an ECM under constant remodeling. Compared to SM that acts like elastic rubber bands, myofibroblast tissues rather behave visco-elastic, like modeling clay on a longer time scale. Such different mechanical boundary conditions may explain the current controversy on how myofibroblasts regulate contraction – like SMCs or like fibroblasts? In both cell types development of contractile force is regulated at the level of MLC phosphorylation. Phosphorylated MLC enables the myosin head to interact with actin filaments and to generate force. In SMCs, increased levels of cytosolic Ca^{2+} enhance the activity of the key enzyme MLC kinase in a Ca^{2+}/calmodulin-mediated pathway; force development is terminated by "constitutive" action of the MLC phosphatase. In fibroblastic cells, MLC phosphatase is proposed to be the key regulatory enzyme (94). Contraction is achieved by inactivation of the MLC phosphatase through the Rho-(associated) kinase (ROCK or ROK), a downstream target of the small GTPase RhoA (95). Hence, changes in cytosolic Ca^{2+} regulate SMC contraction and RhoA tunes baseline force development (96), whereas RhoA activity regulates fibroblast contraction and sufficiently high cytosolic Ca^{2+} levels ensure continued MLC activity (for a review see 91).

A recent study suggests, that instead of relying on either contraction regulation mechanism, myofibroblasts may use both (97). *In vitro*, cytosolic Ca^{2+} mediated small (~400 nm) and weak (~100 pN) cyclic contractions of dorsal stress fibers, engaged with ECM-coated microbeads. Simultaneously, overall cell contraction of several μN was maintained through RhoA/ROCK-mediated contraction of ventral stress fibers, engaged with an elastic rubber substrate (88,97). Experimental data are not yet available on how myofibroblast contraction is regulated at the subcellular level in tissues but the *in vitro* findings provide the molecular basis for an improved "lock-step" model of ECM remodelling (84,97). Overall cell contraction (Rho/ROCK) generates slack and low-tension in collagen fibrils, which become accessible to weak and short-ranged micro-contractions (Ca^{2+}). When gradually raising stress counteracts local fibril translocation, the new fibril configuration will be stabilized by putative collagen remodeling processes. Together, these processes would result in irreversible retractile rather than reversible contractile phenomena (84,97).

Myoepithelial Cells

Myoepithelial cells (MCs) are modified epithelial cells found in sweat, mammary, salivary, lacrimal, and tracheobronchial glands. These cells present some architectural characteristics of SM cells (caveolae, microfilaments, and dense bodies) and display contractile properties that allow ejection of fluids including sweat and milk. Markers of MCs include α-SMA and cytokeratins 5, 14, and 17. Breast tissue is formed from arborescences of ducts and lobules, which evolve during lifetime and particularly during pregnancy and lactation. The mammary gland, which undergoes a cyclical process of hormone-dependent differentiation and dedifferentiation (98), is composed of an inner layer of epithelial cells, surrounded by a layer of MCs, the contraction of which allow milk ejection. In human resting breast the number of glandular structures is rather limited. α-SMA is strongly and homogeneously expressed in all MCs, whereas γ-SMA is only sparsely present. During lactation, when mammary glands are filled with milk and dilated, γ-SMA is upregulated in MCs. These results have been confirmed in a rat model (51).

Myoid Cells

In testis and ovary, myoid cells surround seminiferous tubules (peritubular cells) and mature follicles (theca cells) respectively. Myoid cells express fibroblast and SMC-specific markers such as CD90/Thy-1, CD34, vimentin, desmin, calponin, MHC, and α-SMA (99–101), as well as receptors for endothelin and angiotensin (102,103). In particular, α-SMA is a useful marker for myoid cells *in vivo* and *in vitro* (89,104). Whereas the size of seminiferous tubules remains constant, follicles enlarge during folliculogenesis. Interestingly, myoid cells in testis have only a contractile activity and express only α-SMA, whereas in ovary they are involved in both contraction and dilation and express both α-SMA and γ-SMA (51).

Peritubular myoid cells are not only structural cells bearing the potential to contract (105), but can also actively secrete various paracrine mediators such as growth factors (e.g. IGF-I, bFGF, NGF), MCP-1 and cytokines (IL-6) (106,107). Peritubular myoid cells also synthesize and secrete different ECM components such as fibronectin, laminin, collagen I, IV, and XVIII, proteoglycans, and entactin (108–110). Mast cells and macrophages secrete histamine, tryptase, and TNF-α, which increase, on one side the expression and the secretion of ECM components and molecules by myoid cells, and decrease on the other side the expression of contractile markers by the same cells. This process may result in a local fibrosis, which is the main cause of male infertility.

Pericryptic myoid cells have also been described within the lamina propria surrounding the epithelial layer of crypts in the stomach, intestine, and gallbladder, where they form a syncytium closely connected with the muscularis mucosae and narrow blood vessel pericytes (111). Although they display the typical α-SMA marker, they can usually be distinguished from SMCs by the absence of staining for desmin. They can generate local contractions and they may have, like typical myofibroblasts, a significant role in gastrointestinal protection and wound healing.

CONCLUSION

Over the recent decades, a large number of studies have shown that many cell types are more plastic than previously assumed and that such plasticity is at least in part due to the presence of cells within a given population that are prone to undergo phenotypic modulation. SMC populations exhibit heterogeneity and plasticity features to a high degree both *in vivo* and *in vitro* (Figure 88.4). These features have been particularly studied in VSMCs where they appear crucial for the onset and evolution of adaptative and/or pathological phenomena such as atheromatous plaque formation and restenosis. In the atheromatous plaque, VSMC modulation can evolve into the myofibroblastic phenotype (83). The most reliable tool to investigate the differentiation-dedifferentiation status of SMCs remains the expression level of specific protein content (e.g. actin isoforms, SM-MHCs, S100A4), as identified by proper antibodies.

By the use of isoform specific antibodies, it has been possible to identify the respective distributions of the two SM-actin isoforms: α-SMA is expressed in all SM and SM-like cells, whereas γ-SMA is mainly enteric. α-SMA and γ-SMA may cooperate in a multifunctional SM tissue. Whereas α-SMA is responsible for SM contractile properties, γ-SMA could be responsible for sustaining deformation under strong mechanical constraints. According to this hypothesis, actin isoforms could be better defined as being function-specific instead of tissue-specific. In other words, the two isoforms would have different functions in the same tissue instead of having the same function in different tissues. Investigating SM heterogeneity has been, and still remains, of major importance for understanding the cell mechanisms that are involved in normal and pathological conditions.

ACKNOWLEDGMENTS

The research in the authors' laboratories was supported by the Swiss National Science Foundation (grant no. 310030_125320 to C.C., R.A.), the Heart and Stroke Foundation Ontario (grant no. NA7086 to B.H.), and the Canadian Institutes of Health Research (grant no. 210820 to B.H.).

REFERENCES

1. Bozler E. Smooth muscle physiology, past and future. *Philos Trans R Soc Lond B Biol Sci* 1973;**265**:3–6.
2. Rhodin JA. Fine structure of vascular walls in mammals with special reference to smooth muscle component. *Physiol Rev Suppl* 1962;**5**:48–87.
3. Prosser CL, Burnstock G, Kahn J. Conduction in smooth muscle: comparative structural properties. *Am J Physiol* 1960;**199**:545–52.
4. Harnett KM, Cao W, Biancani P. Signal-transduction pathways that regulate smooth muscle function I. Signal transduction in phasic (esophageal) and tonic (gastroesophageal sphincter) smooth muscles. *Am J Physiol Gastrointest Liver Physiol* 2005;**288**:G407–16.
5. Szymanski PT, Chacko TK, Rovner AS, Goyal RK. Differences in contractile protein content and isoforms in phasic and tonic smooth muscles. *Am J Physiol Cell Physiol* 1998;**275**:C684–92.
6. Sparrow MP, Mohammad MA, Arner A, Hellstrand P, Ruegg JC. Myosin composition and functional properties of smooth muscle from the uterus of pregnant and non-pregnant rats. *Pflugers Arch* 1988;**412**:624–33.
7. Kelley CA, Takahashi M, Yu JH, Adelstein RS. An insert of seven amino acids confers functional differences between smooth muscle myosins from the intestines and vasculature. *J Biol Chem* 1993;**268**:12848–54.
8. Morano I. Tuning smooth muscle contraction by molecular motors. *J Mol Med* 2003;**81**:481–7.
9. Helper DJ, Lash JA, Hathaway DR. Distribution of isoelectric variants of the 17,000-dalton myosin light chain in mammalian smooth muscle. *J Biol Chem* 1988;**263**:15748–53.
10. Chi JT, Rodriguez EH, Wang Z, Nuyten DS, Mukherjee S, van de Rijn M, et al. Gene expression programs of human smooth muscle cells: tissue-specific differentiation and prognostic significance in breast cancers. *PLoS Genet* 2007;**3**:1770–84.
11. Cordes KR, Sheehy NT, White MP, Berry EC, Morton SU, Muth AN, et al. miR-145 and miR-143 regulate smooth muscle cell fate and plasticity. *Nature* 2009;**460**:705–10.
12. Elia L, Quintavalle M, Zhang J, Contu R, Cossu L, Latronico MV, et al. The knockout of miR-143 and -145 alters smooth muscle cell maintenance and vascular homeostasis in mice: correlates with human disease. *Cell Death Differ* 2009;**16**:1590–8.
13. Cheng Y, Liu X, Yang J, Lin Y, Xu DZ, Lu Q, et al. MicroRNA-145, a novel smooth muscle cell phenotypic marker and modulator, controls vascular neointimal lesion formation. *Circ Res* 2009;**105**:158–66.
14. Albinsson S, Suarez Y, Skoura A, Offermanns S, Miano JM, Sessa WC. MicroRNAs are necessary for vascular smooth muscle growth, differentiation, and function. *Arterioscler Thromb Vasc Biol* 2010;**30**:1118–26.

15. Marsh EE, Lin Z, Yin P, Milad M, Chakravarti D, Bulun SE. Differential expression of microRNA species in human uterine leiomyoma versus normal myometrium. *Fertil Steril* 2008;**89**:1771–6.
16. Zavadil J, Ye H, Liu Z, Wu J, Lee P, Hernando E, et al. Profiling and functional analyses of microRNAs and their target gene products in human uterine leiomyomas. *PLoS One* 2010;**5**:e12362.
17. Vandekerckhove J, Weber K. At least six different actins are expressed in a higher mammal: an analysis based on the amino acid sequence of the amino-terminal tryptic peptide. *J Mol Biol* 1978;**126**:783–802.
18. McHugh KM, Crawford K, Lessard JL. A comprehensive analysis of the developmental and tissue-specific expression of the isoactin multigene family in the rat. *Dev Biol* 1991;**148**:442–58.
19. Vandekerckhove J, Weber K. Comparison of the amino acid sequences of three tissue-specific cytoplasmic actins with rabbit skeletal muscle actin [proceedings]. *Arch Int Physiol Biochim* 1978;**86**:891–2.
20. Vandekerckhove J, Weber K. The complete amino acid sequence of actins from bovine aorta, bovine heart, bovine fast skeletal muscle, and rabbit slow skeletal muscle. A protein-chemical analysis of muscle actin differentiation. *Differentiation* 1979;**14**:123–33.
21. Vandekerckhove J, Weber K. Actin typing on total cellular extracts: a highly sensitive protein-chemical procedure able to distinguish different actins. *Eur J Biochem* 1981;**113**:595–603.
22. Gabbiani G, Schmid E, Winter S, Chaponnier C, de Ckhastonay C, Vandekerckhove J, et al. Vascular smooth muscle cells differ from other smooth muscle cells: predominance of vimentin filaments and a specific alpha-type actin. *Proc Natl Acad Sci USA* 1981;**78**:298–302.
23. Fatigati V, Murphy RA. Actin and tropomyosin variants in smooth muscles. Dependence on tissue type. *J Biol Chem* 1984;**259**:14383–8.
24. Skalli O, Vandekerckhove J, Gabbiani G. Actin-isoform pattern as a marker of normal or pathological smooth-muscle and fibroblastic tissues. *Differentiation* 1987;**33**:232–8.
25. Sawtell NM, Lessard JL. Cellular distribution of smooth muscle actins during mammalian embryogenesis: expression of the alpha-vascular but not the gamma-enteric isoform in differentiating striated myocytes. *J Cell Biol* 1989;**109**:2929–37.
26. Kilpinen S, Autio R, Ojala K, Iljin K, Bucher E, Sara H, et al. Systematic bioinformatic analysis of expression levels of 17,330 human genes across 9,783 samples from 175 types of healthy and pathological tissues. *Genome Biol* 2008;**9**:R139.
27. Majesky MW. Developmental basis of vascular smooth muscle diversity. *Arterioscler Thromb Vasc Biol* 2007;**27**:1248–58.
28. Topouzis S, Majesky MW. Smooth muscle lineage diversity in the chick embryo. Two types of aortic smooth muscle cell differ in growth and receptor-mediated transcriptional responses to transforming growth factor-beta. *Dev Biol* 1996;**178**:430–45.
29. Tondeleir D, Vandamme D, Vandekerckhove J, Ampe C, Lambrechts A. Actin isoform expression patterns during mammalian development and in pathology: insights from mouse models. *Cell Motil Cytoskeleton* 2009;**66**:798–815.
30. McHugh KM. Molecular analysis of smooth muscle development in the mouse. *Dev Dyn* 1995;**204**:278–90.
31. Hirai S, Hirabayashi T. Developmental change of protein constituents in chicken gizzards. *Dev Biol* 1983;**97**:483–93.
32. Kocher O, Skalli O, Cerutti D, Gabbiani F, Gabbiani G. Cytoskeletal features of rat aortic cells during development. An electron microscopic, immunohistochemical, and biochemical study. *Circ Res* 1985;**56**:829–38.
33. Saborio JL, Segura M, Flores M, Garcia R, Palmer E. Differential expression of gizzard actin genes during chick embryogenesis. *J Biol Chem* 1979;**254**:11119–25.
34. Owens GK, Thompson MM. Developmental changes in isoactin expression in rat aortic smooth muscle cells in vivo. Relationship between growth and cytodifferentiation. *J Biol Chem* 1986;**261**:13373–80.
35. Glukhova MA, Kabakov AE, Frid MG, Ornatsky OI, Belkin AM, Mukhin DN, et al. Modulation of human aorta smooth muscle cell phenotype: a study of muscle-specific variants of vinculin, caldesmon, and actin expression. *Proc Natl Acad Sci USA* 1988;**85**:9542–6.
36. Franke WW, Schmid E, Vandekerckhove J, Weber K. Permanently proliferating rat vascular smooth muscle cell with maintained expression of smooth muscle characteristics, including actin of the vascular smooth muscle type. *J Cell Biol* 1980;**87**:594–600.
37. Blau HM, Baltimore D. Differentiation requires continuous regulation. *J Cell Biol* 1991;**112**:781–3.
38. Langley LL, Whiteside JA. Mechanism of accommodation and tone of urinary bladder. *J Neurophysiol* 1951;**14**:147–52.
39. Uvelius B, Persson L, Mattiasson A. Smooth muscle cell hypertrophy and hyperplasia in the rat detrusor after short-time infravesical outflow obstruction. *J Urol* 1984;**131**:173–6.
40. Arner A, Malmqvist U, Uvelius B. Metabolism and force in hypertrophic smooth muscle from rat urinary bladder. *Am J Physiol Cell Physiol* 1990;**258**:C923–32.
41. Mannikarottu AS, Changolkar AK, Disanto ME, Wein AJ, Chacko S. Over expression of smooth muscle thin filament associated proteins in the bladder wall of diabetics. *J Urol* 2005;**174**:360–4.
42. Berner PF, Somlyo AV, Somlyo AP. Hypertrophy-induced increase of intermediate filaments in vascular smooth muscle. *J Cell Biol* 1981;**88**:96–100.
43. Shynlova O, Oldenhof A, Dorogin A, Xu Q, Mu J, Nashman N, et al. Myometrial apoptosis: activation of the caspase cascade in the pregnant rat myometrium at midgestation. *Biol Reprod* 2006;**74**:839–49.
44. Jaffer S, Shynlova O, Lye S. Mammalian target of rapamycin is activated in association with myometrial proliferation during pregnancy. *Endocrinology* 2009;**150**:4672–80.
45. Martin L, Finn CA, Trinder G. Hypertrophy and hyperplasia in the mouse uterus after oestrogen treatment: an autoradiographic study. *J Endocrinol* 1973;**56**:133–44.
46. Douglas AJ, Clarke EW, Goldspink DF. Influence of mechanical stretch on growth and protein turnover of rat uterus. *Am J Physiol Endocrinol Metab* 1988;**254**:E543–8.
47. Goldspink DF, Douglas AJ. Protein turnover in gravid and non-gravid horns of uterus in pregnant rats. *Am J Physiol Endocrinol Metab* 1988;**254**:E549–54.
48. Chen J, Chen H, Sanders KM, Perrino BA. Regulation of SRF/CArG-dependent gene transcription during chronic partial obstruction of murine small intestine. *Neurogastroenterol Motil* 2008;**20**:829–42.

49. Cavaille F, Leger JJ. Characterization and comparison of the contractile proteins from human gravid and non-gravid myometrium. *Gynecol Obstet Invest* 1983;**16**:341–53.
50. Shynlova O, Tsui P, Dorogin A, Chow M, Lye SJ. Expression and localization of alpha-smooth muscle and gamma-actins in the pregnant rat myometrium. *Biol Reprod* 2005;**73**:773–80.
51. Arnoldi R, Chaponnier C. Smooth muscle actin isoforms: a tug of war between contraction and compliance. *Eur J Cell Biol* 2012; submitted.
52. Bucher B, Travo P, Stoclet JC. Smooth muscle cell hypertrophy and hyperplasia in the thoracic aorta of spontaneously hypertensive rats. *Cell Biol Int Rep* 1984;**8**:567–77.
53. Johansson B. Structural and functional changes in rat portal veins after experimental portal hypertension. *Acta Physiol Scand* 1976;**98**:381–3.
54. Afting EG, Elce JS. DNA in the rat uterus myometrium during pregnancy and postpartum involution. Measurement of DNA in small pieces of mammalian tissue. *Anal Biochem* 1978;**86**:90–9.
55. Gabella G. Hypertrophy of intestinal smooth muscle. *Cell Tissue Res* 1975;**163**:199–214.
56. Johansson B. Different types of smooth muscle hypertrophy. *Hypertension* 1984;**6**:III64–8.
57. Uvelius B, Arner A, Johansson B. Structural and mechanical alterations in hypertrophic venous smooth muscle. *Acta Physiol Scand* 1981;**112**:463–71.
58. Malmqvist U, Arner A. Isoform distribution and tissue contents of contractile and cytoskeletal proteins in hypertrophied smooth muscle from rat portal vein. *Circ Res* 1990;**66**:832–45.
59. Chaponnier C, Gabbiani G. Pathological situations characterized by altered actin isoform expression. *J Pathol* 2004;**204**:386–95.
60. Lambrechts A, Van Troys M, Ampe C. The actin cytoskeleton in normal and pathological cell motility. *Int J Biochem Cell Biol* 2004;**36**:1890–909.
61. Perrin BJ, Ervasti JM. The actin gene family: function follows isoform. *Cytoskeleton (Hoboken)* 2010;**67**:630–4.
62. Schildmeyer LA, Braun R, Taffet G, Debiasi M, Burns AE, Bradley A, et al. Impaired vascular contractility and blood pressure homeostasis in the smooth muscle alpha-actin null mouse. *FASEB J* 2000;**14**:2213–20.
63. Guo DC, Pannu H, Tran-Fadulu V, Papke CL, Yu RK, Avidan N, et al. Mutations in smooth muscle alpha-actin (ACTA2) lead to thoracic aortic aneurysms and dissections. *Nat Genet* 2007;**39**:1488–93.
64. Owens GK, Kumar MS, Wamhoff BR. Molecular regulation of vascular smooth muscle cell differentiation in development and disease. *Physiol Rev* 2004;**84**:767–801.
65. Jarmolych J, Daoud AS, Landau J, Fritz KE, McElvene E. Aortic media explants. Cell proliferation and production of mucopolysaccharides, collagen, and elastic tissue. *Exp Mol Pathol* 1968;**9**:171–88.
66. Chamley-Campbell J, Campbell GR, Ross R. The smooth muscle cell in culture. *Physiol Rev* 1979;**59**:1–61.
67. Clowes AW, Clowes MM, Kocher O, Ropraz P, Chaponnier C, Gabbiani G. Arterial smooth muscle cells in vivo: relationship between actin isoform expression and mitogenesis and their modulation by heparin. *J Cell Biol* 1988;**107**:1939–45.
68. Owens GK, Loeb A, Gordon D, Thompson MM. Expression of smooth muscle-specific alpha-isoactin in cultured vascular smooth muscle cells: relationship between growth and cytodifferentiation. *J Cell Biol* 1986;**102**:343–52.
69. Schurch W, Skalli O, Seemayer TA, Gabbiani G. Intermediate filament proteins and actin isoforms as markers for soft tissue tumor differentiation and origin. I. Smooth muscle tumors. *Am J Pathol* 1987;**128**:91–103.
70. Trzyna W, McHugh M, McCue P, McHugh KM. Molecular determination of the malignant potential of smooth muscle neoplasms. *Cancer* 1997;**80**:211–7.
71. Hao H, Gabbiani G, Bochaton-Piallat ML. Arterial smooth muscle cell heterogeneity: implications for atherosclerosis and restenosis development. *Arterioscler Thromb Vasc Biol* 2003;**23**:1510–20.
72. Schwartz SM, deBlois D, O'Brien ER. The intima. Soil for atherosclerosis and restenosis. *Circ Res* 1995;**77**:445–65.
73. Murry CE, Gipaya CT, Bartosek T, Benditt EP, Schwartz SM. Monoclonality of smooth muscle cells in human atherosclerosis. *Am J Pathol* 1997;**151**:697–705.
74. Brisset AC, Hao H, Camenzind E, Bacchetta M, Geinoz A, Sanchez JC, et al. Intimal smooth muscle cells of porcine and human coronary artery express S100A4, a marker of the rhomboid phenotype in vitro. *Circ Res* 2007;**100**:1055–62.
75. Gittenberger-de Groot AC, DeRuiter MC, Bergwerff M, Poelmann RE. Smooth muscle cell origin and its relation to heterogeneity in development and disease. *Arterioscler Thromb Vasc Biol* 1999;**19**:1589–94.
76. Frid MG, Kale VA, Stenmark KR. Mature vascular endothelium can give rise to smooth muscle cells via endothelial-mesenchymal transdifferentiation: in vitro analysis. *Circ Res* 2002;**90**:1189–96.
77. Religa P, Bojakowski K, Maksymowicz M, Bojakowska M, Sirsjo A, Gaciong Z, et al. Smooth-muscle progenitor cells of bone marrow origin contribute to the development of neointimal thickenings in rat aortic allografts and injured rat carotid arteries. *Transplantation* 2002;**74**:1310–5.
78. Sata M, Saiura A, Kunisato A, Tojo A, Okada S, Tokuhisa T, et al. Hematopoietic stem cells differentiate into vascular cells that participate in the pathogenesis of atherosclerosis. *Nat Med* 2002;**8**:403–9.
79. Shanahan CM, Weissberg PL. Smooth muscle cell heterogeneity: patterns of gene expression in vascular smooth muscle cells in vitro and in vivo. *Arterioscler Thromb Vasc Biol* 1998;**18**:333–8.
80. Adams LD, Lemire JM, Schwartz SM. A systematic analysis of 40 random genes in cultured vascular smooth muscle subtypes reveals a heterogeneity of gene expression and identifies the tight junction gene zonula occludens 2 as a marker of epithelioid "pup" smooth muscle cells and a participant in carotid neointimal formation. *Arterioscler Thromb Vasc Biol* 1999;**19**:2600–8.
81. Jahn L, Kreuzer J, von Hodenberg E, Kubler W, Franke WW, Allenberg J, et al. Cytokeratins 8 and 18 in smooth muscle cells. Detection in human coronary artery, peripheral vascular, and vein graft disease and in transplantation-associated arteriosclerosis. *Arterioscler Thromb* 1993;**13**:1631–9.
82. Bea F, Bar H, Watson L, Blessing E, Kubler W, Kreuzer J, et al. Cardiac alpha-actin in smooth muscle cells: detection in umbilical cord vessels and in atherosclerotic lesions. *Basic Res Cardiol* 2000;**95**:106–13.
83. Hao H, Gabbiani G, Camenzind E, Bacchetta M, Virmani R, Bochaton-Piallat ML. Phenotypic modulation of intima and media

smooth muscle cells in fatal cases of coronary artery lesion. *Arterioscler Thromb Vasc Biol* 2006;**26**:326–32.

84. Tomasek JJ, Gabbiani G, Hinz B, Chaponnier C, Brown RA. Myofibroblasts and mechano-regulation of connective tissue remodelling. *Nat Rev Mol Cell Biol* 2002;**3**:349–63.
85. Hinz B, Phan SH, Thannickal VJ, Galli A, Bochaton-Piallat ML, Gabbiani G. The myofibroblast: one function, multiple origins. *Am J Pathol* 2007;**170**:1807–16.
86. Wynn TA. Common and unique mechanisms regulate fibrosis in various fibroproliferative diseases. *J Clin Invest* 2007;**117**: 524–9.
87. Hinz B, Desmouliere A, Darby IA, Gabbiani G. The role of the myofibroblast in fibrosis and cancer progression. In: Mueller MM, Fusenig N, editors. *Tumor-associated fibroblasts and their matrix*. New York: Springer;2011.
88. Hinz B, Celetta G, Tomasek JJ, Gabbiani G, Chaponnier C. Alpha-smooth muscle actin expression upregulates fibroblast contractile activity. *Mol Biol Cell* 2001;**12**:2730–41.
89. Benzonana G, Skalli O, Gabbiani G. Correlation between the distribution of smooth muscle or non muscle myosins and alpha-smooth muscle actin in normal and pathological soft tissues. *Cell Motil Cytoskeleton* 1988;**11**:260–74.
90. Chambers RC, Leoni P, Kaminski N, Laurent GJ, Heller RA. Global expression profiling of fibroblast responses to transforming growth factor-beta1 reveals the induction of inhibitor of differentiation-1 and provides evidence of smooth muscle cell phenotypic switching. *Am J Pathol* 2003;**162**: 533–46.
91. Follonier Castella L, Gabbiani G, McCulloch CA, Hinz B. Regulation of myofibroblast activities: calcium pulls some strings behind the scene. *Exp Cell Res* 2010;**316**:2390–401.
92. Grinnell F, Petroll WM. Cell motility and mechanics in three-dimensional collagen matrices. *Annu Rev Cell Dev Biol* 2010;**26**:335–61.
93. Hinz B. The myofibroblast: paradigm for a mechanically active cell. *J Biomech* 2010;**43**:146–55.
94. Katoh K, Kano Y, Amano M, Onishi H, Kaibuchi K, Fujiwara K. Rho-kinase-mediated contraction of isolated stress fibers. *J Cell Biol* 2001;**153**:569–84.
95. Kimura K, Ito M, Amano M, Chihara K, Fukata Y, Nakafuku M, et al. Regulation of myosin phosphatase by Rho and Rho-associated kinase (Rho-kinase). *Science* 273:245–248.
96. Somlyo AP, Somlyo AV. Ca^{2+} sensitivity of smooth muscle and nonmuscle myosin II: modulated by G proteins, kinases, and myosin phosphatase. *Physiol Rev* 2003;**83**:1325–58.
97. Castella LF, Buscemi L, Godbout C, Meister JJ, Hinz B. A new lock-step mechanism of matrix remodelling based on subcellular contractile events. *J Cell Sci* 2010;**123**:1751–60.
98. Neville MC, McFadden TB, Forsyth I. Hormonal regulation of mammary differentiation and milk secretion. *J Mammary Gland Biol Neoplasia* 2002;**7**:49–66.
99. Albrecht M, Ramsch R, Kohn FM, Schwarzer JU, Mayerhofer A. Isolation and cultivation of human testicular peritubular cells: a new model for the investigation of fibrotic processes in the human testis and male infertility. *J Clin Endocrinol Metab* 2006;**91**:1956–60.
100. Kuroda N, Nakayama H, Miyazaki E, Hayashi Y, Toi M, Hiroi M, et al. Distribution and role of CD34-positive stromal cells and myofibroblasts in human normal testicular stroma. *Histol Histopathol* 2004;**19**:743–51.
101. Virtanen I, Kallajoki M, Narvanen O, Paranko J, Thornell LE, Miettinen M, et al. Peritubular myoid cells of human and rat testis are smooth muscle cells that contain desmin-type intermediate filaments. *Anat Rec* 1986;**215**:10–20.
102. Filippini A, Tripiciano A, Palombi F, Teti A, Paniccia R, Stefanini M, et al. Rat testicular myoid cells respond to endothelin: characterization of binding and signal transduction pathway. *Endocrinology* 1993;**133**:1789–96.
103. Rossi F, Ferraresi A, Romagni P, Silvestroni L, Santiemma V. Angiotensin II stimulates contraction and growth of testicular peritubular myoid cells in vitro. *Endocrinology* 2002;**143**:3096–104.
104. Tung PS, Fritz IB. Characterization of rat testicular peritubular myoid cells in culture: alpha-smooth muscle isoactin is a specific differentiation marker. *Biol Reprod* 1990;**42**:351–65.
105. Romano F, Tripiciano A, Muciaccia B, De Cesaris P, Ziparo E, Palombi F, et al. The contractile phenotype of peritubular smooth muscle cells is locally controlled: possible implications in male fertility. *Contraception* 2005;**72**:294–7.
106. Schell C, Albrecht M, Mayer C, Schwarzer JU, Frungieri MB, Mayerhofer A. Exploring human testicular peritubular cells: identification of secretory products and regulation by tumor necrosis factor-alpha. *Endocrinology* 2008;**149**:1678–86.
107. Albrecht M. Insights into the nature of human testicular peritubular cells. *Ann Anat* 2009;**191**:532–40.
108. Skinner MK, Tung PS, Fritz IB. Cooperativity between Sertoli cells and testicular peritubular cells in the production and deposition of extracellular matrix components. *J Cell Biol* 1985;**100**:1941–7.
109. Maekawa M, Kamimura K, Nagano T. Peritubular myoid cells in the testis: their structure and function. *Arch Histol Cytol* 1996;**59**:1–13.
110. Weber MA, Groos S, Aumuller G, Konrad L. Post-natal development of the rat testis: steroid hormone receptor distribution and extracellular matrix deposition. *Andrologia* 2002;**34**:41–54.
111. Powell DW, Mifflin RC, Valentich JD, Crowe SE, Saada JI, West AB. Myofibroblasts. II. Intestinal subepithelial myofibroblasts. *Am J Physiol Cell Physiol* 1999;**277**:C183–201.

Chapter 89

Microcirculation

William F. Jackson
Pharmacology and Toxicology, Michigan State University, East Lansing, MI

INTRODUCTION

The microcirculation is the business end of the cardiovascular system. It is in this branching network of microvessels that transport and exchange of heat, respiratory gases, nutrients, waste products, water and hormones occurs between blood and the body's tissues (1,2). Blood flowing in the microvasculature also carries leukocytes and lymphocytes to their tissue targets, and it is here that trafficking of these inflammatory and immune cells takes place between blood and tissue (3,4). Microvessels also importantly contribute to peripheral vascular resistance (5), vascular capacitance (6), and blood pressure regulation (5), and they are the effectors responsible for the control of blood flow to, and within the body's tissues and organs (1,5,7,). Microvascular smooth muscle cells (1,5,7), or related pericytes (8–12), participate directly or indirectly in all of the listed functions of the microcirculation by controlling vessel diameter and hence local microvascular hemodynamic resistance, pressure, and luminal fluid flow.

ARCHITECTURE OF THE MICROCIRCULATION

The microcirculation begins when a feed artery entering a tissue or organ branches into first-order arterioles. For the purpose of this chapter, what distinguishes a first-order arteriole from a feed artery is its proximity to parenchymal cells to which it supplies blood, and the number of layers of smooth muscle cells in the wall of the vessels: arterioles are embedded in the tissue that they supply, and have one or two layers of smooth muscle cells (see below). Second-order arterioles divergently branch from first-order vessels, and this process continues for 3–5 generations (dependent on the tissue), culminating in terminal arterioles from which capillaries arise (13) (Figure 89.1A). Second-order arterioles through terminal arterioles have a single layer of smooth muscle cells (14).

Each terminal arteriole gives rise to 1–20 capillaries, which are endothelial cell tubes, 5–7 μm in diameter, 100–1000 μm long, surrounded by a basement membrane and lacking a smooth muscle cell layer (14,15) (Figure 89.1A). In skeletal muscle, terminal arterioles and the 10–20 capillaries they supply form a microvascular unit, with changes in terminal arteriolar tone coordinately effecting changes in capillary blood flow within a unit (16). A similar unit structure is observed in other tissues although the number of capillaries comprising the unit may vary. Although lacking smooth muscle cells, capillaries may be invested with pericytes (14,15) that can contract and modulate capillary vascular resistance (see below for more on this issue) (9–12,17).

Two or more capillaries converge to form post-capillary venules, which, in turn, join to form collecting venules. Post-capillary venules, in general, do not have a smooth muscle cell layer, but are covered with pericytes (8,14,15) (Figure 89.1B). Higher-order venules may have 1–2 layers of smooth muscle (14,18). In parallel with the blood microcirculation, there also is the lymphatic microcirculation, which will not be covered in this chapter. The reader is directed to a recent review of this subject for more information (19).

ARTERIOLES AND ARTERIOLAR SMOOTH MUSCLE

Arterioles are a major source of hemodynamic resistance along the cardiovascular system (1,5,20). In skeletal muscle, for example, at least 50% of the vascular resistance of the tissue resides in the arteriolar network (21). Therefore, these microvessels contribute to total peripheral resistance, and hence, the control and regulation of blood pressure (1,5,20). The hemodynamic resistance offered by arterioles determines the blood flow rate to the body's tissues providing convective transfer of oxygen, nutrients, hormones, blood cells, etc. around the body for exchange between blood and extravascular cells (1,2,7). Terminal arterioles, to a large extent, determine the perfusion rate of downstream capillaries impacting not only convective transfer of blood and its components but also the effective surface area available for diffusional exchange in the capillary bed (1,13,16). Arteriolar

Muscle. DOI: http://dx.doi.org/10.1016/B978-0-12-381510-1.00089-2

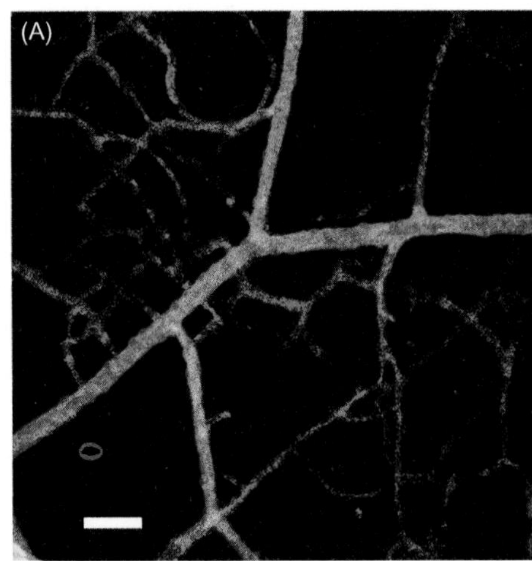

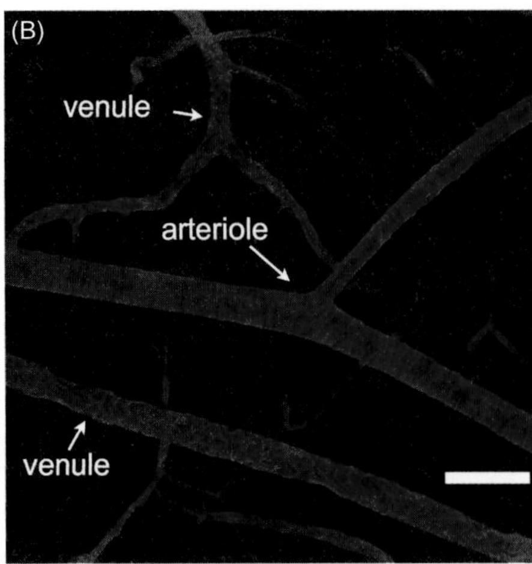

FIGURE 89.1 **Microvascular networks.** (A) Terminal arterioles branch into capillaries. Methanol-fixed, hamster cheek pouch preparation labeled with a mouse monoclonal anti-α-smooth muscle actin antibody (Sigma, St Louis, MO) to stain smooth muscle cells (red), and an anti-CD31 (PECAM-1) antibody (BD Pharmingen, San Diego, CA) to stain endothelial cells (green). Shown is a small fourth-order arteriole branching into terminal arterioles (red and yellow), which then branch into capillaries (green). Scale bar = 50 μm. (B) Smooth muscle cells in arterioles and pericytes in venules. Methanol-fixed hamster cheek pouch preparation labeled with mouse monoclonal anti-α-smooth muscle actin antibody (Sigma, St Louis, MO) to stain smooth muscle cells (circumferential banding pattern on arterioles) and pericytes (web-like pattern on venules). Shown is a second-order arteriole with a third-order branch, parallel with a collecting venule (bottom). At the top of the image, post-capillary venules combine to form a small collecting venule. Scale bar = 100 μm.

resistance also determines the blood pressure transmitted to the capillaries and venules, impacting fluid exchange in these downstream segments of the microcirculation (1,2,7). It also should be noted that small arteries upstream from the microcirculation (resistance arteries) contribute substantially to vascular resistance, and coordination of vasomotor responses between arterioles in the microcirculation and upstream resistance arteries is required for proper regulation of blood flow to active tissue (16,22) (see Chapter 94 for more information on cell–cell communication). Smooth muscle cells in the wall of these microvessels are the effectors of all of the listed functions of arterioles (1,7).

Arterioles are permeable to oxygen and carbon dioxide, and substantial precapillary exchange of these respiratory gasses occurs at this level of the circulation (7,23). Thus, arterioles also participate in the exchange function of the microcirculation. Arterioles often run parallel with, and adjacent to venules (Figure 89.1B), allowing diffusional exchange of oxygen and carbon dioxide between these microvessels (24). Also, diffusion of vasoactive substances from venules adjacent to arterioles has been proposed to contribute to the regulation of arteriolar smooth muscle tone (7,16,25–32).

Arterioles are composed of an endothelial cell tube surrounded by their basal lamina, an internal elastic lamina, overlying smooth muscle cells and adventitial connective tissue (14,15). The laminae are periodically perforated allowing projections from endothelial cells or smooth muscle cells to come into close contact with the membrane of the other cell type, forming myoendothelial junctions (14,33). These junctions may contain connexins, the proteins that form gap junctions, providing the potential for direct electrical and small molecule communication between smooth muscle cells and underlying endothelial cells (14,33–35). There also may be gap junctional communication between adjacent smooth muscle cells (14,15,35) (see Chapter 94 for more information on cell–cell communication).

Smooth muscle cells appear to be more-or-less circumferentially oriented around the arteriolar lumen (Figure 89.1B). Studies of enzymatically isolated smooth muscle cells from second- and third-order arterioles from rat and hamster cremaster muscles suggest that these fusiform cells are at least 100 μm long and about 7 μm wide near the cell nucleus (36). Similar-sized, relaxed smooth muscle cells also have been isolated from porcine coronary arterioles (37). These length values are consistent with early scanning electron microscopy studies of smooth muscle cell morphology in rat intestinal submucosal arterioles (38). However, other scanning electron microscopy studies of pressure-fixed, maximally dilated arterioles from rat small intestine suggest that in situ, the smooth muscle cells are likely 50% longer than estimated from enzymatic dissociation of vessels (39). Regardless, in vessels with maximal diameters less than 50 μm, the smooth muscle cells likely completely encircle the arterioles, and in smaller arterioles, wrap more that once around the arteriole circumference. Relatively modest shortening of the smooth muscle cells is required to produce substantial changes in luminal diameter and arteriolar vascular resistance. Because of the strong, fourth-power relationship between luminal diameter and resistance to blood flow, even small changes in microvascular diameter have large effects on resistance and hence blood pressure and blood flow (5). The smooth muscle cells in terminal arterioles may lose their spindle shape, have multiple processes and appear more pericyte-like than in larger arterioles, at least in the cerebral cortex (40).

Details of the mechanisms responsible for contraction and relaxation of arteriolar smooth muscle remain incomplete. However, from what is known, many of the processes involved appear to be similar to those described in other smooth muscle (see other chapters in this volume), with some exceptions as will be outlined below. A hallmark feature of arterioles is their response to changes in, and steady-state levels of pressure in the lumen of these microvessels (7,41–43) (Figure 89.2). The response to changes in luminal pressure is referred to as the "myogenic response" (Figure 89.2A), whereas the steady-state level of contraction of smooth muscle in pressurized vessels is "myogenic tone" (Figure 89.2B) (7,41–43). These processes are intrinsic to smooth muscle, although they can be modulated by input from hormones, parenchymal cells, nerves and endothelial cells (7,41–43). The myogenic response and myogenic tone contribute to the autoregulation of blood flow that is observed in the brain (44), heart (45,46), kidney (47), eye (48), intestine (49), and skeletal muscle (50), a process that helps reduce changes in tissue blood flow during changes in blood pressure (7,41). Myogenic tone also provides a basal level of smooth muscle activity such that arterioles are capable of substantial dilation and constriction around their resting diameters allowing maintenance of cardiovascular homeostasis and matching of tissue blood flow to the metabolic demands of parenchymal cells (1,7).

The signaling pathways responsible for the myogenic response and myogenic tone in arterioles are still under investigation. Intravascular pressure appears to be transduced into smooth muscle contraction through mechanisms involving stress on, or strain of membrane proteins including integrins, ion channels and membrane-bound enzymes (see 7, 42, 43, 51 and Chapter 93). *In vitro* studies of isolated smooth muscle and pressurized arterioles support a role for membrane depolarization, activation of voltage-gated Ca^{2+} channels, and an increase in intracellular Ca^{2+} as consistent downstream events (7,42,43,51), As in other smooth muscles, the increase in Ca^{2+} results in calmodulin-dependent activation of myosin light-chain kinase, phosphorylation of the 20 kD myosin light chains, actin–myosin cross-bridge formation/cycling and contraction (52–54), with the Ca^{2+} sensitivity of this process being determined by the relative

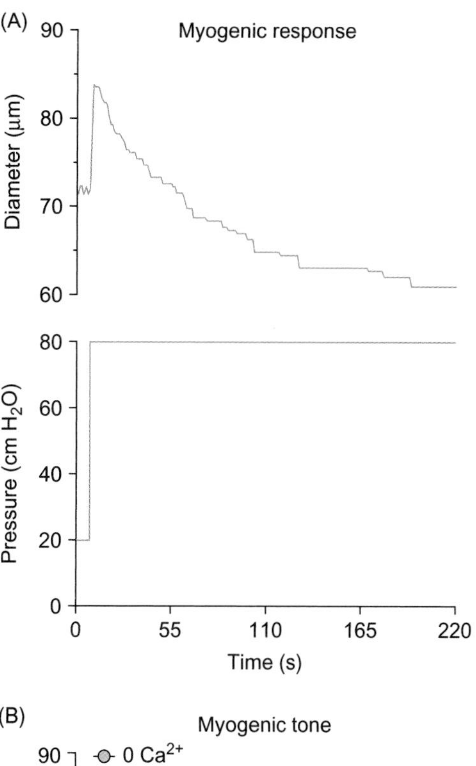

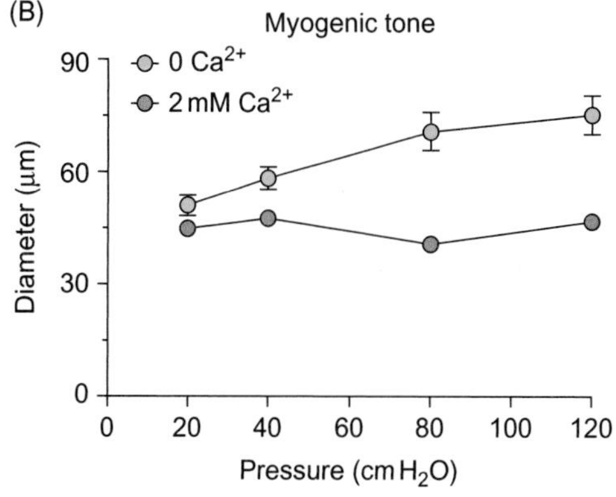

FIGURE 89.2 **The myogenic response and myogenic tone in arterioles.** (A) Myogenic response in a cannulated hamster cremasteric arteriole, *in vitro* prepared as described previously (59–61). Shown in the upper panel is a digitized diameter record of the response of a second-order arteriole to a step-increase in luminal pressure from 20 to 80 cm H_2O as depicted in the lower panel. At the onset of the pressure step, arteriolar diameter increases due to passive distention of the vessel. As the smooth muscle responds and begins to contract, diameter recovers to a new steady-state diameter that is slightly less than the diameter at 20 cmH_2O. This behavior is the myogenic response. (B) Myogenic tone in cannulated hamster cremaster arterioles. Shown are the steady-state diameters of arterioles at different pressures in the absence of extracellular Ca^{2+} (passive) and presence of 2 mM Ca^{2+} (active). As can be seen, at pressures greater than 20 cmH_2O, arterioles develop significant myogenic tone (i.e., steady-state pressure-induced constriction). (Data in panel (B) replotted from reference 61.)

activities of myosin light-chain kinase (MLCK) and myosin light-chain phosphatase (MLCP) (55). However, differences in the details of the pathways involved have clouded our understanding this process.

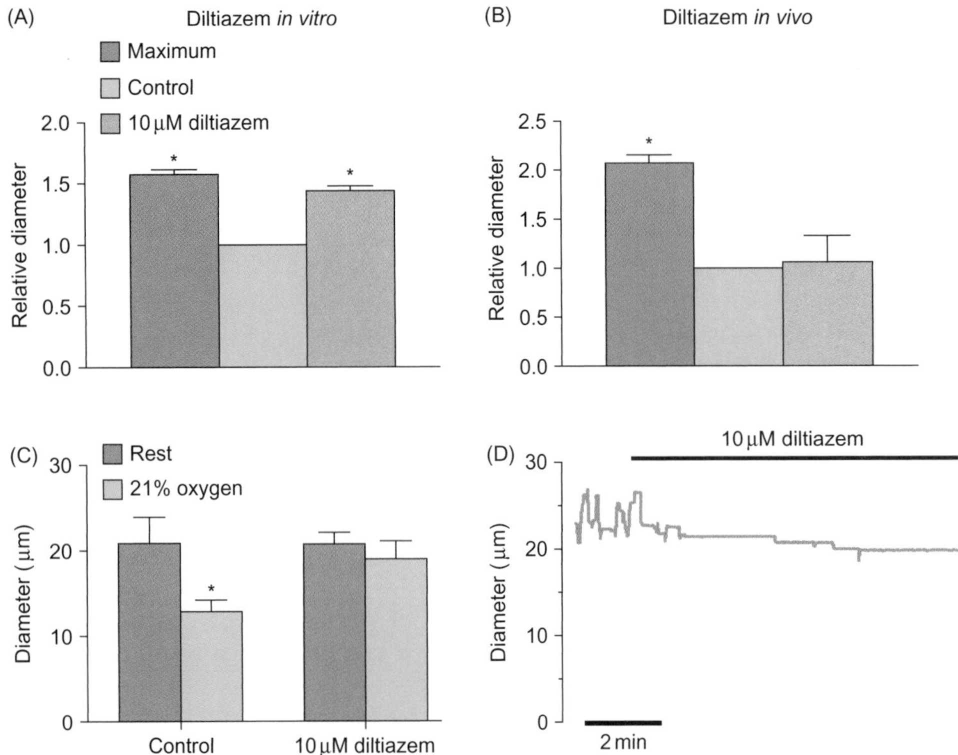

FIGURE 89.3 Blockade of L-type voltage-gated Ca^{2+} channels inhibits arteriolar myogenic tone *in vitro*, but not *in vivo*. (A) Data are relative diameters ± SE (n = 4) of cannulated hamster cremaster arterioles pressurized to 80 cmH_2O at 34 °C at rest (Control = open bar), after removal of extracellular Ca^{2+} (Maximum = black bar), or in the presence of 10 μM diltiazem (grey bar), as indicated. Note that the vessels developed myogenic tone (Control diameters less than Maximum), and that diltiazem caused significant dilation of the arterioles. * = significantly different from Control, $p < 0.05$. (B) Data are relative diameters ± SE (n = 4) of arterioles in superfused hamster cremaster muscles studied by intravital microscopy as described in references 56,57,58. Legend as in panel (A), except that maximum diameters were obtained by topical application of the endothelium-dependent dilator, methacholine (10 μM). Arterioles *in vivo* also develop substantial myogenic tone, however, diltiazem had no significant effect on the steady-state diameters of the arterioles. * = significantly different from Control, $p < 0.05$. (C) Data are mean diameters ± SE (n = 4) of hamster cremaster muscle arterioles studied by intravital microscopy, as in panel (B). Shown are arteriolar diameters at rest and in the presence of elevated superfusate O_2 tension, before (Control) and during superfusion with diltiazem, as indicated. As described previously (56,57,72), under control conditions, elevated O_2 tension caused significant arteriolar constriction. However, this response was abolished by diltiazem. These data demonstrate the efficacy of diltiazem in this preparation. * = significantly different from Rest, $p < 0.05$. (D) Shown is a digitized trace of arteriolar internal diameter in hamster cremaster studied by intravital microscopy before and during superfusion with diltiazem as indicated. As shown, the arteriole displayed vasomotion, the oscillatory diameter shown at the beginning of the trace. This behavior was abolished when the muscle was superfused with diltiazem. These data also demonstrate the efficacy of diltiazem in this preparation.

For example, the role played by L-type, voltage-gated Ca^{2+} channels in myogenic tone may not be the same, *in vivo* and *in vitro*. Hamster cremaster arterioles studied *in vivo* (56–58) or as cannulated, pressurized segments, *in vitro* (59–61), develop substantial myogenic tone (Figures 89.2 and 89.3). However, exposure of these preparations to the L-type Ca^{2+} channel antagonist diltiazem (10 μM), leads only to steady-state arteriolar dilation, *in vitro* (59) (Figure 89.3A): myogenic tone of hamster cremaster arterioles, *in vivo*, is resistant to the effects of this Ca^{2+} channel antagonist (Figure 89.3B). This does not appear to be due to a lack of efficacy of the blocker, *in vivo*, because diltiazem (10 μM) abolishes oxygen-induced arteriolar constriction (Figure 89.3C) and eliminates vasomotion (Figure 89.3D). A lack of effect of Ca^{2+} channel blockers on myogenic tone of cremaster arterioles, studied *in vivo*, also has been reported by Hill and Meininger (51) in rat preparations. Similarly, Welsh et al. (62) found that neither diltiazem nor nifedipine significantly altered steady-state diameters of hamster cheek pouch arterioles, *in vivo*, whereas these Ca^{2+} channel antagonists elicit robust dilation of cannulated, pressurized cheek pouch arterioles, *in vitro* (Figure 89.4A). Such differences might be reconciled if the smooth muscle cells expressed voltage-gated Ca^{2+} channels other than L-type, as has been reported in renal arterioles (63) and small mesenteric arteries (64,65). However, patch clamp studies of smooth muscle cells isolated from hamster cremaster arterioles (66) and hamster cheek pouch arterioles (Figure 89.4B) demonstrate that the smooth muscle cells

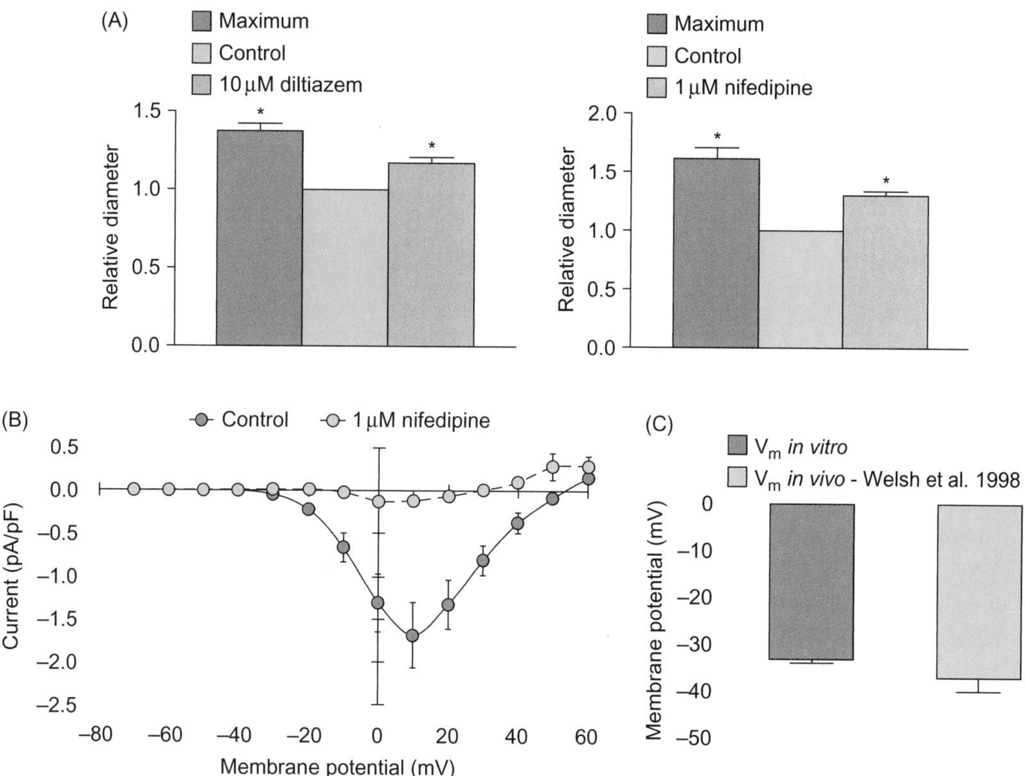

FIGURE 89.4 Role of L-type Ca^{2+} channels in smooth muscle cells from hamster cheek pouch arterioles. (A) Left panel: data are relative diameters ± SE (n = 6) of cannulated, pressurized hamster cheek pouch arterioles (maximum diameter = 95 ± 5 μm) pressurized to 60 cmH_2O at rest (Control, white bar), in the absence of Ca^{2+} (Maximum) and in the presence of diltiazem, as indicated. The arterioles display myogenic tone that is significantly reduced by diltiazem. * = significantly different from Control, $p < 0.05$. Right panel: as in left panel, but using nifedipine to inhibit L-type Ca^{2+} channels. (B) Barium (10 mM) currents recorded from smooth muscle cells enzymatically isolated from hamster cheek pouch arterioles using the perforated patch technique as previously described (36,66). Cells were held at −80 mV and stepped to membrane potentials as indicated and peak currents recorded in the absence (Control) and presence of nifedipine, as indicated. Currents were normalized to cell capacitance. Data are mean current densities ± SE (n = 5). Only high-voltage, dihydropyridine-sensitive Ba^{2+} currents were observed indicating functional expression of L-type Ca^{2+} channels in these cells. (C) Comparison of resting membrane potential in smooth muscle cells of hamster cheek pouch arterioles in isolated, cannulated arterioles, *in vitro* compared with membrane potential measurements recorded in cheek pouch arterioles, *in vivo* by Welsh et al. (62). Resting diameters of vessels studied, *in vitro* = 49 ± 3 (n = 8). *In vivo* diameters were reported as 58 ± 5 μm (n = 10) (62). There was no significant difference in membrane potential ($p > 0.05$).

from these preparations exclusively display high voltage-activated, dihydropyridine-sensitive Ca^{2+} channel currents. The differences between arterioles studied *in vivo* and *in vitro* also do not appear to be due to differences in smooth muscle membrane potential (Figure 89.4C) or myoplasmic Ca^{2+} levels (67), as these parameters appear to be similar under the two experimental conditions. These data suggest that the mechanisms underlying myogenic tone may vary, and that further research will be required to firmly establish the signaling pathways involved in myogenic mechanisms in the microcirculation.

There also appear to be differences in mechanisms that modulate myogenic tone between arterioles and upstream arteries, and between arterioles from different regions of the body. For example, the source of Ca^{2+} used by large-conductance Ca^{2+}-activated K^+ (BK_{Ca}) channels in the negative feedback regulation of myogenic tone appears to differ between arteries and at least some arterioles. These voltage- and Ca^{2+}-activated channels provide a major negative feedback signal during pressure- and agonist-induced activation of vascular smooth muscle (7,68–74). As originally proposed by Nelson and colleagues (69), BK_{Ca} channels in smooth muscle cells of myogenically active cerebral arteries are regulated by Ca^{2+} release from intracellular stores through ryanodine receptors (RyR) in the form of Ca^{2+} sparks, and this coupling between RyR and BK_{Ca} channels participates in the negative feedback regulation of myogenic and agonist-induced smooth muscle tone. Recent studies of small feed arteries supplying the cremaster muscle are consistent with these original findings: RyR appear to participate in Ca^{2+} signaling underlying myogenic tone, and to be functionally coupled to BK_{Ca} channels contributing to the negative feedback regulation of myogenic tone (61). In contrast, however, RyR in downstream, second-order cremaster arterioles are silent and do not contribute to regulation of Ca^{2+} signals or myogenic tone in these microvessels. Instead, BK_{Ca} channels are controlled by Ca^{2+} from another source, such as Ca^{2+} influx through voltage-gated Ca^{2+} channels (61). Consistent with this latter hypothesis, BK_{Ca} channels appear to be silent in arteriolar smooth muscle cells at rest, *in vivo* (72), under the same conditions where voltage-gated Ca^{2+} channels also appear to be silent (Figure 89.3B). In addition, BK_{Ca} channels in cremaster arteriolar smooth muscle cells have a high Ca^{2+} setpoint (the Ca^{2+} threshold for Ca^{2+}-dependent activation of the channels) (72) that appears, in part, to be due to a lower expression of the modulatory β_1-subunit of these channels compared to smooth muscle cells from arteries (75). Thus, there appear to be significant differences in mechanisms modulating myogenic tone in arterioles compared with upstream arteries.

There also appear to be regional differences in the function of RyR in the microcirculation. In contrast to the apparent silence of RyR in cremaster arterioles, RyR in renal arterioles appear to participate in the positive feedback regulation of myogenic tone and vasoconstrictor activity acting to amplify Ca^{2+} signals from other sources through Ca^{2+}-induced-Ca^{2+}-release (CICR) (76–79). Thus, artery vs. arteriole and arteriole vs. arteriole differences in the mechanisms modulating myogenic tone are present and impair our understanding of the signaling pathways involved in this process in the microcirculation.

CAPILLARIES AND PERICYTES

Capillaries that branch off terminal arterioles lack smooth muscle cells, but may be invested with pericytes that are capable of contraction and changing the luminal diameter of capillaries (8,11,12,17,80). Pericytes are elongated cells with multiple branches that envelop the underlying endothelial cell tube (8), much like a hand with fingers grasping a cylinder. Unlike vascular smooth muscle cells, pericytes are enclosed by the basement membrane that surrounds the endothelial cells (8,14,15). However, like vascular smooth muscle cells, pericytes form gap junctions with endothelial cells and other pericytes, forming an electrical syncytium (81,82). Pericytes participate in a range of functions in the microcirculation including angiogenesis and vascular remodeling, regulation of microvascular permeability, and control of local vascular resistance (8–12,17,80,83–85). The focus of this review will be on the latter topic.

The majority of evidence supporting a vasomotor role for pericytes in the regulation of capillary perfusion comes from studies of the retinal microcirculation where the ratio of pericytes to endothelial cells is nearly 1:1 (8). Studies of cultured retinal pericytes (8), isolated retinal capillaries (86–88), and whole retina preparations (85) demonstrate that retinal pericytes respond to a variety of vasoactive agents with contraction or relaxation, producing capillary constriction or dilation, respectively. Similarly, in the brain, pericytes are capable of responding to neurotransmitters and autacoids to produce changes in capillary diameter and hence local alterations in capillary vascular resistance (83–85). Contraction of brain capillary pericytes appears to play a role in the augmented vascular resistance (the so-called "no-reflow" phenomenon) after cerebral ischemia (83). Although recent studies using two-photon confocal microscopy to image the living microcirculation in mouse brain suggest that pericytes may not participate in the increase in cerebral blood flow associated with bicuculine-induced increases in neuronal activity [84], the potential for pericyte-mediated changes in capillary vascular resistance during physiological and pathological conditions in the brain remains. In the kidney, mesangial cells in the glomerulus (89) and pericytes surrounding capillaries in descending vasa recta (10) appear to play a major role in renal physiology. Vasoactive substances, locally applied to capillaries in skeletal muscle, have been demonstrated to cause changes in capillary perfusion that have been presumed to result from conduction of signals from capillary endothelial cells to upstream arterioles (90). The role of pericytes in this phenomenon has not been addressed, partly because the density of pericytes may be low in this capillary bed (14). However, given the gap junction coupling between pericytes, endothelial cells and arteriolar smooth muscle observed in other systems (82), it seems likely that pericytes also are involved in the regulation of capillary flow in skeletal muscle microcirculation.

Pericytes express a variety of proteins in common with vascular smooth muscle cells including α-smooth muscle actin (91), smooth muscle myosin (91), SM22-α (92), and proteins involved in RhoA-Rho kinase signaling (11). Electrophysiological studies of both retinal and renal vasa recta pericytes have demonstrated functional expression of voltage-gated Ca^{2+} channels (86,93,94), Ca^{2+}-activated Cl^- channels (86,95–97), inward rectifier K^+ channels (98,99), and ATP-sensitive K^+ channels (97,100–102). In retinal pericytes, currents identified as being carried by large-conductance Ca^{2+}-activated K^+ channels (103,104), voltage-gated K^+ channels (103), and non-selective cation channels (93) also have been recorded. Agents, such as angiotensin II and endothelin-1, contract retinal and renal pericytes associated with an increase in intracellular Ca^{2+} (93,94,96,97). This increase in Ca^{2+} appears to result from receptor-mediated release of Ca^{2+} from internal stores, concomitant with activation of cation-influx through non-selective cation channels and Ca^{2+}-activated Cl^- channels, and inhibition of

K^+ channels, all of which depolarize the pericytes (93,94,96,97). This depolarization then activates L-type voltage gated Ca^{2+} channels, which add to, and sustain the agonist-induced increase in intracellular Ca^{2+}. Vasodilators such as adenosine, dopamine, prostacyclin, and isoproterenol that act through the adenylate cyclase-cAMP signaling, in contrast, appear to relax retinal pericytes by activation of K^+ channels, membrane hyperpolarization, and decreased activity of voltage-gated Ca^{2+} channels (100,101,103,104). Similarly, glomerular mesangial cells appear to express a variety of ion channels and display Ca^{2+} signaling pathways similar to smooth muscle (89).

VENULES

Capillaries drain into post-capillary venules, which then join to form collecting venules. These vessels consist of an endothelial cell tube surrounded by a near complete coat of pericytes (Figure 89.2), rather than smooth muscle cells (8,14,15,18). Larger, muscular venules may have 1–2 layers of circumferentially oriented smooth muscle cells (14,18). Post-capillary and collecting venules, along with upstream capillaries, are major sites for exchange of solutes and water in the microcirculation (1,2). They are also important sites for inflammatory cell adhesion and transmigration (3,4). Muscular venules and larger veins (6,18) importantly contribute to venous capacitance, and hence cardiovascular homeostasis. Venular hemodynamic resistance is lower than arteriolar resistance due to the greater number of venules of a given size, relative to comparably sized arterioles (5,13). However, changes in venular resistance can have a major effect on capillary and post-capillary venular hydrostatic pressure, which strongly impacts water exchange in these microvessels (7).

There is considerable evidence that muscular venules, vessels $>30\,\mu m$ in diameter, respond to a variety of vasoconstrictors (18,105,106) supporting a role for venular smooth muscle in the regulation of venular diameter, and hence venular capacitance and resistance. Also, these larger venules appear to be innervated by the sympathetic nervous system (18,107). However, the vasomotor role of pericytes that invest post-capillary and collecting venules is less clear. These vessels do not appear to be innervated by the sympathetic nervous system (18). However, studies in the hamster cheek pouch suggest that small venules that are likely to have pericytes, rather than smooth muscle cells (Figure 89.2), display active tone, and show venular constriction when activated by elevated oxygen tensions or norepinephrine (108). These data suggest that pericyte contraction may importantly impact venular hemodynamic function. Nonetheless, the vasomotor function of venular pericytes has not been studied *per se*. Given the evidence from pericytes on retinal (86–88), brain (83–85) and renal capillaries (10), it seems likely that venular pericytes also have the capacity to contract and produce changes in venular diameter, resistance and capacitance. As post-capillary and collecting venules also are important sites for solute exchange in the microcirculation (2), and are importantly involved in inflammation-induced changes in macomolecular permeability (2) and leukocyte transmigration (3), a role for pericytes in the regulation of venular permeability also is likely.

SUMMARY AND CONCLUSIONS

Smooth muscle cells and pericytes serve as important effectors in the functions of the microcirculation. While much has been gleaned about the mechanisms involved, additional research will be required to define the cellular and molecular pathways that operate in smooth muscle and pericytes in the microcirculation, and to determine how these pathways become deranged during diseases, pathologies and aging.

ACKNOWLEDGMENTS

Supported by Public Health Service grants HL 32469, HL086483, and PO1 HL070687. Thanks to Erica Goodwin and Erika Westcott for their technical assistance and to Erika Westcott for proofreading the manuscript.

REFERENCES

1. Renkin EM. Control of microcirculation and blood–tissue exchange. In: Renkin EM, Michel CC, editors. *Handbook of physiology, Section 2: The cardiovascular system, Vol. IV, Microcirculation, part 2*. Bethesda, MD: American Physiological Society;1984. p. 627–87.
2. Durán WN, Sánchez FA, Breslin JW. Microcirculatory exchange function. *Compr Physiol* 2011; **Suppl 9**: Handbook of physiology: The cardiovascular system, Microcirculation: 81–124. First published in print 2008, doi: 10.1002/cphy.cp020404.
3. Ley K. The microcirculation in inflammation. *Compr Physiol* 2011; **Suppl 9**: Handbook of physiology: The cardiovascular system, Microcirculation: 387–448. First published in print 2008, doi: 10.1002/cphy.cp020409.
4. Kogan AN, von Andrian UH. Lymphocyte trafficking. *Compr Physiol* 2011; **Suppl 9**: Handbook of physiology: The cardiovascular system, Microcirculation: 449–482. First published in print 2008, doi: 10.1002/cphy.cp020410.
5. Zweifach BW, Lipowsky HH. Pressure-flow relations in blood and lymph micocirculation. In: Renkin EM, Michel CC, editors. *Handbook of physiology, Section 2: The cardiovascular system, Vol. IV, Microcirculation, part 1*. Bethesda, MD: The American Physiological Society;1984. p. 251–305.
6. Rothe CF. Venous system: physiology of the capacitance vessels. *Compr Physiol* 2011; **Suppl 8**: Handbook of physiology: The cardiovascular system, Peripheral circulation and organ blood

flow: 397–452. First published in print 1983. doi: 10.1002/cphy.cp020313.

7. Davis MJ, Hill MA, Kuo L. Local regulation of microvascular perfusion. *Compr Physiol* 2011; **Suppl 9**: Handbook of physiology: The cardiovascular system, Microcirculation: 161–284. First published in print 2008. doi: 10.1002/cphy.cp020406.
8. Shepro D, Morel NML. Pericyte physiology. *FASEB J* 1993;**7**:1031–8.
9. Krueger M, Bechmann I. CNS pericytes: concepts, misconceptions, and a way out. *Glia* 2010;**58**:1–10.
10. Pallone TL, Zhang Z, Rhinehart K. Physiology of the renal medullary microcirculation. *Am J Physiol Renal Physiol* 2003;**284**: F253–66.
11. Kutcher ME, Herman IM. The pericyte: cellular regulator of microvascular blood flow. *Microvasc Res* 2009;**77**:235–46.
12. Puro DG. Physiology and pathobiology of the pericyte-containing retinal microvasculature: new developments. *Microcirculation* 2007;**14**:1–10.
13. Wiedeman MP. Architecture. In: Renkin EM, Michel CC, editors. *Handbook of physiology, Sect. 2: The cardiovascular system, Vol. IV, Microcirculation, part 1*. Bethesda, MD: American Physiological Society;1984. p. 11–40.
14. Rhodin JAG, Terjung R. Architecture of the vessel wall. *Compr Physiol* 2011; **Suppl 7**: Handbook of physiology: The cardiovascular system, Vascular smooth muscle: 1–31. First published in print 1980. doi: 10.1002/cphy.cp020201.
15. Simionescu M, Simionescu N. Ultrastructure of the microvascular wall: functional correlations. In: Renkin EM, Michel CC, editors. *Handbook of physiology, Sect. 2: The cardiovascular system, Vol. IV, Microcirculation, part 2*. Bethesda, MD: The American Physiological Society;1984. p. 41–101.
16. Segal SS. Regulation of blood flow in the microcirculation. *Microcirculation* 2005;**12**:33–45.
17. Hamilton NB, Attwell D, Hall CN. Pericyte-mediated regulation of capillary diameter: a component of neurovascular coupling in health and disease. *Front Neuroenergetics* 2010;**2**:5.
18. Altura BM. Pharmacology of venular smooth muscle: new insights. *Microvasc Res* 1978;**16**:91–117.
19. Zawieja DC, von der Weid P-Y, Gashev AA. Microlymphatic biology. *Compr Physiol* 2011; **Suppl 9**: Handbook of physiology: The cardiovascular system, Microcirculation: 125–158. First published in print 2008. doi: 10.1002/cphy.cp020405.
20. Pries AR, Secomb TW. Blood flow in microvascular networks. *Compr Physiol* 2011; **Suppl 9**: Handbook of physiology: The cardiovascular system, Microcirculation: 3–36. First published in print 2008. doi: 10.1002/cphy.cp020401.
21. Fronek K, Zweifach BW. Microvascular pressure distribution in skeletal muscle and the effect of vasodilation. *Am J Physiol* 1975;**228**:791–6.
22. Segal SS, Duling BR. Communication between feed arteries and microvessels in hamster striated muscle: segmental vascular responses are functionally coordinated. *Circ Res* 1986;**59**:283–90.
23. Duling BR, Berne RM. Longitudinal gradients in periarteriolar oxygen tension. *Circ Res* 1970;**27**:669–78.
24. Johnson PC. Introduction. *Compr Physiol* 2011; **Suppl 9**: Handbook of physiology: The cardiovascular system, Microcirculation: xi–xxiv. First published in print 2008. doi: 10.1002/cphy.cp0204fm02.
25. Falcone JC, Bohlen HG. EDRF from rat intestine and skeletal muscle venules causes dilation of arterioles. *Am J Physiol Heart Circ Physiol* 1990;**258**:H1515–23.
26. Hester RL. Venular-arteriolar diffusion of adenosine in hamster cremaster microcirculation. *Am J Physiol Heart Circ Physiol* 1990;**258**:H1918–24.
27. Hester RL. Uptake of metabolites by postcapillary venules: mechanism for the control of arteriolar diameter. *Microvasc Res* 1993;**46**:254–61.
28. Saito Y, Eraslan A, Hester RL. Importance of venular flow in control of arteriolar diameter in hamster cremaster muscle. *Am J Physiol Heart Circ Physiol* 1993;**265**:H1294–300.
29. Saito Y, Eraslan A, Lockard V, Hester RL. Role of venular endothelium in control of arteriolar diameter during functional hyperemia. *Am J Physiol Heart Circ Physiol* 1994;**267**:H1227–31.
30. Hester RL. Venular endothelium: metabolic sensors? *News Physiol Sci* 1995;**10**:50–1.
31. McKay MK, Gardner AL, Boyd D, Hester RL. Influence of venular prostaglandin release on arteriolar diameter during functional hyperemia. *Hypertension* 1998;**31**:213–7.
32. Hester RL, Hammer LW. Venular-arteriolar communication in the regulation of blood flow. *Am J Physiol Regul Integr Comp Physiol* 2002;**282**:R1280–5.
33. Sandow SL, Hill CE. Incidence of myoendothelial gap junctions in the proximal and distal mesenteric arteries of the rat is suggestive of a role in endothelium-derived hyperpolarizing factor-mediated responses. *Circ Res* 2000;**86**:341–6.
34. Little TL, Beyer EC, Duling BR. Connexin43 and connexin40 gap junctional proteins are present in arteriolar smooth muscle and endothelium in vivo. *Am J Physiol* 1995;**268**:H729–39.
35. Little TL, Xia J, Duling BR. Dye tracers define differential endothelial and smooth muscle coupling patterns within the arteriolar wall. *Circ Res* 1995;**76**:498–504.
36. Jackson WF, Huebner JM, Rusch NJ. Enzymatic isolation and characterization of single vascular smooth muscle cells from cremasteric arterioles. *Microcirculation* 1997;**4**:35–50.
37. Wu X, Davis MJ. Characterization of stretch-activated cation current in coronary smooth muscle cells. *Am J Physiol Heart Circ Physiol* 2001;**280**:H1751–61.
38. Gattone 2nd VH, Miller BG, Evan AP. Microvascular smooth muscle cell quantitation from scanning electron microscopic preparations. *Anat Rec* 1986;**216**:443–7.
39. Connors BA, Bohlen HG, Evan AP. Vascular endothelium and smooth muscle remodeling accompanies hypertrophy of intestinal arterioles in streptozotocin diabetic rats. *Microvasc Res* 1995;**49**: 340–9.
40. Moore SA, Bohlen HG, Miller BG, Evan AP. Cellular and vessel wall morphology of cerebral cortical arterioles after short-term diabetes in adult rats. *Blood Vessels* 1985;**22**:265–77.
41. Johnson PC. The myogenic response. In: Bohr DF, Somlyo AP, Sparks HV, editors. *Handbook of physiology, Sect 2: The cardiovascular system, Vol. II, Vascular smooth muscle*. Bethesda, MD: American Physiological Society;1980. p. 409–42.
42. Davis MJ, Hill MA. Signaling mechanisms underlying the vascular myogenic response. *Physiol Rev* 1999;**79**:387–423.
43. Hill MA, Zou H, Potocnik SJ, Meininger GA, Davis MJ. Invited review: arteriolar smooth muscle mechanotransduction: Ca(2+)

signaling pathways underlying myogenic reactivity. *J Appl Physiol* 2001;**91**:973–83.

44. Tuma RF. The cerebral microcirculation. *Compr Physiol* 2011; **Suppl 9**: Handbook of physiology: The cardiovascular system, Microcirculation: 485–520. First published in print 2008. doi: 10.1002/cphy.cp020411.
45. Laughlin MH, Korthuis RJ, Duncker DJ, Bache RJ. Control of blood flow to cardiac and skeletal muscle during exercise. In: Rowell LB, Shepherd JT, editors. *Exercise regulation and integration of multiple systems*. New York: Oxford University Press;1996. p. 705–69.
46. Zhang C, Rogers PA, Merkus D, Muller-Delp JM, Tiefenbacher CP, Potter B, et al. Regulation of coronary microvascular resistance in health and disease. *Compr Physiol* 2011; **Suppl 9**: Handbook of physiology: The cardiovascular system, Microcirculation: 521–549. First published in print 2008. doi: 10.1002/cphy.cp020412.
47. Navar LG, Arendshorst WJ, Pallone TL, Inscho EW, Imig JD, Bell PD. The renal microcirculation. *Compr Physiol* 2011; **Suppl 9**: Handbook of physiology: The cardiovascular system, Microcirculation: 550–683. First published in print 2008. doi: 10.1002/cphy.cp020413.
48. Riva CE, Schmetterer L. Microcirculation of the ocular fundus. *Compr Physiol* 2011; **Suppl 9**: Handbook of physiology: The cardiovascular system, Microcirculation: 735–765. First published in print 2008. doi: 10.1002/cphy.cp020416.
49. Granger DN, Kvietys PR, Korthuis RJ, Premen AJ. Microcirculation of the intestinal mucosa. *Compr Physiol* 2011; **Suppl 16**: Handbook of physiology: The gastrointestinal system, Motility and circulation: 1405–1474. First published in print 1989. doi: 10.1002/cphy.cp060139.
50. Shepherd JT. Circulation to skeletal muscle. In: Shepherd JT, Abboud FM, editors. *Handbook of physiology, Sect. 2: The cardiovascular system, Vol. III*. Bethesda, MD: American Physiological Society;1983. p. 319–70.
51. Hill MA, Meininger GA. Calcium entry and myogenic phenomena in skeletal muscle arterioles. *Am J Physiol Heart Circ Physiol* 1994;**267**:H1085–92.
52. Zou H, Ratz PH, Hill MA. Temporal aspects of Ca(2+) and myosin phosphorylation during myogenic and norepinephrine-induced arteriolar constriction. *J Vasc Res* 2000;**37**:556–67.
53. Zou H, Ratz PH, Hill MA. Role of myosin phosphorylation and [Ca2 +]i in myogenic reactivity and arteriolar tone. *Am J Physiol Heart Circ Physiol* 1995;**269**:H1590–6.
54. Takeya K, Loutzenhiser K, Shiraishi M, Loutzenhiser R, Walsh MP. A highly sensitive technique to measure myosin regulatory light chain phosphorylation: the first quantification in renal arterioles. *Am J Physiol Renal Physiol* 2008;**294**:F1487–92.
55. Lai EY, Fahling M, Ma Z, Kallskog O, Persson PB, Patzak A, et al. Norepinephrine increases calcium sensitivity of mouse afferent arteriole, thereby enhancing angiotensin II-mediated vasoconstriction. *Kidney Int* 2009;**76**:953–9.
56. Jackson WF. Prostaglandins do not mediate arteriolar oxygen reactivity. *Am J Physiol Heart Circ Physiol* 1986;**250**:H1102–8.
57. Jackson WF. Regional differences in mechanism of action of oxygen on hamster arterioles. *Am J Physiol Heart Circ Physiol* 1993;**265**:H599–603.
58. Jackson WF. Arteriolar tone is determined by activity of ATP-sensitive potassium channels. *Am J Physiol Heart Circ Physiol* 1993;**265**:H1797–803.
59. Burns WR, Cohen KD, Jackson WF. K^+-induced dilation of hamster cremasteric arterioles involves both the Na^+/K^+-ATPase and inward-rectifier K^+ channels. *Microcirculation* 2004;**11**:279–93.
60. Jackson WF, Boerman EM, Lange EJ, Lundback SS, Cohen KD. Smooth muscle alpha(1D)-adrenoceptors mediate phenylephrine-induced vasoconstriction and increases in endothelial cell Ca(2+) in hamster cremaster arterioles. *Br J Pharmacol* 2008;**155**: 514–24.
61. Westcott EB, Jackson WF. Heterogeneous function of ryanodine receptors, but not IP3 receptors in hamster cremaster muscle feed arteries and arterioles. *Am J Physiol Heart Circ Physiol* 2011;**300**:H1616–30.
62. Welsh DG, Jackson WF, Segal SS. Oxygen induces electromechanical coupling in arteriolar smooth muscle cells: a role for L-type Ca^{2+} channels. *Am J Physiol Heart Circ Physiol* 1998;**274**:H2018–24.
63. Hansen PB, Jensen BL, Andreasen D, Skott O. Differential expression of T- and L-type voltage-dependent calcium channels in renal resistance vessels. *Circ Res* 2001;**89**:630–8.
64. Gustafsson F, Andreasen D, Salomonsson M, Jensen BL, Holstein-Rathlou N. Conducted vasoconstriction in rat mesenteric arterioles: role for dihydropyridine-insensitive Ca(2+) channels. *Am J Physiol Heart Circ Physiol* 2001;**280**:H582–90.
65. Morita H, Cousins H, Onoue H, Ito Y, Inoue R. Predominant distribution of nifedipine-insensitive, high voltage- activated Ca^{2+} channels in the terminal mesenteric artery of guinea pig [see comments]. *Circ Res* 1999;**85**:596–605.
66. Cohen KD, Jackson WF. Hypoxia inhibits contraction but not calcium channel currents or changes in intracellular calcium in arteriolar muscle cells. *Microcirculation* 2003;**10**:133–41.
67. Brekke JF, Jackson WF, Segal SS. Arteriolar smooth muscle Ca^{2+} dynamics during blood flow control in hamster cheek pouch. *J Appl Physiol* 2006;**101**:307–15.
68. Nelson MT, Patlak JB, Worley JF, Standen NB. Calcium channels, potassium channels, and voltage dependence of arterial smooth muscle tone. *Am J Physiol Cell Physiol* 1990;**259**:C3–18.
69. Nelson MT, Cheng H, Rubart M, Santana LF, Bonev AD, Knot HJ, et al. Relaxation of arterial smooth muscle by calcium sparks [see comments]. *Science* 1995;**270**:633–7.
70. Nelson MT, Quayle JM. Physiological roles and properties of potassium channels in arterial smooth muscle. *Am J Physiol Cell Physiol* 1995;**268**:C799–822.
71. Jackson WF. Potassium channels and regulation of the microcirculation. *Microcirculation* 1998;**5**:85–90.
72. Jackson WF, Blair KL. Characterization and function of Ca^{++}-activated K^+ channels in hamster cremasteric arteriolar muscle cells. *Am J Physiol Heart Circ Physiol* 1998;**274**:H27–34.
73. Jackson WF. Ion channels and vascular tone. *Hypertension* 2000;**35**(1.Pt2):173–8.
74. Jackson WF. Potassium channels in the peripheral microcirculation. *Microcirculation* 2005;**12**:113–27.
75. Yang Y, Murphy TV, Ella SR, Grayson TH, Haddock R, Hwang YT, et al. Heterogeneity in function of small artery smooth muscle BKCa: involvement of the beta1-subunit. *J Physiol* 2009;**587**: 3025–44.

76. Thai TL, Fellner SK, Arendshorst WJ. ADP-ribosyl cyclase and ryanodine receptor activity contribute to basal renal vasomotor tone and agonist-induced renal vasoconstriction in vivo. *Am J Physiol Renal Physiol* 2007;**293**:F1107–14.

77. Fellner SK, Arendshorst WJ. Voltage-gated Ca^{2+} entry and ryanodine receptor Ca^{2+}-induced Ca^{2+} release in preglomerular arterioles. *Am J Physiol Renal Physiol* 2007;**292**:F1568–72.

78. Balasubramanian L, Ahmed A, Lo CM, Sham JS, Yip KP. Integrin-mediated mechanotransduction in renal vascular smooth muscle cells: activation of calcium sparks. *Am J Physiol Regul Integr Comp Physiol* 2007;**293**:R1586–94.

79. Fellner SK, Arendshorst WJ. Angiotensin II Ca^{2+} signaling in rat afferent arterioles: stimulation of cyclic ADP ribose and IP3 pathways. *Am J Physiol Renal Physiol* 2005;**288**:F785–91.

80. Hirschi KK, D'Amore PA. Pericytes in the microvasculature. *Cardiovasc Res* 1996;**32**:687–98.

81. Oku H, Kodama T, Sakagami K, Puro DG. Diabetes-induced disruption of gap junction pathways within the retinal microvasculature. *Invest Ophthalmol Vis Sci* 2001;**42**:1915–20.

82. Wu DM, Minami M, Kawamura H, Puro DG. Electrotonic transmission within pericyte-containing retinal microvessels. *Microcirculation* 2006;**13**:353–63.

83. Yemisci M, Gursoy-Ozdemir Y, Vural A, Can A, Topalkara K, Dalkara T. Pericyte contraction induced by oxidative-nitrative stress impairs capillary reflow despite successful opening of an occluded cerebral artery. *Nature Med* 2009;**15**:1031–7.

84. Fernandez-Klett F, Offenhauser N, Dirnagl U, Priller J, Lindauer U. Pericytes in capillaries are contractile in vivo, but arterioles mediate functional hyperemia in the mouse brain. *Proc Natl Acad Sci USA* 2010;**107**:22290–5.

85. Peppiatt CM, Howarth C, Mobbs P, Attwell D. Bidirectional control of CNS capillary diameter by pericytes. *Nature* 2006;**443**: 700–4.

86. Sakagami K, Wu DM, Puro DG. Physiology of rat retinal pericytes: modulation of ion channel activity by serum-derived molecules. *J Physiol* 1999;**521**(Pt3):637–50.

87. Kawamura H, Sugiyama T, Wu DM, Kobayashi M, Yamanishi S, Katsumura K, et al. ATP: a vasoactive signal in the pericyte-containing microvasculature of the rat retina. *J Physiol* 2003;**551**: 787–99.

88. Wu DM, Kawamura H, Sakagami K, Kobayashi M, Puro DG. Cholinergic regulation of pericyte-containing retinal microvessels. *Am J Physiol Heart Circ Physiol* 2003;**284**:H2083–90.

89. Stockand JD, Sansom SC. Glomerular mesangial cells: electrophysiology and regulation of contraction. *Physiol Rev* 1998;**78**:723–44.

90. Dietrich HH, Tyml K. Microvascular flow response to localized application of norepinephrine on capillaries in rat and frog skeletal muscle. *Microvasc Res* 1992;**43**:73–86.

91. Herman IM, D'Amore PA. Microvascular pericytes contain muscle and nonmuscle actins. *J Cell Biol* 1985;**101**:43–52.

92. Ding R, Darland DC, Parmacek MS, D'Amore PA. Endothelial-mesenchymal interactions in vitro reveal molecular mechanisms of smooth muscle/pericyte differentiation. *Stem Cells Dev* 2004;**13**:509–20.

93. Kawamura H, Kobayashi M, Li Q, Yamanishi S, Katsumura K, Minami M, et al. Effects of angiotensin II on the pericyte-containing microvasculature of the rat retina. *J Physiol* 2004;**561**: 671–83.

94. Zhang Z, Lin H, Cao C, Khurana S, Pallone TL. Voltage-gated divalent currents in descending vasa recta pericytes. *Am J Physiol Renal Physiol* 2010;**299**:F862–71.

95. Zhang Z, Huang JM, Turner MR, Rhinehart KL, Pallone TL. Role of chloride in constriction of descending vasa recta by angiotensin II. *Am J Physiol Regul Integr Comp Physiol* 2001;**280**:R1878–86.

96. Zhang Q, Cao C, Zhang Z, Wier WG, Edwards A, Pallone TL. Membrane current oscillations in descending vasa recta pericytes. *Am J Physiol Renal Physiol* 2008;**294**:F656–66.

97. Kawamura H, Oku H, Li Q, Sakagami K, Puro DG. Endothelin-induced changes in the physiology of retinal pericytes. *Invest Ophthalmol Vis Sci* 2002;**43**:882–8.

98. Cao C, Goo JH, Lee-Kwon W, Pallone TL. Vasa recta pericytes express a strong inward rectifier K^+ conductance. *Am J Physiol Regul Integr Comp Physiol* 2006;**290**:R1601–7.

99. Matsushita K, Puro DG. Topographical heterogeneity of KIR currents in pericyte-containing microvessels of the rat retina: effect of diabetes. *J Physiol (Lond)* 2006;**573**:483–95.

100. Li Q, Puro DG. Adenosine activates ATP-sensitive K(+) currents in pericytes of rat retinal microvessels: role of A1 and A2a receptors. *Brain Res* 2001;**907**:93–9.

101. Wu DM, Kawamura H, Li Q, Puro DG. Dopamine activates ATP-sensitive K^+ currents in rat retinal pericytes. *Vis Neurosci* 2001;**18**:935–40.

102. Cao C, Lee-Kwon W, Silldorff EP, Pallone TL. KATP channel conductance of descending vasa recta pericytes. *Am J Physiol Renal Physiol* 2005;**289**:F1235–45.

103. Quignard JF, Harley EA, Duhault J, Vanhoutte PM, Feletou M. K^+ channels in cultured bovine retinal pericytes: effects of beta-adrenergic stimulation. *J Cardiovasc Pharmacol* 2003;**42**: 379–88.

104. Burnette JO, White RE. PGI2 opens potassium channels in retinal pericytes by cyclic AMP-stimulated, cross-activation of PKG. *Exp Eye Res* 2006;**83**:1359–65.

105. Faber JE. In situ analysis of alpha-adrenoceptors on arteriolar and venular smooth muscle in rat skeletal muscle microcirculation. *Circ Res* 1988;**62**:37–50.

106. Muldowney SM, Faber JE. Preservation of venular but not arteriolar smooth muscle α-adrenoceptor sensitivity during reduced blood flow. *Circ Res* 1991;**69**:1215–25.

107. Rosell S. Neuronal control of microvessels. *Ann Rev Physiol* 1980;**42**:359–71.

108. Damon DN, Duling BR. Venular reactivity in the hamster cheek pouch and cremaster muscle. *Microvasc Res* 1986;**31**:379–83.

Chapter 90

Uterine Smooth Muscle

Susan Wray and Sarah Arrowsmith
Department of Cellular and Molecular Physiology, University of Liverpool, Liverpool, UK

EXCITATION–CONTRACTION COUPLING IN THE MYOMETRIUM

Overview

The myometrium is a spontaneously active smooth muscle (myogenic): it is able to produce regular contractions without hormonal or nervous input (1). Like many visceral smooth muscles, contractions of the myometrium are phasic in nature; they show maintenance of a resting tone with cycles of discrete, intermittent contractions of varying frequency, amplitude, and duration. It is these parameters of uterine contractile activity that are varied to equip it for its main physiological functions and which must be well controlled if problems such as preterm or dysfunctional labors are to be avoided. An example of *in vitro* contractility of human myometrium is shown in Figure 90.1. A similar pattern of activity would be recorded *in vivo* via an intra-uterine pressure catheter.

As in all smooth muscles, for contraction to take place there needs to be significant interaction between actin and myosin myofilaments and this is also true of the myometrium. Uterine contractions are triggered by transient increases in intracellular calcium concentration ($[Ca^{2+}]_i$), which in turn are initiated and controlled by myometrial action potentials (2). Figure 90.1(A) shows the Ca^{2+} transients reported by the fluorescent, Ca^{2+}-sensitive indicator Indo-1, which underlie the simultaneously recorded force changes. The sequence of events between action potential generation and contraction initiation is known as excitation–contraction (EC) coupling (ECC). The free $[Ca^{2+}]_i$ is key for controlling the uterine contractions as it is the rise in intracellular Ca^{2+} and its subsequent binding to calmodulin which activates myosin light chain kinase (MLCK). This enzyme is responsible for myosin phosphorylation, enabling acto-myosin cross-bridge cycling, hydrolysis of ATP and promotion of force. A variety of mechanisms residing in the plasma and sarcoplasmic reticular membranes control the level of intracellular Ca^{2+} in the myometrium (discussed later). Myocyte membrane voltage plays the most important role in controlling the entry of Ca^{2+} into the cell, through gating L-type Ca^{2+} channels. The effects on contractions and Ca^{2+} transients of removing external Ca^{2+} can clearly be seen in Figure 90.1(B) – both are abolished. In turn, the changes in membrane voltage and resting membrane potential are controlled by a number of ion channels and transport mechanisms residing in the plasma membrane that are responsible for cell excitability.

Excitability and Contraction in the Myometrium

Myometrial tissue is spontaneously active in that it contracts *in vivo* and *in vitro* without the need for external stimuli. Rather, its activity is initiated and co-ordinated by the muscle cells themselves (as in the heart). Contraction depends upon the spontaneous generation of action potentials, a rise in $[Ca^{2+}]_I$, and the presence of a conducting system between neighboring cells in the form of gap junctions (3). An example of the close apposition between myocytes within a muscle bundle that facilitates cell–cell coupling is shown in Figure 90.2. The resting membrane potential of uterine smooth muscle has been recorded to be between −35 mV and −80 mV (4) and varies with species, gestational status, and muscle layer (5). Low voltage (~10 mV) rhythmic oscillations of membrane potential, termed slow waves, have been recorded in myometrium and may help trigger action potentials at their peak (least depolarized), but this remains to be confirmed. Both simple spike and complex action potentials have been demonstrated. It is considered that spontaneous changes in the ionic permeability (particularly to Ca^{2+}, Na^+, K^+, and Cl^-) of the myocyte membrane leads to the threshold for action potential generation being reached, which results in depolarization of the cell membrane, Ca^{2+} entry, and contraction (see Figure 90.3).

Different combinations of ionic currents contribute to the different patterns of electrical activity observed (6). Simple spike-like action potentials involve a rapid depolarization followed by rapid repolarization; the current is

Muscle. DOI: http://dx.doi.org/10.1016/B978-0-12-381510-1.00090-9

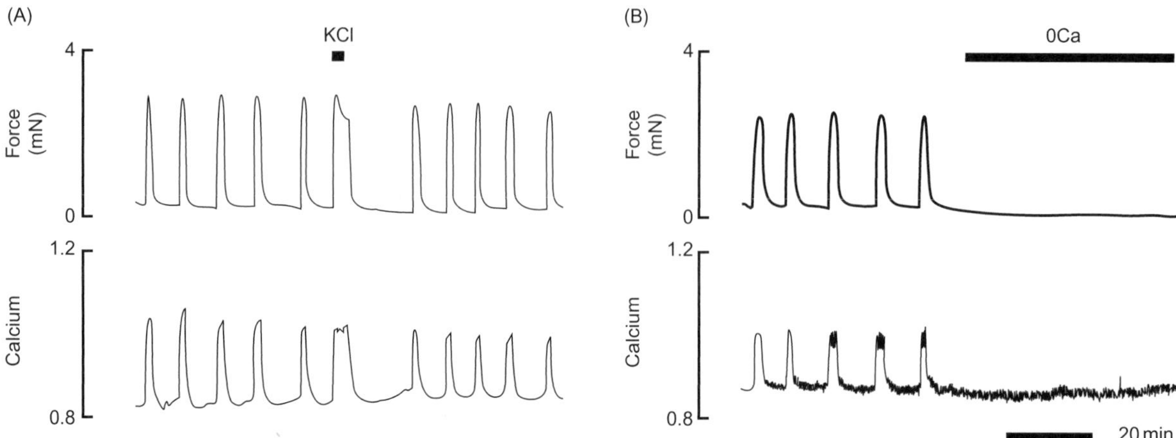

FIGURE 90.1 Simultaneous measurement of force (*black trace*) and calcium (*red trace*) measured using the fluorometric indicator indo-1 in spontaneously contracting strips of human myometrium. In (A), strips were superfused with PSS (pH7.4, 37°C) followed by high potassium (40 mM KCl) depolarization (KCl, black bar). In (B), the effect of removing external calcium (0Ca, black bar) on inhibition of spontaneous contractions can be clearly seen.

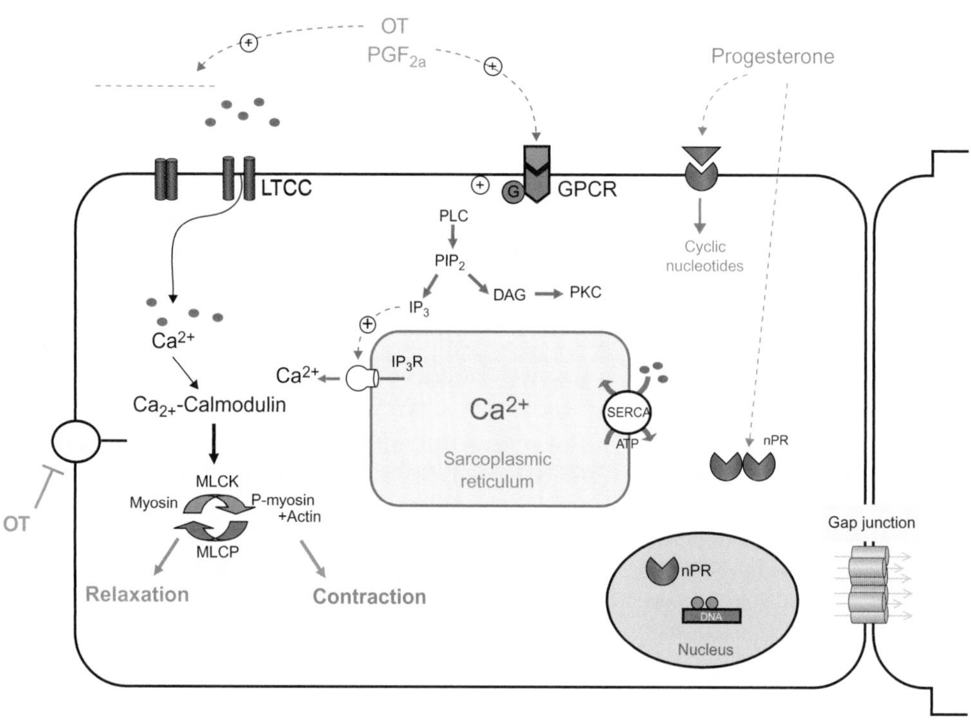

FIGURE 90.2 Schematic to show the excitation–contraction coupling pathway in the myometrium (black arrows) and the major mechanisms of action by the hormones oxytocin, prostaglandin $F_{2\alpha}$ and progesterone. Red arrows and bars show pathways that when activated lead to stimulation of contraction whilst blue arrows and bars show those pathways leading to suppression of contraction. *(Figure adapted from Arrowsmith, Kendrick and Wray, 2010 (45), with permission.)*

predominantly mediated by Ca^{2+}. Individual spikes can often be grouped into bursts, with the number and frequency of spikes within each burst determining the amplitude, speed, and duration of contraction (7). The complex action potential involves an initial spike-like depolarization followed by a sustained plateau of depolarization between −30 and −20 mV, lasting approximately 1 minute, which may involve a weak K^+ but strong Ca^{2+} conductance. The duration of the plateau determines the duration of contraction. Gap junctions ensure propagation of action potentials throughout the myometrium, prompting contraction synchronicity at the whole organ level, and are thus, along

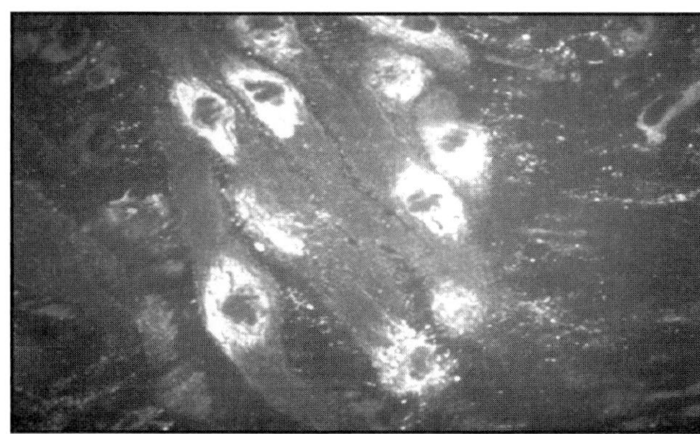

FIGURE 90.3 In situ confocal *x-y* images of intact strips of myometrium loaded with the Ca^{2+}-sensitive indicator Fluo-4, captured using ×60 objective. Uterine muscle bundles and cells can be clearly seen. Note the close apposition between cells within the muscle bundle.

with ionic conductance changes, a central point in changing uterine activity from quiescent to laboring.

Pacemakers

The ionic nature of spontaneous depolarizations and how they are triggered in the myometrium is still unclear. The slow depolarization preceding action potential discharge in some smooth muscles is attributed to the activities of cells described as pacemakers. In smooth muscle cells of the urethra, gastrointestinal tract and urinary bladder, it is specialized interstitial cells of Cajal (ICC) or ICC-like cells (ILC) which give rise to the rhythmical activity observed. This occurs by the regular generation of depolarizing potentials, which are thought to initiate slow waves in adjacent smooth muscle cells (8). Thus, in the myometrium focal pacemaker regions or ILC capable of slowly depolarizing a group of cells to threshold and generating action potentials have been sought. It is clear, however, that there is no anatomically defined pacemaker region in the uterus. Even in human myometrium there is no evidence for electrical activity initiating in the upper segment.

There is, however, evidence in human and rat myometrium for ILC (9), but whether they contribute to a role in pacemaking in the myometrium is not certain. As we could detect little inward current in these cells we considered it very unlikely that ILC were acting as pacemakers. Rather, as outward current was large, we suggested these cells may even have an inhibitory role (9). Care is needed when trying to identify ILC in that they are distinguished from other mesenchymal cell types, and often electrophysiological evidence, the acid test for pacemaking, is absent in descriptive papers.

We have posited that the ability to generate spontaneous depolarizing potentials is an intrinsic property of most smooth cells in the uterus (10). Interestingly, whilst some (~25%) freshly isolated *rat* myometrial cells can generate spontaneous electrical activity, this has not been observed in preparations of human myometrium (11). However, human uterine myocytes are still able to generate action potentials under supra-threshold stimulation, suggesting that perhaps the pacemaking mechanism in human myometrium, unlike some rodent models, may be extracellular to the uterine myocytes.

Myometrial Calcium Channels

Depolarization of the myometrial cell membrane from around −55 to −40 mV leads to the opening of voltage-operated Ca^{2+} channels (VOCCs). The incoming Ca^{2+} contributes substantially to the rising phase of the action potential as well as being the fundamental factor responsible for mediating uterine myocyte contraction. In the myometrium, contractions are abolished in the absence of external Ca^{2+} (as shown in Figure 90.1B). It is L-type, ($Ca_{v1.2}$) rather than T-type, Ca^{2+} channels in the myometrium that predominate and through which the majority, if not all, of the Ca^{2+} current is carried. Nifedipine-blockade of L-type channels abolishes uterine contractions. There is some evidence to suggest that a rapidly activating and inactivating Ca^{2+} current via T-type channels exists and may contribute to Ca^{2+} entry in pregnant myometrium, and that depolarization is contributed to by fast Na channels (12). Current knowledge of EC coupling in the myometrium is compatible with the following: Calcium ion entry is governed by the opening of L-type Ca^{2+} channels. Calmodulin molecules at the myofibrils and plasma-membrane bind four Ca^{2+} ions, and this complex activates MLCK. When activated, MLCK is specifically responsible for the phosphorylation of serine 19 on the regulatory light chains of myosin. This in turn triggers the interaction of phosphorylated myosin with actin myofilaments. The subsequent cross-bridge cycling that generates force development then ensues (see Figure 90.3) (see Chapter 87). The activity of MLCK is central to uterine smooth muscle contraction as its inhibition by wortmanin abolishes contractions, re-affirming that phosphorylation of myosin is essential for force production in the uterus and that MLCK is a major contributor to this force-producing pathway (13). The conformational change in actin and myosin requires ATP hydrolysis and occurs following phosphorylation of its regulatory light chains. Relaxation of the myometrium and restoration of the resting state requires the lowering of $[Ca^{2+}]_i$ to favor dephosphorylation of myosin light chains by myosin light chain phosphatase (MLCP). Return to resting membrane potential (via K^+ efflux) and channel inactivation, limit further Ca^{2+} entry.

Calcium Sensitization

Under physiological conditions, the Ca^{2+}-calmodulin-MLCK pathway is essential for force production, however a number of these steps can be regulated by processes such as phosphorylation and dephosphorylation reactions, or the binding of accessory proteins that alter the activities of the various components in the EC pathway (see Chapter 83). Calcium entry and efflux are the major pathways of myometrial contraction/relaxation in the myometrium. Agonists by binding to their receptors on the membrane can augment or inhibit this pathway, for example by promoting depolarization or reducing Ca^{2+} entry or efflux. However, agonists can also initiate other intracellular pathways and these signals may also influence force, e.g. via changes in enzyme and channel activity. Thus, studies in other smooth muscles have demonstrated that the activity of MLCK and MLCP can be modulated, such that a change in the level contraction then occurs without altering $[Ca^{2+}]_i$. In this way, the relationship between the myofilaments and Ca^{2+}, i.e. calcium sensitivity, is altered (14); a process referred to as Ca^{2+} (de) sensitization. Although it has been sought, especially in relation to agonist stimulation of the myometrium, there is little direct evidence for Ca^{2+} sensitization in the uterus and it may not be an important feature of this tissue (15). Direct evidence was found following altered pH but this was in chemically skinned myometrial preparations and thus how applicable to *in vivo* situations may be questioned (16). Data produced by inhibiting major sensitization pathways (Rho-Rho kinase) in the uterus found little if any effect on $[Ca^{2+}]$ or force (17). Thus, in myometrium, agonists clearly act to affect Ca^{2+} entry and exit across SR and plasma membranes, and may stimulate store-operated Ca^{2+} entry, all discussed next, but may not alter the Ca^{2+} sensitivity of the myofilaments.

Calcium Homeostasis and Calcium Signaling in Myometrium

Control of $[Ca^{2+}]_i$ is of primary importance in the process of EC coupling in the myometrium; an increase in $[Ca^{2+}]_i$ from 10^{-7} M to 10^{-6} M is needed for contractions to take place. This occurs from either Ca^{2+} influx into the cell from the extracellular space and/or Ca^{2+} release from the internal store; the sarcoplasmic reticulum (SR). As discussed above, Ca^{2+} influx via voltage-dependent L-type Ca^{2+} channels is the predominant method for Ca^{2+} entry and is essential for spontaneous activity in the uterus. However, agonists can augment Ca^{2+} entry into myometrial cells through two other ion channels, receptor-operated calcium channels (ROCCs) (which are usually non-selective cation channels) and store-operated calcium channels (SOCC, also termed capacitative calcium entry). Extrusion of Ca^{2+} occurs by the reverse processes; sequestration into SR and/or extrusion through the cell membrane by plasma membrane Ca^{2+}-ATPase (PMCA) and/or the Na^+ Ca^{2+} exchanger (NCX). It is these extrusion mechanisms that help enforce the strong electrochemical gradient for Ca^{2+} entry that exists between the intra-and extracellular space.

For the myometrial cell to be in steady state, i.e. Ca^{2+} balance, the equivalent amount of Ca^{2+} that enters the cell across the plasma membrane must be extruded, and that Ca^{2+} which is released from the SR must be taken back up into the SR (see Figure 90.3).

Ca^{2+} Signaling and the Sarcoplasmic Reticulum

A variety of techniques, including electron and confocal microscopy and fluorescent tags to SR membrane proteins, have shown the myometrium to possess an SR that ramifies extensively throughout each myocyte. The SR is a system of tubules and cisternae within the cytoplasm and occupies ~5% of the total myometrial cell volume. The SR is particularly abundant around the nucleus and there is a close apposition between the SR and plasma membrane, particularly in areas of the plasma membrane containing caveolae (see later). The SR is analogous to the ER in non-muscle cells and undertakes roles in protein synthesis. Both smooth and rough SR is present in the uterus, with the latter shown to increase in volume with pregnancy, probably reflecting the increase in protein synthesis. Classically, the SR in excitable cells is considered to act as a Ca^{2+} store and sink, with Ca^{2+} release augmenting the Ca^{2+} available for contraction and SR uptake promoting relaxation. However more recent evidence has added a role in controlling plasma membrane excitability to the list of SR functions in smooth muscle. Its role in the uterus is still to be fully elucidated but some important points have been established.

The uterine SR actively takes up and stores Ca^{2+} using the sarcoplasmic/endoplasmic reticulum Ca^{2+} ATPase (SERCA), and luminal Ca^{2+} buffers, e.g. calsequestrin. Thus, the SR helps to maintain a relatively low cytosolic $[Ca^{2+}]$. To date three different genes have been identified encoding for three isoforms of SERCA pumps; SERCA 1–3, which can be further spliced to give other variants of the pump. In the uterus, SERCA 2a and 2b (also known as the housekeeping SERCA) and SERCA 3, have been identified and changes in SERCA isoform expression in laboring myometrium has also been reported (18,19). It therefore suggests that SERCA and the SR have a functional importance in the control of uterine contractility in pregnancy, but little detail is known about this.

Release of Ca^{2+} from uterine SR has been demonstrated in both human and animal myometrium (20,21). The uterine SR has two types of Ca^{2+}-release channels; the inositol 1,4,5-trisphosphate (IP_3) receptors (IP_3R) which are activated by agonists that stimulate IP_3 production, but are also modulated by Ca^{2+}, and ryanodine receptors (RyR), which are activated by an increase in the local [Ca^{2+}] but can be pharmacologically manipulated by caffeine or ryanodine. As to whether there are distinct pools of releasable intracellular Ca^{2+} within the SR and preferred Ca^{2+} release sites (hot spots) is the subject of on-going research and is discussed in details elsewhere in this book (see Chapter 86).

IP_3Rs play a central role in the mobilization of Ca^{2+} by agonists in a variety of cell types. Stimulation by agonists leads to the formation of IP_3 and diacylglycerol (DAG) from the hydrolysis of phosphoinositide-bisphosphate (PIP_2) (see Figure 90.3). The major effect of IP_3 is to trigger Ca^{2+} release from the SR via the IP_3Rs. Direct measurements of SR Ca^{2+} have shown a decrease in luminal content when IP_3-generating agonists are applied, followed by a rapid, SERCA-dependent re-uptake of Ca into the SR (22). No changes occurred during spontaneous activity, although intracellular [Ca^{2+}] rises considerably. There are three IP_3R isoforms (types 1–3) with different sensitivities to IP_3 and Ca^{2+} and all three have been found in non-pregnant and pregnant myometrium. There is no evidence to suggest that receptor isoform expression alters in labor, and thus the functional significance for expressing different IP_3Rs in the uterus, or indeed other smooth muscles, remains unclear.

All three types of RyRs have also been demonstrated in the uterus. However, based upon measurements of Ca^{2+} and force in a variety of species, RyRs in the intact myometrium appear to have very little, if any, effect on function (21,23). This conundrum was recently made less puzzling by the discovery that myometrial cells express a splice variant of RyR that is non-functional, i.e. does not transport Ca^{2+}, and which also acts as a dominant negative, inhibiting activity of RyR (24). This also explains why Ca-induced Ca release (CICR), a prominent process in cardiac muscle, is absent in intact myometrium. Furthermore the small SR Ca^{2+}-release events known as Ca^{2+} sparks, which arise from RyRs, and have been shown to activate Ca^{2+}-sensitive, large conductance (BK_{Ca}) K^+ channels, are also absent in the myometrium (see Chapter 86). In addition, although BK_{Ca} channels are expressed in the uterus, their contribution to K^+ efflux in the myometrium is now thought not to be of major importance, as their inhibition has little functional effect (25). Thus the Ca^{2+} sparks-STOCs feedback mechanism is not apparent in myometrium.

It is known that the SR limits uterine contraction under normal physiological conditions. Thus Ca^{2+} signaling and contractility are increased if SR Ca^{2+} release is inhibited, whilst inhibition of SERCA using cyclopiazonic acid (CPA) is associated with enhancement of uterine activity and increased Ca^{2+} signals (26). The mechanism is currently unknown but we speculate it may be that low luminal levels of SR Ca^{2+} may cause cation entry through store or receptor operated channels.

Ca^{2+} Efflux

As discussed above, studies of SR structure and localization within uterine myocytes has shown there to be a close apposition between the SR and the plasma membrane. This facilitates the activities of the membrane bound NCX and PMCA. The Ca^{2+} taken up into the SR can be released into the sub-plasmalemmal space and then extruded from the cell, by a process termed "vectorial Ca^{2+} release". The SR therefore contributes to the decay of the myometrial Ca^{2+} signal, as well as aiding relaxation by maintaining low [Ca^{2+}] in the myocytes at rest. Further details on Ca^{2+} efflux can be found in Floyd and Wray (27).

Caveolae and Ca^{2+} Signaling

The Ω-shaped caveolae are cholesterol-rich inpocketings containing the protein caveolin (see Chapter 83) which are present in high density in the myometrial plasma membrane (28). The uterine caveolae have been shown to be involved in a number of signaling pathways in the myometrium, including the integration of extracellular signals with intracellular effectors such as during agonist-induced contraction. Many cell signaling components, including elements of Ca^{2+} signaling, and BK_{Ca} are located within these cholesterol-rich microdomains.

All three isoforms of caveolin have been identified in the uterus and caveolae may increase in number towards the end of pregnancy as well as be hormonally regulated (29). The estrogen receptor is thought to localize to caveolae and the oxytocin receptor (OTR, discussed later) is also targeted to lipid rafts and caveolae. The activity of OTR is reduced if lipid rafts are disrupted. Gimpl et al. (30) suggest that the receptor exists in a high affinity state only when located to caveolae, suggesting that oxytocin binding is dependent upon the cholesterol content of the membrane.

Disruption of uterine caveolae using methyl-β-cyclodextrin (to sequester cholesterol from membranes) causes increased phasic contractions and increased Ca^{2+} signaling (31–33). Studies of rat myometrium showed this to be mediated through BK_{Ca} channel activity. Depletion of cholesterol caused decreased membrane capacitance, receptor internalization and reduced the outward K^+ current. Therefore in the uterus, BK_{Ca} channel activity is regulated in part by incorporation or exclusion into membrane caveolae and thus, in turn, is sensitive to changes in membrane cholesterol. A change in myometrial membrane cholesterol content therefore has direct consequences for myometrial function; elevated myometrial cholesterol is inhibitory towards force (31–33).

EFFECTS OF FEMALE HORMONES ON THE MYOMETRIUM

The spontaneous contractile activity of uterine smooth muscle can be altered by nervous but primarily hormonal activity via a number of mechanisms that may be excitatory or inhibitory. Hormones may directly affect the underlying myogenic mechanisms producing contraction, i.e. alter the frequency and duration of action potentials, or modulate $[Ca^{2+}]_I$, i.e. by affecting Ca^{2+} entry/efflux/SR release, as well as initiating other signaling pathways that can influence force. Changes during the estrous cycle have been the subject of a recent review and are not discussed further (28). Although many agents may be able to produce some effects on the myometrium, the four main hormones to affect its function are: oxytocin, prostaglandins and estrogen, which are uterine stimulants, and progesterone, which is an inhibitor of myometrial contraction. We consider each of these next.

Oxytocin

Oxytocin (OT) is classically known for its stimulatory actions on myometrial contraction and having a key role in parturition (as well as roles in lactation and female behavior). Upon OT binding to its receptor, phospholipase-C β is activated, which hydrolyses phosphatidylinositol bisphosphate (PIP_2) leading to the formation of two second messengers: IP_3 and diacylglycerol (DAG). As discussed above, IP_3 leads to the mobilization of Ca^{2+} from the SR, whilst DAG can activate protein kinase C (see Figure 90.3), whose role in modulating myometrial contraction is not yet clear. Oxytocin also has a stimulatory effect upon Ca^{2+} entry as well as inhibition of Ca^{2+} efflux, and may inhibit MLCP. The net effect is a powerful enhancement of force and slowing relaxation. This can be seen in Figure 90.4(A) along with the requirement for Ca^{2+} influx (see Figure 90.4B).

In rodents OT is believed necessary to initiate and maintain labor. Oxytocin binding sites in myometrial membranes rapidly increase and there is a rapid increase in circulating OT concentration at the onset of delivery in rats. Interestingly, however, in the mouse, OT and OTR do not appear to be an essential part of labor onset or the process of parturition since OT and OTR null-mice deliver normally. This may, however, result from other pathways compensating for loss of OT. In humans,

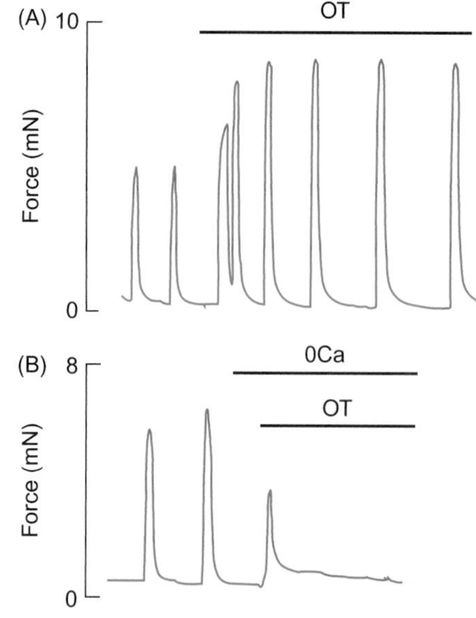

FIGURE 90.4 The stimulatory effect of oxytocin (OT, 10 nM) in the presence (A) and absence (B) of external Ca^{2+} on contractions in human myometrium. Application of OT in the presence of calcium causes significant increase in contraction amplitude, which persists for the duration of OT application. In the absence of extracellular calcium, OT is only capable of initiating one small contraction, indicating that Ca^{2+} influx is a major contributor to the stimulatory effect OT.

circulating OT does not seem essential in parturition as there is no good evidence for an increase in maternal OT concentrations with labor onset. Instead it is proposed that local (uterine or decidual) increases in OT initiate labor onset and that changes in the receptor expression or function, rather than the peptide, are important for labor onset (34). In the myometrial tissues of humans, OTR mRNA levels and OTR density increase at labor onset, which is thought to mediate an increase in sensitivity of the myometrium to oxytocin at term and produce direct contractile effects.

Prostaglandins (PGs)

PGs are bioactive lipids derived from arachidonic acid acting as signaling messengers for many biochemical pathways. Their availability within the different tissues depends upon the presence and activity of the different enzymes that convert their common precursor into the various end products. $PGF_{2\alpha}$ and PGE are the two major PGs known to modulate myometrial activity and play a central role in labor initiation and its progression in most mammalian species studied (35). Prostaglandins are also responsible for uterine contractions during menstruation. PGs have been shown to act in either a paracrine or autocrine manner, mediating their functions by binding to different G-protein-coupled receptors (GPCRs). PGF_{2a}

functions by increasing $[Ca^{2+}]_i$ thus allowing for greater acto-myosin cross-bridge cycling. This can be via IP_3-mediated SR Ca^{2+} release, increasing Ca^{2+} entry due to changes in action potential frequency and/or activation of non-specific cation-channels facilitating Ca^{2+} entry (36) and possibly by Ca^{2+} sensitization (15). PGE can cause relaxation of the myometrium as well as its contraction. This is because there are multiple (four) isoforms of its receptor, some of which couple to Ca^{2+} mobilization pathways or participate in downregulating inhibitory pathways and are therefore uterotonic, whilst other receptors stimulate pathways involving cAMP and protein kinase A, which are relaxatory in the uterus.

Estrogen

Estrogen is known for its role during the menstrual cycle where its levels are highest before ovulation. It increases the motility of the Fallopian tubes, potentially aiding conception, and also stimulates myometrial contractions. In particular, towards the end of pregnancy, estrogen is thought to increase expression of gap junction proteins to facilitate cell–cell coupling and increase responsiveness of the uterus to oxytocin. In most mammals parturition is associated with increasing circulating estrogen levels. However, in humans, serum estrogen levels remain high throughout pregnancy with some evidence to suggest that they increase towards term and are greatest in the final few weeks before labor. Despite the expression of the estrogen receptor (ERα) being increased in the myometrium from laboring women, there is no difference in estrogen levels before and during labor. As with oxytocin, this suggests a functional activation of estrogen rather than changes in the circulating hormone levels *per se*.

Progesterone

The steroid hormone progesterone is known as being a "progestational" agent having a significant role in the myometrium in maintaining the pregnant state and promoting myometrial quiescence. Progesterone also has a role during the menstrual cycle where it inhibits uterine contraction and so encourages implantation. The primary action of progesterone is thought to be mediated by its interaction with the intracellular nuclear progesterone receptor (nPR). Recently, however, there is evidence to support a role for plasma membrane progesterone receptors (mPR) (37,38). As a steroid hormone, one of the main actions of progesterone is to alter gene expression and bring about long-term changes in the contractile phenotype of the myometrium. *In vitro*, progesterone is known to have direct effects on the ECC pathway by directly modulating $[Ca^{2+}]_I$, e.g. by inhibiting Ca^{2+} entry and SR Ca^{2+} release, as well as causing membrane hyperpolarization via activation of K^+ channels.

The pregnant myometrium is often described as being under a progesterone "block" and it is argued that progesterone withdrawal is a prerequisite of pregnancy termination. In species that depend upon the corpus luteum as the principal source of progesterone, e.g. rats, rabbits, mice, circulating levels of progesterone fall shortly before the onset of labor due to the degradation of the corpus luteum. In humans, however, no decrease in maternal circulating progesterone levels is observed and progesterone remains high even during labor until the placenta is expelled. Administration of the progesterone receptor (PR) antagonist mifepristone (RU486), can be used to induce labor by softening the cervix and increasing uterine sensitivity to uterotonic agents (39), suggesting that progesterone withdrawal does have some role in the onset of human parturition. In the absence of a fall in circulating progesterone, it has been suggested that a "functional progesterone withdrawal" precedes labor onset in humans. This functional withdrawal has been postulated to occur through several mechanisms that decrease progesterone activity, including local metabolism of progesterone, altered expression of the different forms of PR, changes in PR cofactor expression and antagonism of the PR receptor by nuclear factor κB (NF-κB) (38).

PARTURITION

Labor is a state in which the uterus contracts frequently and forcefully and is a process whereby the products of conception (fetus, placenta, and membranes) are expelled from the genital tract. Classically, the process of labor is divided into three stages: first stage, from the onset of uterine contractions to full dilation of the cervix; second stage, from full dilation of the cervix and ending with delivery of the fetus; and the third stage, which ends with the delivery of the placenta. The myometrium plays a fundamental role in each of the three stages. However, the events of pregnancy leading to parturition begin many weeks beforehand, which for the uterus, begins with a period of adaptation to pregnancy. This is a period characterized by significant development and differentiation of the uterine myocytes involving significant hyperplasia followed by hypertrophy.

Importantly, during pregnancy the uterus is maintained in a relatively quiescent state to allow for fetal growth and development. Low level expression of gap junctions between smooth muscle cells provided inefficient cell-to-cell coupling and there is minimal contractile activity in the uterine smooth muscle as gestation progresses, despite the influence of stretch. However, the somewhat "relaxed" uterus must transition to an active state, with the ability to generate labor contractions of sufficient power to deliver the fetus. The ability of the myometrium to propagate its electrical activity is a prerequisite for the effectiveness of these labor contractions. This transitional period involves a shift in the components favoring myometrial relaxation to components of the contraction pathways.

In 1994, Challis and Lye proposed a unifying hypothesis that as labor approaches, a group or cassette of genes encoding key "contraction-associated proteins" (CAPs) in the myometrium, is activated. CAPs are necessary to augment the response to uterotonins including oxytocin and prostaglandins, to initiate excitation and increase the frequency and amplitude of myometrial contractions (40). CAPs identified and best characterized include: the oxytocin receptor (OTR), corticotrophin-releasing hormone (CRH) receptor, gap junction protein connexin43 (Cx43), and the cyclo-oxygenase (COX)-2 enzyme responsible for the synthesis of PGs. Upregulation of these genes is thought to shift the balance in the myometrium from the components of the relaxatory system towards components of the contractile pathways. Changes in the functional activity of a number of ion channels and Ca^{2+} homeostatic mechanisms are also likely to be involved in the increased contractile activity in labor (4,18).

It is believed that a combination of hormonal, chemical, and mechanical signals interact gradually to downregulate quiescent mechanisms and upregulate contractile pathways as term and delivery approaches. Uterine stimulants such as prostaglandins and oxytocin (discussed above) also aid forceful, rhythmic, and regular uterine contractions and the initiation of labor onset. These hormones are often used clinically to aid cervical dilation and augment slowly progressing labors. Following parturition there is a period of involution, which involves extensive myometrial tissue remodeling.

Problems in Labor Associated with Smooth Muscle

The regulation of myometrial contraction is of absolute importance for maintenance of pregnancy and for parturition. Disruption of these processes can lead to complications such as preterm labor where contractions occur too early in pregnancy, or dystocia, where contractions are un-coordinated and of poor power (see Figure 90.5). Dysfunctional (dystocic) labor is estimated to affect up to 4% of all labors but is more common in first labors (10%). It is the most common cause of emergency Cesarean section delivery. The only treatment of dystocia is administration of oxytocin; however this is only effective in around 50% of labors.

The most likely cause of inefficient uterine contractions is due to underlying abnormalities within the cellular and molecular components of the uterine myocytes. This may reflect either a lack of adequate stimulation to contract or the presence of a strong inhibitory control over contraction, whist defective intracellular signaling and propagation of contractions as well as changes in myometrial pH are thought to also contribute to weaker, uncoordinated myometrial contractions and labor dystocia (41,42). Quenby et al. found that women laboring dysfunctionally had a more acidic (lactic acid) uterine environment than women laboring normally, with acidification linked to myometrial hypoxia (43). Measurement of high lactic acid (lactate) in amniotic fluid may be predictive of dysfunctional labor (44).

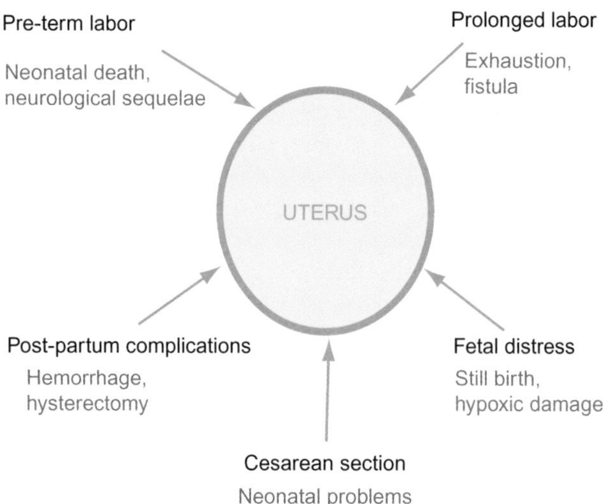

FIGURE 90.5 Schematic to show complications of labor and their associated risks, all of which can result from aberrant uterine activity.

Post-partum hemorrhage is also associated with poor uterine contractility. After delivery of the placenta, the uterus must shift to a more tonic or maintained level of contraction to clamp on blood vessels and allow clotting to occur. This can be induced by uterotonic drugs, usually ergometrine derivatives or prostaglandins.

Prevention of pre-term delivery is the focus of much research as its consequences can be so devastating; it is the largest killer of newborn babies in the developed world. There is a consensus that some events can trigger the parturition cascade, e.g. infection and over-distension of the uterus, such as that which occurs in multiple births, but very many cases are of unknown etiology. Blockers and competitors of L-type Ca^{2+} channels, β_2-mimetics and progesterone form the mainstay of pharmacologic approaches used in clinical practice today (45). If we had a better understanding of uterine pacemaking and ECC, we might be better placed to tackle this aberrant uterine activation.

CONCLUSIONS

In this chapter we have given an overview of our increased understanding of myometrial physiology. The complexity of studying a smooth muscle that undergoes fundamental functional changes and is regulated by both hormonal and mechanical interplay means that there remains much to do before we fully understand these processes. The goals of improving fertility, reducing conditions such as endometriosis and recurrent miscarriage and improving labor outcome for women and babies, mean that increased resource and effort are urgently required. We would highlight at the basic science end the need to understand how myogenic/pacemaking activity arises, what cellular changes occur to trigger labor and elucidation of SR function, to be a critical questions to be resolved. The development of better tocolytics and a reduction in pre-term delivery should follow from this, as the most important clinical priority.

REFERENCES

1. Wray S. Uterine contraction and physiological mechanisms of modulation. *Am J Physiol* 1993;**264**:C1–18.
2. Burdyga T, Wray S, Noble K. In situ calcium signaling: no calcium sparks detected in rat myometrium. *Ann NY Acad Sci* 2007;**1101**:85–96.
3. Garfield RE, Sims S, Daniel EE. Gap junctions: their presence and necessity in myometrium during parturition. *Science* 1977;**198**: 958–60.
4. Sanborn BM. Relationship of ion channel activity to control of myometrial calcium. *J Soc Gynecol Invest* 2000;**7**:4–11.
5. Parkington HC, Tonta MA, Brennecke SP, Coleman HA. Contractile activity, membrane potential, and cytoplasmic calcium in human uterine smooth muscle in the third trimester of pregnancy and during labor. *Am J Obstet Gynecol* 1999;**181**:1445–51.
6. Khan RN, Matharoo-Ball B, Arulkumaran S, Ashford ML. Potassium channels in the human myometrium. *Exp Physiol* 2001;**86**:255–64.
7. Burdyga T, Borisova L, Burdyga AT, Wray S. Temporal and spatial variations in spontaneous Ca events and mechanical activity in pregnant rat myometrium. *Eur J Obstet Gynecol Reprod Biol* 2009;**144**(Suppl. 1):S25–32.
8. Sergeant GP, Hollywood MA, McCloskey KD, Thornbury KD, McHale NG. Specialised pacemaking cells in the rabbit urethra. *J Physiol* 2000;**526**(Pt2):359–66.
9. Duquette RA, Shmygol A, Vaillant C, Mobasheri A, Pope M, Burdyga T, et al. Vimentin-positive, c-kit-negative interstitial cells in human and rat uterus: a role in pacemaking? *Biol Reprod* 2005;**72**:276–83.
10. Wray S, Jones K, Kupittayanant S, Li Y, Matthew A, Monir-Bishty E, et al. Calcium signaling and uterine contractility. *J Soc Gynecol Invest* 2003;**10**:252–64.
11. Shmygol A, Blanks AM, Bru-Mercier G, Gullam JE, Thornton S. Control of uterine Ca^{2+} by membrane voltage: toward understanding the excitation-contraction coupling in human myometrium. *Ann NY Acad Sci* 2007;**1101**:97–109.
12. Young RC, Smith LH, McLaren MD. T-type and L-type calcium currents in freshly dispersed human uterine smooth muscle cells. *Am J Obstet Gynecol* 1993;**169**:785–92.
13. Longbottom ER, Luckas MJ, Kupittayanant S, Badrick E, Shmigol T, Wray S. The effects of inhibiting myosin light chain kinase on contraction and calcium signaling in human and rat myometrium. *Pflugers Arch* 2000;**440**:315–21.
14. Somlyo AP, Somlyo AV. Signal transduction by G-proteins, rho-kinase and protein phosphatase to smooth muscle and non-muscle myosin II. *J Physiol* 2000;**522**(Pt 2):177–85.
15. Woodcock NA, Taylor CW, Thornton S. Prostaglandin F2alpha increases the sensitivity of the contractile proteins to Ca^{2+} in human myometrium. *Am J Obstet Gynecol* 2006;**195**:1404–6.
16. Crichton CA, Taggart MJ, Wray S, Smith GL. Effects of pH and inorganic phosphate on force production in alpha-toxin-permeabilized isolated rat uterine smooth muscle. *J Physiol* 1993;**465**: 629–45.
17. Kupittayanant S, Burdyga T, Wray S. The effects of inhibiting Rho-associated kinase with Y-27632 on force and intracellular calcium in human myometrium. *Pflugers Arch* 2001;**443**:112–4.
18. Tribe RM, Moriarty P, Poston L. Calcium homeostatic pathways change with gestation in human myometrium. *Biol Reprod* 2000;**63**:748–55.
19. Khan I, Tabb T, Garfield RE, Jones LR, Fomin VP, Samson SE, et al. Expression of the internal calcium pump in pregnant rat uterus. *Cell Calcium* 1993;**14**:111–7.
20. Luckas MJ, Taggart MJ, Wray S. Intracellular calcium stores and agonist-induced contractions in isolated human myometrium. *Am J Obstet Gynecol* 1999;**181**:468–76.
21. Taggart MJ, Wray S. Contribution of sarcoplasmic reticular calcium to smooth muscle contractile activation: gestational dependence in isolated rat uterus. *J Physiol* 1998;**511**(Pt 1):133–44.
22. Shmygol A, Wray S. Modulation of agonist-induced Ca^{2+} release by SR Ca^{2+} load: direct SR and cytosolic Ca^{2+} measurements in rat uterine myocytes. *Cell Calcium* 2005;**37**:215–23.
23. Noble K, Matthew A, Burdyga T, Wray S. A review of recent insights into the role of the sarcoplasmic reticulum and Ca entry in uterine smooth muscle. *Eur J Obstet Gynecol Reprod Biol* 2009;**144**(Suppl. 1):S11–9.
24. Dabertrand F, Fritz N, Mironneau J, Macrez N, Morel JL. Role of RYR3 splice variants in calcium signaling in mouse nonpregnant and pregnant myometrium. *Am J Physiol Cell Physiol* 2007;**293**: C848–54.
25. Noble K, Floyd R, Shmygol A, Mobasheri A, Wray S. Distribution, expression and functional effects of small conductance Ca-activated potassium (SK) channels in rat myometrium. *Cell Calcium* 2010;**47**:47–54.
26. Kupittayanant S, Luckas MJ, Wray S. Effect of inhibiting the sarcoplasmic reticulum on spontaneous and oxytocin-induced contractions of human myometrium. *Br J Obstet Gynecol* 2002;**109**: 289–96.
27. Floyd R, Wray S. Calcium transporters and signaling in smooth muscles. *Cell Calcium* 2007;**42**:467–76.
28. Wray S, Noble K. Sex hormones and excitation-contraction coupling in the uterus: the effects of oestrous and hormones. *J Neuroendocrinol* 2008;**20**:451–61.
29. Turi A, Kiss AL, Mullner N. Estrogen downregulates the number of caveolae and the level of caveolin in uterine smooth muscle. *Cell Biol Int* 2001;**25**:785–94.

30. Gimpl G, Burger K, Fahrenholz F. Cholesterol as modulator of receptor function. *Biochemistry* 1997;**36**:10959–74.
31. Smith RD, Babiychuk EB, Noble K, Draeger A, Wray S. Increased cholesterol decreases uterine activity: functional effects of cholesterol alteration in pregnant rat myometrium. *Am J Physiol Cell Physiol* 2005;**288**:C982–8.
32. Shmygol A, Noble K, Wray S. Depletion of membrane cholesterol eliminates the Ca^{2+}-activated component of outward potassium current and decreases membrane capacitance in rat uterine myocytes. *J Physiol* 2007;**581**:445–56.
33. Zhang JZ, Kendrick A, Quenby S, Wray S. Contractility and calcium signaling of human myometrium are profoundly affected by cholesterol manipulation: implications for labor? *Reprod Sci* 2007;**14**:456–66.
34. Blanks AM, Thornton S. The role of oxytocin in parturition. *Br J Obstet Gynecol* 2003;**110**(Suppl. 20):46–51.
35. Challis JRG, Matthews SG, Gibb W, Lye SJ. Endocrine and paracrine regulation of birth at term and preterm. *Endocr Rev* 2000;**21**:514–50.
36. Hertelendy F, Zakar T. Prostaglandins and the myometrium and cervix. *Prostaglandins Leukot Essent Fatty Acids* 2004;**70**:207–22.
37. Gellersen B, Fernandes MS, Brosens JJ. Non-genomic progesterone actions in female reproduction. *Hum Reprod Update* 2009;**15**: 119–38.
38. Mesiano S, Welsh TN. Steroid hormone control of myometrial contractility and parturition. *Semin Cell Dev Biol* 2007;**18**:321–31.
39. Hapangama D, Neilson JP. Mifepristone for induction of labor. *Cochrane Database Syst Rev* 2009; CD002865
40. Challis JRG. Mechanism of parturition and preterm labor. *Obstet Gynecol Surv* 2000;**55**:650–60.
41. Parratt J, Taggart M, Wray S. Abolition of contractions in the myometrium by acidification in vitro. *Lancet* 1994;**344**:717–8.
42. Garfield RE. Cellular and molecular bases for dystocia. *Clin Obstet Gynecol* 1987;**30**:3–18.
43. Quenby S, Pierce SJ, Brigham S, Wray S. Dysfunctional labor and myometrial lactic acidosis. *Obstet Gynecol* 2004;**103**:718–23.
44. Wiberg-Itzel E, Pettersson H, Andolf E, Hansson A, Winbladh B, Akerud H. Lactate concentration in amniotic fluid: a good predictor of labor outcome. *Eur J Obstet Gynecol Reprod Biol* 2010;**152**:34–8.
45. Arrowsmith S, Kendrick A, Wray S. Drugs acting on the pregnant uterus. *Obstet, Gynaecol Reprod Med* 2010;**20**:241–7.

Section C

Adaptations and Response

Chapter 91

Oxidative Stress, Endothelial Dysfunction, and Its Impact on Smooth Muscle Signaling

Thomas Münzel and Tommaso Gori
II Medical Clinic for Cardiology and Angiology, Mainz, Germany

INTRODUCTION

The role traditionally attributed to the vascular endothelium was that of a selective barrier to prevent the indiscriminate diffusion of macromolecules from the vessel lumen to the interstitial space. During the past twenty years, numerous additional roles have been identified such as regulation of vascular tone, modulation of inflammation, promotion as well as inhibition of vascular growth and modulation of platelet aggregation and coagulation. Endothelial dysfunction is a characteristic feature of patients with coronary atherosclerosis. Although the mechanisms underlying endothelial dysfunction are likely very complex and multifactorial, there is a growing body of evidence that increased production of reactive oxygen species (ROS) may contribute considerably to this phenomenon. ROS production has been demonstrated to occur in the endothelial cell layer, but also within the media and adventitia, all of which may impair nitric oxide (NO) signaling within vascular tissues, and therefore the vascular reactivity in response to endothelium-dependent, but also endothelium independent, vasodilators. This review will briefly address mechanisms underlying endothelial dysfunction with focus on oxidative stress, and, finally, the prognostic implications of endothelial dysfunction.

THE L-ARGININE/NO/CGMP PATHWAY IN VASCULAR TISSUE

The endothelium, a single-layered continuous cell sheet lining the luminal vessel wall, separates the intravascular (blood) from the interstitial compartment and the vascular smooth muscle. Our understanding of the role of this tissue in cardiovascular regulation completely changed with the discovery of endothelial autacoids like prostacyclin (PGI_2) (1) and NO (2), as well as with the discovery of integrins and other surface signals (3). It is now evident that the endothelium is not only a means of communication between blood and tissue cells, and that it actively controls the function of surrounding cells by a plethora of signaling routes. One of the prominent signaling lines is established by the so-called L-arginine-NO-cyclic GMP pathway (4). This molecular cascade starts with endothelial NO synthase (eNOS, NOSIII), which generates NO and L-citrulline from L-arginine and O_2 in response to receptor-dependent agonists (bradykinin, acetylcholine, ATP) and physicochemical stimuli (shear, stretch) (5) (Figure 91.1).

NO diffuses to the adjacent smooth muscle where it interacts with different receptor molecules, of which the soluble guanylyl cyclase (sGC) is the best characterized and presumably most important one with regard to control of vessel tone and smooth muscle proliferation. Activation by NO requires sGC heme-iron to be in the ferrous (II) state. Upon binding with NO, cGMP formation increases substantially. cGMP activates the cGMP-dependent kinase I which in turn increases the open probability of Ca^{2+}-activated $K^+(B_K)$-channels, thereby inducing a hyperpolarization of the smooth muscle cells and inhibition of agonist-induced Ca^{2+} influx. In addition, activated cGK-Iβ phosphorylates the inositol trisphosphate (IP_3)-receptor-associated G-kinase substrate (IRAG), thereby inhibiting agonist-induced Ca^{2+} release and smooth muscle contraction. Another cGK-I substrate found in many cell types is the 46/50 kD vasodilator-stimulated phosphoprotein (VASP). cGK-I phosphorylates VASP specifically at serine 239, and this reaction can be exploited as a biochemical monitor for the integrity and activity of the NO-cGMP pathway (6).

Muscle. DOI: http://dx.doi.org/10.1016/B978-0-12-381510-1.00091-0

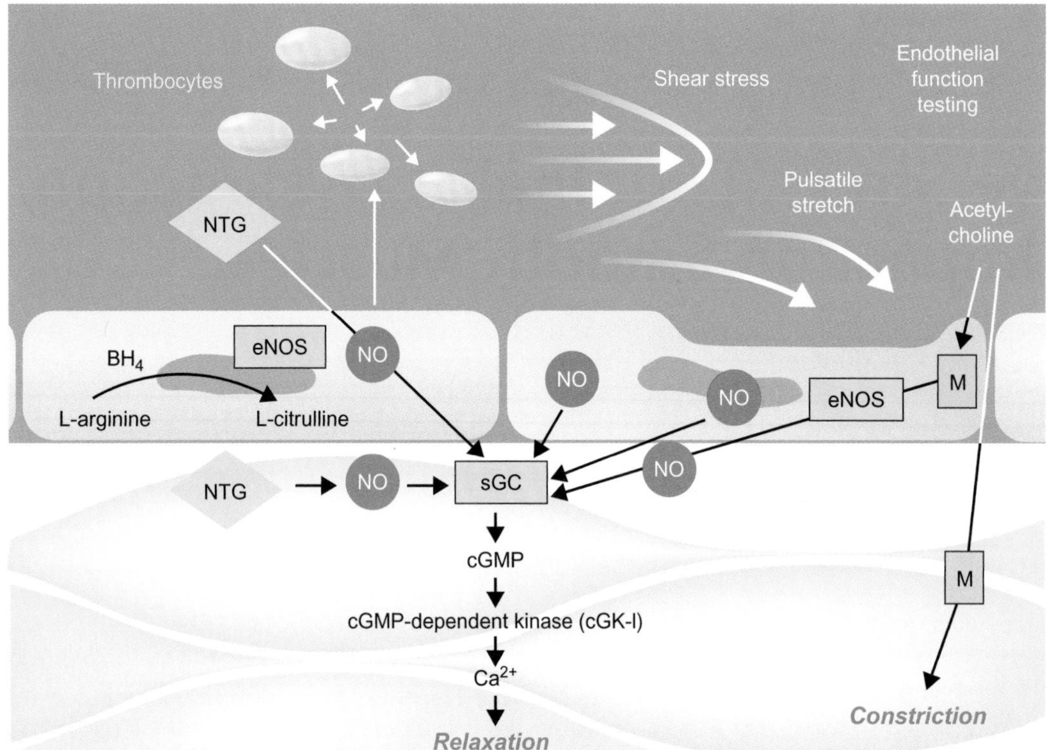

FIGURE 91.1 **Regulation of vascular tone by the endothelium.** The endothelial nitric oxide synthase (eNOS) synthesizes NO by a two-step oxidation of the amino acid L-arginine thereby leading to the formation of L-citrulline. NO is released into the bloodstream thereby inhibiting platelet aggregation and the release of vasoconstricting factors such as ADP and thromboxane. NO diffuses also into the media and activates the soluble guanylate cyclase (sGC). The resulting second messenger cGMP in turn activates the cGMP-dependent kinase, which mediates decreases in intracellular Ca^{2+} concentrations thereby causing vasorelaxation. The physiological stimuli to release NO are shear stress and pulsatile stretch. Intraarterial infusion is used in the clinics to assess endothelial function. Infused into the forearm (brachial artery) ACh causes a dose-dependent vasodilation. In the coronary artery the response (vasoconstriction vs. vasodilation) strictly depends on the functional integrity of the endothelium. In the presence of cardiovascular risk factors and endothelial dysfunction ACh will cause vasoconstriction due to stimulation of muscarinergic receptors in the media.

OXIDATIVE STRESS AND ENDOTHELIAL DYSFUNCTION

The endothelium-derived relaxing factor, which in the 1980s was identified as nitric oxide (NO) (2) or a closely related compound (7), has potent anti-atherosclerotic properties. NO released from endothelial cells works in concert with prostacyclin to inhibit platelet aggregation (8), the attachment of neutrophils to endothelial cells, and the expression of adhesion molecules. NO in high concentrations also inhibits the proliferation of smooth muscle cells (9). Therefore, it is our understanding that the process of atherosclerosis is initiated or accelerated under all conditions where an absolute or relative NO deficit is encountered. The half-life of NO and therefore its biological activity is decisively determined by the bioavailability of oxygen-derived free radicals such as superoxide (10), as these molecules rapidly react with NO to form the highly reactive intermediate peroxynitrite (ONOO) (11), thus quenching NO. The rapid bimolecular reaction (rate constant: $5-10 \times 10^9\,M^{-1}\,s^{-1}$) is about 3–4 times faster than the dismutation of superoxide by the superoxide dismutase, the enzyme that physiologically controls the vascular bioavailability of superoxide. In case of an excess superoxide production, peroxynitrite formation represents a major potential pathway. Peroxynitrite in high concentrations is cytotoxic and may cause oxidative damage to proteins, lipids, and DNA (12). Recent studies also indicate that peroxynitrite may have deleterious effects on activity and function of the prostacyclin synthase (13) and the endothelial NOS (14,15). Other ROS such as the dismutation product of superoxide, hydrogen peroxide, and hypochlorous acid released by activated neutrophils, are not free radicals, but have a powerful oxidizing capacity that will further contribute to oxidative stress within vascular tissues.

ENDOTHELIAL DYSFUNCTION AND CARDIOVASCULAR RISK FACTORS

Endothelial dysfunction is a common feature of cardiovascular diseases and is invariably found in the presence

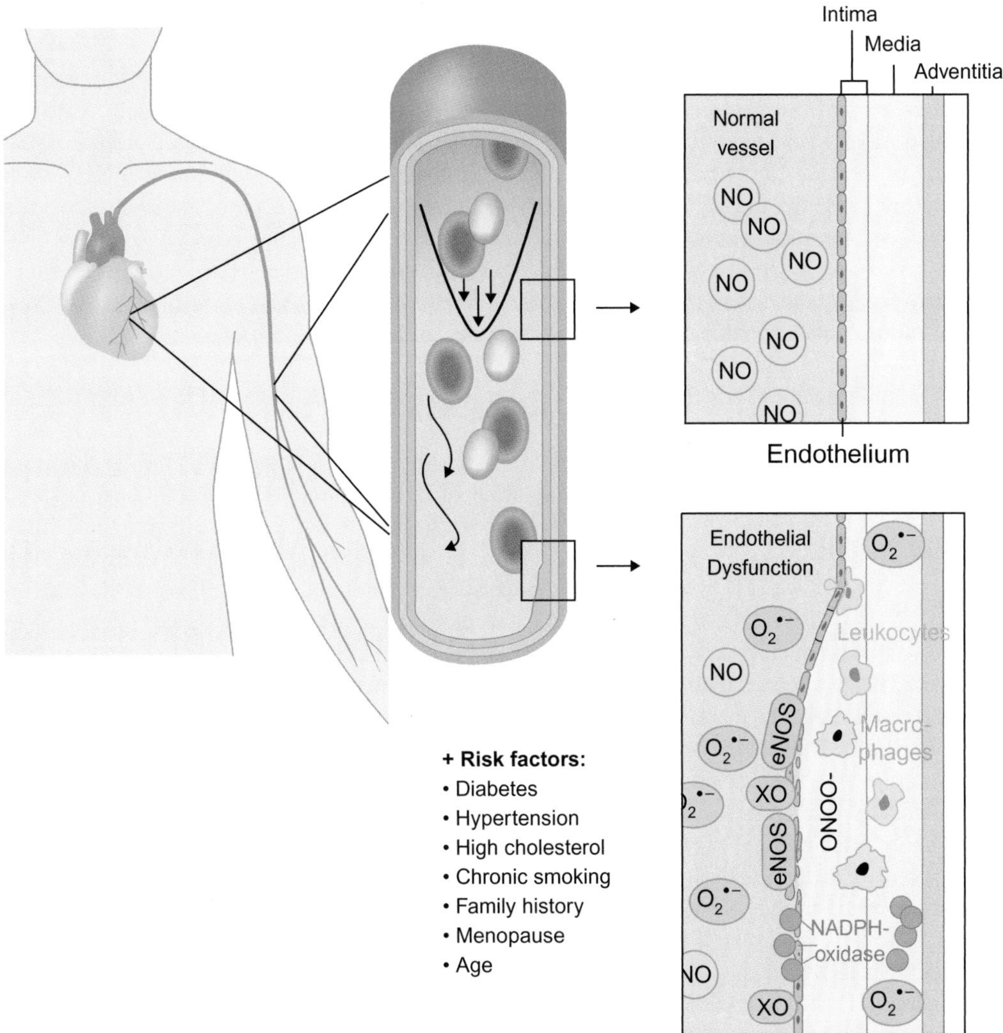

FIGURE 91.2 **Mechanisms underlying endothelial dysfunction and the functional consequences of decreased vascular bioavailability of nitric oxide (NO).** In the presence of cardiovascular risk factors such as smoking, hypertension, diabetes mellitus, age, menopause, familiar history of cardiovascular disease, and hypercholesterolemia, vascular superoxide producing enzymes such as the vascular NADPH oxidase, the xanthine oxidase (XO), and an uncoupled endothelial nitric oxide synthase (eNOS) produce large amounts of superoxide ($O_2^{\cdot-}$), which will metabolize NO. The consequences are increased production of the highly reactive intermediate peroxynitrite ($ONOO^-$) and subsequently adhesion and infiltration of the vascular wall with inflammatory cells such as macrophages and neutrophils and a subsequent intima proliferation. There are some reports demonstrating a close relationship between peripheral and coronary endothelial dysfunction (16).

of all cardiovascular risk factors (Figure 91.2). The list of diseases and conditions that are associated with endothelial dysfunction has now reached more than 200 entries, and impaired endothelium-dependent vasomotor function has been shown for chronic smokers, patients with increased LDL levels, for patients with diabetes type I and II, for hypertensive patients, and for patients with metabolic syndrome. It is important to note that cardiovascular risk factors synergistically impair endothelial function: for instance, we previously showed that chronic smoking causes an endothelial dysfunction that is as analogous to that caused by high LDL levels, but that the combination of both risk factors drastically impairs receptor-dependent increases in forearm blood flow in response to ACh.

What is the key mechanism underlying endothelial dysfunction in patients with cardiovascular risk factors or established coronary artery disease? There are several potential abnormalities that could account for reductions in endothelium-dependent vascular relaxation, including changes in the activity and/or expression of the eNOS, decreased sensitivity of vascular smooth muscle cells to NO, or increased degradation of NO via its interaction with ROS such as superoxide. Among different mechanisms, the concept that increased superoxide bioavailability might lead to NO degradation is the most convincing since in the presence of cardiovascular risk factors endothelial dysfunction is markedly improved by the acute administration of the antioxidant vitamin C (17–20). These findings provide support for the hypothesis that the source of the superoxide is the vasculature *per se*, and that this increased superoxide in turn reduces NO bioavailability by degrading NO and by forming the highly toxic NO/superoxide reaction product peroxynitrite. Among the other implications, this would also inhibit downstream signaling at the level of smooth muscle cells, as the activity of the soluble guanylate cyclase is reduced by oxidation of its Fe^{2+} to the Fe^{3+}, thereby making sGC nonresponsive to NO (21).

VASCULAR SUPEROXIDE SOURCES

Role of the NADPH-Oxidase

The NADPH-oxidase is a superoxide-producing enzyme first characterized in neutrophils (22) and whose activity in endothelial as well as smooth muscle cells is increased upon stimulation with angiotensin II (23). Thus, in the presence of an activated renin-angiotensin system (local or circulating), vascular dysfunction due to increased vascular superoxide production is likely to be expected. Interestingly, there is growing body of evidence that the local renin-angiotensin system is activated in the setting of hypercholesterolemia. In vessels from hypercholesterolemic animals (24) as well as in platelets from hypercholesterolemic patients (25), there is an increase in the expression of the angiotensin II receptor subtype AT_1. Experimental hypercholesterolemia has been shown to be associated with an activation of the NADPH-oxidase (24) and the activity of this enzyme in human saphenous veins in patients with coronary artery disease (26) varies according to the presence of risk factors and in parallel with endothelial function. In atherosclerotic arteries, there is evidence that expression of the NADPH-oxidase subunit gp91phox and nox4 is particularly pronounced in the shoulder of atherosclerotic plaques, all of which may trigger a plaque rupture (27).

Thus, both experimental and clinical studies have provided evidence for stimulation of the renin-angiotensin system in atherosclerosis and simultaneously for an activation of the NADPH-oxidase in the arterial wall. Similar evidence for an activation of this enzyme in the vasculature has been provided from experimental animal models of different forms of hypertension such as angiotensin II infusion (28,29) and in spontaneously hypertensive rats (30) as well as in different forms of diabetes mellitus (31).

The proof of concept that superoxide produced by the NADPH-oxidase may indeed trigger eNOS uncoupling was provided by Harrison's group in the experimental animal model of desoxycorticosterone acetate (DOCA)-salt hypertension (32). With these studies the authors showed that superoxide-induced by DOCA-salt treatment caused increased vascular superoxide production, which was significantly reduced by an inhibitor of eNOS such as L-NAME. Treatment of p47phox knockout animals with DOCA-salt caused markedly reduced levels of oxidative stress and abolished superoxide effects of NOS inhibition compatible with a prevention of eNOS uncoupling (32).

Role of the Xanthine Oxidase

Xanthine oxido-reductase catalyzes the sequential hydroxylation of hypoxanthine to yield xanthine and uric acid. The enzyme can exist in two forms that differ primarily in their oxidizing substrate specificity. The dehydrogenase form preferentially utilizes NAD^+ as an electron acceptor but is also able to donate electrons to molecular oxygen. By proteolytic breakdown as well as thiol oxidation xanthine dehydrogenase from mammalian sources can be converted to the oxidase form that readily donates electrons to molecular oxygen, thereby producing superoxide and hydrogen peroxide, but does not reduce NAD^+. Compatible with an increase in the expression or activity of xanthine oxidase in early hypercholesterolemia, oxypurinol, an inhibitor of xanthine oxidoreductase, has been shown to reduce superoxide production and to improve endothelium-dependent vascular relaxations to acetylcholine in vessels from hyperlipidemic animals (33). The mechanisms underlying such a phenomenon remain unclear, however it has been demonstrated that certain cytokines can stimulate the expression of xanthine oxidase by the endothelium, or alternatively, that increased cholesterol levels may cause the release of xanthine oxidase (e.g. from the liver) into the circulation where it binds to endothelial glycosaminoglycans (34). The results of human studies concerning the efficacy of xanthine oxidase inhibition on endothelial dysfunction are somewhat contradictory. While Panza et al. (35,36) showed that endothelial dysfunction in hypercholesterolemic patients and hypertensive diabetics is improved by acute inhibition of xanthine oxidase with oxypurinol and allopurinol, other groups failed to show similar efficacy for allopurinol (37). Its role in mediating increased oxidative stress in the setting of hypertension is not quite clear. Oxypurinol has blood pressure-lowering effects comparable to heparin binding superoxide dismutase in spontaneously hypertensive rats (38), but fails to demonstrate a positive effect on endothelial dysfunction in hypertensive patients (35). More recent studies in patients with chronic congestive heart failure clearly failed to demonstrate any prognostic benefit when oxypurinol was added to conventional heart failure treatment (39).

Uncoupled eNOS

The coenzyme tetrahydrobiopterin (BH_4) appears to be essential for the function of the NOS as it stabilizes the NOS dimer and it increases the affinity of NOS for L-arginine. Limited availability of BH_4 will inevitably result in increased superoxide formation at the expense of NO formation, i.e. it will uncouple NOS.

Whether BH_4 depletion occurs *in vivo* is a more complex question. *In vitro* studies proposed that native LDL (40) and oxidized LDL (41) are able to stimulate endothelial superoxide production and that this phenomenon is inhibited by the NOS inhibitor L-NAME, suggesting NOS uncoupling in this setting, possibly associated with peroxynitrite-induced oxidation of BH_4 to inactive molecules such as BH_2 (42,43) or to a BH3-radical (15). Thus, NOS uncoupling might require a priming event such as superoxide produced by the NADPH oxidase and/or the xanthine oxidase (so-called "kindling radicals") leading via increased formation of peroxynitrite to eNOS uncoupling.

Notably, reduced pteridines *per se* have strong antioxidant properties, and it has been argued that nonspecific superoxide scavenging effects, rather than a specific regeneration of the coenzyme activity, might be responsible for the improvement in endothelial function associated with the administration of BH_4. To address this issue Heitzer et al. (44) tested *in vitro* the antioxidant capacity of BH_4 and tetrahydroneoptrin on superoxide produced *in vitro* via the xanthine/xanthine oxidase reaction. Although both compounds quenched the superoxide signal to a similar extent *in vitro*, BH_4, but not NH_4, improved endothelial dysfunction in chronic smokers suggesting that indeed prevention of eNOS uncoupling rather than nonspecific antioxidant effects of BH_4 represents the underlying mechanism of the reversal of endothelial dysfunction (44).

The mechanism underlying eNOS uncoupling have recently been discussed in detail (for review see 45). Other studies have established the crucial role of the BH_4 synthesizing enzyme GTP-cyclohydrolase I. Indeed in the setting of diabetes mellitus, nitrate tolerance and angiotensin II hypertension, this BH_4 regenerating enzyme is downregulated, leading to eNOS uncoupling. Pharmacological interventions such as statins or AT1-receptor blockers were able to upregulate the activity and expression of the enzyme and to recouple the eNOS.

Mitochondria

The mitochondrial respiratory chain is a major source of superoxide, which may then be converted to H_2O_2. Molecular O_2 serves as the final electron acceptor for the cytochrome C oxidase complex (IV), the terminal component of the respiratory chain and is ultimately reduced to H_2O_2. Up to 1−4% of O_2 may be incompletely reduced, resulting in O_2^-, mainly at complex I and complex III of the respiratory chain. In the presence of transitional metal ions, the toxic hydroxyl radicals ($OH^\cdot$) radicals may be also formed. Several conditions where metabolism is altered, such as in hyperglycemia or in the presence of high levels of the adipokinine leptin, appear to be associated with mitochondrial uncoupling and increased O_2^- formation in endothelial cells. An increased superoxide production also leads to opening of the mitochondrial permeability transition pore, loss of mitochondrial membrane potential and further respiratory uncoupling, leading to cellular death in the setting of ischemia and reperfusion injury (46).

More recently, the existence of a crosstalk between mitochondria and the NADPH oxidase has been established for the model of angiotensin II infusion and nitrate tolerance (47,48). In this mechanism, an increased superoxide production in the mitochondria would lead to activation of the membrane oxidases, leading to endothelial dysfunction. Accordingly, mitochondria-targeted antioxidant delivery was able to normalize endothelial dysfunction in these models of nitrate tolerance and hypertension (49).

Asymmetric Dimethylarginine (ADMA) and Endothelial Dysfunction

ADMA is an inactive substrate for eNOS, and when present in high concentrations, it may reduce NO production. There is also some evidence that ADMA may even cause eNOS uncoupling. Increased ADMA levels have been demonstrated in patients with risk factors such as hypertension, in chronic smokers, patients with hypercholesterolemia and in patients with diabetes and renal insufficiency. More recent data from our group indicate (50) that ADMA has a prognostic value that is additive to that of traditional risk factors and novel biomarkers such as brain natriuretic peptide. It is important to note that the enzymes synthesizing and degrading ADMA are regulated in a redox-sensitive fashion (51). Thus, in all conditions where oxidative stress within the vasculature is increased, increased cellular/circulating levels of ADMA are expected, and, in line with this, angiotensin II is able to increase ADMA levels in smooth muscle cells by preventing its degradation, by increasing its formation and by decreasing extracellular extrusion (52). The functional consequences remain obscure but it is tempting to speculate that ADMA formed in smooth muscle cells may be able to reduce NO production in adjacent endothelial cells (52).

EFFECTS OF REACTIVE OXYGEN SPECIES ON THE ACTIVITY AND EXPRESSION OF THE sGC AND THE cGK-I

Oxidative Stress and Consequences for the Activity and Expression of the Soluble Guanylate Cyclase

It is well established that endothelial dysfunction caused by increased oxidative stress affects the endothelial, but also the smooth muscle and adventitial, cell layers (53,54). It is important to note that the activity of the heterodimeric hemoprotein-soluble guanylate cyclase is also redox-dependent: while NO stimulates cGMP formation by several hundred-fold, superoxide inhibits basal and stimulated sGC activity. Actually, there is evidence that sGC activity is not only indirectly diminished due to reduced vascular NO-bioavailability, but also that the enzyme is directly inhibited by superoxide (55). In addition, sGC activity has been shown to be inhibited by the NO/superoxide reaction product $ONOO^-$.

Besides these direct effects, oxidative stress may also affect sGC activity by altering the expression of sGC subunits. sGC expression is controlled at the post-transcriptional level by NO and cyclic nucleotides, thereby opening a pathway for superoxide to indirectly modify sGC expression: cAMP-eliciting agonists decrease the expression of sGC mRNA and protein by destabilization of the mRNA in various cell types (56). This effect is mimicked by the activation of the cGMP-signaling pathway, e.g. application of NO donors, stimulation of the particulate GC by atrialnatriuretic factor and by stimulation of the cGK-I by the stable analogue 8-chlorophenythio-cGMP (57).

The molecular mechanism underlying this phenomenon was recently identified. The 3′ untranslated regions (3′UTR) of the rat $sGCa_1$ and β_1 mRNA contain several AUUUA- or AUUUUA-motifs (AU-rich elements, AREs) which target these mRNAs for rapid degradation and for trans-acting factors for regulation of mRNA stability (58). One of these factors is the ubiquitous 34 kDa protein HuR, also known as HuA. HuR binds to AREs present in the 3′UTR of target mRNAs, thereby protecting these mRNA from accelerated decay. The decisive role of HuR for regulation of sGC expression was proven by siRNA-induced knock-down of HuR in rat aortic smooth muscle cells, which led to a concomitant decrease in sGC expression (59). Furthermore, prolonged (6 h) sGC-activation by YC-1 decreased the expression of HuR protein and HuR-binding activity for sGCa1 mRNA in rat aortic smooth muscle cells and isolated aorta. Consequently, the expression of the sGCa1 subunit was decreased (Figure 91.3). All these effects could be blocked by an inhibitor of YC-1-stimulated sGC activity,

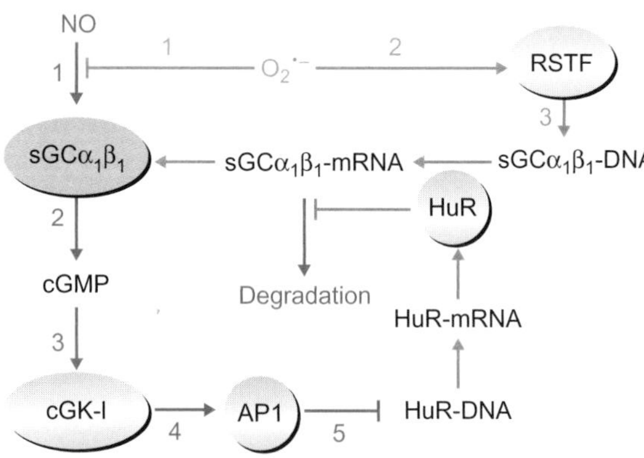

FIGURE 91.3 Hypothetical scheme illustrating the effects of increased NO or superoxide levels on the expression of sGC. Constitutive expression of sGC subunits α_1 and β_1 is the net result of "house keeping" transcription and mRNA stability regulated by the mRNA protecting HuR. Increased NO levels via route 1 to 5 (red) decrease HuR expression via cGMP/cGK-I/SP-1 activation dependent mechanism, promoting degradation of sGC subunit mRNAs and thereby reducing sGC protein synthesis. Conversely, increased superoxide levels via steps 2 to 4 (blue) activate redox sensitive transcription factors (RSTF), increase transcription of sGC subunits, thereby leading to increased sGC protein expression. In addition, increased superoxide also increases sGC protein synthesis by inhibiting cGMP formation and stabilizing sGC mRNA via route 1–5.

NS 2028, indicating that they were caused by an increased sGC activity/cGMP formation. Similarly, the cAMP-induced decrease in sGC expression is accomplished by the same mechanisms, i.e., a cAMP-induced decrease of HuR expression leads to destabilization of sGC mRNA (60). Collectively, these findings suggest the existence of a negative feedback loop formed by sGC and HuR, e.g. increased sGC activity will decrease HuR expression, thereby leading to downregulation of sGC and reduced cGMP formation. Conversely, inhibition of NO/cGMP- and PGI2/cAMP-signaling by superoxide/peroxynitrite will elicit opposite effects, i.e. upregulation of sGC. Though this hypothesis is compatible with the finding of increased sGC expression in superoxide-generating vascular tissue (61,62) it warrants further experimental verification.

OXIDATIVE STRESS AND CONSEQUENCES FOR THE ACTIVITY AND EXPRESSION OF THE cGMP-DEPENDENT KINASE I

Previous studies with cGK-I-deficient mice have demonstrated that the absence of this enzyme leads to a complete disruption of the NO/cGMP signaling pathway in the vascular smooth muscle (63). Therefore, the activity and/or expression of the cGK-I critically modulates NO-dependent vasodilation. cGKI activity in vascular cells can be assessed by immunodetection of phosphorylation

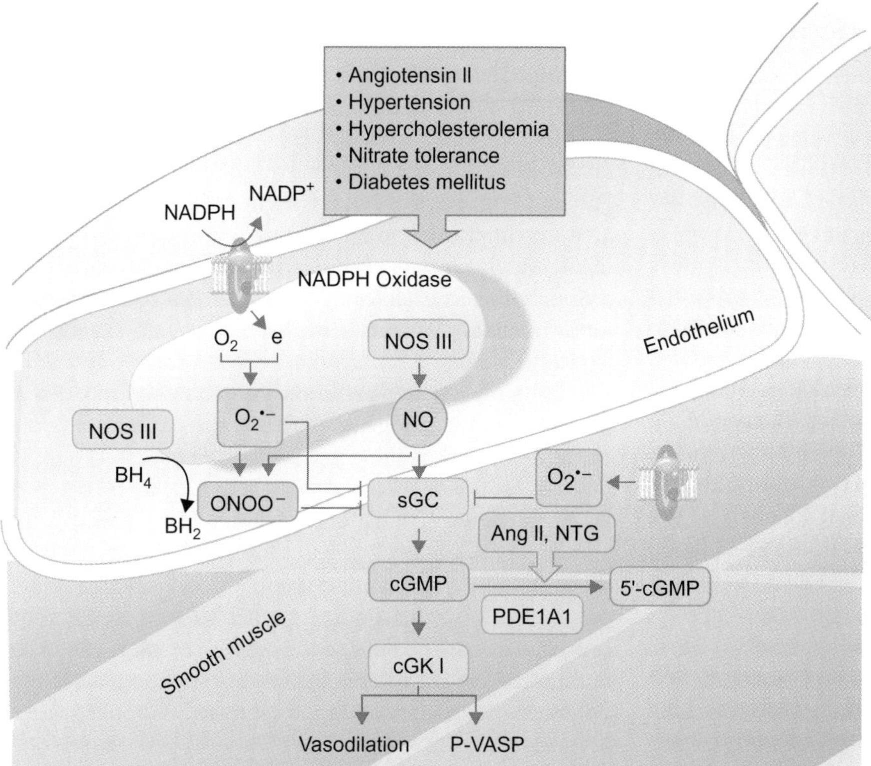

FIGURE 91.4 Schematic representation of the NO/cGMP/cGKI pathway of vascular smooth muscle relaxation and mechanisms of its inactivation by endothelial dysfunction. Also illustrated is the analysis of NO/cGMP/cGKI action and endothelial function by monitoring cGKI phosphorylation of Ser239 of the substrate protein VASP. Under normal conditions, nitric oxide (NO), synthesized by nitric oxide synthase (NOS) III, stimulates soluble guanylate cyclase (sGC), increasing cGMP and thus stimulation of cGMP-dependent protein kinase I (cGKI) and vasorelaxation. This pathway can, however, be inhibited at several sites. Angiotensin II, hypertension, hypercholesterolemia, and nitrate tolerance enhance vascular superoxide ($O_2^{\cdot -}$) production, which inactivates NO, diminishing cGKI action. Both $O_2^{\cdot -}$ and the NO/$O_2^{\cdot -}$ reaction product peroxynitrite ($ONOO^-$) potently inhibit sGC. Peroxynitrite can also uncouple NOSIII by oxidizing the NOSIII cofactor tetrahydrobiopterin (BH_4) to the $BH_3^{\cdot}$ Radical and subsequently to dihydrobiopterin (BH_2) and/or by oxidizing Zn thiolate complexes within NOSIII. Angiotensin II and nitroglycerin (NTG) therapy stimulate the activity and expression of phosphodiesterase PDE1A1, thus decreasing cGKI action and endothelium-dependent and -independent vasodilation while inducing supersensitivity to vasoconstrictors. Interventions that reduce vascular oxidative stress such as therapy with statins, Ang II receptor (AT_1 subtype) blockers, ACE inhibitors, or vitamins improves NO bioavailability by reducing vascular superoxide production. In all cases, P-VASP served as a reliable monitor of the NO/cGMP/cGKI pathway and endothelial dysfunction (6).

at Ser239 of the cGKI substrate protein VASP (P-VASP, Figure 91.4). This approach has been shown to be a reliable surrogate parameter of the integrity of the NO/cGMP signaling pathway in platelets, cultured endothelial and smooth muscle cells (64), and as shown more recently also in intact vascular tissues (6,65). The P-VASP assay appears to be sufficiently sensitive to monitor basal NO release in endothelium-intact arteries. For example, incubation of vessels with NOS inhibitors such as NG-nitro-L-arginine (L-NNA) or with its methylester L-NAME, strongly decreased P-VASP levels (6,65). Likewise, NO donors such as SNP and NTG markedly increased P-VASP in vessels in the absence and presence of an intact endothelium (6,65). Mechanical removal of the endothelium in rat and rabbit aorta almost completely abolished "basal" VASP phosphorylation, whereas total VASP levels (phosphorylated and non-phosphorylated) were reduced by about 40–50 % (6,65). These findings indicate that VASP Ser239 phosphorylation clearly depends on the presence of a functional endothelium, and that the endothelial cell layer in aortic vessels contains a considerable amount of VASP, which is lost upon removal of the endothelium. P-VASP analysis also appears suitable to monitor oxidative stress within vascular tissue. Incubation of isolated endothelium-intact vessels with diethylthiocarbamate (DETC), an inhibitor of Cu/Zn superoxide dismutase (SOD), markedly reduced P-VASP levels (6). Concomitantly, basal endothelial NO formation was decreased and formation of superoxide was increased (6).

ENDOTHELIAL FUNCTION AND PROGNOSIS

Increased oxidative stress within the vasculature has been recently demonstrated to have prognostic implications. For instance, in the setting of coronary artery disease, Volker Schächinger from Zeiher's group has shown that patients who respond to intracoronary ACh with vasodilation have subsequently many fewer cardiovascular events defined as death due to myocardial infarction, coronary and peripheral artery revascularization, and stroke as compared to patients who responded to intracoronary ACh with vasoconstriction (66). As described above, the prognostic relevance of endothelial function assessment at the level of peripheral vessels (while being logistically more feasible) is comparable to that of the study of coronary endothelial function. It has been shown that an improved flow-mediated dilation (FMD) is an independent marker of good prognosis in postmenopausal hypertensive women, even after correction for blood pressure or type of antihypertensive therapy (67). Peripheral endothelial function assessed with FMD of the brachial artery has also been proven to be a good tool in the stratification of the risk of cardiovascular events in patients undergoing peripheral or coronary bypass surgery (68). In this study, Cox proportional hazards model showed that the independent predictors for events were age, renal insufficiency, no carotid surgery and lower flow-dependent dilation of the brachial artery. When an FMD cut-off of 8.1% was used, endothelial function had a sensitivity of 95%, specificity of 37%, and a negative predictive value of 98% to predict incident events. These findings suggest measurement of endothelial function in the brachial artery may provide information about plaque stability in coronary arteries. Gokce et al. (69) further showed that in 199 patients with peripheral artery disease and before elective bypass surgery, patients having postoperatively cardiovascular events had a clearly depressed flow mediated dilation of the brachial artery ($4.4 \pm 2.8\%$) vs. patients without any event ($7.0 \pm 4.9\%$).

Further studies revealed a strong association between endothelial dysfunction and prognosis in patients with chronic congestive heart failure (70) and essential hypertension (71). Similarly, it has been shown that a worsening in FMD is a negative prognostic factor for the development of in-stent restenosis (72). However, a major limitation to the clinical applicability of FMD remains the fact that, while being a valid predictor of future cardiovascular events in a number of settings, large studies suggest that this method adds approximately only 1% to the prognostic accuracy of traditional cardiovascular risk scores in older adults (73). From this perspective, the development of tools that provide additional information – and accuracy – to the study of endothelial function as a technique for cardiovascular screening would be a welcome addition. The development of so-called low-flow-mediated vasoconstriction is an effort in this direction (74,75).

More recently we were able to show that *peripheral* endothelial function also has prognostic meaning (74). Patients with cardiovascular events had a clearly attenuated maximal forearm blood flow in response to intrabrachial infusion of the endothelium-dependent vasodilator acetylcholine as established with the forearm plethysmography method. Patients with cardiovascular events such as death due to cardiovascular disease, stroke, myocardial infarction or revascularization procedures responded to acute vitamin C challenges clearly more strongly as compared to patients with no cardiovascular events.

We also demonstrated that the prognosis of those patients whose endothelial function is improved by the antioxidant vitamin C (i.e., those who have oxidative stress-induced endothelial dysfunction) have a worse prognosis (76). This finding further strengthens the concept that oxidative stress indeed is the key player in determining the degree of endothelial dysfunction but also the prognosis in patients with established coronary artery disease.

CONCLUSION

Methods that allow simple and reliable assessment of endothelial function and dysfunction in coronary and peripheral arteries have been available for almost 20 years. The mechanisms underlying endothelial dysfunction are complex and multifactorial but predominantly involve the production of ROS, not just in endothelial but also in smooth muscle cells. Increased oxidative stress produced by the NADPH-oxidase may lead to eNOS uncoupling, thereby switching a NO to a superoxide-producing enzyme. In addition, increased ROS production in smooth muscle cells adversely affects activity and expression of important NO signaling enzymes such as soluble guanylyl cyclase, the cGMP-dependent protein kinase, and the phosphodiesterases.

Studies with patients with established coronary artery disease and cardiovascular risk factors and congestive heart failure clearly demonstrated that endothelial dysfunction has fundamental prognostic implications. The ability to measure endothelial function non-invasively has helped us to understand the pathophysiologic processes underlying the development of subclinical atherosclerosis. In addition, patients will get important feedback information about the status of their vessels and how lifestyle changes and/or medical treatment favorably influence their vessel function, which in turn will improve patient compliance substantially.

REFERENCES

1. Moncada S, Korbut R, Bunting S, Vane JR. Prostacyclin is a circulating hormone. *Nature* 1978;**273**:767–8.
2. Palmer RM, Ferrige AG, Moncada S. Nitric oxide release accounts for the biological activity of endothelium-derived relaxing factor. *Nature* 1987;**327**:524–6.
3. Stupack DG, Cheresh DA. Integrins and angiogenesis. *Curr Top Dev Biol* 2004;**64**:207–38.
4. Busse R, Fleming I. Regulation of NO synthesis in endothelial cells. *Kidney Blood Press Res* 1998;**21**:264–6.
5. Fleming I, Busse R. Molecular mechanisms involved in the regulation of the endothelial nitric oxide synthase. *Am J Physiol Regul Integr Comp Physiol* 2003;**284**:R1–12.
6. Oelze M, Mollnau H, Hoffmann N, et al. Vasodilator-stimulated phosphoprotein serine 239 phosphorylation as a sensitive monitor of defective nitric oxide/cGMP signaling and endothelial dysfunction. *Circ Res* 2000;**87**:999–1005.
7. Myers PR, Minor Jr RL, Guerra Jr. R, Bates JN, Harrison DG. Vasorelaxant properties of the endothelium-derived relaxing factor more closely resemble S-nitrosocysteine than nitric oxide. *Nature* 1990;**345**:161–3.
8. Radomski MW, Palmer RM, Moncada S. The anti-aggregating properties of vascular endothelium: interactions between prostacyclin and nitric oxide. *Br J Pharmacol* 1987;**92**:639–46.
9. Garg UC, Hassid A. Nitric oxide-generating vasodilators and 8-bromo-cyclic guanosine monophosphate inhibit mitogenesis and proliferation of cultured rat vascular smooth muscle cells. *J Clin Invest* 1989;**83**:1774–7.
10. Gryglewski RJ, Moncada S, Palmer RM. Bioassay of prostacyclin and endothelium-derived relaxing factor (EDRF) from porcine aortic endothelial cells. *Br J Pharmacol* 1986;**87**:685–94.
11. Beckman JS. Oxidative damage and tyrosine nitration from peroxynitrite. *Chem Res Toxicol* 1996;**9**:836–44.
12. Beckman JS, Koppenol WH. Nitric oxide, superoxide, and peroxynitrite: the good, the bad, and ugly. *Am J Physiol* 1996;**271**: C1424–37.
13. Zou MH, Ullrich V. Peroxynitrite formed by simultaneous generation of nitric oxide and superoxide selectively inhibits bovine aortic prostacyclin synthase. *FEBS Lett* 1996;**382**:101–4.
14. Zou MH, Shi C, Cohen RA. Oxidation of the zinc-thiolate complex and uncoupling of endothelial nitric oxide synthase by peroxynitrite. *J Clin Invest* 2002;**109**:817–26.
15. Kuzkaya N, Weissmann N, Harrison DG, Dikalov S. Interactions of peroxynitrite, tetrahydrobiopterin, ascorbic acid, and thiols: implications for uncoupling endothelial nitric-oxide synthase. *J Biol Chem* 2003;**278**:22546–54.
16. Duffy SJ, Gokce N, Holbrook M, et al. Effect of ascorbic acid treatment on conduit vessel endothelial dysfunction in patients with hypertension. *Am J Physiol Heart Circ Physiol* 2001;**280**: H528–34.
17. Levine GN, Frei B, Koulouris SN, Gerhard MD, Keaney Jr. JF, Vita JA. Ascorbic acid reverses endothelial vasomotor dysfunction in patients with coronary artery disease. *Circulation* 1996;**93**:1107–13.
18. Heitzer T, Just H, Munzel T. Antioxidant vitamin C improves endothelial dysfunction in chronic smokers. *Circulation* 1996;**94**:6–9.
19. Ting HH, Timimi FK, Boles KS, Creager SJ, Ganz P, Creager MA. Vitamin C improves endothelium-dependent vasodilation in patients with non-insulin-dependent diabetes mellitus. *J Clin Invest* 1996;**97**:22–8.
20. Munzel T, Genth-Zotz S, Hink U. Targeting heme-oxidized soluble guanylate cyclase: solution for all cardiorenal problems in heart failure? *Hypertension* 2007;**49**:974–6.
21. Bastian NR, Hibbs Jr. JB. Assembly and regulation of NADPH oxidase and nitric oxide synthase. *Curr Opin Immunol* 1994;**6**:131–9.
22. Griendling KK, Sorescu D, Ushio-Fukai M. NAD(P)H oxidase: role in cardiovascular biology and disease. *Circ Res* 2000;**86**:494–501.
23. Warnholtz A, Nickenig G, Schulz E, et al. Increased NADH-oxidase-mediated superoxide production in the early stages of atherosclerosis: evidence for involvement of the renin-angiotensin system. *Circulation* 1999;**99**:2027–33.
24. Nickenig G, Baumer AT, Temur Y, Kebben D, Jockenhovel F, Bohm M. Statin-sensitive dysregulated AT1 receptor function and density in hypercholesterolemic men. *Circulation* 1999;**100**:2131–4.
25. Guzik TJ, West NE, Black E, et al. Vascular superoxide production by NAD(P)H oxidase: association with endothelial dysfunction and clinical risk factors. *Circ Res* 2000;**86**:E85–90.
26. Sorescu D, Weiss D, Lassegue B, et al. Superoxide production and expression of nox family proteins in human atherosclerosis. *Circulation* 2002;**105**:1429–35.
27. Fukui T, Ishizaka N, Rajagopalan S, et al. p22phox mRNA expression and NADPH oxidase activity are increased in aortas from hypertensive rats. *Circ Res* 1997;**80**:45–51.
28. Rajagopalan S, Kurz S, Munzel T, et al. Angiotensin II-mediated hypertension in the rat increases vascular superoxide production via membrane NADH/NADPH oxidase activation. Contribution to alterations of vasomotor tone. *J Clin Invest* 1996;**97**:1916–23.
29. Morawietz H, Weber M, Rueckschloss U, Lauer N, Hacker A, Kojda G. Upregulation of vascular NAD(P)H oxidase subunit gp91phox and impairment of the nitric oxide signal transduction pathway in hypertension. *Biochem Biophys Res Commun* 2001;**285**:1130–5.
30. Hink U, Li H, Mollnau H, et al. Mechanisms underlying endothelial dysfunction in diabetes mellitus. *Circ Res* 2001;**88**:E14–22.
31. Landmesser U, Dikalov S, Price SR, et al. Oxidation of tetrahydrobiopterin leads to uncoupling of endothelial cell nitric oxide synthase in hypertension. *J Clin Invest* 2003;**111**:1201–9.
32. Ohara Y, Peterson TE, Harrison DG. Hypercholesterolemia increases endothelial superoxide anion production. *J Clin Invest* 1993;**91**:2546–51.
33. White CR, Darley-Usmar V, Berrington WR, et al. Circulating plasma xanthine oxidase contributes to vascular dysfunction in hypercholesterolemic rabbits. *Proc Natl Acad Sci USA* 1996;**93**:8745–9.
34. Cardillo C, Kilcoyne CM, Cannon III RO, Quyyumi AA, Panza JA. Xanthine oxidase inhibition with oxypurinol improves endothelial vasodilator function in hypercholesterolemic but not in hypertensive patients. *Hypertension* 1997;**30**:57–63.
35. Butler R, Morris AD, Belch JJ, Hill A, Struthers AD. Allopurinol normalizes endothelial dysfunction in type 2 diabetics with mild hypertension. *Hypertension* 2000;**35**:746–51.

36. O'Driscoll JG, Green DJ, Rankin JM, Taylor RR. Nitric oxide-dependent endothelial function is unaffected by allopurinol in hypercholesterolaemic subjects. *Clin Exp Pharmacol Physiol* 1999;**26**:779–83.
37. Nakazono K, Watanabe N, Matsuno K, Sasaki J, Sato T, Inoue M. Does superoxide underlie the pathogenesis of hypertension? *Proc Natl Acad Sci USA* 1991;**88**:10045–8.
38. Cleland JG, Coletta AP, Clark AL. Clinical trials update from the Heart Failure Society of America meeting: FIX-CHF-4, selective cardiac myosin activator and OPT-CHF. *Eur J Heart Fail* 2006;**8**:764–6.
39. Pritchard Jr. KA, Groszek L, Smalley DM, et al. Native low-density lipoprotein increases endothelial cell nitric oxide synthase generation of superoxide anion. *Circ Res* 1995;**77**:510–8.
40. Vergnani L, Hatrik S, Ricci F, et al. Effect of native and oxidized low-density lipoprotein on endothelial nitric oxide and superoxide production: key role of L-arginine availability. *Circulation* 2000;**101**:1261–6.
41. Laursen JB, Somers M, Kurz S, et al. Endothelial regulation of vasomotion in apoE-deficient mice: implications for interactions between peroxynitrite and tetrahydrobiopterin. *Circulation* 2001;**103**:1282–8.
42. Milstien S, Katusic Z. Oxidation of tetrahydrobiopterin by peroxynitrite: implications for vascular endothelial function. *Biochem Biophys Res Commun* 1999;**263**:681–4.
43. Heitzer T, Krohn K, Albers S, Meinertz T. Tetrahydrobiopterin improves endothelium-dependent vasodilation by increasing nitric oxide activity in patients with Type II diabetes mellitus. *Diabetologia* 2000;**43**:1435–8.
44. Forstermann U, Munzel T. Endothelial nitric oxide synthase in vascular disease: from marvel to menace. *Circulation* 2006;**113**:1708–14.
45. Gori T, Di Stolfo G, Sicuro S, et al. Nitroglycerin protects the endothelium from ischaemia and reperfusion: human mechanistic insight. *Br J Clin Pharmacol* 2007;**64**:145–50.
46. Doughan AK, Harrison DG, Dikalov SI. Molecular mechanisms of angiotensin II-mediated mitochondrial dysfunction: linking mitochondrial oxidative damage and vascular endothelial dysfunction. *Circ Res* 2008;**102**:488–96.
47. Wenzel P, Mollnau H, Oelze M, et al. First evidence for a crosstalk between mitochondrial and NADPH oxidase-derived reactive oxygen species in nitroglycerin-triggered vascular dysfunction. *Antioxid Redox Signal* 2008;**10**:1435–47.
48. Dikalova AE, Bikineyeva AT, Budzyn K, et al. Therapeutic targeting of mitochondrial superoxide in hypertension. *Circ Res* 2010;**107**:106–16.
49. Schnabel R, Blankenberg S, Lubos E, et al. Asymmetric dimethylarginine and the risk of cardiovascular events and death in patients with coronary artery disease: results from the AtheroGene Study. *Circ Res* 2005;**97**:e53–9.
50. Cooke JP. Does ADMA cause endothelial dysfunction? *Arterioscler Thromb Vasc Biol* 2000;**20**:2032–7.
51. Luo Z, Teerlink T, Griendling K, Aslam S, Welch WJ, Wilcox CS. Angiotensin II and NADPH oxidase increase ADMA in vascular smooth muscle cells. *Hypertension* 2011;**56**:498–504.
52. Munzel T, Afanas'ev IB, Kleschyov AL, Harrison DG. Detection of superoxide in vascular tissue. *Arterioscler Thromb Vasc Biol* 2002;**22**:1761–8.
53. Munzel T, Daiber A, Ullrich V, Mulsch A. Vascular consequences of endothelial nitric oxide synthase uncoupling for the activity and expression of the soluble guanylyl cyclase and the cGMP-dependent protein kinase. *Arterioscler Thromb Vasc Biol* 2005;**25**:1551–7.
54. Mulsch A, Bauersachs J, Schafer A, Stasch JP, Kast R, Busse R. Effect of YC-1, an NO-independent, superoxide-sensitive stimulator of soluble guanylyl cyclase, on smooth muscle responsiveness to nitrovasodilators. *Br J Pharmacol* 1997;**120**:681–9.
55. Papapetropoulos A, Marczin N, Mora G, Milici A, Murad F, Catravas JD. Regulation of vascular smooth muscle soluble guanylate cyclase activity, mRNA, and protein levels by cAMP-elevating agents. *Hypertension* 1995;**26**:696–704.
56. Ujiie K, Hogarth L, Danziger R, et al. Homologous and heterologous desensitization of a guanylyl cyclase-linked nitric oxide receptor in cultured rat medullary interstitial cells. *J Pharmacol Exp Ther* 1994;**270**:761–7.
57. Chen CY, Shyu AB. AU-rich elements: characterization and importance in mRNA degradation. *Trends Biochem Sci* 1995;**20**:465–70.
58. Kloss S, Furneaux H, Mulsch A. Post-transcriptional regulation of soluble guanylyl cyclase expression in rat aorta. *J Biol Chem* 2003;**278**:2377–83.
59. Kloss S, Srivastava R, Mulsch A. Down-regulation of soluble guanylyl cyclase expression by cyclic AMP is mediated by mRNA-stabilizing protein HuR. *Mol Pharmacol* 2004;**65**:1440–51.
60. Mulsch A, Oelze M, Kloss S, et al. Effects of in vivo nitroglycerin treatment on activity and expression of the guanylyl cyclase and cGMP-dependent protein kinase and their downstream target vasodilator-stimulated phosphoprotein in aorta. *Circulation* 2001;**103**:2188–94.
61. Laber U, Kober T, Schmitz V, et al. Effect of hypercholesterolemia on expression and function of vascular soluble guanylyl cyclase. *Circulation* 2002;**105**:855–60.
62. Pfeifer A, Klatt P, Massberg S, et al. Defective smooth muscle regulation in cGMP kinase I-deficient mice. *EMBO J* 1998;**17**:3045–51.
63. Smolenski A, Burkhardt AM, Eigenthaler M, et al. Functional analysis of cGMP-dependent protein kinases I and II as mediators of NO/cGMP effects. *Naunyn Schmiedebergs Arch Pharmacol* 1998;**358**:134–9.
64. Ibarra-Alvarado C, Galle J, Melichar VO, Mameghani A, Schmidt HH. Phosphorylation of blood vessel vasodilator-stimulated phosphoprotein at serine 239 as a functional biochemical marker of endothelial nitric oxide/cyclic GMP signaling. *Mol Pharmacol* 2002;**61**:312–9.
65. Schachinger V, Britten MB, Zeiher AM. Prognostic impact of coronary vasodilator dysfunction on adverse long-term outcome of coronary heart disease. *Circulation* 2000;**101**:1899–906.
66. Modena MG, Bonetti L, Coppi F, Bursi F, Rossi R. Prognostic role of reversible endothelial dysfunction in hypertensive postmenopausal women. *J Am Coll Cardiol* 2002;**40**:505–10.
67. Gokce N, Keaney Jr. JF, Hunter LM, Watkins MT, Menzoian JO, Vita JA. Risk stratification for postoperative cardiovascular events via noninvasive assessment of endothelial function: a prospective study. *Circulation* 2002;**105**:1567–72.
68. Gokce N, Keaney Jr. JF, Hunter LM, et al. Predictive value of non-invasively determined endothelial dysfunction for long-term

cardiovascular events in patients with peripheral vascular disease. *J Am Coll Cardiol* 2003;**41**:1769–75.

69. Heitzer T, Baldus S, von Kodolitsch Y, Rudolph V, Meinertz T. Systemic endothelial dysfunction as an early predictor of adverse outcome in heart failure. *Arterioscler Thromb Vasc Biol* 2005;**25**:1174–9.
70. Perticone F, Ceravolo R, Pujia A, et al. Prognostic significance of endothelial dysfunction in hypertensive patients. *Circulation* 2001;**104**:191–6.
71. Kitta Y, Nakamura T, Kodama Y, et al. Endothelial vasomotor dysfunction in the brachial artery is associated with late in-stent coronary restenosis. *J Am Coll Cardiol* 2005;**46**:648–55.
72. Yeboah J, Folsom AR, Burke GL, et al. Predictive value of brachial flow-mediated dilation for incident cardiovascular events in a population-based study: the multi-ethnic study of atherosclerosis. *Circulation* 2009;**120**:502–9.
73. Heitzer T, Schlinzig T, Krohn K, Meinertz T, Munzel T. Endothelial dysfunction, oxidative stress, and risk of cardiovascular events in patients with coronary artery disease. *Circulation* 2001;**104**:2673–8.
74. Gori T, Muxel S, Damaske A, et al. Endothelial function assessment: flow-mediated dilation and constriction provide different and complementary information on the presence of coronary artery disease. *Eur Heart J* 2012;**33(3)**:363–71.
75. Gori T, Parker JD, Münzel T. Flow-mediated constriction: further insight into a new measure of vascular function. *Eur Heart J* 2011;**32(7)**:784–7.
76. Anderson TJ, Uehata A, Gerhard MD, et al. Close relation of endothelial function in the human coronary and peripheral circulations. *J Am Coll Cardiol* 1995;**26**:1235–41.

Chapter 92

Hemodynamic Control of Vascular Smooth Muscle Function

Eileen M. Redmond[1], Caitriona Lally[2] and Paul A. Cahill[3]

[1]Department of Surgery, University of Rochester Medical Center, Rochester, NY, [2]School of Mechanical and Manufacturing Engineering, Dublin City University, [3]School of Biotechnology, Faculty of Science and Health, Dublin City University, Dublin, Ireland

INTRODUCTION

Hemodynamic forces associated with the flow of blood within the vascular compartment are established modifiers of endothelial (EC) (1) and vascular smooth muscle cell (vSMC) (2) structure and function and orchestrate complex cellular and molecular responses in combination with contributions from the extracellular matrix (ECM), growth factors (e.g., EGF, and TGF-β) and cell adhesion receptors (e.g., integrins) (3). This phenomenon, termed mechanotransduction, is an integral part of vascular cell physiology where it has a profound impact on the development of the vasculature during embryogenesis and contributes to the progression of various human vascular disease states if disrupted during adulthood (4). Within the cardiovascular system, blood pressure is carefully regulated through multiple mechanisms to ensure the precise control of blood flow and maintenance of hemodynamic mechanical forces. These forces include fluid shear stress, the frictional force per unit area from flowing blood, which acts on the ECs that line the vessel wall. Blood pressure, which drives fluid flow, causes circumferential and axial stretching of the vessel wall on both the ECs and the vSMC. Hydrostatic pressure also alters cellular physiology, but it is thought less important than shear stress or stretch. In addition, the myogenic response, a mechanism intrinsic to arterial smooth muscle, regulates local blood flow on a time scale of seconds, shielding capillary beds from acute changes in pressure. Disruption of these forces are key prognostic factors in disease states such as hypertension, atherosclerosis, and in-stent restenosis, which, despite the systemic nature of the major risk factors, occur mainly in regions within vessels that experience significant disturbances in blood flow and pressure/strain, respectively. Therefore, while many have focused on important endothelial mechanotransducers that mediate responses to blood flow and shear stress, the direct effect of pressure and strain changes on vSMC function and integrity has revealed a parallel mechanosensitive role for vSMC mechanotransducers in determining vascular cell fate, growth, and function in vascular disease states.

MECHANICAL FORCES IN VESSEL PHYSIOLOGY

Understanding the molecular basis for mechanotransduction requires knowledge of the magnitude and distribution of forces throughout the vasculature at the molecular scale. The periodic contractions of the heart cause large, pulsatile changes in blood pressure on the arterial side of the circulation. The resultant cyclic stretching of the arterial wall promotes and maintains a quiescent, contractile state in which vSMC express a full range of vSMC differentiation and contractile markers (5). While vSMC actively respond to acute changes in blood pressure through a myogenic mechanism, if pressure remains elevated over longer periods, vessels remodel and cause the vascular wall to thicken to resist these forces according to a simple physical law, *La Place's law*, that describes the relationship between the transmural pressure difference and the tension, radius, and thickness of the vessel wall (5):

$$T = (P * R)/M$$

where T is the tension in the walls, P is the pressure difference across the wall, R is the radius of the cylinder, and M is the thickness of the wall. However, under pathological conditions in which pressures are disrupted, this arterial remodeling can eventually compromise vessel elasticity, which decreases their ability to accommodate sudden changes in pressure.

Within the vessel wall, "physiologic stress" is manifested as a tensile strain on vSMC and EC that is perpendicular to the lumen of the vessel and cyclic in nature, while in the lumen, EC cells are subjected to a shear

Muscle. DOI: http://dx.doi.org/10.1016/B978-0-12-381510-1.00092-2

stress, a frictional force at the apical surface produced by blood flow (5). Vascular SMC are subjected to three primary mechanical stresses (6): (i) a blood flow induced wall shear stress τ_w following endothelial denudation (Eq. 1); (ii) a blood pressure-induced circumferential wall stress σ_θ (Eq. 2); and (iii) an axial wall stress σ_z (Eq. 3), that appears to arise during development and to persist into maturity due to the long half-life of elastin. Mean values of these three components of stress (i.e., forces acting over oriented areas) can be calculated as follows:

$$\tau_w = \frac{4\,\mu Q}{\pi a^3} \qquad \text{(Eq. 1)}$$

$$\sigma_\theta = \frac{\text{Pa}}{h} \qquad \text{(Eq. 2)}$$

$$\sigma_z = \frac{-f}{\pi h(2a + h)} \qquad \text{(Eq. 3)}$$

where μ is the blood viscosity, Q the mean volumetric flow rate, a and h the luminal radius and wall thickness in any pressurized configuration, P the transmural pressure (with low perivascular pressure), and f the axial force that maintains the axial "pre-stretch" (which is appreciated via the axial retraction of a transected artery). These relationships reveal the importance of the thickness:lumen ratio (h/a) and the importance of wall cross-sectional area, which is often reported with regard to "eutrophic" vs. "hypertropic" remodeling. Larger arteries maintain these stresses near homeostatic values (e.g., on the order of 1.5 Pa for τ_w and 100 kPa for both σ_θ and σ_z in specific arteries, where 1 kiloPascal (kPa) equals 7.5 mmHg) (6).

All three indices of vessel geometry (radius, thickness, length) are strongly associated with the primary measures of wall stress (wall shear, circumferential, axial). Hence, the biomechanical response of resident vSMC is uniquely sensitive to all three primary stresses (5). In this context, strain-mediated growth and remodeling requires coordinated changes in luminal radius a and wall thickness h based directly on percent perturbations in hemodynamics from their original values. Moreover, if luminal radius and wall thickness are dictated by flow and pressure, then restoring σ_z (Eq. 3) to its normal value requires a change in axial force f, which typically would cause a change in length (e.g., possible tortuosity). The cellular production of vasoactive molecules, growth factors, cytokines, matrix proteins, and proteases in response to these stresses depends often in a sigmoidal manner on changes in these primary stresses. Changes in vessel geometry in response to altered strain depends on (i) coupled elastic deformations (i.e., nonlinear wall properties), (ii) acute and chronic myogenic changes in vascular tone (i.e., smooth muscle contraction or relaxation), and (iii) reorganization or turnover of cells and matrix (i.e., growth and remodeling).

While vSMC normally reside in the tunica media of the arterial wall and are not exposed directly to shear stress associated with blood flow, they can be exposed directly when the intima and internal elastic lamina (IEL) are damaged in procedures such as angioplasty or in the anastomotic region of vascular grafts (7). Furthermore, the most superficial layer of vSMC, lying directly beneath the IEL, can be exposed to higher levels of shear stress due to the funneling of flow through the fenestral pores in the IEL, in the order of 10–50 dyn/cm^2 (8).

MECHANOSENSITIVE GENE EXPRESSION NETWORKS IN VSMC

Genomic profiling studies have identified altered gene expression in a binary fashion using human and animal tissues and cultured vSMC *in vitro* exposed to mechanical loads where vSMC display an altered transcriptome following mechanical stimulation *in vitro* and *in vivo* (12). DNA microarray analysis and gene profiling studies have primarily focused on gene discovery (9). In this context, several discoveries have established that mechanical properties of the cellular microenvironment such as its rigidity, geometry, and external stresses play an important role in determining vascular gene expression. Many different structurally dissimilar molecules (e.g., vasoactive substances, growth factors, cytokines, proteinases, coagulation factors) (10) and extracellular matrix constituents (e.g., fibronectin, elastin, collagens, proteoglycans) (10) are produced by vSMC in response to altered mechanical loads.

Determining the functional importance of these novel mechanosensitive genes *in vitro* has provided important insights into understanding vascular biology with one important caveat; numerous *in vivo* mechanosensitive genes appear to be lost or dysregulated during culture. In addition, these transcriptional profiles may underestimate the number of mechanically induced genes for several reasons. First, only certain time points are examined and some changes may occur at different time points. Second, various thresholds (normally 2.5-fold change in steady-state mRNA levels) have been adopted and expression of some proteins may be importantly changed with smaller changes in steady-state mRNA. Thirdly, as the artery is a mechanically anisotropic 3D structure, *in vitro* deformation methods cannot completely mimic the complex *in vivo* mechanical microenvironment. Finally, vSMCs are heterogeneous both *in vivo* and *in vitro*, and therefore one cannot exclude the possibility that a specific subpopulation of cells accounts for most of the molecular responses reported *in vivo* (i.e., EC, vSMC, mesenchymal stem cells, fibroblasts, smooth muscle adventitial progenitor cells).

The initial transcriptional profile of mechanically induced genes in pure vSMC cultures *in vitro* suggests a response of defense against excessive deformation. Using

TABLE 92.1 Summary of Changes in Cell Fate and Known Mechanotransducers Following Biomechanical Activation of Vascular Smooth Muscle Cells

vSMC Fate	Mechanotransducers
Differentiation	Integrins
Alignment	ROS
Proliferation	Small G-protein
Apoptosis	Ion channels
Migration	Developmental gene regulatory networks

DNA microarray technology cyclic strain causes increases in gene expression for PAI-1 and cyclooxygenase-1, and decreases for P-selectin glycoprotein ligand, interstitial collagenase, and interleukin-1β precursor (12) Furthermore, genomic analysis in vessels from animal models of mechanical force-induced vascular injury and human specimens has also revealed differential gene expression profiles within these vessels. In atherosclerotic lesions, there are 201 genes that showed exclusively differential expression in apoE$^{-/-}$ mice related to atherosclerotic processes, such as cell adhesion, proliferation, differentiation, motility, cell death, lipid metabolism, and immune responses (13,14) (Table 92.1). Indeed, changes in medial stress following carotid artery ligation stimulate PDGF-BB and thrombomodulin (TM) co-expression in the media and neointima, an effect mediated by Ets-1 via the Src kinase/PI3-kinase/Akt/mTOR signaling pathway (15).

An interesting integrative genomics approach was recently used to determine the role of nuclear factor of activated T cells (NFAT) family of transcription factors in mechanical induced vascular pathology and describes Down Syndrome Candidate Region 1 (DSCR) as a novel NFAT-dependent, injury-inducible, early gene that may serve to negatively regulate vSMC phenotypic switching (16). Comparison between vehicle and phenotypic modulatory stimuli identified 63 species-conserved, upregulated genes. Integration of the 63 upregulated genes with an *in silico* NFAT-ome (a species-conserved list of gene promoters containing at least one NFAT binding site) identified 18 putative NFAT-dependent genes. Further intersection of these 18 potential NFAT target genes with a murine *in vivo* vascular injury microarray identified four putative NFAT-dependent, injury-responsive genes.

Genes Related to vSMC Inflammatory Responses

DNA microarrays suggest the involvement of biomechanical forces in driving inflammation responses (17). There is evidence that vSMC may take on a "proinflammatory" phenotype, whereby cells secrete cytokines and express cell adhesion molecules, e.g. IL-8, IL-6, and VCAM-1, respectively, which may functionally regulate monocyte and macrophage adhesion and other processes during atherosclerosis. Among all the interleukins, IL-1β was upregulated when cyclic strain was combined with growth factors, such as bFGF or TGF-β (18). IL-6 was also induced ~2-fold in cells exposed to both cyclic strain and TGF-β compared to those of static controls. High levels of cyclic strain (up to 20% strain) have been shown to induce the expression of IL-6 (18), but not other interleukins (IL-1α, IL-1β, IL-10, IL-12, and IL-18) in previous studies (17). In addition to ILs, a five-fold increase in PTGS2 (prostaglandin-endoperoxide synthase 2), a gene involved in inflammatory response and cell motility as well as in glucose homeostasis, has been observed when vSMC are exposed to both cyclic strain and growth factor TGF-β or both cyclic strain and growth factor PDGF-AB (18). Among the relatively restricted subset of genes induced by biomechanical stimuli of 4% biaxial strain is the hyaluronan-binding protein, TSG6. This hyaluronan-linking protein is primarily known as a pro-inflammatory response gene that is induced by cytokines, but it is intensely overexpressed in mechanically injured arteries (19).

Further analysis has confirmed that cyclic strain regulates many genes involved in cytokine/inflammatory signal transduction pathways such as suppressors of cytokine signaling (SOCS2 and SOCS3) along with STAT1 (20). The Janus kinase (Jak)/signal transducer and activator of transcription (STAT) pathway is one of the key signaling cascades utilized by vSMC to regulate cellular functions, such as migration and proliferation. This pathway is regulated by a family of the suppressors of cytokine signaling (SOCS) that control activation of the Jak/Stat signaling in a feedback loop. Both SOCS and STAT are involved in intracellular signaling cascade and anti-apoptosis and are repressed following strain. Inhibition of SOCS-1 expression in vSMC in response to mechanical strain is mediated via association and functional crosstalk of uPAR and integrins linked to lipid rafts and is independent of the Jak/Stat pathway. Mechanical strain leads to the abrogation of this control via uPAR association with the RGD-dependent integrins, thus resulting in SOCS-1 downregulation that, in turn, affects polyubiquitination and degradation of FAK (20).

Genes Involved in vSMC Cytoskeleton, ECM, and Cell Adhesion

The cytoskeleton is composed of three major types of protein filaments: microtubules, microfilaments, and intermediate filaments, and provides a structural framework for the vSMC to transmit mechanical forces between its luminal, abluminal, and junctional surfaces, as well as its interior, including the focal adhesion sites, the cytoplasm, and the nucleus (21). Beyond the structural modifications incurred, mechanical forces can initiate complex signal transduction cascades leading to functional changes within the cell, often triggered by the activation of integrins but also by stimulation of other structures such as caveolae (22), G-protein receptors (23), ion channels (24), and the distribution and activation of the Rho family GTPases that require changes in the state of microtubule polymerization (25).

Using DNA microarrays, several novel mechanosensitive gene networks associated with the extracellular matrix (ECM) have been established for vSMC (26–28). In particular, gene profiling in vSMC has established a prominent role for proteoglycans in development and maintenance of arterial structure (29). Vascular SMC are the primary source of arterial ECM, including collagens, elastic fibers, and several proteoglycans, versican, also known as PG-M, chondroitin sulfate proteoglycan, decorin, and biglycan (3). The major proteoglycans bind hyaluronan and contribute to tissue mechanical properties, providing a hydrated sponge-like matrix that resists or cushions against deformation. In addition, blood vessels contain perlecan, which is a heparan sulfate proteoglycan associated with basal lamina surrounding vSMC (3).

A potentially more informative approach has been adopted by correlating the levels of gene expression with quantitative physiological parameters (29). Two distinct groups of genes, those associated with cell signaling and those associated with the mechanical regulation of vascular structure (cytoskeletal–cell membrane–extracellular matrix) were revealed. Prominent among the repertoire of mechanically induced fibrosis-promoting proteins implicated in vascular proliferative disease are the matricellular proteins plasminogen activator inhibitor inhibitor-1 (PAI-1, SERPINE1) and connective tissue growth factor (CTGF). Importantly, the transcriptional control networks for both genes are exquisitely sensitive to cytoskeletal perturbations due to changes in hemodynamic stimuli that alter cytoskeletal dynamics, organization, and associated signaling pathways (29). Recent studies also document a complex network of unique signaling control elements leading to the induction of PAI-1 and CTGF in response to modifications in cell shape due to mechanical stimulation (30). Additionally, evidence now suggests that growth factor receptors (such as EGFR) are activated by changes in the cytoarchitecture of vSMC so that the modulatory role of certain signaling proteins (e.g., SMAD, and Rho-GEFs) is maintained by sequestration on cell structural networks (30). Functional repression can be relieved by cytoskeletal perturbations resulting in activation of signaling cascades (e.g., Rho, and MAPK) with associated changes in downstream gene expression (27).

Genes Regulating vSMC Proliferation and Apoptosis

The role of cyclic strain in controlling vSMC growth (balance of proliferation and apoptosis) *in vitro* remains controversial. However, it now appears that vSMC can either increase or decrease their proliferative capacity in response to biomechanical stimuli depending on the species of vSMC, the phenotype studied, the extracellular matrix environment, the cell cycle status (whether quiescent or cycling), and the type of strain regime applied (31). Cell cycle progression is controlled by several cyclin-dependent protein kinases (CDKs), which can associate with activating subunits, the cyclins, and with CDK inhibitory proteins (CKIs). Cyclins p27 and p21CIP1 (p21) are related CKIs that associate with CDK2-, CDK4-, CDK6-, and CDC2-containing complexes, thereby abrogating their catalytic activity leading to growth arrest. Following exposure to physiological strain levels, the proliferative effect of serum growth factors is blocked (18). Flow cytometric analysis revealed that cyclic stretch increased the fraction of vSMC in the G0/G1 phase of the cell cycle. Stretch-inhibited G1/S phase transition was associated with a decrease in retinoblastoma protein phosphorylation and with a selective increase in the cyclin-dependent kinase inhibitor p21, but not p27 (32). These results demonstrate that cyclic stretch inhibits vSMC growth by blocking cell cycle progression and suggests that physiological levels of cyclic stretch contribute to vascular homeostasis by inhibiting the proliferative pathway of vSMC. Gene array analysis confirms that vSMC on exposure to cyclic strain exhibit a decrease in cell proliferation while concomitantly reducing SOCS and STAT, which are involved in intracellular signaling cascade of cell apoptosis. Under cyclic strain, a 2- to 3-fold downregulation in the expression of anti-apoptotic genes SERPINB9 and FAIM2 was also observed (18).

In contrast, pathological strain levels *in vitro* and after balloon angioplasty *in vivo* demonstrate that extracellular matrix/integrin interactions activate Akt which in turn phosphorylates and inactivates AFX-like forkhead transcription factors, leading to transcriptional repression of the G0 phase gatekeeper, p27Kip1 (33). This sequence of events is growth-factor-independent and initiates cell cycle entry and progression, as indicated by Cdk2 activation, RB hyper-phosphorylation and subsequent increased DNA synthesis and mitosis. Pathological stretch has also been shown to initiate signalling pathways of nuclear factor-kappa B (NF-κB) and reactive oxygen species (ROS), leading to vSMC proliferation, stress-induced inflammation and apoptosis (34). Gene profiling confirmed that cyclic strain with growth factors enhanced the expression of important genes involved with cell proliferation and apoptosis such as vascular endothelial growth factor (VEGF), EREG (a gene encoding epiregulin, a member of the epidermal growth factor family), and heat shock proteins (HSP) (18). Interestingly, exposure of vSMC to pathological forces similar to those exerted during balloon angioplasty using an *in vitro* concurrent shear and tensile forces simulator (cyclic tension [5%] and shear [0.1−0.5 dyn/cm^2]) following simulated angioplasty injury (12% stretch), resulted in increased vSMC proliferation, apoptosis, and cell hypertrophy compared to cells exposed to strain alone (35). One major reason for difference in proliferative properties of vSMC is the role of the ECM (36). It has also been suggested that fibronectin (FN)−cell interactions are important for transducing strain into non-proliferative signals, since the RGD peptide or soluble FN can inhibit neonatal rat vSMC proliferation in response to strain (37). Many studies have adopted these results as a rationale for mechanical stimulation of tissue-engineered blood vessels (TEBVs) (38). In addition to the role of cyclic, circumferential mechanical strain, there also is evidence that vSMC may respond to uniaxial strain (39). Increasing the axial strain of rabbit carotid arteries from 62% to 92% increased vSMC proliferation dramatically, while also causing ECM deposition to increase and remain elevated over a 12-week period. *Ex vivo* engineered vessels that were elongated by 50% over 9 days under both physiological and sub-physiological perfusion conditions showed significant increases in proliferation and collagen mass, and exhibited similar viability and appearance of native tissue (40). These data suggest that there are substantial interactions between cyclic strain conditions and axial strain that modulates arterial remodeling. The full extent to which these effects alter expression of contractile vSMC phenotype is not known.

Several studies have reported increased vSMC apoptosis *in vitro* (41) and *in vivo* (42,43) in response to strain or pressure. Cyclic strain increased p53 protein expression and transcriptional activity as well as a significant increase of apoptotic vSMC. Apoptosis was prevented by the p53 inhibitor pifithrin and by p53 antisense oligonucleotides, indicating dependency of force-induced apoptosis on p53. Changes in wall tension as produced by changes in flow or by angioplasty cause apoptosis especially of medial Vsmc (44). The occurrence of apoptosis after balloon angioplasty has been well established in both animal models and humans. However, the mechanism of mechanically induced vSMC apoptosis and its role for the development of neointima and restenosis have not yet been elucidated conclusively. It has been hypothesized the early wave of apoptosis, occurring within hours of the injury and resulting in a marked decrease in vessel wall cellularity, may exacerbate late neointima formation by provoking a greater wound healing response (45). Apoptosis at later time points seems confined to vSMC of the developing neointima. Although the contribution of cellular aspartate-specific cysteinyl proteases (caspases) in apoptosis has clearly been demonstrated, recent attention has been given to the cysteine protease, calpain since its activity is increased by mechanical strain (44). Calpain counteracts mechanically induced excessive vSMC apoptosis through its p53-degrading properties, which identifies calpain as a key regulator of mechanosensitive remodelling processes of the vascular wall. Artery cuffing has been shown to increase apoptosis leading to atrophy of the vessel (46). Gene profiling studies have demonstrated different apoptotic genes, CASP1, CASP8, various tumor protein family genes and CARD10 were down-regulated three to five times, while genes encoding the anti-apoptotic factors, such as Bcl-2-related protein A1 (Bcl-2A1), were upregulated following strain. Bcl-2A1 is a member of the BCL-2 family and has been shown to retard apoptosis in various cell lines. Several interleukins, which are known for their proliferative effects on vSMC including interleukin-1α (IL-1α), interleukin-1β (IL-1β), interleukin-6 (IL-6), and interleukin-8 (IL-8), were also upregulated (18).

A novel mechanism involving microRNAs (miRNAs) for understanding strain-induced changes in pro- and anti-proliferative and apoptotic stimuli has recently been reported (47). Pri-miRNAs appear to be transcriptionally regulated in a similar manner as the transcription of mRNA. Mice homozygous for a hypomorphic allele of Dicer, an enzyme essential for the biogenesis of most microRNAs, develop gross abnormalities during blood vessel development in the embryo (48). The transcriptional factor NF-κB is activated upon cyclic strain and transcriptionally activates the expression of miR-146a (49). MicroRNAs are also phenotypic regulators of vSMC since miR-146a targets the Krüppel-like factor 4 (KLF4) 3′ untranslated region (UTR) and has an important role in promoting vSMC proliferation *in vitro* and vascular neointimal hyperplasia *in vivo*. Using both gain-of-function and loss-of-function approaches, miR-146a promotes vSMC proliferation *in vitro* while transfection of anti-sense miR-146a oligonucleotide into balloon-injured rat carotid arteries markedly decreased neointimal hyperplasia. Therefore, miR-146a and KLF4 may form a feedback loop to regulate each other's expression and vSMC proliferation in response to mechanical strain. Coincidentally, miRNA microarrays have been used to analyze the difference in miRNA expression between vSMCs of SHR and WKY rats to reveal let-7d microRNA through its interaction with RAS (50).

Veins exist in a lower pressure environment and are therefore not subjected to arterial forces. However, when veins are arterialized and subjected to a high-stress environment, such as after coronary artery bypass graft (CABG) procedure, the primary response is extensive intimal hyperplasia (IH) followed by fibrosis and atherosclerosis that may eventually lead to graft failure (51). A group of functionally related genes called arterial intima-enriched (AIE) genes based on expression that is limited to the intimal vSMC of large arteries has been reported (52). The AIE genes include sciellin, periplakin, Small Proline-Rich Protein 3 (SPRR3), galectin 7, and plakoglobin (11). These gene products have been previously characterized in stratified epithelia where they contribute to the ability of the tissues to withstand chemical and biomechanical stresses. A novel role for several human AIE genes in the vSMC response to arterialization and extended cyclic strain has been proposed (11). Sciellin and periplakin are upregulated in saphenous vein coronary artery bypass grafts after arterialization, but were absent in non-arterialized saphenous veins. Sciellin, SPRR3, and periplakin transcripts were also all upregulated by prolonged exposure to cyclic strain, but not at earlier time points (11).

Genes Regulating vSMC Phenotype

Cyclic strain has significant effects on the phenotype of vSMC (53) but its role in controlling vSMC differentiation remains controversial. Phenotypic responses of vSMC exposed to cyclic stretch *in vitro* include increased expression of contractile and cytoskeletal proteins (myosin light chain kinase, smooth muscle myosin heavy chains, desmin, *h*-caldesmon) and increased expression of thrombin receptor PAR1 in vascular smooth muscle cells (54). Under physiologic conditions, vSMC exhibit a contractile phenotype characterized by abundant contractile proteins. In 2D culture, vSMC switch to a synthetic phenotype characterized by a loss of smooth muscle myosin, increases in ECM and protein synthesis, and a proliferative state (55,56). Cyclic stretching of intact rat vessel segments in an axial direction around their *in vivo* lengths causes alignment of vSMC perpendicular to the direction of strain (57) which is in contrast to the parallel alignment resulting from stretching vSMC in 3D collagen gels. Cyclic uniaxial stretch causes vSMC cultured in type I collagen sponges to exhibit a contractile phenotype, but causes vSMC cultured in polyglycolic acid physically bonded with poly(l-lactic acid) to exhibit a synthetic phenotype (58). These studies highlight the importance of the geometry and environment in modulating the effects of mechanical stretch on vSMC structure and function. Under pathological conditions, exposure of vSMC to pathological forces similar to those exerted during balloon angioplasty resulted in a decrease in contractile protein expression and significantly greater expression of the synthetic vSMC marker vimentin when compared to cells exposed to strain alone (59).

Shear Stress and vSMC Gene Expression

Vascular SMC are not the primary cell exposed to fluid shear stress (FSS) but three-dimensional simulations have shown that vSMCs immediately underlying the internal elastic lamina (IEL) can be exposed to FSS through IEL fenestrations (8). Following iatrogenic endothelial denudation and in the healing response to injury, vSMC are exposed to FSS as they migrate across the IEL in the process of intimal hyperplasia (IH). Whereas the effects of hemodynamic forces on endothelial cells are explored in detail, the influence of FSS on vSMC function is poorly characterized. Microarray analysis following exposure of vSMC to laminar FSS of arterial level (14 dyn/cm^2) for 24 hours identified tissue factor pathway inhibitor-2 (TFPI-2) as one of the genes most altered by FSS. TFPI-2 was also expressed in luminal, FSS-exposed SMCs together with caspase-3 in the rat carotid neointima after balloon injury. Functionally, TFPI-2 may play a role in vessel wall repair by regulating vSMC proliferation and survival (60).

MECHANOTRANSDUCERS IN VSMC

Integrins

Mechanical strain stimulates conformational activation of cell integrins and increases cell binding to the extracellular matrix. The dynamic formation of new integrin–ligand connections is required for stretch-induced mechanotransduction, as blocking unoccupied extracellular matrix ligand sites with isotype-specific antibodies or RGD peptides (RGD being the principal amino acid sequence on extracellular matrix proteins to which integrins bind) inhibits intracellular signaling induced by mechanical forces. Barring a few exceptions, the cytoplasmic domain of integrins is functionally linked to various intracellular proteins that constitute the cytoskeleton and numerous kinases including focal adhesion kinase (FAK), a key regulator of biochemical cascades initiated by mechanical forces (Figure 92.1).

Integrins exist as $\alpha\beta$ pairings that interact with extracellular matrix components including fibronectin (ligand for $\alpha5\beta1$ and $\alpha v\beta3$), vitronectin (ligand for $\alpha v\beta3$), and laminin (ligand for $\alpha6\beta1$) (3). The capacity of cells to sense mechanical forces and the ensuing responses therefore depend on specific integrin–extracellular matrix interactions (36). The available evidence also suggests that integrins are mobilized to orchestrate cellular responses following strain in coordination with (i) growth factor receptors (e.g., those that bind epidermal growth

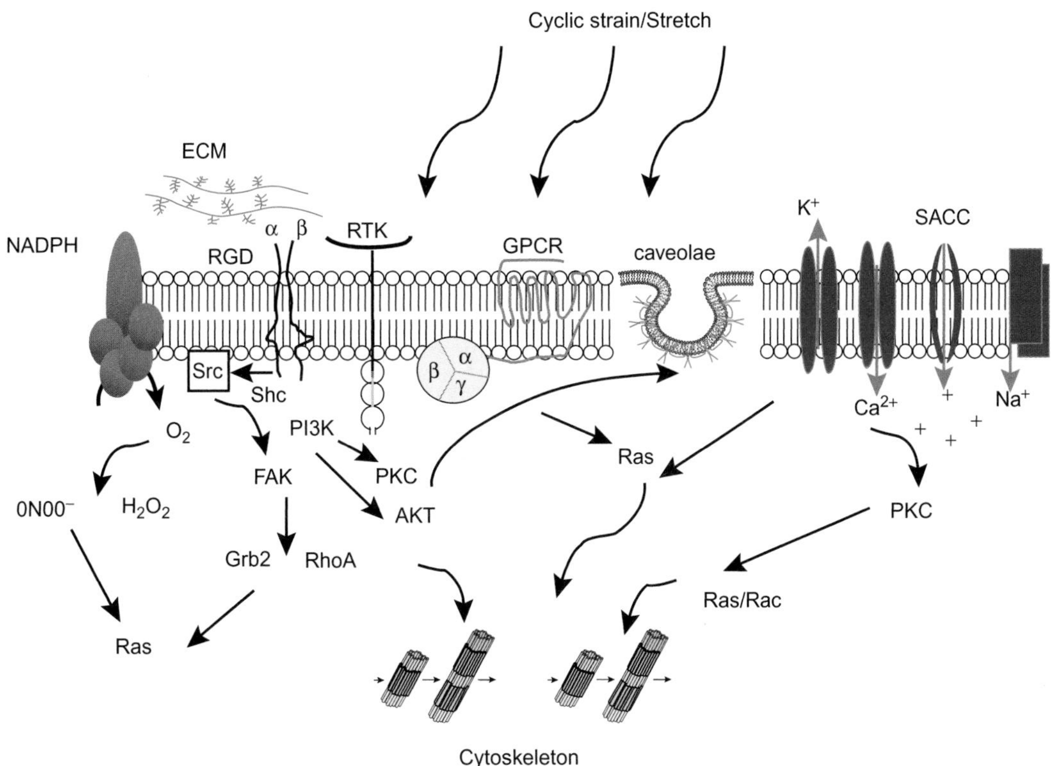

FIGURE 92.1 **Schematic of biomechanical signaling pathways in vSMC.** ECM: extracellular matrix; RTK, receptor tyrosine kinase; RGD, integrins; GPCR, G-protein-coupled receptor; SAAC, swelling-activated anion channels.

factor [EGFR], transforming growth factor-β [TGF-βR], vascular endothelial growth factor [VEGFR] family ligands), (ii) cadherin junctional complexes, and (iii) clues from the ECM. Integrins are the focal points for recruitment of several signaling molecules (e.g., focal adhesion kinase [FAK]) to extracellular matrix (ECM) contact sites in strain-induced vSMC alignment (61). The functional and spatial associations between non-receptor tyrosine kinases (e.g., pp125FAK, pp60c-src) increase with mechanical stimulation reminiscent of those induced by integrin-mediated cell adhesion. Since these same signaling molecules (pp125FAK, pp60c-src) also lie in the main path for mechanical force transfer (i.e., regions enriched in the cytostructural proteins paxcillin, actin, and tensin), it has been proposed that focal adhesion complexes potentially translate mechanical stresses into specific biological responses as a consequence of this cytoskeletal interaction. Indeed, mobilization of FAK, pp60c-src, and Grb2, to focal adhesions under conditions of varying force stimulation engages downstream cascades (i.e., involving mitogen-activated protein (MAP) kinases and the small GTPases Ras, Rac, and Rho) similar to those stimulated by integrin-mediated matrix attachment (4). Mechanical forces may effectively cluster, or initiate conformational changes to, integrin receptors with recruitment of structural proteins at the focal adhesion complex. As part of this response, pp125FAK partitions to the cytoskeletal framework and is tyrosine phosphorylated at Tyr-397 leading to recruitment of pp60c-src, a key kinase in strain-dependent signal transduction.

The pp60c-src kinase is also activated by mechanical stimuli, albeit with different kinetics than that induced by growth factors such as EGF (62). The association of pp60c-src with pp125FAK at focal adhesions further stimulates pp125FAK phosphorylation at Tyr-925, creating a binding site for Grb2 (63). The adaptor protein Shc is tyrosine phosphorylated and binds to Grb2 by an SH2-dependent mechanism facilitating the assembly of a tripartite Shc/Grb2/Sos complex resulting in subsequent Ras GTPase activation. MAP kinase pathways in vSMC similarly function via pp125FAK/pp60c-src/Grb2 interactions with Ras as a downstream target. This has important adaptive consequences as both the extracellular signal-regulated kinase (ERK) and c-Jun-associated kinase (JNK) pathways are activated in a FAK-dependent manner in response to mechanical stimulation (30). Cyclic stretch also rapidly activates p38 MAP kinase in vSMC that requires both the small GTPases Ras and Rac since expression of dominant-negative Ras or Rac constructs attenuates p38 phosphorylation as well as stretch-mediated VSMC migration/proliferation. Stretch-related ERK activation may further modulate cellular mechanical properties by regulating caldesmon, suggesting a direct effect on the contractile properties of the vascular wall (30).

Small GTPases

Mechanical stimulation also activates small GTPases such as Rho, Rac or Cdc42 (25). Indeed, the Rho kinases (Rho-associated coiled-coil forming kinases; ROCK1/2 which are the major immediate downstream targets of RhoA) and mDia are particularly important elements and impact critical functions including cytoskeletal organization, contractility, motility, and gene expression (27) (Figure 92.1). Rho GTPases cycle between active GTP-bound and inactive GDP-bound states which are regulated by guanine nucleotide exchanges factors (GEF) and GTPases-activating proteins (GAPs). The temporal/spatial activation of Rho GTPases likely provides for the physiological adjustment to different cycles or amplitude of mechanical forces commonly encountered by vSMC (64). The complex molecular details of mechanotransduction leading to Rho GTPase signaling, however, are only partially understood.

Reactive Oxygen Species (ROS)

Several lines of evidence suggest that hemodynamic forces can either directly or indirectly activate vascular NAD(P)H oxidase-derived ROS production (2) (Figure 92.1). Hence mitochondria may function as mechanotransducers in vSMC by increasing ROS signaling that may be required for strain-induced increase in NF-κB. However, cells may also modulate this adverse milieu by increasing the expression of glucose-6-phosphate dehydrogenase (G6PDH) to maintain or restore intracellular glutathione (GSH) levels (65). Cyclic strain elicits a rapid increase in intracellular NADH/NADPH oxidase in vSMC concomitant with a rapid and robust phosphorylation of ERK1/2, JNK1/2, and p38 MAPK (66), an effect that was almost completely blocked with DPI (66). Cyclic strain stimulates downstream MMP-2 mRNA and VEGF expression in a NADPH/ROS-dependent manner (67,68). The underlying mechanisms by which strain elicits NAD(P)H oxidase activation probably involve increases in $[Ca^{2+}]i$ and phosphorylation and activation of PKCα (69). PKC-dependent serine phosphorylation of the regulatory p47phox subunit results in its translocation from the cytosol to the membrane oxidase subunits, activating NAD(P)H oxidase function (70). Activation of Nox-1 and Nox-4 in response to hemodynamic forces may differ. Nox-4 does not seem to be regulated by PKC phosphorylation of p47phox, and Nox-1 and Nox-4 are likely to be expressed in different cellular compartments (69,71).

Ion Channels

The discovery of the involvement of stretch-activated ion channels in Ca^{2+} influx in vSMC as mechanosensors began with a nonselective cation channel that is permeable to K^+, Na^+, and Ca^{2+} (Figure 92.1). More recent experiments have shown that the stretch-induced increase of cytosolic Ca^{2+} concentration in vSMC results from the release of intracellular Ca^{2+} stores via a stretch-activated Ca^{2+} channel (72). Notably, cyclic strain activation of Na^+ and Ca^{2+} channels is greater in vSMC isolated from spontaneously hypertensive rats (SHR) when compared to those from normotensive control rats (73). The active transport of ions via membrane-bound ion transport pumps has also been explored. Stretching of vSMC causes an increase in the mRNA expression the α-subunit of Na^+, K^+-ATPase in 6 h (74) and an increase in its protein expression after 4 days (75). Among the classical transient receptor potential (TRPC) subfamily, TRPCs are described as a mechanosensitive and store-operated channel proposed to be activated by hypo-osmotic cell swelling and positive pipette pressure as well as regulated by the filling status of intracellular $Ca(^{2+})$ stores (76). Cyclic stretch significantly decreases transient receptor potential cation channel, subfamily C, member 4 (TRPC4) protein expression and capacitative Ca^{2+} entry in SMC (24). The mechanosensing properties of TRPC channels highly expressed in vSMC are likely to play a key role in regulating myogenic tone in vascular tissue.

RECAPITULATION OF VASCULAR DEVELOPMENTAL SIGNALING

Vascular development is an orchestrated sequence of events whereby different vascular beds form and then adapt to external stimuli applied by cellular interactions as well as the physical forces and signals generated by blood flow (77). During vascular morphogenesis, the maturation of the aortic trunk and its branches results from adaptative mechanisms involving shear and tensile stress (78). One important characteristic of this development process is the number of circumferential layers of vSMC in arteries as determined by ~E14 in mice (see Chapter 82). This unique adaptation in wall structure suggests developmental remodeling in response to altered mechanics and hemodynamics (79). Since this is the time window when the vSMC accumulate around developing arteries, it is tempting to speculate that this gradual increase in pressure (i.e., albeit at low pressures compared with later development) may be a critical stimulus for this vSMC circumferential accumulation.

In this context, there is now compelling evidence to suggest that this vSMC cell-fate decision involves a complex interaction of several developmental gene regulatory networks. The differentiation of arterial and venous endothelial cells in zebrafish is a requisite step for normal blood vessel formation to occur and involves Notch, hedgehog, VEGF and Ephrins pathways (80). The Notch signaling pathway is an evolutionarily conserved, intercellular signaling mechanism that plays a central role in the development of most vertebrate organs. Studies have shown that Notch signaling is required downstream of VEGF to induce arterial differentiation. Moreover, *Notch3* is a cell-autonomous regulator of arterial differentiation and maturation of vSMC in mice since in adult Notch3$^{-/-}$ mice distal arteries exhibit structural defects and arterial myogenic responses are defective (81). In cerebral autosomal dominant arteriopathy with subcortical infarcts and leukoencephalopathy (CADASIL), a systemic vascular disease caused by Notch 3 gene mutations, morphometric analysis of skin vessels using electron microscopy revealed relative absence of stenosis but marked destruction of vSMC resulting in decrease of vessel wall thickness and loss of extracellular matrix area, producing vessel wall weakness. Similar changes were also observed in brain arterioles from five patients with CADASIL (82). In addition, mutant Notch3 impairs selectively the response of resistance arteries to flow and pressure (83). *In vitro* studies have since confirmed that Notch and upstream hedgehog signaling pathways are mechanosensitive in adult vSMC (42,84).

Another developmental pathway implicated in hemodynamic modulation of vSMC function has recently been addressed. Activation of β-catenin signaling, as a result of dismantling of N-cadherin–mediated cell–cell contacts, induced vSMC proliferation *in vitro* via modulation of the expression of the cell cycle genes cyclin D1 and p21. Moreover, similar dismantling of cadherin:β-catenin complexes occurs *in vivo* following balloon-injured rat carotid arteries suggesting a possible mechanosensitive regulation of this pathway in adult vSMC *in vivo*. This is corroborated by the detection of elevated levels of β-catenin after balloon injury in rat carotid arteries (85). The Wnt family (comprised of 19 secreted, lipid-modified glycoproteins) plays a crucial role not only in the regulation of embryogenesis and development, but also in cell proliferation, differentiation, polarity, migration, and invasion. There is also evidence that activation of the Wnt pathway induces vSMC proliferation (86). Although these studies provided evidence for the involvement of the Wnt/β-catenin pathway in vSMC proliferation and intimal thickening following mechanical-induced injury, it is only recently that Wnt/β-catenin signaling was observed in proliferating vSMC during intimal thickening as a result of Wnt4 upregulation (87,88). It is clear that Wnt/β-catenin signaling pathways involved in embryonic development can be reactivated in adults.

Bone morphogenetic protein-2 and -4 (BMP-2/4) are TGF-β superfamily cytokines that are expressed by vSMC and regulate a number of cellular processes involved in atherogenesis, including vascular calcification and endothelial activation (71). BMPs are yet another pathway involved in embryonic and adult blood vessel formation. In particular, the involvement of the BMP-regulated Id family of helix–loop–helix transcription factors in angiogenesis has been investigated extensively. Nevertheless, some controversy exists regarding differences between BMP-2 and BMP-4 on vascular cell proliferation and the different roles that these BMPs may play in vSMC physiology. Despite this, it is clear such BMP-dependent signaling pathways involved in embryonic development can be reactivated in adults and may thus contribute to the neointimal proliferative disease following mechanical-induced injury.

CONCLUSION

During the past three decades, major advancements have emerged in our collective understanding of how hemodynamic forces regulate vascular homeostasis. Changes in hemodynamic forces acting on vSMC activate discrete cellular signaling pathways that translate biomechanical stimuli into specific biological responses. These mechanotransducers are operational under normal and pathological conditions. The predominant mechanical force influencing vSMC structural organization and signaling is cyclic stretch/strain. During normal vascular homeostasis physiological levels of cyclic strain maintain a quiescent vSMC phenotype in normal healthy vessels. In contrast, adverse changes in the hemodynamic microenvironment of vSMC (mean strain, frequency and amplitude) can elicit phenotypic changes favoring vascular remodeling. Strain modulates cell shape, cytoplasmic organization and intracellular processes leading to changes in migration, proliferation, and apoptosis of vSMC. Recapitulation of mechanosensitive signaling pathways involved in embryonic vascular development has presented novel targets for investigation and may present new therapies for the treatment of neointimal proliferative disease following mechanical force-induced injury. Drug therapy directed at the components of the mechanotransducer signaling pathways influenced by strain may ultimately prevent several cardiovascular pathologies associated with intimal hyperplasia.

REFERENCES

1. Califano JP, Reinhart-King CA. Exogenous and endogenous force regulation of endothelial cell behavior. *J Biomech* 2010;**43**:79–86.
2. Birukov KG. Cyclic stretch, reactive oxygen species, and vascular remodeling. *Antioxid Redox Sign* 2009;**11**:1651–67.
3. Gupta V, Grande-Allen KJ. Effects of static and cyclic loading in regulating extracellular matrix synthesis by cardiovascular cells. *Cardiovasc Res* 2006;**72**:375–83.

4. Lehoux S, Castier Y, Tedgui A. Molecular mechanisms of the vascular responses to haemodynamic forces. *J Intern Med* 2006;**259**:381–92.
5. Humphrey JD. Vascular mechanics, mechanobiology, and remodeling. *J Mech Med Biol* 2009;**9**:243–57.
6. Humphrey JD. Mechanisms of arterial remodeling in hypertension: coupled roles of wall shear and intramural stress. *Hypertension* 2008;**52**:195–200.
7. Wang DM, Tarbell JM. Modeling interstitial flow in an artery wall allows estimation of wall shear stress on smooth muscle cells. *J Biomech Eng* 1995;**117**:358–63.
8. Tada S, Tarbell JM. Flow through internal elastic lamina affects shear stress on smooth muscle cells (3D simulations). *Am J Physiol Heart Circ Physiol* 2002;**282**:H576–84.
9. Tromp G, Kuivaniemi H. Developments in genomics to improve understanding, diagnosis and management of aneurysms and peripheral artery disease. *Eur J Vasc Endovasc Surg* 2009;**38**:676–82.
10. Cheng J, Wang Y, Ma Y, Chan BT, Yang M, Liang A, et al. The mechanical stress-activated serum-, glucocorticoid-regulated kinase 1 contributes to neointima formation in vein grafts. *Circ Res* 2010;**107**:1265–74.
11. Pyle AL, Li B, Maupin AB, Guzman RJ, Crimmins DL, Olson S, et al. Biomechanical stress induces novel arterial intima-enriched genes: implications for vascular adaptation to stress. *Cardiovasc Pathol* 2010;**19**:e13–20.
12 Feng Y, Yang JH, Huang H, Kennedy SP, Turi TG, Thompson JF, et al. Transcriptional profile of mechanically induced genes in human vascular smooth muscle cells. *Circ Res* 1999;**85**:1118–23.
13. Van Assche T, Hendrickx J, Crauwels HM, Guns PJ, Martinet W, Fransen P, et al. Transcription profiles of aortic smooth muscle cells from atherosclerosis-prone and -resistant regions in young apolipoprotein E-deficient mice before plaque development. *J Vasc Res* 2011;**48**:31–42.
14. Yoshida T, Komuro I. [Effect of mechanical stress on blood vessels]. *Nippon Rinsho* 2004;**62**(Suppl. 3):29–32.
15. Lo IC, Lin TM, Chou LH, Liu SL, Wu LW, Shi GY, et al. Ets-1 mediates platelet-derived growth factor-BB-induced thrombomodulin expression in human vascular smooth muscle cells. *Cardiovasc Res* 2009;**81**:771–9.
16. Lee MY, Garvey SM, Baras AS, Lemmon JA, Gomez MF, Schoppee Bortz PD, et al. Integrative genomics identifies DSCR1 (RCAN1) as a novel NFAT-dependent mediator of phenotypic modulation in vascular smooth muscle cells. *Hum Mol Genet* 2010;**19**:468–79.
17. Orr AW, Hastings NE, Blackman BR, Wamhoff BR. Complex regulation and function of the inflammatory smooth muscle cell phenotype in atherosclerosis. *J Vasc Res* 2010;**47**:168–80.
18. Kona S, Chellamuthu P, Xu H, Hills SR, Nguyen KT. Effects of cyclic strain and growth factors on vascular smooth muscle cell responses. *Open Biomed Eng J* 2009;**3**:28–38.
19. Ye L, Mora R, Akhayani N, Haudenschild CC, Liau G. Growth factor and cytokine-regulated hyaluronan-binding protein TSG-6 is localized to the injury-induced rat neointima and confers enhanced growth in vascular smooth muscle cells. *Circ Res* 1997;**81**:289–96.
20. Dangers M, Kiyan J, Grote K, Schieffer B, Haller H, Dumler I. Mechanical stress modulates SOCS-1 expression in human vascular smooth muscle cells. *J Vasc Res* 2010;**47**:432–40.
21. Li C, Xu Q. Mechanical stress-initiated signal transduction in vascular smooth muscle cells in vitro and in vivo. *Cell Signal* 2007;**19**:881–91.
22. Albinsson S, Nordstrom I, Sward K, Hellstrand P. Differential dependence of stretch and shear stress signaling on caveolin-1 in the vascular wall. *Am J Physiol Cell Physiol* 2008;**294**:C271–9.
23. Nakayama K, Obara K, Tanabe Y, Saito M, Ishikawa T, Nishizawa S. Interactive role of tyrosine kinase, protein kinase C, and Rho/Rho kinase systems in the mechanotransduction of vascular smooth muscles. *Biorheology* 2003;**40**:307–14.
24. Lindsey SH, Tribe RM, Songu-Mize E. Cyclic stretch decreases TRPC4 protein and capacitative calcium entry in rat vascular smooth muscle cells. *Life Sci* 2008;**83**:29–34.
25. Putnam AJ, Cunningham JJ, Pillemer BB, Mooney DJ. External mechanical strain regulates membrane targeting of Rho GTPases by controlling microtubule assembly. *Am J Physiol Cell Physiol* 2003;**284**:C627–39.
26. Yang R, Amir J, Liu H, Chaqour B. Mechanical strain activates a program of genes functionally involved in paracrine signaling of angiogenesis. *Physiol Genomics* 2008;**36**:1–14.
27. Chapados R, Abe K, Ihida-Stansbury K, McKean D, Gates AT, Kern M, et al. ROCK controls matrix synthesis in vascular smooth muscle cells: coupling vasoconstriction to vascular remodeling. *Circ Res* 2006;**99**:837–44.
28. Yang JH, Briggs WH, Libby P, Lee RT. Small mechanical strains selectively suppress matrix metalloproteinase-1 expression by human vascular smooth muscle cells. *J Biol Chem* 1998;**273**:6550–5.
29. Durier S, Fassot C, Laurent S, Boutouyrie P, Couetil JP, Fine E, et al. Physiological genomics of human arteries: quantitative relationship between gene expression and arterial stiffness. *Circulation* 2003;**108**:1845–51.
30. Samarakoon R, Goppelt-Struebe M, Higgins PJ. Linking cell structure to gene regulation: signaling events and expression controls on the model genes PAI-1 and CTGF. *Cell Signal* 2010;**22**:1413–9.
31. Hahn C, Schwartz MA. Mechanotransduction in vascular physiology and atherogenesis. *Nat Rev Mol Cell Biol* 2009;**10**:53–62.
32. Chapman GB, Durante W, Hellums JD, Schafer AI. Physiological cyclic stretch causes cell cycle arrest in cultured vascular smooth muscle cells. *Am J Physiol Heart Circ Physiol* 2000;**278**:H748–54.
33. Sedding DG, Seay U, Fink L, Heil M, Kummer W, Tillmanns H, et al. Mechanosensitive p27Kip1 regulation and cell cycle entry in vascular smooth muscle cells. *Circulation* 2003;**108**:616–22.
34. Matsushita H, Lee KH, Tsao PS. Cyclic strain induces reactive oxygen species production via an endothelial NAD(P)H oxidase. *J Cell Biochem Suppl* 2001;**Suppl 36**:99–106.
35. Acampora KB, Nagatomi J, Langan EM, LaBerge M. Increased synthetic phenotype behavior of smooth muscle cells in response to in vitro balloon angioplasty injury model. *Ann Vasc Surg* 2010;**24**:116–26.
36. Wilson E, Sudhir K, Ives HE. Mechanical strain of rat vascular smooth muscle cells is sensed by specific extracellular matrix/integrin interactions. *J Clin Invest* 1995;**96**:2364–72.
37. Sun Z, Martinez-Lemus LA, Hill MA, Meininger GA. Extracellular matrix-specific focal adhesions in vascular smooth muscle produce mechanically active adhesion sites. *Am J Physiol Cell Physiol* 2008;**295**:C268–78.

38. Heydarkhan-Hagvall S, Esguerra M, Helenius G, Soderberg R, Johansson BR, Risberg B. Production of extracellular matrix components in tissue-engineered blood vessels. *Tissue Eng* 2006;**12**:831–42.
39. Asanuma K, Magid R, Johnson C, Nerem RM, Galis ZS. Uniaxial strain upregulates matrix-degrading enzymes produced by human vascular smooth muscle cells. *Am J Physiol Heart Circ Physiol* 2003;**284**:H1778–84.
40. Beamish JA, He P, Kottke-Marchant K, Marchant RE. Molecular regulation of contractile smooth muscle cell phenotype: implications for vascular tissue engineering. *Tissue Eng Part B Rev* 2010;**16**:467–91.
41. Wernig F, Mayr M, Xu QB. Mechanical stretch-induced apoptosis in smooth muscle cells is mediated by beta(1)-integrin signaling pathways. *Hypertension* 2003;**41**:903–11.
42. Morrow D, Sweeney C, Birney YA, Cummins PM, Walls D, Redmond EM, et al. Cyclic strain inhibits notch receptor signaling in vascular smooth muscle cells in vitro. *Circ Res* 2005;**96**:567–75.
43. Cappadona C, Redmond EM, Theodorakis NG, McKillop IH, Hendrickson R, Chhabra A, et al. Phenotype dictates the growth response of vascular smooth muscle cells to pulse pressure in vitro. *FASEB J* 1999;**13** A1020-A1020.
44. Sedding DG, Homann M, Seay U, Tillmanns H, Preissner KT, Braun-Dullaeus RC. Calpain counteracts mechanosensitive apoptosis of vascular smooth muscle cells in vitro and in vivo. *FASEB J* 2008;**22**:579–89.
45. Wernig F, Mayr M, Xu Q. Mechanical stretch-induced apoptosis in smooth muscle cells is mediated by beta1-integrin signaling pathways. *Hypertension* 2003;**41**:903–11.
46. Bayer IM, Adamson SL, Langille BL. Atrophic remodeling of the artery-cuffed artery. *Arterioscler Thromb Vasc Biol* 1999;**19**:1499–505.
47. Cheng Y, Liu X, Yang J, Lin Y, Xu DZ, Lu Q, et al. MicroRNA-145, a novel smooth muscle cell phenotypic marker and modulator, controls vascular neointimal lesion formation. *Circ Res* 2009;**105**:158–66.
48. Fish JE, Santoro MM, Morton SU, Yu S, Yeh RF, Wythe JD, et al. miR-126 regulates angiogenic signaling and vascular integrity. *Dev Cell* 2008;**15**:272–84.
49. Kuang W, Tan J, Duan Y, Duan J, Wang W, Jin F, et al. Cyclic stretch induced miR-146a upregulation delays C2C12 myogenic differentiation through inhibition of Numb. *Biochem Biophys Res Commun* 2009;**378**:259–63.
50. Yu ML, Wang JF, Wang GK, You XH, Zhao XX, Jing Q, et al. Vascular smooth muscle cell proliferation is influenced by let-7d microRNA and its interaction with KRAS. *Circ J* 2011;**75**:703–9.
51. Coffman JD. Pathophysiology of obstructive arterial disease. *Herz* 1988;**13**:343–50.
52. Young PP, Modur V, Teleron AA, Ladenson JH. Enrichment of genes in the aortic intima that are associated with stratified epithelium: implications of underlying biomechanical and barrier properties of the arterial intima. *Circulation* 2005;**111**:2382–90.
53. Riha GM, Lin PH, Lumsden AB, Yao Q, Chen C. Roles of hemodynamic forces in vascular cell differentiation. *Ann Biomed Eng* 2005;**33**:772–9.
54. Owens GK. Role of mechanical strain in regulation of differentiation of vascular smooth muscle cells. *Circ Res* 1996;**79**:1054–5.
55. Birukov KG, Bardy N, Lehoux S, Merval R, Shirinsky VP, Tedgui A. Intraluminal pressure is essential for the maintenance of smooth muscle caldesmon and filamin content in aortic organ culture. *Arterioscler Thromb Vasc Biol* 1998;**18**:922–7.
56. Reusch P, Wagdy H, Reusch R, Wilson E, Ives HE. Mechanical strain increases smooth muscle and decreases nonmuscle myosin expression in rat vascular smooth muscle cells. *Circ Res* 1996;**79**:1046–53.
57. Sipkema P, van der Linden PJ, Westerhof N, Yin FC. Effect of cyclic axial stretch of rat arteries on endothelial cytoskeletal morphology and vascular reactivity. *J Biomech* 2003;**36**:653–9.
58. Kim BS, Mooney DJ. Scaffolds for engineering smooth muscle under cyclic mechanical strain conditions. *J Biomech Eng* 2000;**122**:210–5.
59. Acampora KB, Nagatomi J, Langan III EM, LaBerge M. Increased synthetic phenotype behavior of smooth muscle cells in response to in vitro balloon angioplasty injury model. *Ann Vasc Surg* 2010;**24**:116–26.
60. Ekstrand J, Razuvaev A, Folkersen L, Roy J, Hedin U. Tissue factor pathway inhibitor-2 is induced by fluid shear stress in vascular smooth muscle cells and affects cell proliferation and survival. *J Vasc Surg* 2010;**52**:167–75.
61. Liu B, Qu MJ, Qin KR, Li H, Li ZK, Shen BR, et al. Role of cyclic strain frequency in regulating the alignment of vascular smooth muscle cells in vitro. *Biophys J* 2008;**94**:1497–507.
62. Plopper GE, McNamee HP, Dike LE, Bojanowski K, Ingber DE. Convergence of integrin and growth factor receptor signaling pathways within the focal adhesion complex. *Mol Biol Cell* 1995;**6**:1349–65.
63. Eliceiri BP, Puente XS, Hood JD, Stupack DG, Schlaepfer DD, Huang XZ, et al. Src-mediated coupling of focal adhesion kinase to integrin alpha(v)beta5 in vascular endothelial growth factor signaling. *J Cell Biol* 2002;**157**:149–60.
64. Onoue N, Nawata J, Tada T, Zhulanqiqige D, Wang H, Sugimura K, et al. Increased static pressure promotes migration of vascular smooth muscle cells: involvement of the Rho-kinase pathway. *J Cardiovasc Pharmacol* 2008;**51**:55–61.
65. Leopold JA, Loscalzo J. Cyclic strain modulates resistance to oxidant stress by increasing G6PDH expression in smooth muscle cells. *Am J Physiol Heart Circ Physiol* 2000;**279**:H2477–85.
66. Chen Q, Li W, Quan Z, Sumpio BE. Modulation of vascular smooth muscle cell alignment by cyclic strain is dependent on reactive oxygen species and P38 mitogen-activated protein kinase. *J Vasc Surg* 2003;**37**:660–8.
67. Grote K, Flach I, Luchtefeld M, Akin E, Holland SM, Drexler H, et al. Mechanical stretch enhances mRNA expression and proenzyme release of matrix metalloproteinase-2 (MMP-2) via NAD(P)H oxidase-derived reactive oxygen species. *Circ Res* 2003;**92**:e80–6.
68. Mata-Greenwood E, Grobe A, Kumar S, Noskina Y, Black SM. Cyclic stretch increases VEGF expression in pulmonary arterial smooth muscle cells via TGF-beta1 and reactive oxygen species: a requirement for NAD(P)H oxidase. *Am J Physiol Lung Cell Mol Physiol* 2005;**289**:L288–9.
69. Ungvari Z, Csiszar A, Huang A, Kaminski PM, Wolin MS, Koller A. High pressure induces superoxide production in isolated arteries via protein kinase C-dependent activation of NAD(P)H oxidase. *Circulation* 2003;**108**:1253–8.

70. Bedard K, Krause KH. The NOX family of ROS-generating NADPH oxidases: physiology and pathophysiology. *Physiol Rev* 2007;**87**:245–313.
71. Csiszar A, Lehoux S, Ungvari Z. Hemodynamic forces, vascular oxidative stress, and regulation of BMP-2/4 expression. *Antioxid Redox Sign* 2009;**11**:1683–97.
72. Mohanty MJ, Li X. Stretch-induced Ca(2+) release via an IP(3)-insensitive Ca(2+) channel. *Am J Physiol Cell Physiol* 2002;**283**: C456–62.
73. Ohya Y, Adachi N, Nakamura Y, Setoguchi M, Abe I, Fujishima M. Stretch-activated channels in arterial smooth muscle of genetic hypertensive rats. *Hypertension* 1998;**31**:254–8.
74. Sevieux N, Alam J, Songu-Mize E. Effect of cyclic stretch on alpha-subunit mRNA expression of Na^+-K^+-ATPase in aortic smooth muscle cells. *Am J Physiol Cell Physiol* 2001;**280**:C1555–60.
75. Songu-Mize E, Sevieux N, Liu X, Jacobs M. Effect of short-term cyclic stretch on sodium pump activity in aortic smooth muscle cells. *Am J Physiol Heart Circ Physiol* 2001;**281**:H2072–8.
76. Dietrich A, Kalwa H, Storch U, Mederos y Schnitzler M, Salanova B, Pinkenburg O, et al. Pressure-induced and store-operated cation influx in vascular smooth muscle cells is independent of TRPC1. *Pflugers Arch* 2007;**455**:465–77.
77. Davis GE. The development of the vasculature and its extracellular matrix: a gradual process defined by sequential cellular and matrix remodeling events. *Am J Physiol Heart Circ Physiol* 2010;**299**: H245–7.
78. Lucitti JL, Visconti R, Novak J, Keller BB. Increased arterial load alters aortic structural and functional properties during embryogenesis. *Am J Physiol Heart Circ Physiol* 2006;**291**:H1919–26.
79. Faury G, Pezet M, Knutsen RH, Boyle WA, Heximer SP, McLean SE, et al. Developmental adaptation of the mouse cardiovascular system to elastin haploinsufficiency. *J Clin Invest* 2003;**112**:1419–28.
80. Lawson ND, Weinstein BM. Arteries and veins: making a difference with zebrafish. *Nat Rev Genet* 2002;**3**:674–82.
81. Domenga V, Fardoux P, Lacombe P, Monet M, Maciazek J, Krebs LT, et al. Notch3 is required for arterial identity and maturation of vascular smooth muscle cells. *Genes Dev* 2004;**18**:2730–5.
82. Brulin P, Godfraind C, Leteurtre E, Ruchoux MM. Morphometric analysis of ultrastructural vascular changes in CADASIL: analysis of 50 skin biopsy specimens and pathogenic implications. *Acta Neuropathol* 2002;**104**:241–8.
83. Dubroca C, Lacombe P, Domenga V, Maciazek J, Levy B, Tournier-Lasserve E, et al. Impaired vascular mechanotransduction in a transgenic mouse model of CADASIL arteriopathy. *Stroke* 2005;**36**:113–7.
84. Morrow D, Sweeney C, Birney YA, Guha S, Collins N, Cummins PM, et al. Biomechanical regulation of hedgehog signaling in vascular smooth muscle cells in vitro and in vivo. *Am J Physiol Cell Physiol* 2007;**292**:C488–96.
85. Wang X, Xiao Y, Mou Y, Zhao Y, Blankesteijn WM, Hall JL. A role for the beta-catenin/T-cell factor signaling cascade in vascular remodeling. *Circ Res* 2002;**90**:340–7.
86. Mao C, Malek OT, Pueyo ME, Steg PG, Soubrier F. Differential expression of rat frizzled-related frzb-1 and frizzled receptor fz1 and fz2 genes in the rat aorta after balloon injury. *Arterioscler Thromb Vasc Biol* 2000;**20**:43–51.
87. Corada M, Nyqvist D, Orsenigo F, Caprini A, Giampietro C, Taketo MM, et al. The Wnt/beta-catenin pathway modulates vascular remodeling and specification by upregulating Dll4/Notch signaling. *Dev Cell* 2010;**18**:938–49.
88. Tsaousi A, Williams H, Lyon CA, Taylor V, Swain A, Johnson JL, George SJ. Wnt4/{beta}-catenin signaling induces VSMC proliferation and is associated with intimal thickening. *Circ Res* 2011;**108**:427–36.

Chapter 93

Myogenic Tone and Mechanotransduction

Michael A. Hill and Gerald A. Meininger
Dalton Cardiovascular Research Center and the Department of Medical Pharmacology and Physiology, University of Missouri, Columbia, MO

MYOGENIC TONE AND MECHANOTRANSDUCTION

Mechanotransduction refers to the process by which a mechanical stimulus is converted into a set of biochemical reactions and a cellular response. Importantly, the ability to respond to mechanical stimuli is a property of all cells and is not simply limited to cells classically viewed as mechanoreceptors (for example hair cells, baroreceptors, skin, skeletal muscle mechanosenors). Thus cells, in general, use environmentally-provided mechanical signals in the regulation of many events, including positional location and adhesion, contractile activation, responsiveness to shear stress and development/growth. This chapter will restrict its consideration of mechanotransduction to how arteriolar smooth muscle interprets and responds to changes in intraluminal pressure (referred to as myogenic responsiveness or reactivity) and in doing so contributes to the control of local hemodynamics through the acute modulation of vessel caliber (Figure 93.1). It is acknowledged that even in the context of a vascular smooth muscle cell's (SMC's) response to a change in intravascular pressure, that this mechanical stimulus likely simultaneously activate multiple signaling pathways. For example, in addition to contraction these include pathways contributing to gene expression and both short- and longer-term synthetic and phenotypic changes leading to remodeling. (For more general reviews on mechanotransduction the reader is referred to references 1–3.)

THE MYOGENIC RESPONSE IN MICROCIRCULATORY CONTROL

Brief Introduction, Historical Context, and Physiological Significance

The arteriolar myogenic response is typically viewed as the vasoconstriction that occurs in response to an increase in intraluminal pressure or the vasodilation that follows a decrease in intraluminal pressure. The pressure-induced response has been demonstrated to occur independently of the endothelium and does not require neurohumoral input. Instead, intraluminal pressure exerts its direct mechanical effects on the vascular smooth muscle cells to elicit a degree of contractile activation. The expression of basal vascular tone is viewed as resulting from a partial degree of tonic activation resulting from vascular distension brought about by the level of intravascular pressure. Thus, viewed collectively, the myogenic properties of a blood vessel manifest as either a dynamic change in contractile activation responding to an acute alteration in intravascular pressure or as a more static level of activation state (tone) (Figure 93.2).

The first description of the vascular myogenic response is generally attributed to Bayliss in 1902 (4). Bayliss observed an increase in the volume of the hindlimb following transient occlusion of the aorta and attributed this to be a pressure- or stretch-dependent relaxation response of the vascular smooth muscle. In support of this, he further observed pressure-induced contraction in isolated carotid artery segments from dogs. Following the work of Bayliss, metabolic theories of blood flow control dominated until the studies of Folkow (5,6) resurrected interest (7) in the myogenic response. Folkow showed that denervated preparations developed pressure-dependent vascular tone (5) and that autoregulation of blood flow was partly explained by non-neural, pressure-dependent mechanisms (6). In the 1960s and 1970s the development of *in vivo* preparations and video microscopy for quantitative study of the microcirculation enabled myogenic responsiveness to be directly studied at the tissue level (8–10). Following this, the development of myographs (11) and the ability to isolate and cannulate single arterioles (12) allowed pressure-induced vasoconstriction to be studied in single vessels. The availability of fluorescent indicators (for example, Ca^{2+} sensitive indicators, fura 2 (13) and fluo 4 (14)), pharmacological inhibitors, sharp electrode recordings (15), and microbiochemical approaches (16–18) subsequently enabled more direct

Muscle. DOI: http://dx.doi.org/10.1016/B978-0-12-381510-1.00093-4

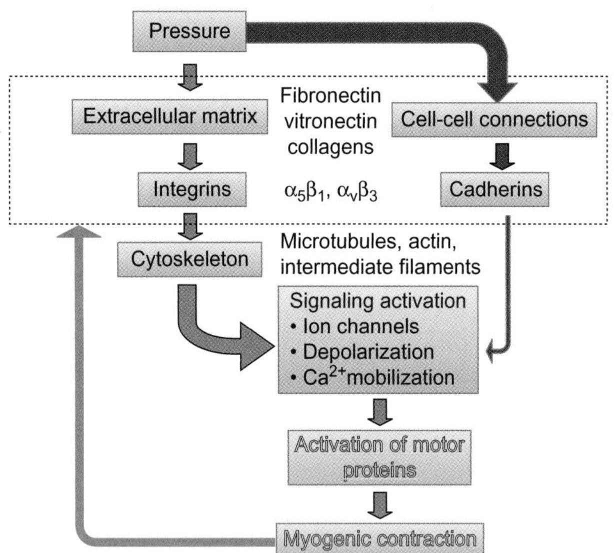

FIGURE 93.1 Block diagram illustrating basic steps underlying myogenic vasoconstriction. Mechanosensory events initiate a series of reactions that transduce the extracellular mechanical stimulus across the plasma membrane to ultimately result in activation of the contractile process. The resultant myogenic vasoconstriction feeds back to reduce the pressure-induced mechanical stimulus (e.g. an increase in wall tension or stretch/deformation of a putative mechanosensor).

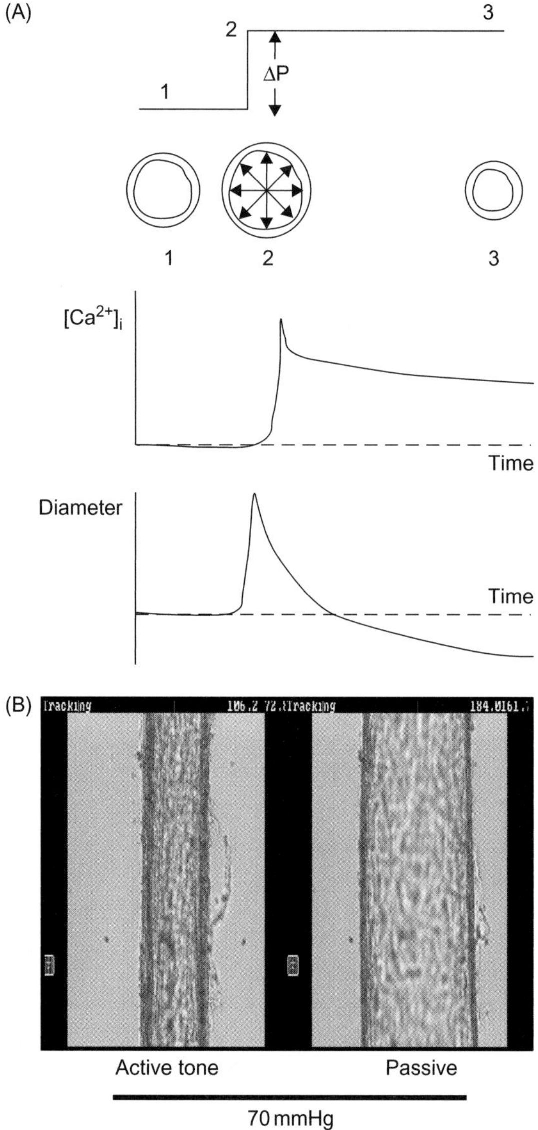

FIGURE 93.2 (A) Schematically demonstrates the temporal relationships between global intracellular Ca^{2+} and vessel diameter in response to an acute increase in intraluminal pressure. From a baseline pressure (1) an acute pressure step is imposed causing radial distension of the arteriole (2). This passive response is followed by a Ca^{2+}-dependent constriction to a new steady-state diameter (3). Importantly, the response is reversible with dilation occurring in response to a decrease in intraluminal pressure. (B) Isolated and cannulated cremaster muscle arteriole at 70 mmHg intraluminal pressure under active (left) and passive (right) conditions.

studies of underlying cellular signaling mechanisms. Many of the intact vessel studies were later complemented by single cell studies using sophisticated approaches such as patch clamping (19) and atomic force microscopy (20).

The overall contribution of the myogenic response to cardiovascular control, and its physiological significance, lies in its role in setting basal peripheral vascular resistance (21). A basal level of vascular tone provides a base state of contractile activation, and hence partial contraction, on which vasodilator or vasoconstrictor stimuli can act to modulate peripheral resistance. This type of fine-tuning of vascular resistance is important for matching blood flow with metabolic requirements and contributing to the control of blood pressure. In relation to matching tissue perfusion with metabolic demand, myogenic responsiveness is considered to play a key role in local blood flow autoregulation where, under conditions of constant metabolic demand, flow is maintained relatively constant across a range of perfusion pressures (22). An additional consequence of myogenic constriction is the regulation of capillary pressure, as pressure-induced arteriolar constriction limits the transfer of an increase in systemic pressure to the exchange vessels preventing excessive fluid leakage and edema formation. This action of the myogenic response may also be protective against physical damage caused by high pressures, particularly in the renal vascular bed where this has been suggested to exert priority over blood flow regulation (23). However, in general, evidence suggests a closer relationship between myogenic responsiveness and autoregulation of blood flow as compared to active capillary pressure regulation (21). Collectively, the various roles played by the myogenic response underscore its fundamental significance in local vasoregulation.

Interactions Between the Myogenic Response and Other Vasoregulatory Mechanisms in Affecting Local Control of Hemodynamics

While being prominent in the setting of basal vascular tone, myogenic responsiveness does not exist in isolation and is modulated by several vasoregulatory mechanisms. For example, adrenergic receptor stimulation enhances myogenic vasoconstriction in some vascular beds through downstream interaction of signaling mechanisms (24). Conversely, the prevailing level of myogenic tone often influences the effectiveness of these other regulatory mechanisms. This has been clearly illustrated in *in vivo* studies of the hindquarter and splanchnic circulations of rats. In these studies, when either of the vasoconstrictors angiotensin II or phenylephrine were infused to induce systemic hypertension, the local increases in hindquarter or splanchnic vascular resistance could be markedly attenuated by protecting the vascular beds from the pressure increase (25). Thus, despite the presence of the circulating agonist, in the absence of an additional pressure stimulus, the vasoconstriction was significantly reduced. It was concluded that pressure-dependent autoregulatory events are activated during agonist-induced contractile activation such that the myogenic mechanism responds to the changes in vascular pressure that result from the direct receptor-mediated response to the agonist. Thus, the net effects on local vascular resistance were a composite effect of both neurohumoral and myogenic components.

Although it is now accepted that myogenic responsiveness occurs independently of the endothelium (26,27), it is clear that endothelial cells modulate pressure-induced myogenic tone. Using cannulated arterioles, under controlled flow and pressure conditions, Kuo et al. (28) demonstrated that luminal flow causes an upward shift in the pressure–diameter relationship such that myogenic tone was attenuated at each level of intraluminal pressure studied. Such interactions largely occur through the release of endothelial-derived paracrine factors (for example, nitric oxide) and the direct coupling of endothelial and smooth muscle cells via myoendothelial gap junctions (MEGJs) (29,30). Collectively, these mechanisms enable the vessel to exhibit integrated phenomena such as conducted and flow-dependent vasomotor responses that allow syncitial-like behavior and coupling along the vascular tree.

Detailed consideration of interactions occurring between these vascular control mechanisms, metabolic factors, and the resultant network behavior, is beyond the scope of this chapter. They are mentioned, however, to emphasize that myogenic pathways of mechanotransduction exist, particularly in the intact network, in a complex array of physiological control mechanisms.

THE UNDERLYING MECHANISM(S)

Mechanosensors – Detecting Changes in Intraluminal Pressure

A change in intraluminal pressure appears to exert a mechanical force on a cellular component that acts as a mechanosensor, perhaps analogous to a receptor, to initiate the signal transduction process. At present it remains uncertain as to what variable is sensed by the vascular smooth muscle (VSM) cell although support has been provided for pressure-induced changes in wall tension, deformation of cell membrane proteins (for example ion channels); conformational changes in non-membrane proteins, including extracellular matrix (ECM) and cytoskeletal proteins; ECM-mediated integrin activation and activation at the site of other cellular junctions such as cadherins. Possible models for how intraluminal pressure is sensed as part of the myogenic response are shown in Figure 93.3 (similar models can be found in a number of reviews, including 1, 31, 32). While these models are presented as being independent of each other it is conceivable that significant interaction occurs between them – for example, ECM–integrin binding likely contributes to modulation of contractile activation, regulation of the actin cytoskeleton and gene transcription.

Thus, the location of a putative myogenic mechanosensor is likely at the level of the cell membrane, cellular adhesion sites (matrix and/or intercellular junctions) or the cytoskeleton, all of which are conceivably mechanically linked. Each of these is briefly considered in the following.

The Cell Membrane

The mechanical forces exerted by intraluminal pressure are proposed to directly impact either the protein or lipid components of the cell membrane. Deformation of ion channel proteins or other integral membranes proteins (for example, mechanosensitive enzymes) could result in changes of activity that initiate a response to the initial mechanical stimulus.

The involvement of specialized regions of the membrane, such as cholesterol-rich lipid rafts or caveolae, remains intriguing. In particular, this relates to numerous studies demonstrating that they represent a site of concentration for many signaling components, including ion channels and intracellular enzymes whose activity is regulated by associated scaffolding proteins such as caveolin-1 (33). Consistent with a role for caveolae, myogenic constriction is impaired both by genetic deletion of caveolin-1 (34) and acute chemical disruption of caveolae (35). Although a number of underlying mechanisms have been proposed many of these actions would likely

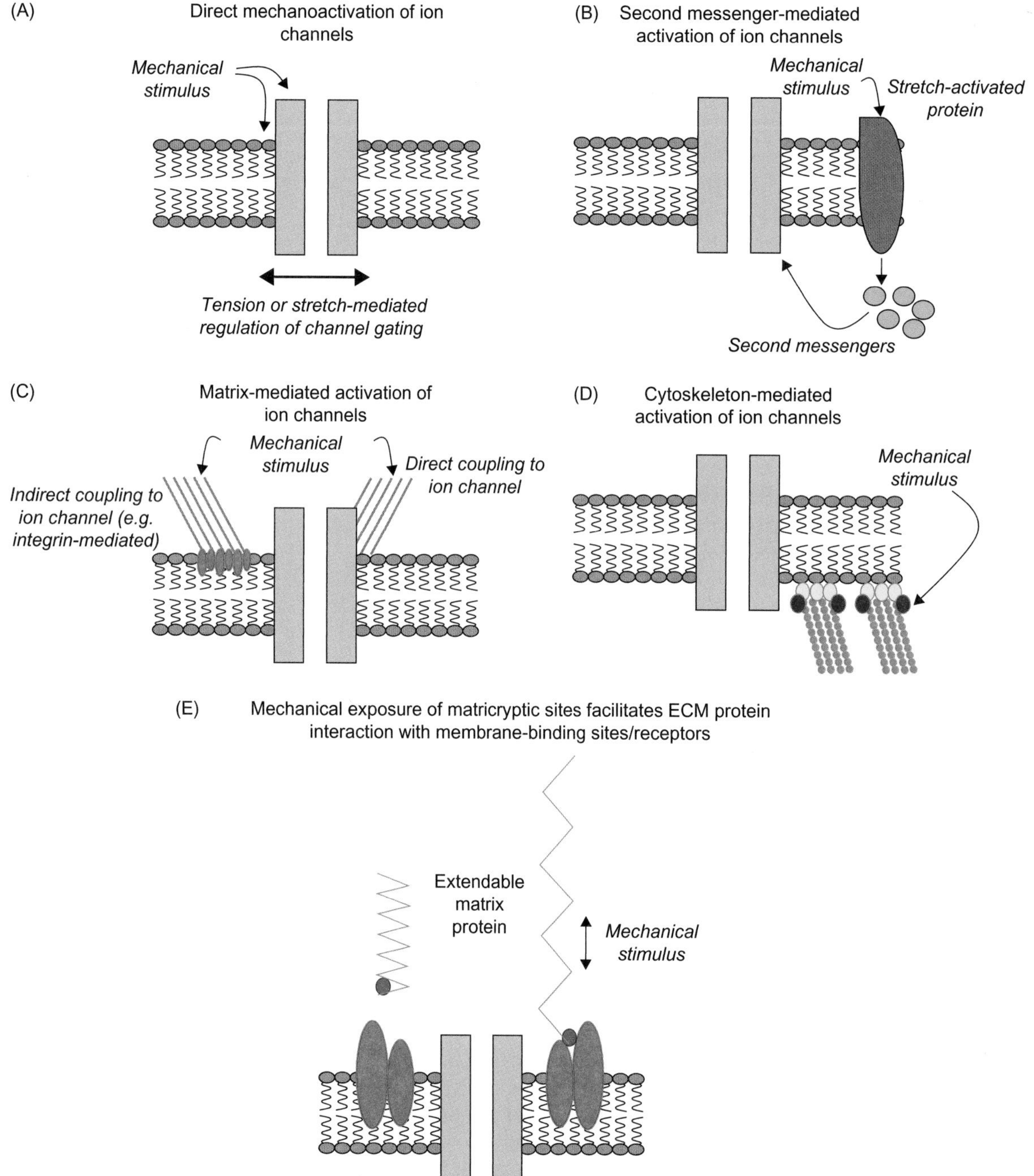

FIGURE 93.3 **Mechanisms by which changes in small artery intraluminal pressure may be sensed in myogenic signaling.** Panel (A) depicts a direct effect of the mechanical stimulus on an ion channel or its local environment with a resultant change in channel opening. Panel (B), involvement of ECM proteins in transmitting mechanical forces to ion channels or other membrane elements. Panel (C), the mechanical stimulus activating second messenger-based pathways with indirect activation of cation channels. Panel (D) depicts the situation where the effect of the pressure increase is transmitted from the cytoskeleton to a population of cation channels that mediate subsequent depolarization. Panel (E), mechanical deformation alters matrix protein conformation to expose previously hidden (matricryptic) binding motifs. While presented as being independent, it is likely that significant interaction occurs between the illustrated mechanisms.

impact contraction, in general, and thus their specific role in myogenic signaling is currently unclear.

Cell Adhesion Sites – Integrins, Novel ECM-Binding Motifs, and Their Receptors

The interaction between ECM proteins and the cell surface provides a direct link from the extracellular matrix environment and a mechanism for transmission of physical force, conveyance of specific matrix protein information, and signal amplification. Physical forces may impact this axis via strain applied to existing linkages or may cause conformational changes in (and unfolding of) ECM proteins to uncover cell membrane binding motifs (Figure 93.3). The latter concept is supported by studies demonstrating the existence of matricryptic sites buried in the three-dimensional structure of native matrix proteins (36) and those showing that specific matrix proteins such as fibronectin possess domains that can be extended by the application of force (37).

A major pathway for VSMC–ECM protein interaction occurs through the cell surface integrins. Integrins are an extensive family of heterodimeric receptors (comprised of alpha and beta subunits) of which some 13 distinct forms (including $\alpha_5\beta_1$, $\alpha_v\beta_3$, $\alpha_4\beta_1$) have been demonstrated in vascular smooth muscle (38). The integrin dimer has an extracellular domain that binds ECM in a cation-dependent manner, and a short cytoplasmic tail, which while lacking intrinsic kinase activity associates with a number of focal adhesion proteins that include various kinases and cytoskeletal proteins. Substantial evidence now exists to support the concept of integrins acting as a mechanism for transmission of mechanical force across the cell membrane to initiate intracellular signaling and subsequent responses including organization of focal adhesions, cytoskeletal remodeling, activation of phosphorylation cascades, and regulation of gene expression (2).

Specifically implicating a vascular role for the integrins are the observations that integrin-recognizing synthetic RGD peptides lower VSMC intracellular Ca^{2+} and cause vasodilation in isolated and pressurized arterioles (39,40). Importantly, these actions were prevented by function-blocking antibodies directed at the β_3 integrin subunit (39). Strong support for integrins as putative sensors for the myogenic response was similarly provided by studies of isolated arterioles showing that blockade of either $\alpha_v\beta_3$ or $\alpha_5\beta_1$ integrins abolishes myogenic constriction to acute step increases in intraluminal pressure (41). Further support for integrins, particularly $\alpha_v\beta_3$ and $\alpha_5\beta_1$, being upstream events that modulate arteriolar mechanotransduction, is that integrin activation leads to phosphorylation and activation of ion channels (including VGCCs and BKCa) important to myogenic responsiveness (42,43).

Atomic force microscopy (AFM) has been used to demonstrate a novel role for fibronectin in integrin-mediated myogenic-like behavior of single VSMC focal adhesion sites (20). In this study, nanoscale forces were applied to focal adhesion sites via fibronectin-functionalized AFM probes. On binding the fibronectin-coated tip to the cell, a focal adhesion was formed with the AFM probe. The co-localization of submembranous actin, integrins, and focal-adhesion-related proteins (FAK and paxillin) at the adhesion site was consistent with focal adhesion formation. Controlled retraction of the AFM probe caused local membrane stretch to which the cells subsequently responded with a localized "contraction" that effectively counteracted the applied stretch. Importantly, this myogenic-like cellular response was inhibited by a myosin light chain MLC kinase inhibitor (ML-7), cytochalasin D or function-blocking antibodies to $\alpha_5\beta_1$- and $\alpha_v\beta_3$-integrins (20). Interestingly, these actions appeared relatively specific to fibronectin, as probes similarly functionalized with other ECM proteins (including collagen, vitronectin and laminin) did not elicit similar localized contractions.

Intercellular Junctions Cadherins

Although mechanosensitivity can be demonstrated at the level of a single VSMC, evidence from a number of systems suggests that mechanotransduction can be enhanced in multicellular preparations demonstrating cell–cell junctions (2). In relation to this, particular interest has evolved in the cadherins, a super family of calcium-dependent, transmembrane cell–cell adhesion proteins that form adherens junctions. This superfamily of cell-to-cell adhesion proteins plays a major role in many multicellular activities requiring a degree of coordination between neighboring cells. Cadherin molecules bind cadherins on neighboring cells and are coupled to catenins on the cytoplasmic side of the membrane. The cadherin–catenin complex directly interacts with the actin cytoskeleton and provides a nucleation site for scaffolding with a variety of signaling molecules (44). Thus this pathway has many of the features that the integrin–extracellular matrix pathway possesses, making it an attractive pathway of mechanotransduction.

As discussed with regard to integrins, it is conceivable that involvement of cadherins in smooth muscle mechanotransduction could be a primary event (that is, being involved in the initial mechanosensory steps) or may be secondarily (inside-out signaling) activated to reinforce the mechanical response, for example, to a change in intraluminal pressure. In recent studies, the role of N-cadherin in arteriolar myogenic responses has been considered using function blocking antibodies and inhibitory peptides (45). Using both approaches myogenic responsiveness of cannulated cremaster muscle arterioles was attenuated. In contrast, pressure-induced changes in $Ca^{2+}{}_i$ were not altered. This latter observation raises questions as to where N-cadherins are involved in the signaling cascade. As cadherins link to the actin cytoskeleton via catenins it is conceivable that their involvement lies in events controlling Ca^{2+} sensitivity or inside-out signaling directed at acutely strengthening/remodeling of cell–cell adhesions. Interestingly, function blocking antibodies directed at either β_1 or β_3 integrins similarly blocked myogenic constriction without inhibiting pressure-induced changes in $Ca^{2+}{}_i$ (45). While in a myogenic signaling context it is uncertain why blockade of either N-cadherins or specific integrins blocks constriction it has been proposed that these junctional molecules maintain tissue homeostasis through cooperative cytoskeleton-based mechanisms (46).

The Cytoskeleton

While a contribution of cytoskeletal elements to mechanotransduction processes has long been suggested, its actual role in arteriolar myogenic constriction has remained somewhat uncertain. This, in part, reflects current limitations for the dynamic study of the cytoskeleton in functional arteriole preparations. Initial studies in this area relied on the use of pharmacological agents that either disrupt or stabilize the actin cytoskeleton. For example, Cipolla and colleagues showed that rat cerebral small arteries were less able to withstand the distending forces exerted by intraluminal pressure following treatment with the actin depolymerizing agent, cytochalasin B (47) while stabilization of actin, with jasplakinolide, enhanced myogenic tone (48). Using confocal fluorescence microscopy Flavahan et al. (49) showed myogenic constriction of isolated rat tail arteries to be associated with G- to F-actin transition. Further, as intraluminal pressure was increased from 10 mmHg to 60 and 90 mmHg, actin redistributed from cell periphery (that is adjacent to the plasma membrane) to the cell interior. Both the redistribution of the actin fibers and myogenic constriction was prevented by the actin depolymerizing agent cytochalasin D. Phenylephrine vasoconstriction was inhibited by the cytochalasin treatment at an intraluminal pressure of 60 mmHg while at 10 mmHg cytochalasin was ineffective and the agonist did not cause actin redistribution. These data appear to demonstrate that the actin cytoskeleton forms an important mechanism for resisting the distending forces imparted by intraluminal pressure and are, therefore, important in facilitating myogenic responsiveness.

In recent studies, El-Yazbi et al. (50) have made the intriguing observation that under certain conditions acute arteriolar myogenic constriction can be dissociated from a change in levels of myosin 20 kD regulatory light chain phosphorylation (pMLC20). Thus, in the presence of serotonin to achieve maximal levels of pMLC20 (approximately 50% of total MLC20) an acute increase in pressure could still elicit myogenic contraction. This effect could be prevented by latrunculin B (marine toxin which binds actin monomers and prevents polymerization) implicating a critical role for the actin cytoskeleton in this form of myogenic contraction.

An alternate hypothesis for cytoskeletal involvement in myogenic constriction is via linkages to critical mechanosensory or mechanotransducing elements. As mentioned earlier, and is discussed below in regard to certain transient receptor potential-like (Trp) proteins, the actin cytoskeleton may couple to ion channels by linker proteins such as filamin A (51). Relevant to this, disruption of the actin cytoskeleton enhances pressure-induced depolarization and Ca^{2+} entry via nifedipine-sensitive VGCCs (52).

It is also conceivable that other cytoskeletal elements play a role in myogenic signaling or, similarly, facilitate its occurrence. Microtubules, for example, provide a resistive force in many cell types (53). Depolymerization of microtubules causes vasoconstriction that in some studies seems to involve Rho-A-dependent Ca^{2+} sensitization without an overt increase in $Ca^{2+}{}_i$ (54). Vimentin- and desmin-deficient mice show normal myogenic responses despite alterations in other vasomotor properties (agonist sensitivity and impaired flow-dependent dilation) (55,56).

Mechanotransduction – Transferring Mechanosensory Events to Contractile Proteins

Key events following the pressure-induced mechanosensory steps involve membrane depolarization, Ca^{2+} signaling and the activation of the contractile proteins via a myosin light chain kinase-mediated mechanism (Figure 93.4). These mechanisms are complemented by pathways including those modulating Ca^{2+} sensitivity of the contractile proteins, remodeling of the cytoskeleton and perhaps inside-out signaling mechanisms that affect alterations in cell–cell and cell–matrix adhesion. (As a number of these steps have formed the basis for recent reviews the reader is also referred to references 21, 57, and 58.)

In general, depolarization could be initiated by activation of non-selective cation channels, which subsequently leads to opening of voltage-gated Ca^{2+} channels. Alternatively, SMC depolarization might occur via closure of K^+ channels (such as closure of BK_{Ca} by pressure-induced generation of arachidonic acid metabolites) or conceivably as a result of opening of a Cl^- channel. The pressure-induced mechanical stimulus is currently proposed to modulate the activity of membrane

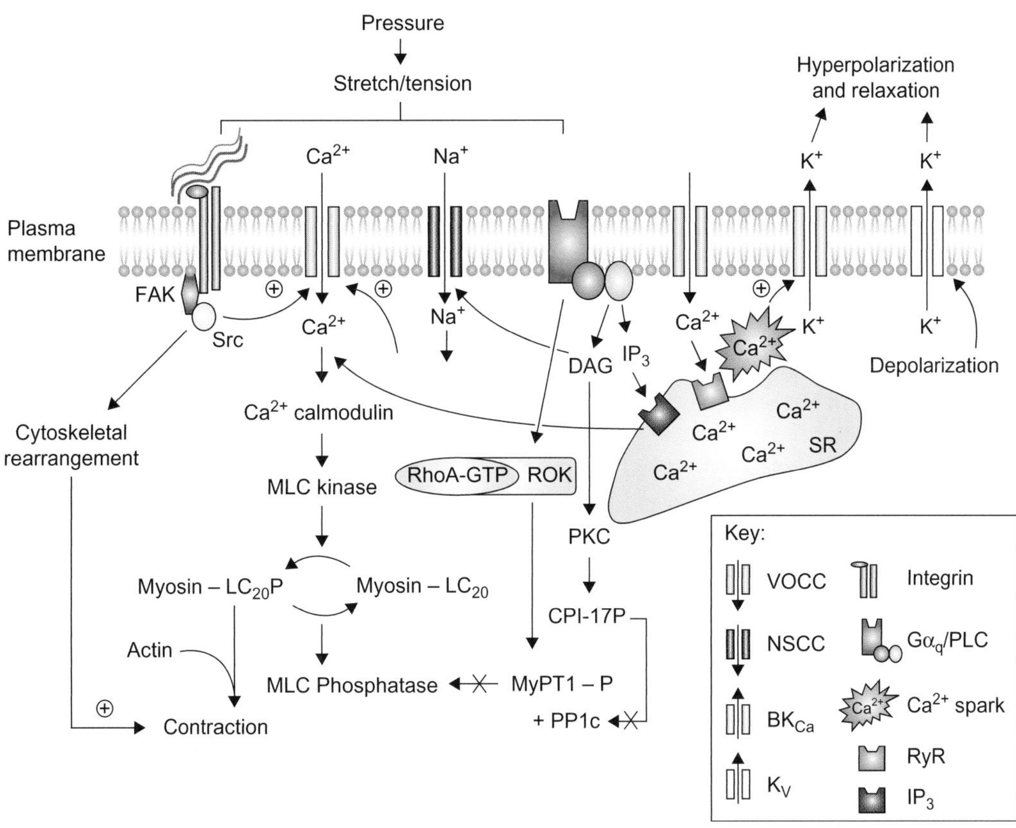

FIGURE 93.4 **Intracellular signaling pathways implicated in myogenic vasoconstriction.** Central to myogenic constriction membrane depolarization leads to opening of VGCCs, Ca^{2+}/calmodulin-mediated activation of myosin light chain kinase and the phosphorylation of the 20 kD myosin regulatory light chain (MLC20). Phosphorylation of MLC_{20} ($MLC_{20}P$) allows acto-myosin interaction, cross-bridge cycling and contraction. Complementing this pathway, Ca^{2+} sensitization via RhoA/Rho kinase-mediated myosin phosphatase inhibition potentiates $MLC_{20}P$ and enhances contraction. Further, the mechanical stimulus activates cytoskeletal rearrangement through mechanisms likely to be dependent on integrin-mediated activation of focal adhesions. Ca^{2+} release from the SR may serve several distinct spatiotemporally confined roles including the regulation of Ca^{2+}-activated ion channels, production of Ca^{2+} waves and provision of activator Ca^{2+}. *(From Hill et al., 2009 (57).)*

channels directly (stretch sensitive or mechanogated) but it could alternately occur via secondary pathways by generation of signaling molecules that modulate ion channel gating.

Membrane Potential (Roles of Stretch/Non-selective Cation/Trp Channels)

A central role for changes in VSMC membrane potential (Em) in myogenic constriction has long been accepted. Using sharp glass electrodes in cat cerebral artery preparations Harder demonstrated that increasing intraluminal pressure was associated with graded membrane depolarization (15). Similar relationships were later demonstrated in other vascular preparations, including small arteries isolated from the rat cerebral and cremaster muscle circulations (59,60). In myogenically active arterioles basal Em, at physiological pressures, is in the range of approximately −45 to −30 mV compared to more hyperpolarized levels (< − 60 mV) in unpressurized vessels. Although available data are more limited, *in vivo* measurements with glass microelectrodes support similar levels of Em (61).

Arguments have been raised to question whether a pressure-induced change in Em is an absolute requirement for myogenic constriction. These arguments are often based on myogenic responsiveness persisting in the presence of high extracellular K^+ (shifting the K^+ equilibrium potential towards 0 mV) and a plateauing of Em vs. myogenic tone relationships at higher intraluminal pressures. However, it is of interest to note that permeabilized preparations (lacking a transmembrane potential difference) do not show myogenic reactivity although these preparations can be used to demonstrate pharmacomechanical coupling and modulation of Ca^{2+} sensitivity. In regard to the curvilinear nature of the myogenic tone vs. Em relationship this phase is not observed until after pressure-induced depolarization has contributed to the development of tone, indirectly suggesting that other mechanisms support maintenance of myogenic tone.

Patch clamp techniques have provided key information as to how smooth muscle cell membrane deformation/strain (e.g. due to suction, directly applied stretch, membrane deformation secondary to osmotic changes) leads to the activation of cation currents (19,62) that presumably leads to membrane depolarization and a subsequent opening of voltage-gated Ca^{2+} channels (VGCC). Although stretch could conceivably activate VGCCs directly this does not occur at a level sufficient to account for the extent of Ca^{2+} entry (63). In contrast to direct stretch activation, it is likely that VGCC-mediated Ca^{2+} entry is further modulated by channel phosphorylation subsequent to the mechanical stimulus (43,64). Moreover, membrane depolarization to stretch persists in the presence of calcium channel blockers including nifedipine and nisoldipine (59,60). Collectively, these observations strongly support opening of VGCCs being secondary to the mechanosensory events and subsequent membrane depolarization.

Stretch-activated channels (SACs), for which gating is modulated by physiological levels of stretch (as might occur during an increase in intraluminal pressure), have been shown to be present in a variety of tissues, including smooth muscle cells from porcine coronary arteries (19). The opening of these SACs has been shown to result in a Na^+ dominated current that causes the membrane depolarization (19,65). Membrane stretch also activates BK_{Ca} channels (64), producing a hyperpolarizing current that may limit the extent of depolarization and, hence, in the intact vessel, myogenic constriction; this conceivably serves as an important negative feedback mechanism to limit the effects of additional myogenic contraction resulting from pressure-induced vasoconstriction of downstream arterioles. The current lack of specific tools to examine the roles of SACs in the myogenic response, together with incomplete understanding of their molecular identity, makes it difficult to appreciate their precise roles in myogenic contraction.

Trp channels represent a diverse family of cation channels that have been implicated in a variety of sensory events including mechanosensation and responsiveness to changes in temperature and osmolality (66). Trp proteins are also implicated in store depletion-mediated Ca^{2+} entry and receptor activation (66). Of potential importance to myogenic signaling, these channels exhibit a spectrum of permeability characteristics from that of non-selective cation channels to some that show a high Ca^{2+} selectivity. In mammals approximately 30 Trp channel genes give rise to sub-families, which have been designated canonical (TrpC), vanilloid (TrpV), and melastatin (TrpM). In addition, related subfamilies are the mucolipins (TrpML), polycystins (TrpP), and ankyrin (TrpA). The active channel exists as a tetramer and evidence exists to support both homo- and extensive hetero-multimerization.

Initial interest in the contribution of Trp channels in myogenic signaling was provided by Welsh et al. (67), who used *in vitro* anti-sense oligonucleotide approaches to examine the role of TrpC6 in isolated cerebral small arteries. Decreased expression of TrpC6 resulted in marked attenuation of both pressure-induced depolarization and myogenic constriction. Further, the oligonucleotide treatment decreased activation of cation channels in isolated cerebral artery SMC in response to a hyperosmotic challenge. Earley et al. later demonstrated that oligonuceotide knockdown of TrpM4 expression similarly impaired pressure-induced membrane depolarization and vasoconstriction. Reduction of the closely related TrpM5 using a similar approach did not, however, affect membrane depolarization or subsequent myogenic constriction, suggesting a degree of specificity. The importance of TrpM4 in myogenic signaling was also suggested *in vivo* as antisense oligonucleotide treatment resulted in impaired cerebral blood flow autoregulation (68).

The properties of TrpM4 channels are consistent with a role in myogenic signaling as they are selective for monovalent cations and are activated by both Ca^{2+} and PKC. However, TrpM4 is not inherently mechanosensitive, suggesting that its role lies downstream of the initial mechanosensory events. Earley suggested that the mechanosensitive TrpC6 may be positioned upstream providing stretch-induced Ca^{2+} entry as an activator of TrpM4. Arguing against this scenario is that the $TrpC6^{-/-}$ genetically-modified mouse shows enhanced basal VSMC membrane depolarization and exhibits slightly elevated systemic blood pressure (116 ± 1 vs. 123 ± 1 mmHg) as measured by telemetry (69). Observations in this genetic model are, however, possibly complicated by an increased expression of TrpC3 (69).

Polycystins (encoded by the PKD1 and PKD2 genes) have been implicated in polycystic renal disease and have been shown to play a mechanosensory role in ductal cilia. They have further been shown to mediate Ca^{2+} entry and release in response to fluid flow. At a molecular level, the extracellular region of polycystins both resembles fibronectin (70) and has been shown, using single molecule force spectroscopy, to undergo stretch-induced changes in conformation that restore when the applied force is removed (71). In a recent study, the presence of polycystins in arteriolar smooth muscle has been confirmed and a novel role in myogenic signaling has been proposed. Rather than acting as an ion channel, *per se*, TrpPP2 has been suggested to be a regulatory molecule for (yet to be molecularly characterized) stretch-activated channels. Sharif-Naeini et al. further showed that TrpP2 (PKD2) was linked to the underlying actin cytoskeleton by filamin A (51). Consistent with this, either knockdown of filamin A or disruption of F-actin prevented the inhibitory effect of TrpP2 on the SAC current (51).

Interestingly, in addition to SACs, polycystins associate with other elements implicated in myogenic signaling, for example cadherins, G-proteins, and cyoskeletal proteins (72). The polycystins have also been shown to associate with focal adhesions and, therefore, the ECM via integrins (72). It is, therefore, conceivable that the polycystins form part of a larger mechanosensory complex located in intercellular junctions. This may provide a "tethering-based" mechanism by which mechanical stimuli are transmitted both intra- and inter-cellularly. Such observations may also explain, in part, why blocking individual components of the putative mechanosensory complex (for example integrins or cadherins) negates myogenic contraction (45).

Overall, it is evident that Trp channel proteins form ion channels that are of fundamental importance to vascular wall function. In terms of smooth muscle contraction, Trp channels appear to contribute to signaling via receptor-mediated activation, store depletion-mediated Ca^{2+} entry and mechanotransduction. In addition, classes of Trp channels underlie vasodilator responses, for example, mediated by Ca^{2+} spark-induced activation of BK_{Ca} and endothelial-dependent hyperpolarization (73). This complexity, together with likely hetero-multimerization indicates the need for further research, particularly to ascertain their direct role in myogenic signaling.

An additional cation channel that has been implicated in myogenic signaling is the epithelial sodium channel, ENaC (74). ENaC was initially described as playing a mechanosensory role in *C. elegans* (75) being linked to shear-stress-mediated mechanotransduction in oocytes and in renal tubule epithelial cells (76). ENaC associates with both the ECM and cytoskeleton, thus serving as a possible link to other candidate mechanosensory elements such as integrins, although this is yet to be specifically demonstrated in VSMCs. Recent data from Drummond et al. have suggested that ENaC might be an important component of the myogenic responses in rat cerebral arterioles and mouse renal interlobular arteries (74). Similarly, Inscho and colleagues, on the basis of pharmacological inhibitor studies, have demonstrated a role for ENaC in the myogenic responsiveness of rat afferent arterioles (77). While substantial work is required to firmly establish ENaC as a myogenic mechanosensor in arteriolar smooth muscle, it is of interest to note that the β-ENaC-deficient mouse shows impaired renal autoregulation (78) together with renal inflammation and chronically raised blood pressure (79).

G-proteins and Membrane Located Effectors

Early studies implicating a role for trimeric G-proteins in small artery myogenic reactivity were largely indirect relying on the use of inhibitors of PLC and measurements of the downstream production/accumulation of signaling molecules (80,81). Thus, Osol et al. showed myogenic responsiveness of cannulated rat posterior cerebral arteries to be attenuated by the PLC inhibitor, U-73122, while Narayanan et al. showed in dog renal vessels that an increase in intraluminal pressure led to the time-dependent accumulation of inositol trisphosphate and diacylglycerol.

Recently, GPCRs, particularly the AT1 receptor, have been shown to be mechanosensitive leading to the activation of $G\alpha_{q/11}$-proteins and downstream phospholipases. The direct mechanical effect on the receptors was shown to be agonist-independent, although in the case of the AT1 receptor pressure-induced activation of $G\alpha_{q/11}$ could be prevented by the receptor blocker losartan. It is proposed that mechanical force directly alters the conformation of the receptor such that it is placed in an activated configuration. Interestingly, this mode of mechanical activation is not limited to the AT1 receptor as it could also be demonstrated for several other GPCRs, including those for histamine and vasopressin. The effect is, however, not totally non-selective as mechanical activation of the Gs-coupled β_2 adrenoceptor could not be demonstrated.

To fully understand the involvement of GPCRs in myogenic constriction it will be critical to determine how these receptors are "coupled" to mechanical deformation. In this regard, Mederos y Schnitzler et al. recently discussed the applicability of tethered (mediated by connection to ECM and/or cytoskeletal proteins) and membrane-based (lateral mechanical forces impacting the membrane lipid bilayer to affect changes in integral membrane protein conformation) models (82). Related to this, Yasuda et al. reported that membrane stretch causes a rotational shift in a transmembrane segment of the AT1 receptor resulting in an active conformation distinct from that dependent on ligand binding (83). The mechanical effect was, however, prevented by the inverse agonist candesartan. This, again, provides links between the mechanical activation of GPCRs and signaling molecules previously implicated in myogenic signaling.

The mechanical activation of G-proteins is an attractive mechanism as the initiation of phospholipase-based signaling has been linked to activation of TrpC6 channels. TrpC6 current would then conceivably lead to membrane depolarization, opening of VGCC, and myogenic contraction thus linking a number of earlier observations. An obvious question concerning this scenario is whether the kinetics of such a series of reactions are consistent with the speed at which myogenic contraction occurs. Although considerable differences exist with regard to speed of contraction in various vascular preparations (both between vascular beds and along a network) G-protein signaling occurs on a time frame of milliseconds (84), suggesting that such a mechanism could, indeed, be consistent with myogenic constriction. A caveat is whether membrane tension-induced changes in G-protein/GPCR conformation occur on this time frame and whether the largely single cell-based observations are applicable to the intact vessel.

Mobilization of Ca^{2+} (Contributions from Entry and Release)

Entry of Ca^{2+} into arteriolar SMCs occurs early in the temporal sequence of signaling events underlying myogenic contraction. Inhibitors of L-type voltage-gated Ca^{2+} channels (including nifedipine and nisoldipine) eliminate active myogenic constriction in most vascular preparations (59,60). As mentioned earlier, opening of L-type Ca^{2+} channels follows pressure-induced SMC membrane. Direct evidence for contributions from other voltage-gated Ca^{2+} channels is, currently, relatively sparse. A relatively minor contribution from Ca^{2+} entry via non-voltage-gated Ca^{2+}-entry pathways to direct contractile regulation may also occur (85). However, Ca^{2+} entry via these sources may participate in the regulation of ion channels and SR Ca^{2+} dynamics. An additional consideration relates to possible regional heterogeneity which could explain disparate results between preparations such as the observations that the myogenic response in small arterioles ($<25\ \mu m$ in diameter) is relatively insensitive to L-type Ca^{2+} channel blockers (86) and afferent arteriolar constriction is sensitive to Ca^{2+} antagonists while the efferent arterioles are not (87).

The role of Ca^{2+} release from the sarcoplasmic reticulum (SR) in myogenic signaling (particularly as relates to contractile activation) is hampered by both technical limitations and the multiple roles played by the SR in smooth muscle cells. Thus, as many pharmacological approaches that alter SR function also affect basal arteriolar tone, such studies have proved difficult to interpret and have provided limited mechanistic information. Dynamic aspects of SR Ca^{2+} release appear to contribute to the regulation of myogenic behavior through an action on ion channels and frequency encoded control of cytoplasmic Ca^{2+} levels; for example, through spatiotemporally localized Ca^{2+} events including Ca^{2+} sparks and waves. Thus, Nelson and colleagues (88) proposed that Ca^{2+} sparks modulate BK_{Ca} channel activity and act as a negative feedback mechanism to prevent excessive depolarization as pressure-induced constriction occurs.

An additional SR release-driven Ca^{2+} transient is evident in the form of cyclical Ca^{2+} waves. The frequency of propagating and asynchronous intracellular Ca^{2+} waves increases with arteriolar intraluminal pressure (89,90), suggesting a possible relationship with the mechanical force related to distension or myogenic contraction *per se*. While at present it is uncertain whether myogenic reactivity is specifically modulated by the presence of cytosolic Ca^{2+} waves, Welsh and colleagues (58,91) have suggested that the waves do, indeed, facilitate the development of myogenic tone (especially at pressures <60 mmHg) via Ca^{2+}-dependent phosphorylation of MLC_{20}.

Kinases and Phosphatases

Myosin Light Chain Kinase and Myosin Phosphatase

A number of protein phosphorylation events have been suggested to be involved in myogenic signaling. As with agonist-induced contraction of smooth muscle, direct measurements have shown that increased arteriolar intraluminal pressure, and active myogenic constriction, is associated with an increase in the phosphorylation of the 20 kDa myosin regulatory light chain (58,92). Further, the light chain is phosphorylated at serine 19 (58). This phosphorylation occurs via a Ca^{2+} and calmodulin-dependent mechanism. The extent of phosphorylation has been shown to be directly related to the instantaneous level of wall tension as calculated by the LaPlace relationship (92). A causative relationship between myosin light chain phosphorylation and myogenic contraction was suggested by the observation that an increase in intraluminal pressure failed to elicit contraction in the presence of the inhibitor ML-7, despite a mechanically-induced increase in intracellular Ca^{2+} (92).

Studies have demonstrated that the net level of myosin phosphorylation is critically dependent on the activity of myosin phosphatase. While the phosphatase was once thought to be unregulated it is clear that its activity is modulated by both Rho kinase and protein kinase C (PKC). Rho kinase phosphorylation of the myosin targeting subunit of the phosphatase (MYPT1) at threonine 855 inhibits binding to the activated myosin molecule thereby decreasing its dephosphorylation (58). PKC phosphorylates CPI-17 that acts as an inhibitor of the phosphatase. Using a sensitive three-step Western blotting approach, Cole et al. (18,93) have shown in cerebral arteries that increasing pressure (10 to 60 and 100 mmHg) leads to Rho kinase-dependent phosphorylation of MYPT1 at Thr 855 while PKC-mediated phosphorylation of CPI-17 was not apparent.

Protein Kinase C

A possible role for PKC in myogenic signaling was initially suggested on the basis of inhibitor studies where pharmacological blockade was shown to attenuate myogenic constriction (94). A number of these studies were, however, limited by the selectivity of the available inhibitors (many of which target the ATP binding site of the kinase), an inability to distinguish between the multiple PKC isoforms, a lack of knowledge of the targets for phosphorylation and the pleiotropic actions of the kinase. For example, with respect to the multiple actions of PKC it has also been shown to activate membrane channels (for example, VGCC, TrpC isoforms, BK_{Ca}) and other kinases (e.g. p42/44 MAP kinase), both of which could impact contractile function. More specific support, however, has been given to a role for PKCα, which has been shown to translocate to the plasma membrane (consistent with activation) in response to increased arteriolar pressure (95). Further, isozyme-specific inhibition of PKCα attenuates myogenic reactivity (95).

The finding that PKC modulates Ca^{2+} sensitization through activation of CPI-17 and inhibition of MYPT1 provided another possible role for the enzyme in myogenic signaling. Consistent with this, direct activation of PKC in permeabilized mesenteric arteries led to increased MLC_{20} phosphorylation despite fixed intracellular Ca^{2+} levels (96). However, direct measurements have not shown pressure-induced changes in CPI-17 phosphorylation (18,58).

Sphingosine Kinase

Membrane sphingomyelin-derived sphingosine has been shown to be phosphorylated in a number of cell types to sphingosine-1-phosphate (S-1P) and act as a second messenger acting via receptors coupled to G-proteins, phospholipase C, and Rho kinase. Bolz and colleagues have implicated S-1P in myogenic constriction on the basis that it is activated by depolarization and subsequently stimulates both SR Ca^{2+} release and Rho-A-mediated Ca^{2+} sensitization. Overexpression of sphingosine kinase in isolated gracilis muscle arterioles enhanced myogenic reactivity via a Rho A-dependent mechanism while a dominant negative construct prevented myogenic constriction (17). A current difficulty in understanding the exact role of S-1P is that it is has also been reported to be involved in contractile responses to agonists (97), suggesting it may not be specific to myogenic contractility. Further, its function is complicated by affecting both smooth muscle and endothelial cells and having both extra- and intracellular actions (97).

Tyrosine Phosphorylation

A variety of mechanical stimuli initiate protein tyrosine phosphorylation, including pathways involving focal adhesion kinase, cSRC, and p42/44 MAP kinase (98). Tyrosine phosphorylation-mediated signaling has been shown to modulate ion channels, transduce integrin-mediated events, reorganize cytoskeletal proteins, and contribute to remodeling of the vascular wall. Doubt in an obligatory role for tyrosine phosphorylation in myogenic responsiveness was initially based on the persistence of pressure-induced contraction in isolated arterioles in the presence of non-selective pharmacological inhibitors (99,100). Further, tyrosine phosphorylation, itself, persists despite inhibition of myogenic contraction by multiple and mechanistically different approaches. While pressure-induced phosphorylation of p44 MAP kinase could be demonstrated in isolated arterioles inhibition with the upstream MEK inhibitor PD98059 did not impact myogenic contraction (99). PD98059 did, however, block p44 MAP kinase phosphorylation. These data, therefore, provide support for changes in intraluminal pressure activating tyrosine phosphorylation events. However, whether it plays a direct or modulatory role in myogenic constriction (for example through remodeling) remains uncertain.

Limiting Myogenic Constriction – Physical Limitations and Feedback Mechanisms

An historical and conceptual difficulty with the myogenic response being an important *in vivo* regulatory mechanism is that it can be viewed as a positive feedback mechanism. Thus, pressure-induced vasoconstriction while decreasing pressure distal to the site of myogenic constriction would increase pressure in the proximal segments stimulating further vasoconstriction. Several factors exist that prevent such a situation arising. Firstly, myogenic constriction occurs only over an optimal range of intraluminal pressures with the vessel behaving passively at very low pressures (approximately <30 mmHg) and at high pressures when the distending force can no longer be opposed by active contraction. In addition to this, not all arterial vessels in a network show equivalent levels of myogenic responsiveness. Thus myogenic responsiveness tends to be greatest in arterioles and declines as vessels increase their caliber. Finally, not all vascular beds display pressure-dependent autoregulation.

In addition to physical limitations on myogenic constriction, cellular negative feedback mechanisms appear to limit myogenic responsiveness. As mentioned, Nelson et al. in studies of cerebral arteries demonstrated that pressure-induced Ca^{2+} entry into the subsarcolemmal space leads to the production of localized Ca^{2+} release events from the adjacent SR (14). These Ca^{2+}-release events, or sparks, raise the localized $[Ca^{2+}]$ to $1-10\,\mu M$ which stimulates large-conductance, Ca^{2+}-activated, K^+ channels (BK_{Ca}). The resulting outward hyperpolarizing current (spontaneously transient outward currents or STOCs) then opposes the pressure-induced depolarization and constriction. Although tight coupling of Ca^{2+} sparks to BK_{Ca} activity and STOCs occurs in cerebral arteries, heterogeneity may exist between tissues (16,60,101).

Heterogeneity in Mechanotransduction Within and Between Tissues

Although a topic of its own, it is important to consider that tissue, network, and cellular heterogeneity likely impacts mechanotransduction processes in small arteries. Presumably this reflects both differences in the local mechanical environment and tissue function. Within a given vascular bed or tissue there is considerable variability in the degree of myogenic reactivity, or gain, exhibited by differing branch orders of arterioles/small arteries (21). This has been demonstrated using both *in vivo* and *in vitro* preparations. In general, myogenic reactivity tends to increase as diameter decreases, although in some tissues the smallest pre-capillary arterioles may be more adapted to respond to metabolic stimuli as opposed to changes in intraluminal pressure (21).

FUTURE CONSIDERATIONS

Although considerable advances in our understanding of myogenic signaling at the cellular level have occurred, the field remains limited by the lack of direct knowledge of the sensed variable and molecular details of the putative mechanosensor/mechanosensory complex. An important consideration is that a pressure change may activate multiple mechanisms that may initiate parallel or interacting signaling pathways. Further, if pressure activates mechanotransduction processes that have common features across cell types, then how are these mechanisms specifically activated in those regions of the circulation that exhibit myogenic behavior? In addition to information relating to the sensor and sensed variable, details of the exact molecular mechanisms affecting pressure-induced depolarization remain to be defined. Consideration also needs to be given to the influence of the three-dimensional environment within which SMCs of the arteriolar wall reside and function. Clearly, the extracellular matrix elements, in addition to potentially acting as myogenic sensors and/or mechanotransducers, also impact structure–function relationships in general. Further, heterogeneity in vessel wall structure likely imparts differences in myogenic signaling between tissues. Specifically, little is currently known as to the exact binding/adhesive interactions between vascular SMCs and matrix elements. Or for that matter, what constitutes the three-dimensional organization of cell–cell adhesions. As these elements differ between tissues, their impact may similarly vary despite the individual SMCs possessing a common myogenic phenotype.

ACKNOWLEDGMENTS

The authors are supported by grants from the National Institutes of Health (HL092241, M.A.H., and HL095486, G.A.M).

REFERENCES

1. Orr AW, Helmke BP, Blackman BR, Schwartz MA. Mechanisms of mechanotransduction. *Dev Cell* 2006;**10**:11–20.
2. Schwartz MA. Integrins and extracellular matrix in mechanotransduction. *Cold Spring Harb Perspect Biol* 2010;**2**:a005066.
3. Ingber DE. From cellular mechanotransduction to biologically inspired engineering: 2009 Pritzker Award Lecture, BMES Annual Meeting October 10, 2009. *Ann Biomed Eng* 2010;**38**:1148–61.
4. Bayliss WM. On the local reactions of the arterial wall to changes of internal pressure. *J Physiol* 1902;**28**:220–31.
5. Folkow B. Intravascular pressure as a factor regulating the tone of the small vessels. *Acta Physiol Scand* 1949;**17**:289–310.
6. Folkow B. A study of the factors influencing the tone of denervated blood vessels perfused at various pressures. *Acta Physiol Scand* 1952;**27**:99–117.
7. Selkurt EE, Johnson PC. Effect of acute elevation of portal venous pressure on mesenteric blood volume, interstitial fluid volume and hemodynamics. *Circ Res* 1958;**6**:592–9.
8. Duling BR. The preparation and use of the hamster cheek pouch for studies of the microcirculation. *Microvasc Res* 1973;**5**:423–9.
9. Intaglietta M, Tompkins WR. On-line measurement of microvascular dimensions by television microscopy. *J Appl Physiol* 1972;**32**:546–51.
10. Johnson PC, Wayland H. Regulation of blood flow in single capillaries. *Am J Physiol* 1967;**212**:1405–15.
11. Mulvany MJ, Halpern W. Mechanical properties of vascular smooth muscle cells in situ. *Nature* 1976;**260**:617–9.
12. Duling BR, Gore RW, Dacey Jr. RG, Damon DN. Methods for isolation, cannulation, and in vitro study of single microvessels. *Am J Physiol Heart Circ Physiol* 1981;**241**:H108–16.
13. Meininger GA, Zawieja DC, Falcone JC, Hill MA, Davey JP. Calcium measurement in isolated arterioles during myogenic and agonist stimulation. *Am J Physiol Heart Circ Physiol* 1991;**261**:H950–9.
14. Nelson MT, Cheng H, Rubart M, Santana LF, Bonev AD, Knot HJ, et al. Relaxation of arterial smooth muscle by calcium sparks. *Science* 1995;**270**:633–7.
15. Harder DR. Pressure-dependent membrane depolarization in cat middle cerebral artery. *Circ Res* 1984;**55**:197–202.
16. Yang Y, Murphy TV, Ella SR, Grayson TH, Haddock R, Hwang YT, et al. Heterogeneity in function of small artery smooth muscle BKCa: involvement of the beta1-subunit. *J Physiol* 2009;**587**:3025–44.
17. Bolz SS, Vogel L, Sollinger D, Derwand R, Boer C, Pitson SM, et al. Sphingosine kinase modulates microvascular tone and myogenic responses through activation of RhoA/Rho kinase. *Circulation* 2003;**108**:342–7.
18. El-Yazbi AF, Johnson RP, Walsh EJ, Takeya K, Walsh MP, Cole WC. Pressure-dependent contribution of Rho kinase-mediated calcium sensitization in serotonin-evoked vasoconstriction of rat cerebral arteries. *J Physiol* 2010;**588**:1747–62.
19. Davis MJ, Donovitz JA, Hood JD. Stretch-activated single-channel and whole cell currents in vascular smooth muscle cells. *Am J Physiol Cell Physiol* 1992;**262**:C1083–8.
20. Sun Z, Martinez-Lemus LA, Hill MA, Meininger GA. Extracellular matrix-specific focal adhesions in vascular smooth

muscle produce mechanically active adhesion sites. *Am J Physiol Cell Physiol* 2008;**295**:C268–78.
21. Davis MJ, Hill MA, Kuo L, editors. *Local regulation of microvascular perfusion.* San Diego, CA: Academic Press;2008.
22. Johnson PC. Autoregulation of blood flow. *Circ Res* 1986;**59**:483–95.
23. Loutzenhiser R, Bidani A, Chilton L. Renal myogenic response: kinetic attributes and physiological role. *Circ Res* 2002;**90**:1316–24.
24. Meininger GA, Faber JE. Adrenergic facilitation of myogenic response in skeletal muscle arterioles. *Am J Physiol Heart Circ Physio* 1991;**l260**:H1424–32.
25. Meininger GA, Trzeciakowski JP. Combined effects of autoregulation and vasoconstrictors on hindquarters vascular resistance. *Am J Physiol Heart Circ Physiol* 1990;**258**:H1032–41.
26. Kuo L, Chilian WM, Davis MJ. Coronary arteriolar myogenic response is independent of endothelium. *Circ Res* 1990;**66**:860–6.
27. Falcone JC, Davis MJ, Meininger GA. Endothelial independence of myogenic response in isolated skeletal muscle arterioles. *Am J Physiol Heart Circ Physiol* 1991;**260**:H130–5.
28. Kuo L, Chilian WM, Davis MJ. Interaction of pressure- and flow-induced responses in porcine coronary resistance vessels. *Am J Physiol Heart Circ Physiol* 1991;**261**:H1706–15.
29. Sandow SL, Tare M, Coleman HA, Hill CE, Parkington HC. Involvement of myoendothelial gap junctions in the actions of endothelium-derived hyperpolarizing factor. *Circ Res* 2002;**90**:1108–13.
30. Dora KA, Gallagher NT, McNeish A, Garland CJ. Modulation of endothelial cell KCa3.1 channels during endothelium-derived hyperpolarizing factor signaling in mesenteric resistance arteries. *Circ Res* 2008;**102**:1247–55.
31. Sharif-Naeini R, Folgering JH, Bichet D, Duprat F, Delmas P, Patel A, et al. Sensing pressure in the cardiovascular system: Gq-coupled mechanoreceptors and TRP channels. *J Mol Cell Cardiol* 2010;**48**:83–9.
32. Patel A, Sharif-Naeini R, Folgering JR, Bichet D, Duprat F, Honore E. Canonical TRP channels and mechanotransduction: from physiology to disease states. *Pflugers Arch* 2010;**460**:571–81.
33. Cohen AW, Hnasko R, Schubert W, Lisanti MP. Role of caveolae and caveolins in health and disease. *Physiol Rev* 2004;**84**:1341–79.
34. Adebiyi A, Zhao G, Cheranov SY, Ahmed A, Jaggar JH. Caveolin-1 abolishment attenuates the myogenic response in murine cerebral arteries. *Am J Physiol Heart Circ Physiol* 2007;**292**:H1584–92.
35. Potocnik SJ, Jenkins N, Murphy TV, Hill MA. Membrane cholesterol depletion with beta-cyclodextrin impairs pressure-induced contraction and calcium signalling in isolated skeletal muscle arterioles. *J Vasc Res* 2007;**44**:292–302.
36. Davis GE. Matricryptic sites control tissue injury responses in the cardiovascular system: relationships to pattern recognition receptor regulated events. *J Mol Cell Cardiol* 2010;**48**:454–60.
37. Erickson HP. Stretching fibronectin. *J Muscle Res Cell Motil* 2002;**23**:575–80.
38. Martinez-Lemus LA, Wu X, Wilson E, Hill MA, Davis GE, Davis MJ, et al. Integrins as unique receptors for vascular control. *J Vasc Res.* 2003;**40**:211–33.
39. Mogford JE, Davis GE, Platts SH, Meininger GA. Vascular smooth muscle alpha vs. beta 3 integrin mediates arteriolar vasodilation in response to RGD peptides. *Circ Res* 1996;**79**:821–6.
40. D'Angelo G, Mogford JE, Davis GE, Davis MJ, Meininger GA. Integrin-mediated reduction in vascular smooth muscle $[Ca^{2+}]i$ induced by RGD-containing peptide. *Am J Physiol Heart Circ Physiol* 1997;**272**:H2065–70.
41. Martinez-Lemus LA, Crow T, Davis MJ, Meininger GA. alphavbeta3- and alpha5beta1-integrin blockade inhibits myogenic constriction of skeletal muscle resistance arterioles. *Am J Physiol Heart Circ Physiol* 2005;**289**:H322–9.
42. Wu X, Yang Y, Gui P, Sohma Y, Meininger GA, Davis GE, et al. Potentiation of large conductance, Ca^{2+}-activated K^+ (BK) channels by alpha5beta1 integrin activation in arteriolar smooth muscle. *J Physiol* 2008;**586**:1699–713.
43. Wu X, Davis GE, Meininger GA, Wilson E, Davis MJ. Regulation of the L-type calcium channel by alpha 5beta 1 integrin requires signaling between focal adhesion proteins. *J Biol Chem* 2001;**276**:30285–92.
44. Aberle H, Schwartz H, Kemler R. Cadherin-catenin complex: protein interactions and their implications for cadherin function. *J Cell Biochem* 1996;**61**:514–23.
45. Jackson TY, Sun Z, Martinez-Lemus LA, Hill MA, Meininger GA. N-cadherin and integrin blockade inhibit arteriolar myogenic reactivity but not pressure-induced increases in intracellular Ca. *Front Physiol* 2010;**1**:165.
46. Brunton VG, MacPherson IR, Frame MC. Cell adhesion receptors, tyrosine kinases and actin modulators: a complex three-way circuitry. *Biochim Biophys Acta* 2004;**1692**:121–44.
47. Cipolla MJ, Osol G. Vascular smooth muscle actin cytoskeleton in cerebral artery forced dilatation. *Stroke* 1998;**29**:1223–8.
48. Cipolla MJ, Gokina NI, Osol G. Pressure-induced actin polymerization in vascular smooth muscle as a mechanism underlying myogenic behavior. *FASEB J* 2002;**16**:72–6.
49. Flavahan NA, Bailey SR, Flavahan WA, Mitra S, Flavahan S. Imaging remodeling of the actin cytoskeleton in vascular smooth muscle cells after mechanosensitive arteriolar constriction. *Am J Physiol Heart Circ Physiol* 2005;**288**:H660–9.
50. El-Yazbi A, Walsh E, Walsh M, Cole W. Potential involvement of actin cytoskeleton reorganization in generation of the arterial myogenic response. *FASEB J* 2011;**25**:1.
51. Sharif-Naeini R, Folgering JH, Bichet D, Duprat F, Lauritzen I, Arhatte M, et al. Polycystin-1 and -2 dosage regulates pressure sensing. *Cell* 2009;**139**:587–96.
52. Gokina NI, Osol G. Actin cytoskeletal modulation of pressure-induced depolarization and Ca(2+) influx in cerebral arteries. *Am J Physiol Heart Circ Physiol* 2002;**282**:H1410–20.
53. Wang N, Butler JP, Ingber DE. Mechanotransduction across the cell surface and through the cytoskeleton. *Science* 1993;**260**:1124–7.
54. Platts SH, Martinez-Lemus LA, Meininger GA. Microtubule-dependent regulation of vasomotor tone requires Rho-kinase. *J Vasc Res* 2002;**39**:173–82.
55. Loufrani L, Matrougui K, Li Z, Levy BI, Lacolley P, Paulin D, et al. Selective microvascular dysfunction in mice lacking the gene encoding for desmin. *FASEB J* 2002;**16**:117–9.
56. Schiffers PM, Henrion D, Boulanger CM, Colucci-Guyon E, Langa-Vuves F, van Essen H, et al. Altered flow-induced arterial

remodeling in vimentin-deficient mice. *Arterioscler Thromb Vasc Biol* 2000;**20**:611–6.

57. Hill MA, Meininger GA, Davis MJ, Laher I. Therapeutic potential of pharmacologically targeting arteriolar myogenic tone. *Trends Pharmacol Sci* 2009;**30**:363–74.
58. Cole WC, Welsh DG. Role of myosin light chain kinase and myosin light chain phosphatase in the resistance arterial myogenic response to intravascular pressure. *Arch Biochem Biophys* 2011;**510**:160–73.
59. Knot HJ, Nelson MT. Regulation of arterial diameter and wall [Ca^{2+}] in cerebral arteries of rat by membrane potential and intravascular pressure. *J Physiol* 1998;**508**(Pt 1):199–209.
60. Kotecha N, Hill MA. Myogenic contraction in rat skeletal muscle arterioles: smooth muscle membrane potential and Ca(2+) signaling. *Am J Physiol Heart Circ Physiol* 2005;**289**:H1326–34.
61. Wolfle SE, Schmidt VJ, Hoepfl B, Gebert A, Alcolea S, Gros D, et al. Connexin45 cannot replace the function of connexin40 in conducting endothelium-dependent dilations along arterioles. *Circ Res* 2007;**101**:1292–9.
62. Welsh DG, Nelson MT, Eckman DM, Brayden JE. Swelling-activated cation channels mediate depolarization of rat cerebrovascular smooth muscle by hyposmolarity and intravascular pressure. *J Physiol* 2000;**527**(Pt 1):139–48.
63. McCarron JG, Crichton CA, Langton PD, MacKenzie A, Smith GL. Myogenic contraction by modulation of voltage-dependent calcium currents in isolated rat cerebral arteries. *J Physiol* 1997;**498**(Pt 2):371–9.
64. Gui P, Chao JT, Wu X, Yang Y, Davis GE, Davis MJ. Coordinated regulation of vascular Ca^{2+} and K^{+} channels by integrin signaling. *Adv Exp Med Biol* 2010;**674**:69–79.
65. Wu X, Davis MJ. Characterization of stretch-activated cation current in coronary smooth muscle cells. *Am J Physiol Heart Circ Physiol* 2001;**280**:H1751–61.
66. Earley S, Brayden JE. Transient receptor potential channels and vascular function. *Clin Sci (Lond)* 2010;**119**:19–36.
67. Welsh DG, Morielli AD, Nelson MT, Brayden JE. Transient receptor potential channels regulate myogenic tone of resistance arteries. *Circ Res* 2002;**90**:248–50.
68. Reading SA, Brayden JE. Central role of TRPM4 channels in cerebral blood flow regulation. *Stroke* 2007;**38**:2322–8.
69. Dietrich A, Mederos YSM, Gollasch M, Gross V, Storch U, Dubrovska G, et al. Increased vascular smooth muscle contractility in TRPC6-/- mice. *Mol Cell Biol* 2005;**25**:6980–9.
70. Vogel V. Mechanotransduction involving multimodular proteins: converting force into biochemical signals. *Annu Rev Biophys Biomol Struct* 2006;**35**:459–88.
71. Qian F, Wei W, Germino G, Oberhauser A. The nanomechanics of polycystin-1 extracellular region. *J Biol Chem* 2005;**280**:40723–30.
72. Drummond IA. Polycystins, focal adhesions and extracellular matrix interactions. *Biochim Biophys Acta* 2011;**1812**:1322–6.
73. Earley S, Heppner TJ, Nelson MT, Brayden JE. TRPV4 forms a novel Ca^{2+} signaling complex with ryanodine receptors and BKCa channels. *Circ Res* 2005;**97**:1270–9.
74. Drummond HA, Grifoni SC, Jernigan NL. A new trick for an old dogma: ENaC proteins as mechanotransducers in vascular smooth muscle. *Physiology (Bethesda)* 2008;**23**:23–31.
75. Fronius M, Clauss WG. Mechano-sensitivity of ENaC: may the (shear) force be with you. *Pflugers Arch* 2008;**455**:775–85.
76. Carattino MD, Sheng S, Kleyman TR. Epithelial Na^{+} channels are activated by laminar shear stress. *J Biol Chem* 2004;**279**:4120–6.
77. Guan Z, Pollock JS, Cook AK, Hobbs JL, Inscho EW. Effect of epithelial sodium channel blockade on the myogenic response of rat juxtamedullary afferent arterioles. *Hypertension* 2009;**54**:1062–9.
78. Grifoni SC, Chiposi R, McKey SE, Ryan MJ, Drummond HA. Altered whole kidney blood flow autoregulation in a mouse model of reduced beta-ENaC. *Am J Physiol Renal Physiol* 2010;**298**:F285–92.
79. Drummond HA, Grifoni SC, Abu-Zaid A, Gousset M, Chiposi R, Barnard JM, et al. Renal inflammation and elevated blood pressure in a mouse model of reduced {beta}ENaC. *Am J Physiol Renal Physiol* 2011;**301**:F443–9.
80. Osol G, Laher I, Kelley M. Myogenic tone is coupled to phospholipase C and G protein activation in small cerebral arteries. *Am J Physiol Heart Circ Physiol* 1993;**265**:H415–20.
81. Narayanan J, Imig M, Roman RJ, Harder DR. Pressurization of isolated renal arteries increases inositol trisphosphate and diacylglycerol. *Am J Physiol Heart Circ Physiol* 1994;**266**:H1840–5.
82. Mederos y Schnitzler M, Storch U, Meibers S, Nurwakagari P, Breit A, Essin K, et al. Gq-coupled receptors as mechanosensors mediating myogenic vasoconstriction. *EMBO J* 2008;**27**:3092–103.
83. Yasuda N, Miura S, Akazawa H, Tanaka T, Qin Y, Kiya Y, et al. Conformational switch of angiotensin II type 1 receptor underlying mechanical stress-induced activation. *EMBO Rep* 2008;**9**:179–86.
84. Yatani A, Brown AM. Rapid beta-adrenergic modulation of cardiac calcium channel currents by a fast G protein pathway. *Science* 1989;**245**:71–4.
85. Potocnik SJ, Hill MA. Pharmacological evidence for capacitative Ca(2+) entry in cannulated and pressurized skeletal muscle arterioles. *Br J Pharmacol* 2001;**134**:247–56.
86. Hill MA, Meininger GA. Calcium entry and myogenic phenomena in skeletal muscle arterioles. *Am J Physiol Heart Circ Physiol* 1994;**267**:H1085–92.
87. Loutzenhiser R, Epstein M. Renal microvascular actions of calcium antagonists. *J Am Soc Nephrol* 1990;**1**:S3–12.
88. Nelson MT, Quayle JM. Physiological roles and properties of potassium channels in arterial smooth muscle. *Am J Physiol Cell Physiol* 1995;**268**:C799–822.
89. Jaggar JH. Intravascular pressure regulates local and global Ca(2+) signaling in cerebral artery smooth muscle cells. *Am J Physiol Cell Physiol* 2001;**281**:C439–48.
90. Ella SR, Davis MJ, Meininger GA, Yang Y, Dora KA, Hill MA. Mechanisms underlying smooth muscle Ca^{2+} waves in cremaster muscle arterioles. *FASEB J* 2009;**23** (Meeting Abstract Supplement):767.8.
91. Mufti RE, Brett SE, Tran CH, Abd El-Rahman R, Anfinogenova Y, El-Yazbi A, et al. Intravascular pressure augments cerebral arterial constriction by inducing voltage-insensitive Ca^{2+} waves. *J Physiol* 2010;**588**:3983–4005.
92. Zou H, Ratz PH, Hill MA. Role of myosin phosphorylation and [Ca^{2+}]i in myogenic reactivity and arteriolar tone. *Am J Physiol Heart Circ Physiol* 1995;**269**:H1590–6.
93. Johnson RP, El-Yazbi AF, Takeya K, Walsh EJ, Walsh MP, Cole WC. Ca^{2+} sensitization owing to Rho kinase-dependent phosphorylation of MYPT1-T855 contributes to myogenic control of

arterial diameter. *J Physiol*. ePub ahead of print April 9, 2009, doi: 101113/physiol.2008.168252.

94. Hill MA, Falcone JC, Meininger GA. Evidence for protein kinase C involvement in arteriolar myogenic reactivity. *Am J Physiol Heart Circ Physiol* 1990;**259**:H1586–94.
95. Dessy C, Matsuda N, Hulvershorn J, Sougnez CL, Sellke FW, Morgan KG. Evidence for involvement of the PKC-alpha isoform in myogenic contractions of the coronary microcirculation. *Am J Physiol Heart Circ Physiol* 2000;**279**:H916–23.
96. Hill MA, Davis MJ, Song J, Zou H. Calcium dependence of indolactam-mediated contractions in resistance vessels. *J Pharmacol Exp Ther* 1996;**276**:867–74.
97. Salomone S, Soydan G, Ip PC, Hopson KM, Waeber C. Vessel-specific role of sphingosine kinase 1 in the vasoconstriction of isolated basilar arteries. *Pharmacol Res* 2010;**62**:465–74.
98. Huang S, Sun Z, Li Z, Martinez-Lemus LA, Meininger GA. Modulation of microvascular smooth muscle adhesion and mechanotransduction by integrin-linked kinase. *Microcirculation* 2010;**17**:113–27.
99. Spurrell BE, Murphy TV, Hill MA. Intraluminal pressure stimulates MAPK phosphorylation in arterioles: temporal dissociation from myogenic contractile response. *Am J Physiol Heart Circ Physiol* 2003;**285**:H1764–73.
100. Murphy TV, Spurrell BE, Hill MA. Tyrosine phosphorylation following alterations in arteriolar intraluminal pressure and wall tension. *Am J Physiol Heart Circ Physiol* 2001;**281**: H1047–56.
101. Jackson WF, Blair KL. Characterization and function of Ca(2+)-activated K^+ channels in arteriolar muscle cells. *Am J Physiol Heart Circ Physiol* 1998;**274**:H27–34.

Chapter 94

Cell–Cell Communication Through Gap Junctions

Cor de Wit
Department of Physiology, University of Lübeck, Lübeck, Germany

COORDINATION OF ORGAN FUNCTION

The function of internal organs requires the activation of many cells, in some cases millions of them, in a timely and spatially coordinated fashion. The most obvious example is the heart, which is able to develop pressure and expulse blood only if the heart muscle cells contract in a precisely determined fashion. Such coordination is achieved by specialized cells that deliver the action potential from the pacemaker cells towards the contracting cardiac muscle cells but additionally by the functional coupling of the cardiac muscle cells themselves. This coupling leads to an initial change of the membrane potential causing an action potential of cardiac muscle cell. The initial depolarization is achieved by means of current transfer which is carried by ion flow along a potential gradient through intercellular channels providing low-resistance connections. In contrast, skeletal muscle cells are activated in a physiologically different way and contract only if they are activated by their corresponding motor nerve. In skeletal muscle force development is mainly controlled by the number of muscle cells activated. Thus tight intercellular coupling between skeletal muscle cells with mutual activation between cells is counterproductive. Consequently, skeletal muscle cells are not coupled through such channels. While this is a hallmark difference between heart and skeletal muscle, most smooth muscle cells resemble in this respect cardiac muscle, i.e. smooth muscle cells are not separately innervated but instead act in concert to achieve organ function through cell coupling. Another example for the necessity of intercellular coupling is secretory glands. The many cells that form the respective gland need to be activated in a concerted manner because the amount of secretion required exceeds the capacity of a single cell. Consequently, intercellular communication through channels is also a requirement in many glands that secrete molecules to the circulation (endocrine secretion) or to the external milieu (exocrine secretion) (1).

The need for a coordinated activation of smooth muscle (and endothelial) cells is further exemplified in the following. The vascular system provides delivery of oxygen and nutrients as well as removal of carbon dioxide and other metabolites, which is achieved by continuous perfusion of the organ. However, blood flow is not constant but perpetually adapted to match tissue needs in order to avoid insufficient, but also excessive perfusion. Since oxygen tissue demand is changing in relation to tissue activity and oxygen delivery is mainly determined by perfusion, the latter needs to be adopted by appropriate changes of vascular diameter, which determines resistance and thereby ultimately blood flow through the tissue. The arterial tree supplying individual organs is composed of small arteries outside of the organ and of arterioles within the tissue itself. Vascular resistance opposing blood flow is generated along this tree due to the small diameter of the supplying arteries and arterioles. The amount of resistance can be calculated by estimation of the pressure drop along the particular vascular segment, which reveals that not only arterioles (also named resistance vessels) but also small arteries exhibit already considerable resistance. Therefore, substantial increases in blood flow require diameter increases (and resistance decrease) along all these vessels. If diameter changes were to be limited to the arterioles just upstream of the capillary bed in which a metabolic stimulus is acting, blood flow would be enhanced, but this increase would be restrained by upstream resistance which becomes flow limiting (2,3). These considerations highlight the need for a communication pathway along the vessel that orchestrates the behavior of vascular cells. Interconnected cells acting in a synchronized fashion or as a single unit to enable organ or in this case vessel function is called a functional syncitium (*syn*: together, *citium*: cytosol). The biological basis of the intercellular connections are named gap junctions (4) and are outlined in more detail in the next paragraph.

Muscle. DOI: http://dx.doi.org/10.1016/B978-0-12-381510-1.00094-6

GAP JUNCTIONS ARE CLUSTERS OF INTERCELLULAR CHANNELS FORMED BY CONNEXINS

Ultrastructural Findings

Cells within a multicellular organ have been known for decades to interact and communicate with their immediate neighbors. Only thereby is the activity of those multiple cells concerted and gives rise to organ function. Molecules that are exchanged include ions and therefore charge. Later the ability to exchange larger molecules and dyes was identified. Such behavior requires the intimate contact of adjacent cells and a pathway to exchange molecules. Initially, Dewey and Barr identified by electron microscopy in canine gut regions in which the plasma membranes of adjacent smooth muscle cells appeared to be fused (5). They named this structure "nexus", and defined the nexus as a region where plasma membranes of adjacent excitable cells are fused. They inferred that these regions would allow electrotonic spread of current from one cell to its neighbor without demonstrating pores or channels through which ion and current flow may occur (6). However, later it became evident that cell membranes are not actually fused but there is a small "gap" between such adjacent cells, which led to the term "gap junction" instead of nexus. In these closely apposed areas of cell contact intercellular channels are clustered which bridge this gap and interconnect adjacent cells. Intercellular gap junction channels are composed of two separate hemichannels that dock face-to-face such that they interconnect their central pore without obstruction. Thus, an intercellular channel is formed which creates a communication pathway between these neighboring cells. Since in these areas hundreds of channels are clustered, the gap junction forms a low resistance connection between adjacent cells (7). Charge is transferred by electrotonic spread of current, which is driven by the difference in membrane potential between interconnected cells. The resistance of the gap junction determines the degree of electrical coupling and thus the decrease of a given membrane potential change initiated somewhere in the syncitium while being conducted. In addition, small metabolites and molecules pass through these channels. These include second messengers like cyclic adenosine monophosphate (cAMP), whose transfer provides another important mechanism to synchronize cell behavior. Importantly, gap junctions are the only structures that allow the direct exchange of molecules between adjacent cells (with the exception of rare true cytoplasmic bridges).

Connexins as the Structural Subunits of Intercellular Channels

Gap junctions are composed of a family of proteins named connexins that are integrated into the plasma membrane. These proteins have four transmembrane-spanning domains named M1 to M4. The N- and C-terminal region reside in the cytoplasm and the connections of the transmembrane domains give rise to one cytoplasmic and two extracellular loops (E1, E2) (Figure 94.1, inset). Within

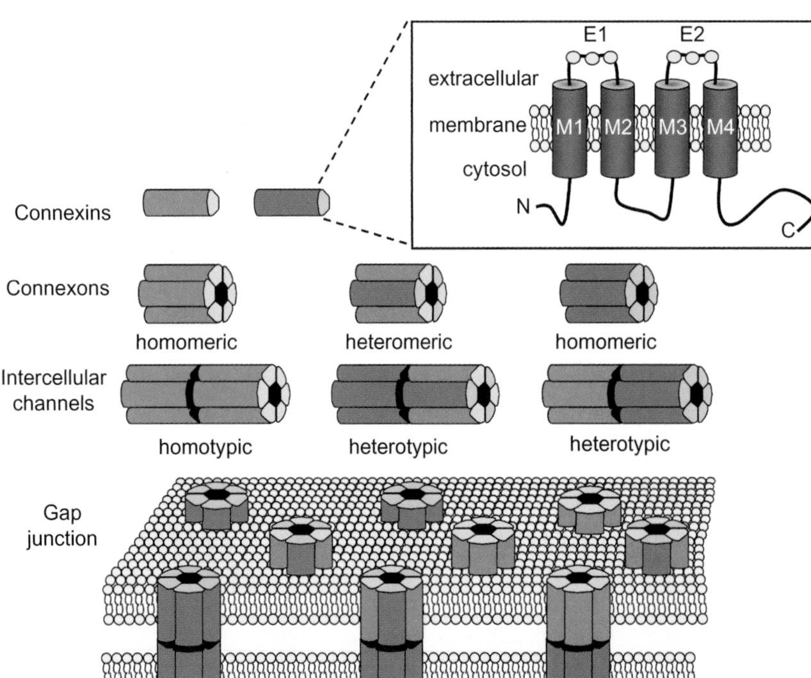

FIGURE 94.1 Assembly of connexins to gap junctions. The modular component of gap junctions are connexins. Inset shows details of a single connexin molecule with four transmembrane domains (M1 to M4), three cysteine residues (C) at each extracellular loop (E1, E2), and the N- and C-terminal end in the cytosol. Six connexins oligomerize to a connexon with a central pore composed of similar (homomeric) or different connexins (heteromeric). Head-to-head docking of two hemichannels from adjacent cells creates a functional intercellular channel consisting of identical or different connexons (homotypic or heterotypic). Channels cluster in a specialized region creating a gap junction. *(Modified from de Wit, 2004 (3), adapted with permission.)*

each extracellular loop three cysteine residues separated by two single amino acids are highly conserved and these cysteine residues may contribute to and stabilize the intercellular connection by forming disulfide bonds (7). Interfering with these extracellular loops by small homologous peptides (connexin mimetic peptides) has been used as a strategy to block gap junctions specifically (8). A hemichannel through the membrane is formed by the oligomerization of six connexins. This hexameric symmetric ring structure is also termed connexon. The central pore is suggested in model systems to be lined by the M3 and M1 transmembrane domains of the connexin (9). Whether a hemichannel also acts by itself as a pure membrane channel connecting the cytoplasm to the extracellular fluid and allows the release of signalling molecules from the cell is a matter of debate (10,11). However, channels made up of a closely related protein (pannexin) may serve this function (12,13). In contrast, it is well established that connexons from adjacent cells dock together, thus forming a channel assembled of 12 protein subunits. The shielding wall against the extracellular environment is created by the extracellular loops E1 and E2, which interact through disulfide bonds generated by the conserved cysteine residues within a single connexin molecule. However, the extracellular loops E1 and E2 also interact between different connexin molecules but this exact interaction is unclear. The two hemichannels are staggered (or rotated) against each other providing a tight docking of the two hemichannels. The aqueous pore in the center of the channel is effectively sealed against the extracellular environment by the rotation and interdigitation, which is a requirement for intercellular communication since it prevents the dilution of exchanged signaling molecules and the loss of ions (and charge) leaking into the extracellular space (7). The size of the pore allows transfer of ions as well as water and other polar molecules up to a size of 1 kilodalton (kDa). Thus, these channels create not only an electrical continuity, but also enable the diffusion of such important molecules as cAMP, inositol trisphosphat (IP_3), or Ca^{2+}-ions (14).

Diversity of Connexin Proteins

The family of connexin genes is comprised of ~20 members (in humans 21, in mice 20) and the proteins are named according to their theoretical molecular mass; for example, connexin40 (Cx40) has a predicted molecular mass of about 40 kDa. The distinct predicted molecular mass and thus the diversity of connexin proteins results from divergencies in the cytoplasmic loop and mostly from differences in the length of the C-terminal cytoplasmic domain. The species from which the respective protein is derived is indicated by a leading small letter, e.g. mCx40 means murine connexin40 and hCX40 human Cx40. In this case, the proteins are orthologous between mice and man and this is also true for the other connexins expressed in the cardiovascular system and smooth muscle (Cx37, Cx40, Cx43, Cx45). However, there are exceptions to this rule (e.g. mCx57 is orthologous to hCX62) and for some human connexins murine orthologs are lacking. A different nomenclature is often used in conjunction with connexin genes. According to sequence identity and the length of the cytoplasmic loop the connexins are divided in groups (α, β, etc.) and then numbered in the order of their discovery. In this terminology a leading Gj (for gap junction) is followed by the subgroup (small letters for mouse, capitals for human) and the respective number, e.g Gja1 is the first mouse connexin of the α-group identified (mCx43) and the human ortholog is named GJA1 or hCX43, respectively (15). The naming of connexins is thus somewhat confusing, even more if other species are considered and a new nomenclature is being developed.

As outlined above, intercellular signalling is functionally important in diverse cell types and tissues. The diversity in the connexin gene family can be partially related to diverse cell types in that specific connexin members serve coupling in specific tissues. Thus, most members of the connexin family are expressed in specific tissues (with some exceptions). However, even in a single cell type within a certain organ multiple connexins have been identified, e.g. in smooth muscle and cardiovascular tissue Cx37, Cx40, Cx43, and Cx45 (16). This diversity generates theoretically a multiplicity of different hemichannels due to their modular design and an even larger diversity of complete intercellular channels considering the fact that a channel is composed of 12 protein subunits. These theoretical interactions can be divided in four groups with respect to the connexins forming the channel (Figure 94.1). A hemichannel composed of six identical connexins is termed homomeric whereas a hemichannel constituted by different connexins is named heteromeric. Analogously, a complete channel constructed by identical hemichannels is named homotypic and a channel made up by nonidentical hemichannels, heterotypic. This nomenclature creates four groups of channels, i.e. homomeric-homotypic (all 12 subunits are identical), homomeric-heterotypic (different hemichannels each composed of six identical subunits), heteromeric-homotypic (two identical hemichannels each composed of more than one connexin), and heteromeric-heterotypic (distinct hemichannels each composed of more than one connexin) (17). Does this diversity indeed exist? Expression of connexins in *Xenopus oocytes* or in cell lines that lack connexins physiologically along with the electrophysiological analysis of coupling between such cells expressing different connexins allows one to verify the theoretical interactions. Of the interesting connexins in the cardiovascular system and smooth muscle mentioned above (Cx37, Cx40, Cx43, Cx45) homomeric-homotypic and homomeric-heterotypic functional channels have all been verified with only one exception reported, namely homomeric Cx40 hemichannels do not form functional channels with homomeric Cx43 hemichannels. However, this view was recently challenged since cells expressing Cx40 and Cx43 form, in addition to homomeric-homotypic, also heteromeric-heterotypic channels (18).

Functionally, this diversity is of utmost importance since conductances, permeabilities, and gating (open vs. closed) characteristics of the intercellular channels varies with the connexins forming them. For example, some connexin channels prefer cations and others, anions. Moreover, conduction and thus capability to transmit electrical impulses ranges from 10 picoSiemens (pS) to more than 300 pS depending on the connexin creating the single channel (14). As mentioned above, the diversity of connexin proteins mainly results from distinct cytoplasmic loops and a different C-terminal cytoplasmic domain. Thus, these domains may also confer unique functional properties to gap junction channels constructed by different connexins specifically with respect to regulatory properties since these sites are subject to phosphorylation. As an example of the possible variation, consider a cell expressing two connexins that assemble under the assumption of a random process into 14 different hemichannels (two of them being homomeric and 12 heteromeric). If such cells pair through an intercellular channel, 196 (14 times 14) different intercellular channels may be found, which exemplifies the tremendous variation theoretically possible.

Regulation of Connexin Channels: Synthesis, Degradation, and Gating

Regulation of cell coupling may involve either alteration in the number of intercellular channels connecting adjacent cells (long term) or modifications in the conductance or open state of existing channels (short term) (4,19). While the first is related to synthesis and implementation of connexins into the membrane as well as degradation, the second requires changes of the connexin molecule in the membrane such that the channel pore or its entrance is modified. This latter may be achieved by ions obstructing the channel mouth as is the case for example in some K^+-channels by Mg^{2+}, however, such a regulatory mechanism has not been demonstrated unequivocally at connexin hemichannels. Instead changes of the pore itself in response to changes of voltage, chemical substances or after phosphorylation are well-known regulatory processes acting on connexins (20). However, the physiological relevance of these regulatory processes in terms of organ function remains mostly obscure. Thus, only major regulatory principles will be discussed in the following paragraphs.

Connexin channels in the membrane experience two different types of voltages, (1) the voltage between the cytoplasm of the two cells they are connecting, termed junctional voltage (V_j) and (2) the voltage between the cytoplasm and the extracellular space which is similar to the voltage across the membrane (V_M) into which they are inserted. Voltage sensitivity of a protein involves charged residues that move in an electrical field. Because the electrical field created by V_j difference is strongest at the intracellular end of the connexin channel, the voltage sensor (charged residue) most likely resides at this location. Conductance through an intercellular homotypic gap junctional channel is indeed dependent on V_j such that conductance is largest at zero V_j and decreases with increasing V_j difference independent of its polarity. Thus, the conductance-voltage relationship of connexin channels is a bell-shaped curve with its maximum at zero V_j and decreasing conductance to both extremes, i.e. at larger negative as well as larger positive V_j (21). This behavior can be explained by charges residing at the cytoplasmic entrance of the pore. Let's assume a negative charge blocks the pore partially on the negative side of a V_j difference since it will be "squeezed" into the pore by the electrical field (Figure 94.2A, left). Thus, conductance will decrease. The same will happen on the other side of the channel if V_j is reversed (Figure 94.2A, right) with the result of the previously explained bell-shaped curve for homotypic gap junctional channels. If the charge that blocks the pore is positive instead of being negative a similar conductance behavior for the overall channel will be observed: blocking will occur at either side of the channel exposed to the positive side of V_j and a bell-shaped curve is formed (Figure 94.2B). The sensitivity of a channel to V_j is lost if certain amino acids in the N-terminal end of connexins are mutated implicating this part of the molecule being involved in voltage gating (22). The gating dependence of homotypic connexin channels on membrane voltage (V_M) is reflected by a deviation of the bell-shaped curve from symmetry.

However, if we now consider a heterotypic channel constructed of hemichannels with a distinct charged residue that obstructs the pore at either side, the channel will be closed at both ends at a certain polarity of V_j (e.g. left negative voltage closes left entrance containing a negative charge and right positive voltage closes right entrance containing a positive charge; Figure 94.2C, left). If now the polarity of V_j is switched, neither entrance will be blocked and conductance is large despite a high V_j (e.g left positive voltage does not close left entrance containing a negative charge and right negative voltage does not close right entrance containing a positive charge;

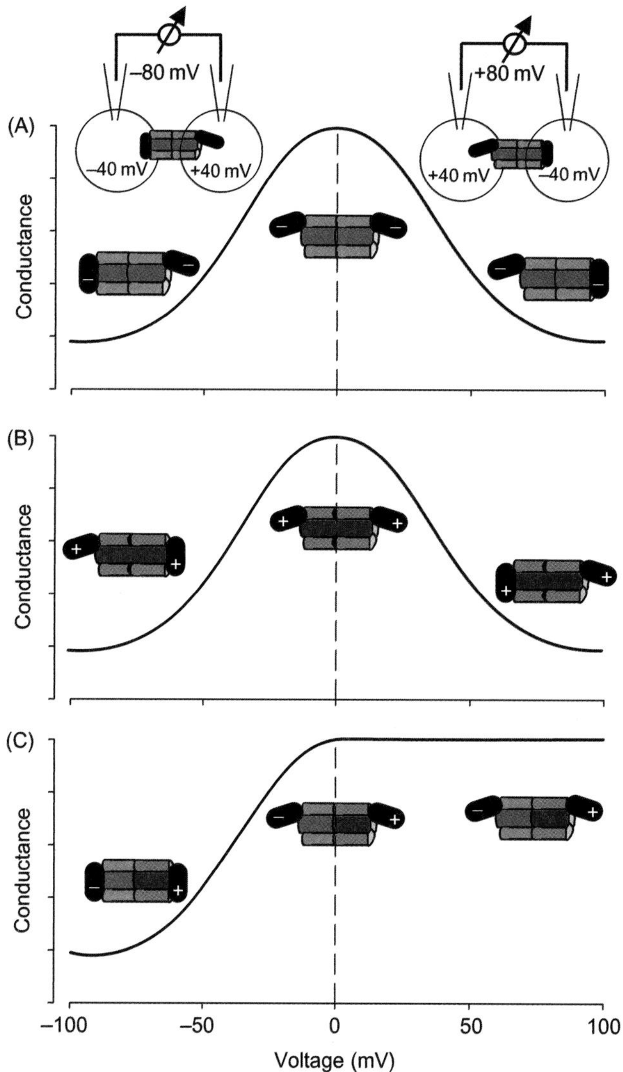

FIGURE 94.2 **Gating of connexin channels in response to transjunctional voltage.** Connexins exhibit charged residues that move in an electric field thereby opening and closing the channel and altering its conductance depending on the voltage difference between adjacent cells (transjunctional voltage, V_j). Homomeric channels exhibit similarly charged residues (negative in (A), positive in (B)) and therefore conductance decreases with enhanced V_j independent of its polarity. In any case, one side of the channel will close giving rise to a symmetric, bell-shaped conductance–voltage relationship. In contrast, in a heterotypic channel both gates will be closed or open depending on the polarity of the difference in V_j which creates a rectifying channel (C).

Figure 94.2C, right). The final result will be that such an heterotypic channel exhibits strong rectification, i.e. conductance is dependent on the polarity of V_j. This may be an important feature considering pacemaker cells, which generate an action potential that can be transmitted to adjacent cells. However, if pacemaker cells exhibit a shorter action potential and are already repolarizing, they will not be affected by a sustained depolarization of these adjacent cells despite the large V_j.

Chemical gating may be important to exclude cell communication to cells in the syncitium that are endangered and have lost their resting potential, for example by a lack of oxygen. This results in intracellular acidification, which in itself is a signal that closes gap junctions. This is best investigated for Cx43 in which intracellular acidification leads to an interaction of sites of the C terminal cytoplasmic domain with the cytosolic loop (23). It has been suggested that the channel closes by a particle-receptor interaction, i.e. a part of the C-terminal end moves to a specific site at the channel mouth.

FUNCTIONAL ASPECTS OF GAP JUNCTIONAL COUPLING IN SMOOTH MUSCLE IN SPECIFIC ORGANS

Gastrointestinal System

In the gastrointestinal system two layers of smooth muscle can be functionally and anatomically distinguished: the outer longitudinal and the inner circular layer separated by a myenteric plexus. In the small intestine the inner circular layer is further subdivided into an inner (smaller, towards the submucosal side) and an outer (larger) division by the deep muscular plexus, a non-ganglionated nerve plexus. These two plexuses harbor neurons and interstitial cells of Cajal (ICC). ICC are spindle-shaped cells with long processes making contact to each other. They are lacking a contractile apparatus, are more frequent in the deep myenteric plexus, and are thought to be involved in pacemaker activity in the intestine (24). Direct coupling between the longitudinal and the circular muscle seems to be non-existent, but they may be functionally coupled indirectly, mediated by the interspersed nervous layer harboring also ICC.

Smooth muscle cells in the circular layers are interconnected by gap junctions mainly composed of Cx43. In contrast, gap junctions are supposedly absent or only occasionally found in the longitudinal layer. Gap junction permeable dye injected into single smooth muscle cells spread to adjacent cells within the circular muscle, indicative of functional cell coupling. Dye spread was also observed in the longitudinal muscle layer, however, at a very slow pace and in a non-uniform pattern (25). The intestinal circular smooth muscle also behaves functionally as a syncitium. If locally activated at any point it contracts in a concentric fashion, suggesting tight electrical coupling. Such synchronous behavior is also observed spontaneously in the form of slow waves, i.e. slow oscillations of the membrane potential, which lead during depolarization to spike potentials accompanied by a spontaneous contraction. Slow waves are not restricted to intestinal smooth muscle cells but can be found also in urinary bladder, ureter, uterus, and in the portal vein. It is assumed that the electrical impulse eliciting the slow waves is generated by pacemaker cells and the slow wave itself conducts along the smooth muscle cells through gap junctions (26). This is reflected by larger and longer waves in the circular compared to the longitudinal layer, which coincides with the number and size of gap junctions detected. Although slow waves are indeed sensitive to blockers of gap junctions, they still persisted at reduced amplitude, duration and frequency during non-specific gap junction blockade, which may reflect insufficient blockade or other mechanisms being involved. The inner division of the circular layer is rather thin and difficult to separate from the outer division in experiments and gap junctions have never been observed in this part (27).

ICC are found in the myenteric plexus and the deep myenteric plexus and are morphologically coupled at their processes through gap junctions. Thus, ICC can be regarded as cellular networks within these two plexus and the gap junctions are constructed likely by Cx43 and Cx45. More questionable is if the ICC form gap junctions with smooth muscle cells. Gap junctions between smooth muscle cells and the ICC located in the myenteric plexus have at best been demonstrated to be rare and only towards the circular but not the longitudinal layer. Other reports suggest that interspersed "fibroblast-like cells", which do not express the specific marker of ICC (c-kit, a tyrosine kinase), do make contact to smooth muscle cells through gap junctions. A different picture emerges regarding ICC in the deep myenteric plexus, which form numerous gap junctions with adjacent smooth muscle cells from the larger outer division of the circular muscle. In accordance with the absence of gap junctions in the inner division of the circular layer, gap junctions are also missing between these cells and adjacent ICC in the deep myentric plexus (27,28). Taken together, ICC are well interconnected and gap junctions between ICC and smooth muscle are mainly found between the deep myenteric plexus and the circular layer. Isolated ICC produce spontaneous depolarizations mediated through a T-type Ca^{2+}-channel, non-specific cation channel, or (in mice) a Ca^{2+}-activated chloride channel, in line with their role to act as pacemaker cells comparable to sinus node cells in the heart (29).

At first glance this supports the concept that ICC control smooth muscle rhythmic spontaneous contraction (slow waves), but the deletion of ICC in mutant mice contrasts with the structural observations. ICC can be abrogated either by application of an antibody directed against the c-kit tyrosine kinase or by introducing a mutation in this protein. Such mice lack ICC in the myenteric plexus, whereas ICC in the deep myenteric plexus are preserved and yet these mice do not exhibit slow waves. This points to ICC of the myenteric plexus as a crucial component of slow waves, which contrasts to the lack of visible gap junctions between these ICC and smooth muscle cells. Despite this controversy, it is well agreed that ICC are required to initiate slow waves in the intestine. The rhythmic depolarization generated by pacemaker ICC changes the excitability of the smooth muscle cells from low to high at a certain pacemaker frequency. While at non-stimulated conditions this will not elicit contractions, it does so at circumstances of stimulation, e.g. after a meal or neural excitation, in that spikes (action potentials) will be generated in smooth muscle cells leading to contraction (slow waves). Different experimental approaches have never been able to elicit slow waves in intestine devoid of ICCs (30). Taken together, these observations indicate that ICC initiate or entrain slow waves in intestinal smooth muscle which are well-coupled to act synchronously and allow propagation of a signal leading to contraction over distances that vary along the gastrointestinal system. The frequency of these slow waves also differs along the gastrointestinal tract and the pace is consequently viewed as being determined by the depolarization generated in ICC. However, it is currently unclear how ICC located in the myenteric plexus transmit the signal to the smooth muscle in the circular layer as gap junctions cannot be identified in these ICC (in the myenteric plexus) that are functionally important. In view of the prominent role of ICC, the term "myogenic activity" needs to be reconsidered as ICC are actually not smooth muscle cells.

Some important aspects of cell-coupling in such a large network need to be considered. The pacemaker generates current flow to adjacent responding cells through its depolarization. However, a large and tightly coupled network exhibits a large capacitance and thus the current generated by the pacemaker may not be sufficient to induce significant depolarization in adjacent coupled cells. This can be overcome by regenerative mechanisms, i.e. the partially depolarized cells produce in response to this initial depolarization an action potential, as is the case, for example, in the myocardium. However, if this occurs the resulting actively generated potential may impose confounding currents onto the pacemaker cells. This latter can be prevented by rectifying gap junction channels which allow current spread in a single direction only (e.g. from a depolarized pacemaker towards adjacent non-depolarized cells) as was envisaged by heterotypic gap junction channels (Figure 94.2).

Interestingly, another connexin has also been identified in the intestine, namely Cx45, at a unique location in the deep muscular plexus that separates the two divisions of the circular smooth muscle (31). Since this plexus also harbors ICC it is interesting to speculate that Cx45 provides a gap junction component that forms heterotypic and thus possibly rectifying channels. Notably, Cx45 is also preferentially expressed in the pacemaker cells of the heart, the sinus node. Whereas in the heart Cx40 is also expressed in the conduction system, Cx40 is only present in vessels in the intestine (see below for vascular gap junctions) (27).

Uterus

Smooth muscle cells in the uterus need to be activated and contract synchronously to deliver the fetus. Garfield discovered the induction of gap junctions in the myometrium in the uterus before parturition and their absence prior to that (32). The most prominent connexin is Cx43 and its expression is hormonally controlled. Progesterone is synthesized in the corpus luteum and the placenta generating high plasma levels during gestation and pregnancy. It effectively suppresses Cx43 expression in the myometrium and prevents synchronous activation of the myometrial smooth muscle cells during pregnancy. Thus, the uterus is kept in a quiescent state disabling preterm labor. Shortly before term, there is a marked surge of estrogen concentrations reversing the relative concentrations of these hormones (33). Estrogen induces Cx43 expression in the myometrium and in rodents the ratio of estrogen/progesterone has been documented to enhance gap junctional communication in the myometrium. This tremendous increase in gap junctions allows the smooth muscle cells to communicate electrotonically and contract in a coordinated manner to ensure labor and delivery of the fetus (34). Cell-specific induced ablation of Cx43 strongly reduced coupling of myometrial cells (assessed by transfer of dye) and led to delayed parturition without altering other processes involved herein (e.g. expression of the oxytocin or the prostaglandin F receptor) verifying the importance of Cx43 in this process (35). Notably, the strategy used (tamoxifen induced gene deletion) was insufficient to abrogate Cx43 expression completely, which may explain why these animals delivered pups at all.

Vascular System

The vascular wall harbors smooth muscle and endothelial cells that form the border and contact site to the flowing blood in the vessel. Located at this strategic position endothelial cells are able to monitor blood flow changes due to the force elicited by the flowing blood, termed shear stress. Shear stress depends on the velocity of the flowing blood and the vessel diameter. Since shear stress elicits a dilation through the endothelial release of mediators acting on the smooth muscle and shear stress decreases with enhanced diameter, a feedback system is established which is able to keep shear stress and thus energy dissipation relatively constant (36). This so-called "flow-induced dilation" is an example of how endothelial cells by releasing vasodilator substances take control over the contractile state of the smooth muscle. This mechanical stimulus serves the purpose of decreasing vascular resistance in arterioles and supplying arteries located further upstream from the site of oxygen exchange, the capillaries. More recently, the old idea of a so-called "ascending dilation" has been revived and resurrected. As outlined in the introduction, the formation of a syncitium by gap junctional coupling ensures that vascular cells act in a concerted fashion. Signals elicited in vessels that are in close contact to the tissue (e.g. capillaries) may spread through such communication pathways against the direction of blood flow to arterioles and arteries located upstream. If these signals are vasodilatory they may underly such an "ascending dilation". Indeed, remote responses exist in the microcirculation and can be experimentally initiated by locally confined stimulation of the vessel. The resulting vessel response is not restricted to the site of stimulation but rather travels or conducts to up- and downstream sites along its length. Such a response (dilation or constriction) is named conducted response and identifies that the vascular cells act in synchrony (up to certain distances) (2,3).

In the search for the underlying mechanism, neural transmission was excluded since conducted responses are not sensitive to substances that block voltage-dependent Na^+-channels (tetrodotoxin). Furthermore, the signal that initiates diameter changes travels along the vessel at considerable velocity, which cannot be exactly resolved by just studying the mechanical response since smooth muscle contraction or relaxation is the rate-limiting step. Most important, not all vasodilators are able to initiate such a conducted response. For example, the endothelial-derived vasodilator nitric oxide (NO) if applied exogenously is unable to do so. Other substances such as acetylcholine, bradykinin, or adenosine have in common that they initiate a dilation by a change of the membrane potential and all are also capable of initiating a conducted response suggesting a necessity for a membrane potential change. In fact, direct measurement of membrane potential in vascular cells using sharp electrodes verified that membrane potential changes spread along the vessel wall. In addition, electrotonic conduction as the spreading mechanism is also supported by its speed.

Is it the endothelial or the smooth muscle cell layer that allows the transmission of an electrotonic signal, or in other words, what is the cable? The easy answer is both, but their properties are different. Destruction of each layer separately did not prevent the spread of the conducted responses and thus one single layer is capable of transmitting the signal through the partially destroyed vessel site. Additional evidence for this comes from animals that are devoid of one of the endothelial connexins (see below). However, in other vessels residing outside of

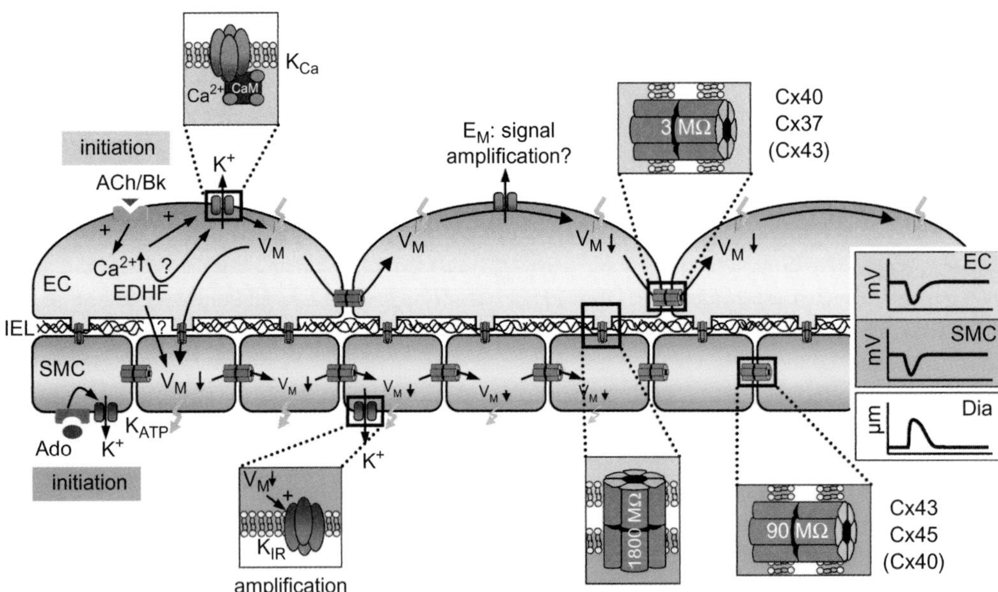

FIGURE 94.3 Gap junctions connect separate cell layers in the vessel wall enabling conducted responses. Local stimulation using agonists (initiation) that act on endothelial cells (EC; acetylcholine, ACh; bradykinin, Bk) or smooth muscle cells (SMC; adenosine, Ado) hyperpolarizes the cell through activation of K^+-channels. The hyperpolarization is transmitted along the vessel wall through gap junctions that couple either EC or SMC homocellularly by different connexins (Cx) as indicated. The conducting signal may be amplified by K^+-channels. In spite of amplification, the signal dissipates with distance, which is most pronounced in SMC, possibly related to higher intercellular resistances (values from reference 37) and a larger number of cell membranes to be crossed. Heterocellular coupling between EC and SMC (myoendothelial) may allow direct current transfer from EC to SMC and provide a molecular substrate for dilations accounted for by an endothelium-derived hyperpolarizing factor (EDHF). However, a distinct EDHF may be present additionally. IEL, internal elastic lamina; V_M, membrane potential; Dia, diameter; K_{Ca}, Ca^{2+}-activated, K_{ATP}, ATP-dependent, and K_{IR}, inwardly rectifying K^+ channel, respectively. *(Modified from de Wit and Griffith, 2010 (38), with permission from Springer Science + Business Media.)*

the tissue the sole destruction of the endothelial cell layer at a restrained site along the pathway abrogated the conduction of a dilation throughout this site. Thus, there are vessels in which aside from the endothelium the smooth muscle layer is also connected by low-resistance gap junctions (Figure 94.3) but this is obviously not the case for all vessels. The reason for this discrepancy is not yet clear but it was suggested that this behavior (i.e. non-coupling of smooth muscle cells) is related to the density of sympathetic innervation, which if dense enough leaves tight gap junctional communication dispensable since most smooth muscle may respond to neurotransmitter release (39).

Gap junctions in the vessel wall are formed by Cx37, Cx40, Cx43, and Cx45 with a cell-specific preference of these connexins. In general, the endothelium expresses Cx37 and Cx40, whereas Cx43 and Cx45 was identified in smooth muscle cells. Although this can be taken as an initial rule there are exceptions, and specifically in renal vessels Cx43 has also been located in endothelial cells. While some reports also suggest that Cx40 is likewise expressed in smooth muscle cells, Cx37 has not been reported to be found in smooth muscle. The situation for Cx45 is not completely clear, mainly due to the lack of a specific antibody.

Deletion of Cx40 results in an attenuation of dilations at remote sites in case the local dilation is elicited by a substance that requires the endothelium (endothelium-dependent dilators, such as actylcholine or bradykinin) (3). Although this highlights the role of the endothelial pathway to conduct dilatory signals along the vessel wall, remote responses are not completely abrogated. Thus, either a remaining endothelial connexin (Cx37) is able to maintain a less efficient conduction pathway or the backup smooth muscle pathway sustains the attenuated dilations at remote sites. Interestingly, the second connexin (Cx37) is also strongly reduced or even lacking in the endothelium if Cx40 is deleted (40). This suggests that the smooth muscle layer is likewise able to transmit conducted responses, although less efficiently. Interestingly, a vasodilator that acts directly on smooth muscle (adenosine) is also able to elicit a conducted response. However, the amplitude of the dilation decreases more strongly with distance, suggesting again that the smooth muscle layer is interconnected and acts as a cable, but that coupling is less effective (Figure 94.3). These experimental data are supported by mathematical modeling, which identifies the endothelial cell layer as the main conducting pathway but the smooth muscle cell layer as a less efficient backup system. This may be in part due to the anatomical positioning of the respective cells. Endothelial cells are oriented longitudinally along the vessel whereas smooth muscle cells are oriented perpendicularly. In the latter case, the number of cell membranes that have to be crossed by a conducted signal (membrane potential change) is fairly larger. Although gap junctions provide low-resistance channels, their resistance is considerably higher than the cytosol, which increases overall resistance along the vessel length considerably (41). Taken together, these data suggest that two conduction pathways exist, an endothelial Cx40-dependent and a (less efficient) smooth muscle pathway in which Cx43 may be functionally important but experimental evidence supporting this idea is currently lacking.

Another site of interesting cell coupling in the vessel wall are the gap junctions that connect endothelial and smooth muscle cells (myoendothelial junctions). These connections have been suggested to be the molecular substrate for the so-called endothelium-derived hyperpolarizing dilations (EDH-type dilations) that are defined as dilations initiated in the endothelium and are independent of nitric oxide and prostaglandins. Moreover, EDH-type dilations are elicited through a smooth muscle cell hyperpolarization, which is followed by dilation possibly due to the closure of voltage-dependent Ca^{2+}-channels. Myoendothelial gap junctions may be able to transfer a hyperpolarization from the endothelium to the smooth muscle by allowing current spread and thus the search for a chemical factor mediating the EDH-type dilation is eventually not necessary. Although there are experiments verifying the need for myoendothelial gap junctions to elicit an EDH-type dilation, other experiments argue against this idea (38). This unsettled issue will have to await further clarification. Needless to say, the connexin subtypes providing these junctions are not clearly identified.

CONCLUSION

In conclustion, the crucial role of gap junctions in converting individual smooth muscle cells into a synchronously contracting or relaxing unit of smooth muscle is well established. Different connexins with distinct properties form those gap junctions and researchers have just begun to unravel differences by investigating organ function in mice lacking specific connexins. This strategy is complicated by the fact that connexins are also critical in embryogenesis and loss of a specific connexin is often lethal. Major efforts are required to uncover the role of the regulation of gap junction permeability in organ function. Despite these hindrances, gap junction physiology is an exciting field that is not limited to muscle cells, a fact that makes it even more attractive.

REFERENCES

1. Bavamian S, Klee P, Allagnat F, Haefliger JA, Meda P. Connexins and secretion. In: Harris AL, Locke D, editors. *Connexins: a guide*. New York: Springer – Humana Press;2009. p. 511–27.
2. Segal SS. Integration of blood flow control to skeletal muscle: key role of feed arteries. *Acta Physiol Scand* 2000;**168**:511–8.
3. de Wit C. Connexins pave the way for vascular communication. *News Physiol Sci* 2004;**19**:148–53.
4. Saez JC, Berthoud VM, Branes MC, Martinez AD, Beyer EC. Plasma membrane channels formed by connexins: their regulation and functions. *Physiol Rev* 2003;**83**:1359–400.
5. Dewey MM, Barr L. Intercellular connection between smooth muscle cells: the nexus. *Science* 1962;**137**:670–2.
6. Barr L, Berger W, Dewey MM. Electrical transmission at the nexus between smooth muscle cells. *J Gen Physiol* 1968;**51**:347–68.
7. Yeager M. Gap junction channel structure. In: Harris AL, Locke D, editors. *Connexins: a guide*. New York: Springer – Humana Press;2009. p. 27–75.
8. Evans WH, Leybaert L. Mimetic peptides as blockers of connexin channel-facilitated intercellular communication. *Cell Commun Adhes* 2007;**14**:265–73.
9. Verselis VK. The connexin channel pore: pore-lining segments and residues. In: Harris AL, Locke D, editors. *Connexins: a guide*. New York: Springer – Humana Press;2009. p. 77–101.
10. Goodenough DA, Paul DL. Beyond the gap: functions of unpaired connexon channels. *Nat Rev Mol Cell Biol* 2003;**4**:285–94.
11. Spray DC, Ye ZC, Ransom BR. Functional connexin "hemichannels": a critical appraisal. *Glia* 2006;**54**:758–73.
12. Scemes E, Spray DC, Meda P. Connexins, pannexins, innexins: novel roles of "hemi-channels". *Pflugers Arch* 2009;**457**:1207–26.
13. Barbe MT, Monyer H, Bruzzone R. Cell–cell communication beyond connexins: the pannexin channels. *Physiology (Bethesda)* 2006;**21**:103–14.
14. Harris AL, Locke D. Permeability of connexin channels. In: Harris AL, Locke D, editors. *Connexins: a guide*. New York: Springer – Humana Press;2009. p. 165–206.
15. Sohl G, Willecke K. Gap junctions and the connexin protein family. *Cardiovasc Res* 2004;**62**:228–32.
16. Johnstone S, Isakson B, Locke D. Biological and biophysical properties of vascular connexin channels. *Int Rev Cell Mol Biol* 2009;**278**:69–118.
17. Koval M. Pathways and control of connexin oligomerization. *Trends Cell Biol* 2006;**16**:159–66.
18. Cottrell GT, Burt JM. Heterotypic gap junction channel formation between heteromeric and homomeric Cx40 and Cx43 connexons. *Am J Physiol Cell Physiol* 2001;**281**:C1559–67.
19. Segretain D, Falk MM. Regulation of connexin biosynthesis, assembly, gap junction formation, and removal. *Biochim Biophys Acta* 2004;**1662**:3–21.
20. Lampe PD, Lau AF. Regulation of gap junctions by phosphorylation of connexins. *Arch Biochem Biophys* 2000;**384**:205–15.
21. Bargiello T, Brink P. Voltage-gating mechanisms of connexin channels. In: Harris AL, Locke D, editors. *Connexins: a guide*. New York: Springer – Humana Press;2009. p. 103–28.
22. Gemel J, Lin X, Veenstra RD, Beyer EC. N-terminal residues in Cx43 and Cx40 determine physiological properties of gap junction channels, but do not influence heteromeric assembly with each other or with Cx26. *J Cell Sci* 2006;**119**:2258–68.

23. Delmar M, Coombs W, Sorgen P, Duffy HS, Taffet SM. Structural bases for the chemical regulation of Connexin43 channels. *Cardiovasc Res* 2004;**62**:268–75.
24. Komuro T. Structure and organization of interstitial cells of Cajal in the gastrointestinal tract. *J Physiol* 2006;**576**:653–8.
25. Farraway L, Ball AK, Huizinga JD. Intercellular metabolic coupling in canine colon musculature. *Am J Physiol Cell Physiol* 1995;**268**:C1492–502.
26. Ward SM, Sanders KM. Involvement of intramuscular interstitial cells of Cajal in neuroeffector transmission in the gastrointestinal tract. *J Physiol* 2006;**576**:675–82.
27. Daniel EE, Wang YF. Gap junctions in intestinal smooth muscle and interstitial cells of Cajal. *Microsc Res Tech* 1999;**47**:309–20.
28. Daniel EE. Communication between interstitial cells of Cajal and gastrointestinal muscle. *Neurogastroenterol Motil* 2004;**16** (Suppl. 1):118–22.
29. Sanders KM. A case for interstitial cells of Cajal as pacemakers and mediators of neurotransmission in the gastrointestinal tract. *Gastroenterology* 1996;**111**:492–515.
30. Huizinga JD, Zarate N, Farrugia G. Physiology, injury, and recovery of interstitial cells of Cajal: basic and clinical science. *Gastroenterology* 2009;**137**:1548–56.
31. Nakamura K, Kuraoka A, Kawabuchi M, Shibata Y. Specific localization of gap junction protein, connexin45, in the deep muscular plexus of dog and rat small intestine. *Cell Tissue Res* 1998;**292**:487–94.
32. Garfield RE, Sims S, Daniel EE. Gap junctions: their presence and necessity in myometrium during parturition. *Science* 1977;**198**:958–60.
33. Young RC. Myocytes, myometrium, and uterine contractions. *Ann NY Acad Sci* 2007;**1101**:72–84.
34. Kidder GM, Winterhagen E. Connexins in the female reproductive system. In: Harris AL, Locke D, editors. *Connexins: a guide*. New York: Springer – Humana Press;2009. p. 481–93.
35. Doring B, Shynlova O, Tsui P, Eckardt D, Janssen-Bienhold U, Hofmann F, et al. Ablation of connexin43 in uterine smooth muscle cells of the mouse causes delayed parturition. *J Cell Sci* 2006;**119**:1715–22.
36. Pohl U, de Wit C. A unique role of NO in the control of blood flow. *News Physiol Sci* 1999;**14**:74–80.
37. Diep HK, Vigmond EJ, Segal SS, Welsh DG. Defining electrical communication in skeletal muscle resistance arteries: a computational approach. *J Physiol* 2005;**568**:267–81.
38. de Wit C, Griffith TM. Connexins and gap junctions in the EDHF phenomenon and conducted vasomotor responses. *Pflugers Arch* 2010;**459**:897–914.
39. Segal SS. Regulation of blood flow in the microcirculation. *Microcirculation* 2005;**12**:33–45.
40. de Wit C. Different pathways with distinct properties conduct dilations in the microcirculation in vivo. *Cardiovasc Res* 2010;**85**:604–13.
41. Tran CHT, Welsh DG. The differential hypothesis: a provocative rationalization of the conducted vasomotor response. *Microcirculation* 2010;**17**:226–36.

Chapter 95

Vascular Smooth Muscle Cell Phenotypic Adaptation

Joseph M. Miano
Aab Cardiovascular Research Institute, University of Rochester School of Medicine and Dentistry, Rochester, New York

Cardiac, skeletal, and smooth muscle cells share similar programs of gene expression during development, but then differentiate into their respective cell types characterized by distinct gene expression profiles necessary to mediate the unique contractile activity each form of muscle exhibits in postnatal life. Adult cardiac and skeletal muscle cells are largely post-mitotic with limited capacity to reenter the cell cycle and engage in new functions. On the other hand, adult vascular smooth muscle cells (VSMC) can undergo a phenotypic switch from the classic contractile phenotype to one of growth and myofilament loss, especially in the context of vascular diseases that elicit neointimal formation (Figure 95.1). Distorted VSMC differentiation was initially referred to as *dedifferentiation* (1). The term dedifferentiation continues to permeate the VSMC literature; however, its use in the context of VSMC phenotypes is restrictive since it does not adequately define the spectrum of phenotypic states that VSMC may display. Another term often used to describe altered VSMC states is *plasticity*, but VSMC plasticity was used in the mid 1960s to describe cell shape changes accompanying mechanical deformation as occurs during stretch. Phenotypic modulation gained popularity in the early 1980s as a definition for the dynamic nature of SMC phenotypes upon cell culture and during vascular disease processes such as atherosclerosis (2). Since then, VSMC have been shown to have enormous adaptability both *in vitro* and *in vivo* with not only a spectrum of phenotypes from contractile to synthetic states, but the ability to transdifferentiate into other cell types. Here, alterations in molecular, structural, and physiological VSCM phenotype will be referred to as *phenotypic adaptation*. The focus of this chapter will be on the major factors that promote a differentiated VSMC phenotype and conditions in which the normal program of VSMC differentiation changes as a consequence of phenotypic adaptation.

NORMAL DIFFERENTIATED PHENOTYPE OF VSMC

The principal functions of differentiated VSMC are to stabilize blood vessels during embryonic and postnatal development and control the distribution of blood throughout the microcirculation. These operations are facilitated by a number of attributes that collectively distinguish VSMC from all other cells of the body. First, adult VSMC express a number of cell-specific contractile genes such as the smooth muscle isoforms of myosin heavy chain, calponin, and gamma actin (*MYH11*, *CNN1*, and *ACTG2*, respectively)* that encode for proteins necessary to mediate the distinct contractile activity of this muscle cell type (3). A second characteristic of adult VSMC is their low rate (less than 0.1%) of cell division in the normal vessel wall (4). During embryogenesis, VSMC must divide and express a number of contractile genes; however, VSMC replication wanes late in gestation as the fully contractile phenotype is manifest to meet the growing circulatory demands of the body (5). A third feature of adult VSMC is their firm association with a complex and dynamic extracellular matrix that promotes a sessile, non-motile state conducive for cellular contraction (6). Although limited protein synthesis occurs in adult VSMC, they elaborate essentially all surrounding matrix proteins needed for structural support of the vessel wall. At the ultrastructural level, contractile VSMC contain thick (myosin) and thin (actin) myofilaments as well as intermediate filaments (primarily desmin), dense bodies that act as connection points for actin filaments through associations with alpha actinin, pinocytotic vesicles for the transport of materials into the cell, and a basal lamina that serves as a critical interface between the

* Throughout this chapter, official human genome nomenclature committee gene symbols are used. Previous gene/protein aliases may be found in any number of websites (e.g., http://www.ncbi.nlm.nih.gov/mapview/).

Muscle. DOI: http://dx.doi.org/10.1016/B978-0-12-381510-1.00095-8

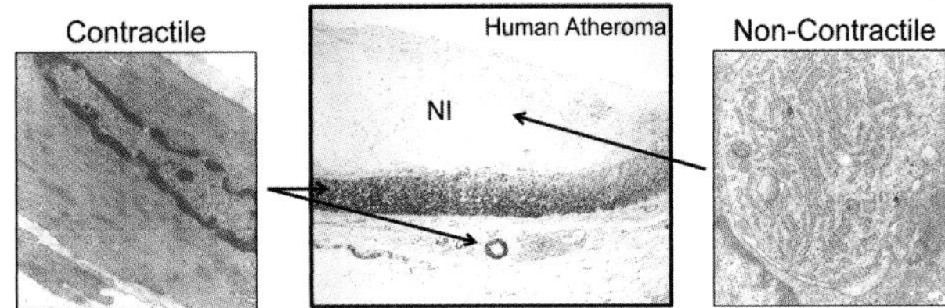

FIGURE 95.1 **VSMC phenotypes in normal and pathological vascular tissue layers.** The normal VSMC contractile phenotype is defined by the presence of myofilaments (electron micrograph at left) and positive immunostaining for proteins associated with myofilaments such as CNN1 (brown staining shown with arrows pointing to tunica media of coronary artery and adventitial arterioles). These characteristics are often lost in VSMC due to phenotypic adaptation to a non-contractile phenotype (electron micrograph at right) permissive for proliferation, migration, and matrix production in neointimal (NI) lesions.

extracellular milieu and various VSMC membrane-associated receptors such as integrin complexes, cadherins, and syndecans that anchor VSMC to the matrix and provide a means through which extracellular signaling cues are transmitted into VSMC via mechano-signal transduction (7). Differentiated VSMC make variable numbers of connections with endothelial cells through myoendothelial junctions that penetrate the internal elastic lamina. These specialized junctions are hypothesized to be important for the transport of solutes and perhaps other molecular mediators between VSMC and the overlying endothelium (8). Differentiated VSMC may therefore be defined as quiescent, non-motile cells that express an array of cell-restricted contractile genes and a number of specialized structures both within the cell itself and at the cell membrane, all of which serve to maintain homeostasis within the medial compartment of the vessel wall where VSMC normally reside.

EFFECTORS OF THE NORMAL VSMC DIFFERENTIATION PROGRAM

Regulatory Effectors

VSMC are defined molecularly by a unique pattern of gene expression found only in this cell type (Table 95.1). Great strides were made over the past 20 years in understanding the transcriptional control processes underlying this distinct program of gene expression. A common finding among many of these genes' regulatory regions is the presence of a 10 base pair *cis* element known as a CArG box (consensus is CCW_6GG, where W can be either A or T). The CArG box is one of the best understood regulatory elements in the genome. There are more than a thousand sequence permutations of CArG throughout the genome, collectively referred to as the CArGome (9). These CArG sequences are recognized and bound by serum response factor (SRF), a ubiquitously expressed transcription factor controlling many cytoskeletal and contractile genes across all three muscle types (10). More than half of the genes restricted to VSMC are dependent upon SRF (Table 95.1). Thus, when SRF is genetically inactivated in VSMC, there are profound reductions in many VSMC contractile genes which likely undermine normal contractile activity of the vessel wall (11).

Together, CArG-SRF orchestrate cell- and context-specific programs of gene expression. How this nucleoprotein complex achieves such specificity in gene expression was a mystery until it became clear that SRF recruits a number of coactivators (currently numbering 63) that modulate the binding of CArG-SRF around those genes whose expression is requisite for maintaining cellular homeostasis. One such coactivator is myocardin (MYOCD), a cardiac- and VSMC-restricted gene that selectively transactivates CArG-containing contractile

TABLE 95.1 Genes Expressed Primarily in Differentiated VSMC

SRF-dependent Genes			SRF-independent Genes	
ACTA2	*DMD*	*MYLKv7 (Telokin)*	*AEBP1*	*ITGA8*
ACTG2	*FHL2*	*MYOCD**	*APEG1*	*MEOX2*
ACTN1	*ITGA1*	*SMTNA*	*ARID2*	*NOTCH3*
BARX2	*KCNMB1*	*SRF*	*CACNA1C*	*PGM5*
CALD1	*LPP*	*TAGLN1 (SM22α)*	*CCN3*	*PTK2 (FRNK)*
CNN1	*MIR-143/145*	*TPM1*	*ELN*	*SMTNB*
CSRP1	*MYH11*	*TPM2*	*GLMN*	
DES	*MYLK*		*HRC*	

Common gene aliases are indicated in parentheses. The asterisk signifies that MYOCD *does not have a known functional CArG element, but is nevertheless dependent on SRF for expression (see text).*

genes through a physical association with the MADS domain of SRF (12). SRF-MYOCD is most highly active over cardiac and VSMC genes containing multiple CArG elements (13,14) although there appears to be some preference for consensus CArG sites that often are functionally integrated with adjacent regulatory sites (15). Importantly, the presence of multiple CArG sites does not always indicate functionality in SRF-MYOCD because the *EGR1* promoter, harboring five CArG elements, is only weakly responsive to MYOCD transactivation (16). This implies the existence of additional coding information in DNA that attenuates SRF-MYOCD transcriptional activation, probably through structural changes in CArG-SRF leading to sub-optimal MYOCD binding. It will be informative to elucidate all of the sequence information in and around CArG elements that enhance or minimize MYOCD binding to SRF.

There is much genetic evidence supporting an important role for MYCOD in establishing and maintaining the differentiated phenotype of VSMC. For example, deletion of MYOCD in mice results in mid-embryonic arrest, presumably because VSMC do not fully differentiate around developing blood vessels (17). Knocking out MYOCD in a subset of VSMC derived from neural crest causes a decrease in myofilaments and key contractile genes as the cells phenotypically adapt to a more synthetic state (18). Conversely, ectopic expression of MYOCD in skeletal myoblasts is sufficient to induce several SRF-dependent VSMC genes and reduces cell growth *in vitro* (14). In fact, essentially any non-VSMC type overexpressing MYOCD is biochemically and structurally converted into a VSMC-like state (Figure 95.2). Further, MYOCD induces VSMC myofilament formation (but not cardiac sarcomeres) at the ultrastructural level in the BC_3H1 cell line. These cells also show VSMC contractile competence following agonist stimulation (19). Thus MYOCD, in conjunction with CArG-SRF, is sufficient for the biochemical, ultrastructural, and physiological attributes associated with VSMC differentiation. In this regard, MYOCD may arguably be considered the VSMC equivalent of MYOD1 in skeletal muscle. There are two other related myocardin genes (MRTFA and MRTFB) that have similar SRF-dependent functions but are widely expressed and are under different control processes than MYOCD (20). As discussed below, VSMC phenotypic adaptation to various perturbations often results in reduced expression of MYOCD which has consequences for the expression of many VSMC differentiation genes and, by extension, the contractile phenotype these cells normally display. Collectively, the available data support the idea of SRF-MYOCD acting as a transcriptional switch for the VSMC differentiated phenotype (Figure 95.3).

microRNAs (miRs) represent another class of regulatory effectors of VSMC differentiation. These non-coding RNAs function as molecular rheostats by lowering protein levels through imperfect Watson–Crick base pairing of target mRNAs resulting in mRNA degradation, mRNA deadenylation, or translational repression. In some contexts, a miR can enhance mRNA/protein expression (21). Several miRs have been defined in VSMC but the major

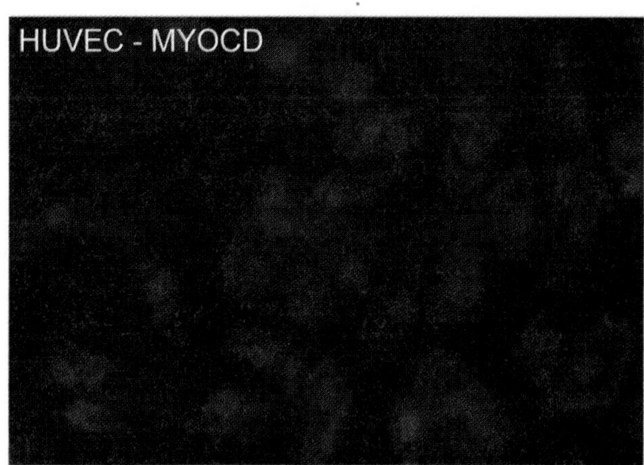

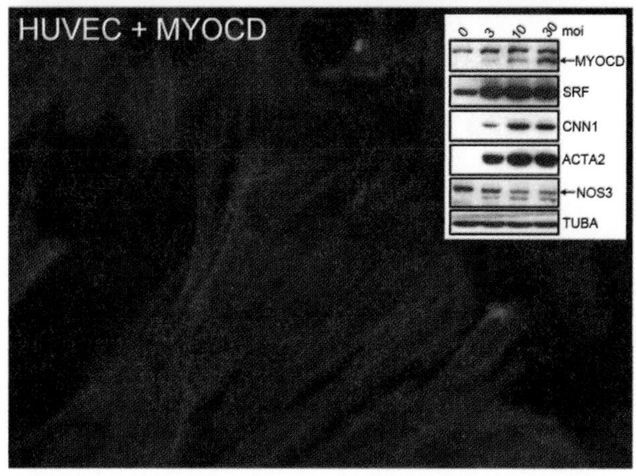

FIGURE 95.2 Myocardin-mediated conversion of endothelial cells into VSMC. Upon MYOCD expression, the normal cobblestone-like morphology of human umbilical vein endothelial cells (HUVEC) shows abundant stress fibers reflecting filamentous actin as indicated with phalloidin stain. Increasing amounts of MYOCD (in moi) induce expression of several VSMC markers as endothelial nitric oxide synthase (NOS3) levels decrease (Western blot inset).

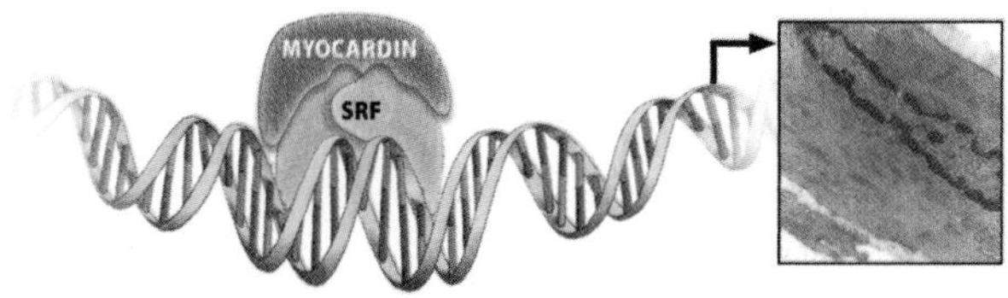

FIGURE 95.3 SRF-MYOCD acts as a molecular switch for the VSMC contractile phenotype. SRF bound to CArG elements directs a VSMC differentiated state through the MYOCD coactivator.

regulatory effector for VSMC differentiation is the miR-143/145 bicistronic cluster. Interestingly, the miR-143/145 gene is a direct target of SRF-MYOCD (22,23) (Table 95.1). miR-145 appears to be the dominant miR in directing VSMC differentiation because ectopic expression in non-VSMC or VSMC that have phenotypically adapted to another state, is sufficient to turn on several VSMC differentiation genes while reducing the proliferative response to growth factors (22). Although the full spectrum of miR-145 targets in VSMC has yet to be determined, known mRNA targets implicated in VSMC differentiation include KLF4 and KLF5 (22,23). To summarize, SRF-MYOCD promotes VSMC differentiation directly through binding to CArG elements and the activation of the corresponding gene and indirectly through the repressive action of miR-145 (and perhaps other miRs) on key target genes that in turn modulate VSMC differentiation processes.

As evident in Table 95.1, there are a number of VSMC differentiation genes whose expression is independent of CArG-SRF. This implies the existence of parallel circuits of transcriptional (or post-transcriptional) control of the VSMC differentiated state. For example, the histidine-rich calcium-binding protein (HRC) gene lacks functional CArG elements but contains a conserved binding site for the MEF2 family of transcription factors. This MEF2 site is required for HRC promoter activity in transgenic mice demonstrating one example of a factor working independently of SRF to control a VSMC-restricted gene (24). MYOCD itself is regulated through a distal MEF2 site in transgenic mice (25), although levels of myocardin mRNA are reduced when SRF is inactivated suggesting that SRF may also control MYOCD expression indirectly, perhaps through a microRNA. In addition to MEF2, there are a number of other regulatory factors that may positively effect VSCM differentiation, including HAND2, intracellular Notch receptor domains, SMADs and a large number of ill-defined zinc finger-containing transcription factors. Some of these factors (e.g., SMAD3) are convergent points of critical signaling pathways that control VSMC differentiation. Perhaps the best example of the latter is TGF-β_1 signaling which has been shown in numerous model systems to direct VSMC differentiation, presumably through SMAD-responsive elements. Other members of the TGF-β superfamily of signaling proteins include BMP2 and BMP4, which may also direct VSMC differentiation through similar SMAD transcriptional activators (26). It will be important to define the SRF-MYOCD independent control of such highly VSMC-specific genes as *NOTCH3* and *SMTNB* to gain a more complete understanding of the transcriptional effectors of VSMC differentiation and how such circuits are perturbed under conditions of VSMC phenotypic adaptation.

Mechano-Signaling Effectors

Adult VSMC are embedded in a matrix composed of collagen type III, elastin, and various proteoglycans that not only serves to anchor the cell for optimal contractile activity, but continuously feeds signaling input from the immediate exterior milieu to the VSMC's interior through integrin complexes and other membrane-associated proteins that bridge the extracellular matrix to the actin cytoskeleton. A constant source of mechano-signaling transmitted by the matrix to VSMC stems from the pulsatile action of blood flow, which comprises shear and tangential forces related to stretch. Laminar shear stress positively impacts the overlying endothelium through this cell's secretion of nitric oxide and the latter's diffusion into subjacent VSMC. Upon entry into VSMC, nitric oxide stimulates guanylate cyclase resulting in elevations in the second messenger cyclic GMP, which activates protein kinase G, a known effector of VSMC differentiation (27). Cyclical stretch directly deforms VSMC and this has been modeled in various two- and three-dimensional model systems of VSMC differentiation. In general, stretching VSMC promotes a differentiated phenotype as measured by the expression of various contractile genes, particularly those that are dependent on SRF-MYOCD (28). A dynamic interplay exists between key membrane-bound proteins, such as integrin complexes and ion channels that "sense" mechanical stretch, and the actin cytoskeleton to facilitate signals that promote a more differentiated VSMC state. In this context, the ITGA8 integrin subunit has been shown to promote VSMC differentiation *in vitro* although it is unclear whether such signaling converges on SRF-MYOCD or is responsive to stretch-induced stimulation (29). Further work is needed to recapitulate as many elements of the normal vessel wall as possible in organ culture, including the dimension of time, to tease apart additional mechano-signaling effectors of VSMC differentiation.

CONDITIONS OF VSMC PHENOTYPIC ADAPTATION

VSMC in Culture

Essentially all of the initial knowledge of factors controlling VSMC differentiation arose from experiments performed in cell culture. Such studies were initiated by the elegant work of Campbell and Chamley-Campbell (reviewed in 30), followed by work in the laboratory of Thyberg (reviewed in 31). These studies and others showed that when VSMC are cultivated in a dish, they initially exhibit characteristics of a contractile cell with expression of myosin and actin and the ability to contract upon agonist stimulation. With time, however, cultured

VSMC from a variety of species, including human, lose their expression of myosin (MYH11), acquire an elaborate rough endoplasmic reticulum/Golgi system, and begin to proliferate. This was shown to coincide with not only reductions in VSMC contractile genes, but also elevations in cytoskeletal proteins such as non-muscle myosin and vinculin as well as alterations in the compartmentalization of contractile versus cytoskeletal proteins. The growth state of VSMC is also associated with reduced expression of various ion channels (32) and, with that, loss in excitation-transcriptional coupling involving SRF-MYOCD dependent genes (33). Decreases in other VSMC genes and microRNAs such as miR-143/145 ensue as cultured VSMC assume a less contractile phenotype. Importantly, expression of MYOCD is consistently reduced in several *in vitro* models of VSMC when compared to fresh aortic tissue (14). Ectopic MYOCD expression in these and other phenotypically modified VSMC results in partial reconstitution of the VSMC differentiated state (above). Thus, the >40-year-old phenomenon of VSMC phenotypic modulation (or adaptation) appears mainly to be a function of reduced MYOCD expression. We currently have little insight into the molecular mechanisms underlying attenuated MYOCD expression *in vitro* but it likely involves direct transcriptional and/or post-transcriptional processes. In addition to changes in gene expression, cultured VSMC show increased growth when plated on fibronectin, but not laminin or fibrillar collagen, highlighting the fact that the repertoire of membrane-associated integrin complexes changes when VSMC adapt to an *in vitro* environment. Although cultured VSMC exhibit variable degrees of phenotypic adaptation, they are useful for examining various molecular aspects of VSMC biology.

Mechanical Injury to the Vessel Wall

Early studies showed that medial VSMC undergo dramatic ultrastructural phenotypic adaptations following mechanical injury to the vessel wall (1). These changes in VSMC are very similar to those observed when VSMC are placed in a culture dish (e.g., reduced myofilaments and increases in rough endoplasmic reticulum). The ultrastructural adaptations were further confirmed in other species such as rabbit, pig, and monkey using various methods of injury including balloon catheter dilation of the vessel wall. Immediately following balloon catheter injury to the vessel wall, the normal matrix–integrin–actin cytoskeleton axis is perturbed resulting in defective organization of cytoskeletal-contractile proteins, VSMC death, and release of VSMC- and matrix-associated growth factors. At the same time, plasma- and platelet-derived factors permeate the vessel wall and flood the immediate milieu of surviving VSMC (34). Platelet-derived factors play a pivotal role in reprogramming the normal VSMC contractile program of gene expression to one of hyper-secretion, motility, and proliferation through binding and activation of surface receptors displayed on VSMC. Not surprisingly, VSMC that have undergone this phenotypic adaptation lose normal contractile competence. Together, these structural, molecular, and physiological changes in VSMC are considered pivotal to the development of neointimal lesions following mechanical injury to the vessel wall.

Interestingly, levels of SRF do not appreciably change in VSMC following arterial injury (Figure 95.4). The absence of significant changes in SRF expression after mechanical injury to the vessel wall reflects this factor's association with different coactivators (such as ELK1) that direct new programs of gene expression. For example, within 15 minutes following arterial injury, several SRF-dependent immediate early genes are upregulated in medial VSMC (35). Normally, these genes are not expressed in adult VSMC because SRF is bound to MYOCD, which recognizes the same domain of SRF as ELK1 (36). Induction of immediate early genes, many of which encode for transcription factors, result in the secondary activation of delayed response genes, including growth factors that act in an autocrine/intracrine fashion to stimulate VSMC cell cycle entry and migration.

In contrast to the lack of change in SRF expression after mechanical injury to the vessel wall, sharp decreases in myocardin mRNA occur following wire injury to the mouse carotid artery (37). miR-143/145 levels are also reduced following balloon injury to the vessel wall in rat (38) as well as ligation injury to the mouse carotid artery (22). Much of the decrease in VSMC contractile gene expression following vascular injury likely results from a decrease in MYOCD and miR-145. The reduction in MYOCD coupled with injury-induced signals that stabilize ELK1 binding to SRF highlight the "toggling" of SRF from a pro VSMC differentiation factor in the normal vessel wall to a pro growth/migratory factor in a vessel undergoing repair and thus requiring phenotypic

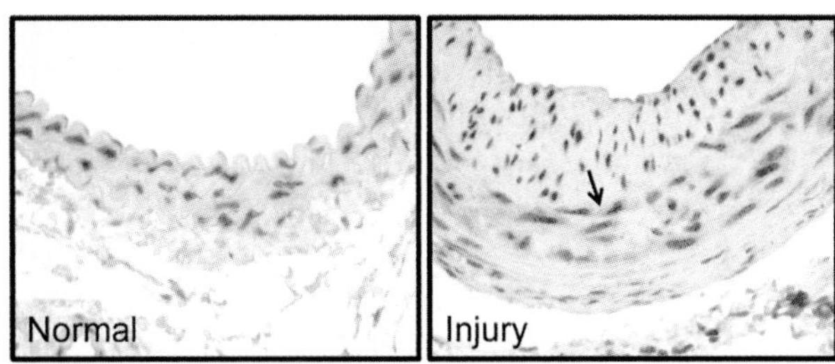

FIGURE 95.4 **SRF expression in the vessel wall.** Immunostaining for SRF (red nuclear stain) in normal and injured carotid artery of the mouse. Note that all cells throughout the medial and neointimal layers of the injured vessel stain positive for SRF. The arrow indicates the internal elastic lamina that demarcates the medial layer of the vessel wall from the overlying neointima.

adaptation of VSMC. Thus, SRF in neointimal cells most likely engages a set of CArG-dependent genes different from those in medial VSMC (Figure 95.4). In this context, expression profiling of normal adult VSMC versus neointimal cells (derived in part from medial VSMC that have undergone phenotypic adaptation following arterial injury) has revealed distinct molecular phenotypes between these two cell populations. The general consensus is that at least a subset of differentiated VSMC reverts to a more primitive phenotype characterized by the expression of so-called "embryonic" genes (e.g., tropoelastin, osteopontin, PDGF-BB) that effect growth and migratory attributes characteristic of an evolving neointima (39,40). Whether local inhibition of SRF or acute over-expression of MYOCD mitigates VSMC phenotypic adaptation following vascular injury is currently unknown.

Hundreds of studies have been done over the past 25 years testing various interventions in the context of mechanical injury to the vessel wall. These studies included various gene therapies ranging from antisense oligonucleotides against cell cycle regulators to gain-of-function protein expression and pharmaceutical interventions with drugs that have shown promise in other hyper-proliferative conditions such as retinoids and immunosuppressants (e.g., rapamycin). The latter intervention is the principal therapeutic to combat neointimal formation following clinical interventions to increase vascular luminal area. Whether rapamycin has any influence on SRF-MYOCD expression and/or activity is unknown.

Atherosclerosis

Atherosclerosis is a chronic inflammatory disease characterized by distinct pathologic stages involving multiple cells that are recruited to focal regions of large and medium-sized arteries subjected to an array of stressors such as altered blood flow and hyperlipidemia. Resident VSMC contribute to the pathogenesis of atherosclerosis through phenotypic adaptations that arise at essentially every stage of the disease from fatty streak to complicated plaque. For example, while monocyte/macrophages are well known for their early involvement in lipid ingestion within the intima of arteries, medial VSMC are equal to the task and can readily form foam cells as well, a concept that was recognized as early as the 1960s (41). In fact, "intermediate" VSMC types have been described in atherosclerotic lesions with some cells showing little lipid uptake and others much more lipids with a reduction in the content of myofilaments and increases in rough endoplasmic reticulum (42). These early studies provided unequivocal evidence for a role of VSMC in early fatty streak formation and the expansion of a neointima through cell proliferation and migration. The conversion of normal contractile VSMC into foam cells of atherosclerotic lesions suggests a transdifferentiation process exists in the vessel wall (43). Indeed, there is evidence for VSMC transdifferentiation into a number of cell types that could make their way into an atherosclerotic lesion, including osteoblasts, chondrocytes, and endothelial cells (44–46). It is unclear whether VSMC directly transdifferentiate into another cell type or first revert to a more embryonic cell permissive for subsequent differentiation into a distinct cell.

More recently, phenotypic adaptation was noted in VSMC stimulated with various oxidized phospholipids known to be present in atherosclerotic lesions. These cells exhibit reductions in MYOCD and, consequently, a diminution in contractile gene expression as well (47). Lipid-ingesting macrophages release an array of growth factors and cytokines that stimulate medial VSMC to enter the cell cycle and become motile, thus further augmenting intimal expansion, fatty streak formation and the deposition of a neointimal matrix. Interestingly, as the atheroma expands and the amount of cellular and extracellular material increases, local cells (presumably former contractile VSMC) phenotypically adapt to the changing environment by partially reverting to differentiated VSMC with the formation of a fibrous cap. The fibrous cap is thought to confer stability to an otherwise unstable plaque susceptible to physical breaches and catastrophic thrombosis. Thus, VSMC might serve a dual role in atherogenesis by contributing to early pathology via foam cell formation and then functioning later in the creation of a protective fibrous cap.

In addition to lipid as a stimulus for VSMC phenotypic adaptation, changes in blood flow at sites of predilection for atherosclerosis may impact on the cyto-contractile apparatus in adult VSMC thus promoting a less differentiated state. Moreover, there likely exist periodic bursts of VSMC stimulation from local cells or biological agents (e.g., microorganisms) known to reside in atherosclerotic lesions. Further, elevated glucose and advanced glycation end products may impact VSMC phenotype in the context of type II diabetes. The development of genetic models to directly evaluate the role of SRF-MYOCD in atherogenesis and diabetes is a worthy endeavor.

An accelerated form of atherosclerosis occurs in vessels of transplanted organs. Such transplant arteriopathy is also associated with VSMC phenotypic adaptation with similar changes in growth and migration as observed in lipid-associated atherosclerosis. An outstanding question in this context is whether the immune response to transplantation, typically controlled with immunosuppressant drugs such as cyclosporine A, has any effects on the expression or activity of SRF-MYOCD or key miRs such as miR-145.

Aneurysms

Dilation of the vessel wall either through advanced atherosclerosis or genetic mutations in proteins such as fibrillin may involve VSMC phenotypic adaptation. For example, in an elastase-induced model of aortic aneurysms, VSMC were shown to exhibit decreases in TAGLN1 and ACTA2 with a concomitant increase in matrix metalloproteinases (48). The increase in matrix metalloproteinases is of interest since they are thought to contribute to vessel wall weakening through matrix degradation. There is also clinical evidence for VSMC phenotypic adaptation in cerebral vascular aneurysms (49). Whether changes in VSMC phenotype associated with clinical or experimental aneurysm formation stems from altered SRF-MYOCD or miR expression and activity is presently unclear. However, a recent clinical study demonstrated attenuated miR-143/145 expression in thoracic aortic dissections as compared to age-matched control aortic samples (50).

Varicose Veins

Another disease involving dilation of the vessel wall is varicose veins. The adaptation of VSMC to this condition is similar to aneurysms with increases in cytokines and MMPs at the expense of VSMC contractile markers (51). Again, however, there have been no reported studies examining expression or activity of SRF-MYOCD in the context of varicose veins.

Hypertension

The development of hypertension, like atherosclerosis, is complex and multi-factorial. Whether the underlying etiology is genetic or environmental, VSMC play a prominent role and they do so through phenotypic adaptations similar to those described above, including changes in growth, migration, and secretory capacity (52). However, in the microcirculation particularly, there may be manifestations of VSMC phenotypic adaptation that include elevations in contractile elements resulting in hypercontractility. In this context, a common model for experimental hypertension, the spontaneously hypertensive rat, has a genetic insertion adjacent to a CArG box in the promoter region of the *MYLK* gene resulting in enhanced SRF binding and expression of MYLK; no such mutation or expression change was seen in the control rat strain (53). Interestingly, a recent clinical study of patients with essential hypertension showed increases in myocardin mRNA in peripheral blood leukocytes (54). Although no studies could be done in vascular samples, the finding of MYOCD as a biomarker for essential hypertension warrants deeper analysis, including a determination of any genetic variants in or around the *MYOCD* locus that could explain its elevated expression.

Alzheimer's Disease

Recent studies have implicated both SRF and MYOCD in two important aspects of Alzheimer's disease (AD): namely cerebral hypoperfusion and cerebral amyloid angiopathy. The mechanisms underlying cerebral hypoperfusion include VSMC phenotypic adaptation to a hyper-contractile state through increases in both SRF and MYOCD. Such hyper-contractility can be normalized by knocking down SRF in AD VSMC. Conversely, ectopic expression of MYOCD in control VSMC phenocopies the AD hyper-contractile state both *in vitro* and *in vivo* (55). The other aspect of AD where SRF-MYOCD may exert some influence is with the aggregation of amyloid beta in and around blood vessels of the brain. Specifically, SRF-MYOCD appears to inhibit amyloid beta clearance from VSMC through a transcriptional pathway involving activation of the CArG-containing sterol regulatory element binding transcription factor 2 and this factor's subsequent repression of the major amyloid beta clearance receptor, low density lipoprotein receptor-related protein 1 (56). Collectively, these results highlight conditions of VSMC phenotypic adaptation involving *elevations* in SRF-MYOCD as opposed to the more common diminution seen in various other vascular pathologies. What the underlying mechanism is for increases in SRF-MYOCD in AD is unclear, but one possibility is local hypoxia due to upstream atherosclerotic disease, which is a known risk factor for AD (56). It will be of interest to determine whether other conditions of elevated SRF-MYOCD exist where a super-differentiated VSMC phenotype is present (e.g., asthma).

PERSPECTIVE

Phenotypic adaptation is pervasive throughout development and disease processes. In the vasculature, progenitor cells are recruited to an endothelial tube and traverse intermediate stages of phenotypic adaptation from embryonic to adult VSMC (Figure 95.5). Related progenitor cells likely remain in the vessel wall throughout life with the potential to become other cell types within the local vascular milieu (Figure 95.5). Evidence exists to support circulating progenitor cells homing to sites of vascular pathology with subsequent differentiation into various cells (Figure 95.5). It is equally plausible that adult VSMC transdifferentiate into other cell types of vascular lesions either directly or, more likely, through an intermediate embryonic VSMC cell. The genome of an embryonic VSMC may be more permissive for differentiation into other cell types in vascular disease than a

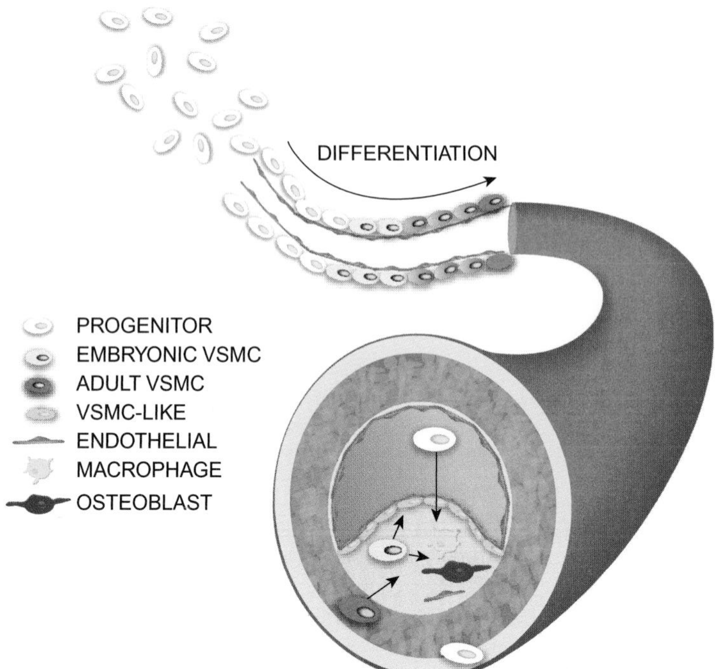

FIGURE 95.5 **VSMC phenotypic adaptations in the vessel wall.** Schematic illustrating the role of progenitor cells in embryonic and adult VSMC differentiation and their differentiation into cells of neointimal lesions. Note that adult VSMC may contribute to neointimal cells either directly or indirectly through an embryonic VSMC-like phenotype which itself may have potential to become other cell types, including VSMC-like cells of the fibrous cap. See text for further details.

differentiated VSMC. Further, the embryonic VSMC might revert back to a quasi-differentiated VSMC as occurs in a fibrous cap of an atheroma (Figure 95.5). A major driver of phenotypic adaptation will be the relative level of various transcriptional and post-transcriptional regulatory effectors in VSMC such as SRF, MYOCD, and miR-145 versus other lineage-restricted regulatory effectors (e.g., RUNX2, MSX2) that can be induced in vascular cells under conditions of vascular injury. It will be informative to dissect these and other molecular events that an adult or embryonic VSMC must interpret before locking into a new specific cell type with distinct functions unrelated to contractility.

REFERENCES

1. Murray M, Schrodt GR, Berg HF. Role of smooth muscle cells in healing of injured arteries. *Arch. Pathol* 1966;**82**:138–46.
2. Campbell GR, Chamley-Campbell JH. Smooth muscle phenotypic modulation: role in atherogenesis. *Med. Hypotheses* 1981;**7**:729–35.
3. Owens GK, Kumar MS, Wamhoff BR. Molecular regulation of vascular smooth muscle cell differentiation in development and disease. *Physiol. Rev.* 2004;**84**:767–801.
4. Goldberg ID, Stemerman MB, Schnipper LE, Ransil BJ, Crooks GW, Fuhro RL. Vascular smooth muscle cell kinetics: a new assay for studying patterns of cellular proliferation in vivo. *Science* 1979;**205**:920–1.
5. Cook CL, Weiser MCM, Schwartz PE, Jones CL, Majack RA. Developmentally timed expression of an embryonic growth phenotype in vascular smooth muscle cells. *Circ Res* 1994;**74**:189–96.
6. Wagenseil JE, Mecham RP. Vascular extracellular matrix and arterial mechanics. *Physiol Rev* 2009;**89**:957–89.
7. Moiseeva EP. Adhesion receptors of vascular smooth muscle cells and their function. *Cardiovasc Res* 2001;**52**:372–86.
8. Heberlein KR, Straub AC, Isakson BE. The myoendothelial junction: breaking through the matrix? *Microcirculation* 2009;**16**:307–22.
9. Sun Q, Chen G, Streb JW, Long X, Yang Y, Stoeckert Jr CJ, et al. Defining the mammalian CArGome. *Genome Res* 2006;**16**:197–207.
10. Miano JM, Long X, Fujiwara K. Serum response factor: master regulator of the actin cytoskeleton and contractile apparatus. *Am J Physiol Cell Physiol* 2007;**292**:C70–81.
11. Miano JM, Ramanan N, Georger MA, de Mesy-Bentley KL, Emerson RL, Balza Jr RO, et al. Restricted inactivation of serum response factor to the cardiovascular system. *Proc Natl Acad Sci USA* 2004;**101**:17132–7.
12. Wang D-Z, Chang PS, Wang Z, Sutherland L, Richardson JA, Small E, et al. Activation of cardiac gene expression by myocardin, a transcriptional cofactor for serum response factor. *Cell* 2001;**105**:851–62.
13. Wang Z, Wang D-Z, Pipes GCT, Olson EN. Myocardin is a master regulator of smooth muscle gene expression. *Proc Natl Acad Sci USA* 2003;**100**:7129–34.
14. Chen J, Kitchen CM, Streb JW, Miano JM. Myocardin: a component of a molecular switch for smooth muscle differentiation. *J Mol Cell Cardiol* 2002;**34**:1345–56.
15. Sun Q, Taurin S, Sethakorn N, Long X, Imamura M, Wang DZ, et al. Myocardin-dependent activation of the CArG box-rich smooth muscle gamma actin gene: Preferential utilization of a single CArG element through functional association with the NKX3.1 homeodomain protein. *J Biol Chem* 2009;**284**:32582–90.
16. Zhou J, Herring BP. Mechanisms responsible for the promoter-specific effects of myocardin. *J Biol Chem* 2005;**280**:10861–9.

17. Li S, Wang D-Z, Richardson JA, Olson EN. The serum response factor coactivator myocardin is required for vascular smooth muscle development. *Proc Natl Acad Sci USA* 2003;**100**:9366–70.
18. Huang J, Cheng L, Li J, Chen M, Zhou D, Lu MM, et al. Myocardin regulates expression of contractile genes in smooth muscle cells and is required for closure of the ductus arteriosus in mice. *J Clin Invest* 2008;**118**:515–25.
19. Long X, Bell RD, Gerthoffer WT, Zlokovic BV, Miano JM. Myocardin is sufficient for a SMC-like contractile phenotype. *Arterioscler Thromb Vasc Biol* 2008;**28**:1505–10.
20. Pipes GCT, Creemers EE, Olson EN. The myocardin family of transcriptional coactivators: versatile regulators of cell growth, migration, and myogenesis. *Genes Dev* 2006;**20**:1545–56.
21. Carthew RW, Sontheimer EJ. Origins and mechanisms of miRNAs and siRNAs. *Cell* 2009;**136**:642–55.
22. Cordes KR, Sheehy NT, White MP, Berry EC, Morton SU, Muth AN, et al. miR-145 and miR-143 regulate smooth muscle cell fate and plasticity. *Nature* 2009;**460**:705–10.
23. Xin M, Small EM, Sutherland LB, Qi X, McAnally J, Plato CF, et al. MicroRNAs miR-143 and miR-145 modulate cytoskeletal dynamics and responsiveness of smooth muscle cells to injury. *Genes Dev* 2009;**23**:2166–78.
24. Anderson JP, Dodou E, Heidt AB, de Val SJ, Jaehnig EJ, Greene SB, et al. HRC is a direct transcriptional target of MEF2 during cardiac, skeletal, and arterial smooth muscle development in vivo. *Mol Cell Biol* 2004;**24**:3757–68.
25. Creemers EE, Sutherland LB, McNally J, Richardson JA, Olson EN. Myocardin is a direct transcriptional target of Mef2, Tead and Foxo proteins during cardiovascular development. *Development* 2006;**133**:4245–56.
26. Bobik A. Transforming growth factor-betas and vascular disorders. *Arterioscler Thromb Vasc Biol* 2006;**26**:1712–20.
27. Boerth NJ, Dey NB, Cornwell TL, Lincoln TM. Cyclic GMP-dependent protein kinase regulates vascular smooth muscle cell phenotype. *J Vasc Res* 1997;**34**:245–59.
28. Beamish JA, He P, Kottke-Marchant K, Marchant RE. Molecular regulation of contractile smooth muscle cell phenotype: implications for vascular tissue engineering. *Tissue Eng Part B Rev* 2010;**16**:467–91.
29. Zargham R, Touyz RM, Thibault G. a8 integrin overexpression in de-differentiated vascular smooth muscle cells attenuates migratory activity and restores the characteristics of the differentiated phenotype. *Atherosclerosis* 2007;**195**:303–12.
30. Chamley-Campbell J, Campbell GR, Ross R. The smooth muscle cell in culture. *Physiol Rev* 1979;**59**:1–61.
31. Thyberg J. Differentiated properties and proliferation of arterial smooth muscle cells in culture. *Int Rev Cytol* 1996;**169**:183–265.
32. Cidad P, Moreno-Dominguez A, Novensa L, Roque M, Barquin L, Heras M, et al. Characterization of ion channels involved in the proliferative response of femoral artery smooth muscle cells. *Arterioscler Thromb Vasc Biol* 2010;**30**:1203–11.
33. Wamhoff BR, Bowles DK, Owens GK. Excitation–transcription coupling in arterial smooth muscle. *Circ Res* 2006;**98**:868–78.
34. Goldberg ID, Stemerman MB, Handin RI. Vascular permeation of platelet factor four following endothelial injury. *Science* 1980;**209**:611–2.
35. Miano JM, Vlasic N, Tota RR, Stemerman MB. Localization of Fos and Jun proteins in rat aortic smooth muscle cells after vascular injury. *Am J Pathol* 1993;**142**:715–24.
36. Wang Z, Wang D-Z, Hockemeyer D, McNally J, Nordheim A, Olson EN. Myocardin and ternary complex factors compete for SRF to control smooth muscle gene expression. *Nature* 2004;**428**:185–9.
37. Hendrix JA, Wamhoff BR, McDonald OG, Sinha S, Yoshida T, Owens GK. 5′ CArG degeneracy in *smooth muscle α-actin* is required for injury-induced gene suppression in vivo. *J Clin Invest* 2005;**115**:418–27.
38. Cheng Y, Liu X, Yang J, Lin Y, Xu DZ, Lu Q, et al. MicroRNA-145, a novel smooth muscle cell phenotypic marker and modulator, controls vascular neointimal lesion formation. *Circ Res* 2009;**105**:158–66.
39. Majesky MW, Giachelli CM, Reidy MA, Schwartz SM. Rat carotid neointimal smooth muscle cells reexpress a developmentally regulated mRNA phenotype during repair of arterial injury. *Circ Res* 1992;**71**:759–68.
40. Weiser-Evans MCM, Schwartz PE, Grieshaber NA, Quinn BE, Grieshaber SC, Belknap JK, et al. Novel embryonic genes are preferentially expressed by autonomously replicating rat embryonic and neointimal smooth muscle cells. *Circ Res* 2000;**87**:608–15.
41. Wissler RW. The arterial medial cell, smooth muscle, or multifunctional mesenchyme? *Circulation* 1967;**36**:1–4.
42. Scott RF, Jones R, Daoud AS, Zumbo O, Coulston F, Thomas WA. Experimental atherosclerosis in rhesus monkeys. II. Cellular elements of proliferative lesions and possible role of cytoplasmic degeneration in pathogenesis as studied by electron microscopy. *Exp. Mol. Pathol.* 1967;**7**:34–57.
43. Rong JX, Shapiro M, Trogan E, Fisher EA. Transdifferentiation of mouse aortic smooth muscle cells to a macrophage-like state after cholesterol loading. *Proc Natl Acad Sci, USA* 2003;**100**:13531–6.
44. Liu Y, Shanahan CM. Signalling pathways and vascular calcification. *Front Biosci* 2011;**16**:1302–14.
45. Speer MY, Yang HY, Brabb T, Leaf E, Look A, Lin WL, et al. Smooth muscle cells give rise to osteochondrogenic precursors and chondrocytes in calcifying arteries. *Circ Res* 2009;**104**:733–41.
46. Wang H, Yan S, Chai H, Riha GM, Li M, Yao Q, et al. Shear stress induces endothelial transdifferentiation from mouse smooth muscle cells. *Biochem Biophys Res Commun* 2006;**346**:860–5.
47. Pidkovka NA, Cherepanova OA, Yoshida T, Alexander MR, Deaton RA, Thomas JA, et al. Oxidized phospholipids induce phenotypic switching of vascular smooth muscle cells in vivo and in vitro. *Circ Res* 2007;**101**:792–801.
48. Ailawadi G, Moehle CW, Pei H, Walton SP, Yang Z, Kron IL, et al. Smooth muscle phenotypic modulation is an early event in aortic aneurysms. *J Thorac Cardiovasc Surg* 2009;**138**:1392–9.
49. Nakajima N, Nagahiro S, Sano T, Satomi J, Satoh K. Phenotypic modulation of smooth muscle cells in human cerebral aneurysmal walls. *Acta Neuropathol* 2000;**100**:475–80.
50. Liao M, Zou S, Weng J, Hou L, Yang L, Zhao Z, et al. A microRNA profile comparison between thoracic aortic dissection and normal thoracic aorta indicates the potential role of microRNAs in contributing to thoracic aortic dissection pathogenesis. *J Vasc Surg* 2011;**53**:1341–9.
51. Xiao Y, Huang Z, Yin H, Lin Y, Wang S. In vitro differences between smooth muscle cells derived from varicose veins and normal veins. *J Vasc Surg* 2009;**50**:1149–54.

52. Pauletto P, Sarzani R, Rappelli A, Chiavegato A, Pessina AC, Sartore S. Differentiation and growth of vascular smooth muscle cells in experimental hypertension. *Am J Hypertens* 1994;**7**:661–74.
53. Han Y-J, Hu W-Y, Chernaya O, Antic N, Gu L, Gupta M, et al. Increased myosin light chain kinase expression in hypertension: regulation by serum response factor via an insertion mutation in the promoter. *Mol Biol Cell* 2006;**17**:4039–50.
54. Kontaraki JE, Marketou ME, Zacharis EA, Parthenakis FI, Vardas PE. Early cardiac gene transcript levels in peripheral blood mononuclear cells in patients with untreated essential hypertension. *J Hypertens* 2011;**29**:791–7.
55. Chow N, Bell RD, Deane R, Streb JW, Chen J, Brooks A, et al. Serum response factor and myocardin mediate arterial hypercontractility and cerebral blood flow dysregulation in Alzheimer's phenotype. *Proc Natl Acad Sci USA* 2007;**104**:823–8.
56. Bell RD, Deane R, Chow N, Long X, Sagare A, Singh I, et al. SRF and myocardin regulate LRP-mediated amyloid-beta clearance in brain vascular cells. *Nat Cell Biol* 2009;**11**:143–53.

Chapter 96

Molecular Pathways of Smooth Muscle Disease

Alejandra San Martín, Lula Hilenski, and Kathy K. Griendling
Department of Medicine, Division of Cardiology, Emory University, Atlanta, GA

INTRODUCTION

The normal contractile function of smooth muscle cells (SMCs) can be compromised in pathological situations, thereby contributing to the development of disease. External environmental stimuli can influence smooth muscle phenotype such that cells lose their contractile properties and become migratory, proliferative, secretory, and sometimes proinflammatory (see Chapter 95) (1). Although these responses are adaptive and required for normal physiology, they also represent the beginning of many pathological conditions. As a result, phenotypically modulated SMCs contribute to lesion formation and vessel occlusion in atherosclerosis (2), increased pulmonary vascular resistance in pulmonary hypertension (3), increased airway smooth muscle mass in asthma (4), and colitis (5). By understanding the molecular processes underlying these functions of smooth muscle, we are better able to design targeted therapeutics to interfere specifically with the pathological aspects of smooth muscle behavior.

MIGRATION

Cell migration is fundamental to any life form. In humans, tissue formation during development, as well as wound healing and immune responses in the adult, all require the movement of cells in particular directions to specific locations. It should be noted that all cells are constantly in motion. However, there is a clear distinction between motility (nondirectional cell movement), chemotaxis and directed cell migration (movement of a cell from one region to another). Migration of SMCs from their original site of residence (e.g. vessel media) to an atypical location (e.g. intima) is an important response to injury (e.g. mechanical injury during angioplasty), but unchecked can lead to pathology (in this case vessel occlusion). Our knowledge of the molecular mechanisms of migration stems largely from wound-healing studies in fibroblasts, although in recent years, more work on SMCs has been undertaken and will be highlighted here.

SMCs migrate in response to a number of stimuli, including peptide growth factors, extracellular matrix components and cytokines (6). Migration is also influenced by physical factors such as shear stress, stretch, and matrix stiffness. Platelet-derived growth factor (PDGF)-BB, basic fibroblast growth factor (bFGF) and sphingosine-1-phosphate (S1P) are some of the most potent promigratory stimuli for SMCs. Intracellular signals initiated by these agonists act in concert with those activated by integrin receptor interaction with extracellular matrix (ECM) to mediate the migratory response. Matrix surrounding the migrating cell must be degraded by matrix metalloproteinases (MMPs) to create a path into which the cell can protrude.

Growth Factor Signaling to Lamellipodia

PDGF is one of the best-understood migratory stimuli for SMCs (4,7); it will be used here therefore as a paradigm to describe the molecular mechanisms underlying the migratory response in general. PDGF is produced by platelets, monocytes/macrophages, endothelial cells and vascular SMCs (VSMCs), and has paracrine promigratory and proproliferative effects on the surrounding cells (8). There are three isoforms of PDGF, PDGF-AA, -AB and -BB, which are all disulphide linked homo- or hetero-dimers (9). PDGF-AB or -BB usually have similar efficacies, but PDGF-AA has generally been reported to possess lower mitogenic activity (10).

The PDGF receptor is composed of two monomeric receptor subunits, PDGFR-α and PDGFR-β (11,12). *In vivo* migration of VSMCs is primarily the consequence of the activation of PDGFR-β by PDGF-BB (9). When PDGF-BB binds to PDGF receptors, receptor autophosphorylation creates binding sites for phospholipase Cγ, which increases intracellular calcium and activates protein kinase C (PKC), in turn stimulating NADPH oxidases

Muscle. DOI: http://dx.doi.org/10.1016/B978-0-12-381510-1.00096-X

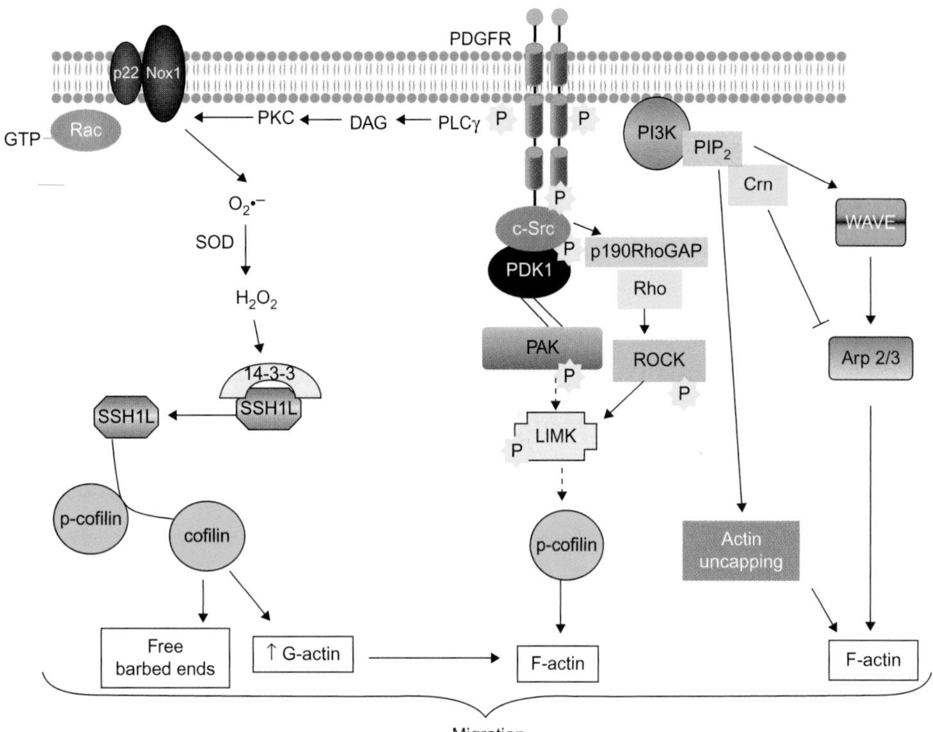

FIGURE 96.1 **Signaling pathways at the leading edge of migrating cells.** Different ROS-dependent and -independent signaling pathways participate in actin dynamics. Both extension of F-actin and a constant supply of G-actin are required to maintain the migration process. See text for details.

to generate reactive oxygen species (ROS); the small molecular weight G-protein Ras, which stimulates the mitogen-activated protein kinase (MAPK) cascade; and phosphatidylinositol 3-kinase (PI3K), which forms the membrane-targeting lipid phosphatidylinositol 4,5-bisphosphate (PIP_2) that by facilitating the uncapping of actin filaments and activating the WAVE/Arp2/3 pathway increases the rate of F-actin formation in the cell (13). Each of these pathways contributes to migration by coordinated regulation of the actin cytoskeleton (Figure 96.1).

Reorganization of the actin cytoskeleton is dynamic and requires specialized signaling domains at the front and rear of the cell (14–16). Migration begins when a cell senses a gradient (e.g. an increased concentration of PDGF) and establishes polarity (17). Plasma membrane is extended in the direction of eventual movement in the form of extended F-actin-rich protrusions or lamellipodia (18). The characteristics of such a protrusion are mainly governed by the identity of the small molecular weight GTPases activated. G-proteins are inactive when bound to GDP, but bind to their effector proteins when in the GTP-bound active state (19). All three major classes of these molecules play a role in migration: Rho regulates F-actin elongation/focal complexes, cdc42 triggers the formation of filopodia (cellular structures containing long, unbranched, parallel bundles of actin filaments), and Rac regulates the polymerization of actin, in part by activation of p21-activated kinase (PAK)-mediated phosphorylation of actin-binding proteins, to produce lamellipodia (20) (Figure 96.1).

Extension of these actin-rich protrusions in moving cells requires cycles of actin polymerization and depolymerization (17). Nucleation of new actin filaments at the leading edge is initiated from existing filaments by dissociation of actin capping proteins, many of which are regulated by PIP_2; binding of nucleation promoting factors verprolin–homologous protein (WAVE) and Wiskott–Aldrich syndrome protein (WASP) to actin-related protein ARP2/3; and phosphorylation of the actin binding coronin (Crn). The extension of the plus end of the actin filament, which binds ATP and displays a higher rate of polymerization, is regulated by formins (mDia1 and mDia2) and profilin. Regulation of mDia occurs largely via conformational changes induced by RhoA and cdc42. Profilin increases nucleotide exchange on G-actin monomers, thus enhancing actin polymerization. Severing of existing actin filaments is a consequence of activation of gelsolin and cofilin, which limit the length of filaments and initiate turnover of existing filaments (21).

Cofilin is of particular importance because, by virtue of its actin-severing capabilities, it produces a continuous supply of actin monomers for polymerization and rapid turnover of actin filaments (22). The activity of cofilin is negatively regulated by the LIM kinase (LIMK) family of serine/threonine kinases through phosphorylation at a conserved serine-3 of cofilin (23–25). Suppression of cofilin activity in different cell types by LIMK overexpression abolishes both lamellipodium formation and polarized cell migration (26,27). The Ser-3-phosphorylated cofilin is dephosphorylated and therefore reactivated by protein phosphatases 1 and 2A (28), chronophin (29) and the slingshot family of protein phosphatases (30). One of the members of this family, Slingshot 1L (SSH1L), has been shown to play a major role in PDGF-induced VSMC migration *in vitro* (31) and *in vivo* (32). As lamellipodia protrude and retract, cofilin must be turned on and off. This is accomplished by a tight regulation of its activators/inhibitors. LIMKs are activated through Rho family small GTPases, Rho, Rac, and Cdc42, and their downstream protein kinases, such as Rho-associated kinase (ROCK) and PAK (33,34). The mechanisms of SSH1L activation require ROS produced by NADPH oxidases (35,36) and include the disruption of an inhibitory complex with 14-3-3 proteins (37).

In fact, ROS may play multiple roles in migration. Sundaresan et al. (38) showed that incubation of VSMC with the hydrogen peroxide catabolist catalase prevents mitogen-activated protein kinase (MAPK) activation and migration. Subsequently, ROS were shown to activate the tyrosine kinase Src, the Akt kinase phosphoinositide-dependent kinase-1 (PDK1) and PAK (39,40). The bulk of the evidence suggests that ROS are derived from PDGF- or bFGF-mediated activation of NADPH oxidases, particularly Nox1, in VSMCs (32,41,42).

Matrix Degradation

In order to move through the ECM, migrating cells must create a path. They do so by secreting MMPs and simultaneously inhibiting tissue inhibitors of metalloproteinases (TIMPs). MMP activity is regulated by transcriptional and post-transcriptional mechanisms. ROS have been shown to be major regulators of MMP activity and expression: they downregulate the activity of MMP-1, -2, -14 and -7 (43,44), but can also activate MMP-9 (45,46).

In smooth muscle, the secretion of MMPs is thought to be coordinated by podosomes. Podosomes are actin-based structures that act as sites of cell adhesion and active ECM remodeling (47). Their formation is usually induced when cells are migrating, although they are not required for cell migration (48). Similar to the invadopodia present in carcinoma cells, podosomes establish tight contact with the substrate and are capable of degrading components of the ECM (49). Like focal adhesions, they can also function as mechanosensors capable of generating traction in response to differential substrate stiffness (50). Among the extracellular triggers for podosome formation are cytokines and growth factors (49). Once podosomes have attached and activated integrins, activation of tyrosine kinase receptors initiates intracellular cascades that induce the activation of PKC, c-Src, and the Rho family of GTPases (49). In VSMCs, the protein p53, a known regulator of the cell cycle, seems to be a key regulator of podosome formation. The relationship between p53 and migration is not clear, but data obtained in other cell types suggest that p53 negatively regulates Rac1 and Cdc42 (51). In this regard, studies performed in A7r5 VSMCs have indicated that Src transformed cells produce podosomes spontaneously (52), and p53 suppresses Src-induced podosome formation (53) by a mechanism that involves caldesmon (a prominent component of VSMC podosomes) and phosphatase and tensin homolog (PTEN) (54).

Focal Adhesion Turnover

In addition to lamellipodial protrusion, migration requires that these protrusions attach to the substratum by creating focal complexes, which later mature into focal adhesions, and that focal adhesions in the rear of the cell detach to allow forward progression (55). Focal adhesions are highly specialized cell structures through which the cell communicates with the ECM. They are intimately related to the microtubular network, but evolve and mature as they increase the number and complexity of adhesion proteins. Signaling at focal adhesions is coordinated by integrins, a family of transmembrane receptors that bind most ECM proteins. Integrins consist of a large extracellular domain, a single transmembrane domain and a short C-terminal domain. The distortion of an integrin bound to a matrix protein as the cell attempts to migrate creates intracellular signals that regulate focal adhesion turnover.

There is abundant evidence that integrin-mediated signaling is critical to vascular remodeling. Smooth muscle-specific deletion of β_1 integrins leads to postnatal lethality due to failure of cytoskeletal alignment in SMCs, gaps between cells, and ultimately aneurysm formation (56). Moreover, α_v, β_3 and β_5 integrin expression is increased 14 days after balloon injury of the rat carotid artery (57), while α_8 and β_1 integrin expression is decreased for up to 4 weeks, changes that appear to be obligatory for PDGF-induced migration (58).

Integrin interaction with the matrix leads to integrin clustering and the activation of a series of protein tyrosine kinases, including integrin-linked kinase (ILK), focal adhesion kinase (FAK) and Src, as well as interaction with the cortical F-actin cytoskeleton (6). Phosphorylation of focal adhesion components including FAK and paxillin occurs during SMC migration, as does turnover of focal adhesion proteins by membrane-type metalloproteinases.

Migration is particularly dependent on dynamic focal adhesion turnover. Focal adhesions have to form and mature under the cell extension, and to dissolve at the rear end. Rho activity (59) and the Poldip2/Nox4 (60) pathway have been demonstrated to be required for the

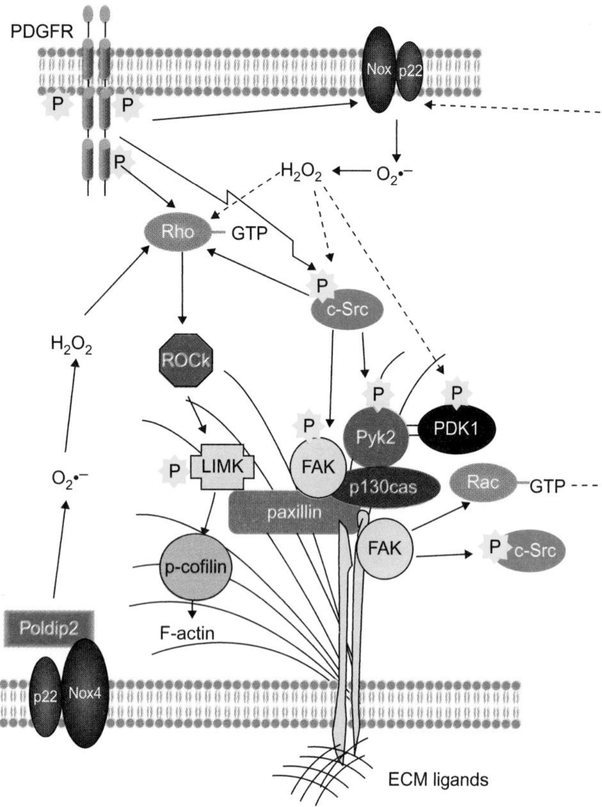

FIGURE 96.2 Regulation of focal adhesion turnover during migration. Focal adhesion maturation and dissolution are required to allow cellular migration. Frequently, tyrosine kinase receptor and integrin-initiated signaling are coordinated in order to properly maintain focal adhesion dynamics. See text for details.

maintenance of focal adhesion maturation and turnover (Figure 96.2).

Cell Body Contraction

The final major phase of cell migration is contraction of the cell body. Matrix interaction induces VSMC contraction through calcium-mediated activation of myosin light chain kinase and myosin light chain phosphorylation in the same way that differentiated cells respond to contractile agents (see Chapters 83 and 87). RhoA and Rho kinase may also be involved, because inhibition of Rho kinase blocks migration as well (61).

PROLIFERATION

In the course of lesion formation, either in atherogenesis or during postangioplasty restenosis, vein bypass graft failure and transplant failure (62), VSMCs not only migrate to the intimal region of the vessel wall, but they also proliferate. Proliferation can be initiated by a variety of growth factors, such as PDGF, insulin-like growth factor-1 (IGF1), bFGF, transforming growth factor-beta (TGF-β), and epidermal growth factor (EGF), that act through receptor tyrosine kinases, or via G-protein-coupled receptors that transactivate receptor tyrosine kinases, some of which, like angiotensin II and endothelin, regulate contraction when the cells are differentiated (63).

Growth of smooth muscle is initiated by activation of sequential, branching signaling cascades of tyrosine kinases, Ser/Thr kinases, and GTPases. Among the most universal early pathways are those involving the MAPKs, roughly divided into Ras/MAPK:ERK kinase (MEK)/Erk, MAP kinase kinase (MKK)3/6/p38MAPK, and MKK4/Jnk pathways, which ultimately lead to activation of transcription factors including Elk-1, ATF-2, and c-jun. In addition, as noted above for PDGF in migration, many growth factors activate NADPH oxidases, which generate ROS that are required for a full proliferative response (Figure 96.3). Downstream of ROS is the Ser/Thr kinase Akt, which is activated by PI3K and ROS and in turn induces cyclin D1 expression (64). Tyrosine phosphatases are also important regulators of growth-related signaling that can vary according to the stimulus. For example, Src homology 2-containing protein tyrosine phosphatase 2 (SHP2) dephosphorylates tyrosine residues on target proteins in response to growth factors (65). In VSMCs, SHP2 positively regulates IGF-1-induced MAPK signaling pathways, but has negative effects on EGF- and Ang II-induced Akt signaling.

Part of the growth response is an increase in protein synthesis. In fully proliferative cells, this is accompanied by DNA duplication (see below for discussion of the cell cycle). However, VSMCs in large arteries in hypertensive animals and SMCs in some types of colitis undergo hypertrophy instead (5,66). Translation initiation, the rate-limiting step for protein synthesis, is regulated by the binding of mRNA to the ribosome and the initiation of mRNA translation. Ribosomal binding is mediated by ribosomal p70S6 kinase, which is downstream of PI3K and phosphorylates the ribosomal S6 protein (RPS6), enabling the binding of mRNA to the ribosome (67). Translation initiation depends upon eukaryotic initiation factor eIF4F, a protein complex containing an ATP-dependent helicase (eIF4A), a larger subunit of unknown function, and eIF4E, which allows the complex to bind to the mRNA cap structure (68). eIF4E activity is upregulated upon treatment with growth factors (69). An important integrator of translation is mTOR (mammalian target of rapamycin), a protein kinase that regulates translation initiation through p70S6 kinase and eIF4E. Inhibition of mTOR by rapamycin, an immunosuppressive macrolide antibiotic, abrogates protein synthesis leading to cell cycle arrest (2). Rapamycin (sirolimus) has been employed effectively as a coating for stents to reduce postangioplasty restenosis rates in interventional cardiology (70).

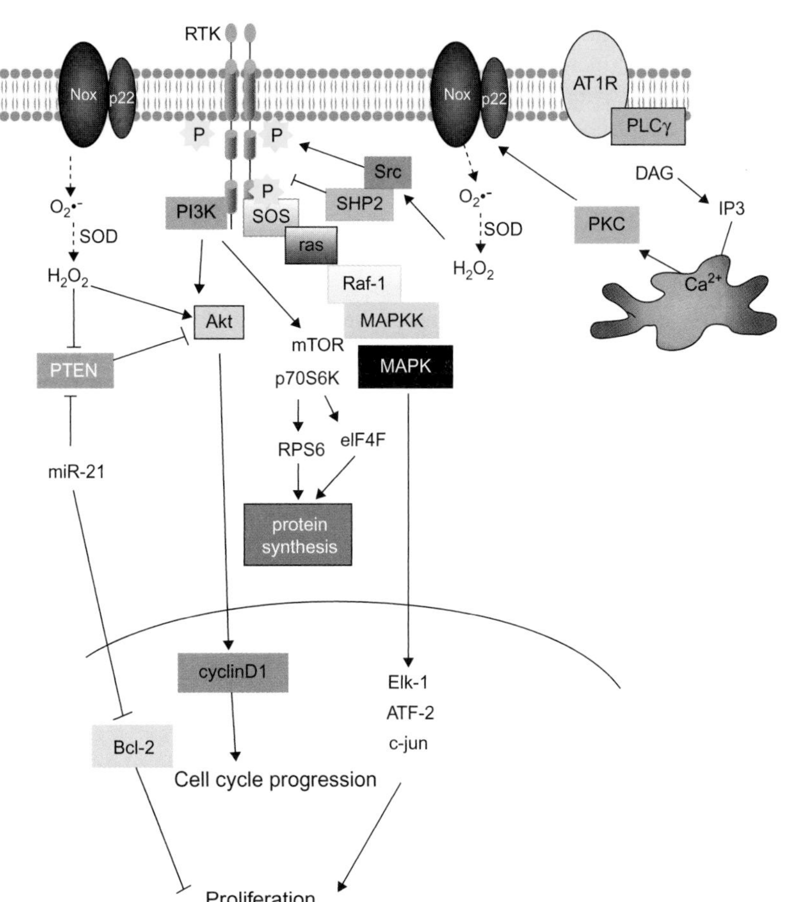

FIGURE 96.3 Molecular mechanisms of smooth muscle proliferation. Agonist-mediated signals transduced by tyrosine kinase and seven-transmembrane receptors participate in the induction of smooth muscle proliferation. Signals that lead to protein synthesis and cell cycle progression are also in place to achieve cell growth. ROS-mediated signaling pathways are of critical importance during smooth muscle proliferation.

In dividing cells, growth factor initiated signaling ultimately converges onto the cell cycle (2). The cell cycle consists of four distinct phases: (i) Gap 1 (G1), in which factors necessary for DNA replication are assembled; (ii) DNA replication or S phase; (iii) Gap 2 (G2), in preparation for mitosis; and (iv) mitosis or M phase. Cell cycle progression is heavily regulated at restriction points, which occur at transitions between G1/S and G2/M. Progression through these restriction points is regulated by cyclin-dependent kinases (CDKs) and their regulatory cyclin subunits. Cyclins D/E and CDK2, -4 and -5 are active in G1, cyclin A and CDK2 control the S phase along with the DNA polymerase cofactor PCNA, and cyclins A/B and CDK1 regulate the M phase. Cell cycle progression is also heavily dependent upon the activity of cyclin-dependent kinase inhibitors (CDKIs). For example, induction of CDKIs $p27^{KIP1}$ and $p21^{CIP1}$ arrests cells in G1. In general, CDK activity is controlled by the levels of expression of cyclins, the phosphorylation status of CDKs, and the nuclear translocation of cyclin-CDK complexes. Thus, transcription factors responsible for regulating the expression of CDKs and CDKIs can strongly affect cell cycle progression. One important regulator of transcription is the retinoblastoma protein Rb, which regulates E2F transcription factors to control the G1/S transition (2).

Calcium, magnesium, and potassium transport via ion channels is also important for VSMC proliferation. Transient increases in Ca^{2+} concentration in response to growth factors are absolutely required for proliferation (71,72). Not only does calcium regulate immediate early activation of protein kinases, but it is also required for the G1 to S transition (73). Elevated Mg^{2+} levels induce cyclin D1 and CDK4 expression and decrease activation of $p21^{CIP1}$ and $p27^{KIP1}$ via an ERK1/2-dependent pathway (74). Changes in VSMC K^+ channel expression and activity also affect cell cycle progression (75). Intermediate-conductance Ca^{2+}-activated K^+ (IK_{Ca})-type channels, the predominant Ca^{2+}-sensitive K^+ channel in proliferating VSMCs, are activated by growth factor-induced release of Ca^{2+} (76). In addition, expression of voltage-gated K^+ channels $K_V1.3$ (77) and $K_V3.4$ (78) is increased in proliferating VSMCs. Inhibition of these Ca^{2+}-activated and voltage-gated K^+ channels reduces proliferation and abrogates injury-induced remodeling in rodents (79).

Telomerase activity is also required for VSMC proliferation. Telomeres cap and stabilize chromosomes (80) and are regulated by telomerase, an enzyme that consists of an RNA component and two proteins, one of which is TERT (telomerase reverse transcriptase). In VSMCs, phosphorylation of TERT is associated with telomerase activation, and telomerase levels and activity correlate with proliferation (80). Telomerase activation and telomere maintenance are associated with excessive VSMC growth in both animal and human vascular injury and disease (80), but disruption of telomerase activity reduces this proliferative response.

Many other signaling pathways also impinge on VSMC proliferation. One example is Notch proteins (81), which repress the CDKIs $p27^{KIP1}$ and $p21^{CIP1}$ and enhance Akt signaling, resulting in VSMC proliferation. Notch1 has been shown to mediate neointimal formation and remodeling after vascular injury (82). Another important pathway involves PPARs (peroxisome proliferator-activated receptors), nuclear hormone receptors that inhibit proliferation and neointimal formation in atherosclerosis and postangioplasty restenosis (83). Thiazolidinediones, PPARγ agonists used in the clinic to treat type 2 diabetes mellitus, decrease VSMC proliferation and prevent atherosclerosis in mouse models (83). Finally, cyclic adenosine 3′,5′-monophosphate (cAMP) and cyclic guanosine 3′,5′-monophosphate (cGMP) act as antagonists to mitogenic signaling pathways and inhibit cell cycle progression (84,85).

Very recent data implicate microRNAs (miRNAs) as important regulators of VSMC growth. In balloon-injured rat carotid arteries, several miRNAs, most notably miR-21, are upregulated (86). miR-21 is a pro-proliferative and anti-apoptotic regulator of VSMCs that downregulates PTEN, and upregulates B-cell lymphoma 2 (Bcl-2). PTEN modulates VSMC growth by regulating the PI3K/Akt pathway (87), while Bcl-2 alters AP-1 activity.

It should be noted that the milieu in which VSMCs exist is critically important to proliferation (64). In the vessel wall, VSMCs are surrounded by and interact with polymerized collagen type 1 fibrils through $\alpha_2\beta_1$ integrins, are arrested in the G1 phase of the cell cycle and are generally refractory to mitogenic stimuli. In contrast, VSMCs on monomeric collagen matrices are responsive to growth factors. Thus, degradation of the collagen matrix to monomeric collagen in vascular lesions may contribute to altered VSMC proliferation and neointimal formation (88).

INFLAMMATION

In addition to the contractile and synthetic phenotypes, smooth muscle can also express markers of an inflammatory phenotype. Inflammatory SMCs, found, for example, in the vascular media, express both markers of differentiation and inflammatory genes such as vascular cell adhesion molecule (VCAM-1), and display activated nuclear factor kappa B (NF-κB) signaling (89). Various stimuli, including self-secreted cytokines, circulating cytokines, changes in matrix composition, and oxidized low-density lipoprotein (oxLDL), induce expression of inflammatory cytokines and VCAM-1. Because inflammation plays a major role in the pathophysiology of asthma and chronic obstructive pulmonary disease (COPD) (90) as well as in the progression of atherosclerosis (91), this phenotype, produced in response to inflammatory stimuli or itself producing inflammatory cytokines, can have a profound effect on disease development.

In smooth muscle and other cell types, the expression of inflammatory genes is largely due to the activation of the stress-activated protein kinase p38MAPK/C/EBPβ pathway (92) and regulation by proinflammatory transcription factors such as NF-κB and **S**ignal **T**ransducer and **A**ctivator of **T**ranscription 1/3 (STAT1/3) (93), both of which are activated by ROS. The NF-κB pathway is key for the transcriptional regulation of many, if not most, proinflammatory genes. The transactivating factors p65 and p50 are located in the cytosol in resting cells bound to IκBα. Upon exposure to proinflammatory stimuli, IκBα is phosphorylated and degraded, and the p50-p65 heterodimer is translocated to the nucleus, where it binds to NF-κB-containing elements to increase proinflammatory gene transcription. Similarly, regulation of gene expression by STATs results from tyrosine kinase receptor activation of Janus kinase (JAK) and subsequent phosphorylation of STAT, followed by translocation to the nucleus and binding to specific DNA sequences.

In atherosclerotic plaques, VSMCs secrete collagen I and collagen III, and, as a result of NF-κB activation, express MMP-1, MMP-3, and MMP-9, which degrade ECM. Many ECM proteins are in turn capable of promoting the expression of inflammatory genes such as VCAM-1 (94), producing a positive feedback effect. The matrix receptor CD44 also stimulates VCAM-1 expression (95) when bound to hyaluronic acid present in the matrix, implicating it in the transition to the proinflammatory phenotype (95).

In the vasculature, many stimuli have been shown to upregulate inflammatory genes in VSMCs. Angiotensin II (via AT1R) induces the secretion of IL-6 by VSMC (96), while advanced glycation end-products induce the expression of iNOS (97). Additionally, oxLDL and other cytokines such as tumor necrosis factor-α (TNF-α) and interleukin-1β (IL-1β) stimulate expression of adhesion molecules such as ICAM-1, VCAM-1, and CCR-2, the receptor for MCP-1, and increase expression of chemokine (C-X-C motif) ligand 1 (CXCL1), monocyte chemotactic protein-1 (MCP-1), and TNF-α. Many of these molecules in turn activate NF-κB, resulting in a positive feedback loop that exacerbates the local inflammatory response (Figure 96.4).

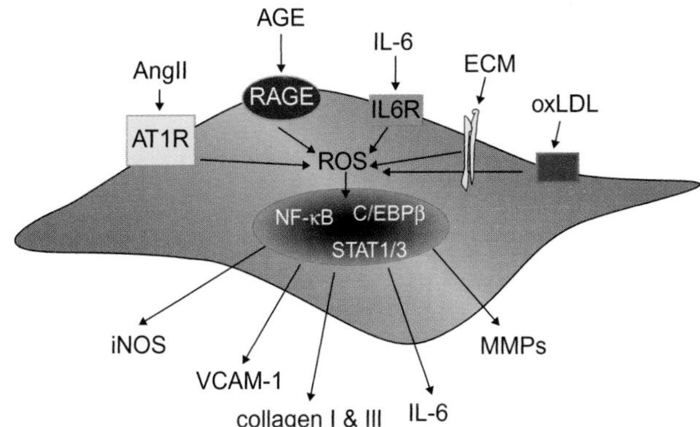

FIGURE 96.4 Establishment of the inflammatory phenotype. Smooth muscle plasticity also can lead this cell type to adopt an inflammatory phenotype. This phenotype is produced in response to inflammatory cytokines or by agonists that stimulate the production of cytokines by smooth muscle.

CONCLUSION

The ability of adult SMCs to phenotypically modulate increases their adaptability, but also their propensity to contribute to disease progression. Proliferation, migration, and inflammation are hallmarks of many disease processes, and understanding the molecular basis of these functions of synthetic SMCs is key to developing therapeutic strategies to permit physiological wound healing, but inhibit excessive pathological responses.

REFERENCES

1. Owens GK, Kumar MS, Wamhoff BR. Molecular regulation of vascular smooth muscle cell differentiation in development and disease. *Physiol Rev* 2004;**84**:767–801.
2. Dzau VJ, Braun-Dullaeus RC, Sedding DG. Vascular proliferation and atherosclerosis: new perspectives and therapeutic strategies. *Nat Med* 2002;**8**:1249–56.
3. Tajsic T, Morrell NW. Smooth muscle cell hypertrophy, proliferation, migration and apoptosis in pulmonary hypertension. *Compr Physiol* 2011;**1**:295–317.
4. Hirota JA, Ask K, Farkas L, Smith JA, Ellis R, Rodriguez-Lecompte JC, et al. In vivo role of platelet derived growth factor-BB in airway smooth muscle proliferation in mouse lung. *Am J Respir Cell Mol Biol* 2011;**45**:566–72.
5. Nair DG, Han TY, Lourenssen S, Blennerhassett MG. Proliferation modulates intestinal smooth muscle phenotype in vitro and in colitis in vivo. *Am J Physiol Gastrointest Liver Physiol* 2011;**300**: G903–13.
6. Gerthoffer WT. Mechanisms of vascular smooth muscle cell migration. *Circ Res* 2007;**100**:607–21.
7. Jawien A, Bowen-Pope DF, Lindner V, Schwartz SM, Clowes AW. Platelet-derived growth factor promotes smooth muscle migration and intimal thickening in a rat model of balloon angioplasty. *J Clin Invest* 1992;**89**:507–11.
8. Hughes AD, Clunn GF, Refson J, Demoliou-Mason C. Platelet-derived growth factor (PDGF): actions and mechanisms in vascular smooth muscle. *Gen Pharmacol* 1996;**27**:1079–89.
9. Raines EW. PDGF and cardiovascular disease. *Cytokine Growth Factor Rev* 2004;**15**:237–54.
10. Sachinidis A, Locher R, Vetter W, Tatje D, Hoppe J. Different effects of platelet-derived growth factor isoforms on rat vascular smooth muscle cells. *J Biol Chem* 1990;**265**:10238–43.
11. Heldin CH, Backstrom G, Ostman A, Hammacher A, Ronnstrand L, Rubin K, et al. Binding of different dimeric forms of PDGF to human fibroblasts: evidence for two separate receptor types. *EMBO J* 1988;**7**:1387–93.
12. Hart CE, Forstrom JW, Kelly JD, Seifert RA, Smith RA, Ross R, et al. Two classes of PDGF receptor recognize different isoforms of PDGF. *Science* 1988;**240**:1529–31.
13. Logan MR, Mandato CA. Regulation of the actin cytoskeleton by PIP2 in cytokinesis. *Biol Cell* 2006;**98**:377–88.
14. Ballestrem C, Hinz B, Imhof BA, Wehrle-Haller B. Marching at the front and dragging behind: differential alphavbeta3-integrin turnover regulates focal adhesion behavior. *J Cell Biol* 2001;**155**:1319–32.
15. Carpenter CL. Actin cytoskeleton and cell signaling. *Crit Care Med* 2000;**28**:N94–9.
16. Raftopoulou M, Hall A. Cell migration: Rho GTPases lead the way. *Dev Biol* 2004;**265**:23–32.
17. Lauffenburger DA, Horwitz AF. Cell migration: a physically integrated molecular process. *Cell* 1996;**84**:359–69.
18. Small JV, Stradal T, Vignal E, Rottner K. The lamellipodium: where motility begins. *Trends Cell Biol* 2002;**12**:112–20.
19. Schiller MR, Chakrabarti K, King GF, Schiller NI, Eipper BA, Maciejewski MW. Regulation of RhoGEF activity by intramolecular and intermolecular SH3 domain interactions. *J Biol Chem* 2006;**281**:18774–86.
20. Nobes CD, Hall A. Rho, rac, and cdc42 GTPases regulate the assembly of multimolecular focal complexes associated with actin stress fibers, lamellipodia, and filopodia. *Cell* 1995;**81**:53–62.
21. Condeelis J. How is actin polymerization nucleated in vivo? *Trends Cell Biol* 2001;**11**:288–93.
22. Chen H, Bernstein BW, Bamburg JR. Regulating actin-filament dynamics in vivo. *Trends Biochem Sci* 2000;**25**:19–23.
23. Arber S, Barbayannis FA, Hanser H, Schneider C, Stanyon CA, Bernard O, et al. Regulation of actin dynamics through phosphorylation of cofilin by LIM-kinase. *Nature* 1998;**393**:805–9.
24. Toshima J, Toshima JY, Amano T, Yang N, Narumiya S, Mizuno K. Cofilin phosphorylation by protein kinase testicular protein kinase 1 and its role in integrin-mediated actin reorganization and focal adhesion formation. *Mol Biol Cell* 2001;**12**:1131–45.
25. Yang N, Higuchi O, Ohashi K, Nagata K, Wada A, Kangawa K, et al. Cofilin phosphorylation by LIM-kinase 1 and its role in Rac-mediated actin reorganization. *Nature* 1998;**393**:809–12.
26. Dawe HR, Minamide LS, Bamburg JR, Cramer LP. ADF/cofilin controls cell polarity during fibroblast migration. *Curr Biol* 2003;**13**:252–7.
27. Zebda N, Bernard O, Bailly M, Welti S, Lawrence DS, Condeelis JS. Phosphorylation of ADF/cofilin abolishes EGF-induced actin nucleation at the leading edge and subsequent lamellipod extension. *J Cell Biol* 2000;**151**:1119–28.
28. Ambach A, Saunus J, Konstandin M, Wesselborg S, Meuer SC, Samstag Y. The serine phosphatases PP1 and PP2A associate with

and activate the actin-binding protein cofilin in human T lymphocytes. *Eur J Immunol* 2000;**30**:3422–31.
29. Gohla A, Birkenfeld J, Bokoch GM. Chronophin, a novel HAD-type serine protein phosphatase, regulates cofilin-dependent actin dynamics. *Nat Cell Biol* 2005;**7**:21–9.
30. Niwa R, Nagata-Ohashi K, Takeichi M, Mizuno K, Uemura T. Control of actin reorganization by Slingshot, a family of phosphatases that dephosphorylate ADF/cofilin. *Cell* 2002;**108**:233–46.
31. San Martin A, Lee MY, Williams HC, Mizuno K, Lassegue B, Griendling KK. Dual regulation of cofilin activity by LIM kinase and Slingshot-1L phosphatase controls platelet-derived growth factor-induced migration of human aortic smooth muscle cells. *Circ Res* 2008;**102**:432–8.
32. Lee MY, San Martin A, Mehta PK, Dikalova AE, Garrido AM, Lyons E, et al. Mechanisms of vascular smooth muscle NADPH oxidase 1 (Nox1) contribution to injury-induced neointimal formation. *Arterioscler Thromb Vasc Biol* 2009;**29**:480–7.
33. Ohashi K, Nagata K, Maekawa M, Ishizaki T, Narumiya S, Mizuno K. Rho-associated kinase ROCK activates LIM-kinase 1 by phosphorylation at threonine 508 within the activation loop. *J Biol Chem* 2000;**275**:3577–82.
34. Dan C, Kelly A, Bernard O, Minden A. Cytoskeletal changes regulated by the PAK4 serine/threonine kinase are mediated by LIM kinase 1 and cofilin. *J Biol Chem* 2001;**276**:32115–21.
35. Kim JS, Huang TY, Bokoch GM. Reactive oxygen species regulate a slingshot-cofilin activation pathway. *Mol Biol Cell* 2009;**20**:2650–60.
36. San Martin A, Lee MY, Griendling KK. Novel Nox1-mediated mechanism of SSH1L activation in VSMC: Role in cell migration. *Atheroscler Thromb Vasc Biol* 2008;**28**:e109.
37. Sarmiere PD, Bamburg JR. Regulation of the neuronal actin cytoskeleton by ADF/cofilin. *J Neurobiol* 2004;**58**:103–17.
38. Sundaresan M, Yu ZX, Ferrans VJ, Irani K, Finkel T. Requirement for generation of H_2O_2 for platelet-derived growth factor signal transduction. *Science* 1995;**270**:296–9.
39. Taniyama Y, Weber DS, Rocic P, Hilenski L, Akers ML, Park J, et al. Pyk2- and Src-dependent tyrosine phosphorylation of PDK1 regulates focal adhesions. *Mol Cell Biol* 2003;**23**:8019–29.
40. Weber DS, Taniyama Y, Rocic P, Seshiah PN, Dechert MA, Gerthoffer WT, et al. Phosphoinositide-dependent kinase 1 and p21-activated protein kinase mediate reactive oxygen species-dependent regulation of platelet-derived growth factor-induced smooth muscle cell migration. *Circ Res* 2004;**94**:1219–26.
41. Rodriguez AI, Gangopadhyay A, Kelley EE, Pagano PJ, Zuckerbraun BS, Bauer PM. HO-1 and CO decrease platelet-derived growth factor-induced vascular smooth muscle cell migration via inhibition of Nox1. *Arterioscler Thromb Vasc Biol* 2010;**30**:98–104.
42. Schroder K, Helmcke I, Palfi K, Krause KH, Busse R, Brandes RP. Nox1 mediates basic fibroblast growth factor-induced migration of vascular smooth muscle cells. *Arterioscler Thromb Vasc Biol* 2007;**27**:1736–43.
43. Fu X, Kassim SY, Parks WC, Heinecke JW. Hypochlorous acid oxygenates the cysteine switch domain of pro-matrilysin (MMP-7). A mechanism for matrix metalloproteinase activation and atherosclerotic plaque rupture by myeloperoxidase. *J Biol Chem* 2001;**276**:41279–87.
44. Elliot S, Catanuto P, Stetler-Stevenson W, Cousins SW. Retinal pigment epithelium protection from oxidant-mediated loss of MMP-2 activation requires both MMP-14 and TIMP-2. *Invest Ophthalmol Vis Sci* 2006;**47**:1696–702.
45. Rajagopalan S, Meng XP, Ramasamy S, Harrison DG, Galis ZS. Reactive oxygen species produced by macrophage-derived foam cells regulate the activity of vascular matrix metalloproteinases in vitro. Implications for atherosclerotic plaque stability. *J Clin Invest* 1996;**98**:2572–9.
46. Moon SK, Kang SK, Kim CH. Reactive oxygen species mediates disialoganglioside GD3-induced inhibition of ERK1/2 and matrix metalloproteinase-9 expression in vascular smooth muscle cells. *FASEB J* 2006;**20**:1387–95.
47. Gimona M, Buccione R, Courtneidge SA, Linder S. Assembly and biological role of podosomes and invadopodia. *Curr Opin Cell Biol* 2008;**20**:235–41.
48. Quintavalle M, Elia L, Condorelli G, Courtneidge SA. MicroRNA control of podosome formation in vascular smooth muscle cells in vivo and in vitro. *J Cell Biol* 2010;**189**:13–22.
49. Linder S. The matrix corroded: podosomes and invadopodia in extracellular matrix degradation. *Trends Cell Biol* 2007;**17**:107–17.
50. Collin O, Na S, Chowdhury F, Hong M, Shin ME, Wang F, et al. Self-organized podosomes are dynamic mechanosensors. *Curr Biol* 2008;**18**:1288–94.
51. Guo F, Zheng Y. Involvement of Rho family GTPases in p19Arf- and p53-mediated proliferation of primary mouse embryonic fibroblasts. *Mol Cell Biol* 2004;**24**:1426–38.
52. Mak AS. p53 regulation of podosome formation and cellular invasion in vascular smooth muscle cells. *Cell Adh Migr* **5**:144–9.
53. Mukhopadhyay UK, Eves R, Jia L, Mooney P, Mak AS. p53 suppresses Src-induced podosome and rosette formation and cellular invasiveness through the upregulation of caldesmon. *Mol Cell Biol* 2009;**29**:3088–98.
54. Mukhopadhyay UK, Mooney P, Jia L, Eves R, Raptis L, Mak AS. Doubles game: Src-Stat3 versus p53-PTEN in cellular migration and invasion. *Mol Cell Biol* **30**:4980–95.
55. Anthony TE, Mason HA, Gridley T, Fishell G, Heintz N. Brain lipid-binding protein is a direct target of Notch signaling in radial glial cells. *Genes Dev* 2005;**19**:1028–33.
56. Abraham S, Kogata N, Fassler R, Adams RH. Integrin beta1 subunit controls mural cell adhesion, spreading, and blood vessel wall stability. *Circ Res* 2008;**102**:562–70.
57. Kappert K, Blaschke F, Meehan WP, Kawano H, Grill M, Fleck E, et al. Integrins alphavbeta3 and alphavbeta5 mediate VSMC migration and are elevated during neointima formation in the rat aorta. *Basic Res Cardiol* 2001;**96**:42–9.
58. Zargham R, Thibault G. alpha8beta1 Integrin expression in the rat carotid artery: involvement in smooth muscle cell migration and neointima formation. *Cardiovasc Res* 2005;**65**:813–22.
59. Nobes CD, Hall A. Rho GTPases control polarity, protrusion, and adhesion during cell movement. *J Cell Biol* 1999;**144**:1235–44.
60. Lyle AN, Deshpande NN, Taniyama Y, Seidel-Rogol B, Pounkova L, Du P, et al. Poldip2, a novel regulator of Nox4 and cytoskeletal integrity in vascular smooth muscle cells. *Circ Res* 2009;**105**:249–59.
61. Seasholtz TM, Majumdar M, Kaplan DD, Brown JH. Rho and Rho kinase mediate thrombin-stimulated vascular smooth muscle cell DNA synthesis and migration. *Circ Res* 1999;**84**:1186–93.

62. Fuster JJ, Fernandez P, Gonzalez-Navarro H, Silvestre C, Nabah YN, Andres V. Control of cell proliferation in atherosclerosis: insights from animal models and human studies. *Cardiovasc Res* 2010;**86**:254–64.
63. Berk BC. Vascular smooth muscle growth: autocrine growth mechanisms. *Physiol Rev* 2001;**81**:999–1030.
64. Schwartz MA, Assoian RK. Integrins and cell proliferation: regulation of cyclin-dependent kinases via cytoplasmic signaling pathways. *J Cell Sci* 2001;**114**:2553–60.
65. Kandadi MR, Stratton MS, Ren J. The role of Src homology 2 containing protein tyrosine phosphatase 2 in vascular smooth muscle cell migration and proliferation. *Acta Pharmacol Sin* 2010;**31**:1277–83.
66. Owens GK, Rabinovitch PS, Schwartz SM. Smooth muscle cell hypertrophy versus hyperplasia in hypertension. *Proc Natl Acad Sci USA* 1981;**78**:7759–63.
67. Giasson E, Meloche S. Role of p70 S6 kinase in angiotensin II-induced protein synthesis in vascular smooth muscle cells. *J Biol Chem* 1995;**270**:5225–31.
68. Graves L, Bornfeldt K, Argast G, Krebs E, Kong X, Lin T, et al. cAMP and rapamycin sensitive regulation of the association of eIF-4E and PHAS-1 in aortic smooth muscle. *Procl Natl Acad Sci* 1995;**92**:7222–6.
69. Donaldson R, Hagedorn C, Cohen S. Epidermal growth factor or okadaic acid stimulates the phosphorylation of eucaryotic initiation factor 4F. *J Biol Chem* 1991;**266**:3162–6.
70. Abizaid A. Sirolimus-eluting coronary stents: a review. *Vasc Health Risk Manag* 2007;**3**:191–201.
71. Kahl CR, Means AR. Regulation of cell cycle progression by calcium/calmodulin-dependent pathways. *Endocr Rev* 2003;**24**: 719–36.
72. Mahn K, Ojo OO, Chadwick G, Aaronson PI, Ward JP, Lee TH. Ca(2+) homeostasis and structural and functional remodelling of airway smooth muscle in asthma. *Thorax* **65**:547–52.
73. Koledova VV, Khalil RA. Ca^{2+}, calmodulin, and cyclins in vascular smooth muscle cell cycle. *Circ Res* 2006;**98**:1240–3.
74. Touyz RM, Yao G. Modulation of vascular smooth muscle cell growth by magnesium – role of mitogen-activated protein kinases. *J Cell Physiol* 2003;**197**:326–35.
75. Burg ED, Remillard CV, Yuan JXJ. Potassium channels in the regulation of pulmonary artery smooth muscle cell proliferation and apoptosis: pharmacotherapeutic implications. *Br J Pharmacol* 2008;**153**:S99–111.
76. Neylon CB. Potassium channels and vascular proliferation. *Vasc Pharmacol* 2002;**38**:35–41.
77. Cidad P, Moreno-Dominguez A, Novensa L, Roque M, Barquin L, Heras M, et al. Characterization of ion channels involved in the proliferative response of femoral artery smooth muscle cells. *Arterioscler Thromb Vasc Biol* 2010;**30**:1203–11.
78. Miguel-Velado E, Perez-Carretero FD, Colinas O, Cidad P, Heras M, Lopez-Lopez JR, et al. Cell cycle-dependent expression of Kv3.4 channels modulates proliferation of human uterine artery smooth muscle cells. *Cardiovasc Res* 2010;**86**:383–91.
79. Jackson WF. KV1.3: a new therapeutic target to control vascular smooth muscle cell proliferation. *Arterioscler Thromb Vasc Biol* 2010;**30**:1073–4.
80. Fuster JJ, Andres V. Telomere biology and cardiovascular disease. *Circ Res* 2006;**99**:1167–80.
81. Gridley T. Notch signaling in the vasculature. *Curr Top Dev Biol* 2010;**92**:277–309.
82. Li Y, Takeshita K, Liu P-Y, Satoh M, Oyama N, Mukai Y, et al. Smooth muscle Notch1 mediates neointimal formation after vascular injury. *Circulation* 2009;**119**:2686–92.
83. Gizard F, Bruemmer D. Transcriptional control of vascular smooth muscle cell proliferation by peroxisome proliferator-activated receptor-gamma: therapeutic implications for cardiovascular diseases. *PPAR Res* 2008;**2008**:429123.
84. Fukumoto S, Koyama H, Hosoi M, Yamakawa K, Tanaka S, Morii H, et al. Distinct role of cAMP and cGMP in the cell cycle control of vascular smooth muscle cells: cGMP delays cell cycle transition through suppression of cyclin D1 and cyclin-dependent kinase 4 activation. *Circ Res* 1999;**85**:985–91.
85. Stewart AG, Harris T, Fernandes DJ, Schachte LC, Koutsoubos V, Guida E, et al. Beta2-adrenergic receptor agonists and cAMP arrest human cultured airway smooth muscle cells in the G(1) phase of the cell cycle: role of proteasome degradation of cyclin D1. *Mol Pharmacol* 1999;**56**:1079–86.
86. Cheng Y, Zhang C. MicroRNA-21 in cardiovascular disease. *J Cardiovas Trans Res* 2010;**3**:251–5.
87. Mitra AK, Jia G, Gangahar DM, Agrawal DK. Temporal PTEN inactivation causes proliferation of saphenous vein smooth muscle cells of human CABG conduits. *J Cell Mol Med* 2009;**13**:177–87.
88. Koyama H, Raines EW, Bornfeldt KE, Roberts JM, Ross R. Fibrillar collagen inhibits arterial smooth muscle proliferation through regulation of Cdk2 inhibitors. *Cell* 1996;**87**:1069–78.
89. Landry DB, Couper LL, Bryant SR, Lindner V. Activation of the NF-kappa B and I kappa B system in smooth muscle cells after rat arterial injury. Induction of vascular cell adhesion molecule-1 and monocyte chemoattractant protein-1. *Am J Pathol* 1997;**151**:1085–95.
90. Westergren-Thorsson G, Larsen K, Nihlberg K, Andersson-Sjoland A, Hallgren O, Marko-Varga G, et al. Pathological airway remodelling in inflammation. *Clin Respir J* 2010;**4**(Suppl. 1):1–8.
91. Orr AW, Hastings NE, Blackman BR, Wamhoff BR. Complex regulation and function of the inflammatory smooth muscle cell phenotype in atherosclerosis. *J Vasc Res* 2010;**47**:168–80.
92. Roth M, Tamm M. Airway smooth muscle cells respond directly to inhaled environmental factors. *Swiss Med Wkly* 2010;**140**:w13066.
93. Sprague AH, Khalil RA. Inflammatory cytokines in vascular dysfunction and vascular disease. *Biochem Pharmacol* 2009;**78**:539–52.
94. Orr AW, Lee MY, Lemmon JA, Yurdagul Jr A, Gomez MF, Schoppee Bortz PD, et al. Molecular mechanisms of collagen isotype-specific modulation of smooth muscle cell phenotype. *Arterioscler Thromb Vasc Biol* 2009;**29**:225–31.
95. Cuff CA, Kothapalli D, Azonobi I, Chun S, Zhang Y, Belkin R, et al. The adhesion receptor CD44 promotes atherosclerosis by mediating inflammatory cell recruitment and vascular cell activation. *J Clin Invest* 2001;**108**:1031–40.
96. Kranzhofer R, Schmidt J, Pfeiffer CA, Hagl S, Libby P, Kubler W. Angiotensin induces inflammatory activation of human vascular smooth muscle cells. *Arterioscler Thromb Vasc Biol* 1999;**19**:1623–9.
97. San Martin A, Foncea R, Laurindo FR, Ebensperger R, Griendling KK, Leighton F. Nox1-based NADPH oxidase-derived superoxide is required for VSMC activation by advanced glycation end-products. *Free Radic Biol Med* 2007;**42**:1671–9.

Section D

Smooth Muscle Disease

Chapter 97

Genetic Variants in Smooth Muscle Contraction and Adhesion Genes Cause Thoracic Aortic Aneurysms and Dissections and Other Vascular Diseases

Dianna M. Milewicz and Callie S. Kwartler

Department of Internal Medicine, University of Texas Health Science Center at Houston, Houston, TX

INTRODUCTION

Smooth muscle cells (SMC) lack the characteristic cross-striations of cardiac and skeletal muscle, but contain contractile proteins organized in contractile units (1). Although smooth muscle cells line all hollow organs in the body, including the arteries, gastrointestinal tract, bladder, and uterus, genetic mutations that disrupt SMC-specific isoforms of contractile proteins, along with the mutations in the kinase that controls SMC contraction, lead primarily to vascular diseases. The major vascular disease resulting from these mutations is aortic aneurysm involving the ascending thoracic aorta immediately above the heart. These aneurysms predispose to a life-threatening complication, acute aortic dissections.

THORACIC AORTIC ANEURYSMS AND DISSECTIONS

The major disease affecting the ascending thoracic aorta is aortic aneurysm, defined as a localized, permanent dilatation of an artery, and acute aortic dissection (Figure 97.1) (2). The natural history of thoracic aortic aneurysms located just above the heart is to asymptomatically enlarge over time until an acute tear in the intimal layer leads to an ascending aortic dissection (type A dissections based on the Stanford classification) or, rarely, an aortic rupture. Collectively, thoracic aortic aneurysms and their complications are designated as TAAD. With dissection, blood penetrates into the medial layer, separating the aortic layers and causing tearing through the adventitia (rupture) or other complications. Type A aortic dissections cause sudden death in up to 50% of individuals; survivors of the acute event have a 1% per hour death rate until they undergo emergent surgical repair. TAAD are a common cause of premature deaths, ranking as high as the 15th leading cause of death in the United States (3). Less-deadly aortic dissections can also originate in the descending thoracic aorta just distal to the branching of the subclavian artery (Stanford type B dissections) and are a further part of the TAAD disease spectrum. Although medical treatments can slow the enlargement of an aneurysm, the mainstay of treatment to prevent dissections and premature deaths is surgical repair of the thoracic aortic aneurysm before an aortic dissection occurs. This is typically recommended when the aneurysm reaches 5.0–5.5 cm in diameter; however, studies on patients presenting with acute type A dissections indicate that up to 60% present with aneurysms smaller than 5.5 cm (4). Studies to identify genetic causes of TAAD have determined that the specific gene can both identify individuals at risk for the disease and predict at what aortic diameter a dissection may occur, thereby optimizing the timing of aortic surgery.

Risk factors for TAAD include poorly controlled hypertension and congenital cardiovascular abnormalities, such as a bicuspid aortic valve (BAV) and aortic coarctation. In addition, genetic predisposition plays a prominent role in the etiology of TAAD. Thoracic aortic disease is inherited in families in an autosomal dominant manner in the presence or absence of syndromic features. Marfan syndrome (MFS), caused by mutations in *FBN1,* is an example of a genetic syndrome in which essentially all affected individuals have TAAD, in addition to skeletal and ocular complications (see Chapter 71) (5). Studies using mice engineered with a heterozygous *Fbn1* missense mutation known to cause MFS have suggested that defects in *Fbn1* lead to excessive active transforming

Muscle. DOI: http://dx.doi.org/10.1016/B978-0-12-381510-1.00097-1

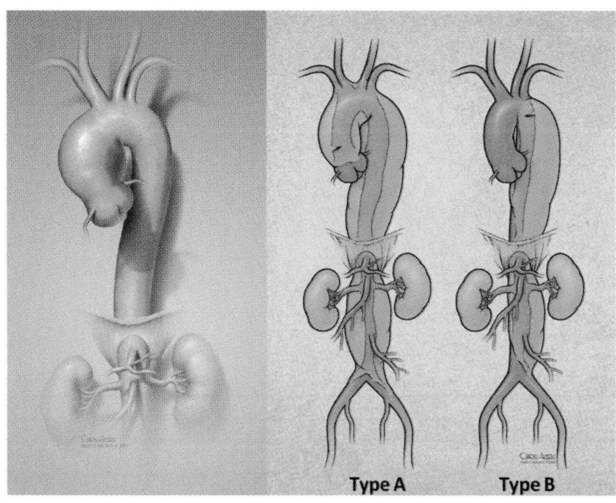

FIGURE 97.1 **Classification of thoracic aortic aneurysms and dissections.** A thoracic ascending aortic aneurysm is a permanent, localized dilation of the ascending aorta immediately above the heart. An aortic dissection is a tear in the intimal layer of the aorta allowing blood to penetrate the medial layer and dissect along this layer. Dissections in the aorta are classified by their location: Stanford Type A dissections are dissections in which the intimal tear is in the ascending aorta, while Stanford Type B dissections are dissections in which the intimal tear is in the descending thoracic aorta just distal to the left subclavian artery.

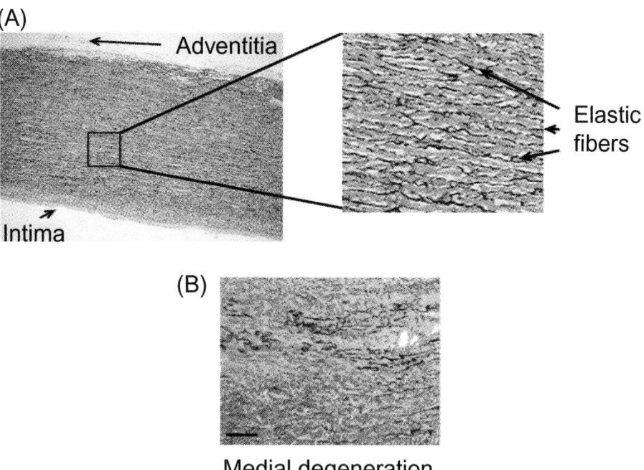

FIGURE 97.2 **Thoracic ascending aortic wall structure and pathology associated with thoracic aortic aneurysms and dissections.** (A) The medial layer of the healthy aorta stained with Movat's pentachrome stain. The wall is comprised of layers of elastic lamellae separated by layers of smooth muscle cells. In the vessel wall, the lamellae are arranged concentrically, and in large elastic arteries like the aorta, a single layer of smooth muscle cells separates each layer of elastin. (B) Aortic tissue from the surgical repair of an aortic aneurysm stained with Movat's pentachrome stain. Medial degeneration is characteristic of the diseased aorta, and includes fragmentation of the elastic fibers, focal areas of smooth muscle cell loss, focal areas of smooth muscle cell hyperplasia, and accumulation of proteoglycans within the medial layer.

growth factor-β (TGF-β) being released from stores in the microfibrils (6,7). The identification of mutations in the TGF-β receptors type I and II (*TGFBR1* and *TGFBR2*) as a cause of another syndrome predisposing to TAAD, Loeys–Dietz syndrome (LDS), further implicate a role for altered TGF-β signaling in the pathogenesis of syndromic TAAD (8–10).

Family aggregation studies indicate that up to one-fifth of TAAD patients who lack features of a genetic syndrome have family histories of TAAD (11,12). TAAD in these families is typically inherited in an autosomal dominant manner, with decreased penetrance, particularly in women (familial disease is designated FTAAD) (13). FTAAD families demonstrate variable expression of TAAD, including varying age of disease onset, severity of presentation, and whether the aneurysm involves the aortic root or ascending aorta. Additionally, phenotypic variability between families is evident by the characterization of a subset of FTAAD families whose members experience aortic dissections with little to no enlargement of the ascending aorta, whereas other families present with large, stable aneurysms that are not prone to dissection. Clinical heterogeneity appears in other features inherited by subsets of families, which can include intracranial aneurysms (ICAs), bilateral iliac artery aneurysms, occlusive vascular diseases such as early onset strokes and coronary artery disease (defined as age of onset less than 55 years of age in men and 60 years in women), abdominal aortic aneurysms (AAAs), bicuspid aortic valve (BAV), and patent ductus arteriosus (PDA). Along with informing management of aortic disease, the specific gene causing FTAAD in a given family can determine the risk for vascular disease beyond TAAD and associated congenital heart defects, such as BAV and PDA.

The aorta is comprised of three layers: a thin inner layer, the tunica intima; a thick middle layer, the tunica media; and a thin outer layer, the tunica adventitia. The tensile strength and elasticity of a normal aorta reside in the medial layer, which contains concentrically arranged elastic fibers and SMCs (Figure 97.2A). The SMCs are longitudinally oriented and dispersed among the circular elastic fibers. Contractile filaments composed of thick and thin filaments within the SMCs are linked up to elastin fibers through connections between focal adhesions on the cell surface and bundles of elastin-associated microfibrils in the matrix. Together, these form a continuous structure called the "elastin-contractile unit", which provides the basis for uniform force generation (14). Humans have between 40–50 layers of elastin lamellae and SMCs in the ascending aorta. Aortic SMCs contract in response to pulsatile blood flow but, unlike the small muscular arteries, this contraction does not regulate blood flow and pulse pressure in the large diameter aorta. In fact, data indicate that the elasticity of the ascending aorta is due to the elastic fibers with little to no contribution from SMC contraction (15,16).

The aortic pathology associated with TAAD is medial degeneration, previously termed "cystic medial degeneration". Medial degeneration is characterized by loss and fragmentation of elastic fibers, accumulation of proteoglycans in the aortic media, and focal regions of the aortic media depleted of SMCs (Figure 97.2B). Although there are areas of SMC loss, there are also often adjacent areas of SMC hyperplasia. Debate persists as to whether SMC loss or hyperplasia is more important to the pathology, but more recent studies provide data to suggest that there is overall SMC hyperplasia in the aortic media with aneurysm progression (17). Inflammatory cells often accompany medial degeneration, but the role of inflammation in disease progression remains to be defined (18,19).

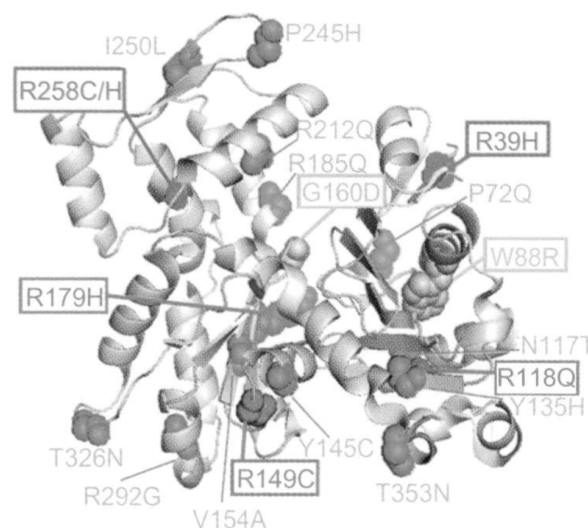

FIGURE 97.3 Distribution of identified *ACTA2* mutations. The structure of the smooth muscle α-actin protein is represented; residues identified to harbor mutations are highlighted. Mutations represented in green (R258 and R39) are associated with a clinical presentation of thoracic aortic disease and early onset stroke (including Moyamoya disease). Mutations represented in red (R149, R118) are associated with a clinical presentation of thoracic aortic disease and early onset coronary artery disease. Mutations in yellow (W88 and G160) are only associated with thoracic aortic disease. The mutation in pink (R179) is associated with global smooth muscle cell dysfunction. For mutations shown in blue, insufficient data are available to characterize the clinical phenotype.

MUTATIONS IN GENES FOR SMC CONTRACTION PROTEINS CAUSE FAMILIAL THORACIC AORTIC DISEASE

The clinical heterogeneity of FTAAD described above is due to underlying genetic heterogeneity, i.e., many genes can be altered to cause aortic disease to be inherited in families and the specific causative genetic alteration in a family leads to a particular disease presentation and associated features. Six FTAAD genes have been identified and are responsible for disease in 20% of families. Three of the genes are the genes responsible for MFS and LDS: *FBN1*, *TGFBR1*, and *TGFBR2*. In FTAAD families with mutations in these genes, the affected family members have no or minimal syndromic features of MFS or LDS and the onset of the thoracic aortic disease is later in life (9,20). The three additional genes that cause FTAAD, *MYH11*, *ACTA2*, and *MYLK*, all encode proteins critical for SMC contractile function and provide the focus of this chapter.

Mutations in *ACTA2*, which encodes the SMC-specific α-actin (SM α-actin), a component of the contractile complex and the most abundant protein in vascular SMCs, are the most common cause of FTAAD identified to date (21,22). Thirty-three *ACTA2* missense mutations, one in-frame deletion, and a splice site mutation deleting the second to last exon (exon 8) of the gene have been identified in TAAD patients (21,23–25). The penetrance of TAAD in family members heterozygous for *ACTA2* mutations is low, with only approximately 50% of the mutation carriers experiencing aortic disease. In a subset of families, *ACTA2* mutations segregate with a skin rash caused by dermal capillary and small artery occlusion referred to as livedo reticularis. Other features present in some families with *ACTA2* mutations include iris flocculi, PDA, and BAV.

ACTA2 mutations are heterozygous missense mutations predicted to produce a mutant α-actin monomer. These heterozygous mutations are located in all four subdomains of actin and are predicted to produce structurally-altered actin monomers (Figure 97.3). Over 100 *ACTA1* mutations, primarily missense mutation, have been identified to cause congenital myopathies (see Chapter 74). Similarly, *ACTAC* missense mutations cause either hypertrophic or dilated cardiomyopathies (see Chapter 33). As described in Chapter 33, characterization of *ACTA1* mutations has provided genetic evidence for a dominant negative pathogenesis of these mutations. Preliminary assessment of the effect of *ACTA2* missense mutations performed by visualizing all cellular polymerized actin in filaments with phalloidin, and SM α-actin-specific filaments using a specific monoclonal antibody (21). SMCs explanted from the aortas of unaffected individuals demonstrated abundant SM α-actin in stress fibers that extended across the cell. In contrast, SMCs explanted from individuals heterozygous for *ACTA2* missense mutations had no SM α-actin-containing filaments extending across the cell. These observations suggest that missense mutations perturb SM α-actin incorporation into filaments or stability of assembled filaments in aortic SMCs, implicating a dominant negative pathogenesis of *ACTA2* mutations, similar to the findings with *ACTA1* mutations.

ACTA2 missense mutations known to cause FTAAD have been engineered into yeast actin and the effect on actin function assessed (26). *ACTA2* missense mutations N117T and R118Q were both introduced into yeast and led to reduced growth and abnormal mitochondrial

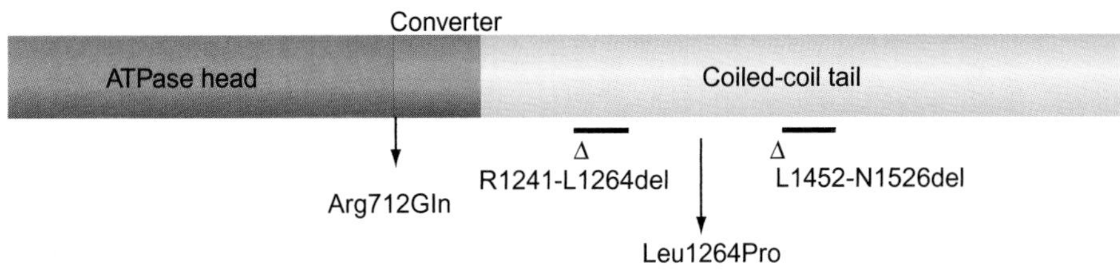

FIGURE 97.4 Location of *MYH11* mutations on a graphic representation of the β-myosin heavy chain.

morphology. Additionally, both mutant actins exhibited altered thermostability and nucleotide exchange rates as well as abnormalities during polymerization, but exact results differed between the N117T and R118Q mutations.

A large French family with TAAD associated with patent ductus arteriosus was used to map and identify mutations in *MYH11* as a cause of FTAAD (27). *MYH11* encodes the SMC-specific myosin heavy chain, a major component of the contractile unit in SMCs. Further studies determined that *MYH11* mutations were responsible for 1% of FTAAD, and were specifically seen in families with TAAD associated with PDA (28). The spectrum of *MYH11* mutations identified for the familial TAAD/PDA phenotype is limited to four mutations: a small deletion, a splice site mutation, and two missense mutations (Figure 97.4). The deletion and the splice site mutation cause removal of 24 and 71 amino acids respectively from the coiled-coil tail domain of the myosin heavy chain (27). Both of these mutations are likely to result in protein products that are either unstable or unable to assemble into polymerized filaments. A coiled-coil modeling tool predicts that both deletions would decrease the probability of coiled-coil formation, and wild-type and mutant rod domain constructs could not co-immunoprecipitate, suggesting altered interactions between the myosin monomers (27). These mutations likely result in a dominant negative effect on filament formation, similar to that observed with the *ACTA2* mutations described above.

A *MYH11* missense mutation results in the substitution of a proline for a leucine at amino acid 1264, also in the coiled-coil domain. This substitution likely disrupts the formation of the coiled-coil as predicted by the *in silico* modeling analysis, and may affect filament assembly in a similar fashion to the deletion mutations.

Only one motor domain mutation has been linked to aortic aneurysms: a missense mutation R712Q. This residue lies in the crucial SH1 helix, which links the enzymatic region of the molecule with the converter domain that functions as a lever and actively moves the rest of the head domain. An equivalent mutation in *MYH9*, the nonmuscle myosin heavy chain II, causes syndromic deafness (29,30). When engineered into a *Dictyostelium* myosin background, alteration of this arginine caused a decrease in the velocity of actin movement along the myosin filament, but did not affect the enzymatic ATPase activity of the motor (29). These results suggest that the R712Q mutation likely disrupts force generation by the mutant myosin heavy chains.

Heterozygous mutations in the gene for myosin light chain kinase (*MYLK*) have also been reported as a cause of FTAAD (31). Cell signaling events that increase intracellular $[Ca^{2+}]_i$ in SMCs, such as the opening of stretch-activated Ca^{2+} channels, stimulate the Ca^{2+}/calmodulin-dependent myosin light chain kinase (MLCK) (see Chapter 87). The kinase then phosphorylates a specific site on the N-terminus of the regulatory light chain (RLC) of myosin polymerized in thick filaments. RLC phosphorylation is sufficient to activate the myosin motor, and thereby affect cellular contraction. MLCK appears to be the only known kinase for this function and the only known physiological substrate for MLCK is myosin RLC; thus, it is a dedicated protein kinase (32–34). The aortic phenotype in FTAAD families with *MYLK* mutation is characterized by presentation with an acute aortic dissection with little to no enlargement of the aorta (35). Mice with SMC-specific knockdown of *Mylk* demonstrate altered gene expression and pathology consistent with medial degeneration of the aorta, though as with the human patients no dilation of the vessel was apparent (31).

MYLK mutations lead to a loss of enzymatic function of MLCK: one mutation is a nonsense mutation, R1480X, that leads to a truncated protein lacking the kinase- and calmodulin-binding domains, while the other, S1759P, alters amino acids in the α-helix of the calmodulin-binding sequence. The latter alteration disrupts MLCK binding to calmodulin as shown by immunoprecipitation. An *in vitro* kinase assay also showed decreased enzymatic activity (decreased Vmax and increased Km) (31).

The identification of mutations in the major structural proteins of the SMC contractile unit, along with mutations in the kinase controlling SMC contraction, as causes of FTAAD implicate disruption of the "elastin-contractile unit" as a factor that predisposes to TAAD (Figure 97.5). The major protein in microfibrils in fibrillin-1, and mutations in the gene for this protein, *FBN1*, also lead to a genetic predisposition to TAAD in patients with MFS and FTAAD as described above (36–38). Therefore, these data suggest that aortic SMCs may act as sensors for

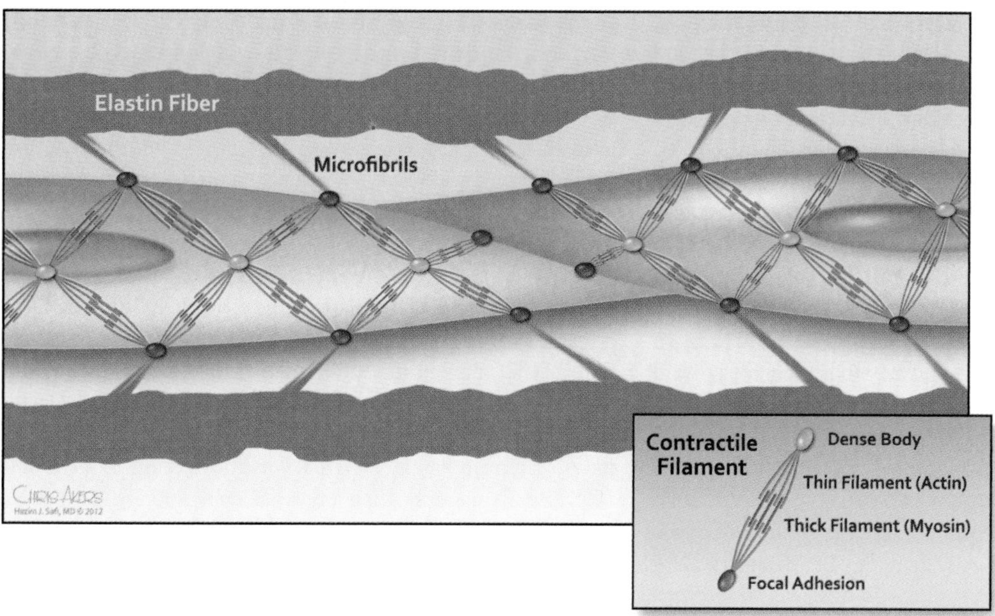

FIGURE 97.5 **Diagram of the "elastin-contractile unit".** Contractile proteins like α-actin and β-myosin are assembled into filaments that comprise the contractile unit of a smooth muscle cell. These units are then linked to integrin-containing focal adhesions at the cell surface, and the integrins in these adhesions form connections with microfibrils in the extracellular matrix. These fibers connect the cells to the large elastic fibers in the vessel wall. These "elastin-contractile units" connect all cells to the elastic fibers, allowing the aortic wall to contract coordinately.

biomechanical stress on the ascending aorta and that intact SMC "elastin-contractile units" serve as a critical component for this sensor function. The aortic SMCs respond to aberrant forces on this unit by activating cellular signaling pathways in an attempt to repair and remodel the wall to withstand these stressors. If SMCs continually respond to increased forces or stresses, resulting either from genetically-mediated disruption of the elastin-contractile unit or from the increased pressures of poorly controlled hypertension, these cell signaling pathways may be continuously activated, leading to medial degeneration and TAAD. Analysis of human TAAD aortas and mouse models of thoracic aortic disease have implicated the following to be some of the signaling pathways leading to TAAD: proteoglycan accumulation, increased metalloproteinases (MMPs) activity, including MMP-2 (39,40), hyperplastic medial SMC cellular proliferation (17), increased TGF-β signaling (7,41,42), increased expression of insulin-like growth factor-1 (IGF-1), and evidence of increased angiotensin (AngII) signaling (28,43).

Although many of the genes that predispose to TAAD directly encode proteins found in the "elastin-contractile unit," how mutations in the TGF-β receptors could disrupt this unit is not immediately obvious. Heterozygous mutations in *TGFBR1* and *TGFBR2* cause both FTAAD and LDS. The causative mutations are missense mutations in the intracellular kinase domain of the receptor that are predicted, and for a few of the missense mutations proven, to disrupt the kinase activity of the receptors (44,45). Therefore, these mutations are predicted to disrupt TGF-β-driven cellular signaling that is activated with ligand binding, and those same signaling pathways regulate the expression of contractile proteins by vascular SMCs (46). Explanted aortic SMCs from FTAAD patients with *TGFBR2* missense mutations have intact canonical Smad signaling but decreased expression and protein levels of contractile proteins, including SM α-actin, β-myosin, and calponin, when compared with control SMCs. In contrast to control SMCs that have SM α-actin filaments extending across the cells, aortic SMCs from *TGFBR2* mutant patients have no incorporation of SM α-actin into filaments, similar to the phenotype observed in SMCs with *ACTA2* missense mutations. Analysis of proteins isolated from aortic tissue also showed decreased expression of contractile proteins in *TGFBR2* patients compared with controls. Dermal fibroblasts from *TGFBR2* patients similarly demonstrated defective trans-differentiation into myofibroblasts with TGF-β exposure when compared to control fibroblasts, a finding that may help explain the poor wound healing and atrophic scarring observed in these patients (45). These results suggest that heterozygous missense mutations in the TGF-β type II receptor intracellular kinase domain disrupt TGF-β signaling such that SMCs and fibroblasts fail to fully express contractile proteins that mark differentiation and trans-differentiation of these cells into contractile SMCs and myofibroblasts, respectively. Animal models of these mutations, along with further cellular studies, are needed to determine if the cellular defects described in *TGFBR2* mutant cells also disrupt contractile properties of SMCs. Finally, there is also genetic evidence that disruption of the connection between α-actin filaments and cell surface integrin receptors also predisposes to thoracic aortic disease. Filamin A is a large, multi-domain, homodimeric actin-binding protein that interacts with the actin cytoskeleton and integrin receptors, thereby regulating various aspects of cell shape, motility, and function. Mutations in filamin A (*FLNA*) result in X-linked inheritance of a brain malformation known as periventricular heterotopia (47). The disorder occurs mostly in females and affected women have an increased number of miscarriages of male fetuses, suggesting that hemizygous males die perinatally. In addition, *FLNA* mutations also cause aortic dissections in women with periventricular heterotopias (48). The identification of thoracic aortic disease in women with *FLNA* mutations further highlights a potential role for filamin A in the "elastin-contractile unit".

GENETIC VARIANTS CONTRIBUTING TO SPORADIC THORACIC AORTIC DISEASE DISRUPT SMOOTH MUSCLE CELL CONTRACTION AND ADHESION

The majority of patients with TAAD do not report a family history of the condition: their disease is classified as sporadic TAAD (STAAD) and accounts for approximately 80% of thoracic aortic disease (11,49). Identification of patients at risk for TAAD via a genetic strategy could potentially prevent sudden deaths due to acute aortic dissections. Initial studies have begun to identify the genetic variants that predispose to disease in STAAD patients and have highlighted a role for genomic copy number variants (CNVs) in predisposing individuals to STAAD. CNVs are large regions of the genome that are either deleted or duplicated in the population. They can encompass multiple genes or involve regions that contain no genes, leading to decreased or increased gene dosage. They may also disrupt the structure of genes at the boundaries of the affected region. CNVs have been shown to confer increased risk for common multifactorial diseases such as autism and schizophrenia, as well as congenital cardiovascular disorders such as tetralogy of Fallot (50–52). The findings in these studies support a genetic model wherein any of a large number of individually rare copy number mutations contribute to disease causation or predisposition (53). This model is supported by the observation that CNVs for neuropsychiatric conditions are enriched for genes involved in neuronal function and activity (54,55).

Through the analysis of over 750 STAAD patients, the CNV burden in these patients was found to be significantly increased when compared with a control population (56,57). Furthermore, ontology, expression profiling, and network analysis showed that genes within and disrupted by the CNVs in patients with STAAD regulate SMC focal adhesions and contractility, and many of the CNV-involved genes encode proteins that interact with SM α-actin and β-myosin. Therefore, the CNVs in patients with STAAD disrupt the ability of the SMC to adhere and contract, once again implicating the "elastin-contractile unit" in the maintenance of the integrity of the ascending aorta.

It is notable that a recurrent CNV involving duplications of chromosome 16p13.1 was more commonly found in STAAD patients than controls (p value $= 1.4 \times 10^{-8}$, Odds Ratio 10.7 [Confidence Interval 5.1–21.1]) (58). Nine genes are in the chromosome 16p13.1 duplicated region, including *MYH11*. Since *MYH11* mutations cause FTAAD, increased gene dosage of *MYH11* may be responsible for the increased risk for thoracic aortic disease associated with this duplication. Increased *MYH11* gene expression was found in aortic tissues from TAAD patients with the 16p13.1 duplications when compared either with unaffected aortas or aortas from patients without the 16p13.1 duplication. Studies in *C. elegans* have shown that a precise ratio of β-myosin to its cellular chaperone, UNC45, is required for proper folding of myosin and its assembly into thick filaments, and an imbalance in this ratio causes the degradation of myosin heavy chain protein and dysfunction of the contractile complex (59). Further studies are needed to determine if overexpression of *MYH11* in aortic SMCs similarly leads to an imbalance of β-myosin to its chaperone, leading to degradation of β-myosin and dysfunction of the SMC contractile unit.

ACTA2 MUTATIONS CAUSE OCCLUSIVE VASCULAR DISEASES IN ADDITION TO FTAAD

Analysis of families with inherited heterozygous mutations *ACTA2* determined that these mutations predispose not only to TAAD but also to occlusive vascular diseases, including early onset coronary artery disease (CAD), early onset strokes, and Moyamoya disease (23). The investigation into occlusive vascular diseases in FTAAD patients with *ACTA2* mutations was initiated when it was observed that, as described above, in some families with *ACTA2* mutations, mutation carriers had livedo reticularis (21). Interestingly, the rash was present in mutation carriers whether or not they had aortic disease. Subsequent pathologic studies of the *vasa vasorum* in the outer layers of the aorta in *ACTA2* mutation patients identified occlusion or stenosis of these arteries due to thickening of the medial layer. Further linkage analysis and association studies from 20 families with *ACTA2* mutations began to uncover a concurrent predisposition among mutation carriers for occlusive vascular diseases, including greater-than-expected incidences of early-onset ischemic stroke and CAD. Additionally, a recurrent mutation in TAAD families, *ACTA2* R258C, was associated with an unusual number of cases of primary Moyamoya disease (23). Moyamoya disease is a rare cerebrovascular syndrome often leading to ischemic stroke at a young age. Diagnostic features on angiography of Moyamoya disease include bilateral occlusion or stenosis of the terminal internal carotid artery and the formation of collateral vessel networks at the base of the brain, the so-called "Moyamoya vessels". These occlusive lesions occur in young and middle-aged mutation carriers despite minimal risk factors for vascular disease such as hyperlipidemia, smoking, or diabetes. These data demonstrated that diffuse vascular diseases, resulting from either occluded or dilated arteries, can be caused by a mutation in a single gene.

Analysis of the mutated sites along the SM α-actin sequence suggested that different vascular diseases were associated with specific *ACTA2* missense mutations (21). *ACTA2* mutations R118Q and R149C are significantly associated with CAD and are less frequently associated with strokes. In contrast, mutations that alter R258 are primarily associated with strokes, including Moyamoya disease, and not with CAD.

The thickened medial layer of the *vasa vasorum* in the arteries of *ACTA2* patients appeared to be composed of increased numbers of SMCs, suggesting that excessive SMC proliferation might be the mechanism of occlusive lesion formation in these patients. Occlusive diseases due to unchecked SMC hyperplasia were further suggested by the observation that atherosclerotic coronary artery lesions in *ACTA2* mutation carriers were SMC-rich and lipid-poor (60). Interestingly, the occlusive lesions in the distal internal carotids of Moyamoya disease patients have also been described as SMC-rich and lipid-poor (61). Given the evidence of hyperplasia of SMCs in vascular lesions in *ACTA2* mutation patients, it was not surprising that SMCs and myofibroblasts from *ACTA2* mutation carriers proliferate more rapidly *in vitro* than matched control cells (21). Based on these data, it is hypothesized that *ACTA2* mutations lead to a "gain of function" in SMC, specifically an excessive hyperplasia in response to vascular injuries, in addition to the "loss of" contractile function leading to the thoracic aortic disease. Extensive evidence has linked polymerization of G actin monomers into F actin filaments to differentiation and proliferation of SMCs through serum response factor (SRF), an axis that may be responsible for the increased proliferation of SMCs harboring *ACTA2* mutations (reviewed in Chapter 95). Actin polymerization leads to the translocation of myocardin-related transcription factors (MRTF; myocardin, MRTF1 and MRTF2) to the nucleus and co-activation with SRF for the transcription of genes encoding SMC-restricted contractile proteins, which marks the differentiation of these cells (62–67). Dedifferentiation of SMCs is associated with the nuclear export of MRTF-A/B and downregulation of contractile protein expression, allowing for the binding of SRF to ternary complex factors (TCFs, members of the Ets family of transcription factors) (68,69). The TCF–SRF complex activates a subset of SRF-regulated growth responsive genes, leading to cellular proliferation.

Why *ACTA2* mutations lead to dilation of the aorta but occlusion of smaller arteries may be related to one or more of the following: (i) the differences between large elastic arteries and smaller muscular arteries, including the different developmental origins of SMCs in the ascending aorta versus other arteries and the organization of elastin fibers in relation to SMCs (70,71); (ii) differences in force experienced by these two types of arteries may activate different pathways (23); or (iii) differential response of SMCs to the underlying mutation. This differential SMC response may result from two roles for α-actin in SMCs: force generation and mechanotransduction (linking mechanical stresses to transcription) (62–64). The differential response of elastic versus muscular arteries to *ACTA2* mutations is in part suggested by the observation that occlusive lesions in the distal internal carotid arteries in Moyamoya disease patients stereotypically form in the region where the distal carotid artery transitions from an elastic to a muscular artery (72).

SYNDROME OF GLOBAL SMOOTH MUSCLE DYSFUNCTION DUE TO A *DE NOVO ACTA2* MUTATION

ACTA2 mutations have also been found in a rare syndrome that is characterized by global SMC dysfunction (25). Recurrent mutations in *ACTA2* altering R179H have been identified *de novo* in seven children with this syndrome. Children heterozygous for this *ACTA2* missense mutation are diagnosed with TAAD and have cerebrovascular lesions diagnostic or similar to Moyamoya disease under the age of 20 years. Interestingly, these patients also form fusiform aneurysms of the carotid artery proximal to the MMD occlusive lesions in the distal carotids. Therefore, these children have earlier onset of the vascular diseases found in FTAAD patients with *ACTA2* mutations. Additional phenotypic features in these children indicate that the R179H mutation disrupts more than just the vascular SMCs and leads to global SMC contractile failure. The children have fixed and dilated pupils (congenital mydriasis), which is most likely due to loss of function of the SMCs responsible for contraction of the pupil. Affected children have hypotonic bladders diagnosed shortly after birth and a subset of patients also have hypoperistalsis of the gut. Another complication observed in these children is primary pulmonary hypertension, which occurs due to occlusion or stenosis of pulmonary arteries due to SMC hyperplasia. The severity and onset of clinical complications at a young age, along with the identification of this mutation *de novo* in patients, indicates that this is the most clinically severe *ACTA2* mutation identified to date. Similar to what is observed with *ACTA2* mutations leading to TAAD and other occlusive vascular diseases, there is a significant phenotype to genotype correlation with the *ACTA2* R179H mutation.

CONCLUSION

Identification of genes that when mutated predispose to thoracic aortic disease has uncovered a previously unconsidered mechanism for aortic disease pathogenesis: disruption of the smooth muscle cell "elastin-contractile unit". Disease-causing mutations have been identified in the genes encoding the smooth muscle-specific isoforms of α-actin and β-myosin, as well as the kinase governing the contractile function of myosin, myosin light chain kinase. SMCs harboring *TGFBR2* mutations failed to express and assemble contractile proteins, suggesting that a loss of contractile function may underlie aortic disease in these patients as well. Analysis of CNVs in STAAD patients also points to defects in SMC contractility and adhesion as predisposing to disease. Taken together, the results of all these inquiries suggest that an intact "elastin-contractile unit" in the medial layer of the aortic wall is crucial to maintaining vessel integrity and preventing aneurysm formation.

Furthermore, the identification of both occlusive vascular diseases and aneurysms in *ACTA2* mutation carriers signifies a shift in the paradigm for vascular disease, i.e., one gene can cause diverse and diffuse vascular disease. Given that vascular SMCs line the arteries throughout the body, it is perhaps not surprising that SMC-specific gene mutations can cause such a diffuse vasculopathy. Further studies are needed to confirm that SMC hyperplasia in response to *ACTA2* missense mutations is responsible for the occlusive diseases in these patients and to identify the link between the mutant α-actin and the SMC proliferative response.

REFERENCES

1. Small JV. Contractile units in vertebrate smooth muscle cells. *Nature* 1974;**249**:324–7.
2. Hiratzka LF, Bakris GL, Beckman JA, Bersin RM, Carr VF, Casey Jr DE, et al. ACCF/AHA/AATS/ACR/ASA/SCA/SCAI/SIR/STS/SVM Guidelines for the Diagnosis and Management of Patients With Thoracic Aortic Disease: Executive Summary. A Report of the American College of Cardiology Foundation/American Heart Association Task Force on Practice Guidelines, American Association for Thoracic Surgery, American College of Radiology, American Stroke Association, Society of Cardiovascular Anesthesiologists, Society for Cardiovascular Angiography and Interventions, Society of Interventional Radiology, Society of Thoracic Surgeons, and Society for Vascular Medicine. *Circulation* 2010; ePub ahead of print March 16, 2010, doi:10.1161/CIR.0b013e3181d4739e.
3. Hoyert DL, Arias E, Smith BL, Murphy SL, Kochanek KD. Deaths: final data for 1999. *Natl Vital Stat Rep* 2001;**49**:1–113.
4. Pape LA, Tsai TT, Isselbacher EM, Oh JK, O'Gara PT, Evangelista A, et al. Aortic diameter >or = 5.5 cm is not a good predictor of type A aortic dissection: observations from the International Registry of Acute Aortic Dissection (IRAD). *Circulation* 2007;**116**:1120–7.
5. Pyeritz RE, McKusick VA. The Marfan syndrome: diagnosis and management. *N Engl J Med* 1979;**300**:772–7.
6. Neptune ER, Frischmeyer PA, Arking DE, Myers L, Bunton TE, Gayraud B, et al. Dysregulation of TGF-beta activation contributes to pathogenesis in Marfan syndrome. *Nat Genet* 2003;**33**:407–11.
7. Habashi JP, Judge DP, Holm TM, Cohn RD, Loeys BL, Cooper TK, et al. Losartan, an AT1 antagonist, prevents aortic aneurysm in a mouse model of Marfan syndrome. *Science* 2006;**312**:117–21.
8. Loeys BL, Schwarze U, Holm T, Callewaert BL, Thomas GH, Pannu H, et al. Aneurysm syndromes caused by mutations in the TGF-beta receptor. *N Engl J Med* 2006;**355**:788–98.
9. Pannu H, Fadulu V, Chang J, Lafont A, Hasham SN, Sparks E, et al. Mutations in transforming growth factor-beta receptor type II cause familial thoracic aortic aneurysms and dissections. *Circulation* 2005;**112**:513–20.
10. Tran-Fadulu V, Pannu H, Kim DH, Vick III GW, Lonsford CM, Lafont AL, et al. Analysis of multigenerational families with thoracic aortic aneurysms and dissections due to TGFBR1 or TGFBR2 mutations. *J Med Genet* 2009;**46**:607–13.
11. Biddinger A, Rocklin M, Coselli J, Milewicz DM. Familial thoracic aortic dilatations and dissections: a case control study. *J Vasc Surg* 1997;**25**:506–11.
12. Albornoz G, Coady MA, Roberts M, Davies RR, Tranquilli M, Rizzo JA, et al. Familial thoracic aortic aneurysms and dissections – incidence, modes of inheritance, and phenotypic patterns. *Ann Thorac Surg* 2006;**82**:1400–5.
13. Milewicz DM, Chen H, Park ES, Petty EM, Zaghi H, Shashidhar G, et al. Reduced penetrance and variable expressivity of familial thoracic aortic aneurysms/dissections. *Am J Cardiol* 1998;**82**:474–9.
14. Davis EC. Smooth muscle cell to elastic lamina connections in developing mouse aorta. Role in aortic medial organization. *Lab Invest* 1993;**68**:89–99.
15. Wagenseil JE, Mecham RP. Vascular extracellular matrix and arterial mechanics. *Physiol Rev* 2009;**89**:957–89.
16. Berry CL, Greenwald SE, Rivett JF. Static mechanical properties of the developing and mature rat aorta. *Cardiovasc Res* 1975;**9**:669–78.

17. Tang PC, Coady MA, Lovoulos C, Dardik A, Aslan M, Elefteriades JA, et al. Hyperplastic cellular remodeling of the media in ascending thoracic aortic aneurysms. *Circulation* 2005;**112**:1098–105.
18. Tang PC, Yakimov AO, Teesdale MA, Coady MA, Dardik A, Elefteriades JA, et al. Transmural inflammation by interferon-gamma-producing T cells correlates with outward vascular remodeling and intimal expansion of ascending thoracic aortic aneurysms. *FASEB J* 2005;**19**:1528–30.
19. He R, Guo DC, Estrera AL, Safi HJ, Huynh TT, Yin Z, et al. Characterization of the inflammatory and apoptotic cells in the aortas of patients with ascending thoracic aortic aneurysms and dissections. *J Thorac Cardiovasc Surg* 2006;**131**:671–8.
20. Brautbar A, LeMaire SA, Franco LM, Coselli JS, Milewicz DM, Belmont JW. FBN1 mutations in patients with descending thoracic aortic dissections. *Am J Med Genet A* 2010;**152A**:413–6.
21. Guo DC, Pannu H, Papke CL, Yu RK, Avidan N, Bourgeois S, et al. Mutations in smooth muscle alpha-actin (ACTA2) lead to thoracic aortic aneurysms and dissections. *Nat Genet* 2007;**39**:1488–93.
22. Fatigati V, Murphy RA. Actin and tropomyosin variants in smooth muscles. Dependence on tissue type. *J Biol Chem* 1984;**259**:14383–8.
23. Guo DC, Papke CL, Tran-Fadulu V, Regalado ES, Avidan N, Johnson RJ, et al. Mutations in smooth muscle alpha-actin (ACTA2) cause coronary artery disease, stroke, and moyamoya disease, along with thoracic aortic disease. *Am J Hum Genet* 2009;**84**:617–27.
24. Morisaki H, Akutsu K, Ogino H, Kondo N, Yamanaka I, Tsutsumi Y, et al. Mutation of ACTA2 gene as an important cause of familial and nonfamilial nonsyndromatic thoracic aortic aneurysm and/or dissection (TAAD). *Hum. Mutat* 2009;**30**:1406–11.
25. Milewicz DM, Ostergaard JR, la-Kokko LM, Khan N, Grange DK, Mendoza-Londono R, et al. De novo ACTA2 mutation causes a novel syndrome of multisystemic smooth muscle dysfunction. *Am J Med Genet A* 2010;**152A**:2437–43.
26. Bergeron SE, Wedemeyer EW, Lee R, Wen KK, McKane M, Pierick AR, et al. Allele-specific effects of thoracic aortic aneurysm and dissection {alpha}-smooth muscle actin mutations on actin function. *J Biol Chem* 2011;**286**:11356–69.
27. Zhu L, Vranckx R, Khau Van KP, Lalande A, Boisset N, Mathieu F, et al. Mutations in myosin heavy chain 11 cause a syndrome associating thoracic aortic aneurysm/aortic dissection and patent ductus arteriosus. *Nat Genet* 2006;**38**:343–9.
28. Pannu H, Tran-Fadulu V, Papke CL, Scherer S, Liu Y, Presley C, et al. MYH11 mutations result in a distinct vascular pathology driven by insulin-like growth factor 1 and angiotensin II. *Hum. Mol. Genet* 2007;**16**:3453–62.
29. Iwai S, Hanamoto D, Chaen S. A point mutation in the SH1 helix alters elasticity and thermal stability of myosin II. *J. Biol. Chem* 2006;**281**:30736–44.
30. Lalwani AK, Goldstein JA, Kelley MJ, Luxford W, Castelein CM, Mhatre AN. Human nonsyndromic hereditary deafness DFNA17 is due to a mutation in nonmuscle myosin MYH9. *Am J Hum Genet* 2000;**67**:1121–8.
31. Wang L, Guo DC, Cao J, Gong L, Kamm KE, Regalado E, et al. Mutations in myosin light chain kinase cause familial aortic dissections. *Am J Hum Genet* 2010;**87**:701–7.
32. Kamm KE, Stull JT. Dedicated myosin light chain kinases with diverse cellular functions. *J Biol Chem* 2001;**276**:4527–30.
33. He WQ, Peng YJ, Zhang WC, Lv N, Tang J, Chen C, et al. Myosin light chain kinase is central to smooth muscle contraction and required for gastrointestinal motility in mice. *Gastroenterology* 2008;**135**:610–20.
34. Zhang WC, Peng YJ, Zhang GS, He WQ, Qiao YN, Dong YY, et al. Myosin light chain kinase is necessary for tonic airway smooth muscle contraction. *J Biol Chem* 2010;**285**:5522–31.
35. Elefteriades JA, Tranquilli M, Darr U, Cardon J, Zhu BQ, Barrett P. Symptoms plus family history trump size in thoracic aortic aneurysm. *AnnThorac Surg* 2005;**80**:1098–100.
36. Dietz HC, Pyeritz RE. Mutations in the human gene for fibrillin-1 (FBN1) in the Marfan syndrome and related disorders. *Hum Mol Genet* 1995;**4 Spec No.**, 1799–1809
37. Francke U, Berg MA, Tynan K, Brenn T, Liu WG, Aoyama T, et al. A Gly1127Ser mutation in an Egf-like domain of the fibrillin-1 gene is a risk factor for ascending aortic-aneurysm and dissection. *Am J Hum Genet* 1995;**56**:1287–96.
38. Milewicz DM, Michael K, Fisher N, Coselli JS, Markello T, Biddinger A. Fibrillin-1 (FBN1) mutations in patients with thoracic aortic aneurysms. *Circulation* 1996;**94**:2708–11.
39. LeMaire SA, Wang X, Wilks JA, Carter SA, Wen S, Won T, et al. Matrix metalloproteinases in ascending aortic aneurysms: bicuspid versus trileaflet aortic valves. *J Surg Res* 2005;**123**:40–8.
40. Ikonomidis JS, Jones JA, Barbour JR, Stroud RE, Clark LL, Kaplan BS, et al. Expression of matrix metalloproteinases and endogenous inhibitors within ascending aortic aneurysms of patients with bicuspid or tricuspid aortic valves. *J Thorac Cardiovasc Surg* 2007;**133**:1028–36.
41. Matt P, Schoenhoff F, Habashi J, Holm T, Van EC, Loch D, et al. Circulating transforming growth factor-beta in Marfan syndrome. *Circulation* 2009;**120**:526–32.
42. Carta L, Smaldone S, Zilberberg L, Loch D, Dietz HC, Rifkin DB, et al. MAPKp38 is an early determinant of promiscuous Smad2/3 signaling in the aortas of fibrillin-1 (Fbn1) null mice. *J Biol Chem* 2009;**284**:5630–6.
43. Tieu BC, Lee C, Sun H, Lejeune W, Recinos III A, Ju X, et al. An adventitial IL-6/MCP1 amplification loop accelerates macrophage-mediated vascular inflammation leading to aortic dissection in mice. *J Clin Invest* 2009;**119**:3637–51.
44. Mizuguchi T, Collod-Beroud G, Akiyama T, Abifadel M, Harada N, Morisaki T, et al. Heterozygous TGFBR2 mutations in Marfan syndrome. *Nat Genet* 2004;**36**:855–60.
45. Inamoto S, Kwartler CS, Lafont AL, Liang YY, Fadulu VT, Duraisamy S, et al. TGFBR2 mutations alter smooth muscle cell phenotype and predispose to thoracic aortic aneurysms and dissections. *Cardiovasc Res* 2010;**88**:520–9.
46. Grainger DJ, Metcalfe JC, Grace AA, Mosedale DE. Transforming growth factor-beta dynamically regulates vascular smooth muscle differentiation in vivo. *J Cell Sci* 1998;**111**(Pt 19):2977–88.
47. Fox JW, Lamperti ED, Eksioglu YZ, Hong SE, Feng Y, Graham DA, et al. Mutations in filamin 1 prevent migration of cerebral cortical neurons in human periventricular heterotopia. *Neuron* 1998;**21**:1315–25.
48. Sheen VL, Jansen A, Chen MH, Parrini E, Morgan T, Ravenscroft R, et al. Filamin A mutations cause periventricular heterotopia with Ehlers–Danlos syndrome. *Neurology* 2005;**64**:254–62.

49. Coady MA, Davies RR, Roberts M, Goldstein LJ, Rogalski MJ, Rizzo JA, et al. Familial patterns of thoracic aortic aneurysms. *Arch Surg* 1999;**134**:361–7.
50. Sebat J, Lakshmi B, Malhotra D, Troge J, Lese-Martin C, Walsh T, et al. Strong association of de novo copy number mutations with autism. *Science* 2007;**316**:445–9.
51. Kirov G, Grozeva D, Norton N, Ivanov D, Mantripragada KK, Holmans P, et al. Support for the involvement of large copy number variants in the pathogenesis of schizophrenia. *Hum Mol Genet* 2009;**18**:1497–503.
52. Greenway SC, Pereira AC, Lin JC, DePalma SR, Israel SJ, Mesquita SM, et al. De novo copy number variants identify new genes and loci in isolated sporadic tetralogy of Fallot. *Nat Genet* 2009;**41**:931–5.
53. Schork NJ, Murray SS, Frazer KA, Topol EJ. Common vs. rare allele hypotheses for complex diseases. *Curr Opin Genet Dev* 2009;**19**:212–9.
54. Elia J, Gai X, Xie HM, Perin JC, Geiger E, Glessner JT, et al. Rare structural variants found in attention-deficit hyperactivity disorder are preferentially associated with neurodevelopmental genes. *Mol Psychiatry* 2010;**15**:637–46.
55. Raychaudhuri S, Korn JM, McCarroll SA, Altshuler D, Sklar P, Purcell S, et al. Accurately assessing the risk of schizophrenia conferred by rare copy-number variation affecting genes with brain function. *PLoS Genet* 2010;**6**(9) pii:e1001097
56. Prakash S, LeMaire SA, Bray M, Milewicz DM, Belmont JW. Large deletions and uniparental disomy detected by SNP arrays in adults with thoracic aortic aneurysms and dissections. *Am J Med Genet A* 2010;**152A**:2399–405.
57. Prakash SK, LeMaire SA, Guo DC, Russell L, Regalado ES, Golabbakhsh H, et al. Rare copy number variants disrupt genes regulating vascular smooth muscle cell adhesion and contractility in sporadic thoracic aortic aneurysms and dissections. *Am J Hum Genet* 2010;**87**:743–56.
58. Kuang S-Q, Guo DC, Prakash SK, McDonald ML, Johnson RJ, Wang M, et al. The GenTAC Investigators. Recurrent chromosome 16p13.1 duplications are a risk factor for aortic dissection. *PLoS Genet.* ePub June 16, 2011, e1002118.
59. Landsverk ML, Li S, Hutagalung AH, Najafov A, Hoppe T, Barral JM, et al. The UNC-45 chaperone mediates sarcomere assembly through myosin degradation in *Caenorhabditis elegans*. *J Cell Biol* 2007;**177**:205–10.
60. Stary HC, Chandler AB, Dinsmore RE, Fuster V, Glagov S, Insull Jr W, et al. A definition of advanced types of atherosclerotic lesions and a histological classification of atherosclerosis. A report from the Committee on Vascular Lesions of the Council on Arteriosclerosis, American Heart Association. *Arterioscler Thromb Vasc Biol* 1995;**15**:1512–31.
61. Haltia M, Iivanainen M, Majuri H, Puranen M. Spontaneous occlusion of the circle of Willis (Moyamoya syndrome). *Clin Neuropathol* 1982;**1**:11–22.
62. Wang DZ, Li S, Hockemeyer D, Sutherland L, Wang Z, Schratt G, et al. Potentiation of serum response factor activity by a family of myocardin-related transcription factors. *Proc Natl Acad Sci USA* 2002;**99**:14855–60.
63. Owens GK, Kumar MS, Wamhoff BR. Molecular regulation of vascular smooth muscle cell differentiation in development and disease. *Physiol Rev* 2004;**84**:767–801.
64. Parmacek MS. Myocardin-related transcription factors: critical coactivators regulating cardiovascular development and adaptation. *Circ Res* 2007;**100**:633–44.
65. Miano JM, Carlson MJ, Spencer JA, Misra RP. Serum response factor-dependent regulation of the smooth muscle calponin gene. *J Biol Chem* 2000;**275**:9814–22.
66. Miano JM. Serum response factor: toggling between disparate programs of gene expression. *J Mol Cell Cardiol* 2003;**35**: 577–93.
67. Yoshida T, Sinha S, Dandre F, Wamhoff BR, Hoofnagle MH, Kremer BE, et al. Myocardin is a key regulator of CArG-dependent transcription of multiple smooth muscle marker genes. *Circ Res* 2003;**92**:856–64.
68. Posern G, Sotiropoulos A, Treisman R. Mutant actins demonstrate a role for unpolymerized actin in control of transcription by serum response factor. *Mol Biol Cell* 2002;**13**:4167–78.
69. Zaromytidou AI, Miralles F, Treisman R. MAL and ternary complex factor use different mechanisms to contact a common surface on the serum response factor DNA-binding domain. *Mol Cell Biol* 2006;**26**:4134–48.
70. Majesky MW. Developmental basis of vascular smooth muscle diversity. *Arterioscler Thromb Vasc Biol* 2007;**27**:1248–58.
71. Stoller JZ, Epstein JA. Cardiac neural crest. *Semin Cell Dev Biol* 2005;**16**:704–15.
72. Masuoka T, Hayashi N, Hori E, Kuwayama N, Ohtani O, Endo S. Distribution of internal elastic lamina and external elastic lamina in the internal carotid artery: possible relationship with atherosclerosis. *Neurol Med Chir (Tokyo)* 2010;**50**:179–82.

Chapter 98

Vascular Smooth Muscle Cell Remodeling in Atherosclerosis and Restenosis

Elaine Smolock and Bradford C. Berk

Aab Cardiovascular Research Institute, University of Rochester School of Medicine and Dentistry, Rochester, NY

PATHOGENESIS OF ATHEROSCLEROSIS AND VASCULAR REMODELING

Vascular Remodeling: Glagov Phenomenon

Vascular remodeling is a physiological response of the vascular wall to compensate for hemodynamic changes, as seen in atherosclerosis. Fluid dynamics, dictated by Reynold's number ($N_R = \rho VD/\eta$), Poiseuille's law ($\tau = 4\eta\pi r_{lumen}^{3}$) and LaPlace's law ($T = Pr$), are crucial determinants of vessel wall homeostasis. The primary physical properties inherent to these equations are fluid density (ρ), velocity (V), viscosity (η), flow (Q), pressure (P) and vessel diameter (D) and radius (r). Low N_R values (<2000) are representative of laminar, steady state flow, while high N_R values (>3000) are indicative of turbulent blood flow. Laminar flow produces a frictional force, termed shear stress, which is atheroprotective when steady and of sufficient force (>10 dyn/cm^2), maintaining vascular wall homeostasis. However, turbulent flow and/or low shear stress (LSS) (<1 dyn/cm^2) occur with atherosclerosis progression and result in wall remodeling.

Mulvaney and colleagues described remodeling as being either inward (vessel diameter narrows) or outward (vessel diameter enlarges) and further characterized it to include either increases (hypertrophic), decreases (atrophic) or no changes (eutrophic) in vessel wall mass (1) (Figure 98.1). Vascular remodeling in response to changes in blood flow is dependent on the presence of an intact endothelium (2,3). Conventional thinking prior to the late 1980s was that inward remodeling with stenosis was directly related to plaque formation. This dogma was contradicted when an important aspect of vascular remodeling was observed by Glagov (4). Glagov's study of human coronary arteries demonstrated that the vessel wall compensates by initially undergoing outward remodeling. The vessel's response to outwardly remodel and enlarge, termed "Glagov phenomenon", preserves lumen diameter and maintains blood flow (Figure 98.1). If stenosis from the developing plaque is <40% the lumen diameter is preserved and there is an increase in the vessel wall mass and external radius. Once plaque stenosis reaches limits of >40%, the result is "vascular failure" (5) with significant inward remodeling and decreased lumen diameter (4,6).

Mechanism of Vascular Remodeling

The mechanisms responsible for Glagov's phenomenon have been elucidated by animal models of flow-dependent vascular remodeling. Carotid ligation, either by fully or partially restricting blood flow through the left carotid artery, results in stenosis. In terms of a developing atheroma, the partial carotid ligation model, where flow is not completely restricted but significantly reduced, is an optimal model of remodeling. Partial ligation of the left carotid results in an ~90% reduction in flow with a ~50% flow increase in the right carotid artery (7–9). The degree of stenosis associated with flow-dependent vascular remodeling is in part genetically determined (6). Studies using various mouse strains demonstrate the genetic propensity to remodel to varying extents (8) and several gene candidates were highlighted as likely mediators of remodeling: neuronal nitric oxide synthase (nNOS), P2X type ATP receptors, vimentin, inducible nitric oxide synthase (iNOS), toll-like receptor 4 (TLR4), matrix metalloproteinase (MMP-9), t-ACE, dopamine–hydroxylase, and p22^{phox} (10). Upon further examination of the biochemical pathways involving these genes it was found that there were alterations in responses to oxidative stress (11–14), changes in ECM proteins (15) and plasminogen activators (16,17), and inflammatory signaling through TLR4 (10). The role of oxidative stress, ECM, and inflammation will be discussed in further detail in the context of VSMC response in vascular remodeling.

Muscle. DOI: http://dx.doi.org/10.1016/B978-0-12-381510-1.00098-3

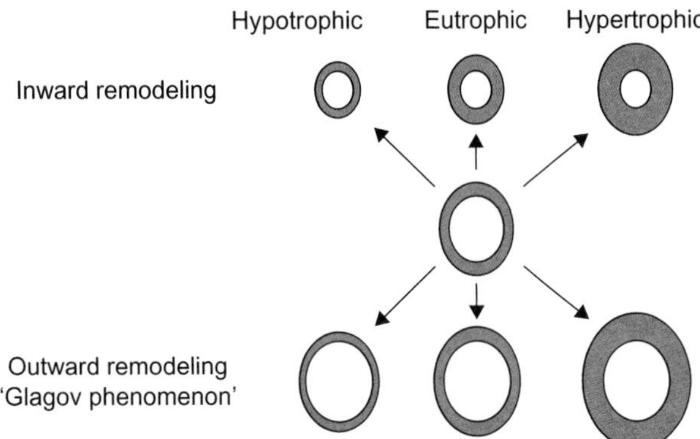

FIGURE 98.1 **Vessels respond to changes in blood flow by either inward or outwardly remodeling.** In both types of remodeling, the vessel wall can change to compensate for the altered blood flow: hypotrophic (decrease in wall mass), eutrophic (no change) or hypertrophic (increase). Inward remodeling typically involves a narrowing of the lumen diameter while outwards remodeling, termed "Glagov phenomenon", occurs to maintain the lumen size.

Pathogenesis of Restenosis

Treatment of atherosclerotic arteries commonly involves angioplasty to reopen occluded vessels or surgical replacement of diseased arteries. Interventional therapies are complicated by restenosis, which is a consequence of increased inflammation, ECM remodeling, and VSMC migration and proliferation.

Percutaneous Transluminal Angioplasty (PCTA) and Vein Grafts

PCTA has been the predominant intervention for restoring blood flow in stenotic arteries since 1977. Acutely, PCTA is highly beneficial. However, the vessel is unable to maintain lumen diameter following the mechanical dilation and restenosis occurs. A number of factors regarding the atheroma contribute to restenosis, including the degree and distribution of plaque formation, plaque rupture, neointimal disturbance, hemorrhage, and thrombosis. Another primary factor is the vessel wall's capacity to remodel (18). IMT is a major consequence of inward remodeling that occurs when VSMC undergo phenotypic modulation, migrate and proliferate forming a neointima. Until Glagov's phenomenon of outward remodeling was defined, restenosis was attributed to inward remodeling and intima formation. Glagov's observations of outward remodeling are also important in restenosis (6). As in atherosclerosis development, a vessel will initially attempt to outwardly remodel after PCTA, but following PCTA the capacity of the vessel wall to outwardly remodel is diminished. Mechanistically this impairment is due to increased ECM deposition by VSMC. In particular, an increase in fibrin formation inhibits the compensatory remodeling. Therefore, even in the absence of intima formation, the lumen diameter decreases and flow is again restricted (19).

Coronary artery bypass grafting (CABG) is often used to treat patients who have severely atherosclerotic coronaries. In most cases the saphenous vein is surgically implanted to replace the diseased artery. The short-term effects of CABG are positive. However, the long-term success significantly decreases within one year. A major disadvantage of vein grafting is the inability of the vessel to remain patent. Despite evidence that Glagov's phenomenon occurs in the early stages following engraftment, inward remodeling and occlusion are prominent. As early as one week post implant there is a measurable wall thickening and remodeling. Commonly the regions distal to the surgical placement of the graft are laden with lesions that are still capable of potentiating infiltration of inflammatory cells, ECM deposition, and VSMC migration and proliferation, leading to neointima formation and vessel occlusion (20).

Cellular and Molecular Mechanisms of Atherosclerosis and Vascular Remodeling

Vascular remodeling is mediated in large part by endothelial cells (EC) and VSMC responses to changes in blood flow. As discussed, blood flow is an important determinant of vascular wall homeostasis. Under normal physiological conditions blood flow exerts a shear stress on the vascular wall that is sensed by EC, which in turn signal and maintain VSMC in a contractile phenotype. At regions of vessel bifurcation, curvature or branching blood flow is disturbed. As a result, VSMC phenotypically modulate and assume a myofibroblast phenotype that is migratory, proliferative and associated with secretion of factors that contribute to neointima and atheroma development. There are numerous cellular and molecular mechanisms that promote VSMC phenotypic modulation that involve EC and changes in ECM composition.

Secretion of Soluble Growth Factors

Growth factors are key mediators of VSMC phenotype. The most well characterized secreted growth factors include: epidermal growth factor (EGF), fibroblast growth factor (FGF), growth arrest specific gene-6 (Gas6), hepatocyte growth factor (HGF), insulin growth factor-1 (IGF-1), platelet derived growth factor (PDGF), angiotensin II (AngII), catecholamines, endothelin-1 (ET-1), thrombin, interleukins (ILs), natriuretic peptides, transforming growth factor (TGF)-β, macroglobulins, cholesterol esters, cyclophilins (CyPs), and heat shock proteins (21). Depending on the pathological conditions and stimulus, growth factors can promote VSMC migration,

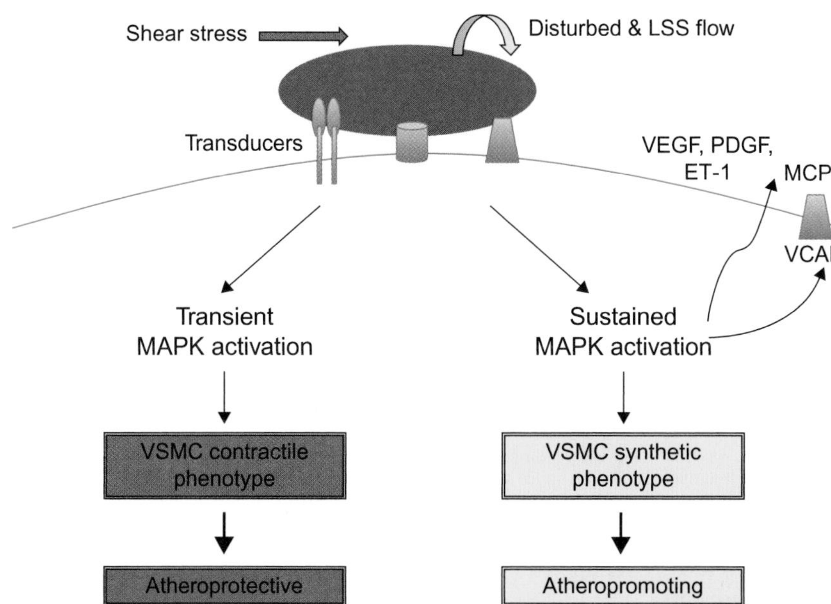

FIGURE 98.2 **Blood flow is an important determinant of VSMC remodeling.** Endothelial cells (EC = green circle) are the primary sensors for changes in blood flow. Various sensors on EC transduce mechanical signals into biochemical signals in VSMC. Fluid shear stress is atheroprotective and results in a transient activation of MAPK and the contractile phenotype of VSMC. Turbulent blood flow, as well as low shear stress, is atheropromoting which results in sustained MAPK activation and phenotypic modulation of VSMC from contractile to synthetic.

proliferation or apoptosis, which will be described in subsequent sections.

Monocyte-Derived Cytokines

LSS or turbulent blood flow results in injury of the vascular endothelium, initiating an inflammatory response. Increased expression of intracellular adhesion molecule-1 (ICAM-1) and vascular cell adhesion molecule-1 (VCAM-1) by EC and VSMC recruits circulating monocytes and promotes their adherence to the endothelium, followed by transendothelial migration into the developing neointima and media. These monocytes interact with resident cells in the vascular wall and secrete factors such as vascular endothelial growth factor (VEGF), monocyte chemoattractant protein-1 (MCP-1), ILs and various chemokines, all of which promote VSMC phenotypic modulation to a synthetic state and enhance plaque formation.

Endothelial Injury and VSMC Remodeling

EC exist in a monolayer interfacing with the circulation and are primary sensors of blood flow. Several proteins are important in transducing force in EC, including integrins, connexins, platelet endothelial cell adhesion molecule-1 (PECAM-1), tyrosine kinase receptors, VEGF receptor-2 (VEGFR2), G-proteins, and ion channels. Structural components of the endothelium also play a role in mechanosensing: caveolae, gap junctions, primary cilium, membrane lipids, and glycocalyx. Shear stress modulates these mechanosensors and transiently activates mitogen activated protein kinases (MAPK) and induces expression of VSMC atheroprotective genes (22,23). However, LSS or persistent disturbed flow sustains MAPK activation and atheroprotective gene expression is reduced (24,25). LSS upregulates VSMC mitogens, including PDGF, ET-1, and VEGF. Endothelium injury also results in enhanced expression of MCP-1 and inflammatory cell adhesion marker, VCAM-1, which plays a role in the recruitment of circulating monocytes. All of these responses to EC injury signal the VSMC to phenotypically modulate and promote VSMC migration and proliferation in the neointima (24,26) (Figure 98.2).

Direct Cell–Cell Interaction

Neointima and atherosclerotic plaque development are largely dependent on VSMC interaction with resident vascular cells, ECM components, and circulating and infiltrating cells.

EC and VSMC interaction, both physical and biochemical, is crucial to vascular wall homeostasis. Proper EC function and interaction maintains VSMC in the contractile phenotype. Gap junctions consisting of connexins aid in sensing changing blood flow and facilitate alterations in membrane potential of both EC and VSMC. *In vitro* co-culture systems have demonstrated that EC stimulate phosphatidylinositol-3 (PI-3) kinase and Akt signaling which promotes the VSMC contractile phenotype (27,28). *In vivo* models of EC injury have shown that without an intact endothelium VSMC undergo phenotypic modulation, becoming more migratory and proliferative (29). These changes are mediated by multiple molecules secreted by EC, including NO and prostacyclin, as well as the redox state of the vessel (30).

Vascular remodeling involves reorganization of the ECM (8). The ECM is a milieu of proteins consisting of collagen, laminin, elastin, fibronectin, and vitronectin that provide structural support in the vascular wall. ECM components interact with VSMC primarily via integrin and cadherin expression on the VSMC membrane. In response to varying stimuli, including growth factors and cytokines, the interaction with the ECM stimulates VSMC to increase expression of MMPs, which are upregulated in atherosclerotic lesions. MMPs are classified by their ECM substrate: interstitial collagenases (MMP-1, -8 and -13), gelatinases (MMP-2 and -9), stromelysins/matrilysins (MMP-3 and -7), and membrane type MMP-14 and -17, and a metalloelastase (MMP-12) (31–33). VSMC also synthesize and secrete plasminogen activators (PAs) which contribute to ECM remodeling (34). The two most studied PAs in vascular disease are the serine proteases tissue plasminogen activator (tPA) and urokinase-type plasminogen activator (uPA). tPA acts on fibrin in the ECM and has potent fibrinolytic activity. uPA acts in an autocrine manner to bind to uPA receptors on the VSMC membrane (31). MMPs and PAs are important regulators of VSMC migration, proliferation and apoptosis and will be discussed further in later sections pertaining to these properties.

Interaction of monocytes with VMSC is evident in developing plaques. Monocyte recruitment to the injured vessel wall occurs primarily through VCAM-1 expression on VSMC. *In vitro* studies indicate that monocytes can directly interact with migratory VSMC and increase release of VEGF. The exact mechanism by which this happens is not completely understood but evidence suggests that direct contact of the monocyte and VSMC cell membranes stimulates a cellular mechanism that enhances VEGF release mediated by IL-6, PDGF, and/or TGF-β (35).

Oxidative Stress and VSMC Remodeling

Increased production of reactive oxygen species (ROS) in the vascular wall is an early determinant of atherosclerosis development. Exogenous superoxide (O_2^-) directly stimulates EC apoptosis and augments production of intracellular ROS in the form of peroyxnitrite and hydrogen peroxide. Endogenous ROS production in EC, VSMC, and infiltrating inflammatory cells is attributed to activation of xanthine oxidase (XO), endothelial nitric oxidase synthase (eNOS), inducible nitric oxidase synthase (iNOS), NADPH oxidases, and myeloperoxidase (MPO). Under physiological conditions eNOS activation and production of nitric oxide (NO) results in cGMP-mediated atheroprotection (36). In the atherosclerotic wall, ROS generation results in VSMC DNA damage and G_1 cell cycle arrest (37). Multiple stimuli increase ROS production: mechanical stretch, VEGF, PDGF, elevated glucose, TNFα, oxidized LDL, AngII and lipopolysaccharide (LPS). Ang II- and PDGF-mediated ROS production in VSMC directly activates MAPK signaling pathways necessary for migration and proliferation and p53 signaling in apoptosis (26,38). Pathological blood flow exposes VSMC to increased mechanical stress, which in turn generates ROS production and increased MMP mRNA expression (39). ROS also stimulate VSMC secretion of cyclophilin A (CyPA) which augments the oxidative stress response in VSMC (40). The primary effect of sustained ROS production in the vascular wall is enhanced in VSMC migration, growth or apoptosis depending on the type and concentration of ROS.

THE ROLE OF VSMC IN ATHEROMA EVOLUTION AND COMPLICATIONS

As atheromas develop the vascular wall significantly remodels to compensate for the reduced lumen size. Several important VSMC processes occur during remodeling. The first involves migration of VSMC from the medial layer to the developing neointima. The second is VSMC proliferation in the developing plaque. Finally, VSMC undergo apoptosis eventually contributing to plaque rupture (Figure 98.3). These processes are governed by the molecular and cellular mechanisms previously discussed for remodeling and are described in more detail below.

VSMC Migration and Atherosclerotic Lesions

VSMC migration from the media to the newly developing intima is a primary stage in atherosclerosis development. Migration occurs in response to stimuli including growth factors EGF, IGF-1, PDGF, and in some reports TGF-β (41). Models of vessel injury in carotids induced by balloon injury indicate that VSMC replicate in the media and migrate inward in response to increased platelet adherence to the vascular wall and release of PDGF (5). The effect of PDGF is ROS-dependent such that inhibiting NADPH oxidase decreases ROS production and VSMC chemotaxis (26,42). Activated inflammatory cells in the injured vessel also secrete factors, such as eicosanoids, that induce VSMC migration. Leukotriene B_4 (LTB_4) secreted from infiltrating leukocytes induces ROS production and VSMC chemotaxis. LTB_4 secretion exacerbates VSMC migration and intima hyperplasia because it increases MMP-2 and MMP-9 production (43). Stimulated upregulation and release of MMPs is important since MMPs degrade matrix components and allow VSMC passage into the neointima. The gelatinase MMPs are predominantly responsible for mediating VSMC migration. *In vitro* and *in vivo* experimental models where MMP-2 and MMP-9 expression have been decreased emphasize the importance on these enzymes on neointimal formation (44,45).

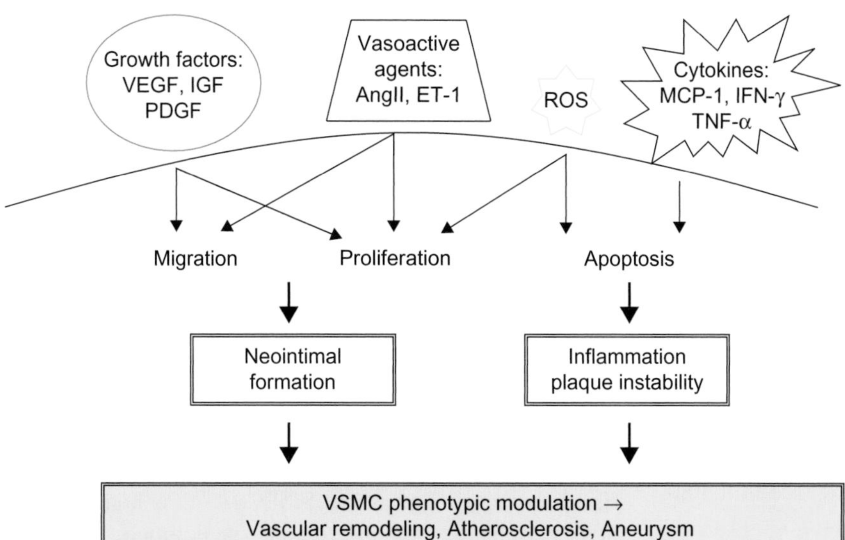

FIGURE 98.3 VSMC phenotypic modulation occurs in response to a number of stimuli in addition to changes in blood flow. Growth factors, vasoactive agents, ROS, and cytokines promote VSMC proliferation, migration, and apoptosis leading to increased vessel wall remodeling and pathological conditions.

VSMC Proliferation and the Development of the Lesion

Markers of cellular proliferation have been identified in human atheromas. While monocytes and macrophages are the primary proliferative cell type, VSMC are the second most abundant cell found in atherosclerotic plaques (46). Multiple stimuli induce proliferation of VSMC, including growth factors and cytokines, ROS, vasoactive agents, and ECM proteins (41). Growth factors are expressed by resident vascular cells and infiltrating inflammatory cells in atherosclerotic lesions. Those shown to increase VSMC proliferation include EGF, basic FGF, IGF-1, interferon-γ (IFN-γ), IL-6, PDGF, thrombin, TGF-α, and tumor necrosis factor-α (TNF-α). Cytokine, EC, and VSMC production of MCP-1 has been shown to increase expression of proliferation activating nuclear antigen (PCNA) and cyclin A (47). VSMC proliferation in response to thrombin and PDGF is ROS-dependent such that inhibition of H_2O_2 production inhibits proliferation (42,48). MMPs and PAs also increase VSMC proliferation. In the balloon catheter injury model uPA stimulates VSMC proliferation and increases neointima formation (49). uPA has also been shown to increase proliferation by potentiating ROS production and recruiting inflammatory cells (17,49,50). Vasoactive agents such as AngII, ET-1, catecholamines, and substance P also induce VSMC proliferation. AngII has received much attention as a stimulus of protein synthesis in VSMC since activation of its receptors on the cell membrane results in increased production of H_2O_2, MAPK signaling, and VSMC-mediated neointimal formation (51).

Cell proliferation is regulated by cell cycle-dependent kinases (CDKs), CDK inhibitor proteins (CKIs), CDK-interacting proteins ($p27^{Kip}$ and $p21^{Cip}$), and p53. Studies using the balloon injury model have demonstrated the time course of cell cycle gene expression following injury. In the initial hours post injury there is a rapid increase in protooncogene expression of *c-fos*, *c-jun*, and *c-myc,* which is followed by an increase in DNA synthesis. There is also a decrease in $p27^{Kip}$ and $p21^{Cip}$, disinhibiting the CDKs and allowing cell cycle progression from G_0/G_1 to S. In the media and intima there is also an increase in PCNA and cyclins E and A markers of increased cell proliferation. However, following 1 day of injury there is an increase in cell cycle inhibitors p53 and $p21^{Cip}$, presumably to compensate for the initial increase in proliferation (52).

VSMC Apoptosis and Plaque Rupture

A balance of pro-apoptotic and anti-apoptotic pathways in VSMC is integral to vascular wall homeostasis. Upon injury, pro-apoptotic signaling is increased. Ligands such as FasL, oxidized LDL, IFN-γ, TNF-α, serum derived factor-1α (SDF-1α), TGF-β, ROS, and NO stimulate VSMC apoptosis (53). Acute VSMC apoptosis in early atheroma formation is considered beneficial. As an example, inhibiting Bcl-x expression in neointimal cells induces apoptosis and results in lesion regression (54). However, chronic levels of apoptosis negatively affect lesion development. In a mouse model where VSMC apoptosis was specifically induced, vessels exhibited accelerated atherosclerosis, intimal calcification, medial degeneration, and medial expansion (55). In atherosclerotic vessels VSMC apoptosis is particularly important since these cells synthesize the proteins necessary to maintain the integrity of the fibrous cap. In late stages of atherosclerosis, VSMC present in the fibrous cap develop granulovesicular degeneration and increased Bax, caspace

3 expression and TUNEL positive staining. These cells are flattened in morphology and have a decreased ability to produce ECM, specifically collagen type I which can be mediated by increased MMP activation via FasL stimulation (31). Furthermore, uPA increases NADPH oxidase expression which in turn enhances VSMC apoptosis (49,50). These factors weaken the fibrous cap and under conditions of chronic inflammation the fibrous cap thins and ruptures, exposing the contents of the necrotic lipid core (NLC) to the circulation (37).

Aneurysm Formation

Aneurysm formation is a particularly common vascular abnormality in elderly humans. The exact mechanisms remain uncertain, but clearly involve increased inflammation and VSMC apoptosis resulting in disruption of lamellae and medial thinning (56). The infrarenal abdominal aorta is more susceptible to aneurysm and occlusive plaques in comparison to the thoracic aorta (57). Aortic enlargement and lesion development are correlative. Atherosclerotic plaques that develop in the abdominal aorta typically consist of larger NLCs and are prone to rupture, promoting further vessel enlargement, medial weakening and increased abdominal aortic aneurysm (AAA) susceptibility (57). The thinning of the medial wall is attributed to degeneration of the elastic properties due in large part to VSMC senescence and apoptosis (58). The environment in the vessel is highly inflammatory which stimulates proapoptotic signaling in the VSMC, evident by elevated levels of p53 and p21 in the vascular wall (59). Increased apoptosis leads to a decrease in matrix protein secretion, including matrix MMP9 and MMP2, diminishing tissue repair (60). With the increased apoptosis there are elevated levels of ROS (61,62) which promote release of cytokines including CyPA (40). The secretion of CyPA potentiates the response to oxidative stress and augments VSMC apoptosis, increasing AAA susceptibility.

ROLE OF ADULT PROGENITOR CELLS IN VSMC REMODELING DURING ATHEROSCLEROSIS

It is well accepted that VSMC are integral in the manifestation of vascular wall repair and pathology. However, VSMC progenitor cells have been given increasingly greater attention with regard to their role in atherosclerosis development. Multipotent vascular stem cell progenitors, mesenchymal stem cells, circulating vascular smooth muscle progenitor cells, vascular wall resident smooth muscle progenitor cells and extravascular non-bone marrow smooth muscle cells are found in the vascular wall (63). These progenitor cells have the ability to differentiate into VSMC but their precise contribution in atherosclerosis has not been completely elucidated.

A primary early event in atheroma development is the accumulation of VSMC in the neointima and fibrous cap of plaques. The source of these VSMC is believed to be not only from migratory medial VSMC, but also from VSMC generated from smooth muscle progenitor cells (SMPC) (64). In atherosclerotic lesions in ApoE-deficient mice transplanted with bone marrow from GFP-expressing mice there was a population of cells found in the developing intima that were not derived from medial VSMC, indicating that bone marrow-derived SMPC contribute to lesion development (65). Bone marrow-derived SMPC secrete growth factors and cytokines but do not actually reside in the fibrous cap of the plaque. This evidence strongly suggests that SMPC from the bone marrow and peripheral blood promote neointimal formation (66,67).

ROLE OF GENETICS IN VSMC REMODELING LEADING TO ATHEROSCLEROSIS

Genetics plays a major role in atherosclerosis development. A highly predictive factor for subclinical atherosclerosis in humans is carotid IMT, which is measured by intravascular ultrasound and is a genetically determined trait involving VSMC remodeling (68–70). Microarray analyses have identified candidate genes that regulate VSMC-mediated vascular remodeling. As discussed, oxidative stress plays a significant role in atherosclerosis development. Microarrays performed on VSMC from wild-type and NADPH oxidase-deficient mice demonstrated that NAD(P)H oxidase-mediated regulation of ROS dependent genes CD44, BMP4, Id1, and Id3 was important in VSMC remodeling in atherosclerosis and restenosis (71). Id3 was also identified in human IMT as an important regulator of atherosclerosis (72). Thrombospondin-1 (TSP-1), an ECM protein and potent inducer of VSMC migration and proliferation, has been shown to be upregulated in diabetic models. A microarray in VSMC stimulated with TSP-1 identified 10 genes associated with atherosclerosis development (UGDH, TGFβ2, HAS2, SLC2A1, TIMP3, THBS1, Serpine1, GART, and SRF) (73). Microarray analysis of SJL/J and C3H/FeJ mice, which vary significantly in the IMT response to low flow, demonstrated increased expression of inflammatory factors, IL18 and macrophage inhibitory factor (MIF) (74).

FUTURE DIRECTIONS

Vascular remodeling is a complex process that involves physical, biochemical and genetic components. Biological and physiological studies have greatly elucidated the mechanisms by which VSMC undergo phenotypic modulation and promote neointima formation. As genetic technologies advance, this already large body of literature will expand. While our understanding of the genetic basis of vascular remodeling increases, the future challenges will require systems biology approaches. Specifically, gene profiling now enables the transcriptome to be analyzed and mass spectrometry enables the proteome to be characterized. However, many diseases involve complex interactions among proteins mediated by post-translational modifications (e.g., acylation, glycation, nitrosylation, oxidation, phosphorylation, SUMOylation, ubiquitination). Finally, alterations in key metabolic products (the metabolome) play critical roles in the vasculature. Furthermore, alterations in ECM and cell–cell interactions within the wall are critical determinants of vascular remodeling. It is likely that recruitment of pluripotent stem cells also contributes to vascular remodeling. In summary, our understanding of the multiple mechanisms involved in VSMC vascular remodeling should facilitate development of therapies to treat aneurysms, atherosclerosis, and restenosis.

REFERENCES

1. Mulvany MJ, Baumbach GL, Aalkjaer C, Heagerty AM, Korsgaard N, Schiffrin EL, et al. Vascular remodeling. *Hypertension* 1996;**28**: 505–6.
2. Langille BL, O'Donnell F. Reductions in arterial diameter produced by chronic decreases in blood flow are endothelium-dependent. *Science* 1986;**231**:405–7.
3. Langille BL, Reidy MA, Kline RL. Injury and repair of endothelium at sites of flow disturbances near abdominal aortic coarctations in rabbits. *Arteriosclerosis* 1986;**6**:146–54.
4. Glagov S, Weisenberg E, Zarins CK, Stankunavicius R, Kolettis GJ. Compensatory enlargement of human atherosclerotic coronary arteries. *N Engl J Med* 1987;**316**:1371–5.
5. Schwartz SM, Geary RL, Adams LD. Vascular failure: a hypothesis. *Curr Atheroscler Rep* 2003;**5**:201–7.
6. Korshunov VA, Schwartz SM, Berk BC. Vascular remodeling: hemodynamic and biochemical mechanisms underlying Glagov's phenomenon. *Arterioscler Thromb Vasc Biol* 2007;**27**:1722–8.
7. Ibrahim J, Miyashiro JK, Berk BC. Shear stress is differentially regulated among inbred rat strains. *Circ Res* 2003;**92**:1001–9.
8. Korshunov VA, Berk BC. Flow-induced vascular remodeling in the mouse: a model for carotid intima-media thickening. *Arterioscler Thromb Vasc Biol* 2003;**23**:2185–91.
9. Miyashiro JK, Poppa V, Berk BC. Flow-induced vascular remodeling in the rat carotid artery diminishes with age. *Circ Res* 1997;**81**:311–9.
10. Hollestelle SC, De Vries MR, Van Keulen JK, Schoneveld AH, Vink A, Strijder CF, et al. Toll-like receptor 4 is involved in outward arterial remodeling. *Circulation* 2004;**109**:393–8.
11. Khatri JJ, Johnson C, Magid R, Lessner SM, Laude KM, Dikalov SI, et al. Vascular oxidant stress enhances progression and angiogenesis of experimental atheroma. *Circulation* 2004;**109**:520–5.
12. Rudic RD, Bucci M, Fulton D, Segal SS, Sessa WC. Temporal events underlying arterial remodeling after chronic flow reduction in mice: correlation of structural changes with a deficit in basal nitric oxide synthesis. *Circ Res* 2000;**86**:1160–6.
13. Yamamoto K, Sokabe T, Matsumoto T, Yoshimura K, Shibata M, Ohura N, et al. Impaired flow-dependent control of vascular tone and remodeling in P2X4-deficient mice. *Nature Med* 2006;**12**:133–7.
14. Yogo K, Shimokawa H, Funakoshi H, Kandabashi T, Miyata K, Okamoto S, et al. Different vasculoprotective roles of NO synthase isoforms in vascular lesion formation in mice. *Arterioscler Thromb Vasc Biol* 2000;**20**:E96–100.
15. Hilgers RH, Schiffers PM, Aartsen WM, Fazzi GE, Smits JF, De Mey JG. Tissue angiotensin-converting enzyme in imposed and physiological flow-related arterial remodeling in mice. *Arterioscler Thromb Vasc Biol* 2004;**24**:892–7.
16. Korshunov VA, Massett MP, Carey RM, Berk BC. Role of angiotensin-converting enzyme and neutral endopeptidase in flow-dependent remodeling. *J Vascular Res* 2004;**41**:148–56.
17. Korshunov VA, Solomatina MA, Plekhanova OS, Parfyonova YV, Tkachuk VA, Berk BC. Plasminogen activator expression correlates with genetic differences in vascular remodeling. *J Vasc Res* 2004;**41**:481–90.
18. Cox JL, Gotlieb AI. Restenosis following percutaneous transluminal angioplasty: clinical, physiologic and pathological features. *CMAJ* 1986;**134**:1129–32.
19. Courtman DW, Schwartz SM, Hart CE. Sequential injury of the rabbit abdominal aorta induces intramural coagulation and luminal narrowing independent of intimal mass: extrinsic pathway inhibition eliminates luminal narrowing. *Circ Res* 1998;**82**:996–1006.
20. Murphy GJ, Angelini GD. Insights into the pathogenesis of vein graft disease: lessons from intravascular ultrasound. *Cardiovasc Ultrasound* 2004;**2**:8.
21. Berk BC. Vascular smooth muscle growth: autocrine growth mechanisms. *Physiol Rev* 2001;**81**:999–1030.
22. Berk BC. Atheroprotective signaling mechanisms activated by steady laminar flow in endothelial cells. *Circulation* 2008;**117**:1082–9.
23. Pan S. Molecular mechanisms responsible for the atheroprotective effects of laminar shear stress. *Antioxid Redox Signal* 2009;**11**:1669–82.
24. Chatzizisis YS, Coskun AU, Jonas M, Edelman ER, Feldman CL, Stone PH. Role of endothelial shear stress in the natural history of coronary atherosclerosis and vascular remodeling: molecular, cellular, and vascular behavior. *J Am Coll Cardiol* 2007;**49**: 2379–93.
25. Chien S. Effects of disturbed flow on endothelial cells. *Ann Biomed Eng* 2008;**36**:554–62.
26. Taniyama Y, Griendling KK. Reactive oxygen species in the vasculature: molecular and cellular mechanisms. *Hypertension* 2003;**42**:1075–81.
27. Brown DJ, Rzucidlo EM, Merenick BL, Wagner RJ, Martin KA, Powell RJ. Endothelial cell activation of the smooth muscle cell phosphoinositide 3-kinase/Akt pathway promotes differentiation. *J Vasc Surg* 2005;**41**:509–16.
28. Brown DJ, Schermerhorn ML, Powell RJ, Fillinger MF, Rzucidlo EM, Walsh DB, et al. Mesenteric stenting for chronic mesenteric ischemia. *J Vasc Surg* 2005;**42**:268–74.

29. Fingerle J, Au YP, Clowes AW, Reidy MA. Intimal lesion formation in rat carotid arteries after endothelial denudation in absence of medial injury. *Arteriosclerosis* 1990;**10**:1082–7.
30. Redmond EM, Cahill PA, Sitzmann JV. Flow-mediated regulation of endothelin receptors in cocultured vascular smooth muscle cells: an endothelium-dependent effect. *J Vasc Res* 1997;**34**:425–35.
31. Garcia-Touchard A, Henry TD, Sangiorgi G, Spagnoli LG, Mauriello A, Conover C, et al. Extracellular proteases in atherosclerosis and restenosis. *Arterioscler Thromb Vasc Biol* 2005;**25**:1119–27.
32. Newby AC. Matrix metalloproteinases regulate migration, proliferation, and death of vascular smooth muscle cells by degrading matrix and non-matrix substrates. *Cardiovasc Res* 2006;**69**:614–24.
33. Newby AC, Pauschinger M, Spinale FG. From tadpole tails to transgenic mice: metalloproteinases have brought about a metamorphosis in our understanding of cardiovascular disease. *Cardiovasc Res* 2006;**69**:559–61.
34. Bobik A, Tkachuk V. Metalloproteinases and plasminogen activators in vessel remodeling. *Curr Hypertens Rep* 2003;**5**:466–72.
35. Hojo Y, Ikeda U, Maeda Y, Takahashi M, Takizawa T, Okada M, et al. Interaction between human monocytes and vascular smooth muscle cells induces vascular endothelial growth factor expression. *Atherosclerosis* 2000;**150**:63–70.
36. Sarkar R, Webb RC. Does nitric oxide regulate smooth muscle cell proliferation? A critical appraisal. *J Vasc Res* 1998;**35**:135–42.
37. Kockx MM, Herman AG. Apoptosis in atherosclerosis: beneficial or detrimental? *Cardiovasc Res* 2000;**45**:736–46.
38. Dimmeler S, Zeiher AM. Reactive oxygen species and vascular cell apoptosis in response to angiotensin II and pro-atherosclerotic factors. *Regulatory Peptides* 2000;**90**:19–25.
39. Grote K, Flach I, Luchtefeld M, Akin E, Holland SM, Drexler H, et al. Mechanical stretch enhances mRNA expression and proenzyme release of matrix metalloproteinase-2 (MMP-2) via NAD(P)H oxidase-derived reactive oxygen species. *Circ Res* 2003;**92**:e80–86.
40. Satoh K, Nigro P, Berk BC. Oxidative stress and vascular smooth muscle cell growth: a mechanistic linkage by cyclophilin A. *Antioxid Redox Signal* **12**:675–682.
41. Raines EW, Ross R. Smooth muscle cells and the pathogenesis of the lesions of atherosclerosis. *Br Heart J* 1993;**69**(1 Suppl):S30–7.
42. Sundaresan M, Yu ZX, Ferrans VJ, Irani K, Finkel T. Requirement for generation of H_2O_2 for platelet-derived growth factor signal transduction. *Science* 1995;**270**:296–9.
43. Hlawaty H, Jacob MP, Louedec L, Letourneur D, Brink C, Michel JB, et al. Leukotriene receptor antagonism and the prevention of extracellular matrix degradation during atherosclerosis and in-stent stenosis. *Arterioscler Thromb Vasc Biol* 2009;**29**:518–24.
44. Galis ZS, Khatri JJ. Matrix metalloproteinases in vascular remodeling and atherogenesis: the good, the bad, and the ugly. *Circ Res* 2002;**90**:251–62.
45. Pyo R, Lee JK, Shipley JM, Curci JA, Mao D, Ziporin SJ, et al. Targeted gene disruption of matrix metalloproteinase-9 (gelatinase B) suppresses development of experimental abdominal aortic aneurysms. *J Clin Invest* 2000;**105**:1641–9.
46. Fuster JJ, Fernandez P, Gonzalez-Navarro H, Silvestre C, Nabah YN, Andres V. Control of cell proliferation in atherosclerosis: insights from animal models and human studies. *Cardiovascular Research* **86** (2):254–264.
47. Selzman CH, Miller SA, Zimmerman MA, Gamboni-Robertson F, Harken AH, Banerjee A. Monocyte chemotactic protein-1 directly induces human vascular smooth muscle proliferation. *Am J Physiol* 2002;**283**:H1455–61.
48. Patterson C, Ruef J, Madamanchi NR, Barry-Lane P, Hu Z, Horaist C, et al. Stimulation of a vascular smooth muscle cell NAD(P)H oxidase by thrombin. Evidence that p47(phox) may participate in forming this oxidase in vitro and in vivo. *J Biol Chem* 1999;**274**:19814–22.
49. Plekhanova O, Parfyonova Y, Bibilashvily R, Domogatskii S, Stepanova V, Gulba DC, et al. Urokinase plasminogen activator augments cell proliferation and neointima formation in injured arteries via proteolytic mechanisms. *Atherosclerosis* 2001;**159**:297–306.
50. Plekhanova OS, Men'shikov MY, Bashtrykov PP, Berk BC, Tkachuk VA, Parfenova EV. Urokinase induces ROS production in vascular smooth muscle cells. *Bull Exp Biol Med* 2006;**142**:304–7.
51. Schmidt-Ott KM, Kagiyama S, Phillips MI. The multiple actions of angiotensin II in atherosclerosis. *Regul Peptides* 2000;**93**:65–77.
52. Braun-Dullaeus RC, Mann MJ, Dzau VJ. Cell cycle progression: new therapeutic target for vascular proliferative disease. *Circulation* 1998;**98**:82–9.
53. Korshunov VA, Berk BC. Smooth muscle apoptosis and vascular remodeling. *Curr Opin Hematol* 2008;**15**:250–4.
54. Pollman MJ, Hall JL, Mann MJ, Zhang L, Gibbons GH. Inhibition of neointimal cell bcl-x expression induces apoptosis and regression of vascular disease. *Nature Med* 1998;**4**:222–7.
55. Clarke MC, Littlewood TD, Figg N, Maguire JJ, Davenport AP, Goddard M, et al. Chronic apoptosis of vascular smooth muscle cells accelerates atherosclerosis and promotes calcification and medial degeneration. *Circ Res* 2008;**102**:1529–38.
56. Daugherty A, Cassis LA. Mechanisms of abdominal aortic aneurysm formation. *Curr Atheroscler Rep* 2002;**4**:222–7.
57. Zarins CK, Xu C, Glagov S. Atherosclerotic enlargement of the human abdominal aorta. *Atherosclerosis* 2001;**155**:157–64.
58. Kunieda T, Minamino T, Katsuno T, Tateno K, Nishi J, Miyauchi H, et al. Cellular senescence impairs circadian expression of clock genes in vitro and in vivo. *Circ Res* 2006;**98**:532–9.
59. Thompson RW, Liao S, Curci JA. Vascular smooth muscle cell apoptosis in abdominal aortic aneurysms. *Coron Artery Dis* 1997;**8**:623–31.
60. Thompson RW, Baxter BT. MMP inhibition in abdominal aortic aneurysms. Rationale for a prospective randomized clinical trial. *Ann NY Acad Sci* 1999;**878**:159–78.
61. Griendling KK, FitzGerald GA. Oxidative stress and cardiovascular injury: Part II: animal and human studies. *Circulation* 2003;**108**:2034–40.
62. Griendling KK, FitzGerald GA. Oxidative stress and cardiovascular injury: Part I: basic mechanisms and in vivo monitoring of ROS. *Circulation* 2003;**108**:1912–6.
63. Orlandi A, Bennett M. Progenitor cell-derived smooth muscle cells in vascular disease. *Biochem Pharmacol* **79**:1706–1713.
64. Qian H, Yang Y, Li J, Huang J, Dou K, Yang G. The role of vascular stem cells in atherogenesis and post-angioplasty restenosis. *Ageing Res Rev* 2007;**6**:109–27.
65. Sata M. Circulating vascular progenitor cells contribute to vascular repair, remodeling, and lesion formation. *Trends Cardiovasc Med* 2003;**13**:249–53.

66. Saiura A, Sata M, Hirata Y, Nagai R, Makuuchi M. Circulating smooth muscle progenitor cells contribute to atherosclerosis. *Nature Med* 2001;**7**:382–3.
67. Sata M, Saiura A, Kunisato A, Tojo A, Okada S, Tokuhisa T, et al. Hematopoietic stem cells differentiate into vascular cells that participate in the pathogenesis of atherosclerosis. *Nature Med* 2002;**8**:403–9.
68. Davis PH, Dawson JD, Riley WA, Lauer RM. Carotid intimal-medial thickness is related to cardiovascular risk factors measured from childhood through middle age: the muscatine study. *Circulation* 2001;**104**:2815–9.
69. Lorenz MW, Markus HS, Bots ML, Rosvall M, Sitzer M. Prediction of clinical cardiovascular events with carotid intima-media thickness: a systematic review and meta-analysis. *Circulation* 2007;**115**:459–67.
70. Sacco RL, Blanton SH, Slifer S, Beecham A, Glover K, Gardener H, et al. Heritability and linkage analysis for carotid intima-media thickness: the family study of stroke risk and carotid atherosclerosis. *Stroke* 2009;**40**:2307–12.
71. Vendrov AE, Madamanchi NR, Hakim ZS, Rojas M, Runge MS. Thrombin and NAD(P)H oxidase-mediated regulation of CD44 and BMP4-Id pathway in VSMC, restenosis, and atherosclerosis. *Circ Res* 2006;**98**:1254–63.
72. Doran AC, Lehtinen AB, Meller N, Lipinski MJ, Slayton RP, Oldham SN, et al. Id3 is a novel atheroprotective factor containing a functionally significant single-nucleotide polymorphism associated with intima-media thickness in humans. *Circ Res* **106**:1303–1311.
73. Maier KG, Han X, Sadowitz B, Gentile KL, Middleton FA, Gahtan V. Thrombospondin-1: a proatherosclerotic protein augmented by hyperglycemia. *J Vasc Surg* **51**:1238–1247.
74. Korshunov VA, Nikonenko TA, Tkachuk VA, Brooks A, Berk BC. Interleukin-18 and macrophage migration inhibitory factor are associated with increased carotid intima-media thickening. *Arterioscler Thromb Vasc Biol* 2006;**26**:295–300.

Chapter 99

Arterial Hypertension

Rhian M. Touyz[1] and Ernesto L. Schiffrin[2]

[1]*Kidney Research Centre, Ottawa Hospital Research Institute, University of Ottawa, Ontario, Canada,* [2]*Lady Davis Institute for Medical Research and Department of Medicine, Sir Mortimer B. Davis-Jewish General Hospital, McGill University, Montreal, Canada*

INTRODUCTION

Small arteries (lumen diameter <300 μm) are responsible for blood pressure (BP) control and regional distribution of blood flow, through effects on vascular resistance (1). Based on Poiseuille's law, vessel resistance is inversely proportional to the radius (lumen diameter) to the fourth power (r^4) and accordingly small changes in lumen size result in marked changes in resistance (2). The lumen diameter of resistance arteries is a function of vasomotor tone (vasoconstriction/vasodilation) and the structural characteristics of the vessel. Vasomotor control underlies acute rapid adaptation of vessel diameter, due mainly to vasoconstriction exerted by the active contraction of vascular smooth muscle cells (VSMC) in the vessel media, whereas alterations in structure constitute a dynamic process occurring in response to chronic hemodynamic variations. Initially structural changes are adaptive, but subsequently become maladaptive resulting in alterations in media thickness and lumen diameter (2,3). This process, called vascular remodeling, contributes to the pathophysiology of vascular diseases, including hypertension (4,5).

Acute regulation of vascular diameter depends on the activation/deactivation of the contractile machinery involving actin–myosin interaction in VSMCs. Changes in intracellular calcium concentration, ion fluxes, and membrane potential lead to calcium–calmodulin-mediated phosphorylation of the regulatory myosin light chains and actin–myosin cross-bridge cycling with consequent rapid VSMC contraction (3). Calcium-independent mechanisms associated with changes in calcium sensitization and actin filament remodeling contribute to intermediate and more chronic processes regulating vascular lumen diameter (2).

The lumen diameter of resistance arteries is governed not only by the magnitude of vasoconstriction, but also by the structural characteristics of the vessel wall, influenced by vascular remodeling processes (3). At the molecular and cellular levels remodeling involves changes in cytoskeletal organization, cell-to-cell connections, and altered growth/apoptosis, senescence, calcification, inflammation, and rearrangement of VSMCs (2,6). At the extracellular level, remodeling is influenced by changes in matrix protein composition and reorganization of proteoglycans, collagens (type I and III), and fibronectin, which provide tensile strength, and elastin, responsible for vascular elasticity (7). These sub-cellular, cellular, and extracellular matrix (ECM) events manifest as structural changes with modifications in lumen diameter, wall thickness, and media and adventitia cross-sectional areas, processes that define remodeling. With respect to resistance arteries, the most widely used classification of vascular remodeling is that described by Mulvany et al. (8), where changes in the passive luminal diameter may be increased (outward) or decreased (inward) and media mass (cross-sectional area) may be increased, unchanged or reduced (hypertrophic, eutrophic, hypotrophic respectively) (8,9) (Figure 99.1). Whether increased pressure itself or other factors are responsible for the initiation of vascular remodeling remains unclear, but the endothelium probably plays an important role as it is a sensor of hemodynamic and humoral factors and is a moderator of signals to underlying VSMCs critically involved in the remodeling process (10). Remodeling allows arteries to withstand an increased pressure load and under physiological conditions (e.g., aging and exercise) is adaptive. Pathological remodeling occurs when the adaptive process is overwhelmed, resulting in rigid, stiff, and poorly compliant vessels, typically observed in hypertension. Molecular and cellular mechanisms implicated in changes in vasomotor tone and structural remodeling in hypertension involve multiple cell types, complex signaling pathways, and multiple local and circulating factors. The present chapter focuses on the role of VSMCs in the regulation of vascular function (contraction) and structure (remodeling) in hypertension.

Muscle. DOI: http://dx.doi.org/10.1016/B978-0-12-381510-1.00099-5

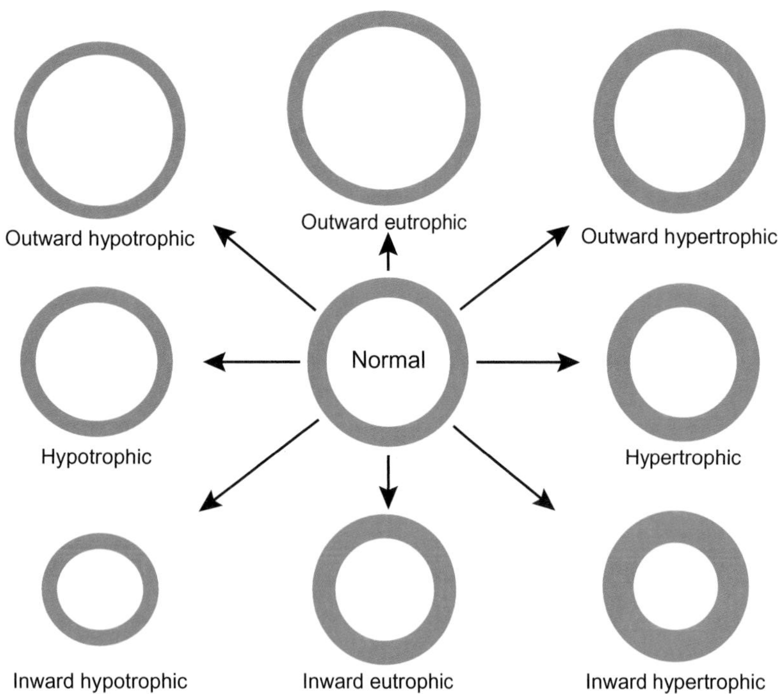

FIGURE 99.1 **Remodeling of vessels.** Changes in lumen diameter and media mass (cross-sectional area) define the different patterns of vascular remodeling (5,8,9). Vessel narrowing with increased wall thickness occurs in chronic hypertension (hypertrophic remodeling), while mild hypertension is associated with smaller lumen and no increase in cross-sectional area (eutrophic remodeling).

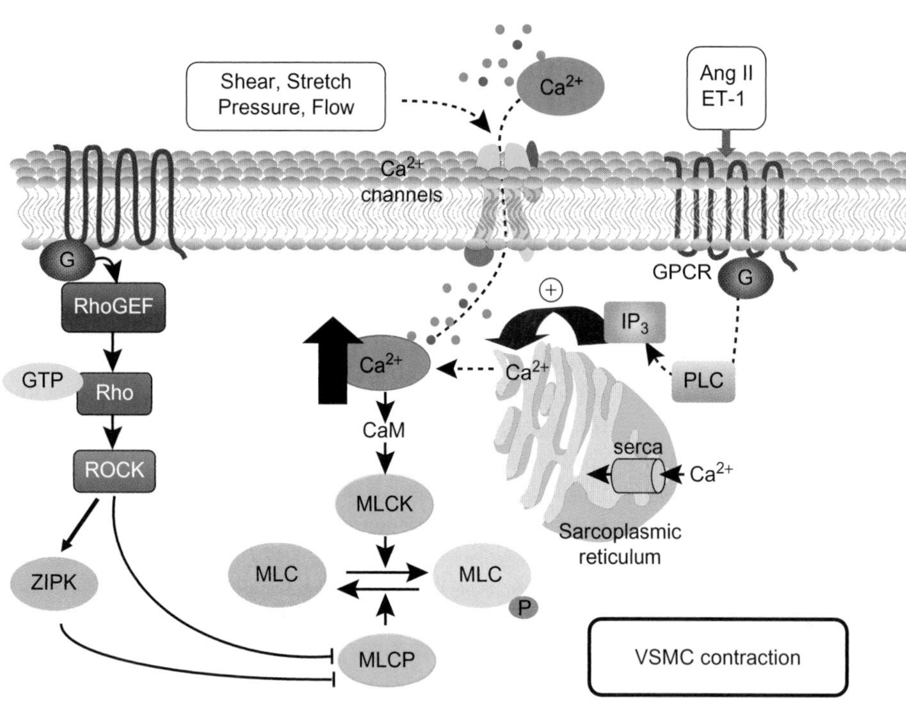

FIGURE 99.2 **Signaling pathways that regulate VSMC contraction.** VSMC is activated by phosphorylation of myosin light chain (MLC) by MLC kinase (MLCK) activated by Ca^{2+}/calmodulin (CaM). Ligand-receptor binding induces G-protein-coupled receptor (GPCR) activation and stimulation of PLC-IP_3-induced release of Ca^{2+} from sarcoplasmic reticulum (SR) and activation of SERCA (SR ATPase). Activation of the RhoA/ROCK pathway and stimulation of ZIP kinase (ZIPK) leads to MLC phosphatase (MLCP) inhibition and increased Ca^{2+} sensitization. These pathways are upregulated in hypertension.

VASCULAR SMOOTH MUSCLE AND VASCULAR FUNCTIONAL CHANGES IN HYPERTENSION

Smooth muscle cells constitute the bulk of the arterial wall, playing a key function in vascular resistance and blood flow. Basal vascular tone and contractility are increased in hypertension. The contractile machinery of vascular smooth muscle, actin and myosin, is activated in a Ca^{2+}-dependent and Ca^{2+}-independent manner (Figure 99.2). The key event in VSMC excitation–contraction coupling is an increase in intracellular free Ca^{2+} concentration ($[Ca^{2+}]_i$) in response to agonist-induced activation of receptors coupled to phopholipase C

(PLC), responses that are upregulated in experimental and human hypertension (3,11–13) (see Chapter 86 on calcium homeostasis and Chapter 87 on regulation of smooth muscle contraction). In addition to VSMC-derived factors regulating tone, endothelium-derived factors, such as prostacyclin, PGH_2, and thromboxane A_2 act as endothelium-derived contracting factors (EDCF) that counteract the vasodilator effect of nitric oxide (NO) (14). Increased generation of EDCFs has been demonstrated in human essential hypertension (15,16) and in spontaneously hypertensive rats (SHR) (14), and further contributes to increased vascular tone in hypertension.

Smooth muscle myosin can also be phosphorylated in a Ca^{2+}-independent manner by additional kinases like Rho kinase (ROCK) (17), integrin-linked kinase (ILK) (18), and zipper-interacting protein kinase (ZIPK) (19) (see Chapter 87). These Ca^{2+}-independent processes influence contraction by increasing Ca^{2+} sensitization and by actin filament remodeling. Rho kinases (ROCK1 and ROCK2) are serine/threonine kinases and are downstream effectors of the small GTPase RhoA. RhoA is abundantly expressed in VSMC and is rapidly activated by vasoconstrictors, such as Ang II via the $G_{12/13}$ family of G proteins and G_q (20). RhoGEFs, which catalyze exchange of GDP for GTP on RhoA, are sensitive to $G_{12/13}$ such as Arhgef1 (p115RhoGEF), Arhgef12 (LARG), and Arhgef11 (PDZ-RhoGEF), and hence play an important role in RhoA activation (21). Increased RhoA/Rho kinase activity leads to decreased MLCP activation and consequent sustained vasoconstriction and blood pressure elevation.

Ang II-induced hypertension in rodents exhibits increased vascular RhoA/Rho kinase activation, without changes in expression (22). This is associated with increased activity of Arhgef1, implicated to be important in RhoA hyperactivation, vasoconstriction, and hypertension (23). Pharmacological inhibition of Rho kinase with fasudil or Y27632 suppresses acute pressor responses of Ang II, but does not reduce BP chronically, supporting the role of RhoA/Rho kinase in acute vasoconstriction, rather than in mechanisms associated with adaptive vascular remodeling in hypertension that occur chronically with Ang II infusion (23–25). Clinical studies have demonstrated beneficial effects of ROCK inhibitors. The isoquinoline derivative fasudil has been used clinically since 1995 and proven to be successful in preventing vasospasm associated with subarachnoid hemorrhage (26), acute ischemic stroke (27), angina pectoris (28), coronary artery spasm, pulmonary arterial hypertension (29), atherosclerosis (30), and in the regulation of vascular tone in hypertensive renal transplant recipients (31). Therapeutic use of ROCK inhibitors in human essential hypertension is not yet approved, but may be an interesting therapeutic strategy.

In addition to the Ca^{2+}-dependent and -independent modulation of MLC_{20} phosphorylation, changes in organization of actin filaments, intermediate filaments, and microtubules play an important role in the acute phase of VSMC contraction. Increased polymerization of actin, tyrosine phosphorylation of paxillin, activation of small GTP-binding proteins Rho and Cdc42 and conformational changes in focal adhesion sites result in stiffening and reorganization of the cytoskeleton (6). This dynamic arrangement of the actin cytoskeleton is key in maintaining vascular tone and plasticity, especially important in the regulation of vascular diameter related to pressure-dependent myogenic tone.

VASCULAR SMOOTH MUSCLE AND VASCULAR STRUCTURAL CHANGES IN HYPERTENSION

In hypertension, resistance arteries undergo vascular remodeling characterized by reduced vascular lumen with increased media thickness (2,5,32). Myogenic tone, the intrinsic ability of vessels to constrict in response to increased intraluminal pressure, contributes to structural alterations within the arterial wall. On the other hand, structural narrowing of the lumen may amplify vasoconstriction. Eutrophic vascular remodeling, characterized by reduced outer diameter and lumen with no change in media mass and cross-sectional area (32,33), is observed in patients with mild–moderate hypertension. With chronic vasoconstriction and longstanding or severe hypertension, blood vessels develop hypertrophy in response to increased wall stress. Chronic vasoconstriction associated with deposition of extracellular matrix which characterizes hypertensive vascular remodeling may lead to a smaller lumen as the constricted state becomes embedded in the newly deposited extracellular matrix (33). Changes in the interaction between extracellular matrix components and integrins on the cell membrane of smooth muscle cells may also contribute to the remodeling of arteries in hypertension (34). Other mechanisms that may participate include inward growth encroaching on the lumen associated with apoptosis of cells in the periphery of the vessel wall. Some studies have implicated tissue transglutaminases that participate in the interactions of fibrillar components in extracellular matrix (ECM) that attach to smooth muscle cells and play a role in signal transduction. VSMC growth may predominate over apoptosis, and in this scenario, remodeling may be hypertrophic (32–35). This type of vascular remodeling is characterized by an increased media cross-section and media to lumen ratio (M/L). The process of remodeling is dynamic and eutrophic and hypertrophic remodeling may occur simultaneously in different vascular beds. Hypertrophic remodeling of resistance arteries is more common in renovascular hypertension, diabetes, acromegaly, and hyperaldosteronism (36–38). Inflammation and extracellular matrix deposition are critically involved in these processes and activation of the RAS also plays a role in the development of hypertension-induced vascular remodeling (39).

MOLECULAR AND CELLULAR MECHANISMS OF VASCULAR REMODELING

Molecular mechanisms underlying vascular remodeling are complex and multifactorial, but activation of the RAS, stimulation of growth signaling pathways, induction of pro-inflammatory responses and modification of ECM components appear to be most important. VSMCs are dynamic, plastic, multifunctional cells, which contribute to arterial remodeling through various processes, including growth (hyperplasia and hypertrophy), apoptosis, cell elongation, reorganization, realignment and inflammation (39,40) (Figure 99.3). Their content in the media increases with decreasing diameter, and constitutes up to 85% in small arteries. Agonist-stimulated growth and profibrotic effects are modulated, in part, by endogenous production of mitogenic factors, such as TGF-β, PDGF, EGF, IGF-1 and ET-1 (39,41). Of these, TGF-β, a multifunctional cytokine, appears to be especially important. TGF-β increases extracellular matrix biosynthesis, downregulates matrix degradative enzymes, and influences integrin receptors (42). TGF-β, synthesized by macrophages, lymphocytes, fibroblasts, and VSMCs, elicits effects by interacting with two signaling receptors, a type II TGF-β receptor and a type I receptor (ALK-5). Major downstream profibrogenic mediators of TGF-β include p38MAPK, ERK1/2. TGF-β is

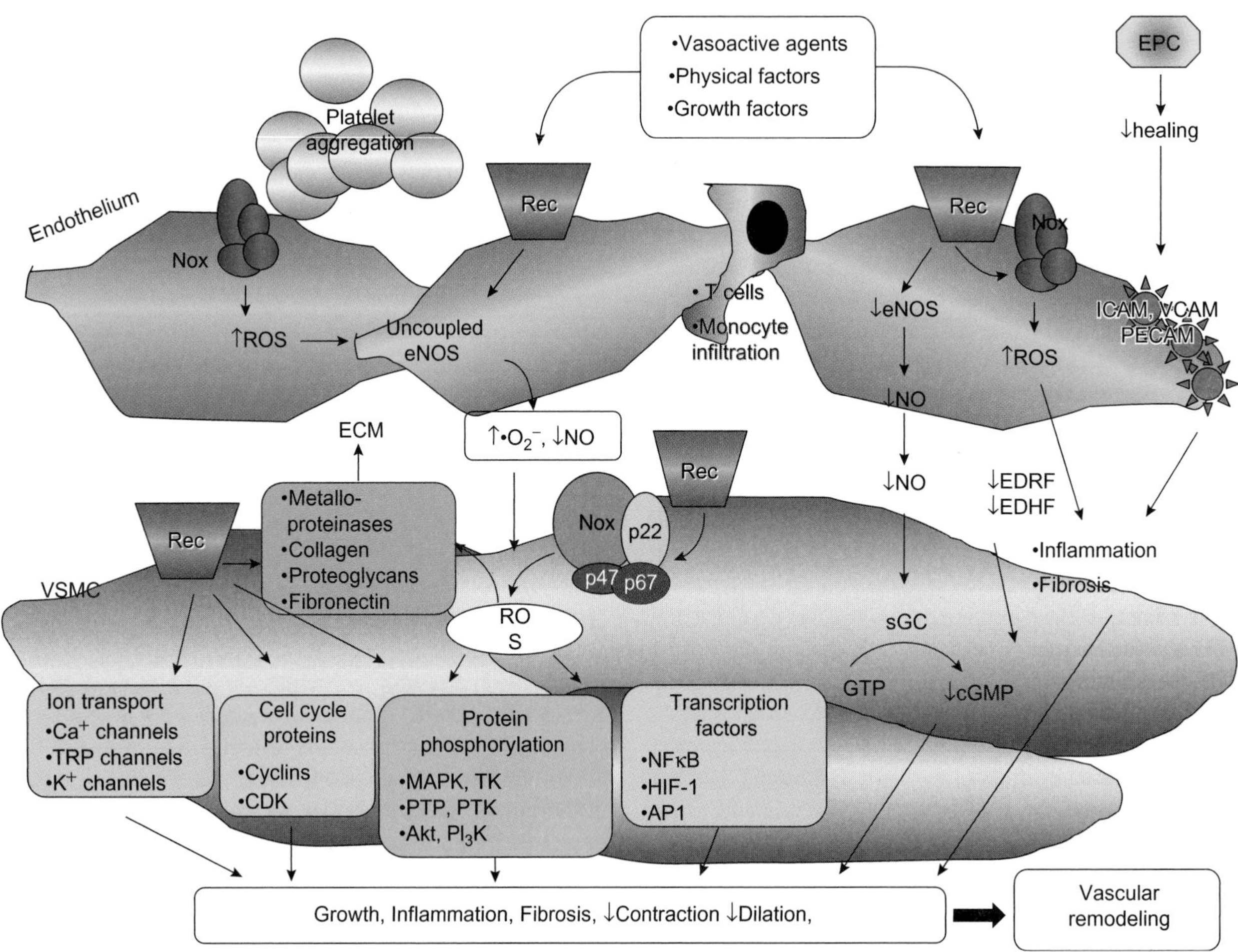

FIGURE 99.3 Molecular events regulating vascular remodeling in hypertension. Increased activation of endothelial and VSMC receptors (Rec) by multiple mechanisms leads to decreased NO bioavailability, activation of Nox (NADPH oxidase) and increased reactive oxygen species (ROS) production. Pathways that stimulate cell growth, inflammation, dedifferentiation, and contraction are stimulated. Increased deposition of extracellular matrix proteins (ECM) contributes to vascular fibrosis. These processes lead to vascular remodeling in hypertension. ICAM, VCAM, PECAM, adhesion molecules; EPC, endothelial progenitor cells.

overexpressed in many cardiovascular disorders associated with hypertension (42).

Arterial stiffness is associated with fibrosis, which involves accumulation of ECM proteins, such as collagen, elastin, fibrillin, fibronectin, and proteoglycans in the vascular wall. VSMC hypertrophy and proliferation and deposition of collagen and other components of the ECM contribute to media thickening in hypertrophic remodeling of resistance arteries (39,43). Cell growth and ECM deposition may result from blood pressure elevation or from growth-promoting factors including Ang II and ET-1. Increased ECM may also result from diminished activity of matrix metalloproteinases (MMPs), leading to accumulation of collagen type IV and V and fibronectin in resistance arteries (44). MMP-1 and MMP-3 activity is reduced in SHR before hypertension is established (45). In hypertensive patients with increased vascular type I collagen, serum concentrations of MMP-1 are reduced. In large arteries, polymorphisms of isoforms of MMP-3 and MMP-9 may be important determinants of vascular remodeling and age-related arterial stiffening (46), and polymorphisms in the AT1 angiotensin receptor have also been implicated.

Apoptosis also contributes to structural remodeling (6). Apoptosis influences fine-tuning of media growth, and is increased in some vascular beds and decreased in others in hypertension (6). The exact role of apoptosis in arterial remodeling remains unclear and it is unknown whether apoptosis is a growth-associated compensatory and adaptive process or a primary event. However, an imbalance between growth and apoptosis could be important. Detachment of VSMCs and endothelial cells (anoikis), increased microparticles and decreased endothelial progenitor cells may further contribute to vascular dysfunction and remodeling in hypertension.

VASCULAR SMOOTH MUSCLE, ENDOTHELIAL FUNCTION, AND HYPERTENSION-ASSOCIATED VASCULAR CHANGES

Endothelial cells normally regulate vascular tone by releasing relaxing and constricting factors such as NO, arachidonic acid metabolites, ROS, and vasoactive agents. They also produce endothelial-derived hyperpolarizing factors (EDHF) that induce endothelium-dependent relaxation through hyperpolarization of underlying VSMCs independently of NO. EDHF-mediated responses are important in hypertension, where they provide a vasorelaxation reserve for endothelial dysfunction due to decreased NO bioavailability (14). Endothelial dysfunction is a hallmark of hypertension and may reflect the premature aging of the intima exposed to chronic blood pressure increase. It is characterized by impaired vasomotor responses, VSMC proliferation and migration, ECM protein deposition, platelet activation, vascular permeability, and a pro-inflammatory and prothrombotic phenotype (39,47,48).

Of the many factors important in the protection of the endothelium are endothelial progenitor cells (EPCs). EPCs are bone marrow-derived cells capable of developing into mature endothelial cells (49). They contribute to vascular homeostasis through direct cell-to-cell contact and through autocrine and paracrine actions. EPCs mobilize out of the bone marrow in response to peripheral tissue hypoxia and injury and release EPC-activation factors, such as hypoxia-inducible factor-1 (HIF-1), VEGF, erythropoietin and NO to facilitate endothelial healing, regeneration, and reendothelialization after vascular damage (50). The multidrug resistance-related protein-1 (MRP1) has been identified as a negative regulator of EPC function and survival and MRP1 inhibition has been suggested as a novel strategy to increase EPC survival (51). The number of circulating EPCs may reflect endothelial function since decreased numbers are associated with reduced arterial elasticity, and decreased endothelial integrity (52). Circulating EPCs are reduced in hypertension (51,52). Studies in cultured EPCs suggest that ROS are involved in Ang II-mediated EPC senescence (53).

In addition to EPCs, microparticles have been considered as biomarkers of vascular status. Microparticles are tiny fragments of cellular membranes that are generated from activated or apoptotic cells (54). Microparticles circulate in healthy individuals and their levels increase in cardiovascular and athero-thrombotic diseases (54). In patients with hypertension plasma levels of microparticles correlated with systolic and diastolic blood pressure (55). In patients with diabetes, endothelial microparticle levels are a strong predictor of myocardial infarction and correlate with arterial stiffness and endothelium-mediated vasodilation (56). They also relate to the extent and severity of coronary stenosis in patients with coronary syndromes (56). *In vitro* endothelial microparticles are released in response to inflammatory stimuli such as TNF-α, thrombin, uremic toxins, ROS, and PAI-1, which are increased in hypertension. Although the precise mechanism leading to *in vivo* generation of microparticles is not fully understood, there is evidence that endothelial nitric oxide synthase (NOS) uncoupling and low shear stress (57), which are features of endothelial dysfunction in hypertension, enhance their production. They in turn may contribute to some extent to endothelial dysfunction through ROS production (55–57). The exact role of microparticles in vascular remodeling awaits clarification, but it is possible that they may be more than biomarkers of endothelial dysfunction. They interfere with target cell responses by transferring chemokines and adhesion molecules to endothelial cells leading to monocyte adhesion and hence have the potential to directly contribute to vascular injury in hypertension.

VASCULAR SMOOTH MUSCLE, INFLAMMATION, AND VASCULAR REMODELING IN HYPERTENSION

Low grade inflammation in the vascular wall is increasingly recognized as an important contributor to the pathophysiology of hypertension (58), to the initiation and progression of atherosclerosis, and to the development of cardiovascular disease (CVD). Inflammation participates in vascular remodeling (59) and may contribute to accelerated vascular damage in cardiovascular diseases and in aging. Whether Ang II or BP elevation itself, through effects on adhesion molecules, chemokines, and cytokines, or through neo-antigen formation induced by cyclic mechanical strain, are associated with the inflammatory response in hypertension, is unclear. Inflammation contributes to vascular remodeling promoting cell growth and proliferation of VSMCs. Greater expression of adhesion molecules (VCAM-1, ICAM-1) on the endothelial cell membrane, accumulation of monocyte/macrophages, dendritic cells, natural killer cells, and B and T lymphocytes are some of the mechanisms that participate in the inflammatory response in the vascular wall (59). Activators of nuclear receptors, such as PPARs, downregulate the vascular inflammatory response in experimental animals and decrease serum markers of inflammation in humans (60). Thus, PPARs and vasoactive substances may be endogenous modulators of the inflammatory process involved in vascular structural changes occurring in hypertension. Innate immunity has been implicated to contribute to the low-grade inflammatory response in hypertension where different subsets of T lymphocytes may be involved in processes leading to inflammation. An imbalance exists between the pro-inflammatory Th1, Th2, and Th17, and the anti-inflammatory T regulatory (Treg) subsets of T lymphocytes (59,61). Mice deficient in T and B lymphocytes have a blunted hypertensive response to Ang II and DOCA salt and vascular remodeling in response to Ang II (61,62). Effector T cell, but not B lymphocyte adoptive transfer, corrected the lack of response to Ang II. The central and pressor effects of Ang II are also critical for T-cell activation and development of vascular inflammation (63,64). One of the mechanisms whereby T lymphocytes participate in hypertension and peripheral inflammation is in response to increased oxidative stress (63,64). An imbalance between T effector lymphocytes and T regulatory lymphocytes may contribute to remodeling of blood vessels, if the protective action of T regulatory cells is impaired as has been suggested in Dahl salt-sensitive rats (65) or in response to Ang II in mice (66).

VASCULAR AGING, REMODELING, AND HYPERTENSION

The age-associated changes in blood vessels that occur in healthy individuals include increased arterial wall thickness, reduced compliance, increased stiffness, and decreased lumen diameter – typical features of the hypertensive vascular phenotype (67). These structural changes are associated with impaired endothelial function, caused by decreased production of vasodilators, such as NO and prostacyclins, and increased bioavailability of ROS (67). Consistent with a dysfunctional endothelium is increased vascoconstriction and decreased fibrinolysis. Arterial aging is a predominant risk factor for the onset of cardiovascular diseases, such as hypertension, and is associated with activation of the RAS, increased vascular stiffness, intima-media thickening, calcification, and a proinflammatory phenotype (67). Moreover, vascular repair systems become progressively impaired with aging. These features are characteristic of the vascular phenotype in hypertension and in fact hypertension is considered a critically important factor in accelerated aging of the vasculature. Cellular and molecular mechanisms underlying age-associated changes of the vascular system are unclear, but cardiovascular cells, including stem and/or progenitor cells, undergo senescence. Senescent cells enter irreversible growth arrest, exhibit a flattened and enlarged phenotype and express genes, such as negative cell cycle regulators p53 and p16, that differ from those normally expressed (68). Factors implicated in cellular senescence include decreased telomerase activity and telomere shortening, DNA damage, and genomic instability. These processes are modulated by Ang II and are redox-sensitive. There are now extensive data indicating that ROS bioavailabilty and RAS activation are increased in aging, as well as in hypertension (69).

Increased aortic stiffness, typical of vascular changes associated with aging and hypertension, has been correlated with the expression of genes involved in increased vascular tone and remodeling. These include protein phosphatase-1, the catalytic subunit of myosin light chain phosphatase, members of the family of A kinase anchor protein and PKCbeta-1, involved in long-term sustained contraction (67). There are relationships also between extracellular matrix molecules and aortic stiffness. Expression of proteoglycans and integrins $\alpha 2b$ and $\alpha 6$ is increased in the remodeled stiff aorta of aging.

VASCULAR CALCIFICATION

Vascular calcification is associated with mineralization of the internal elastic lamina and elastic fibers within the media resulting in stiffened vessels and increased pulse pressure. Arterial calcification is not uncommon in aging, chronic kidney disease, diabetes, atherosclerosis, and hypertension, and is related to cardiovascular morbidity and mortality (70). Vascular calcification is a tightly regulated process similar to bone formation and VSMCs play a critical role in the process (71). VSMCs have a remarkable capacity to undergo phenotypic differentiation. Factors that trigger and promote VSMC osteogenic induction include abnormalities in mineral metabolism, particularly hyperphosphatemia and hypercalcemia. This is driven by upregulation of transcription factors such as cbfa1 (core-binding factor 1α)/Runx2, MSX-2 and bone morphogenetic protein 2 (BMP-2), involved in normal bone development, and which control the expression of osteogenic proteins, including osteocalcin, osteonectin, alkaline phosphatase, collagen-1, and bone sialoprotein (72). Another mechanism contributing to vascular mineralization is loss of calcification inhibitors, such as fetuin-A, matrix Gla protein, pyrophosphate, and osteopontin (70,72). Molecular processes underlying this remain to be fully defined but vasoactive agents, such as Ang II, ET-1, and urotensin, may be important modulators of vascular calcification. Ang II influences calcification by redox-sensitive pathways that stimulate expression of BMP2 and the osteoblast transcription factor Runx2/Cbfa1 (73), and through modulation of Ca^{2+} and Mg^{2+} transport through cation channels, such as TRPM7 (74). AT_1R blockade can inhibit arterial calcification by disrupting vascular osteogenesis, suggesting that patients with vascular calcification may benefit therapeutically from Ang II receptor blockers.

CONCLUSIONS

Regulation of blood flow includes adaptation of vascular tone and structure of small arteries. Increased blood pressure leads to vascular structural modifications so that vessels adapt to hemodynamic changes. Decompensation of these processes is associated with remodeling of small arteries, characterized by a reduced lumen size and an increase in wall thickness. Initial factors contributing to this process involve increased transmural pressure, changes in blood flow, and endothelial dysfunction. The subsequent alterations of VSMC growth, migration, differentiation, calcification, inflammation, and production of ECM proteins are then responsible for the resulting vascular remodeling. Critical to these events is the plastic nature of VSMCs that have the capacity to undergo phenotypic modification. At the level of the vascular cells, receptors are activated by vasoactive agents and mechanical forces triggering intracellular signaling via PLC-PKC, MAP kinases, tyrosine kinases, RhoA/ROCK and TGFβ, and generation of ROS. These signaling events promote VSMC dedifferentiation, realignment, and growth and stimulate inflammation, fibrosis, and osteogenic transformation, which together with increased ECM deposition contribute to thickening of the vascular wall. Such plasticity of VSMCs is key to arterial remodeling in hypertension, a process that may be reversible with antihypertensive treatment.

ACKNOWLEDGMENTS

Studies performed by R.M.T. and E.L.S. were supported by grants from the Canadian Institutes of Health Research (CIHR). R.M.T. and E.L.S. are supported through Canada Research Chair/Canadian Foundation for Innovation awards.

REFERENCES

1. Christensen KL, Mulvany MJ. Location of resistance arteries. *J Vasc Res* 2001;**38**:1–12.
2. Martinez-Lemus LA, Hill MA, Meininger GA. The plastic nature of the vascular wall: a continuum of remodeling events contributing to control of arteriolar diameter and structure. *Physiology* 2009;**24**:45–57.
3. Fisher SA. Vascular smooth muscle phenotypic diversity and function. *Physiol Genomics* 2010;**42A**:169–87.
4. Gibbons GH, Dzau VJ. The emerging concept of vascular remodeling. *N Eng J Med* 1994;**330**:1431–8.
5. Mulvany MJ. Small artery remodeling and significance in the development of hypertension. *News Physiol Sci* 2002;**17**:105–9.
6. Intengan HD, Schiffrin EL. Review: vascular remodeling in hypertension. Roles of apoptosis, inflammation and fibrosis. *Hypertension* 2001;**38**:581–7.
7. Lemarié CA, Tharaux PL, Lehoux S. Extracellular matrix alterations in hypertensive vascular remodeling. *J Mol Cell Cardiol* 2010;**48**:433–9.
8. Mulvany MJ, Baumbach GL, Aalkjaer C, Heagerty AM, Korsgaard N, Schiffrin EL, et al. Vascular remodeling. *Hypertension* 1996;**28**: 505–6.
9. Schiffrin EL. Remodeling of resistance arteries in essential hypertension and effects of antihypertensive treatment. *Am J Hypertens* 2004;**17**:1192–200.
10. Xu S, He Y, Vokurkova M, Touyz RM, et al. Endothelial cells negatively modulate reactive oxygen species generation in vascular smooth muscle cells: role of thioredoxin. *Hypertension* 2009;**54**:427–33.
11. Wynne BM, Chiao CW, Webb RC. Vascular smooth muscle cell signaling mechanisms for contraction to angiotensin II and endothelin-1. *J Am Soc Hyperten* 2009;**3**:84–95.
12. Touyz RM, El Mabrouk M, He G, Wu XH, Schiffrin EL. Mitogen-activated protein/extracellular signal-regulated kinase inhibition attenuates angiotensin II-mediated signaling and contraction in spontaneously hypertensive rat vascular smooth muscle cells. *Circ Res* 1999;**84**:505–15.
13. de Campos Grifoni S, Bendhack LM. Functional study of the $[Ca^{2+}]_i$ signaling pathway in aortas of L-NAME-hypertensive rats. *Pharmacology* 2004;**70**:160–8.
14. Félétou M, Verbeuren TJ, Vanhoutte PM. Endothelium-dependent contractions in SHR: a tale of prostanoid TP and IP receptors. *Br J Pharmacol* 2009;**156**:563–74.
15. Virdis A, Ghiadoni L, Taddei S. Human endothelial dysfunction: EDCFs. *Pflugers Arch* 2010;**459**:1015–23.

16. Versari D, Daghini E, Virdis A, Ghiadoni L, Taddei S. Endothelium-dependent contractions and endothelial dysfunction in human hypertension. *Br J Pharmacol* 2009;**157**:527–36.
17. Wirth A. Rho kinase and hypertension. *Biochim Biophys Acta* 2010;**1802**:1276–84.
18. Deng JT, Van Lierop JE, Sutherland C, Walsh MP. Ca^{2+}-independent smooth muscle contraction. a novel function for integrin-linked kinase. *J Biol Chem* 2001;**276**:16365–73.
19. Endo A, Surks HK, Mochizuki S, Mochizuki N, Mendelsohn ME. Identification and characterization of zipper-interacting protein kinase as the unique vascular smooth muscle myosin phosphatase-associated kinase. *J Biol Chem* 2004;**279**:42055–61.
20. Seko T, Ito M, Kureishi Y, Okamoto R, Moriki N, Onishi K, et al. Activation of RhoA and inhibition of myosin phosphatase as important components in hypertension in vascular smooth muscle. *Circ Res* 2003;**92**:411–8.
21. Gohla A, Schultz G, Offermanns S. Role for G12/G13 in agonist-induced vascular smooth muscle cell contraction. *Circ Res* 2000;**87**:221–7.
22. Loirand G, Pacaud P. The role of Rho protein signaling in hypertension. *Nature Rev Cardiol* 2010;**7**:637–47.
23. Uehata M, Ishizaki T, Satoh H, Ono T, Kawahara T, Morishita T, et al. Calcium sensitization of smooth muscle mediated by a Rho-associated protein kinase in hypertension. *Nature* 1997;**389**:990–4.
24. Komers R, Oyama TT, Beard DR, Anderson S. Effects of systemic inhibition of Rho kinase on blood pressure and renal haemodynamics in diabetic rats. *Br J Pharmacol* 2011;**162**:163–74.
25. Chan CK, Mak JC, Man RY, Vanhoutte PM. Rho kinase inhibitors prevent endothelium-dependent contractions in the rat aorta. *J Pharmacol Exp The* 2009;**329**:820–6.
26. Zhao J, Zhou D, Guo J, Ren Z, Zhou L, Wang S. Effect of fasudil hydrochloride, a protein kinase inhibitor, on cerebral vasospasm and delayed cerebral ischemic symptoms after aneurysmal subarachnoid hemorrhage. *Neurol Med Chir* 2006;**46**:421–8.
27. Fukumoto Y, Mohri M, Inokuchi K, Ito A, Hirakawa Y, Masumoto A. Anti-ischemic effects of fasudil, a specific Rho-kinase inhibitor, in patients with stable effort angina. *J Cardiovasc Pharmacol* 2007;**49**:117–21.
28. Masumoto A, Mohri M, Shimokawa H, Urakami L, Usui M, Takeshita A. Suppression of coronary artery spasm by the Rho-kinase inhibitor fasudil in patients with vasospastic angina. *Circulation* 2002;**105**:1545–7.
29. Fujita H, Fukumoto Y, Saji K, Sugimura K, Demachi J, Nawata J, et al. Acute vasodilator effects of inhaled fasudil, a specific Rho-kinase inhibitor, in patients with pulmonary arterial hypertension. *Heart Vessels* 2010;**25**:144–9.
30. Nohria A, Grunert ME, Rikitake Y, Noma K, Prsic A, Ganz P. Rho kinase inhibition improves endothelial function in human subjects with coronary artery disease. *Circ Res* 2006;**99**:1426–32.
31. Büssemaker E, Herbrig K, Pistrosch F, Palm C, Passauer J. Role of rho-kinase in the regulation of vascular tone in hypertensive renal transplant recipients. *Atherosclerosis* 2009;**207**:567–72.
32. Schiffrin EL. The vascular phenotypes in hypertension: relation to the natural history of hypertension. *J Am Soc Hypertens* 2007;**1**:56–67.
33. van der Akker J, Schoorl MJ, ENTP Bakker, vanBavel E. Small artery remodeling: current concepts and questions. *J Vasc Res* 2010;**47**:183–202.
34. Brassard P, Amiri F, Schiffrin EL. Combined angiotensin II type 1 and type 2 receptor blockade on vascular remodeling and matrix metalloproteinases in resistance arteries. *Hypertension* 2005;**46**:598–606.
35. Touyz RM, Yao G, Schiffrin EL. c-Src induces phosphorylation and translocation of p47phox role in superoxide generation by Ang II in human vascular smooth muscle cells. *Arterioscler Thromb Vasc Biol* 2003;**23**:981–7.
36. Rizzoni D, Porteri E, Guelfi D, Piccoli A, Castellan M, Pasini GM, et al. Cellular hypertrophy in subcutaneous small arteries of patients with renovascular hypertension. *Hypertension* 2000;**25**:931–5.
37. Endemann DH, Pu Q, De Ciuceis C, Savoia C, Virdis A, Neves MF, et al. Persistent remodeling of resistance arteries in type 2 diabetic patients on antihypertensive treatment. *Hypertension* 2004;**43**:399–404.
38. Rizzoni D, Porteri E, Giustina A, De Ciuceis C, Sleiman I, Boari GEM, et al. Agromegalic patients show the presence of hypertrophic remodeling of subcutaneous small resistance arteries. *Hypertension* 2004;**43**:561–5.
39. Savoia C, Burger D, Nishigaki N, Montezano A, Touyz RM. Angiotensin II and the vascular phenotype in hypertension. *Expert Rev Mol Med* 2011;**13**:e11–20.
40. Touyz RM, Schiffrin EL. Signal transduction mechanisms mediating the physiological and pathophysiological actions of angiotensin II in vascular smooth muscle cells. *Pharmacol Rev* 2000;**52**:639–72.
41. Sarkar S, Sarkar S, Vellaichamy E, Young D, Sen S. Influence of cytokines and growth factors in Ang II-mediated collagen upregulation by fibroblasts in rats: role of myocytes. *Am J Physiol Heart Cell Physiol* 2004;**287**:H107–17.
42. Popovic N, Bridenbaugh EA, Neiger JD, Hu JJ, Vannucci M, Mo Q, et al. Transforming growth factor-beta signaling in hypertensive remodeling of porcine aorta. *Am J Physiol Heart Cell Physiol* 2009;**297**:H2044–53.
43. Intengan HD, Deng LY, Li JS, Schiffrin EL. Mechanics and composition of human subcutaneous resistance arteries in essential hypertension. *Hypertension* 1999;**33**:569–74.
44. Tayebjee MH, MacFadyen RJ, Lip GY. Extracellular matrix biology: a new frontier in linking the pathology and therapy of hypertension? *J Hypertens* 2003;**21**:2211–8.
45. Intengan HD, Schiffrin EL. Structure and mechanical properties of resistance arteries in hypertension role of adhesion molecules and extracellular matrix determinants. *Hypertension* 2000;**36**:312–8.
46. Medley TL, Kingwell BA, Gatzka CD, Pillay P, Cole TJ. Matrix metalloproteinase-3 genotype contributes to age-related aortic stiffening through modulation of gene and protein expression. *Circ Res* 2003;**92**:1254–61.
47. Schiffrin EL. Review: Beyond blood pressure: the endothelium and atherosclerosis progression. *Am J Hypertens* 2002;**15**(Suppl. 1): S115–22.
48. Endemann DH, Schiffrin EL. Endothelial dysfunction. *J Am Soc Nephrol.* 2004;**15**:1983–92.
49. Hill JM, Zalos G, Halcox JP, Schenke WH, Waclawiw MA, Quyyumi AA, et al. Circulating endothelial progenitor cells, vascular function, and cardiovascular risk. *N Engl J Med* 2003;**348**:593–600.
50. Sen S, McDonald SP, Coates PT, Bonder CS. Endothelial progenitor cells: novel biomarker and promising cell therapy for cardiovascular disease. *Clin Sci (Lond)* 2011;**120**:263–83.

51. Mueller CF, Afzal S, Becher UM, Wassmann S, Nickenig G, Wassmann K. Role of the multidrug resistance protein-1 (MRP1) for endothelial progenitor cell function and survival. *J Mol Cell Cardiol* 2010;**49**:482–9.
52. Urbich C, Dimmeler S. Endothelial progenitor cells: characterization and role in vascular biology. *Circ Res* 2004;**95**:343–53.
53. Salguero G, Akin E, Templin C, Kotlarz D, Doerries C, Landmesser U, et al. Renovascular hypertension by two-kidney one-clip enhances endothelial progenitor cell mobilization in a p47phox-dependent manner. *J Hypertens* 2008;**26**:257–68.
54. Boulanger CM. Microparticles, vascular function and hypertension. *Curr Opin Nephrol Hypertens* 2010;**19**:177–80.
55. Preston RA, Jy W, Jimenez JJ. Effects of severe hypertension on endothelial and platelet microparticles. *Hypertension* 2003;**41**:211–7.
56. Chironi GN, Boulanger CM, Simon. Endothelial microparticles in diseases. *Cell Tissues Res* 2009;**355**:143–51.
57. Boulanger C, Amabile N, Guerin AP. In vivo shear stress determines circulating levels of endothelial microparticles in end-stage renal disease. *Hypertension* 2007;**49**:1–7.
58. De Ciuceis C, Amiri F, Brassard P, Endemann DH, Touyz RM, Schiffrin, et al. Reduced vascular remodeling, endothelial dysfunction, and oxidative stress in resistance arteries of angiotensin II-infused macrophage colony-stimulating factor-deficient mice: evidence for a role in inflammation in angiotensin-induced vascular injury. *Arterioscler Thromb Vasc Biol* 2005;**25**: 2106–13.
59. Schiffrin EL. T lymphocytes: a role in hypertension? *Curr Opin Nephrol Hypertens* 2010;**19**:181–6.
60. Sigmund CD. Endothelial and vascular muscle PPARgamma in arterial pressure regulation: lessons from genetic interference and deficiency. *Hypertension* 2010;**55**:437–44.
61. Guzik TJ, Hoch NE, Brown KA. Role of T cell in the genesis of angiotensin II induced hypertension and vascular dysfunction. *J Exp Med* 2007;**204**:2449–60.
62. Marvar PJ, Thabet SR, Guzik TJ, Lob HE, McCann LA, Weyand C, et al. Central and peripheral mechanisms of T-lymphocyte activation and vascular inflammation produced by angiotensin II-induced hypertension. *Circ Res* 2010;**107**:263–70.
63. Touyz RM, Briones AM. Reactive oxygen species and vascular biology: implications in human hypertension. *Hypertens Res* 2011;**34**:5–14.
64. Lob HE, Marvar PJ, Guzik TJ, Sharma S, McCann LA, Weyand C, et al. Induction of hypertension and peripheral inflammation by reduction of extracellular superoxide dismutase in the central nervous system. *Hypertension* 2010;**55**:277–83.
65. Viel EC, Lemarié CA, Benkirane K, Paradis P, Schiffrin EL. Immune regulation and vascular inflammation in genetic hypertension. *Am J Physiol Heart Circ Physiol* 2010;**298**:H938–44.
66. Barhoumi T, Kasal DAB, Li MW, Shbat L, Laurant P, Fritsch Neves M, et al. T regulatory lymphocytes prevent angiotensin II-induced hypertension and vascular injury. *Hypertension* 2011;**57**:469–76.
67. Camici GG, Sudano I, Noll G, Tanner FC, Lüscher TF. Molecular pathways of aging and hypertension. *Curr Opin Neph Hypertens* **18**:134–37.
68. Kortlever RM, Brummelkamp TR, van Meeteren LA, Moolenaar WH, Bernards R. Suppression of the p53-dependent replicative senescence response by lysophosphatidic acid signaling. *Mol Cancer Res* 2008;**6**:1452–60.
69. Nilsson PM, Lurbe E, Laurent S. The early life origins of vascular ageing and cardiovascular risk: the EVA syndrome. *J Hypertens* 2008;**26**:1049–57.
70. Rosito GA, Massaro JM, Hoffmann U, Ruberg FL, Mahabadi AA, Vasan RS, et al. Pericardial fat, visceral abdominal fat, cardiovascular disease risk factors, and vascular calcification in a community-based sample: the Framingham heart study. *Circulation* 2008;**117**:605–13.
71. Serrano CV, Oranges M, Brunaldi V, de M, Soeiro A, Torres TA, et al. Skeletonized coronary arteries: pathophysiological and clinical aspects of vascular calcification. *Vasc Health Risk Man* 2011;**7**:143–51.
72. Alam MU, Kirton JP, Wilkinson FL, Towers E, Sinha S, Rouhi M, et al. Calcification is associated with loss of functional calcium-sensing receptor in vascular smooth muscle cells. *Cardiovasc Res* 2009;**81**:260–8.
73. Trebak M, Ginnan R, Singer HA, Jourd'heuil D. Interplay between calcium and reactive oxygen/nitrogen species: an essential paradigm for vascular smooth muscle signaling. *Antioxid Redox Signal* 2010;**12**:657–74.
74. Montezano AC, Zimmerman D, Yusuf H, Chignalia AZ, Wadhera V, Touyz RM. Vascular smooth muscle cell differentiation to an osteogenic phenotype involves TRPM7 modulation by magnesium. *Hypertension* 2010;**56**:453–62.

Chapter 100

Diabetic Vascular Disease

Adam Whaley-Connell[1], Hanrui Zhang[2], Cuihua Zhang[2,3] and James R. Sowers[1,4,5]

[1]Harry S Truman VA Medical Center and the University of Missouri-Columbia School of Medicine, Department of Internal Medicine, Division of Nephrology and Hypertension, [2]Dalton Cardiovascular Research Center, [3]Division of Cardiovascular Medicine, Department of Internal Medicine, Department of Medical Pharmacology & Physiology, [4]MU Diabetes and Cardiovascular Center, [5]Department of Medical Pharmacology & Physiology, University of Missouri-Columbia, Columbia, MO

INTRODUCTION

Diabetes mellitus represents the sixth leading cause of mortality in adults in the United States (US) and is present in 6.3% of the population, approximately 18.2 million individuals (1,2). Prevalent diabetes is highest in those above 65 years; however, the greatest increase in the last decade is occurring in younger individuals (below 45 years) (3,4). Although prevalent diabetes is highest in the US, the rapid expansion of diabetes is occurring globally driven by growth in Southeast Asia and the Middle East and the number of persons with diabetes is predicted to expand to over 300 million (1,2). The importance of diabetes in the US is highlighted by the fact it is now the leading cause of end-stage kidney disease (ESKD) and non-traumatic amputations (5,6). However, cardiovascular disease (CVD) is the leading cause of premature mortality in those with type 2 diabetes, a finding amplified in the presence of hypertension (7–11).

At least 80% of mortality in type 2 diabetes in the US is attributable to CVD, and the age-adjusted relative risk of a fatal CVD is three times higher than the non-diabetic population (9). Further, the presence of one or more traditional cardiovascular risk factors such as tobacco use, advanced age, hypercholesterolemia, and hypertension convey a significantly higher risk for CVD mortality in patients with diabetes than in non-diabetics (10,11). The presence of hypertension and obesity are especially powerful co-morbid risk factors in the diabetic population (11–14). Indeed, the presence of hypertension markedly increases the risk for CVD in patients with type 2 diabetes (8–10). There is increasing concern regarding the increasing prevalence of obesity and physical inactivity as it relates to development of diabetes-related CVD in pediatric and adolescent populations, especially among Native Americans, African Americans, and Hispanic American children (1–4).

While the presence of hyperglycemia and endothelial dysfunction contributes significantly to the development of hypertension, recent data suggest that development of obesity-related insulin resistance in early stages of diabetes directly contributes to endothelial dysfunction and early atherosclerosis through impairments in insulin metabolic signaling and reductions in bioavailable NO that alter the integrity of the endothelium. Here, therefore, we will review the importance of insulin resistance as well as hyperglycemia and the mechanisms by which both contribute to the progression of vascular disease in the insulin-resistant, diabetic patient.

ENDOTHELIAL DYSFUNCTION IN DIABETES

The endothelium lines the lumen of the vasculature and serves as an interface between circulating blood and vascular smooth muscle cells (VSMC). Thereby, integrity of the endothelium is needed to maintain the balance between vasodilation and vasoconstriction in order to preserve a sufficient vascular diameter for perfusion of the cardiovascular system (15,16). Impairments in vasorelaxation in states of hyperglycemia and insulin resistance is indicative of endothelial dysfunction long identified as an important component in the development of cardiovascular pathology in those with diabetes (15–20).

The endothelium plays a key role in the function of VSMC through the release of several factors that promote vasodilation. Nitric oxide (NO) is produced in response to a variety of stimuli by the oxidation of L-arginine by the NADPH-dependent enzyme NO synthase (NOS) (15). NO production leads to physiological vasodilation and the relaxation of VSMC. NO acts on smooth muscle cells by stimulating guanylate cyclase and by increasing the intracellular concentration of cyclic guanosine monophosphate (cGMP). cGMP decreases the intracellular Ca^{2+} concentration causing vascular relaxation. In addition to its vasodilating properties, NO further aids in the prevention of

Muscle. DOI: http://dx.doi.org/10.1016/B978-0-12-381510-1.00100-9

atherogenesis through inhibition of platelet aggregation and proliferation of vascular smooth muscle cells (17–19).

In normal functioning endothelium, insulin stimulates NO production through the phosphatidylinositol 3-kinase (PI3K) and protein kinase B (Akt) signaling pathways (18), while it stimulates migration and growth of vascular smooth muscle cells via the mitogen-activated protein kinase (MAPK) pathway (19). Individuals with insulin resistance display a selective defect in the aforementioned PI3K/Akt pathway. This impairment in insulin-dependent metabolic signaling ultimately results in the development of endothelial dysfunction that manifests as hypertension with subsequent development of left ventricular hypertrophy and cardiovascular disease (20).

Over the past several years, we have explored mechanisms by which the renin-angiotensin-aldosterone system (RAAS) contributes to cardiovascular insulin resistance as a mechanism of endothelial dysfunction. Angiotensin (Ang II) exerts pro-oxidative and pro-inflammatory effects and promotes vascular growth/remodeling, proliferation, and fibrosis that lead to endothelial dysfunction and arterial stiffening. Recent work from our laboratory suggests that Ang II contributes to endothelial dysfunction and vascular fibrosis through inhibition of insulin-dependent metabolic signaling, in part, by promoting phosphorylation of the nutrient sensing pathway mammalian target of rapamycin (mTOR)/S6 kinase 1 (S6K1) and downstream insulin receptor substrate one (IRS-1) serine (Ser) phosphorylation (P) (19) (Figure 100.1). Work in cultured endothelial cells (EC), VSMC, and cardiomyocytes as well as in *ex vivo* cardiovascular tissue, suggests that excessive Ser P of IRS-1 interferes with IRS-1/PI3-K docking and the consequent activation of Akt. In cardiomyocytes, insulin activation of the PI3-K/Akt pathway stimulates glucose transporter 4 (GLUT4) recruitment to the plasma membrane resulting in glucose uptake as well as diastolic relaxation of the heart (Figure 100.1). Signaling via this pathway promotes insulin-dependent vasorelaxation through increased endothelial NOS (eNOS) activity and reductions in myosin light chain (MLC) activation in VSMC and decreases in calcium (Ca^{2+}) in cardiac tissue (19).

Numerous insults contribute to reductions in bioavailable NO and endothelial dysfunction. Generation of excess reactive oxygen (ROS) and nitrogen (RNS) species reduce bioavailable NO which plays a seminal role in vascular pathology (20,21) and this increase in oxidative stress has been shown to be elevated during episodes of hyperglycemia and insulin resistance (22). Superoxide anion (O_2^-) is a highly reactive compound produced when oxygen is reduced by a single electron, and may be generated during the normal catalytic function of a number of enzymes. Potential vascular sources of O_2^- in animals and humans include NADPH-dependent oxidases, xanthine oxidase, lipoxygenase, mitochondrial oxidases, and NO synthases. When O_2^- is produced it reacts rapidly with NO, reducing bioavailable NO. Increased ROS also decreases NOS activity in endothelial cells, resulting in decreased production of NO (23). In addition to its effects on NO, increased ROS causes further endothelial damage through pro-atherogenic actions on smooth muscle cell proliferation, and through the recruitment of inflammatory modulators (23,24).

To further complicate vascular and endothelial dysfunction, superoxide dismutase (SOD), an anti-oxidant enzyme that acts as a scavenger of oxygen free radicals, is often suppressed in diabetes. Moreover, plasma levels of asymmetric dimethylarginine (ADMA), an endogenous competitive inhibitor of NOS, are also significantly increased in those with insulin resistance and diabetes (20,25). Endothelial dysfunction occurs as a result of this combination of increased production of free radicals with the decreased ability for their removal in conjunction with reductions in bioavailable NO, creating an environment of increased oxidative stress that ultimately contributes to the development of hypertension and CVD.

THE ROLE OF HYPERGLYCEMIA IN ENDOTHELIAL DYSFUNCTION

Several other mechanisms of endothelial dysfunction in diabetes have also been proposed and center around the development of hyperglycemia. In the face of hyperglycemia, the increased production of diacylglycerol (DAG) through the process of glycolysis increases the level of protein kinase C (PKC) activation (26). PKC activity leads to reduced levels of NOS, as well as producing vasoconstrictive substances such as endothelin-1 (ET-1) (26). In addition, PKC increases the production of growth factors by the endothelium, such as vascular endothelial growth factor (VEGF), epidermal growth factor (EGF), and transforming growth factor (TGF) as well, which contributes to the migration and proliferation of vascular smooth muscle cells (VSMC) (27).

Another perspective has focused on hyperglycemia-induced formation of non-enzymatic advanced glycosylation products (AGE) that tend to accumulate in vascular tissue (28). These products act to neutralize NO and increase the susceptibility of LDL to oxidation. The binding of the AGE to their receptors (RAGE) also activates the receptors for the cytokines interleukin-1 (IL-1), tumor-necrosis factor-alpha (TNF-α), and growth factors, leading to the migration and proliferation of VSMCs (29,30).

Hyperglycemia promotes the formation of AGE through non-enzymatic glycation of proteins and lipids by

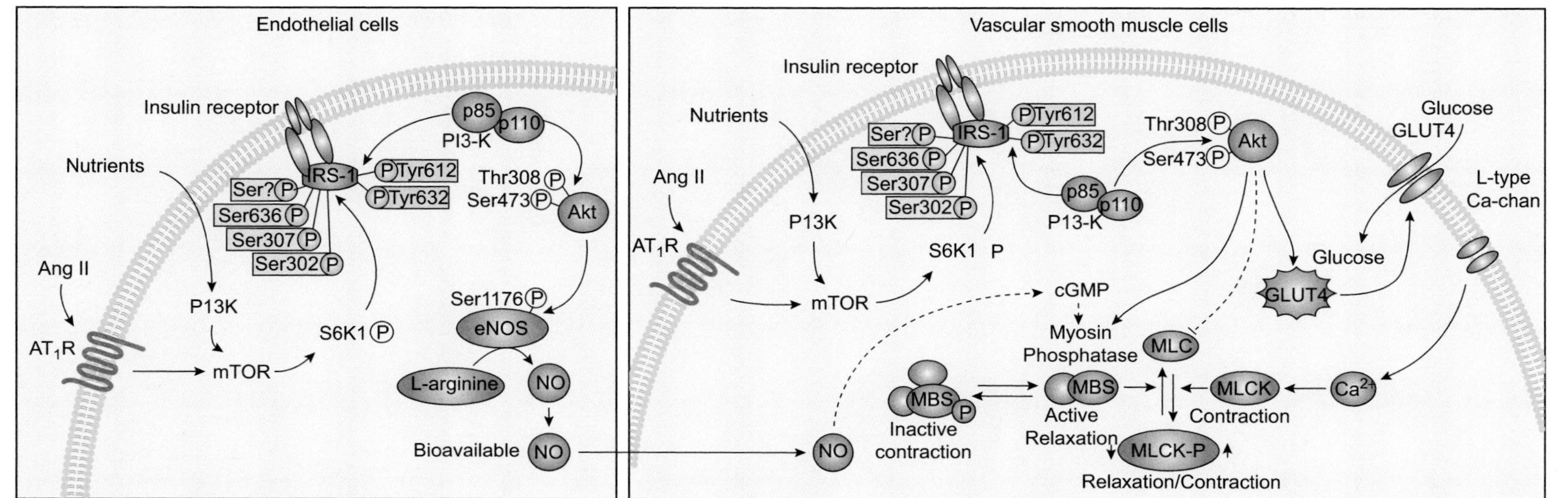

FIGURE 100.1 **The opposing effects of angiotensin (Ang) II and over-nutrition on endothelial and vascular function.** Insulin-dependent metabolic signaling plays a critical role in routine function of the endothelium and in vasorelaxation. Insulin actions on the blood vessel are partially mediated by increased production of nitric oxide (NO) through phosphorylation and secondary activation of endothelial NO synthase (eNOS). Ang type 1 receptor (AT_1R) activation decreases the availability of NO via the induction of resistance to insulin-dependent metabolic signaling, promoting NADPH oxidase-induced ROS production and diminishing eNOS. Thereby, the counter-regulatory effects of Ang II activation of the (AT_1R) and excess nutrition in endothelial cells serve to promote impairments in vasorelaxation and endothelial dysfunction. Abbreviations: Akt, protein kinase B; GLUT, glucose transporter; IRS, insulin receptor substrate; MBS, myosin-bound serine; MLC, myosin light chain; MLCK, MLC kinase; mTOR, mammalian Target of Rapamycin; PI3-K, phosphatidylinositol 3-kinase; PIP, phosphatidylinositol phosphate; PIP2, phosphatidylinositol bisphosphate; PIP3, phosphatidylinositol (3,4,5)-trisphosphate; P, phosphorylation; p70, ribosomal protein S6 kinase 1 (S6K1); Ser, serine; Tyr, tyrosine.

several pathways such as activation of the polyol pathway as well as oxidative stress-induced generation of peroxynitrite ($ONOO^-$) (29–32). This free radical is a NO-derived RNS that not only leads to reductions in bioavailable NO but is also known to contribute to AGE formation. AGE signaling through RAGE can exert deleterious vascular effects in receptor-dependent or receptor-independent pathways (30). AGEs independently contribute to excessive crosslinking of collagen and disruption of extracellular matrix in the vessel wall. However, ligand binding to RAGE activates an inflammatory cascade in endothelial cells, macrophages, and smooth muscle cells with secondary overexpression of pro-inflammatory cytokines, adhesion molecules, and chemokines, increased production of ROS and activation nuclear factor NF-κB (30–32), a cascade of events that enhance formation of atherogenesis and endothelial dysfunction in diabetic vascular disease.

Lastly, increased activity of the polyol pathway resulting in the formation of sorbitol has been studied as well. In this pathway, glucose is reduced into sorbitol by aldose reductase, leading to depletion of NADPH. NADPH co-enzyme is essential for the regeneration of anti-oxidant molecules (20). Reduced NADPH is required for the functioning of many endothelial enzymes, including eNOS and cytochrome P450, as well as for the antioxidant activity of glutathione reductase. Alternatively, a high polyol pathway flux consumes large quantities of ATP and may thus compromise the energy supply required for endothelium-derived relaxation factor (EDRF) production (33).

THE ROLE OF HYPERINSULINEMIA IN ENDOTHELIAL DYSFUNCTION

The reactive hyperinsulinemia in insulin resistance and hyperglycemia also contributes to the development of endothelial dysfunction. Upon binding to specific insulin receptors (IR), insulin activates a number of downstream signaling systems that result in vasorelaxation such as ligand-activation of transmembrane receptors with tyrosine kinase activity, phosphorylation of insulin receptor substrate (IRS) and Shc (34–36). Tyrosine phosphorylation of IRS phosphorylation engages Src Homology 2 (SH2)-domain binding motifs for SH2-domain signaling molecules, including PI3K. When SH2 domains of the p85 regulatory subunit bind to tyrosine-phosphorylated motifs on IRS-1, this activates the pre-associated p110 catalytic subunit to generate 3,4,5-trisphosphate PI(3,4,5) P_3. This molecule then binds to the pleckstrin-homology domain in 3-phosphoinositide-dependent protein kinase-1 (PDK-1) resulting in its phosphorylation and activation of other downstream serine–threonine kinases including Akt and atypical protein kinase C isoforms, which mediate a number of metabolic actions including GLUT-4 translocation to membrane leading to NO production in blood vessels (34,37).

Vascular growth and remodeling responses to insulin involve signal transduction and activation of transcription (STAT) and the MAPK signaling pathways. This involves tyrosine-phosphorylated IRS-1 or Shc binding to the SH2 domain of Grb-2, which results in activation of the pre-associated guanosine triphosphate (GTP) exchange factor son of sevenless (SOS) and the GTP-binding protein Ras, which, phosphorylates/activates extracellular signal-regulated kinase (MEK), and MAPK. Crosstalk from signaling pathways of heterologous receptors, such as the Ang II type 1 receptor (AT_1R), exert enhancing effects on VSMC growth/remodeling signaling pathways while interfering with the metabolic signaling (34–37). Protein tyrosine phosphatases that dephosphorylate the insulin and IGF-1 receptor and IRS-1, as well as lipid phosphatases (i.e. SHIP-2 and PTEN) that dephosphorylate PI (3,4,5) P_3 are involved in the negative regulation of insulin and IGF-1 signaling pathways (38). Inappropriate activation of these phosphatases contributes to insulin resistance in cardiovascular, as well as traditional insulin sensitive tissues such as liver, skeletal muscle, and adipose tissue (34–38).

Vascular relaxation effects of insulin are mediated in part, by endothelial cell production of NO (Figure 100.1) (34,39,40). IR-mediation of PI3-K/PDK-1/Akt phosphorylation/activation leads to stimulation of eNOS enzyme activity to produce NO. Phosphorylated/activated Akt, in turn, phosphorylates human eNOS at Ser^{1177} resulting in enhanced eNOS activity (40). This insulin-mediated activation requires the formation of a ternary eNOS-Heat Shock Protein 90(HSP90)-Akt complex (34,41). Insulin also increases vascular smooth muscle cell production of NO (42). Thus, insulin promotes vascular relaxation, in part, through increases in NO bioavailability. Insulin also promotes vascular relaxation by attenuating agonist-induced increases in cytosolic calcium [Ca^{2+}] and myosin light chain (MLC) kinase activity (41,43,44). By enhancing MLC phosphatase activity, insulin reduces MLC kinase activity and thus [Ca^{2+}]-sensitive contraction.

THE ROLE OF THE RAAS IN ENDOTHELIAL DYSFUNCTION IN DIABETES

The beneficial impact of RAAS inhibition on diabetic-related CVD has clearly delineated a role for the RAAS in the diabetic-related endothelial dysfunction. Ang II is a potent vasoconstrictor with additional pro-inflammatory, pro-oxidative, and pro-atherosclerotic properties that promote endothelial dysfunction in diabetes. Ang II binding to the AT_1R induces production of reactive oxygen species (ROS) through activation of the vascular enzyme complex NADPH oxidase (35,36). In the setting of insulin resistance, Ang II has been shown to also stimulate xanthine oxidase, promote NADH auto-oxidation, and inhibit SOD, as well as stimulate the potent vasoconstrictor endothelin 1 (ET-1) and antagonize the actions of NO (45).

Recent data support that all elements of the RAAS are expressed in adipose tissue (especially visceral) (46). Dysfunction of adipocyte function could then partially explain the overactivity of the RAAS in obese and insulin-resistant patients. Thereby, in conditions of inappropriate activation of the RAAS, such as in obesity and insulin resistance, the normal balance between vasodilator and vasoconstricting properties of the endothelium is impaired (45–47). Increased vascular oxidative stress results in an inflammatory and pro-atherosclerotic vascular milieu, in which there is lipid peroxidation, cellular membranes injury, DNA damage, impairment of gene expression, and endothelial dysfunction (48).

Equally, Ang II promotes coagulation and platelet aggregation through its effect on PAI-1 and generates a pro-thrombotic environment (49,50). PAI-1 impairs matrix metalloproteinases (MMP), hampers extracellular matrix degradation, and promotes proliferation and atherosclerosis. Ang II acts in concert with sustained hyperglycemia to stimulate transforming growth factor-β (TGF-β), a major regulator of vascular remodeling and a known mediator of sclerotic changes found in type 2 diabetic patients (51).

In endothelium, Ang II participates in insulin resistance through interference of the PI3K and its downstream kinase Akt in insulin-dependent glucose utilization and production of NO (45,51). Excess Ang II in conjunction with hyperinsulinemia stimulates MAPK and thereby promotes cell proliferation and migration of vascular smooth muscle cells and endothelial cells as well as production of intracellular adhesion molecule-1 (ICAM-1) and monocyte chemoattractant protein-1 (MCP-1) (52). Therefore, the concept of selective insulin resistance and compensatory hyperinsulinemia is characterized in the vasculature by impairment of normal metabolic and vasorelaxing actions of insulin with a simultaneous stimulation of proliferative, inflammatory, and oxidative pathways that combine to result in endothelial dysfunction and atherosclerosis.

The abnormal endothelial-dependent vasodilation in the insulin-resistant state has been shown to predict CVD in humans and can also be found in first-degree relatives of patients with type 2 diabetes, in aging, and in obese individuals (53). Collectively, these data support that insulin resistance, even without hyperglycemia and a clinical diagnosis of type 2 diabetes, is characterized by impairment of the normal functions of the endothelium.

THE ROLE OF OXIDATIVE STRESS IN DIABETES-RELATED ENDOTHELIAL DYSFUNCTION

Oxidative stress is known to be a critical mechanism in the pathogenesis of diabetes-related endothelial dysfunction (54). Oxidative stress is due to excessive production of ROS including O_2^-, hydrogen peroxide (H_2O_2), and $ONOO^-$. There are multiple cellular sources of O_2^-, including NAD(P)H oxidase, xanthine oxidase, the mitochondrial respiratory chain, the arachidonic acid cascade (including lipoxygenase and cycloxygenase), and uncoupled endothelial nitric oxide synthase (eNOS) (55). NADPH oxidase serves as a key source of O_2^- in the vasculature (56). Ample evidence suggests that activation of NADPH oxidase contributes to vascular oxidative stress in virtually every forms of experimental diabetes (57,58). Furthermore, inhibition of O_2^- generation by genetic deletion of $gp91^{phox}$, by administration of dominant-negative Rac1, or by structurally different pharmacological inhibitors of NADPH oxidase also remarkably attenuates vascular O_2^- production in diabetes (54,57–59). NADPH oxidase activity and O_2^- production are elevated in coronary microvessels and aortas of type 2 diabetic mice (db/db), accompanied by impaired endothelium-dependent vasodilation (54,59). NADPH inhibitor, apocynin, ameliorates endothelial dysfunction in type 2 diabetic mice. Uncoupled eNOS and mitochondria are also frequently observed sources of vascular O_2^- in diabetic vasculature (60). Diabetes is associated with eNOS uncoupling and decreased tetrahydrobiopterin levels. Tetrahydrobiopterin supplementation improves NO production and endothelial function in type 2 diabetic patients (61). Although physiological levels of mitochondria-derived ROS functions in normal signaling, e.g. contributing to endothelium-dependent dilation in response to shear stress in specific vascular beds (62), increased levels exert pathological effects in diabetes (55).

The increase in vascular O_2^- production initiates prominent oxidative/nitrative stress. On the one hand, inactivation of NO by O_2^- anion is known to be a key mechanism underlying the reduction of NO bioavailability and the development of endothelial dysfunction (63). The interaction of O_2^- and NO produces $ONOO^-$, which leads to protein tyrosine nitration and the generation of nitrotyrosine (64). Nitrotyrosine was initially considered as a specific marker of peroxynitrite generation, but now is generally regarded as an index of RNS. Accumulating evidence supports the view that diabetes is associated with increased nitrosative stress and $ONOO^-$ formation (65). N-Tyr protein content is increased in both coronary and aortic vasculature of type 2 diabetic mice (54,59). Toxic effects of $ONOO^-$ and/or nitrotyrosine on the cardiovascular system are also supported by the fact that the degree of cell death and/or dysfunction correlates with levels of nitrotyrosine in endothelial cells, myocytes, and fibroblasts from diabetic patients (66,67). On the other hand, O_2^- can be dismutased spontaneously or by the catalytic effects of superoxide dismutase (SOD) to produce H_2O_2 (68), which is significantly increased in the serum of type 2 diabetic mice (54,59).

Thus, oxidative stress is clearly a contributing mechanism to diabetes-associated endothelial dysfunction and these findings may have important implications for prevention and management of vascular disease in diabetes mellitus by antioxidants and/or strategies designed to inhibit enzymatic sources of reactive oxygen species (60).

CONCLUSIONS

It is evident that diabetes increases cardiovascular risk. However, it is increasingly recognized that obesity-related insulin resistance contributes significantly to cardiovascular disease independent of the contribution of diabetes. The compensatory hyperinsulinemia associated with insulin resistance contributes significantly to a pro-inflammatory, pro-oxidative milieu that contributes to endothelial dysfunction through alterations in insulin metabolic signaling and reductions in bioavailable NO that alter the integrity of the endothelium. The importance of over-nutrition and obesity are increasingly recognized as critical in initiating the sequence of events that lead to endothelial dysfunction manifesting as hypertension and leading to CVD.

REFERENCES

1. *National Diabetes Fact Sheet: General Information and National Estimates on Diabetes in the United States.* <http://www.cdc.gov/diabetes/pubs/pdf/ndfs_2007.pdf>; 2007.
2. Wild S, Roglic G, Green A, Sicree R, King H. Global prevalence of diabetes: estimates for the year 2000 and projections for 2030. *Diabetes Care* 2004;**27**:1047–53.
3. Fagot-Campagna A, Saaddine JB, Flegal KM, Beckles GL. Diabetes, impaired fasting glucose and elevated HbA1c in U.S. adolescents: the Third National Health and Nutrition Examination Survey. *Diabetes Care* 2001;**24**:834–7.
4. Sinha R, Fisch G, Teague B, Tamborlane WV, Banyas B, Allen K, et al. Prevalence of impaired glucose tolerance among children and adolescents with marked obesity. *N Engl J Med* 2002;**346**:802–10.
5. Selby JV, Ray GT, Zhang D, Colby CJ. Excess costs of medical care for patients with diabetes in a managed care population. *Diabetes Care* 1997;**20**:1396–402.
6. Krop JS, Powe NR, Weller WE, Shaffer TJ, Saudek CD, Anderson GF. Patterns of expenditure and use of services among older adults with diabetes. *Diabetes Care* 1998;**21**:747–52.
7. Nichols GA, Glauber HS, Brown JB. Type 2 diabetes: incremental medical care costs during the first 8 years preceding diagnosis. *Diabetes Care* 2000;**23**:1654–9.
8. Gress TW, Nieto FJ, Shahar E, Wofford MR, Brancati FL. Hypertension and antihypertensive therapy as risk factors for type 2 diabetes mellitus: Atherosclerotic Risk in Communities Study. *N Engl J Med* 2000;**342**:905–12.
9. Haffner SM, Lehto S, Rönnemaa T, Pyörälä K, Laakso M. Mortality from coronary heart disease in subjects with type 2 diabetes mellitus in patients with myocardial infarction and in non-diabetic subjects with and without prior history of myocardial infarction. *N Engl J Med* 1998;**339**:229–34.
10. Stamler J, Vaccaro O, Neaton JD, Wentworth D. Diabetes, other risk factors and 12-year cardiovascular mortality for men screened in the Multiple Risk Factor Intervention Trial. *Diabetes Care* 1993;**16**:434–44.
11. Sowers JR. Diabetes mellitus and cardiovascular disease. *Arch Intern Med* 1998;**158**:617–21.
12. Davis TM, Millems H, Stratten JM, et al. Risk factors for stroke in type 2 diabetes mellitus: United Kingdom Prospective Diabetes Study (UKPDS) 29. *Arch Intern Med* 1999;**159**:1097–103.
13. Steinberg HO, Chaker H, Leaming R, Johnson A, Brechtel G, Baron AD. Obesity/insulin resistance is associated with endothelial dysfunction: implications for the syndrome of insulin resistance. *J Clin Invest* 1996;**97**:2601–10.
14. McFarlane SI, Jacober SJ, Winer N, Kaur J, Castro JP, Wui MA, et al. Control of cardiovascular risk factors in patients with diabetes and hypertension at urban academic medical centers. *Diabetes Care* 2002;**25**:718–23.
15. Guerci B, Böhme P, Kearney-Schwartz A, Zannad F, Drouin P. Endothelial dysfunction and type 2 diabetes (Part 1). *Diabetes Metab* 2001;**27**:425–34.
16. Moncada S, Higgs A. The L-Arginine-nitric oxidase pathway. *N Engl J Med* 1993;**329**:2002–12.
17. Garg UC, Hassid A. Nitric oxide-generating vasodailators and 8-bromo-cyclic guanosine monophosphate inhibit mitogenesis and proliferation of cultured rat vascular smooth muscle cells. *J Clin Invest* 1989;**83**:1774–7.
18. Kuboki K, Jiang ZY, Takahara N, Ha SW, Igarashi M, Yamauchi T, et al. Regulation of endothelial constitutive nitric oxide synthase gene expression in endothelial cells in vivo: a specific vascular action of insulin. *Circulation* 2000;**101**:676–81.
19. Whaley-Connell A, Pulakat L, DeMarco VG, Hayden MR, Habibi J, Henrikson E, et al. Over-nutrition and the Cardiorenal Syndrome (CRS): use of a rodent model to examine mechanism. *Cardiorenal Med* 2011;**1**:23–30.
20. Cooper SA, Whaley-Connell A, Habibi J, Wei Y, Lastra G, Manrique C, et al. Renin-angiotensin-aldosterone system and oxidative stress in cardiovascular insulin resistance. *Am J Physiol Heart Circ Physiol* 2007;**293**:H2009–23.
21. Guzik TJ, Mussa S, Gastaldi D, Sadowski J, Ratnatunga C, Pillai R, et al. Mechanisms of increased vascular superoxide production in human diabetes mellitus. *Circulation* 2002;**105**:1656.
22. Cosentino F, Hishikawa K, Katusic ZS, Lüscher TF. High glucose increases nitric oxide synthase expression and superoxide anion generation in human aortic endothelial cells. *Circulation* 1997;**86**:25–8.
23. Peterson TE, Poppa V, Ueba H, Wu A, Yan C, Berk BC. Opposing effects of reactive oxygen species and cholesterol on endothelial nitric oxide synthase and endothelial cell caveolae. *Circ Res* 1999;**85**:29–37.

24. Wolin MS. Interactions of oxidants with vascular signaling systems. *Arterioscler Thromb Vasc Biol* 2000;**20**:1430–42.
25. Williams SB, Cusco JA, Roddy MA, Johnstone MT, Creager MA. Impaired nitric oxide-mediated vasodilation in patients with non-insulin-dependent diabetes mellitus. *J Am Coll Cardiol* 1996;**27**:567–74.
26. Tesfamariam B, Brown ML, Cohen RA. Elevated glucose impairs endothelium-dependent relaxation by activating protein kinase. *Clin Invest* 1991;**87**:1643–8.
27. Williams B. Factors regulating the expression of vascular permeability/vascular endothelial growth human vascular tissues. *Diabetologia* 1997;**40**:S118–20.
28. Steinberg HO, Chaker H, Leaming R, Johnson A, Brechtel G, Baron AD. Obesity/insulin resistance is associated with endothelial dysfunction: implications for the syndrome of insulin resistance. *J Clin Invest* 1996;**97**:2601–10.
29. Cooper ME, El-Osta A. Mechanisms and implications for diabetic complications. *Circ Res* 2010;**107**:1403–13.
30. Yan SF, Ramasamy R, Naka Y, Schmidt AM. Glycation, inflammation, and RAGE: A scaffold for the macrovascular complications of diabetes and beyond. *Circ Res* 2003;**93**:1159–69.
31. Nishikawa T, Edelstein D, Du XL, Yamagishi S, Matsumura T, Kaneda Y, et al. Normalizing mitochondrial superoxide production blocks three pathways of hyperglycaemic damage. *Nature* 2000;**404**:787–90.
32. Yao D, Brownlee M. Hyperglycemia-induced reactive oxygen species increase expression of the receptor for advanced glycation end products (RAGE) and RAGE ligands. *Diabetes* 2010;**59**:249–55.
33. De Vriese AS, Verbeuren TJ, Van de Voorde J, Lameire NH, Vanhoutte PM. Endothelial dysfunction in diabetes. *Br J Pharmacol* 2000;**130**:963–74.
34. Muniyappa R, Montagnani M, Kon Koh K, Quon MJ. Cardiovascular actions of insulin. *Endocr Rev* 2007;**28**:463–91.
35. Sowers JR. Hypertension, angiotensin II, and oxidative stress. *N Engl J Med* 2002;**346**(25):1999–2001.
36. Sowers JR. Insulin resistance and hypertension. *Am J Physiol Heart Circ Physiol* 2004;**286**:H1597–602.
37. Taniguchi CM, Emanuelli B, Kahn CR. Critical nodes in signaling pathways: insights into insulin action. *Nat Rev Mol Cell Biol* 2006;**7**:85–96.
38. Vinciguerra M, Foti M. PTEN and SHIP2 pPhosphoinositide phosphatasis as negative regulators of insulin signaling. *Arch Physiol Biochem* 2006;**442**:89–104.
39. Walsh MF, Barazi M, Sowers JR. IGF-1 diminishes in vivo and in vitro vascular contractility: role of vascular nitric oxide. *Endocrinology* 1996;**137**:1798–803.
40. Zeng G, Nystrom FH, Ravichandran LV, Cong LN, Kirby M, Mostowski H, et al. Roles for insulin receptor, PI-3 kinase and Akt in insulin-signaling pathways related to production of nitric oxide in human vascular endothelial cells. *Circulation* 2000;**101**:1539–45.
41. Takahasi S, Mendelsohn ME. Synergistic activation of endothelial nitric-oxide synthase (eNOS) by HSP90 and Akt: calcium-independent eNOS activation involves formation of an HSP90-Akt-CaM-bound eNOS complex. *J Biol Chem* 2003;**278**:30821–7.
42. Bergandi L, Silvagno F, Russo I, Riganti C, Anfossi G, Aldieri E, et al. Insulin stimulates glucose transport via nitric oxide 1 cyclic GMP pathway in human vascular smooth muscle cells. *Arterioscler Thromb Vasc Biol* 2003;**23**:2215–21.
43. Standley PR, Zhang F, Ram JL, Sowers JR. Insulin attenuates vasopressin-induced calcium transients and a voltage-dependent calcium response in rat vascular smooth muscle cells. *J Clin Invest* 1991;**88**:1230–6.
44. Saito F, Hori MT, Fittingoff M, Hino T, Tuck ML. Insulin attenuates agonist-mediated calcium mobilization in cultured rat vascular smooth muscle cells. *J Clin Invest* 1993;**92**:1161–7.
45. Sowers JR, Whaley Connell A, Hayden MR. The role of overweight and obesity in the cardiorenal syndrome. *Cardiorenal Med* 2011;**1**:5–12.
46. Cooper SA, Whaley-Connell A, Habibi J, Wei Y, Lastra G, Manriquem C, et al. Role of renin-angiotensin-aldosterone system-induced oxidative stress in cardiovascular insulin resistance. *Am J Physiol Heart Circ Physiol* 2007;**293**:H2009–23.
47. Steimberg HO, Chaker H, Leaming R, Johnson A, Bretchel G. Obesity/insulin resistance is associated with endothelial dysfunction: implications for the syndrome of insulin resistance. *J Clin Invest* 1996;**97**:2601–10.
48. Griendling KK, Minieri CA, Ollerenshaw JD, Alexander RW. Angiotensin II stimulates NADH and NADPH oxidase activity in cultured vascular smooth muscle cells. *Circ Res* 1994;**74**:1141–8.
49. Nickenig G, Harrison DG. The AT1-type angiotensin receptor in oxidative stress and atherogenesis. Part I: Oxidative stress and atherogenesis. *Circulation* 2002;**105**:393–6.
50. Vaughan DE, Lazos SA, Tong K. Angiotensin II regulates the expression of plasminogen activator inhibitor 1 in cultured endothelial cells: a potential link between the renin-angiotensin system and thrombosis. *J Clin Invest* 1995;**95**:995–1001.
51. Pessin JE, Salteil AR. Signaling pathways in insulin action: molecular targets of insulin resistance. *J Clin Invest* 2000;**106**:165–9.
52. Xi XP, Graf K, Goetze S, Fleck E, Hsueh WA, Law RE. Central role of MAPK pathway in ang II-mediated DNA synthesis and migration in rat vascular smooth cells. *Atheroscler Thromb Vasc Biol* 1999;**19**:73–82.
53. Balletshofer BM, Rittig K, Enderle MD, Volk A, Maerker E, Jacob S, et al. Endothelial dysfunction is detectable in young normotensive first-degree relatives of subjects with type 2 diabetes in association with insulin resistance. *Circulation* 2000;**101**:1780–4.
54. Zhang H, Zhang J, Ungvari Z, Zhang C. Resveratrol improves endothelial function: role of TNF{alpha} and vascular oxidative stress. *Arterioscler Thromb Vasc Biol* 2009;**29**:1164–71.
55. Brownlee M. Biochemistry and molecular cell biology of diabetic complications. *Nature* 2001;**414**:813–20.
56. Griendling KK. NADPH oxidases: new regulators of old functions. *Antioxid Redox Signal* 2006;**8**:1443–5.
57. Picchi A, Gao X, Belmadani S, Potter BJ, Focardi M, Chilian WM, et al. Tumor necrosis factor-alpha induces endothelial dysfunction in the prediabetic metabolic syndrome. *Circ Res* 2006;**99**:69–77.
58. Ebrahimian TG, Heymes C, You D, Blanc-Brude O, Mees B, Waeckel L, et al. NADPH oxidase-derived overproduction of reactive oxygen species impairs postischemic neovascularization in mice with type 1 diabetes. *Am J Pathol* 2006;**169**:719–28.
59. Gao X, Belmadani S, Picchi A, Xu X, Potter BJ, Tewari-Singh N, et al. Tumor necrosis factor-alpha induces endothelial dysfunction in Lepr(db) mice. *Circulation* 2007;**115**:245–54.
60. Tabit CE, Chung WB, Hamburg NM, Vita JA. Endothelial dysfunction in diabetes mellitus: molecular mechanisms and clinical implications. *Rev Endocr Metab Disord* 2010;**11**:61–74.

61. Heitzer T, Krohn K, Albers S, Meinertz T. Tetrahydrobiopterin improves endothelium-dependent vasodilation by increasing nitric oxide activity in patients with Type II diabetes mellitus. *Diabetologia* 2000;**43**:1435–8.
62. Liu Y, Zhao H, Li H, Kalyanaraman B, Nicolosi AC, Gutterman DD. Mitochondrial sources of H_2O_2 generation play a key role in flow-mediated dilation in human coronary resistance arteries. *Circ Res* 2003;**93**:573–80.
63. Shah AM, Channon KM. Free radicals and redox signalling in cardiovascular disease. *Heart* 2004;**90**:486–7.
64. Zou MH, Cohen R, Ullrich V. Peroxynitrite and vascular endothelial dysfunction in diabetes mellitus. *Endothelium* 2004;**11**:89–97.
65. Pacher P, Beckman JS, Liaudet L. Nitric oxide and peroxynitrite in health and disease. *Physiol Rev* 2007;**87**:315–424.
66. Frustaci A, Kajstura J, Chimenti C, Jakoniuk I, Leri A, Maseri A, et al. Myocardial cell death in human diabetes. *Circ Res* 2000;**87**:1123–32.
67. Pacher P, Szabo C. Role of peroxynitrite in the pathogenesis of cardiovascular complications of diabetes. *Curr Opin Pharmacol* 2006;**6**:136–41.
68. Papa S, Skulachev VP. Reactive oxygen species, mitochondria, apoptosis and aging. *Mol Cell Biochem* 1997;**174**:305–19.

Chapter 101

Vascular Mechanisms of Hypertension in the Pathophysiology of Preeclampsia

Eric M. George and Joey P. Granger

Department of Physiology and Biophysics and the Center for Excellence in Cardiovascular-Renal Research, University of Mississippi Medical Center, Jackson, MS

PREECLAMPSIA

Preeclampsia is a gestational hypertensive disorder defined by new-onset hypertension, proteinuria, and maternal vascular dysfunction. It typically manifests late in gestation, commonly presenting only after the 20th week of gestation (1). Despite increased awareness and intensive screening, it remains one of the leading causes of fetal and maternal morbidity and mortality, and approximately 15% of all preterm pregnancies can be attributed to preeclampsia (2). While the overall incidence of preeclampsia is approximately 8%, certain subpopulations have significantly higher incidence rates, and the rate of preeclampsia has risen steadily in the past several decades (3–5). Primarily, preeclampsia is seen in nulliparous women with decreased incidence with subsequent pregnancies (6).

Cardiovascular function is severely altered in preeclampsia. In normal pregnancies, there are marked decreases in total vascular resistance and arterial pressure, with concomitant increases in cardiac output and plasma volume (7). In contrast, during preeclampsia the typical high output, low resistance seen in normal pregnancy is reversed to a low output, high resistance phenotype (8). Additionally, normal pregnancy is associated with decreased renal vascular resistance and decreased pressor and vasoconstrictor response (9–11). In preeclampsia, however, there is a marked increase in vascular resistance and pressure with increased Ang II sensitivity (12).

The specific etiology behind these cardiovascular changes is not clear. Recent evidence, however, suggests that it is a combination of enhanced smooth muscle contraction and decreased endothelial-dependent vasorelaxation. The central causative factor, however, lies in abnormal development of the placenta.

PLACENTATION AND THE ORIGIN OF PREECLAMPSIA

There are many effector molecules and systems that are implicated in the pathological phase of preeclampsia, but the central causative agent underlying them all is the placenta itself. This became clear when it was realized that the only totally effective intervention to treat the disorder was delivery of the placenta, and that in cases where the fetus alone was delivered, the maternal syndrome failed to remit (13,14). In a normal healthy pregnancy, there are a number of coordinated events which ensure proper blood supply to both the placenta and the fetus. Typically, fetally-derived trophoblasts migrate to the maternal vasculature and invade the maternal uterine arteries. They then undergo a phenotypic shift in their lineage to an endothelial-like phenotype. The net effect is to convert the maternal spiral arterioles from low capacitance, high resistance, muscular, and reactive vessels into high capacitance, low resistance, and significantly larger vessels (13,15).

In preeclampsia, this process does not proceed normally. Examination of the myometrial segments of the spiral arteries reveals that in preeclampsia there is a failure of this remodeling, leading to significantly smaller, muscular, and elastic vessels (16). Even under normal circumstances, the placenta is a relatively hypoxic environment, but the failure of the spiral arteries to remodel and adequately supply the placenta with blood renders it extremely hypoxic as indicated by a number of hypoxia-regulated gene transcripts (17–19). One important caveat in this mechanism is that there are reported cases in which failure of spiral artery remodeling occurs, but does not lead to a pathological state resembling preeclampsia (20). It still remains to be seen whether there are compounding factors which must be present for the full

Muscle. DOI: http://dx.doi.org/10.1016/B978-0-12-381510-1.00101-0

disease state to manifest itself. Despite this uncertainty, it is now widely recognized that placental hypoxia, and the resulting ischemia, are at the root of many of the secondary factors that produce the maternal syndrome.

PLACENTAL ISCHEMIA AND HYPOXIA

How can hypoxic conditions in the placenta lead to widespread maternal endothelial dysfunction and hypertension? In order to address this question a rodent model known as the reduced uterine perfusion pressure (RUPP) model of pregnancy-induced hypertension has been utilized extensively. As can be seen in Table 101.1, the RUPP model shares many similarities with human preeclampsia, and is a valuable tool for the investigation of the role of placental ischemia in gestational hypertension. Recent research in humans and in experimental models has focused on two types of factors produced in response to placental hypoxia which are believed to have a role in the etiology of the disease: angiogenic factors and oxidative stress. Each of these in turn has significant effects on the maternal vasculature and contributes to the hypertension associated with preeclampsia.

Angiogenic Factors

One of the most promising systems to receive scrutiny in recent preeclampsia research is the vascular endothelial growth factor (VEGF) signaling pathway. VEGF, a powerful pro-angiogenic protein, is an essential factor in the maintenance of endothelial cell health. Additionally, VEGF is necessary for the maintenance of glomerular ultra-structure through the maintenance of glomerular fenestrated endothelium. Transgenic VEGF knockout in glomerular podocytes resulted in proteinuria and glomerular endotheliosis, two common findings in preeclampsia (21). Similar findings are found in cancer patients who have been treated with VEGF monoclonal antibodies, as hypertension and proteinuria are common side effects (22). It is clear then, that proper levels of VEGF are necessary for endothelial and vascular health.

One factor shown to interfere with VEGF signaling is the soluble form of the VEGF receptor Flt-1. sFlt-1 is an alternately spliced variant of the full length receptor in which the transmembrane and cytosolic domains have been excised, leaving only the extracellular recognition domain (23). This recognition domain acts as a VEGF antagonist by binding free VEGF, and making it unavailable for proper signaling, additionally, it can act as a dominant negative receptor, rendering functional full length Flt-1 receptors inert (24). Of particular interest for preeclampsia, sFlt-1 is positively regulated by hypoxia, specifically through the actions of HIF-1α, and has been shown to be produced by both placental trophoblasts and human placental villous explants in response to low oxygen tension (25–27). Analysis of circulating levels of sFlt-1 in preeclamptic patients demonstrates a significant increase compared to normal pregnant controls, sometimes even months prior to the manifestation of the syndrome (28).

Several experimental models have demonstrated a causative role for sFlt-1 in the pathology of preeclampsia. Viral ectopic expression of sFlt-1 in pregnant rats led to a preeclampsia-like state, with hypertension, glomerular endotheliosis, and proteinuria (29). Models of reduced uterine perfusion pressure in both nonhuman primates and rats have shown significant increases in circulating sFlt-1, and concurrent decreases in bioavailable circulating

TABLE 101.1 The RUPP Model of Pregnancy-Induced Hypertension Mirrors Human Preeclampsia, and Is a Useful Model for the Study of Placental Ischemia

Symptom	RUPP	Preeclampsia	Reference
Hypertension	+	+	Alexander et al. (53)
Proteinuria	+	+	Alexander et al. (53)
Decreased renal plasma flow	+	+	Alexander et al. (53)
Decreased GFR	+	+	Alexander et al. (53)
Endothelial dysfunction	+	+	Crews et al. (56)
Angiogenic imbalance	+	+	Gilbert et al. (30)
Enhanced ET-1 expression	+	+	Alexander et al. (67)
Oxidative stress	+	+	Sedeek et al. (43)
Increased inflammatory cytokines	+	+	LaMarca et al. (70), Gadonski et al. (75)
Agonistic AT1-AA production	+	+	LaMarca et al. (79)

VEGF (30,31). In agreement with the viral expression experiments, direct infusion of sFlt-1 into pregnant rats induces preeclamptic-like symptoms, including hypertension, reduced fetal weight, and increases in vascular ROS (32). As with several other experimental forms of hypertension, endothelin is one of the major effector molecules in sFlt-1 induced PIH, as administration of an ET_A receptor antagonist completely normalizes blood pressure (33).

It does not appear that the pathological manifestations seen in sFlt-1 induced PIH are a direct result of circulating sFlt-1 but rather the loss of VEGF. Simultaneous administration of high levels of sFlt-1 and VEGF to pregnant rat results in significantly diminished hypertension and increased renal protection (34,35). Additionally, VEGF administration in rats with placental ischemia restored normal blood pressure, renal function, and vascular activity (36). These and other data have led to the hypothesis that the ratio between sFlt-1 and VEGF is critical to maintain a healthy endothelium and normal vascular activity. The role of these proteins in the development of preeclampsia is a promising avenue in the search for new therapeutics.

Oxidative Stress

There is abundant evidence from the clinical literature that oxidative stress is significantly elevated in the preeclamptic placenta (37,38). Specifically, two important markers of oxidative stress, lipid hydroperoxides and arachadonic acid-derived free isoprostane, are elevated in the placental decidua in preeclamptic women (39–41). Oxidative stress is not confined to the placenta of preeclamptic women, but has been identified systemically. Levels of peroxynitrite in the vascular endothelium are significantly elevated in preeclampsia when compared to normal pregnant women. The presence of vascular oxidative stress can be a significant contributor to endothelial dysfunction by direct detrimental action on the endothelial cells themselves, and indirectly through reduction in the production of vasoactive compounds. Accordingly, the same study that identified oxidative stress in the maternal vascular endothelium also indicated a decreased production of nitric oxide synthase (42). There are also reports indicating that preeclamptic women have suppressed expression of superoxide dismutase in both the vasculature and placenta, indicating an overall decrease in antioxidant activity during preeclampsia (42).

Experimental models of placental ischemia demonstrate the importance of ischemia and hypoxia in the induction of oxidative stress in the placenta. Placental hypoperfusion in the rat significantly increases placental oxidative stress. Significantly, the superoxide dismutase mimetic compound Tempol significantly reduced the hypertension associated with this model, indicating that oxidative stress is an important regulator of hypertension during preeclampsia, presumably through maternal endothelial dysfunction (43). Similar reductions in hypertension in this model have also been shown by inhibition of the NADPH oxidase with apocynin, suggesting the possibility that increased NADPH oxidase activity or production is one of the sources of oxidative stress produced in response to placental ischemia (44). Further research into the manipulation of oxidative stress pathways is warranted, as they may provide a fresh target for treating the disease.

ENDOTHELIAL DYSFUNCTION IN PREECLAMPSIA

One of the most significant recognized symptoms of preeclampsia is widespread maternal endothelial dysfunction, which coincidentally is the major mechanism through which smooth muscle is affected during preeclampsia. There are several important pathological factors that are associated with endothelial dysfunction. Here we will discuss several of the most prominent: decreased nitric oxide, increased endothelin-1 production, increased reactive oxygen, and the maternal inflammatory response.

Nitric Oxide

The preponderance of available data suggests that changes in vascular reactivity mentioned above which occur during normal pregnancy are, at least in part, due to increased levels of endothelial cell-derived nitric oxide (NO) (45–47). Several reports have demonstrated that there is increased nitric oxide synthase (NOS) production in the uterine artery during pregnancy. Coincidentally, levels of the NO secondary messenger cyclic guanosine monophosphate (cGMP) are also up in the circulation, suggesting an increase in NOS activity (48,49). Gestational studies in animals have also demonstrated an increased endothelial derived NO-mediated vasorelaxation with progressivity of pregnancy, and concurrent induction of both tissue NOS synthesis and NO production (50–53).

Given that NO appears to be important for the vasodilation seen during a healthy pregnancy, a logical hypothesis would be that reduced NO bioavailability could be one of the causes of the maternal increase in peripheral resistance which is seen in preeclamptic patients. Accordingly, when compared to normal pregnant women, preeclamptic patients show a significant alteration in the levels of NO metabolites in the umbilical vein and amniotic fluid (54,55). As seen in Figure 101.1, when the vasculature of the RUPP rat model of placental ischemia was examined, there was an impaired vascular relaxation in response to acetylcholine and decreased production of

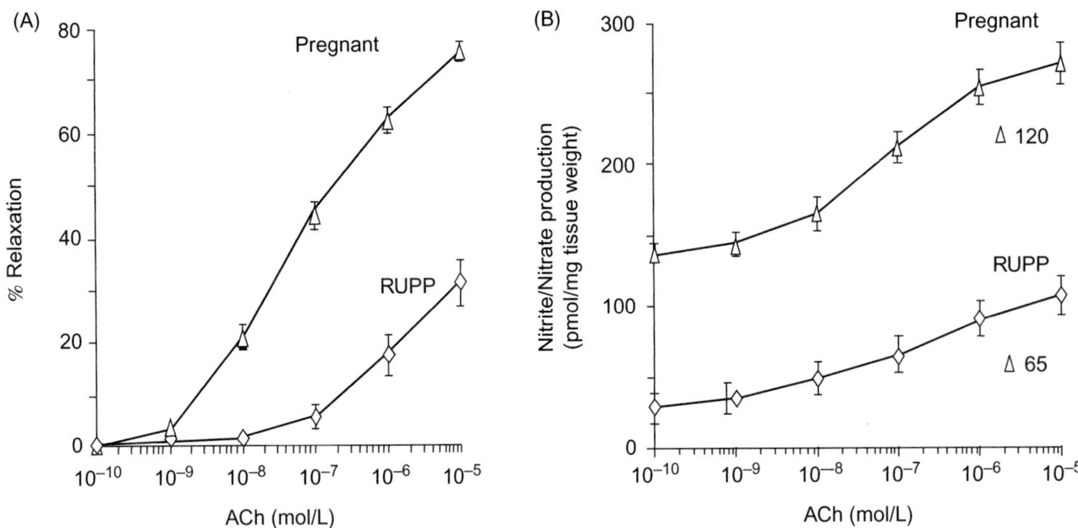

FIGURE 101.1 RUPP rats have a decreased vasorelaxation response to acetylcholine (ACh) when compared to normal pregnant control animals (A). They also exhibit a decreased production of NO when stimulated with ACh (B).

NO metabolites. There is also a differential response to endothelium removal and NOS inhibition when vascular reactivity was measured. This effect was also seen when cGMP production was impaired, suggesting that at least in the RUPP rats, there is a direct correlation between decreased NO/cGMP formation and vascular dysfunction, indicating that NO is important in the endothelial dysfunction resulting from placental ischemia (56).

Strikingly, experimental inhibition of NOS by the L-arginine derivative L-NAME in rodent models also leads to a preeclampsia-like state. This hypertensive effect is markedly enhanced when compared to NOS inhibition in non-pregnant animals (51). In addition to hypertension, this model exhibits fetal growth restriction, proteinuria, and increased renal vasoconstriction (57–59). Additionally vascular reactivity to phenylephrine is significantly increased when compared to normal pregnant animals (51). While not definitively causative, it seems clear that there is an important role for NO bioavailability in the symptomatic phase of preeclampsia.

Endothelin

Perhaps one of the most important factors in the symptomatic phase of preeclampsia is the increase in circulating and tissue levels of the signaling protein endothelin-1 (ET-1). ET-1 was first identified over twenty years ago as one of the most potent vasoconstrictors ever discovered. The active form of ET-1 is a 21 amino acid peptide derived from the two-step degradation from the precursor preproendothelin (preproET-1) (60–62). While not universally observed, the majority of published studies indicate that there is a significant increase in the circulating levels of ET-1 in preeclamptic patients when compared to normal pregnant controls, and that these levels return to normal shortly after birth (63–66). This is consistent with the resolution of preeclampsia-associated hypertension post-partum.

ET-1 expression has also been implicated as an important pathological factor in a number of experimental models of preeclampsia. Perhaps the most well established of these is the rat RUPP model. This model demonstrates increased renal cortical and medullary preproET message levels compared to control pregnant animals. Importantly, the hypertension that is associated with this model can be significantly attenuated by the administration of an endothelin type-A receptor (ET_A) antagonist (67). In a separate model in which tumor necrosis factor-alpha (TNF-α) is infused into pregnant rats to mimic circulating levels seen in preeclamptic women, again, renal levels of preproET-1 message were elevated, but there were also increases in preproET-1 message in the aorta and placenta. ET_A receptor antagonism was especially efficacious in this model, completely normalizing the associated hypertension (68). This was in line with earlier evidence which suggested that preproET-1 transcription is directly regulated by TNF-α signaling in a dosage-dependent manner (69). In a follow-up study which linked these two pathways, blockade of TNF-α by the soluble receptor Etanerecept in the RUPP model led to a significant decrease in the levels of tissue ET-1, and again the associated hypertension was completely normalized (70).

The previously mentioned sFlt-1 infusion model of pregnancy-induced hypertension elevates mean arterial pressure ~15 mmHg in pregnant rats, while having no effect on non-pregnant animals. In this model, preeproET-1 message levels are significantly elevated in the renal cortex. As with the TNF-α infusion model, administration of an ET_A receptor antagonist completely abolished the associated hypertension (33). Finally, ET-1 has been identified as an important pathological factor in the recently established angiotensin-1 autoantibody (AT1-AA) infusion model of pregnancy induced hypertension, discussed in greater detail below. When the agonistic antibodies are administered experimentally in the rat, preeclampsia-like symptoms are observed. As with the other experimental models mentioned above, this includes significant elevations in tissue preproET-1. Furthermore, as with all the other models of pregnancy-induced hypertension discussed here, administration of an ET_A receptor antagonist significantly attenuated the hypertension associated with this model (71). The fact that ET_A receptor antagonism so thoroughly and consistently reduces hypertension in the various models of hypertension in pregnancy argues for a pivotal role of ET-1, specifically through ET_A signaling, in the etiology of preeclampsia.

The Maternal Inflammatory Response

There is a growing interest in the maternal immunity and inflammatory processes as mediators of the clinical manifestations of preeclampsia. Even in normal pregnancies, there is a heightened inflammatory response when compared to non-pregnant women, but in preeclampsia, there is significant elevation of inflammation markers, e.g. IL-6 and TNF-α, when compared to healthy pregnancies (72–74). This is more than correlative, as there are several experimental lines of evidence demonstrating that infusion of these factors leads to states that mimic preeclampsia in animals. In the RUPP model of hypertension, IL-6, and TNF-α are both elevated, just as in the human syndrome, and blockade of TNF-α with the soluble receptor Etanercept attenuated the associated hypertension and decreased tissue ET-1 expression (70,75). Even more convincingly, infusion of either IL-6 or TNF-α to pregnant rats at doses that mimic levels seen in preeclamptic women, is sufficient to produce a hypertensive response, indicating the importance of these inflammatory cytokines in the etiology of the disorder (75,76).

Another factor produced by the maternal immune system that has received a great deal of attention in recent years is the recently identified angiotensin-1 receptor autoantibody (AT1-AA), which has been identified in the circulation of preeclamptic women. These antibodies activate the AT-1 receptor, causing vasoconstriction and are hypothesized to play an important role in preeclampsia-associated hypertension (77,78). Intriguingly, they are also found in the circulation of the RUPP rat, indicating an important link between placental ischemia and autoantibody production (79). Though still in early stages of research, several experimental lines of evidence support an important role for the AT1-AA and suggest it is an important therapeutic target. First, there is evidence that besides its vasoconstriction activity, AT1-AA can upregulate sFlt-1 through the AT-1 receptor, ROS through NADPH oxidase activity, and tissue ET-1 (71,80,81). Infusion of purified AT1-AA into pregnant animals causes significant hypertension, which can be totally normalized by ET_A receptor blockade, indicating that ET-1 signaling is the predominant mechanism through which AT1-AA induces hypertension (71). Future research into the AT1-AA and the maternal inflammatory response are likely to provide a wealth of new insight into the pathological mechanisms underlying preeclampsia.

POTENTIAL THERAPIES FOR THE TREATMENT OF PREECLAMPSIA

Despite our increased understanding of the mechanisms that underlie the pathological symptoms of preeclampsia, and more awareness of the disorder, there remains little in the way of effective therapeutic intervention available to the clinician. The only definitive remediation of the disorder comes from the delivery of the fetus and placenta. While some traditional hypertensive medications can be given in severe cases, they are often ineffective, and normal pressure is rarely achieved. As a consequence, management of preeclampsia focuses on prolonging pregnancy as long as possible without risk to the mother through a combination of bed rest and anticonvulsive therapy. Often, preterm delivery of the fetus results, as the symptoms become dangerous to the mother. New therapies for the management of the disease symptoms would be an important advancement in women's health. In this chapter, we have seen many pathways that could be important targets for therapeutic intervention in preeclampsia.

We have seen in this chapter that reduced NO bioavailability and increased oxidative stress are important mediators of preeclampsia symptoms. One intriguing mechanism by which both of these pathways could be manipulated is through the protein heme oxygenase-1 (HO-1). HO-1 is component of the heme salvage pathway, whose normal function is to convert free heme, a potent pro-oxidant molecule, from degraded proteins into the eventual breakdown products carbon monoxide (CO) and bilirubin. CO, while toxic at high levels in the circulation, is in fact a potent vasodilator produced endogenously. Furthermore, CO has been hypothesized to have a role in the maintenance of vasodilation in placental blood vessels (82). CO functions in a manner quite similar to NO. It is possible then, that extra production of CO by HO-1 could help compensate for the reduced bioavailability of NO in preeclampsia, improving endothelial function, increasing vasodilation, and reducing hypertension. As an added bonus, it has recently been shown that at least in an *in vitro* context, HO-1 or CO alone can downregulate sFlt-1 expression (83).

Bilirubin, the other major byproduct of HO-1, is a powerful antioxidant. As discussed previously, oxidative stress is an important regulator of vascular dysfunction in preeclampsia. Therefore, increased HO-1 activity might be one way to decrease vascular oxidative stress and improve endothelial function. Indeed, HO-1 has been shown to have beneficial effects in diverse models of hypertension which share several common pathways with preeclampsia (84–87). A recent study in the RUPP rodent model showed that induction of HO-1 significantly decreased blood pressure, increased circulating VEGF, and reduced placental superoxide in this model (88). Furthermore, HO-1 infusion had beneficial effects on hypertension in response to sFlt-1 infusion, suggesting that HO-1 induction has additional beneficial properties besides sFlt-1 suppression (89). Together these data suggest that manipulation of the HO-1 pathway might prove an efficacious approach to the treatment of preeclampsia.

A second treatment that has been suggested for the management of preeclampsia is administration of a phosphodiesterase type-5 (PDE5) inhibitor, such as sildenafil. In a normal context, PDE enzymes function in the degradation of the NO secondary messenger cGMP. In consequence, they antagonize vasodilation. Of particular interest to pregnancy and preeclampsia, there are reports in sheep that PDE5 is localized in the uteroplacental unit (90). Several *ex vivo* studies of myometrial arteries taken from preeclamptic or growth-restricted pregnancies have demonstrated that there is an enhanced endothelial-dependent relaxation when the preparations were incubated in the presence of a PDE5 inhibitor (91,92). Despite this promising experimental evidence, the effect of PDE5 inhibition during preeclampsia remains scanty. Phase 2 clinical trials of sildenafil administration have been reported in both normal and preeclamptic pregnancies, with no apparent adverse effects on the mother or offspring. However, there was also no concurrent benefit to sildenafil treatment in the preeclamptic patients (93). The study is not without several caveats, however, as the drug was only given in late pregnancy. The possibility remains then that early administration to counteract the initiation of placental ischemia might prove more efficacious (94). More research is needed to determine whether more targeted dosing might make sildenafil a more potent therapeutic for preeclampsia.

Lastly, one of the most consistently effective agents for the treatment of pregnancy-induced hypertension in a wide variety of models is an ET_A receptor-selective antagonist. The effect of ET_A blockade in humans is not known, nor is the effect of ET_A antagonism. Reluctance to experiment with this treatment in humans has stemmed in large measure from mouse knockouts of the ET_A receptor, which are embryonically lethal due to developmental defects (95). An important caveat however comes from follow-up pharmacological ET_A blockades studies in rats which pinpointed the mid-gestation as the critical role for the teratogenic effects of loss of ET_A signaling (96). More detailed investigations into the safety and efficacy of ET_A antagonism are warranted to explore its potential as a therapeutic.

CONCLUSION

Despite intensive research and aggressive management, preeclampsia remains a serious health concern. While the exact molecular origins of the disease remain unknown, as seen in Figure 101.2, it is now clear that through failure of uteroplacental vascular remodeling, placental hypoxia/ischemia causes the production of factors that lead to widespread endothelial and vascular dysfunction. Continuing efforts to explore these factors and their actions holds the potential to finally find an effective therapeutic to treat this serious malady.

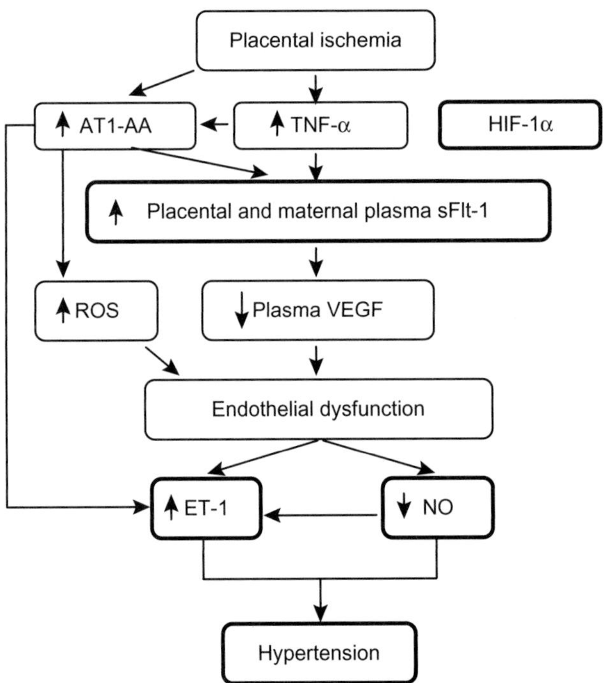

FIGURE 101.2 Placental ischemia initiates numerous pathways in the pathophysiology of preeclampsia. AT1-AA (angiotensin 1 receptor auto antibody), TNF-α (tumor necrosis factor-alpha), HIF-1α (hypoxia inducible factor-1α), ROS (reactive oxygen species), VEGF (vascular endothelial growth factor), sFlt-1 (soluble fms-like tyrosine kinase-1), ET-1 (endothelin-1), NO (nitric oxide).

REFERENCES

1. Roberts JM, Cooper DW. Pathogenesis and genetics of pre-eclampsia. *Lancet* 2001;**357**:53–6.
2. Meis PJ, Goldenberg RL, Mercer BM, Iams JD, Moawad AH, Miodovnik M, et al. The preterm prediction study: risk factors for indicated preterm births. Maternal-Fetal Medicine Units Network of the National Institute of Child Health and Human Development. *Am J Obstet Gynecol* 1998;**178**:562–7.
3. Roberts JM, Pearson G, Cutler J, Lindheimer M. Summary of the NHLBI Working Group on Research on Hypertension During Pregnancy. *Hypertension* 2003;**41**:437–45.
4. Poon LC, Kametas NA, Chelemen T, Leal A, Nicolaides KH. Maternal risk factors for hypertensive disorders in pregnancy: a multivariate approach. *J Hum Hypertens* 2010;**24**:104–10.
5. Paul DA, Mackley A, Locke RG, Ehrenthal D, Hoffman M, Kroelinger C. Increased preeclampsia in mothers delivering very low-birth-weight infants between 1994 and 2006. *Am J Perinatol* 2009;**26**:467–72.
6. Caritis S, Sibai B, Hauth J, Lindheimer M, VanDorsten P, Klebanoff M, et al. Predictors of pre-eclampsia in women at high risk. National Institute of Child Health and Human Development Network of Maternal-Fetal Medicine Units. *Am J Obstet Gynecol* 1998;**179**:946–51.
7. Robson SC, Hunter S, Boys RJ, Dunlop W. Serial study of factors influencing changes in cardiac output during human pregnancy. *Am J Physiol Heart Cell Physiol* 1989;**256**:H1060–5.
8. Visser W, Wallenburg HC. Central hemodynamic observations in untreated preeclamptic patients. *Hypertension* 1991;**17**:1072–7.
9. Davidge ST, McLaughlin MK. Endogenous modulation of the blunted adrenergic response in resistance-sized mesenteric arteries from the pregnant rat. *Am J Obstet Gynecol* 1992;**167**:1691–8.
10. Davison JM, Dunlop W. Renal hemodynamics and tubular function normal human pregnancy. *Kidney Int* 1980;**18**:152–61.
11. Duvekot JJ, Peeters LL. Renal hemodynamics and volume homeostasis in pregnancy. *Obstet Gynecol Surv* 1994;**49**:830–9.
12. Gant NF, Daley GL, Chand S, Whalley PJ, MacDonald PC. A study of angiotensin II pressor response throughout primigravid pregnancy. *J Clin Invest* 1973;**52**:2682–9.
13. Hladunewich M, Karumanchi SA, Lafayette R. Pathophysiology of the clinical manifestations of preeclampsia. *Clin J Am Soc Nephrol* 2007;**2**:543–9.
14. Shembrey MA, Noble AD. An instructive case of abdominal pregnancy. *Aust NZ J Obstet Gynaecol* 1995;**35**:220–1.
15. Khong Y, Brosens I. Defective deep placentation. *Best Pract Res Clin Obstet Gynaecol* 2011;**25**:301–11.
16. Brosens IA, Robertson WB, Dixon HG. The role of the spiral arteries in the pathogenesis of preeclampsia. *Obstet Gynecol Annu* 1972;**1**:177–91.
17. Rodesch F, Simon P, Donner C, Jauniaux E. Oxygen measurements in endometrial and trophoblastic tissues during early pregnancy. *Obstet Gynecol* 1992;**80**:283–5.
18. Rajakumar A, Doty K, Daftary A, Harger G, Conrad KP. Impaired oxygen-dependent reduction of HIF-1alpha and -2alpha proteins in pre-eclamptic placentae. *Placenta* 2003;**24**:199–208.
19. Rajakumar A, Whitelock KA, Weissfeld LA, Daftary AR, Markovic N, Conrad KP. Selective overexpression of the hypoxia-inducible transcription factor, HIF-2alpha, in placentas from women with preeclampsia. *Biol Reprod* 2001;**64**:499–506.
20. Sheppard BL, Bonnar J. An ultrastructural study of utero-placental spiral arteries in hypertensive and normotensive pregnancy and fetal growth retardation. *Br J Obstet Gynaecol* 1981;**88**:695–705.
21. Ballermann BJ. Glomerular endothelial cell differentiation. *Kidney Int* 2005;**67**:1668–71.
22. Zhu X, Wu S, Dahut WL, Parikh CR. Risks of proteinuria and hypertension with bevacizumab, an antibody against vascular endothelial growth factor: systematic review and meta-analysis. *Am J Kidney Dis* 2007;**49**:186–93.
23. Banks RE, Forbes MA, Searles J, Pappin D, Canas B, Rahman D, et al. Evidence for the existence of a novel pregnancy-associated soluble variant of the vascular endothelial growth factor receptor, Flt-1. *Mol Hum Reprod* 1998;**4**:377–86.
24. Wu FT, Stefanini MO, Mac Gabhann F, Kontos CD, Annex BH, Popel AS. A systems biology perspective on sVEGFR1: its biological function, pathogenic role and therapeutic use. *J Cell Mol Med* 2010;**14**:528–52.
25. Nagamatsu T, Fujii T, Kusumi M, Zou L, Yamashita T, Osuga Y, et al. Cytotrophoblasts up-regulate soluble fms-like tyrosine kinase-1 expression under reduced oxygen: an implication for the placental vascular development and the pathophysiology of preeclampsia. *Endocrinology* 2004;**145**:4838–45.
26. Ahmad S, Ahmed A. Elevated placental soluble vascular endothelial growth factor receptor-1 inhibits angiogenesis in preeclampsia. *Circ Res* 2004;**95**:884–91.
27. Nevo O, Soleymanlou N, Wu Y, Xu J, Kingdom J, Many A, et al. Increased expression of sFlt-1 in in vivo and in vitro models of human placental hypoxia is mediated by HIF-1. *Am J Physiol Regul Integr Comp Physiol* 2006;**291**:R1085–93.
28. Levine RJ, Lam C, Qian C, Yu KF, Maynard SE, Sachs BP, et al. Soluble endoglin and other circulating antiangiogenic factors in preeclampsia. *N Engl J Med* 2006;**355**:992–1005.
29. Maynard SE, Min JY, Merchan J, Lim KH, Li J, Mondal S, et al. Excess placental soluble fms-like tyrosine kinase 1 (sFlt1) may contribute to endothelial dysfunction, hypertension, and proteinuria in preeclampsia. *J Clin Invest* 2003;**111**:649–58.
30. Gilbert JS, Babcock SA, Granger JP. Hypertension produced by reduced uterine perfusion in pregnant rats is associated with increased soluble fms-like tyrosine kinase-1 expression. *Hypertension* 2007;**50**:1142–7.
31. Makris A, Thornton C, Thompson J, Thomson S, Martin R, Ogle R, et al. Uteroplacental ischemia results in proteinuric hypertension and elevated sFLT-1. *Kidney Int* 2007;**71**:977–84.
32. Bridges JP, Gilbert JS, Colson D, Gilbert SA, Dukes MP, Ryan MJ, et al. Oxidative stress contributes to soluble fms-like tyrosine kinase-1 induced vascular dysfunction in pregnant rats. *Am J Hypertens* 2009;**22**:564–8.
33. Murphy SR, LaMarca BB, Cockrell K, Granger JP. Role of endothelin in mediating soluble fms-like tyrosine kinase 1-induced hypertension in pregnant rats. *Hypertension* 2010;**55**:394–8.
34. Li Z, Zhang Y, Ying Ma J, Kapoun AM, Shao Q, Kerr I, et al. Recombinant vascular endothelial growth factor 121 attenuates hypertension and improves kidney damage in a rat model of preeclampsia. *Hypertension* 2007;**50**:686–92.
35. Bergmann A, Ahmad S, Cudmore M, Gruber AD, Wittschen P, Lindenmaier W, et al. Reduction of circulating soluble Flt-1 alleviates preeclampsia-like symptoms in a mouse model. *J Cell Mol Med* 2010;**14**:1857–67.

36. Gilbert JS, Verzwyvelt J, Colson D, Arany M, Karumanchi SA, Granger JP. Recombinant vascular endothelial growth factor 121 infusion lowers blood pressure and improves renal function in rats with placental ischemia-induced hypertension. *Hypertension* 2010;**55**:380–5.
37. Burton GJ, Jauniaux E. Placental oxidative stress: from miscarriage to preeclampsia. *J Soc Gynecol Invest* 2004;**11**:342–52.
38. Hung TH, Skepper JN, Charnock-Jones DS, Burton GJ. Hypoxia-reoxygenation: a potent inducer of apoptotic changes in the human placenta and possible etiological factor in preeclampsia. *Circ Res* 2002;**90**:1274–81.
39. Staff AC, Halvorsen B, Ranheim T, Henriksen T. Elevated level of free 8-iso-prostaglandin F2alpha in the decidua basalis of women with preeclampsia. *Am J Obstet Gynecol* 1999;**181**:1211–5.
40. Staff AC, Ranheim T, Khoury J, Henriksen T. Increased contents of phospholipids, cholesterol, and lipid peroxides in decidua basalis in women with preeclampsia. *Am J Obstet Gynecol* 1999;**180**:587–92.
41. Wang Y, Walsh SW, Kay HH. Placental lipid peroxides and thromboxane are increased and prostacyclin is decreased in women with preeclampsia. *Am J Obstet Gynecol* 1992;**167**:946–9.
42. Roggensack AM, Zhang Y, Davidge ST. Evidence for peroxynitrite formation in the vasculature of women with preeclampsia. *Hypertension* 1999;**33**:83–9.
43. Sedeek M, Gilbert JS, LaMarca BB, Sholook M, Chandler DL, Wang Y, et al. Role of reactive oxygen species in hypertension produced by reduced uterine perfusion in pregnant rats. *Am J Hypertens* 2008;**21**:1152–6.
44. Sedeek M, Wang YP, Granger JP. Increased oxidative stress in a rat model of preeclampsia. *Am J Hypertens* 2004;**17**:142A.
45. Anumba DO, Robson SC, Boys RJ, Ford GA. Nitric oxide activity in the peripheral vasculature during normotensive and preeclamptic pregnancy. *Am J Physiol Heart Circ Physiol* 1999;**277**:H848–54.
46. Conrad KP, Joffe GM, Kruszyna H, Kruszyna R, Rochelle LG, Smith RP, et al. Identification of increased nitric oxide biosynthesis during pregnancy in rats. *FASEB J* 1993;**7**:566–71.
47. Cooke CL, Davidge ST. Pregnancy-induced alterations of vascular function in mouse mesenteric and uterine arteries. *Biol Reprod* 2003;**68**:1072–7.
48. Nelson SH, Steinsland OS, Wang Y, Yallampalli C, Dong YL, Sanchez JM. Increased nitric oxide synthase activity and expression in the human uterine artery during pregnancy. *Circ Res* 2000;**87**:406–11.
49. Conrad KP, Vernier KA. Plasma level, urinary excretion, and metabolic production of cGMP during gestation in rats. *Am J Physiol Regul Integr Comp Physiol* 1989;**257**:R847–53.
50. Crews JK, Novak J, Granger JP, Khalil RA. Stimulated mechanisms of Ca^{2+} entry into vascular smooth muscle during NO synthesis inhibition in pregnant rats. *Am J Physiol Regul Integr Comp Physiol* 1999;**276**:R530–8.
51. Khalil RA, Crews JK, Novak J, Kassab S, Granger JP. Enhanced vascular reactivity during inhibition of nitric oxide synthesis in pregnant rats. *Hypertension* 1998;**31**:1065–9.
52. Abram SR, Alexander BT, Bennett WA, Granger JP. Role of neuronal nitric oxide synthase in mediating renal hemodynamic changes during pregnancy. *Am J Physiol Regul Integr Comp Physiol* 2001;**281**:R1390–3.
53. Alexander BT, Kassab SE, Miller MT, Abram SR, Reckelhoff JF, Bennett WA, et al. Reduced uterine perfusion pressure during pregnancy in the rat is associated with increases in arterial pressure and changes in renal nitric oxide. *Hypertension* 2001;**37**:1191–5.
54. Lyall F, Young A, Greer IA. Nitric oxide concentrations are increased in the fetoplacental circulation in preeclampsia. *Am J Obstet Gynecol* 1995;**173**:714–8.
55. Lyall F, Greer IA. The vascular endothelium in normal pregnancy and pre-eclampsia. *Rev Reprod* 1996;**1**:107–16.
56. Crews JK, Herrington JN, Granger JP, Khalil RA. Decreased endothelium-dependent vascular relaxation during reduction of uterine perfusion pressure in pregnant rat. *Hypertension* 2000;**35**:367–72.
57. Danielson LA, Conrad KP. Acute blockade of nitric oxide synthase inhibits renal vasodilation and hyperfiltration during pregnancy in chronically instrumented conscious rats. *J Clin Invest* 1995;**96**:482–90.
58. Molnar M, Suto T, Toth T, Hertelendy F. Prolonged blockade of nitric oxide synthesis in gravid rats produces sustained hypertension, proteinuria, thrombocytopenia, and intrauterine growth retardation. *Am J Obstet Gynecol* 1994;**170**:1458–66.
59. Yallampalli C, Garfield RE. Inhibition of nitric oxide synthesis in rats during pregnancy produces signs similar to those of preeclampsia. *Am J Obstet Gynecol* 1993;**169**:1316–20.
60. Yanagisawa M, Inoue A, Ishikawa T, Kasuya Y, Kimura S, Kumagaye S, et al. Primary structure, synthesis, and biological activity of rat endothelin, an endothelium-derived vasoconstrictor peptide. *Proc Natl Acad Sci USA* 1988;**85**:6964–7.
61. Yanagisawa M, Kurihara H, Kimura S, Goto K, Masaki T. A novel peptide vasoconstrictor, endothelin, is produced by vascular endothelium and modulates smooth muscle Ca^{2+} channels. *J Hypertens Suppl* 1988;**6**:S188–91.
62. Yanagisawa M, Kurihara H, Kimura S, Tomobe Y, Kobayashi M, Mitsui Y, et al. A novel potent vasoconstrictor peptide produced by vascular endothelial cells. *Nature* 1988;**332**:411–5.
63. Taylor RN, Varma M, Teng NN, Roberts JM. Women with preeclampsia have higher plasma endothelin levels than women with normal pregnancies. *J Clin Endocrinol Metab* 1990;**71**:1675–7.
64. Bernardi F, Constantino L, Machado R, Petronilho F, Dal-Pizzol F. Plasma nitric oxide, endothelin-1, arginase and superoxide dismutase in pre-eclamptic women. *J Obstet Gynaecol Res* 2008;**34**:957–63.
65. Nezar MA, el-Baky AM, Soliman OA, Abdel-Hady HA, Hammad AM, Al-Haggar MS. Endothelin-1 and leptin as markers of intrauterine growth restriction. *Indian J Pediatr* 2009;**76**:485–8.
66. Benigni A, Orisio S, Gaspari F, Frusca T, Amuso G, Remuzzi G. Evidence against a pathogenetic role for endothelin in pre-eclampsia. *Br J Obstet Gynaecol* 1992;**99**:798–802.
67. Alexander BT, Rinewalt AN, Cockrell KL, Massey MB, Bennett WA, Granger JP. Endothelin type a receptor blockade attenuates the hypertension in response to chronic reductions in uterine perfusion pressure. *Hypertension* 2001;**37**:485–9.
68. LaMarca BB, Cockrell K, Sullivan E, Bennett W, Granger JP. Role of endothelin in mediating tumor necrosis factor-induced hypertension in pregnant rats. *Hypertension* 2005;**46**:82–6.
69. Marsden PA, Brenner BM. Transcriptional regulation of the endothelin-1 gene by TNF-alpha. *Am J Physiol* 1992;**262**:C854–61.
70. LaMarca B, Speed J, Fournier L, Babcock SA, Berry H, Cockrell K, et al. Hypertension in response to chronic reductions in uterine perfusion in pregnant rats: effect of tumor necrosis factor-alpha blockade. *Hypertension* 2008;**52**:1161–7.

71. LaMarca B, Parrish M, Ray LF, Murphy SR, Roberts L, Glover P, et al. Hypertension in response to autoantibodies to the angiotensin II type I receptor (AT1-AA) in pregnant rats: role of endothelin-1. *Hypertension* 2009;**54**:905–9.
72. Schiessl B. Inflammatory response in preeclampsia. *Mol Aspects Med* 2007;**28**:210–9.
73. Redman CW, Sargent IL. Preeclampsia and the systemic inflammatory response. *Semin Nephrol* 2004;**24**:565–70.
74. Sacks GP, Studena K, Sargent K, Redman CW. Normal pregnancy and preeclampsia both produce inflammatory changes in peripheral blood leukocytes akin to those of sepsis. *Am J Obstet Gynecol* 1998;**179**:80–6.
75. Gadonski G, LaMarca BB, Sullivan E, Bennett W, Chandler D, Granger JP. Hypertension produced by reductions in uterine perfusion in the pregnant rat: role of interleukin 6. *Hypertension* 2006;**48**:711–6.
76. Alexander BT, Cockrell KL, Massey MB, Bennett WA, Granger JP. Tumor necrosis factor-alpha-induced hypertension in pregnant rats results in decreased renal neuronal nitric oxide synthase expression. *Am J Hypertens* 2002;**15**:170–5.
77. Wallukat G, Homuth V, Fischer T, Lindschau C, Horstkamp B, Jupner A, et al. Patients with preeclampsia develop agonistic autoantibodies against the angiotensin AT1 receptor. *J Clin Invest* 1999;**103**:945–52.
78. Herse F, Staff AC, Hering L, Muller DN, Luft FC, Dechend R. AT1-receptor autoantibodies and uteroplacental RAS in pregnancy and pre-eclampsia. *J Mol Med* 2008;**86**:697–703.
79. LaMarca B, Wallukat G, Llinas M, Herse F, Dechend R, Granger JP. Autoantibodies to the angiotensin type I receptor in response to placental ischemia and tumor necrosis factor alpha in pregnant rats. *Hypertension* 2008;**52**:1168–72.
80. Dechend R, Viedt C, Muller DN, Ugele B, Brandes RP, Wallukat G, et al. AT1 receptor agonistic antibodies from preeclamptic patients stimulate NADPH oxidase. *Circulation* 2003;**107**:1632–9.
81. Zhou CC, Ahmad S, Mi T, Abbasi S, Xia L, Day MC, et al. Autoantibody from women with preeclampsia induces soluble Fms-like tyrosine kinase-1 production via angiotensin type 1 receptor and calcineurin/nuclear factor of activated T-cells signaling. *Hypertension* 2008;**51**:1010–9.
82. Bainbridge SA, Farley AE, McLaughlin BE, Graham CH, Marks GS, Nakatsu K, et al. Carbon monoxide decreases perfusion pressure in isolated human placenta. *Placenta* 2002;**23**:563–9.
83. Cudmore M, Ahmad S, Al-Ani B, Fujisawa T, Coxall H, Chudasama K, et al. Negative regulation of soluble Flt-1 and soluble endoglin release by heme oxygenase-1. *Circulation* 2007;**115**:1789–97.
84. Cao J, Inoue K, Li X, Drummond G, Abraham NG. Physiological significance of heme oxygenase in hypertension. *Int J Biochem Cell Biol* 2009;**41**:1025–33.
85. Botros FT, Schwartzman ML, Stier Jr CT, Goodman AI, Abraham NG. Increase in heme oxygenase-1 levels ameliorates renovascular hypertension. *Kidney Int* 2005;**68**:2745–55.
86. Sabaawy HE, Zhang F, Nguyen X, ElHosseiny A, Nasjletti A, Schwartzman M, et al. Human heme oxygenase-1 gene transfer lowers blood pressure and promotes growth in spontaneously hypertensive rats. *Hypertension* 2001;**38**:210–5.
87. Yang L, Quan S, Nasjletti A, Laniado-Schwartzman M, Abraham NG. Heme oxygenase-1 gene expression modulates angiotensin II-induced increase in blood pressure. *Hypertension* 2004;**43**:1221–6.
88. George EM, Cockrell K, Aranay M, Csongradi E, Stec DE, Granger JP. Induction of heme oxygenase 1 attenuates placental ischemia-induced hypertension. *Hypertension* 2011;**57**:941–8.
89. George EM, Arany M, Cockrell K, Storm MV, Stec DE, Granger JP. Induction of heme oxygenase-1 attenuates sFlt-1-induced hypertension in pregnant rats. *Am J Physiol Regul Integr Comp Physiol* 2011;**301**:R1495–500.
90. Coppage KH, Sun X, Baker RS, Clark KE. Expression of phosphodiesterase 5 in maternal and fetal sheep. *Am J Obstet Gynecol* 2005;**193**:1005–10.
91. Wareing M, Myers JE, O'Hara M, Kenny LC, Warren AY, Taggart MJ, et al. Effects of a phosphodiesterase-5 (PDE5) inhibitor on endothelium-dependent relaxation of myometrial small arteries. *Am J Obstet Gynecol* 2004;**190**:1283–90.
92. Wareing M, Myers JE, O'Hara M, Baker PN. Sildenafil citrate (Viagra) enhances vasodilatation in fetal growth restriction. *J Clin Endocrinol Metab* 2005;**90**:2550–5.
93. Samangaya RA, Mires G, Shennan A, Skillern L, Howe D, McLeod A, et al. A randomised, double-blinded, placebo-controlled study of the phosphodiesterase type 5 inhibitor sildenafil for the treatment of preeclampsia. *Hypertens Pregnancy* 2009;**28**:369–82.
94. Downing J. Sildenafil for the treatment of preeclampsia. *Hypertens Pregnancy* 2010;**29**:248–50; author reply 251–2.
95. Clouthier DE, Hosoda K, Richardson JA, Williams SC, Yanagisawa H, Kuwaki T, et al. Cranial and cardiac neural crest defects in endothelin-A receptor-deficient mice. *Development* 1998;**125**:813–24.
96. Taniguchi T, Muramatsu I. Pharmacological knockout of endothelin ET(A) receptors. *Life Sci* 2003;**74**:405–9.

Chapter 102

Erectile Dysfunction

Kelvin P. Davies
Albert Einstein College of Medicine, Bronx, NY

ERECTILE DYSFUNCTION IS AN IMPORTANT MEDICAL CONDITION

A consensus panel of the National Institutes of Health defined erectile dysfunction (ED) as the inability to achieve or maintain an erection sufficient for satisfactory sexual performance. Although in the past ED was relegated to a "quality of life type" disease, primarily of interest to urologists, recent research has attracted a wider group of scientists to investigate the mechanisms underlying its development. The major impetus for this change was the recognition that ED acts as a strong predictor of other vascular diseases. Indeed it is now recommended by the American Medical Association that patients presenting with ED should be investigated for evidence of cardiovascular disease (CVD) (1). It has been suggested that common mechanisms may act in the development of both ED and CVD, and understanding the processes resulting in the development of ED may lead to novel strategies for the treatment of other vascular diseases (2).

Depending on the cause, ED can be broadly classified as organic, psychogenic or mixed. Psychogenic impotence is where an erection or penetration fails due to thoughts or feelings (psychological reasons) rather than physical pathology. Until the late 1960s psychogenic reasons were thought to be the cause of the majority of cases of ED. However, following the development of surgical interventions in the 1950s, and pharmacological treatments in the 1990s that were able to successfully treat ED, this position has been totally reversed. Physiological factors are now considered to be the cause of ED in >80% of patients. Two of the most common risk factors for organic ED are diabetes and aging. Diabetic men are three times as likely to develop ED as non-diabetic men, and men aged 50–90 years have a 10-times greater risk for ED than those younger than 50 years (3). However, there is a multitude of conditions that are associated with the development of ED, as shown in Figure 102.1.

Several lines of evidence demonstrate how important maintaining erectile function is to men. A recent study demonstrated that ED not only affects a man's sex life, but serves as a significant detriment to their overall psychological wellbeing (4). The demand for treatments for ED demonstrates the importance of erectile function to men. For example, in the first six years after FDA approval of Viagra (an oral phosphodiesterase-5 inhibitor used for the treatment for ED), 23 million men worldwide filled prescriptions, with annual sales of about $1 billion, making it one of the most financially successful drugs of all time.

THE ROLE OF SMOOTH MUSCLE IN ERECTILE PHYSIOLOGY

In the penis the smooth muscle of the corpora cavernosa and of the arteriolar and arterial walls play a key role in the erectile process (see Figure 102.2). Normally these smooth muscles are maintained in a state of heightened tone, keeping the penis flaccid. A small amount of arterial blow flow maintains the viability of corporal tissue. Sexual stimulation triggers release of neurotransmitters from the cavernous nerve terminals, initiating relaxation of smooth muscle of the arterioles and arteries resulting in increased blood flow in the penis and engorgement of the corpora cavernosa. The venous outflow of blood is simultaneously reduced by compression of the subtunical venular plexuses between the tunica albuginea and the peripheral sinusoids, reducing the venous outflow. Further stretching of the tunica to its capacity occludes the emissary veins between the inner circular and the outer longitudinal layers, decreasing the venous outflow to a minimum. In humans the duration of a normal erection depends on age, peaking in a man of 21–25 years, where the median duration of an erection is 54.43 minutes (5).

The process of detumesence, returning the penis to the flaccid state, has been studied in detail in dogs (6). There are three stages: a transient intracorporal pressure increase, indicating the beginning of smooth muscle contraction against a closed venous system. This is followed by a slow pressure decrease, suggesting a slow reopening of the venous channels with resumption of the basal level

Muscle. DOI: http://dx.doi.org/10.1016/B978-0-12-381510-1.00102-2

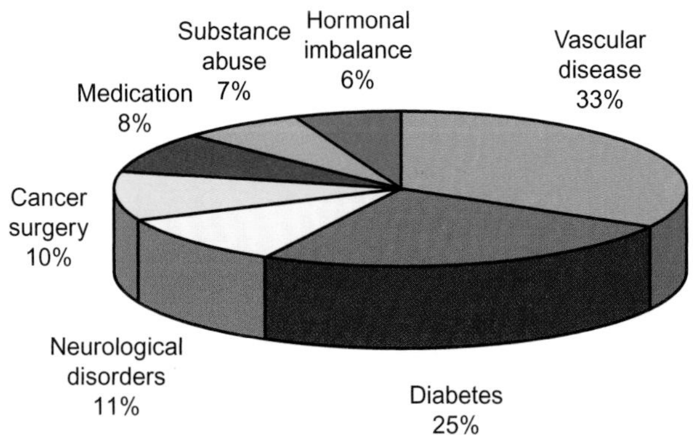

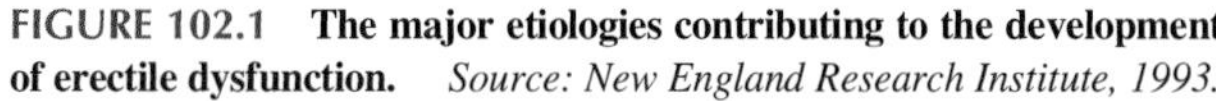
FIGURE 102.1 **The major etiologies contributing to the development of erectile dysfunction.** *Source: New England Research Institute, 1993.*

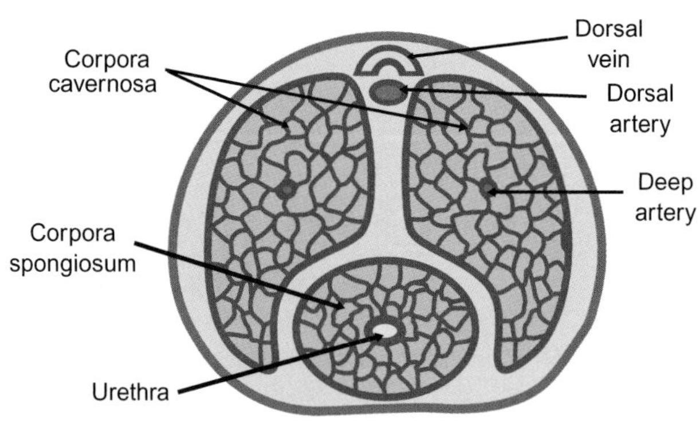

FIGURE 102.2 **Cross-section of the penis.** During an erection the sinusoidal spaces of the corpora cavernosa become engorged with blood.

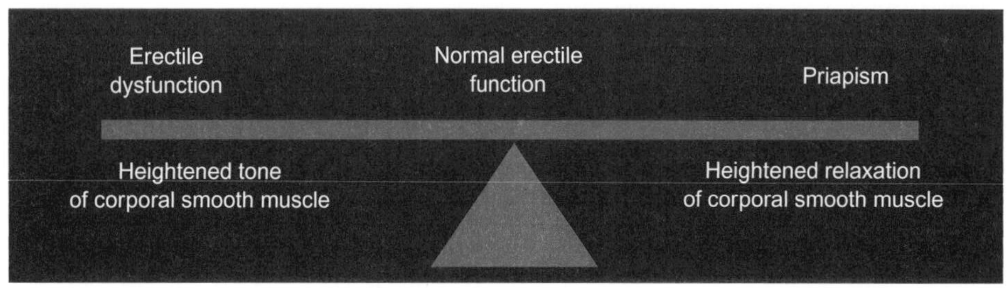

FIGURE 102.3 **Normal erectile function requires relaxation of the tone of the corpora cavernosal smooth muscle tissue.** If there is heightened tone of these tissues then erectile dysfunction occurs because of the inability of the corpora cavernosal sinusoids to become engorged with blood. If there is heightened relaxation of the corpora cavernosal smooth muscle then the penis fails to return to the flaccid state, resulting in a persistent erection called priapism.

of arterial flow. Finally there is a fast pressure decrease with fully restored venous outflow capacity.

The physiological aspects of the erectile process described above demonstrates the central role that smooth muscle tissue, in particular corpora cavernosal smooth muscle (CCSM) tissue plays in the erectile process. Disturbing the regulation of CCSM tone can result in pathology; an inability to relax the CCSM results in ED, whereas an impaired ability of the CCSM to return to its resting state of heightened tone, can result in a persistent, painful, penile erection called priapism (Figure 102.3).

Although pathological disturbance of the regulation of CCSM tone is arguably the key determinant of ED, several research groups have focused on the contribution that endothelial pathology can contribute to ED, which has led to the popular adage ED2: erectile dysfunction = endothelial dysfunction (2). Several conditions associated with ED, such as aging, hypertension, smoking, hypercholesterolemia, and diabetes are known to affect the function of endothelium. However, even when there is endothelial and nerve dysfunction, the ultimate cause of ED is mediated directly or indirectly through changes in the regulation of CSSM tone.

MAINTENANCE OF THE FLACCID STATE

The penis is usually maintained in the flaccid state by maintaining the CCSM in a tonically contracted state. This is achieved mainly through the action of sympathetic nerves releasing noradrenaline which acts on α1- and α2-postsynaptic receptors (7). Activation of these receptors results in higher intracellular Ca^{2+} levels, resulting in heightened tone by mechanisms described below. In addition erectile tissues synthesize several locally acting vasoconstricting agents, such as prostanoids, endothelin-I, and angiotensin-II (7).

α1- and α2-adrenoceptor antagonists (such as prostaglandin E1 (Alprostadil) and phentolamine), have the potential to treat ED based on the rationale that reduced CCSM tone would potentiate an erectile response. Alprostadil is the most widely used intracavernosal agent, with a response rate of >70%, but produces painful erections in up to 30% of cases (8). Intracavernosal injection of phentolamine (in combination with vasoactive intestinal polypeptide) has shown promise in treating ED in clinical trials and is also available as an oral formulation for ED treatment in some non-US (e.g., South American) markets (9).

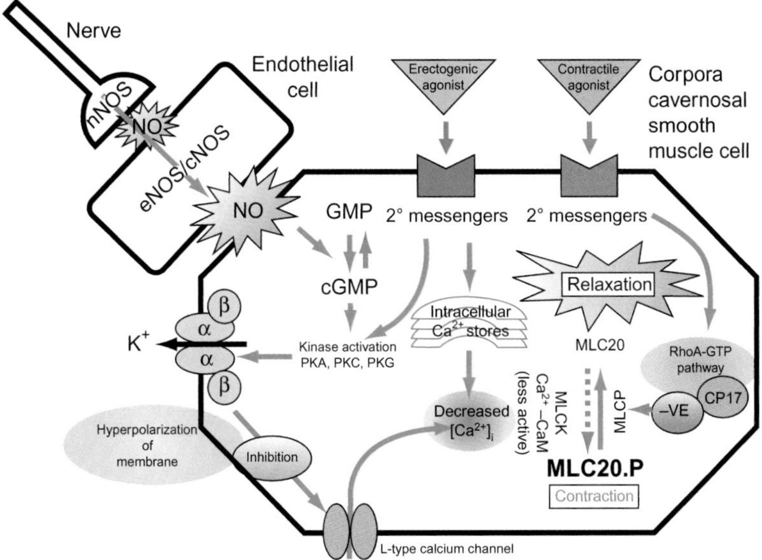

FIGURE 102.4 **The major pathways (shown with green arrows) resulting in relaxation of the corpora cavernosal smooth muscle tissue that occurs with an erection**. Smooth muscle tone is maintained through balancing pathways that either phosphorylate (and cause contraction) or dephosphorylate (and cause relaxation) myosin light chain (MLC). Nitric oxide (NO) produced by neurogenic nitric oxide synthase (nNOS) or endothelial/ constitutive NOS (eNOS/cNOS) diffuse into corporal smooth muscle cells. NO activates guanylate cyclase, raising the levels of cyclic GMP (cGMP), through its action on ion channels and intracellular Ca^{2+} storage sites, lowers intracellular calcium concentrations $[Ca^{2+}]_i$. Lower $[Ca^{2+}]_i$ reduces the activity of MLC kinase (MLCK) which shifts the balance towards unphosphorylated MLC and relaxation. Calcium sensitization pathways (by contractile agonists, such as endothelin-1) result in the activation of the Rho-kinase (ROK) or CPI-17 pathway, causing heightened tone by inhibiting smooth muscle myosin light chain phosphatase (MLCP) either by directly phosphorylating MLCP or by binding to CPI-17.

INITIATION OF AN ERECTION

The initiation of penile erection is controlled by the parasympathetic and sympathetic branches of the autonomic nervous system (7). Peripherally, the balance between contractile and relaxing factors regulates the tone of the CCSM and determines the functional state of the penis. Neurogenic nitric oxide (NO) is considered the most important factor for relaxation of the CCSM and penile vessels. While NO may operate in several ways to direct the relaxation of CCSM, its most significant role is in signal transduction. In this role NO is produced and released from autonomic nerve terminals and endothelial cells where it diffuses into adjacent CCSM cells and binds with intracellular guanylate cyclase (Figure 102.4). This binding induces a conformational change of guanylate cyclase, activating the enzyme so that it catalyzes the conversion of guanosine triphosphate (GTP) to cyclic guanosine monophosphate (cGMP). cGMP then acts through a cGMP-dependent protein kinase to determine the contractile state of the CCSM. cGMP co-ordinates several downstream activities that affect CCSM tone including direct changes in the phosphorylation state of myosin light chain cross-bridging, control of calcium and potassium ion fluxes and stores, interaction with other signal transduction mechanisms, and several other effects on cellular contractile proteins independent of phosphorylation biochemistry. Recent experimental studies suggest that cGMP also inhibits the presynaptic release and contractile effects of the adrenergic contractile neurotransmitter, noradrenaline.

The role of NO in initiating an erection has led to several groups researching treatments of ED based on increasing local levels of NO. Several approaches have been shown to be successful in animal models, such as increasing the levels of nitric oxide synthase (NOS) through gene transfer or increasing the L-arginine concentration (the substrate for NO production) either by direct supplementation or inhibition of arginase (10). A recent development which has proven effective in animal models of ED is to increase local NO concentrations by applying nanoparticles encapsulating NO which are capable of transdermal penetration directly to the dermis of the penis (11).

Breakdown of cGMP in the CCSM is achieved through the action of phosphodiesterase-5 (PDE5). The highly successful oral treatments for ED, Viagra (sildenafil), Cialis (tadalafil), and Levitra (vardenafil), are inhibitors of this enzyme, and result in increased levels of cGMP following sexual stimulation (12). All three seem to have similar efficacy profiles, being effective in 55–85% of patients. Although all these compounds have the same mechanism of action they exhibit different pharmacokinetics. Whereas sildenafil and vardenafil have a half-life of about 4 hours, that of tadalafil is much longer (approximately 17.5 hours) which is associated with a much broader window of efficacy and has led to the nickname "the weekend pill" (13). The realization that there is a large market demand for ED treatments, and that certain patient groups are often refractory to treatment by the PDE5 inhibitors, such as diabetics or patients having undergone radical prostatectomy, has spurred research into pharmacological treatments for ED which target different biochemical pathways.

Recently, Opiorphin and Opiorphin-related peptides, which act as potent neutral endopeptidase inhibitors, have been shown to play a role in erectile physiology (14). The genes encoding Opiorphins are downregulated in the CCSM of animal models of ED, and human patients with ED. Their involvement in erectile physiology is hypothesized to involve the protection of vasoactive peptides that result in smooth muscle relaxation (15). In animal models both intracorporal injection of the peptide or gene transfer of plasmids expressing Opiorphins have demonstrated efficacy in treating ED (15).

BIOCHEMICAL MECHANISMS REGULATING CORPORAL SMOOTH MUSCLE TONE

CSSM tone is achieved by shifting the balance of biochemical pathways that act on myosin-driven actin filament sliding (16), summarized in Figure 102.4. Unlike skeletal muscle, the central regulator of CCSM contraction is the state of myosin light chain (MLC) phosphorylation. In response to a relaxation stimulus, which would initiate an erection, the level of intracellular calcium ($[Ca^{2+}]_i$) is reduced. This inactivates the Ca^{2+}-calmodulin-dependent myosin light chain kinase (MLCK) thereby shifting the ratio of myosin towards a dephosphorylated state through the action of smooth muscle myosin light chain phosphatase (MLCP). Conversely, contractile stimuli result in an increase in intracellular calcium which activates MLCK which phosphorylates the 20 kDa regulatory subunit of smooth muscle MLC at Ser19, correlating with an increase in actin-activated ATP hydrolysis and cross-bridge cycling resulting in increased tone.

From this description it is clear that $[Ca^{2+}]_i$ plays a major role in regulating CSSM tone and therefore erectile function. Although release of calcium from intracellular stores, such as ryanodine-sensitive sarcoplasmic reticulum calcium and IP3, is critical in determining $[Ca^{2+}]_i$, sustained transmembrane calcium flux can largely be attributed to the presence of L-type, voltage-dependent calcium channels (see Figure 102.4). It might be expected that drugs that target L-type calcium channels, through their action of reducing $[Ca^{2+}]_i$, and relaxing CSSM, might help in the treatment of ED. Although there are no reports where a strategy of blocking L-type calcium channels has been used in the treatment of ED, anecdotal reports suggest that when verapamil (an L-type calcium channel blocker) is injected directly into the penis for treatment of Peyronnies disease it can result in transient erections. However, when verapamil (or nifedipine, another L-type calcium channel blocker) is taken orally to treat hypertension, one of the reported side-effects is ED, perhaps due to lowered systemic blood pressure (17).

THE BK CHANNEL INDIRECTLY BLOCKS THE L-TYPE CALCIUM CHANNEL AND IS A TARGET FOR TREATMENT OF ERECTILE DYSFUNCTION

Activation of the BK channel (also referred to as Maxi-K and KCNMA1) leads to efflux of potassium from the cell and hyperpolarization of the membrane, which in turn inhibits the flow of calcium through L-type channels (18). The BK channel consists of at least two non-covalently associated subunits: the pore-forming α-subunit (encoded by the *Slo* gene) and a regulatory β_1-subunit. Although the α-subunit is responsible for the basic ion flux function of BK channels, the regulatory β_1-subunit can dramatically affect channel conduction by changing channel kinetics, voltage/Ca^{2+} sensitivities and pharmacology (19).

The importance of the BK channel to erectile function has been clearly demonstrated in BK knockout mice (20). In the absence of the BK channel the mice suffer from ED. In addition, many studies on the mechanisms by which nitric oxide (NO) and prostaglandin E1 (PGE1) elicit blood vessel relaxation have also highlighted a role for the BK channel in CCSM as a common downstream effector. The BK channel also may serve as a target for endothelium-derived hyperpolarizing factor (EDHF) and the non-NO, non-PGI2 endothelium-derived relaxing factor in some blood vessels (21).

The *Slo* gene can undergo alternative splicing, generating several protein isoforms, each of which has unique biochemical properties. In both aging and diabetes, two conditions that are associated with ED, it has been shown that there are changes in the splicing of the *Slo* gene in CCSM (22,23). In diabetes there appears to be an upregulation of a more active BK variant, which has been proposed to be a compensatory mechanism for other effects of diabetes. Animals develop ED once the effect of diabetes is no longer compensated by the maximal levels of endogenous BK. In the CCSM of aging animals with ED a dominant negative BK variant is expressed, which traps the active BK forms in the cytoplasm. Overall changes in levels of expression of the BK gene and/or alternative splicing of the *Slo* gene can have an impact on CCSM and erectile physiology. The important role of BK in erectile physiology is the basis for several pharmacological strategies utilizing channel openers to treat ED. Several of these channel openers have proven effective in animal models (24). In addition, the use of gene therapy, where intracorporal injection of plasmids increases expression of *hSlo* in the penis, has been shown to improve erectile function in both aging and diabetic models of ED (25,26). These observations are the basis of on-going clinical trials for the use of BK based gene therapy to treat ED (27).

CALCIUM SENSITIZATION OF SMOOTH MUSCLE CELLS

The tone of CSSM can also be regulated independently of changes in $[Ca^{2+}]_i$ through the inhibition of MLCP activity. This process in effect increases the cells' contractility in the presence of $[Ca^{2+}]_i$ and has been termed "calcium sensitization" (28). Two major pathways have been identified which lead to the inactivation of MLCP (see Figure 102.4). The first involves an enzyme known as Rho-kinase (ROK). Binding of a small GTP-binding protein known as RhoA causes ROK to migrate to the cell membrane where it is maximally active. When active, ROK can increase the phosphorylation level of MLC either by directly phosphorylating the myosin (shown only *in vitro*) or indirectly by phosphorylating and consequently inhibiting MLCP, which is responsible for dephosphorylating MLC. A ROK inhibitor (Y-27632) increases CCSM pressure in an *in vivo* rat model, suggesting that inhibition of Rho-kinase may be a potential treatment for ED (29).

Endothelin-1 (ET1) also has been shown to increase the calcium sensitivity of smooth muscle, the mechanism of which is proposed to involve the ROK pathway because this calcium sensitization can be decreased by the ROK antagonist known as Y-27632 (30). The effect of ET1 on calcium sensitization appears to be mediated by the endothelin A receptor (ETA) and the heterotrimeric G-Protein, Gq (31). Thus, alterations in expression of ET-1, ETA or Gq can have significant effects on contractility of CCSM cells in the absence of changes in intracellular calcium concentration.

In addition to the RhoA/ROK pathway described above, a molecule known as CPI-17 can also inhibit MLCP activity and lead to calcium sensitization. CPI-17 is a protein kinase C-potentiated MLCP inhibitory protein of 17 kDa that is expressed predominantly in smooth muscle and that similar to ROK can potentiate contraction at constant $[Ca^{2+}]_i$ (31). Although significantly active in its unphosphorylated form, phosphorylation at Thr38 increases the affinity of CPI-17 for MLCP by more than 1000-fold. By regulating the balance between calcium, MLCK, MLCP, ROK, and CPI-17, a cell can finely tune its contractile state (see Figure 102.4).

REGULATION OF CORPORAL SMOOTH MUSCLE TONE THROUGH CHANGES IN MYOSIN ISOFORM EXPRESSION

Unlike striated muscle, where different genes code for mysosin heavy chain (MHC) isoforms, SM tone can be regulated via alternative splicing of the SM MHC and the SM myosin light chain (SM MLC) pre-mRNAs. Alternative splicing at the 5′ end of the pre-mRNA produces two SM MHC isoforms, MHC-A and MHC-B. The MHC-B isoform contains a 7-amino acid insert near the ATP-binding site (encoded by a 21 nucleotide insert in the mRNA) which is absent in the SM-A isoform (32). A higher expression of MHC-B in smooth muscle tissue correlates with increased actin-activated Mg^{2+}-ATPase activity and velocity of movement of actin filaments *in vitro* compared with smooth muscle that expresses more of the MHC-A isoform. In human smooth muscle the 17 kDa MLC mRNA differ by the presence or absence of an insert of 44 nt (exon 6) located in the 3-region. The two MLC isoforms can be separated by two-dimensional polyacrylamide gel electrophoresis due to their different isoelectric points. The more acidic MLC17 is designated as MLC17a and the more basic as MLC17b.

Recently it was shown that men with clinically diagnosed ED expressed detectable levels of only the MHC-A isoform, which has the lower ATPase activity (33). In all patients the ratio of MLC17b to MLC17a was approximately 1:1 for all patients with the exception of a sub-group of patients with ED who failed conservative therapy with PDE5 inhibitors compared with all others. This group of patients demonstrated a significantly lower relative expression of MLC17b compared with all others. Although more research is needed, and the potential for this observation for clinical translation into a treatment for ED may prove elusive, alternative splicing events in the MHC and 17 kDa MLC pre-mRNA is a possible molecular mechanism for the altered contractility of the CCSM in patients with ED, and may be predictive of which patients are likely to be refractory to treatment with PDE5 inhibitors.

THE ROLE OF ANDROGENS IN ERECTILE FUNCTION

Testosterone is the androgen most studied for its connection to erectile function, although several others such as dihydrotestosterone, dehydrepiandrosterone, and oestrogen are also believed to play a role. There is a well-documented link between ED, hypogonadism, and underlying disorders (such as metabolic syndrome and type 2 diabetes mellitus) (34). In animal studies low testosterone levels can impact both the cytology and biochemistry of corporal smooth muscle tissue. Lower testosterone levels reduce expression of nitric oxide synthase (NOS) isoforms and the expression and activity of PDE5 (35). As described above, both these enzymes play a critical role in erectile function. Low testosterone also results in reduced smooth muscle tissue in the corpora cavernosum and an increase in connective tissue deposition. The smooth muscle cells appear more disorganized and contain a large number of cytoplasmic vacuoles.

In animals the effects of low testosterone can be reversed by testosterone supplementation. However, the role of testosterone in the development of ED, and the ability of testosterone to improve erectile function in men is an area of contention (34). It has proven difficult to dissociate the involvement of testosterone in regulating sexual desire (a psychogenic effect) from a direct organic/physiological effect. Although in animal models of hypogonadism there is clearly a deleterious affect on erectile function, castrated men are still capable of developing an erection, even in the absence of testosterone replacement therapy. Despite several clinical studies the efficacy of this hormone in the treatment of patients with ED has not been clearly demonstrated.

MECHANISMS UNDERLYING PRIAPISM

Priapism is a persistent, often painful, penile erection that continues hours beyond, or is unrelated to, sexual stimulation; it can eventually lead to progressive fibrosis of the erectile tissue and ultimately results in ED (36,37). It is increasingly recognized that in low-flow, ischemic priapism, misregulation of CCSM tone plays a significant role in this disorder, but in contrast to ED, it involves prolonged relaxation of smooth muscle. The development of priapism is associated with the use of pharmacological agents, particularly antipsychotics (38), recreational drugs, drugs for hematological disorders, metabolic disorders, trauma, tumors, neurological disorders and bites from spiders and scorpions (39). Men with sickle cell disease are particularly prone to priapism, where its incidence is about 40% (40,41).

At present there are no approved pharmacological treatments for priapism, however recent progress in understanding the molecular events leading to priapism has identified novel targets for its potential treatment. Somewhat counterintuitively endothelial NOS knock-out ($eNOS^{-/-}$) mice exhibit priapic-like, excessive erectile tendencies (42). Later work demonstrated that in the corpora of the $eNOS^{-/-}$ mice there was reduced PDE-5 expression (43). Following sexual stimulation resulting in increased release of neuronal nitric oxide (NO), large amounts of cyclic guanosine monophosphate (cGMP) were produced because of the lowered levels of PDE-5 resulting in excessive corporal smooth muscle tissue relaxation. It has also been reported that mice lacking adenosine deaminase (ADA), an enzyme necessary for the breakdown of adenosine, display unexpected priapic activity (44). Treatment of these mice with ADA enzyme therapy corrected the priapic-like activity suggesting that it was dependent on elevated adenosine levels. Further genetic and pharmacologic evidence demonstrated that A2B adenosine receptor-mediated (A2BR-mediated) cyclic adenosine monophosphate (cAMP) and cGMP induction was required for elevated adenosine-induced prolonged penile erection. In sickle cell mice elevated adenosine levels and A2BR activation were also associated with the development of priapism. Another mechanism may involve overexpression of Opiorphins in corporal tissue, which occurs in the corpora of sickle cell mice even before they demonstrate priapism (45). Overexpression of Opiorphins can then result in priapism through a mechanism that involves activation of polyamine synthesis (45).

Several novel therapies for treating or preventing priapism are being investigated, such as the use of PDE5 inhibitors, polyethylene glycol-modified ADA or inhibitors of ornithine decarboxylase (45–48). However, these treatments are as yet unproven in a clinical environment, and there remains an urgent need to better understand the molecular events that result in priapism in order to facilitate the development of better treatment regimens. There is increased awareness that oxidative stress in corporal tissue is a contributing factor to the development of ED (49).

CONCLUSION: IS IT EASY TO TREAT ERECTILE DYSFUNCTION?

Understanding the molecular mechanisms that result in erectile dysfunction has led to the investigation of several novel pharmacotherapeutic approaches to treat ED. In addition to the approaches described in this chapter, there are almost weekly descriptions in the research literature of novel therapeutic strategies showing promise in animal models for the treatment of ED. A potential explanation for this is that erectile function, conferring as it does reproductive success, is of central importance to the survival of mammalian species. Therefore, there is a great deal of redundancy built into the pathways leading to an erection. Although multiple pathways probably have to fail for an animal to develop ED, only a single pathway has to be compensated for restoration of erectile function. It might therefore be argued that amongst all the pathologies that result from smooth muscle dysfunction, ED may be the one most amenable to treatment.

REFERENCES

1. Thompson IM, Tangen CM, Goodman PJ, Probstfield JL, Moinpour CM, Coltman CA. Erectile dysfunction and subsequent cardiovascular disease. *Jama* 2005;**294**:2996–3002.
2. Guay AT. ED2: erectile dysfunction = endothelial dysfunction. *Endocrinol Metab Clin North Am* 2007;**36**:453–63.
3. Selvin E, Burnett AL, Platz EA. Prevalence and risk factors for erectile dysfunction in the US. *Am J Med* 2007;**120**:151–7.
4. Jonler M, Moon T, Brannan W, Stone NN, Heisey D, Bruskewitz RC. The effect of age, ethnicity and geographical location on impotence and quality of life. *Br J Urol* 1995;**75**:651–5.
5. Kinsey AC, et al. *Sexual behavior in the human male.* Philadelphia, PA: W.B. Saunders; 1948.
6. Bosch RJ, Benard F, Aboseif SR, Stief CG, Lue TF, Tanagho EA. Penile detumescence: characterization of three phases. *J Urol* 1991;**146**:867–71.
7. Andersson KE, Wagner G. Physiology of penile erection. *Physiol Rev* 1995;**75**:191–236.
8. Chen JK, Hwang TI, Yang CR. Comparison of effects following the intracorporeal injection of papaverine and prostaglandin E1. *Br J Urol* 1992;**69**:404–7.
9. Seftel AD. From aspiration to achievement: assessment and noninvasive treatment of erectile dysfunction in aging men. *J Am Geriatr Soc* 2005;**53**:119–30.
10. Bivalacqua TJ, Usta MF, Champion HC, Adams D, Namara DB, Abdel-Mageed AB, et al. Gene transfer of endothelial nitric oxide synthase partially restores nitric oxide synthesis and erectile function in streptozotocin diabetic rats. *J Urol* 2003;**169**:1911–7.
11. Han G, Tar M, Kuppam DS, Friedman A, Melman A, Friedman J, et al. Nanoparticles as a novel delivery vehicle for therapeutics targeting erectile dysfunction. *J Sex Med* 2010;**7**:224–33.
12. Dorsey P, Keel C, Klavens M, Hellstrom WJ. Phosphodiesterase type 5 (PDE5) inhibitors for the treatment of erectile dysfunction. *Expert Opin Pharmacother* **11**:1109–22.
13. Carson CC, Lue TF. Phosphodiesterase type 5 inhibitors for erectile dysfunction. *BJU Int* 2005;**96**:257–80.
14. Davies KP. The role of opiorphins (endogenous neutral endopeptidase inhibitors) in urogenital smooth muscle biology. *J Sex Med* 2009;**6**(Suppl. 3):286–91.
15. Davies KP, Tar M, Rougeot C, Melman A. Sialorphin (the mature peptide product of Vcsa1) relaxes corporal smooth muscle tissue and increases erectile function in the ageing rat. *BJU Int* 2007;**99**:431–5.
16. Christ GJ, Hodges S. Molecular mechanisms of detrusor and corporal myocyte contraction: identifying targets for pharmacotherapy of bladder and erectile dysfunction. *Br J Pharmacol* 2006;**147**(Suppl. 2):S41–55.
17. Barrett TD, Triggle DJ, Walker MJ, Maurice DH. Mechanism of tissue-selective drug action in the cardiovascular system. *Mol Interv* 2005;**5**:84–93.
18. Ghatta S, Nimmagadda D, Xu X, O'Rourke ST. Large-conductance, calcium-activated potassium channels: structural and functional implications. *Pharmacol Ther* 2006;**110**:103–16.
19. Tanaka Y, Koike K, Alioua A, Shigenobu K, Stefani E, Toro L. Beta1-subunit of MaxiK channel in smooth muscle: a key molecule which tunes muscle mechanical activity. *J Pharmacol Sci* 2004;**94**:339–47.
20. Werner ME, Zvara P, Meredith AL, Aldrich RW, Nelson MT. Erectile dysfunction in mice lacking the large-conductance calcium-activated potassium (BK) channel. *J Physiol* 2005;**567**:545–56.
21. Tanaka Y, Koike K, Toro L. MaxiK channel roles in blood vessel relaxations induced by endothelium-derived relaxing factors and their molecular mechanisms. *J Smooth Muscle Res* 2004;**40**:125–53.
22. Davies KP, Stanevsky Y, Tar MT, Chang JS, Chance MR, Melman A. Ageing causes cytoplasmic retention of MaxiK channels in rat corporal smooth muscle cells. *Int J Impot Res* 2007;**19**:371–7.
23. Davies KP, Zhao W, Tar M, Figueroa JC, Desai P, Verselis VK, et al. Diabetes-induced changes in the alternative splicing of the slo gene in corporal tissue. *Eur Urol* 2007;**52**:1229–37.
24. Kun A, Matchkov VV, Stankevicius E, Nardi A, Hughes AD, Kirkeby HJ, et al. NS11021, a novel opener of large-conductance $Ca(^{2+})$-activated $K(^{+})$ channels, enhances erectile responses in rats. *Br J Pharmacol* 2009;**158**:1465–76.
25. Christ GJ, Day N, Santizo C, Sato Y, Zhao W, Sclafani T, et al. Intracorporal injection of hSlo cDNA restores erectile capacity in STZ-diabetic F-344 rats in vivo. *Am J Physiol Heart Circ Physiol* 2004;**287**:H1544–53.
26. Melman A, Zhao W, Davies KP, Bakal R, Christ GJ. The successful long-term treatment of age related erectile dysfunction with hSlo cDNA in rats in vivo. *J Urol* 2003;**170**:285–90.
27. Melman A, Bar-Chama N, McCullough A, Davies K, Christ G. hMaxi-K gene transfer in males with erectile dysfunction: results of the first human trial. *Hum Gene Ther* 2006;**17**:1165–76.
28. Christ G, Wingard C. Calcium sensitization as a pharmacological target in vascular smooth-muscle regulation. *Curr Opin Investig Drugs* 2005;**6**:920–33.
29. Chitaley K, Wingard CJ, Clinton Webb R, Branam H, Stopper VS, Lewis RW, et al. Antagonism of Rho-kinase stimulates rat penile erection via a nitric oxide-independent pathway. *Nat Med* 2001;**7**:119–22.
30. Mills TM, Lewis RW, Wingard CJ, Chitaley K, Webb RC. Inhibition of tonic contraction – a novel way to approach erectile dysfunction. *J Androl* 2002;**23**:S5–9.
31. Evans AM, Cobban HJ, Nixon GF. ET(A) receptors are the primary mediators of myofilament calcium sensitization induced by ET-1 in rat pulmonary artery smooth muscle: a tyrosine kinase independent pathway. *Br J Pharmacol* 1999;**127**:153–60.
32. Babij P. Tissue-specific and developmentally regulated alternative splicing of a visceral isoform of smooth muscle myosin heavy chain. *Nucl Acids Res* 1993;**21**:1467–71.
33. Koi PT, Milhoua PM, Monrose V, Melman A, DiSanto ME. Expression of myosin isoforms in the smooth muscle of human corpus cavernosum. *Int J Impot Res* 2007;**19**:62–8.
34. Corona G, Maggi M. The role of testosterone in erectile dysfunction. *Nat Rev Urol* **7**: 46–56.
35. Morelli A, Filippi S, Zhang XH, Luconi M, Vignozzi L, Mancina R, et al. Peripheral regulatory mechanisms in erection. *Int J Androl* 2005;**28**(Suppl. 2):23–7.
36. El-Bahnasawy MS, Dawood A, Farouk A. Low-flow priapism: risk factors for erectile dysfunction. *BJU Int* 2002;**89**:285–90.
37. Montague DK, Jarow J, Broderick GA, Dmochowski RR, Heaton JP, Lue TF, et al. American Urological Association guideline on the management of priapism. *J Urol* 2003;**170**:1318–24.

38. Sood S, James W, Bailon MJ. Priapism associated with atypical antipsychotic medications: a review. *Int Clin Psychopharmacol* 2008;**23**:9–17.
39. Nunes KP, Costa-Goncalves A, Lanza LF, Cortes SF, Cordeiro MN, Richardson M, et al. Tx2-6 toxin of the *Phoneutria nigriventer* spider potentiates rat erectile function. *Toxicon* 2008;**51**:1197–206.
40. Fowler Jr JE, Koshy M, Strub M, Chinn SK. Priapism associated with the sickle cell hemoglobinopathies: prevalence, natural history and sequelae. *J Urol* 1991;**145**:65–8.
41. Emond AM, Holman R, Hayes RJ, Serjeant GR. Priapism and impotence in homozygous sickle cell disease. *Arch Intern Med* 1980;**140**:1434–7.
42. Burnett AL, Chang AG, Crone JK, Huang PL, Sezen SE. Noncholinergic penile erection in mice lacking the gene for endothelial nitric oxide synthase. *J Androl* 2002;**23**:92–7.
43. Champion HC, Bivalacqua TJ, Takimoto E, Kass DA, Burnett AL. Phosphodiesterase-5A dysregulation in penile erectile tissue is a mechanism of priapism. *Proc Natl Acad Sci USA* 2005;**102**:1661–6.
44. Mi T, Abbasi S, Zhang H, Uray K, Chunn JL, Xia LW, et al. Excess adenosine in murine penile erectile tissues contributes to priapism via A2B adenosine receptor signaling. *J Clin Invest* 2008;**118**:1491–501.
45. Kanika ND, Tar M, Tong Y, Kuppam DS, Melman A, Davies KP. The mechanism of opiorphin-induced experimental priapism in rats involves activation of the polyamine synthetic pathway. *Am J Physiol Cell Physiol* 2009;**297**:C916–27.
46. Yuan J, Desouza R, Westney OL, Wang R. Insights of priapism mechanism and rationale treatment for recurrent priapism. *Asian J Androl* 2008;**10**:88–101.
47. Burnett AL. Molecular pharmacotherapeutic targeting of PDE5 for preservation of penile health. *J Androl* 2008;**29**:3–14.
48. Dai Y, Zhang Y, Phatarpekar P, Mi T, Zhang H, Blackburn MR, et al. Adenosine signaling, priapism and novel therapies. *J Sex Med* 2009;**6**(Suppl. 3):292–301.
49. Agarwal A, Nandipati KC, Sharma RK, Zippe CD, Raina R. Role of oxidative stress in the pathophysiological mechanism of erectile dysfunction. *J Androl* 2006;**27**:335–47.

Chapter 103

Smooth Muscle in the Normal and Diseased Pulmonary Circulation

Michael E. Yeager, Maria G. Frid, Eva Nozik-Grayck, and Kurt R. Stenmark

University of Colorado Denver, Anschutz Medical Campus, Department of Pediatric Critical Care Medicine and Developmental Lung Biology Laboratory, Aurora, CO

INTRODUCTION: PULMONARY VERSUS SYSTEMIC CIRCULATIONS

The pulmonary and systemic circulatory systems are similar in that both circulate the same blood volume via a pulsatile fluid pump at the same periodicity. However, the pulmonary circulation is a system of low resistance and corresponding pulmonary artery pressures, about one-sixth that of the systemic circulation. This low resistance results in the pulsatility of the pulmonary blood flow extending into, and to some degree throughout, the microvessels of the lung. The right ventricle requires one-fifth of the energy of the left ventricle to move the same amount of blood through the low resistance lung vasculature. The mature right ventricle is less capable than the left ventricle of acutely or chronically increasing its volume and/or pressure output. This requires efficient coupling of the right ventricle to the pulmonary circulation. Thus, and importantly, the material stiffness of large conduit vessels is lower in the pulmonary than systemic circulation and the hydraulic capacitance of the pulmonary circulation is quite significant. This large capacitance allows for the normal pulmonary circulation to accommodate a large range of blood flows with little increase in pulmonary arterial pressure.

The vascular load imposed by the pulmonary circulation on the heart as a result of both downstream hydraulic resistance hemodynamics and coupled vascular capacitance is an important and determinant factor of right ventricular function. The first of these loads, downstream hydraulic resistance, is imposed by the arterioles and capillaries of the lung. In the pulmonary circulation, this resistive load is typically characterized by the measure of pulmonary vascular resistance (PVR). The second of these loads is associated with the hydraulic capacitance provided by the deformation of the conduit arteries during the cardiac cycle. By focusing on these two hydraulic loads, right ventricular (RV) afterload can be reduced to a function of both the steady-state resistance, categorized by PVR, and dynamic compliance, defined by the pulmonary vascular stiffness (PVS) of the conduit pulmonary arteries (PA) (1). Though PVR measurement has been the standard diagnostic tool, ignoring pulmonary vascular stiffness (PVS) is an important omission given the inherently pulsatile nature of cardiac function and the importance of robust ventriculo-vascular coupling in maintaining hemodynamic efficiency through the pulmonary vasculature.

From a pathologic and functional perspective, there are two main categories of pulmonary arteries, elastic and muscular. Large pulmonary arteries are of the elastic type, are located proximal to the heart, and serve both as a conduit for the total pulmonary blood volume and as a hydrodynamic capacitor through artery compliance. The primary resistive structures are the pulmonary arterioles, small muscular arteries whose function is to regulate the hydraulic resistance of the system through vasoreactive changes in inter-luminal diameter and the capillary network of the lung. These resistance vessels are critical for regulating matching of perfusion to ventilation. This regulating system presumably is present to some extent to correct the passive gravity-dependent distribution of blood flow in the lung and is unique to the pulmonary circulation. Hypoxic pulmonary vasoconstriction was in fact first reported by von Euler and Liljestrand, who showed that hypoxia increased resistance to blood flow in the lung in contrast to the hypoxic-induced vasodilation seen in systemic tissues. The hypoxic pulmonary pressure responses are universal in mammals and in birds but with considerable intraspecies and interindividual variability (2). The constrictive response to hypoxia is biphasic and is observed in lungs devoid of nervous connections and in isolated pulmonary arterial smooth muscle cells. The biochemical mechanisms of hypoxic pulmonary vasoconstriction remain incompletely understood.

Muscle. DOI: http://dx.doi.org/10.1016/B978-0-12-381510-1.00103-4

PULMONARY HYPERTENSION

Pulmonary hypertension (PH) is not a disease *per se* but rather a pathophysiological parameter defined by a mean pulmonary arterial pressure exceeding the upper limits of normal, i.e. ≥ 25 mmHg at rest (3). PH occurs in a variety of clinical situations and is associated with a broad spectrum of histological patterns and abnormalities. A classification system for PH has been developed to organize the diseases into categories, based on common clinical parameters, potential etiologic mechanisms, and responses to treatment, because of this diversity. At present, six groups of chronic PH are described (4). Group 1 comprises a number of diverse diseases termed pulmonary arterial hypertension (PAH) that have several pathophysiological, histological, and prognostic features in common. Distinction between the various groups of patients with PH is of significance because they differ in etiology, prognosis, histologic appearance, and response to various therapies. Further, differences in microanatomical site and histologic features of the different vascular lesions in these various conditions, point to differences in pathogenesis, the elucidation of which is key to the design of effective therapeutic strategies.

Although any form of PH can contribute to increases in patient morbidity and mortality, PAH (group 1), is a particularly severe and progressive form that frequently leads to right heart failure and premature death (5,6). Thus, when it is stated that a patient has PAH, this diagnosis must include a series of defined clinical parameters, which extend beyond mere elevations in pulmonary arterial pressures. For instance, diseases categorized as PAH share some common characteristics such as precapillary PH, pulmonary hypertensive arteriopathy (usually with plexiform lesions), slow clinical onset (months/years), and a chronic time course (years) characterized by progressive deterioration. Further, patients with "PAH" often demonstrate similar responses to the currently available treatments (endothelin receptor antagonists (ERAs), phosphodiasterase type-5 inhibitors (iPDE-5)), and prostanoids. However, patients within this group also exhibit some relevant differences, for example in the case of congenital heart disease-associated PAH and pulmonary veno-occlusive disease (PVOD).

PH and specifically PAH must be considered a panvasculopathy since abnormalities are seen in each of the compartments of the pulmonary vessel wall (intima, media, and adventitia). The histologic findings include intimal hyperplasia, medial hypertrophy, adventitial proliferation and fibrosis, occlusion of small pulmonary arteries, thrombosis in situ, and infiltration of the vascular wall, particularly the adventitia, with inflammatory and progenitor cells. The endothelium is clearly abnormal in the setting of pulmonary hypertension and marked changes in the vasodilator/vasoconstrictor ratio have been demonstrated (7). In PAH, enhanced smooth muscle cell (SMC) proliferation and survival as well as hypertrophy in the pulmonary arterial media have been reported. Many factors are thought to drive these responses, as discussed further below, including mutation or downregulation of BMPR2, mitochondrial metabolic abnormalities, de novo expression of anti-apoptotic proteins, increased expression activity of 5-HTT, increased expression activity of PDGF receptor, tyrosine kinase activation, and decreased expression of voltage gated O_2 sensitive potassium channels (8). Adventitial thickening is also commonly observed and the adventitial abnormalities have been reviewed in detail elsewhere (9).

ANIMAL MODELS OF PULMONARY HYPERTENSION

Much of what we know regarding the pathogenesis of PH and specifically PAH is derived from work in animal models. Unfortunately, there is no currently available perfect preclinical model of human PAH. The two most commonly used involve exposure of rodents to chronic hypoxia or injection of the pyrrizolidine alkaloid monocrotaline (10). Each has its own limitations, especially as they relate to PAH. More recently, modifications of these models have been generated, which produce different lesions, some plexiform-like, over different time courses (10). In addition, genetic mouse models are also now in common use. Arguably, there is probably no animal model that accurately reproduces all the clinical pathologic features of any of the groups of human PH. Comparison of the characteristics of some of these models to the human condition is shown in Table 103.1. Despite these limitations, it is also clear that animal models have provided, and will continue to provide, valuable insight into the numerous pathways that contribute to the development and maintenance of PH. For each given biologic pathway studied to date, the relative importance in a specific animal strain appears influenced by not only the inciting stimulus and/or the disease, but also by age, gender, environment, and species-specific counter-regulatory modifications in cells and tissues. Precise comparisons between animal species and the human condition are therefore difficult and the cellular and molecular pathogenesis of even the obstructive vascular lesions described in new animal models may not duplicate that which occurs over time in human PH/PAH. The remainder of this chapter presents a review of the role of changes in SMC and SMC-like cell phenotype as it relates to PH/PAH and pulmonary vascular remodeling.

TABLE 103.1 Comparison of Animal Models to Human PAH with Respect to Physiologic and Pathologic Parameters

Condition/ Characteristic	Precapillary Arteriopathy	Alveolar Hypoxia	Pulmonary Hypertensive Arteriopathy with Plexiformesions	Vascular/ Peri-vascular Inflammation	Slow Clinical Onset (m/y) and Chronic Time-coures (y) with Progressive Deterioration	Simillar Response to Drugs (ERAs, PDE5-Inhibitors, Protanoids)	Response to O_2 Therapy	Conduit Artery Stiffening
Clinical "human" PAH	Y	N	Y	Y	Y	Y	N	Y
Hypoxic PH animal models	Y	Y	N	Y	N	Y	Y	Y
Monocrotaline rat model	Y	N	N	Y	N	Y	?	?
Monocrotaline rat + Pneumonectomy	Y	N	N	Y	N	Y	?	?
Monocrotaline rat + pneumonectomy + Young age	Y	N	Y +/−	Y	N	?	?	?
Sugen 5416 + Hypoxia	Y	Y	N	Y	N	?	N	?
S100A4 overexpressing mice	Y	N	Y +/−	Y	Y	?	?	Y +/−
IL-6 overexpressing mice	Y	Y/N*	Y +/−	Y	Y +/−	?	?	?
Left-to-right shunt in piglets and calves	Y	N	N	Y +/−	N	Y	?	?
SHIV-net Infected macaques	Y	N	Y +/−	Y	N	?	?	?

*Y = Yes/present or similar; N = No or not present; ? = no data available; Y +/− = Yes in the opinion of the authors of the published manuscript, not, however reliably reproduced by multiple investigators; * = both normoxic and hypoxic conditions have seen studied.*

ORIGINS OF PULMONARY SMC IN DEVELOPMENT AND IN PULMONARY HYPERTENSIVE VASCULAR REMODELING

While the proximal part of the pulmonary circulation is derived from the truncus arteriosus, the intrapulmonary arteries appear to be derived from a continuous expansion of the primary capillary plexus that is contained within the mesenchyme, by vasculogenesis. The developmental origins of the SMC and pericytes surrounding blood vessels in the lung are poorly understood (11). In humans, SMCs in the intrapulmonary arteries are said to be derived from three sites in a temporally distinct sequence: the earliest cells come from the bronchial smooth muscle, followed by the mesenchyme surrounding the arteries, and finally from the endothelial cells (12). Despite their different origins, all pulmonary artery SMCs (PA-SMCs) follow the same sequence of expression of smooth muscle (SM)-specific contractile and cytoskeletal proteins with increasing age (12). During the process of vascular remodeling in the adult, PA-SMCs can also potentially originate from other cell types, such as endothelial (via endothelial-to-mesenchymal transdifferentiation, EnMT) (13). Other possibilities have also been raised including the origin of PA-SMC from epithelial cells (via epithelial-to-mesenchymal transition (EMT)), and from SM progenitor cells – either circulating bone marrow-derived or vessel wall resident progenitors (14). However, in contrast to the systemic circulation, where origin of SMCs from progenitor cells is now commonly accepted, there are few studies that have reported accumulation of bone marrow-derived cells within the pulmonary arterial media of animals with experimentally-induced PH (15) or human patients with either COPD (16) or with chronic thromboembolic PH (17). The level of SMC differentiation was never assessed beyond expression of α-SM-actin (which is expressed by myofibroblasts and other cell types), and therefore an origin of "true" (differentiated) SMCs from circulating or resident progenitor cells in pulmonary vascular remodeling remains to be elucidated.

As for cells characterized only by α-SM-actin positivity (SM-like) cells, increased numbers of such cells have been reported to accumulate in the remodeled PAs in virtually all forms of chronic PH (8). Traditionally, it has been thought that the accumulating α-SM-actin-expressing cells were exclusively derived from either the resident vascular SMCs through their dedifferentiation or from adventitial fibroblasts via their differentiation into myofibroblasts. New experimental data suggest alternative sources/origins of these cells, including circulating fibrocytes. Fibrocytes are bone marrow-derived circulating mesenchymal progenitors of a monocytic lineage that could be rapidly recruited to the site of injury, where they differentiate into fibroblast/myofibroblast-like cells (18,19). Differentiation of fibrocytes into mesenchymal cells that are ultrastructurally, phenotypically, and functionally similar to fibroblasts/myofibroblasts is promoted by stimulation with TGF-β or endothelin (19). Accumulation of α-SM-actin expressing fibrocytes occurs in the remodeled pulmonary arteries of chronically hypoxic hypertensive rats and calves (20,21). These cells exhibited highly augmented proliferative, migratory, invasive, and potent promitogenic capabilities, and may contribute to the remodeling process directly through differentiation into myofibroblast-like cells, but also indirectly through secretion of potent pro-mitogenic and pro-inflammatory mediators.

In summary, it needs to be re-emphasized that, contrary to abundant experimental evidence in the systemic circulation, data in the pulmonary circulation presents limited evidence demonstrating contribution of circulating and/or resident progenitor cells to the pool of SMCs and/or SM-like (α-SM-actin expressing) cells.

PHENOTYPIC AND FUNCTIONAL HETEROGENEITY OF PA-SMCS

The vascular media in both pulmonary and systemic arteries is a complex structure, comprised of multiple phenotypically and functionally distinct SMC populations that may subserve distinct cellular functions in health and disease (22–24). For the pulmonary circulation, SMC heterogeneity has been described in both site-specific and regional (along the longitudinal axis) patterns.

In the large conducting portion of the pulmonary circulation, *in vivo* and *in vitro* studies demonstrate that PA-SMCs exhibit functional heterogeneity in growth and matrix-producing capabilities. These findings support the notion that the heterogeneity of PA-SMCs governs, at least in part, the pattern of abnormal cell proliferation and matrix protein synthesis that characterize chronic hypoxic forms of PH. In the bovine main pulmonary artery, four phenotypically distinct SMC populations were described to reside in the subendothelial, middle, and outer compartments of the tunica media (Figure 103.1) (22,24). These cell subpopulations were morphologically distinct, differently oriented within the pulmonary artery wall, exhibited a distinct pattern of SM contractile and cytoskeletal protein expression and distinct matrix-producing capabilities. In severe hypoxia-induced PH, these phenotypically distinct SMC populations displayed markedly different proliferative and matrix-producing responses, so that less differentiated PA-SMCs demonstrated higher indices in proliferative capabilities as well as higher elastogenic responses to chronic hypoxic exposure (Figure 103.2) (25,26). These phenotypically distinct PA-SMC populations, when isolated and maintained in

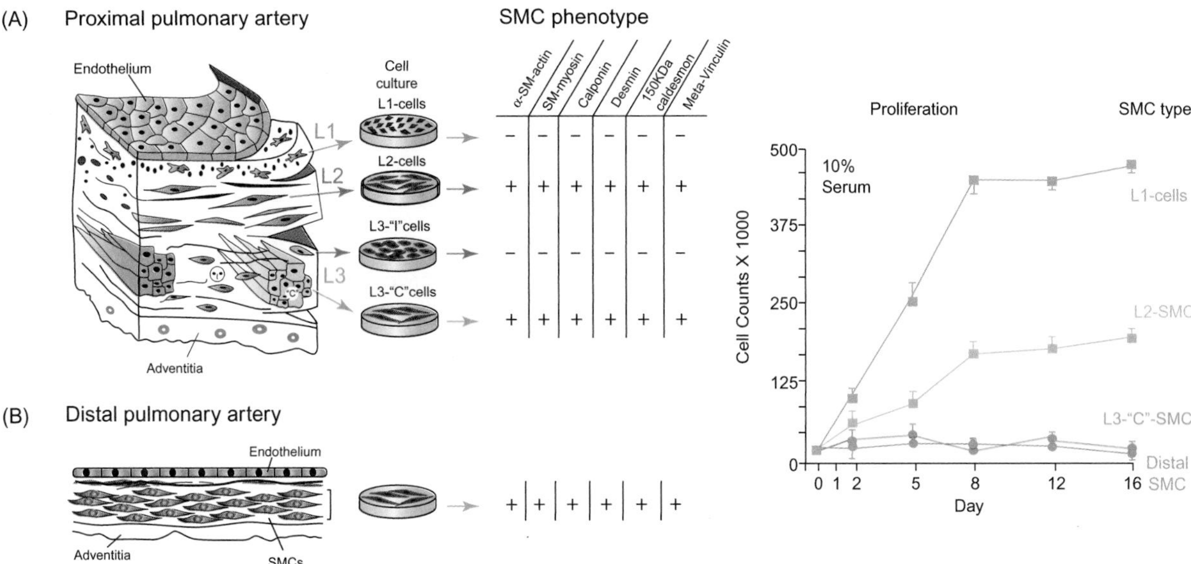

FIGURE 103.1 Media of proximal large elastic pulmonary arteries in the bovine species is comprised of phenotypically distinct SMC populations, in contrast to a phenotypically uniform SMC population in distal pulmonary arteries. In culture, distinct SMC populations isolated from the arterial media of large proximal elastic arteries (A) exhibit stable phenotypic differences in contractile and cytoskeletal protein expression (table "SMC Phenotype") and differences in growth potential (graph "Proliferation", orange, blue, and green growth curves), whereas SMC isolated from the media of distal pulmonary arteries (B) are phenotypically uniform (table "SMC Phenotype") and are growth-resistant (graph "Proliferation", purple growth curve). *(Adapted from Frid et al., 1997 (22), with permission from Wolters Kluwer.)*

culture, exhibited a stable functional phenotype for numerous passages, including distinct growth capabilities in response to serum, growth factors and hypoxia (Figure 103.1) (22,27). Furthermore, production of elastin has been suggested to reflect phenotypic changes in the developing SMCs. Expression of elastin precursor, tropoelastin, by SMCs within the pulmonary artery media has been demonstrated to produce a heterogeneous pattern both during fetal development and in response to hypoxia-induced PH (25). The molecular mechanisms that contributed to *in vitro* differences in hypoxia-induced proliferative responses of distinct PA-SMC populations (i.e. hypoxia-proliferative versus hypoxia-nonproliferative cells) were found to be attributed to differences in responses to G-protein coupled receptor (GPCR) agonists (22) and differences in responses to stimulation of the protein kinase C (PKC), specifically PKC-α pathway (27), where hypoxia-proliferative and less differentiated SMCs exhibited markedly higher responses. These observations raise the possibility that hypoxia-proliferative cells display membrane-bound receptors that are sensitive to hypoxic activation, as well as the capability to engage specific intracellular signaling pathways, which confer unique proliferative responses to these cells.

Differences in phenotype and functional capabilities of PA-SMCs in distal resistance versus large conductance pulmonary arteries have also been described. A progressive increase in phenotypic uniformity and level of PA-SMC differentiation is observed along the proximal-to-distal axis of the pulmonary circulation so that the media of distal (1500−100 μm diameter) pulmonary arteries is composed of a phenotypically uniform population of "well-differentiated" (as identified by a panel of SM-specific antibodies) SMCs (Figure 103.1) (28). When isolated in culture and assessed, distal PA-SMCs represented a phenotypically uniform population of well-differentiated SMCs that were proliferation-resistant and had a substantial capability to hypertrophy in response to growth-promoting stimuli (28). The distinct PA-SMC phenotypes present in distal versus proximal pulmonary arteries may therefore confer distinct response mechanisms during pulmonary vascular remodeling in PH.

Furthermore, significant differences in the ion channel expression exist between SMCs from proximal versus distal pulmonary arteries and have been suggested to represent the differences in pulmonary vasoconstriction between distal and proximal sites of pulmonary circulation (29). PA-SMCs from large proximal vessels are enriched in the large-conductance calcium-sensitive (BK) potassium channels while those from distal, resistance pulmonary arteries have mainly the voltage-dependent (Kv) potassium channels, particularly hypoxia- and 4-aminopyridine (4-AP)-sensitive Kv1.5 and Kv2.1 channels, suggesting an important role for these Kv channels in the resting membrane potential and hypoxic constriction of resistance pulmonary arteries (30). Differences in expression of transient receptor potential proteins and the store- and receptor-operated Ca^{2+} channel between

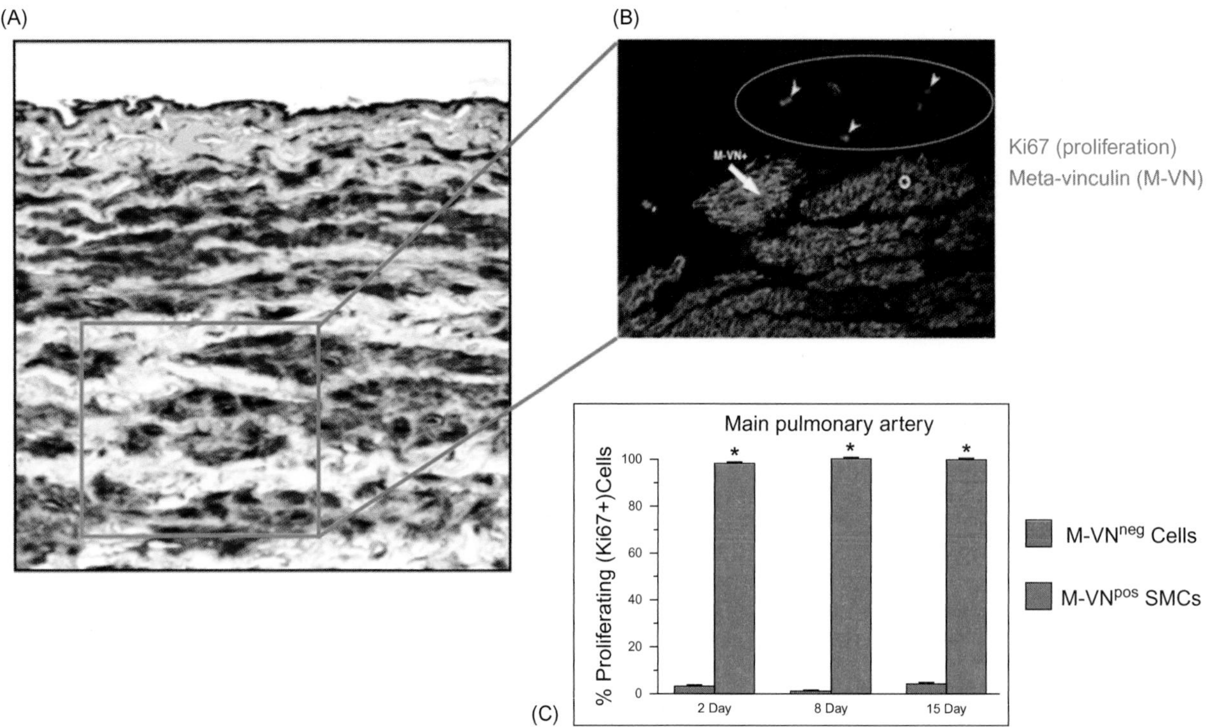

FIGURE 103.2 **Pulmonary arterial media of the large elastic arteries in the bovine species is comprised of phenotypically and functionally distinct SMC populations (*in vivo* analysis).** (A) IHC staining demonstrates that only specific SMC subpopulations express SM-myosin heavy chains (SM-1 and SM-2) isoforms (brown staining), whereas a-SM-actin expression is characteristic of all cells within the arterial media. In the outer media, SMCs expressing SM-myosin (shown in the inset in panel A, brown staining) also co-express meta-vinculin (green fluorescence in panel B). (B) Hypoxia-induced cell proliferation (Ki-67^{+} cell nuclei, red fluorescence) within the pulmonary artery media of hypertensive calves occurs almost exclusively in meta-vinculin-negative cell populations. (C) Time-course evaluation of cell proliferation within the pulmonary artery media of hypoxic hypertensive calves demonstrates that more than 95% of replicating cells are from a population of meta-vinculin-negative SMCs (red bars), whereas meta-vinculin expressing SMCs remain relatively quiescent (green bars). (*Panel (A) adapted from Frid et al., 1994 (24), with permission; panel (C) adapted from Wohrley et al., 1995 (26), with permission from the American Society for Clinical Investigation.*)

PA-SMCs in distal versus proximal pulmonary arteries have also been documented (31).

MECHANISMS INVOLVED IN CONTROL OF SMC (OR SM-LIKE CELL) PHENOTYPE IN PULMONARY VASCULAR DISEASE

A balance between the factors that regulate vasoconstriction and those that regulate vasodilation influence the contractile state of PA-SMCs and thus the tone of the pulmonary circulation in health and disease. Most of these factors also modulate other SMC functions such as proliferation, migration, or apoptosis. Differences in responses to these factors are observed in PA-SMC along the pulmonary vascular tree. There is an overlap between some of the mechanisms regulating PA-SMCs and systemic (i.e. aortic) SMCs, and a number of these regulatory mechanisms are disrupted in PAH, contributing to enhanced pulmonary vasoconstriction and vessel wall remodeling. Here, we summarize the primary factors known to influence PA-SMC function under normal and pathological conditions.

Mechanisms Contributing to Pulmonary Vascular Tone

Vasoactive Peptides

Three extensively studied peptides, endothelin-1 (ET-1), serotonin (5-HT), and angiotensin (AngII), lead to both vasoconstriction and pro-mitogenic effects in PA-SMCs, and contribute to abnormalities in animal models of PH and to human disease. ET-1 acts via G-protein coupled receptors located on PA-SMCs (ET-A receptors) and on pulmonary artery endothelial cells via both ET-A and ET-B) receptors. Blockade of ET-1 signaling has become a mainstay of the therapeutic toolkit for PH. Three ET-1 receptor antagonists approved by the Food and Drug Administration (FDA) are used in World Health Organization-classified PAH patients: bosentan, ambrisentan, and sitaxsentan.

Blockade of ET-1 receptors results in reduced vasoconstriction, largely due to decreased intracellular calcium release. Besides vasoconstriction, ET-1 is a powerful mitogen for many cell types (32). Therapeutic blockade of ET-1 receptors is therefore of critical importance with regard to pulmonary arterial smooth muscle cell proliferation and vasoconstriction.

In the 1960s and again in the 1980s, patients taking the anorexigens aminorex or fenfluramine were identified as having an increased risk of developing PAH. Both aminorex and fenfluramine are serotonin transporter substrates and act by increasing extracellular (5-HT). 5-HT, in turn, causes vasoconstriction and pulmonary vascular remodeling through induction of proliferation of both pulmonary arterial fibroblasts and pulmonary arterial SMCs. Patients with idiopathic PAH have increased circulating 5-HT levels, which persist after heart–lung transplantation. The rate-limiting step in 5-HT biosynthesis is catalyzed by the enzyme tryptophan hydroxylase. Human pulmonary artery endothelial cells produce 5-HT and express the tryptophan hydroxylase-1 isoform, and both are increased in patients with idiopathic PAH compared with controls (33). Mice lacking tryptophan hydroxylase-1 are resistant to both hypoxia- and dexfenfluramine-induced PH (34). 5-HT vasoconstriction of SMCs is primarily mediated by 5-HT receptors 1B, and 2A, while the mitogenic effects of 5-HT require internalization through the serotonin transporter 5-HTT. Drugs that competitively inhibit 5-HTT can block proliferation of SMCs. Fenfluramine and aminorex not only inhibit 5-HT reuptake but also trigger indoleamine release and interact with 5-HTT and -HT receptors (35). 5-HTT is abundantly expressed on PA-SMCs, and increased 5-HTT expression correlates with increased severity of hypoxic PH, and when overexpressed in PASMCs, is sufficient to produce spontaneous PH (36,37).

Angiotensin (Ang)-converting enzyme 2 (ACE2) is a component of the renin-angiotensin system (RAS) that has been implicated in a variety of physiologic and pathophysiologic processes. It is a monocarboxypeptidase homologue of ACE, and it generates Ang-(1–7), which blunts the vasoconstrictive, proliferative, fibrotic, and inflammatory effects of Ang II (38). ACE2 is broadly vasoprotective by offsetting the vasoconstrictive, proliferative, and fibrotic actions of the ACE–Ang II–Ang II type 1 receptor (AT_1R) axis (38,39). Because many of the RAS components are so widely expressed in the lung, ACE2 has been investigated for its putative role(s) in the pathogenesis of lung injury and as a therapeutic target in a number of lung diseases. One potential clue for modulation of the RAS at the level of PASMC comes from *in vitro* studies using hypoxia. Hypoxia can elicit changes in the expression profiles of ACE and ACE2 in human PA-SMCs. HIF-1α can directly and simultaneously upregulate ACE and downregulate ACE2. Furthermore, reduction of ACE2 expression in human PA-SMCs by siRNA interference boosted proliferation and migration under hypoxia (40).

Potassium Channels/Calcium Handling

In PA-SMCs, the free cytosolic Ca^{2+} concentration (Ca^{2+}_{cyt}) modulates contraction, proliferation, and migration. The Ca^{2+}_{cyt} in PA-SMCs can be increased by: (i) Ca^{2+} influx through voltage-dependent, receptor-operated, and store-operated Ca^{2+} channels (41), and (ii) Ca^{2+} release from intracellular stores (42). Conversely, Ca^{2+}_{cyt} in PA-SMCs can be decreased by: (i) Ca^{2+} extrusion by the Ca^{2+}-Mg^{2+} adenosine triphosphatase (Ca^{2+} pump) and by the forward mode of Na^{+}/Ca^{2+} exchanger in the plasma membrane; and (ii) Ca^{2+} sequestration by the Ca^{2+}-Mg^{2+} adenosine triphosphatase in the sarcoplasmic reticulum. Distal PA-SMCs have greater expression of transient receptor potential proteins (TRPC) 1, 6, and 4 and of stromal interacting molecule 1 (STIM1), than proximal PA-SMCs (31). Studies conducted under conditions of extracellular Ca^{2+}-free medium demonstrated that hypoxia-induced $[Ca^{2+}]_i$ elevation through store-operated calcium (SOC) channels was greater in distal than in proximal PA-SMCs, indicating an important role for SOC in hypoxic pulmonary vasoconstriction (43,44).

Abundant evidence has accumulated indicating that PH is associated with reduced PA-SMC expression and function of K^{+} channels in PA-SMCs as well as a decrease in Kv channel subunits (e.g., Kv1.2 and Kv1.5) (45). Interestingly, Kv channel expression and mitochondrial metabolism are functionally linked. More specifically, some forms of PAH seem to exhibit a cancer-like glycolytic phenotype in PA-SMCs that is characterized by mitochondrial abnormalities and a metabolic shift from oxidative phosphorylation to glycolysis (46). The resulting decreases in electron flux and reactive oxygen species production results in normoxic HIF-1 activation and decreased Kv1.5 expression similar to that seen in chronic hypoxia. The rationale for mitochondrial therapy and restoration of Kv1.5 expression and function is supported by the observation that inhibition of pyruvate dehydrogenase kinase by dichloroacetate or Kv1.5 gene therapy partially regresses three distinct rat models of PH (47). As mentioned above (see "Phenotypic and Functional Heterogeneity"), significant differences in the ion channel expression exist between SMCs from proximal versus distal pulmonary arteries and contribute to hypoxic vasoconstriction characteristics of resistance pulmonary arteries (30,48).

Rho-A/Pho-kinase

The triggers for vasoconstriction involve both an increase in cytosolic calcium in the PA-SMCs and increased calcium sensitization. Activation of Rho-A/Rho kinase signaling leads to inhibition of myosin-light chain phosphatase (MLCP), which mediates PA-SMC relaxation when in its dephosphorylated form by leading to actin-myosin cross branch dissociation, through phosphorylation of the MYPT1 regulatory subunit of MLCP (49–51). Inhibition of MLCP by Rho kinase prolongs actin–myosin interaction and sustained SMC contraction at any given level of intracellular calcium. Rho-A/Rho-kinase signaling plays a key role in the pathogenesis of various animal models of PH, including hypoxia-induced, monocrotaline-induced, shunt-induced, bleomycin-induced, spontaneously hypertensive fawn-hooded rats, and hypoxia plus VEGF receptor antagonist, Sugen5416 (49–51). Importantly, in these studies, administration of the Rho kinase inhibitor, fasudil, caused dramatic reductions in pulmonary artery pressure even in animal models of PH where traditional vasodilators such as iNO or prostacyclin had little or no effect (50,51). Furthermore a recent report indicates that there is high Rho-A/Rho-kinase activity in distal pulmonary arteries of humans with PAH (52).

Prostacyclins

Prostacyclin, a member of the endogenous prostanoid family, is produced from arachidonic acid through the actions of prostacyclin synthase and cyclooxygenase. In the pulmonary circulation, prostacyclin is released by pulmonary artery endothelial cells, and on target cells is bound by a cell-surface G-protein-coupled receptor on target cells. Receptor binding and G-protein activation triggers increases in intracellular cAMP, which activates protein kinase A. This causes PA-SMC relaxation and vasodilation, even in the presence of vasoconstrictors. Additionally, prostacyclin inhibits PA-SMC proliferation, particularly when administered in combination with phosphodiesterase inhibitors (53).

Reactive oxygen and nitrogen species

Nitric oxide (NO) is the primary pulmonary vasodilator both produced and released by the endothelium by the enzyme endothelial nitric oxide synthase (eNOS). The primary function of NO is the regulation of vascular tone, inhibition of SMC proliferation, and platelet aggregation. Upon its release by endothelium, NO diffuses into SMCs where it acts to stimulate production of the second messenger cyclic guanosine monophosphate (cGMP) from guanylyl cyclase ultimately leading to dilation of blood vessels *via* dephosphorylation of myosin light chain. Alternatively NO can also react with thiols such as cysteine, and nitrosylated cysteine can be transported by amino acid transporters into the cell to facilitate its intracellular actions. When eNOS is uncoupled, production of NO is decreased and production of the reactive oxygen species peroxynitrite and superoxide are increased, both of which can act directly and indirectly to cause vasoconstriction. Multiple sources of reactive oxygen species, in addition to uncoupled eNOS have been identified and contribute to altered vascular tone as well as intracellular signaling and proliferation. In the pulmonary circulation, other important sources generated within the PA-SMCs as well as other cell types include the mitochondrial electron transport chain, NADPH oxidase, in particular NOX2 and NOX4, and xanthine oxidase. Reactive oxygen species can activate G-protein-coupled receptors and Rho kinase to mediate vasoconstriction and vascular remodeling and antioxidant strategies may modulate PA-SMC function in PH (54–56).

Vasoactive Intestinal Peptide (VIP)

VIP is emerging as a critical regulator of vasodilation and structural remodeling in the pulmonary circulation. Recently it was shown that male mice lacking the gene for VIP spontaneously developed features of moderately severe idiopathic PAH (57). It is also interesting to note that VIP containing nerves, normally plentiful in the pulmonary arteries, were reported absent in the pulmonary arteries of patients with idiopathic PAH.

Adrenomedullin (ADM)

ADM is a potent vasodilator peptide that was originally isolated from human pheochromocytoma. Its vasodilatory effects have been shown to be mediated through cAMP- and NO-dependent mechanisms (58). In addition, ADM has angiogenic, anti-inflammatory, and positive ionotropic activities and is also known to inhibit SMC proliferation and migration (58). The actions of ADM are mediated by calcitonin receptor-like receptor (CRLR), which functions as a selective ADM receptor. Several studies have shown that plasma ADM levels are elevated in proportion to the severity of PH. Most importantly, it has been demonstrated that administration of ADM, either by intravenous or intratracheal routes, significantly decreases pulmonary artery pressure and pulmonary vascular resistance in patients with PAH (58). Recently ADM gene modified endothelial progenitor cells have been demonstrated to incorporate into the lung tissue and attenuate monocrotaline-induced PH in rats (59).

Mechanisms Contributing to Proliferation and Enhanced Survival of PA-SMCs and SM-Like Cells

Pulmonary vascular remodeling is due to the abnormal accumulation of endothelial cells and cells that have been referred to as SMC but that may be better characterized as myofibroblasts or SM-like cells since they have been, for the most part, characterized only by the expression of α-SM-actin. Most of these accumulating cells exhibit high proliferative potential and also may exhibit a relative resistance to apoptosis. In addition these cells often produce excessive amounts of matrix proteins and matrix metalloproteinases (MMPs), and also release factors that are involved in the continued stimulation of pro-proliferative and pro-survival signaling pathways (8,60). As discussed above, the agents that mediate vasoconstriction also in general augment cell proliferation and the anti-apoptotic phenotype, while the vasodilator agents inhibit cell proliferation and promote pro-apoptotic mechanisms. These observations have led to the idea that, in limited ways, the mechanisms involved in vascular remodeling in PH are analogous to neoplasia. It therefore has been hypothesized that agents that can either block cell proliferation and/or migration or induce apoptosis may lead to a regression of the remodeling and to lessening of pulmonary vascular resistance. Many pathways have now been shown, at least in animal models, to contribute to PH through stimulation of proliferation and increases in resistance apoptosis resistance in the PA-SMCs. These include increases in growth factors such as PDGF and EGF; receptor tyrosine kinases such as VEGFR-2, VEGFR-3, PDGF-beta, Flt-3, cKIT, and FGFR1; other protein kinases such as MEK-1, ERK-1, EGFR, or HRT-2; elastase; and phosphodiesterases. Emerging data also indicate that alterations in epigenetic mechanisms including DNA methylation, histone acetylation, and microRNA expression are likely contributing factors in PH. New therapies in development target not only the mediators of vascular tone but also the pathways that lead to a hyperproliferative, anti-apoptotic state.

In culture, bovine SMCs from normal distal pulmonary arteries demonstrate a resistance to traditional growth-promoting stimuli, including platelet-derived growth factor (PDGF)-BB, angiotensin II, and TGF-β1, as well as 5-HT, and ET-1. Importantly, hypoxia also consistently inhibited growth of distal PA-SMCs derived from the distal pulmonary arteries in the presence or absence of serum (28). These responses differ significantly from those described in the far more commonly used bovine SMCs derived from the main (large proximal) pulmonary artery, or rodent SMCs derived from large proximal pulmonary arteries of rats or mice, where PDGF, serotonin, endothelin, and angiotensin stimulate SMC proliferation rather than induce SMC hypertrophy (61,62). Yang et al. reported that serum-stimulated proliferation of SMCs from the main pulmonary arteries of humans was inhibited by TGF-β and bone morphogenetic proteins (BMPs)-2, -4, and -7, whereas in PA-SMCs obtained from distal pulmonary arteries, BMPs-2 and -4 stimulated cell proliferation (63). Studies by Davie et al. also demonstrated regional (proximal versus distal) heterogeneity in human PA-SMC phenotypes by showing that distal pulmonary arteries possessed more ET-1 binding sites and a greater proportion of ET_B receptors than proximal pulmonary arteries, and that, in pulmonary hypertensive patients receptor density in distal pulmonary arteries was twofold greater than in control subjects (64).

Perhaps the most characteristic, yet least understood, change in the pulmonary vasculature seen in all forms of PH is the "muscularization" of the normally partially or non-muscular segments thus converting the precapillary segment into a resistance structure. It is the first cellular event to occur in response to chronic hypoxic exposure, as well as the first to disappear on withdrawal of the hypoxic stimulus. Several mechanisms have been invoked to explain the distal muscularization process, from contribution/recruitment of pericytes and/or "intermediate cells", or interstitial fibroblasts with their subsequent differentiation toward a SM-like cell, to endothelial- and/or epithelial-to-mesenchymal transdifferentiation (EnMT or EMT, respectively), to contribution of mesenchymal precursor cells or circulating monocytic cells (20,65–67).

Role of Inflammation in SMC Phenotype

Inflammation plays a critical yet often under-appreciated role in many forms of human PH. Several types of inflammatory cells, including activated monocytes, macrophages, dendritic cells, and T- and B-lymphocytes, have been documented to accumulate around the pulmonary artery wall in idiopathic forms of PAH (iPAH) (68). Concordantly, pulmonary arteries of patients with idiopathic PAH express IL-1, IL-6, PDGF-BB, RANTES, and macrophage inflammatory protein (MIP)-1α (69). These mediators may have significant effects on the phenotype of PA-SMCs, including increases in proliferation and matrix protein production and changes in the responses to vasoconstricting or vasodilating substances.

Studies in experimental animals, as well as reports in humans showed that acute and chronic exposure to even moderate levels of hypoxia results in the accumulation of leukocytes not only within the lungs but also in perivascular spaces around pulmonary arteries, and, concordantly, increased expression of inflammatory cytokines, chemokines, and adhesion molecules (20,70). Interestingly, at least in animal models, hypoxia-induced perivascular accumulation of mononuclear cells appeared specific to the pulmonary circulation because no monocyte recruitment was noted in systemic vessels (20,70). Influx of inflammatory cells with progenitor-like mRNA expression profile within the arterial media itself was also reported. When isolated in culture, these cells exhibited marked pro-mitogenic effects on medial PA-SMCs (21).

TABLE 103.2 Novel Therapies in Pulmonary Hypertension

Reverse sustained vasoconstriction
1. Rho kinase inhibitors
2. Vasodilator peptides (VIP, adrenomedullin)
3. eNos coupling agents
4. cGMP stimulating agents
Stop/reverse cell growth
5. Kinase inhibitors
6. Akt/mTor inhibitors
7. Anti-inflammatory agents • (nFAT inhibitors, JAK/STAT inhibitors, immune suppressors, etc.)
8. Normalize mitochondrial function • (dichloroacetate)
9. PPAR-γ-agonists
10. Statins
11. TRP channel suppressors
12. Progenitor cells (with or without eNOS)

TREATMENT OF PULMONARY HYPERTENSION

The goals for the treatment of PAH are to reduce pulmonary vascular resistance (PVR) and pulmonary arterial pressure and thereby to reverse the pressure overload on the right ventricle (RV) to prevent its failure and ultimately death of the patient. In addition to adjunctive therapy with anticoagulants, diuretics, ionotropic drugs, and supplemental oxygen, patients with PAH are currently treated with one or a combination of three specific classes of agents, which include prostacyclin analogs, endothelin-1 receptor antagonists, and phosphodiesterase type-5 inhibitors. The rationale for these agents is provided above. The effect of these treatments on function and survival has been assessed in recent meta-analysis of randomized trials in PAH patients, which conclude that the current treatment strategy for PAH patients remains inadequate (71,72). Based on cell studies in animal models and the molecular mechanisms described above, several new therapeutic approaches are currently being considered for human patients (Table 103.2). The drugs are aimed at reversing sustained or abnormal vasoconstriction and/or at stopping or reversing abnormal cell growth and survival (73).

REFERENCES

1. Champion HC, Michelakis ED, Hassoun PM. Comprehensive invasive and noninvasive approach to the right ventricle-pulmonary circulation unit: state of the art and clinical and research implications. *Circulation* 2009;**120**:992–1007.
2. Rhodes J. Comparative physiology of hypoxic pulmonary hypertension: historical clues from brisket disease. *J Appl Physiol* 2005;**98**:1092–100.
3. Badesch BD, Champion HC, Gomez-Sanchez MA, Hoeper M, Loyd J, Manes A, et al. Diagnosis and assessment of pulmonary arterial hypertension. *J Am Coll Cardiol* 2009;**54**:S55–6.
4. Simonneau G, Robbins IM, Beghetti M, Channick RN, Delcroix M, Denton CP, et al. Updated clinical classification of pulmonary hypertension. *J Am Coll Cardiol* 2009;**54**:S43–54.
5. McLaughlin VV, Archer SL, Badesch DB, Barst RJ, Farber HW, Lindner JR, et al. ACCF/AHA 2009 expert consensus document on pulmonary hypertension: a report of the American College of Cardiology Foundation Task Force on Expert Consensus Documents and the American Heart Association developed in collaboration with the American College of Chest Physicians; American Thoracic Society, Inc. and the Pulmonary Hypertension Association. *J Am Coll Cardiol* 2009;**53**:1573–619.
6. Voelkel NF, Quaife RA, Leinwand LA, Barst RJ, McGoon MD, Meldrum DR, et al. Right ventricular function and failure: report of a National Heart, Lung, and Blood Institute working group on cellular and molecular mechanisms of right heart failure. *Circulation* 2006;**114**:1883–91.
7. Humbert M, Montani D, Perros F, Dorfmuller P, Adnot S, Eddahibi S. Endothelial cell dysfunction and cross talk between endothelium and smooth muscle cells in pulmonary arterial hypertension. *Vascul Pharmacol* 2008;**49**:113–8.
8. Humbert M, Morrell NW, Archer SL, Stenmark KR, MacLean MR, Lang IM, et al. Cellular and molecular pathobiology of pulmonary arterial hypertension. *J Am Coll Cardiol* 2004;**43**:13S–24S.
9. Stenmark KR, Nozik-Grayck E, Gerasimovskaya E, Anwar A, Li M, Riddle S, Frid MG. The adventitia: essential role in pulmonary vascular remodeling. *Compr Physiol* 2011;**1**:141–61.
10. Stenmark KR, Meyrick B, Galie N, Mooi WJ, McMurtry IF. Animal models of pulmonary arterial hypertension: the hope for etiological discovery and pharmacological cure. *Am J Physiol Lung Cell Mol Physiol* 2009;**297**:L1013–32.
11. Morrisey EE, Hogan BL. Preparing for the first breath: genetic and cellular mechanisms in lung development. *Dev Cell* 2010;**18**:8–23.
12. Hall SM, Hislop AA, Pierce CM, Haworth SG. Prenatal origins of human intrapulmonary arteries: formation and smooth muscle maturation. *Am J Respir Cell Mol Biol* 2000;**23**:194–203.
13. Frid MG, Kale VA, Stenmark KR. Mature vascular endothelium can give rise to smooth muscle cells via endothelial-mesenchymal transdifferentiation: in vitro analysis. *Circ Res* 2002;**90**:1189–96.
14. Zengin E, Chalajour F, Gehling UM, Ito WD, Treede H, Lauke H, et al. Vascular wall resident progenitor cells: a source for postnatal vasculogenesis. *Development* 2006;**133**:1543–51.
15. Hayashida K, Fujita J, Miyake Y, Kawada H, Ando K, Ogawa S, et al. Bone marrow-derived cells contribute to pulmonary vascular remodeling in hypoxia-induced pulmonary hypertension. *Chest* 2005;**127**:1793–8.
16. Peinado VI, Ramirez J, Roca J, Rodriguez-Roisin R, Barbera JA. Identification of vascular progenitor cells in pulmonary arteries of patients with chronic obstructive pulmonary disease. *Am J Respir Cell Mol Biol* 2006;**34**:257–63.
17. Firth AL, Yao W, Ogawa A, Madani MM, Lin GY, Yuan JX. Multipotent mesenchymal progenitor cells are present in endarterectomized tissues from patients with chronic thromboembolic pulmonary hypertension. *Am J Physiol Cell Physiol* 2010;**298**:C1217–25.
18. Herzog EL, Bucala R. Fibrocytes in health and disease. *Exp Hematol* 2010;**38**:548–56.

19. Pilling D, Fan T, Huang D, Kaul B, Gomer RH. Identification of markers that distinguish monocyte-derived fibrocytes from monocytes, macrophages, and fibroblasts. *PLoS One* 2009;**4**:e7475.
20. Frid MG, Brunetti JA, Burke DL, Carpenter TC, Davie NJ, Reeves JT, et al. Hypoxia-induced pulmonary vascular remodeling requires recruitment of circulating mesenchymal precursors of a monocyte/macrophage lineage. *Am J Pathol* 2006;**168**:659–69.
21. Frid MG, Li M, Gnanasekharan M, Burke DL, Fragoso M, Strassheim D, et al. Sustained hypoxia leads to the emergence of cells with enhanced growth, migratory, and promitogenic potentials within the distal pulmonary artery wall. *Am J Physiol Lung Cell Mol Physiol* 2009;**297**:L1059–72.
22. Frid MG, Aldashev AA, Dempsey EC, Stenmark KR. Smooth muscle cells isolated from discrete compartments of the mature vascular media exhibit unique phenotypes and distinct growth capabilities. *Circ Res* 1997;**81**:940–52.
23. Hao H, Gabbiani G, Bochaton-Piallat ML. Arterial smooth muscle cell heterogeneity: implications for atherosclerosis and restenosis development. *Arterioscler Thromb Vasc Biol* 2003;**23**:1510–20.
24. Frid MG, Moiseeva EP, Stenmark KR. Multiple phenotypically distinct smooth muscle cell populations exist in the adult and developing bovine pulmonary arterial media in vivo. *Circ Res* 1994;**75**:669–81.
25. Durmowicz AG, Frid MG, Wohrley JD, Stenmark KR. Expression and localization of tropoelastin mRNA in the developing bovine pulmonary artery is dependent on vascular cell phenotype. *Am J Respir Cell Mol Biol* 1996;**14**:569–76.
26. Wohrley JD, Frid MG, Moiseeva EP, Orton EC, Belknap JK, Stenmark KR. Hypoxia selectively induces proliferation in a specific subpopulation of smooth muscle cells in the bovine neonatal pulmonary arterial media. *J Clin Invest* 1995;**96**:273–81.
27. Dempsey EC, Das M, Frid MG, Xu Y, Stenmark KR. Hypoxic growth of bovine pulmonary artery smooth muscle cells: dependence on synergy, heterogeneity, and injury-induced phenotypic change. *Chest* 1998;**114**:29S–30S.
28. Stiebellehner L, Frid MG, Reeves JT, Low RB, Gnanasekharan M, Stenmark KR. Bovine distal pulmonary arterial media is composed of a uniform population of well-differentiated smooth muscle cells with low proliferative capabilities. *Am J Physiol Lung Cell Mol Physiol* 2003;**285**:L819–28.
29. Weir EK, Reeve HL, Cornfield DN, Tristani-Firouzi M, Peterson DA, Archer SL. Diversity of response in vascular smooth muscle cells to changes in oxygen tension. *Kidney Int* 1997;**51**:462–6.
30. Bonnet S, Archer SL. Potassium channel diversity in the pulmonary arteries and pulmonary veins: implications for regulation of the pulmonary vasculature in health and during pulmonary hypertension. *Pharmacol Ther* 2007;**115**:56–69.
31. Remillard CV, Yuan JX. TRP channels, CCE, and the pulmonary vascular smooth muscle. *Microcirculation* 2006;**13**:671–92.
32. Pullamsetti SS, Schermuly RT. Endothelin receptor antagonists in preclinical models of pulmonary hypertension. *Eur J Clin Invest* 2009;**39**(Suppl. 2):3–13.
33. Eddahibi S, Guignabert C, Barlier-Mur AM, Dewachter L, Fadel E, Dartevelle P, et al. Cross talk between endothelial and smooth muscle cells in pulmonary hypertension: critical role for serotonin-induced smooth muscle hyperplasia. *Circulation* 2006;**113**:1857–64.
34. Morecroft I, Dempsie Y, Bader M, Walther DJ, Kotnik K, Loughlin L, et al. Effect of tryptophan hydroxylase 1 deficiency on the development of hypoxia-induced pulmonary hypertension. *Hypertension* 2007;**49**:232–6.
35. Guignabert C, Raffestin B, Benferhat R, Raoul W, Zadigue P, Rideau D, et al. Serotonin transporter inhibition prevents and reverses monocrotaline-induced pulmonary hypertension in rats. *Circulation* 2005;**111**:2812–9.
36. Eddahibi S, Hanoun N, Lanfumey L, Lesch KP, Raffestin B, Hamon M, et al. Attenuated hypoxic pulmonary hypertension in mice lacking the 5-hydroxytryptamine transporter gene. *J Clin Invest* 2000;**105**:1555–62.
37. Guignabert C, Izikki M, Tu LI, Li Z, Zadigue P, Barlier-Mur AM, et al. Transgenic mice overexpressing the 5-hydroxytryptamine transporter gene in smooth muscle develop pulmonary hypertension. *Circ Res* 2006;**98**:1323–30.
38. Bradford CN, Ely DR, Raizada MK. Targeting the vasoprotective axis of the renin-angiotensin system: a novel strategic approach to pulmonary hypertensive therapy. *Curr Hypertens Rep* 2010;**12**:212–9.
39. Ferreira AJ, Shenoy V, Yamazato Y, Sriramula S, Francis J, Yuan L, et al. Evidence for angiotensin-converting enzyme 2 as a therapeutic target for the prevention of pulmonary hypertension. *Am J Respir Crit Care Med* 2009;**179**:1048–54.
40. Zhang R, Wu Y, Zhao M, Liu C, Zhou L, Shen S, et al. Role of HIF-1alpha in the regulation ACE and ACE2 expression in hypoxic human pulmonary artery smooth muscle cells. *Am J Physiol Lung Cell Mol Physiol* 2009;**297**:L631–40.
41. Venkatachalam K, van Rossum DB, Patterson RL, Ma HT, Gill DL. The cellular and molecular basis of store-operated calcium entry. *Nat Cell Biol* 2002;**4**:E263–72.
42. Golovina VA, Platoshyn O, Bailey CL, Wang J, Limsuwan A, Sweeney M, et al. Upregulated TRP and enhanced capacitative Ca ($^{2+}$) entry in human pulmonary artery myocytes during proliferation. *Am J Physiol Heart Circ Physiol* 2001;**280**:H746–55.
43. Leung FP, Yung LM, Yao X, Laher I, Huang Y. Store-operated calcium entry in vascular smooth muscle. *Br J Pharmacol* 2008;**153**:846–57.
44. Lu W, Wang J, Shimoda LA, Sylvester JT. Differences in STIM1 and TRPC expression in proximal and distal pulmonary arterial smooth muscle are associated with differences in Ca^{2+} responses to hypoxia. *Am J Physiol Lung Cell Mol Physiol* 2008;**295**:L104–13.
45. Platoshyn O, Yu Y, Golovina VA, McDaniel SS, Krick S, Li L, et al. Chronic hypoxia decreases K(V) channel expression and function in pulmonary artery myocytes. *Am J Physiol Lung Cell Mol Physiol* 2001;**280**:L801–12.
46. Bonnet S, Archer SL, Allalunis-Turner J, Haromy A, Beaulieu C, Thompson R, et al. A mitochondria-K^+ channel axis is suppressed in cancer and its normalization promotes apoptosis and inhibits cancer growth. *Cancer Cell* 2007;**11**:37–51.
47. Bonnet S, Michelakis ED, Porter CJ, Andrade-Navarro MA, Thebaud B, Haromy A, et al. An abnormal mitochondrial-hypoxia inducible factor-1alpha-Kv channel pathway disrupts oxygen sensing and triggers pulmonary arterial hypertension in fawn hooded rats: similarities to human pulmonary arterial hypertension. *Circulation* 2006;**113**:2630–41.
48. Archer SL, Wu XC, Thebaud B, Nsair A, Bonnet S, Tyrrell B, et al. Preferential expression and function of voltage-gated, O_2-sensitive K^+ channels in resistance pulmonary arteries explains regional heterogeneity in hypoxic pulmonary vasoconstriction: ionic diversity in smooth muscle cells. *Circ Res* 2004;**95**:308–18.

49. Fagan KA, Oka M, Bauer NR, Gebb SA, Ivy DD, Morris KG, et al. Attenuation of acute hypoxic pulmonary vasoconstriction and hypoxic pulmonary hypertension in mice by inhibition of Rho-kinase. *Am J Physiol Lung Cell Mol Physiol* 2004;**287**:L656–64.
50. McNamara PJ, Murthy P, Kantores C, Teixeira L, Engelberts D, van Vliet T, et al. Acute vasodilator effects of Rho-kinase inhibitors in neonatal rats with pulmonary hypertension unresponsive to nitric oxide. *Am J Physiol Lung Cell Mol Physiol* 2008;**294**:L205–13.
51. Oka M, Homma N, Taraseviciene-Stewart L, Morris KG, Kraskauskas D, Burns N, et al. Rho kinase-mediated vasoconstriction is important in severe occlusive pulmonary arterial hypertension in rats. *Circ Res* 2007;**100**:923–9.
52. Hemnes AR, Champion HC. Sildenafil, a PDE5 inhibitor, in the treatment of pulmonary hypertension. *Expert Rev Cardiovasc Ther* 2006;**4**:293–300.
53. Phillips PG, Long L, Wilkins MR, Morrell NW. cAMP phosphodiesterase inhibitors potentiate effects of prostacyclin analogs in hypoxic pulmonary vascular remodeling. *Am J Physiol Lung Cell Mol Physiol* 2005;**288**:L103–15.
54. Farrow KN, Lakshminrusimha S, Reda WJ, Wedgwood S, Czech L, Gugino SF, et al. Superoxide dismutase restores eNOS expression and function in resistance pulmonary arteries from neonatal lambs with persistent pulmonary hypertension. *Am J Physiol Lung Cell Mol Physiol* 2008;**295**:L979–87.
55. Chi AY, Waypa GB, Mungai PT, Schumacker PT. Prolonged hypoxia increases ROS signaling and RhoA activation in pulmonary artery smooth muscle and endothelial cells. *Antioxid Redox Signal* 2010;**12**:603–10.
56. Perez-Vizcaino F, Cogolludo A, Moreno L. Reactive oxygen species signaling in pulmonary vascular smooth muscle. *Respir Physiol Neurobiol* 2010;**174**:212–20.
57. Said SI, Hamidi SA, Dickman KG, Szema AM, Lyubsky S, Lin RZ, et al. Moderate pulmonary arterial hypertension in male mice lacking the vasoactive intestinal peptide gene. *Circulation* 2007;**115**:1260–8.
58. Murakami S, Kimura H, Kangawa K, Nagaya N. Physiological significance and therapeutic potential of adrenomedullin in pulmonary hypertension. *Cardiovasc Hematol Disord Drug Targets* 2006;**6**:125–32.
59. Zhao YD, Courtman DW, Deng Y, Kugathasan L, Zhang Q, Stewart DJ. Rescue of monocrotaline-induced pulmonary arterial hypertension using bone marrow-derived endothelial-like progenitor cells: efficacy of combined cell and eNOS gene therapy in established disease. *Circ Res* 2005;**96**:442–50.
60. Michelakis ED, Wilkins MR, Rabinovitch M. Emerging concepts and translational priorities in pulmonary arterial hypertension. *Circulation* 2008;**118**:1486–95.
61. Guldemeester A, Stenmark KR, Brough GH, Stevens T. Mechanisms regulating cAMP-mediated growth of bovine neonatal pulmonary artery smooth muscle cells. *Am J Physiol* 1999;**276**: L1010–7.
62. Liu Y, Fanburg BL. Serotonin-induced growth of pulmonary artery smooth muscle requires activation of phosphatidylinositol 3-kinase/serine-threonine protein kinase B/mammalian target of rapamycin/p70 ribosomal S6 kinase 1. *Am J Respir Cell Mol Biol* 2006;**34**:182–91.
63. Yang X, Long L, Southwood M, Rudarakanchana N, Upton PD, Jeffery TK, et al. Dysfunctional Smad signaling contributes to abnormal smooth muscle cell proliferation in familial pulmonary arterial hypertension. *Circ Res* 2005;**96**:1053–63.
64. Davie N, Haleen SJ, Upton PD, Polak JM, Yacoub MH, Morrell NW, et al. ET(A) and ET(B) receptors modulate the proliferation of human pulmonary artery smooth muscle cells. *Am J Respir Crit Care Med* 2002;**165**:398–405.
65. Jones R, Capen DE, Jacobson M, Cohen KS, Scadden DT, Duda DG. VEGFR^{2+}PDGFRbeta^{+} circulating precursor cells participate in capillary restoration after hyperoxia acute lung injury (HALI). *J Cell Mol Med* 2009;**13**:3720–9.
66. Yamagishi S, Imaizumi T. Pericyte biology and diseases. *Int J Tissue React* 2005;**27**:125–35.
67. Davie NJ, Crossno Jr. JT, Frid MG, Hofmeister SE, Reeves JT, Hyde DM, et al. Hypoxia-induced pulmonary artery adventitial remodeling and neovascularization: contribution of progenitor cells. *Am J Physiol Lung Cell Mol Physiol* 2004;**286**:L668–78.
68. Tuder RM, Marecki JC, Richter A, Fijalkowska I, Flores S. Pathology of pulmonary hypertension. *Clin Chest Med* 2007;**28**:23–42 vii.
69. Dorfmuller P, Perros F, Balabanian K, Humbert M. Inflammation in pulmonary arterial hypertension. *Eur Respir J* 2003;**22**:358–63.
70. Burke DL, Frid MG, Kunrath CL, Karoor V, Anwar A, Wagner BD, et al. Sustained hypoxia promotes the development of a pulmonary artery-specific chronic inflammatory microenvironment. *Am J Physiol Lung Cell Mol Physiol* 2009;**297**:L238–50.
71. Galie N, Manes A, Negro L, Palazzini M, Bacchi-Reggiani ML, Branzi A. A meta-analysis of randomized controlled trials in pulmonary arterial hypertension. *Eur Heart J* 2009;**30**:394–403.
72. Macchia A, Marchioli R, Marfisi R, Scarano M, Levantesi G, Tavazzi L, Tognoni G. A meta-analysis of trials of pulmonary hypertension: A clinical condition looking for drugs and research methodology. *Am Heart J* 2007;**153**:1037–47.
73. Stenmark KR, Rabinovitch M. Emerging therapies for the treatment of pulmonary hypertension. *Pediatr Crit Care Med* 2010;**11**: S85–90.

Chapter 104

Airway Smooth Muscle and Asthma

Susan J. Gunst
Department of Cellular and Integrative Physiology, Indiana University School of Medicine, Indianapolis, IN

STRUCTURE AND FUNCTION OF AIRWAY SMOOTH MUSCLE

Airway smooth muscle is a structural component of the walls of all of the airways within the bronchial tree, from the trachea to the smallest respiratory bronchioles (1,2). In the lung parenchymal tissue, smooth muscle is found within the alveolar ducts that form the entrance to alveolar sacs and may also be dispersed within other areas of the lung parenchyma. In the trachea, the smooth muscle is contained solely within the trachealis membrane that extends along the dorsal side of the trachea where the trachea abuts the esophagus (3). The trachealis membrane, which contains a thin layer of muscle tissue adjacent to the mucosal membrane that lines the entire trachea, connects the ends of the horseshoe-shaped rings of cartilage that form the length of the trachea. In the largest bronchi, bundles of smooth muscle are arranged circumferentially and helically within the airway wall just below the mucosal membrane (4), and are surrounded by rings of cartilage, which make these bronchi stiff and may limit narrowing of the lumen when the airway muscle contracts (1,5,6). As the bronchi divide into successive generations within the lungs, the amount of cartilage diminishes and takes the form of irregular plates. In the more distal generations of intra-parenchymal bronchi (bronchioles), the cartilage entirely disappears from the airway wall, and the smooth muscle layer and associated connective tissue represents the major structural component of the wall (2). Thus in these airways, airway circumference and stiffness is regulated primarily by the smooth muscle tissue. The constriction of the airway smooth muscle in the smaller bronchi and bronchioles can result in airway closure and obstruction of the airway lumen, completely blocking airflow, as occurs in asthma (7).

Airway smooth muscle may be the only smooth muscle tissue in the body for which the normal physiologic function is unknown. Although a number of hypotheses have been advanced for the function of airway smooth muscle, there is considerable debate as to whether it has any beneficial function at all! As the contraction of airway smooth muscle results in airway narrowing and the obstruction of airflow, clearly widespread airway constriction is not beneficial to breathing or health. Indeed, pervasive airway narrowing and airway smooth muscle hyperresponsiveness is considered a cardinal pathophysiologic feature of asthma. The ablation of localized regions of airway smooth muscle through the application of heat is currently being applied as a treatment for asthma (8), and the use of gene therapy to inactivate the contractile mechanism of airway smooth muscle has been proposed as a treatment for asthma (9). The fact that the widespread constriction of airway smooth muscle has pathological consequences has led to the suggestion that airway smooth muscle may in fact be "the appendix of the lung" – in essence, a vestigial organ with no useful function (10)!

If airway smooth muscle does serve a useful function, what might that function be? The normal function of airway smooth muscle has been debated for decades, and a variety of possible functions have been proposed for it (11). One physiologic function that has been traditionally ascribed to airway smooth muscle is that of modulating the distribution of ventilation to optimize ventilation perfusion matching. The contraction of the smooth muscle in the alveolar ducts and small airways can markedly influence the distensibility of the lungs; thus changes in bronchomotor tone might influence ventilation distribution by locally modulating lung compliance, thus improving the homogeneity of lung expansion. An additional mechanism by which airway smooth muscle might regulate the ventilation distribution is through alterations in airway tone induced by changes in CO_2. As CO_2 causes the relaxation of airway smooth muscle (12), inadequate ventilation of local lung units that results in a build-up of CO_2 might lead to airway dilation and thus enhance the ventilation of the lung units that they subserve. Other functions have been proposed for airway smooth muscle, among them: that it protects the airways from overdistension or distortion during breathing (13); that it optimizes anatomic dead space volume (1,14); that it assists in mucous clearance by modulating the location and extent

Muscle. DOI: http://dx.doi.org/10.1016/B978-0-12-381510-1.00104-6

of airway compression during cough (11); that it assists in exhalation or mucous propulsion through peristalsis (15); that it stabilizes the large airways during cough (6). Critics argue that while some of these arguments may be plausible, it is difficult to make a compelling argument for any of them based on the available experimental evidence (10,16).

Recent advances in the study of airway smooth muscle have led to the recognition that it has complex physiologic properties beyond those of simply contracting and relaxing in response to external stimulation – these discoveries may enhance our perspectives on the normal function of the muscle (17–20). The contractility of airway smooth muscle and its material properties are highly malleable and are modulated dynamically in response to forces that are imposed on it (18,19,21). In the lung this may be a critical property, as the process of breathing results in an environment in which the physical forces imposed on the airways are constantly changing, and both airway caliber and stiffness need to be dynamically adjusted to accommodate to changes in lung volume and ventilatory patterns. Furthermore, airway smooth muscle is now widely accepted to be a synthetic organ, capable of producing and secreting immunomodulatory and other compounds in response to a variety of external stimuli (20). Its phenotypic status is also dynamic – airway smooth muscle cells can actively transition between a contractile and a synthetic state in response to multiple cues from the local environment, such as mechanical stimuli and tissue matrix interactions (20,22). Pathophysiologic conditions of the airways such as asthma result in alterations in all of these properties: asthma is associated with the increased hypersensitivity of the airways to contractile stimuli, alterations in its response to mechanical forces during breathing, and enhanced secretion of inflammatory mediators and the modulation of its structural properties. The degree to which alterations in these functions are interrelated and underlie the pathophysiologic features of asthma are the subjects of intensive investigation. No doubt, better understanding of the broad functional properties of airway smooth muscle may provide new insights into the role of airway smooth muscle in normal lung function.

EXCITATION–CONTRACTION COUPLING AND ITS MODULATION IN ASTHMA

The signaling pathways and processes by which diverse physiologic stimuli regulate the activation of actomyosin cross-bridge cycling, tension development, and shortening have been extensively characterized in airway smooth muscle (18,21,23–25). As in other smooth muscle tissues, the phosphorylation of the 20 kD myosin regulatory light chains and the activation of actomyosin cross-bridge cycling is a key event in the regulation of shortening velocity and tension development (23). Myosin light chain phosphorylation can be mediated by the Ca^{2+}-calmodulin mediated activation of myosin light chain kinase, as well as by Ca^{2+}-independent signaling pathways that act primarily to regulate the activity of myosin light chain phosphatase (26). Both RhoA GTPase activity and Rho kinase mediate the inhibition of myosin light chain phosphatase in airway smooth muscle (27); however, the Rho-mediated regulation of myosin light chain phosphorylation may not be of as much physiologic importance in the regulation of the contractility of airway smooth muscle as it is in vascular smooth muscle (28).

A number of studies have reported increases in the velocity of shortening of airways taken from animal models of allergic asthma and studied *ex vivo*, and in human airway smooth muscle cells isolated from asthmatics (29–32). An increase in airway smooth muscle shortening velocity or force generation would be predicted to lead to greater airway smooth muscle shortening and increases airway narrowing. Therefore, possible alterations in the function or regulation of the actomyosin system, long viewed as the primary regulator of force generation and shortening velocity in airway smooth muscle, have been extensively investigated as possible contributing causes of airway hyperresponsiveness associated with asthma (33,34). Although evidence from a number of studies suggests that alterations in the isoforms and expression levels of contractile proteins and their activating molecules may contribute to increased airway contractility and airway hyperresponsiveness, consistent results are not observed among different laboratories. Stephens and colleagues reported increased shortening velocity in cells from asthmatic humans, and found that it correlated with an increase in the gene expression for myosin light chain kinase (29). They reported similar observations in airway smooth muscle tissues from a canine model of allergic asthma (35). However, Woodruff and colleagues found no differences in gene expression of myosin light chain kinase in airway smooth muscle cells taken from asthmatics by bronchial biopsy, although they did observe a significant increase in airway smooth muscle cell number (34).

Alterations in myosin heavy chain isoforms have also been proposed as a mechanism for airway hyperresponsiveness (33). The presence of a 7 amino acid insert in the motor domain of the myosin heavy chain molecule, referred to as SM-B, is associated with a faster rate of actin propulsion in the *in vitro* motility assay than the SM-A isoform, which lacks the insert (36). This insert is associated with a faster rate of myosin ATPase activity and a faster cross-bridge cycling rate (36–38). Fischer rats exhibit an increased expression of the (+) insert myosin heavy chain isoform relative to Lewis rats, and also have relatively greater airway responsiveness (39).

Studies of human airway smooth muscle are mixed: one study (40) reported that the SM-B isoform is expressed in human tracheal smooth muscle; however, another (29) did not detect the myosin SM-B isoform in human airway smooth muscle cells. The possibility of differences in asthmatic and non-asthmatics in the expression of these myosin isoforms remains to be determined.

While the evidence for intrinsic differences in the isoforms or expression levels of contractile or signaling proteins in asthmatics versus non-asthmatics is inconclusive, considerable evidence has accumulated demonstrating that inflammatory mediators associated with airway inflammation and asthma – such as interleukin (IL)-1-β, tumor necrosis factor-alpha (TNF-α), interferon-gamma, and Th2 cytokines IL-13 and IL-5 – enhance the contractility of airway smooth muscle (41–44). Many of these mediators modulate the expression of proteins involved in the regulation of airway smooth muscle contractility: The incubation of airway smooth muscle with IL-13 *in vitro* alters the expression of SmMHC, the small GTPase RhoA, and phospholipase A2 (34,45,46). Both IL-13 and TNF-α modulate the expression of proteins involved in Ca^{2+} signaling and homeostasis and stimulate elevated levels of intracellular Ca^{2+} which could contribute to an increased sensitivity to contractile stimuli (47–50). Both IL-13 and TNF-α also stimulate the synthesis and secretion of inflammatory mediators and cytokines by the airway smooth muscle cells (as well as by fibroblasts and airway epithelial cells), which may activate cellular processes that lead to the proliferation and hypertrophy of airway smooth muscle cells (20,51–53). The amount of airway smooth muscle and the thickness of connective tissue in the airway wall can both increase in asthmatics; thus it has been proposed that the structural changes in airway wall thickness may be of equal or greater importance than alterations in the contractility of airway smooth muscle in causing the airway hyperresponsiveness characteristic of asthma (7,54,55). However, extensive experimental evidence documenting direct effects of inflammatory mediators on airway smooth muscle contractility and changes in excitation–contraction coupling provide convincing support for the argument that hyperresponsiveness of the airway smooth muscle itself is an important contributor to the airway hyperreactivity associated with asthma.

MECHANICAL ADAPTATION OF AIRWAY SMOOTH MUSCLE

During normal breathing, the smooth muscle of the airways is exposed to continuously changing mechanical conditions. Increases and decreases in lung volume that occur with each breath during tidal breathing cause the airways to expand and contract, which stretches and retracts the airway smooth muscle. Airway smooth muscle is also periodically subjected to larger forces of expansion caused by intermittent deep breaths. The oscillations in lung volume and periodic deep breaths that occur during breathing are well-documented to have profound effects on airway tone and airway responsiveness in both humans and experimental animals (7,56–62). The imposition of tidal volume oscillations suppresses airway responsiveness and maintains a low level of airway tone (58,61–66). When the tidal breathing is reduced to low volumes or temporarily stopped, airway responsiveness to a bronchoconstrictor challenge is dramatically increased (62,65). The suppression of periodic deep inspirations can result in an increase in airway responsiveness to levels similar to that observed in asthmatic subjects (61,64,66). Deep inspiration frequently does not result in airway dilation in asthmatic subjects, and may even trigger airway constriction or narrowing (59,60,66). This has led to the suggestion that the airway hyperresponsiveness of asthmatics may result from the absence of the normal response of the airways to mechanical stretch (59,66,67).

Many of the characteristic responses of the airways to volume oscillation that are observed *in vivo* are also seen in isolated strips of airway smooth muscle *in vitro*, which suggests these behaviors reflect inherent properties of the airway smooth muscle cells, rather than responses to reflexes or humoral agents (18,68–73). The responsiveness of isolated airways and airway smooth muscle *in vitro* is reduced by subjecting them to volume/length or pressure/load oscillations (68–70,72,73). Furthermore, the same contractile stimulus may elicit different contractile responses from the airway smooth muscle depending on its mechanical history – how it has been stretched or shortened prior to receiving the stimulus (69,71,73–78). Mechanical history also modulates the stiffness of airway smooth muscle tissue (71,77). All of these observations suggest that airway smooth muscle cell structure or organization is altered by mechanical forces, and that these alterations in structure underlie the physiologic effects of mechanical stimuli on airway smooth muscle properties. Thus the mechanisms by which the smooth muscle of the airways adapts and responds to mechanical forces play a critical role in regulating airway properties that are important to their physiologic or pathophysiologic function (18).

MOLECULAR MECHANISMS FOR MECHANICAL ADAPTATION OF AIRWAY SMOOTH MUSCLE

The mechanisms by which external mechanical forces regulate the properties and contractility of airway smooth muscle have been the subject of extensive investigation.

It has become increasingly evident that airway smooth muscle contraction is comprised of processes far more complex and extensive than just contractile filament activation and actomyosin interaction (18,19,25,79–81). Contractile stimulation elicits processes of cytoskeletal reorganization that include the recruitment of structural and signaling proteins to membrane adhesion junctions, the activation of catalytic processes that regulate dynamic changes in the polymerization state of actin, myosin, and other cytoskeletal filaments, and the activation of membrane adhesion junction proteins that link cytoskeletal filaments to the extracellular matrix (19,25,81). These dynamic cytoskeletal events are essential for force development and tension maintenance in airway smooth muscle in response to a contractile stimulus. Proteins that localize to adhesion and adherens junctions also transduce signals from extracellular stimuli to the smooth muscle cell nucleus, and can thereby alter the phenotype and physiologic function of the airway smooth muscle cell as well as its contractility and stiffness (22,82–84) (Figure 104.1).

Actin polymerization is clearly a critical step in the process of tension development and shortening in airway smooth muscle (25,81). The contractile stimulation of airway smooth muscle triggers an increase in filamentous (F) actin and a decrease in soluble monomeric globular (G) actin. The pool of G actin constitutes approximately 20% of the total actin in the smooth muscle cell in resting tissues, and this pool decreases by 30–40% in response to a contractile stimulus, which means that contractile activation results in an increase in the percentage of F actin by approximately 10%, from about 80% to 90% of the total actin (85). In airway and most other smooth muscle tissues, the inhibition of actin polymerization by pharmacologic or molecular approaches results in the depression of tension development with little or no effect on phosphorylation of the 20 kD regulatory light chain of myosin or on cross-bridge cycling (28,81,85,86). Conversely, myosin light chain phosphorylation can be inhibited without inhibiting agonist-induced actin polymerization (28,87,88). However, the inhibition of either process by itself markedly depresses active tension development,

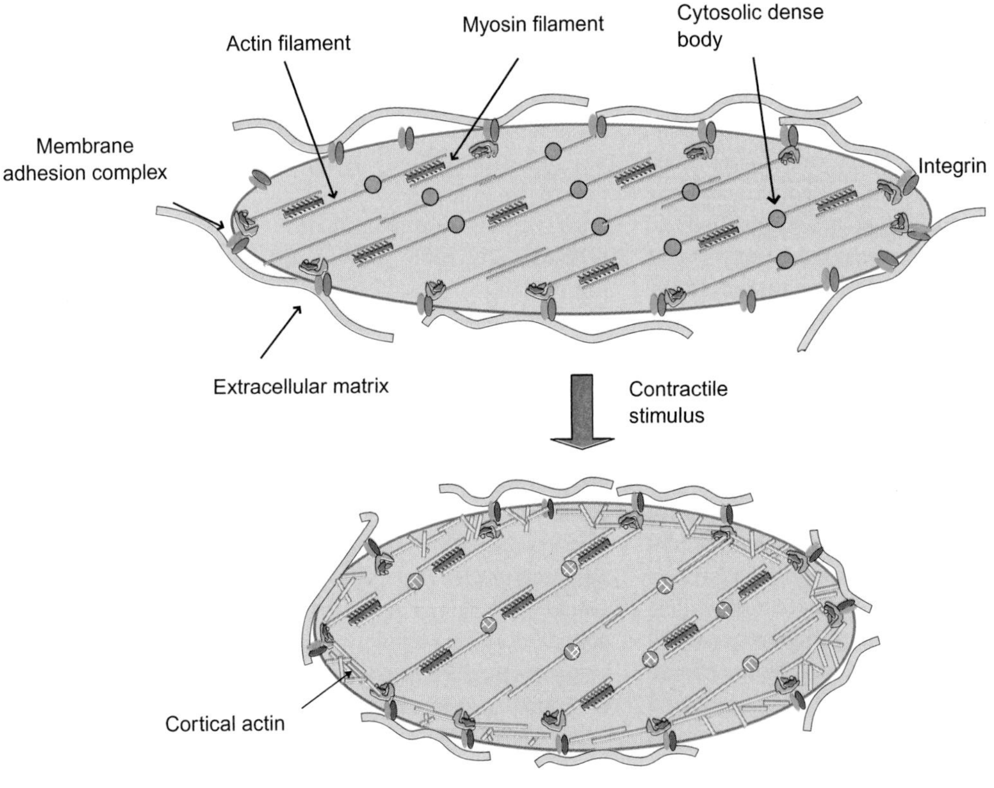

FIGURE 104.1 Cytoskeletal dynamics during smooth muscle contraction. The activation of the smooth muscle cell stimulates the assembly of protein complexes at cell membrane adhesion junctions. These protein complexes initiate signaling pathways that collaborate with receptor activated signals to catalyze the formation of a network of actin filaments at the cell cortex, activate the actomyosin cross-bridge cycling system, and fortify connections between the actin filaments and integrin proteins. The formation of a cortical actin filament network strengthens the membrane for the transmission of force generated by the actomyosin system and enables adaptation of the smooth muscle cell to accommodate to external mechanical forces.

indicating that both actin polymerization and cross-bridge cycling are essential steps in the process of tension development and transmission in airway smooth muscle tissues (28). The fact that a relatively small amount of actin undergoes polymerization during smooth muscle contraction suggests that this pool of actin serves a specialized function that is distinct from that of the actin that interacts with myosin to regulate cross-bridge cycling.

The proteins known to catalyze actin polymerization in airway smooth muscle localize predominantly to the submembranous area of the smooth muscle cell during contractile stimulation (see below and Figure 104.1), suggesting that the actin undergoing polymerization is primarily cortical (81,85). The formation of a submembranous actin network in airway smooth muscle cells could function to modulate the mechanical properties and contractility of the airway smooth muscle through several mechanisms: by enhancing membrane rigidity (89), by connecting the contractile and cytoskeletal filament lattice to the membrane to transmit the tension generated by cross-bridge cycling, and by adapting the smooth muscle cell shape and rigidity to changing external mechanical conditions (17,18,23,79–81).

In airway smooth muscle, actin polymerization in response to a contractile stimulus is catalyzed by the cdc42-mediated activation of neuronal Wiskott–Aldrich Syndrome protein (N-WASp), a member of the WASP family of proteins (81,85), which are well-known activators of the Arp2/3 (actin-related protein) complex (90,91). The Arp2/3 complex, a complex of seven strongly associated protein subunits including Arp2 and Arp3, forms a template for the formation of new actin filaments (92). The contractile stimulation of airway smooth muscle tissues initiates the recruitment of N-WASp to the membrane where it binds to and activates the Arp2/3 complex, initiating the polymerization of new actin filaments (81,85).

The activation of N-WASp and the Arp2/3 complex is regulated by a complex of cytoskeletal proteins that are recruited to membrane adhesion sites at the initiation of the contractile stimulus (17,21,81,93). The proteins in this complex include vinculin, an adhesion junction protein that forms structural links between actin filaments and integrin adhesion junction proteins (94), and paxillin, a scaffolding protein that binds to vinculin and can be tyrosine phosphorylated by focal adhesion kinase (FAK) (95,96). Both paxillin and FAK undergo tyrosine phosphorylation during the contractile activation of airway smooth muscle, and the tyrosine phosphorylation of both proteins is increased by strain or mechanical stimulation (97–101). In airway smooth muscle, paxillin facilitates the cdc42-mediated activation of N-WASp via the SH_2/SH_3 adaptor protein CrkII, which binds to the tyrosine phosphorylated sites on paxillin and to the SH_3 effector binding site on N-WASp (98,102,103). Actin polymerization may also be mechanosensitive; the effectiveness of inhibitors of actin polymerization on contractile force is greater at high than at low levels of mechanical strain, suggesting that actin polymerization may contribute to the mechanosensitivity of airway smooth muscle responsiveness (86,104). Thus mechanical stimuli may modulate the activation of N-WASp-mediated actin polymerization, which could provide a molecular mechanism by which cytoskeletal organization and actin structure could be dynamically modulated to adapt smooth muscle cell shape and stiffness to its environment (Figure 104.2).

The assembly of myosin filaments may also be regulated in airway smooth muscle during contractile stimulation (105). There is structural evidence that the number of myosin filaments is modulated by changes in mechanical length or contractile stimulation of airway smooth muscle cells (106,107). Monomeric myosin smooth muscle myosin II heavy chains can exist in a closed 10S self-inhibited conformation that interacts weakly with actin and has a low myosin ATPase activity (reviewed by Cremo and Hartshorne (108)). A significant pool of myosin exists in the 10S conformation in airway smooth muscle cells, and myosin filament assembly *in vitro* is promoted by MLC phosphorylation; thus 10S myosin has been proposed to exist in cells as an assembly-competent pool in equilibrium with filamentous myosin (109). As 10S myosin only weakly binds to actin it should not compete with filamentous myosin for actin binding. Thus this pool of myosin may enable the assembly of new myosin filaments in response to changing cellular conditions (109). Myosin filament assembly has been proposed as a mechanism for the plastic adaptation of airway smooth muscle cells to mechanical oscillation and altered mechanical conditions (105). However, the molecular mechanisms by which this assembly process is regulated have not been determined.

REGULATION OF AIRWAY SMOOTH MUSCLE FUNCTION BY ADHESION COMPLEX PROTEINS

The mechanism by which airway smooth muscle cells sense and transduce external signals in order to modulate their structure and function in response to changes in their external environment is a key question. The macromolecular protein complexes that associate with the cytoplasmic face of integrin proteins within membrane adhesion junctions mediate the transduction of signals from multiple extracellular sources, including extracellular matrix proteins, cytokines, and other mediators (21,110,111). Proteins within integrin-associated adhesion complexes regulate signaling pathways that control cytoskeletal organization and structure and that signal to the nucleus to

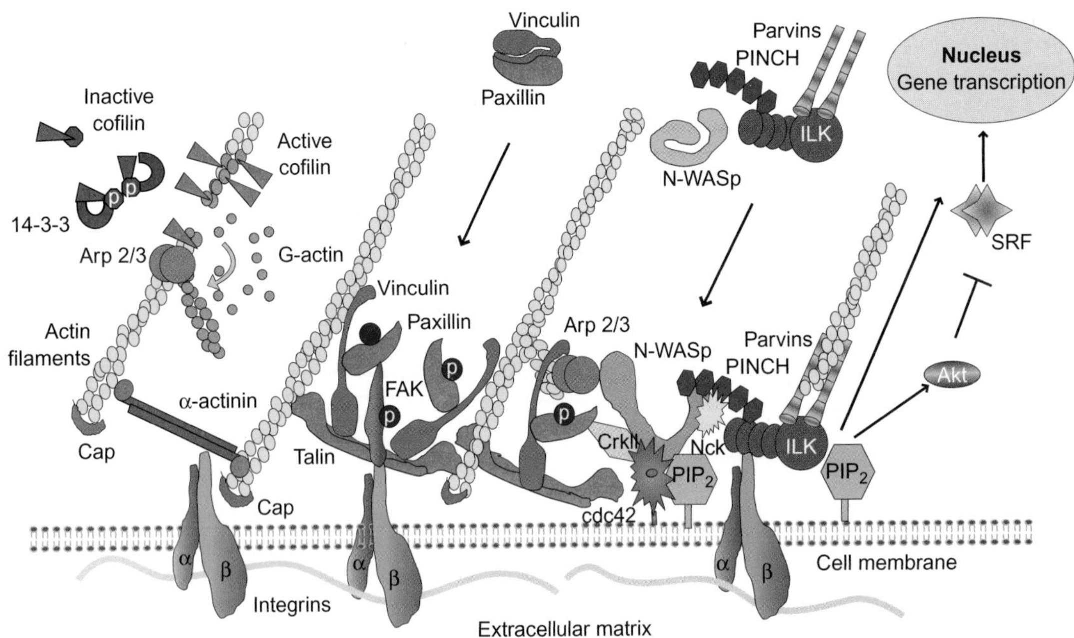

FIGURE 104.2 **Molecular organization of integrin adhesion junctions in smooth muscle.** The assembly of macromolecular signaling complexes at integrin adhesion junctions is regulated by multiple external stimuli. Integrin-associated protein complexes sense and transduce mechanical, pharmacologic, inflammation and extracellular matrix-mediated signals from the local environment. Integrin-associated protein complexes receive signals from other membrane receptors and act collaboratively to regulate cytoskeletal processes such as actin dynamics, cytoskeletal reorganization, actomyosin activation, and nuclear processes such as gene transcription, protein synthesis, and cell proliferation.

modulate cell phenotype and function in response to external signals (Figure 104.2).

Proteins within adhesion complexes are in a constant state of dynamic exchange with their cytoplasmic pools, where they may exist in an inactive state (110–112). In airway smooth muscle, the recruitment and localization of cytoskeletal proteins to adhesion complexes and to the cell cortex is dynamically regulated during contractile stimulation (21,80,83,85,93,113–115). Contractile stimulation of freshly dissociated differentiated airway smooth muscle cells catalyzes the rapid localization of structural and signaling proteins including talin, α-actinin, paxillin, vinculin, FAK, integrin linked kinase (ILK), PINCH, and others to integrin junctions at the membrane. The imposition of mechanical tension or the twisting of integrin proteins bound to magnetic beads on the surface of isolated airway smooth muscle cells also stimulates the recruitment of adhesion complex proteins to the membrane at sites of tension, suggesting that these proteins aggregate at points of mechanical tension (116–118).

The formation of these macromolecular complexes may serve both structural and signaling functions. Talin and α-actinin bind to the β subunit of integrin heterodimers and to actin filaments and can support the formation of links between integrins and actin filaments (110,119). Vinculin can bind to the integrin-binding proteins talin and α-actinin and to filamentous actin when it is in an "activated" conformation and may thereby also support connections between the cytoskeleton and the cell matrix (120). Contractile stimulation of airway smooth muscle catalyzes a change in the conformation of vinculin from an inactive "auto-inhibited" conformation, in which its binding sites with talin and actin are allosterically blocked, to an activated "open" state (115). In airway smooth muscle, vinculin activation in response to acetylcholine stimulation is regulated by a Rho-dependent mechanism, and is necessary for the generation of active contractile tension. However, vinculin also binds tightly to paxillin, a key regulator of actin polymerization, and the recruitment of vinculin to integrin adhesion junctions is necessary for agonist-induced actin polymerization and tension development in airway smooth muscle (115).

Integrin-linked kinase (ILK), a multidomain protein that also binds to the cytoplasmic domain of β_1 integrins, plays a critical role in the assembly of macromolecular signaling complexes at smooth muscle adhesion sites. ILK forms a heterotrimeric complex with PINCH, an adaptor protein that consists of 5 LIM domains, and α-parvin, which binds to actin filaments to form a stable heterotrimeric complex, the ILK/PINCH/α-parvin (IPP complex) (121). The contractile activation of tracheal smooth muscle stimulates the recruitment of the IPP complex to membrane adhesion complexes and increases its interaction with β integrins, paxillin, and

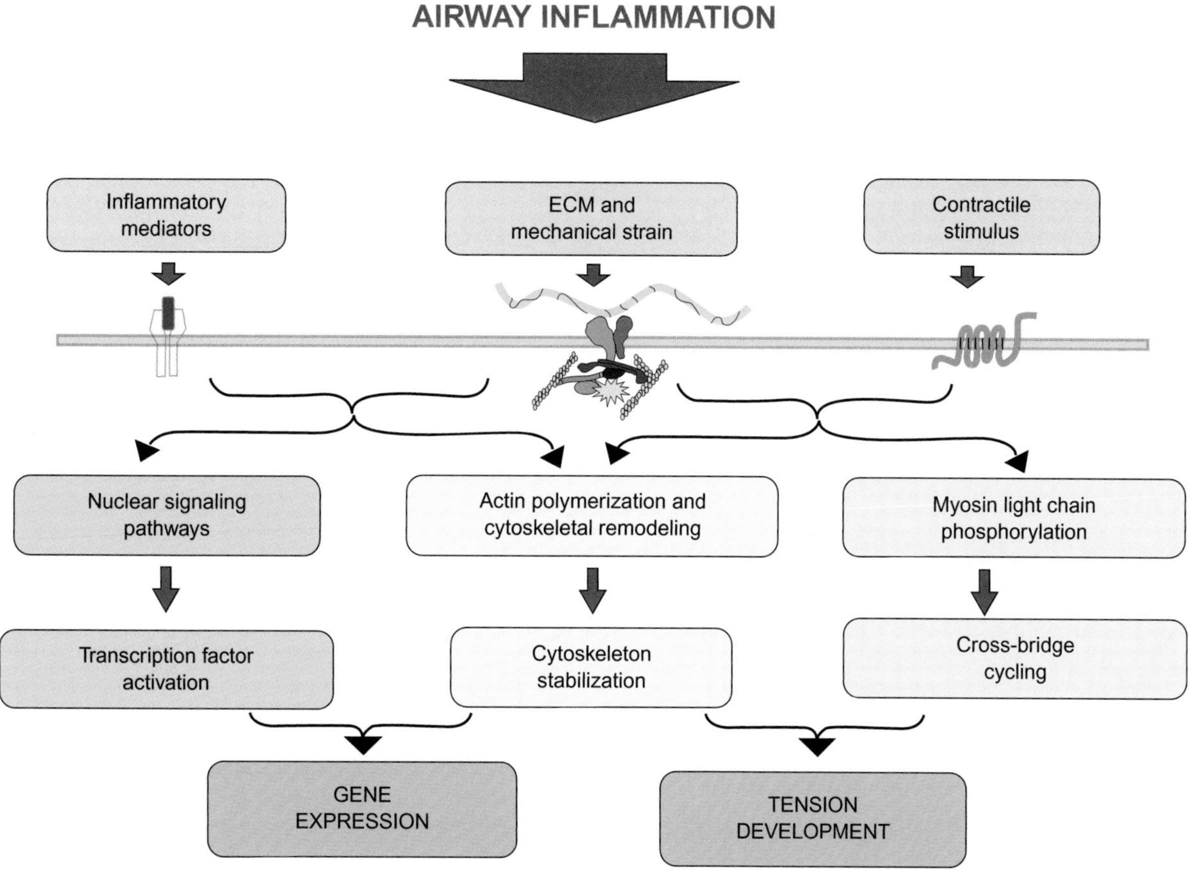

FIGURE 104.3 **Signaling pathways activated by contractile, inflammatory and environmental stimuli collaborate to regulate airway smooth muscle contractility, phenotype, and function.** Airway inflammation alters stimuli to all of these signaling pathways.

vinculin (83). The recruitment of the IPP complex at membrane adhesion sites in tracheal smooth muscle is necessary for tension development and for N-WASp-mediated actin polymerization during contractile activation. The recruitment of proteins to adhesion junctions and the regulation of their activation states may modulate the formation and strength of linkages between actin filaments and integrin adhesion junctions. The reversible formation of these linkages may provide a mechanism for the modulation of airway smooth muscle cell shape and stiffness during the generation of contractile tension or in response to externally imposed mechanical loads (Figure 104.2).

Adhesion junction protein complexes are also capable of regulating changes in the phenotype of airway smooth muscle in response to extracellular signals. ILK is an effector for the phosphatidylinositol-3 kinase (PI3 kinase)-dependent activation of protein kinase B (PKB)/Akt (122). In airway smooth muscle tissues, ILK and the IPP complex mediate the activation of Akt, which inhibits activity of the transcriptional regulator, serum response factor (SRF), thereby suppressing the expression of smooth muscle specific marker proteins (82). Externally applied mechanical loads stimulate the expression of SmMHC and inhibit the IPP-dependent activation of Akt (123).

Proteins that localize to adherens junctions – sites of homophilic cell-to-cell contact – have also been implicated in the regulation of both tension and phenotype in airway smooth muscle (124–126). β-catenin, a membrane-associated protein that is part of the cadherin complex at membrane adherens junctions, contributes to the regulation of actin tension development in response to KCL or methacholine (125). Mitogenic stimulation causes β-catenin to localize in the nucleus where it regulates gene transcription (127,128). Furthermore, caveolins – membrane proteins that localize to the caveolar regions of the smooth muscle cell membrane – are also involved in the regulation of airway smooth muscle phenotype (124,126).

Airway inflammation may modulate stimuli that activate pathways mediated by membrane adhesion and adherens junction complexes, resulting in changes in airway smooth muscle phenotype and contractility. The inflammatory mediator IL-13 activates Akt via the IPP complex, which suppresses the expression of the phenotypic marker protein, SmMHC. IL-13 also upregulates the expression of RhoA protein in murine airway smooth muscle *in vivo* (46), which suggests that it might also modulate Rho-dependent cytoskeletal processes such as actin polymerization, myosin light chain phosphorylation, and the recruitment of cytoskeletal proteins to adhesion junctions. The modulation of airway smooth muscle phenotype, cytoskeletal organization, and activity by inflammatory mediators might thus contribute to alterations in airway contractility and airway remodeling characteristic of asthma.

SUMMARY AND CONCLUSIONS

A broader understanding of the mechanisms for the regulation of airway smooth muscle function by contractile and environmental stimuli can provide novel perspectives to explain the normal physiologic behavior of the airways and pathophysiologic properties of the airways in asthma. Local mediators and contractile stimuli cooperate with environmental stimuli such as extracellular matrix proteins and mechanical forces to modulate signaling pathways mediated by junctional protein complexes that regulate the contractility, compliance, and phenotype of the airway smooth muscle cell. Pathophysiologic processes that disturb normal cytoskeletal dynamics might result in abnormalities in the ability of the airways to regulate their contractility and compliance normally, and modulation of the phenotype and function of the cell (Figure 104.3). Airway hyperresponsiveness and remodeling could be a by-product of such disturbances. However, much remains to be determined regarding the mechanistic basis for the properties of mechanical and physiological adaptation of airway smooth muscle, and the role of dynamic cytoskeletal processes in the regulation of the physiologic properties of airway smooth muscle. A better understanding of these processes will provide novel insights into the basis for the normal physiologic properties of the airways and into disturbances in their function that occur during disease.

REFERENCES

1. Macklin CC. The musculature of the bronchi and lungs. *Physiol Rev* 1929;**9**:1–60.
2. Nagaishi C. *Functional anatomy and histology of the lung*. Baltimore, MD: University Park Press;1972.
3. Miller WS. The trachealis muscle. Its arrangement at the carina tracheae and its probable influence on the lodgement of foreign bodies in the right lower bronchus and lung. *Anatomical Record* 1913;**7**:73–385.
4. Miller WB. *The lung*. Springfield, IL: Thomas;1937.
5. Gunst SJ, Stropp JQ. Pressure-volume and length-stress relationships in canine bronchi in vitro. *J Appl Physiol* 1988;**64**:2522–31.
6. Olsen CR, DeKock MA, Colebatch HJ. Stability of airways during reflex bronchoconstriction. *J Appl Physiol* 1967;**23**:23–6.
7. An SS, Bai TR, Bates JH, Black JL, Brown RH, Brusasco V, et al. Airway smooth muscle dynamics: a common pathway of airway obstruction in asthma. *Eur Respir J* 2007;**29**:834–60.
8. Bel EH. "Hot stuff": bronchial thermoplasty for asthma. *Am J Respir Crit Care Med* 2006;**173**:941–2.
9. Fernandes DJ, McConville JF, Stewart AG, Kalinichenko V, Solway J. Can we differentiate between airway and vascular smooth muscle? *Clin Exper Pharm Physiol* 2004;**31**:805–10.
10. Mitzner W. Airway smooth muscle: the appendix of the lung. *Am J Respir Crit Care Med* 2004;**169**:787–90.
11. Mead J. Point: Airway smooth muscle is useful. *J Appl Physiol* 2007;**102**:1708–9.
12. Duckles SP, Rayner MD, Nadel JA. Effects of CO_2 and pH on drug-induced contractions of airway smooth muscle. *J Pharm Exper Therap* 1974;**190**:472–81.
13. Perez Fontan JJ. On lung nerves and neurogenic injury. *Ann Med* 2002;**34**(4):226–40.
14. Von Hayek H. *The human lung*. New York: Hafner Publishing;1960.
15. Bullowa JGM, Gottlieb C. Additional experimental studies in bronchial function. *Laryngoscope* 1922;**32**:284–9.
16. Seow CY, Fredberg JJ. Historical perspective on airway smooth muscle: the saga of a frustrated cell. *J Appl Physiol* 2001;**91**:938–52.
17. Zhang W, Gunst SJ. Dynamics of cytoskeletal and contractile protein organization: an emerging paradigm for airway smooth muscle contraction. In: Chung KF, editor. *Airway smooth muscle biology and pharmacology*. New York: Wiley;2008.
18. Gunst SJ, Tang DD, Opazo-Saez AM. Cytoskeletal remodeling of the airway smooth muscle cell: a mechanism for adaptation to mechanical forces in the lung. *Respir Physiol Neurobiol* 2003;**137**:151–68.
19. Seow CY, Fredberg JJ. Emergence of airway smooth muscle functions related to structural malleability. *J Appl Physiol* 2011;**110**:1130–5.
20. Tliba O, Panettieri RA. Noncontractile functions of airway smooth muscle cells in asthma. *Annu Rev Physiol* 2009;**71**:509–35.
21. Zhang W, Gunst SJ. Interactions of airway smooth muscle cells with their tissue matrix: implications for contraction. *Proc Am Thorac Soc* 2008;**5**:32–9.
22. Halayko AJ, Solway J. Molecular mechanisms of phenotypic plasticity in smooth muscle cells. *J Appl Physiol* 2001;**90**:358–68.
23. Gunst SJ, Tang DD. The contractile apparatus and mechanical properties of airway smooth muscle. *Eur Respir J* 2000;**15**:600–16.
24. Sanderson MJ, Delmotte P, Bai Y, Perez-Zogbhi JF. Regulation of airway smooth muscle cell contractility by Ca^{2+} signaling and sensitivity. *Proc Am Thorac Soc* 2008;**5**:23–31.
25. Zhang W, Gunst SJ. Interactions of airway smooth muscle cells with their tissue matrix: implications for contraction. *Proc Am Thorac Soc* 2008;**5**:32–9.
26. Somlyo AP, Somlyo AV. Ca^{2+} sensitivity of smooth muscle and nonmuscle myosin II: modulated by G proteins, kinases, and myosin phosphatase. *Physiol Rev* 2003;**83**:1325–58.

27. Liu C, Zuo J, Pertens E, Helli PB, Janssen LJ. Regulation of Rho/ROCK signaling in airway smooth muscle by membrane potential and $[Ca^{2+}]i$. *Am J Physiol Lung Cell Mol Physiol* 2005;**289**: L574–82.
28. Zhang W, Du L, Gunst SJ. The effects of the small GTPase RhoA on the muscarinic contraction of airway smooth muscle result from its role in regulating actin polymerization. *Am J Physiol Cell Physiol* 2010;**299**:C298–306.
29. Ma X, Cheng Z, Kong H, Wang Y, Unruh H, Stephens NL, et al. Changes in biophysical and biochemical properties of single bronchial smooth muscle cells from asthmatic subjects. *Am J Physiol Lung Cell Mol Physiol* 2002;**283**:L1181–9.
30. Fan T, Yang M, Halayko A, Mohapatra SS, Stephens NL. Airway responsiveness in two inbred strains of mouse disparate in IgE and IL-4 production. *Am J Respir Cell Molec Biol* 1997;**17**:156–63.
31. Blanc FX, Coirault C, Salmeron S, Chemla D, Lecarpentier Y. Mechanics and crossbridge kinetics of tracheal smooth muscle in two inbred rat strains. *Eur Respir J* 2003;**22**:227–34.
32. Duguet A, Biyah K, Minshall E, Gomes R, Wang CG, Taoudi-Benchekroun M, et al. Bronchial responsiveness among inbred mouse strains. Role of airway smooth-muscle shortening velocity. *Am J Respir Crit Care Med* 2000;**161**:839–48.
33. Leguillette R, Lauzon AM. Molecular mechanics of smooth muscle contractile proteins in airway hyperresponsiveness and asthma. *Proc Am Thorac Soc* 2008;**5**:40–6.
34. Woodruff PG. Gene expression in asthmatic airway smooth muscle. *Proc Am Thorac Soc* 2008;**5**:113–8.
35. Jiang H, Rao K, Halayko AJ, Liu X, Stephens NL. Ragweed sensitization-induced increase of myosin light chain kinase content in canine airway smooth muscle. *Am J Respir Cell Mol Biol* 1992;**7**:567–73.
36. Rovner AS, Freyzon Y, Trybus KM. An insert in the motor domain determines the functional properties of expressed smooth muscle myosin isoforms. *J Muscle Res Cell Motil* 1997;**18**:103–10.
37. Lauzon AM, Tyska MJ, Rovner AS, Freyzon Y, Warshaw DM, Trybus KM. A 7-amino-acid insert in the heavy chain nucleotide binding loop alters the kinetics of smooth muscle myosin in the laser trap. *J Muscle Res Cell Motil* 1998;**19**:825–37.
38. Kelley CA, Takahashi M, Yu JH, Adelstein RS. An insert of seven amino acids confers functional differences between smooth muscle myosins from the intestines and vasculature. *J Biol Chem* 1993;**268**:12848–54.
39. Gil FR, Zitouni NB, Azoulay E, Maghni K, Lauzon AM. Smooth muscle myosin isoform expression and LC20 phosphorylation in innate rat airway hyperresponsiveness. *Am J Physiol Lung Cell Mol Physiol* 2006;**291**:L932–40.
40. Leguillette R, Gil FR, Zitouni N, Lajoie-Kadoch S, Sobieszek A, Lauzon AM. (+)Insert smooth muscle myosin heavy chain (SM-B) isoform expression in human tissues. *Am J Physiol Cell Physiol* 2005;**289**:C1277–85.
41. Hakonarson H, Grunstein MM. Autocrine regulation of airway smooth muscle responsiveness. *Respir Physiol Neurobiol* 2003;**137**:263–76.
42. Halayko AJ, Amrani Y. Mechanisms of inflammation-mediated airway smooth muscle plasticity and airways remodeling in asthma. *Respir Physiol Neurobiol* 2003;**137**:209–22.
43. Laporte JC, Moore PE, Baraldo S, Jouvin MH, Church TL, Schwartzman IN, et al. Direct effects of interleukin-13 on signaling pathways for physiological responses in cultured human airway smooth muscle cells. *Am J Respir Crit Care Med* 2001;**164**:141–8.
44. Amrani Y, Panettieri Jr RA. Cytokines induce airway smooth muscle cell hyperresponsiveness to contractile agonists. *Thorax* 1998;**53**:713–6.
45. Lee JH, Kaminski N, Dolganov G, Grunig G, Koth L, Solomon C, et al. Interleukin-13 induces dramatically different transcriptional programs in three human airway cell types. *Am J Respir Cell Molec Biol* 2001;**25**:474–85.
46. Chiba Y, Nakazawa S, Todoroki M, Shinozaki K, Sakai H, et al. Interleukin-13 augments bronchial smooth muscle contractility with an up-regulation of RhoA protein. *Am J Respir Cell Mol Biol* 2009;**40**:159–67.
47. Amrani Y, Panettieri Jr RA. Modulation of calcium homeostasis as a mechanism for altering smooth muscle responsiveness in asthma. *Curr Opin Allerg Clin Immunol* 2002;**2**:39–45.
48. Deshpande DA, Walseth TF, Panettieri RA, Kannan MS. CD38/cyclic ADP-ribose-mediated Ca^{2+} signaling contributes to airway smooth muscle hyper-responsiveness. *FASEB J* 2003;**17**:452–4.
49. Moynihan B, Tolloczko B, Michoud MC, Tamaoka M, Ferraro P, et al. MAP kinases mediate interleukin-13 effects on calcium signaling in human airway smooth muscle cells. *Am J Physiol Lung Cell Mol Physiol* 2008;**295**:L171–7.
50. Sathish V, Thompson MA, Bailey JP, Pabelick CM, Prakash YS, Sieck GC. Effect of proinflammatory cytokines on regulation of sarcoplasmic reticulum Ca^{2+} reuptake in human airway smooth muscle. *Am J Physiol Lung Cell Molec Physiol* 2009;**297**: L26–34.
51. Moore PE, Church TL, Chism DD, Panettieri Jr RA, Shore SA. IL-13 and IL-4 cause eotaxin release in human airway smooth muscle cells: a role for ERK. *Am J Physiol Lung Cell Mol Physiol* 2002;**282**:L847–53.
52. Peng Q, Matsuda T, Hirst SJ. Signaling pathways regulating interleukin-13-stimulated chemokine release from airway smooth muscle. *Am J Respir Crit Care Med* 2004;**169**:596–603.
53. Gosens R, Meurs H, Bromhaar MMG, Mckay S, Nelemans SA, Zaagsma J. Functional characterization of serum- and growth factor-induced phenotypic changes in intact bovine tracheal smooth muscle. *Br J Pharmacol* 2002;**137**:459–66.
54. Pare PD, McParland BE, Seow CY. Structural basis for exaggerated airway narrowing. *Can J Physiol Pharmacol* 2007;**85**:653–8.
55. Bosse Y, Riesenfeld EP, Pare PD, Irvin CG. It's not all smooth muscle: non-smooth-muscle elements in control of resistance to airflow. *Annu Rev Physiol* 2010;**72**:437–62.
56. Nadel JA, Tierney DF. Effect of a previous deep inspiration on airway resistance in man. *J Appl Physiol* 1961;**16**:717–9.
57. Gunst SJ, Shen X, Tepper RS. Bronchoprotective and bronchodilatory effects of deep inspiration in rabbits subjected to methacholine challenge. *J Appl Physiol* 2001;**91**:2511–6.
58. Warner DO, Gunst SJ. Limitation of maximal bronchoconstriction in living dogs. *Am Rev Respir Dis* 1992;**145**:553–60.
59. Kapsali T, Permutt S, Laube B, Scichilone N, Togias A. Potent bronchoprotective effect of deep inspiration and its absence in asthma. *J Appl Physiol* 2000;**89**:711–20.

60. Fish JE, Ankin MG, Kelly JF, Peterman VI. Regulation of bronchomotor tone by lung inflation in asthmatic and nonasthmatic subjects. *J Appl Physiol* 1981;**50**:1079–86.
61. King GG, Moore BJ, Seow CY, Pare PD. Time course of increased airway narrowing caused by inhibition of deep inspiration during methacholine challenge. *Am J Respir Crit Care Med* 1999;**160**:454–7.
62. Shen X, Gunst SJ, Tepper RS. Effect of tidal volume and frequency on airway responsiveness in mechanically ventilated rabbits. *J Appl Physiol* 1997;**83**:1202–8.
63. Tepper RS, Shen X, Bakan E, Gunst SJ. Maximal airway response in mature and immature rabbits during tidal ventilation. *J Appl Physiol* 1995;**79**:1190–8.
64. Skloot G, Permutt S, Togias A. Airway hyperresponsiveness in asthma: a problem of limited smooth muscle relaxation with inspiration. *J Clin Invest* 1995;**96**:2393–403.
65. Salerno FG, Shinozuka N, Fredberg JJ, Ludwig MS. Tidal volume amplitude affects the degree of induced bronchoconstriction in dogs. *J Appl Physiol* 1999;**87**:1674–7.
66. Jensen A, Atileh H, Suki B, Ingenito EP, Lutchen KR. Airway caliber in healthy and asthmatic subjects: effects of bronchial challenge and deep inspirations. *J Appl Physiol* 2001;**91**: 506–15.
67. Fredberg JJ, Jones KA, Nathan M, Raboudi S, Prakash YS, Shore SA, et al. Friction in airway smooth muscle: mechanism, latch, and implications in asthma. *J Appl Physiol* 1996;**81**: 2703–12.
68. Shen X, Wu MF, Tepper RS, Gunst SJ. Mechanisms for the mechanical response of airway smooth muscle to length oscillation. *J Appl Physiol* 1997;**83**:731–8.
69. Gunst SJ. Contractile force of canine airway smooth muscle during cyclical length changes. *J Appl Physiol Respirat Environ Exercise Physiol* 1983;**55**:759–69.
70. Gunst SJ, Stropp JQ, Service J. Mechanical modulation of pressure-volume characteristics of contracted canine airways in vitro. *J Appl Physiol* 1990;**68**:2223–9.
71. Gunst SJ, Wu MF. Plasticity of airway smooth muscle stiffness and extensibility: role of length-adaptive mechanisms. *J Appl Physiol* 2001;**90**:741–9.
72. Fredberg JJ, Inouye D, Miller B, Nathan M, Jafari S, Raboudi SH, et al. Airway smooth muscle, tidal stretches, and dynamically determined contractile states. *Am J Respir Crit Care Med* 1997;**156**:1752–9.
73. Wang L, Pare PD, Seow CY. Effects of length oscillation on the subsequent force development in swine tracheal smooth muscle. *J Appl Physiol* 2000;**88**:2246–50.
74. Wang L, Pare PD, Seow CY. Effect of chronic passive length change on airway smooth muscle length-tension relationship. *J Appl Physiol* 2001;**90**:734–40.
75. Gunst SJ, Mitzner W. Mechanical properties of contracted canine bronchial segments in vitro. *J Appl Physiol: Respir Environ Exercise Physiol* 1981;**50**:1236–47.
76. Gunst SJ. Effect of length history on contractile behavior of canine tracheal smooth muscle. *Am J Physiol Cell Physiol* 1986;**250**:C146–54.
77. Gunst SJ, Meiss RA, Wu MF, Rowe M. Mechanisms for the mechanical plasticity of tracheal smooth muscle. *Am J Physiol Cell Physiol* 1995;**268**:C1267–76.
78. Gunst SJ, Wu MF, Smith DD. Contraction history modulates isotonic shortening velocity in smooth muscle. *Am J Physiol Cell Physiol* 1993;**265**:C467–76.
79. Gunst SJ. Applicability of the sliding filament/crossbridge paradigm to smooth muscle. *Rev Physiol Biochem Pharmacol* 1999;**134**:7–61.
80. Gunst SJ, Fredberg JJ. The first three minutes: smooth muscle contraction, cytoskeletal events, and soft glasses. *J Appl Physiol* 2003;**95**:413–25.
81. Gunst SJ, Zhang W. Actin cytoskeletal dynamics in smooth muscle: a new paradigm for the regulation of smooth muscle contraction. *Am J Physiol Cell Physiol* 2008;**295**:C576–87.
82. Wu Y, Huang Y, Herring BP, Gunst SJ. Integrin-linked kinase regulates smooth muscle differentiation marker gene expression in airway tissue. *Am J Physiol Lung Cell Mol Physiol* 2008;**295**: L988–97.
83. Zhang W, Wu Y, Wu C, Gunst SJ. Integrin-linked kinase (ILK) regulates N-WASp-mediated actin polymerization and tension development in tracheal smooth muscle. *J Biol Chem* 2007;**282**:34568–80.
84. Tran T, Halayko AJ. Extracellular matrix and airway smooth muscle interactions: a target for modulating airway wall remodelling and hyperresponsiveness? *Can J Physiol Pharmacol* 2007;**85**:666–71.
85. Zhang W, Wu Y, Du L, Tang DD, Gunst SJ. Activation of the Arp2/3 complex by N-WASp is required for actin polymerization and contraction in smooth muscle. *Am J Physiol Cell Physiol* 2005;**288**:C1145–60.
86. Mehta D, Gunst SJ. Actin polymerization stimulated by contractile activation regulates force development in canine tracheal smooth muscle. *J Physiol* 1999;**519**(Pt 3):829–40.
87. An SS, Laudadio RE, Lai J, Rogers RA, Fredberg JJ. Stiffness changes in cultured airway smooth muscle cells. *Am J Physiol Cell Physiol* 2002;**283**:C792–801.
88. Smith BA, Tolloczko B, Martin JG, Grutter P. Probing the viscoelastic behavior of cultured airway smooth muscle cells with atomic force microscopy: stiffening induced by contractile agonist. *Biophys J* 2005;**88**:2994–3007.
89. Morone N, Fujiwara T, Murase K, Kasai RS, Ike H, Yuasa S, et al. Three-dimensional reconstruction of the membrane skeleton at the plasma membrane interface by electron tomography. *J Cell Biol* 2006;**174**:851–62.
90. Rohatgi R, Ma L, Miki H, Lopez M, Kirchhausen T, Takenawa T, et al. The interaction between N-WASP and the Arp2/3 complex links Cdc42-dependent signals to actin assembly. *Cell* 1999;**97**:221–31.
91. Machesky LM, Insall RH. Signaling to actin dynamics. *J Cell Biol* 1999;**146**:267–72.
92. Pollard TD, Blanchoin L, Mullins RD. Molecular mechanisms controlling actin filament dynamics in nonmuscle cells. *Annu Rev Biophys Biomol Struct* 2000;**29**:545–76.
93. Opazo Saez A, Zhang W, Wu Y, Turner CE, Tang DD, Gunst SJ. Tension development during contractile stimulation of smooth muscle requires recruitment of paxillin and vinculin to the membrane. *Am J Physiol Cell Physiol* 2004;**286**:C433–47.
94. Humphries JD, Wang P, Streuli C, Geiger B, Humphries MJ, Ballestrem C. Vinculin controls focal adhesion formation by direct interactions with talin and actin. *J Cell Biol* 2007;**179**:1043–57.

95. Turner CE. Paxillin interactions. *J Cell Sci* 2000;**113**(Pt 23):4139–40.
96. Schaller MD, Parsons JT. pp125FAK-dependent tyrosine phosphorylation of paxillin creates a high-affinity binding site for Crk. *Mol Cell Biol* 1995;**15**:2635–45.
97. Wang Z, Pavalko FM, Gunst SJ. Tyrosine phosphorylation of the dense plaque protein paxillin is regulated during smooth muscle contraction. *Am J Physiol* 1996;**271**:C1594–602.
98. Tang DD, Turner CE, Gunst SJ. Expression of non-phosphorylatable paxillin mutants in canine tracheal smooth muscle inhibits tension development. *J Physiol* 2003;**553**:21–35.
99. Tang DD, Gunst SJ. Roles of focal adhesion kinase and paxillin in the mechanosensitive regulation of myosin phosphorylation in smooth muscle. *J Appl Physiol* 2001;**91**:1452–9.
100. Smith PG, Garcia R, Kogerman L. Mechanical strain increases protein tyrosine phosphorylation in airway smooth muscle cells. *Exp Cell Res* 1998;**239**:353–60.
101. Tang DD, Mehta D, Gunst SJ. Mechanosensitive tyrosine phosphorylation of paxillin and focal adhesion kinase in tracheal smooth muscle. *Am J Physiol* 1999;**276**:C250–8.
102. Tang DD, Gunst SJ. The small GTPase Cdc42 regulates actin polymerization and tension development during contractile stimulation of smooth muscle. *J Biol Chem* 2004;**279**:51722–8.
103. Tang DD, Zhang W, Gunst SJ. The adapter protein CrkII regulates neuronal Wiskott-Aldrich syndrome protein, actin polymerization, and tension development during contractile stimulation of smooth muscle. *J Biol Chem* 2005;**280**:23380–9.
104. Youn T, Kim SA, Hai CM. Length-dependent modulation of smooth muscle activation: effects of agonist, cytochalasin, and temperature. *Am J Physiol Cell Physiol* 1998;**274**:C1601–7.
105. Seow CY. Myosin filament assembly in an ever-changing myofilament lattice of smooth muscle. *Am J Physiol Cell Physiol* 2005;**289**:C1363–8.
106. Kuo KH, Herrera AM, Wang L, Pare PD, Ford LE, Stephens NL, Seow CY. Structure-function correlation in airway smooth muscle adapted to different lengths. *Am J Physiol Cell Physiol* 2003;**285**: C384–90.
107. Qi D, Mitchell RW, Burdyga T, Ford LE, Kuo KH, Seow CY. Myosin light chain phosphorylation facilitates in vivo myosin filament reassembly after mechanical perturbation. *Am J Physiol Cell Physiol* 2002;**282**:C1298–305.
108. Cremo C, Harteshorne DJ. Smooth muscle myosin II. In: Coluccio LM, editor. *Myosins: a superfamily of molecular motors*. Proteins and Cell Regulation series. Vol. 7, Springer, Dordrecht: Springer; 2008. p. 171–22.
109. Milton DL, Schneck AN, Ziech DA, Ba M, Facemyer KC, Halayko AJ, et al. Direct evidence for functional smooth muscle myosin II in the 10S self-inhibited monomeric conformation in airway smooth muscle cells. *Proc Natl Acad Sci USA* 2011;**108**:1421–6.
110. Critchley DR. Focal adhesions – the cytoskeletal connection. *Curr Opin Cell Biol* 2000;**12**:133–9.
111. Brakebusch C, Fassler R. The integrin–actin connection, an eternal love affair. *EMBO J* 2003;**22**:2324–33.
112. Galbraith CG, Yamada KM, Sheetz MP. The relationship between force and focal complex development. *J Cell Biol* 2002;**159**:695–705.
113. Kim HR, Hoque M, Hai CM. Cholinergic receptor-mediated differential cytoskeletal recruitment of actin- and integrin-binding proteins in intact airway smooth muscle. *Am J Physiol Cell Physiol* 2004;**287**:C1375–83.
114. Zhang WW, Gunst SJ. Dynamic association between alpha-actinin and beta-integrin regulates contraction of canine tracheal smooth muscle. *J Physiol-London* 2006;**572**:659–76.
115. Huang Y, Zhang W, Gunst SJ. Activation of vinculin induced by cholinergic stimulation regulates contraction of tracheal smooth muscle tissue. *J Biol Chem* 2010;**286**:3630–44.
116. Deng L, Fairbank NJ, Cole DJ, Fredberg JJ, Maksym GN. Airway smooth muscle tone modulates mechanically induced cytoskeletal stiffening and remodeling. *J Appl Physiol* 2005;**99**:634–41.
117. Smith PG, Garcia R, Kogerman L. Strain reorganizes focal adhesions and cytoskeleton in cultured airway smooth muscle cells. *Exp Cell Res* 1997;**232**:127–36.
118. Deng L, Fairbank NJ, Fabry B, Smith PG, Maksym GN. Localized mechanical stress induces time-dependent actin cytoskeletal remodeling and stiffening in cultured airway smooth muscle cells. *Am J Physiol Cell Physiol* 2004;**287**:C440–8.
119. Otey CA, Carpen O. Alpha-actinin revisited: a fresh look at an old player. *Cell Motil Cytoskeleton* 2004;**58**:104–11.
120. Bakolitsa C, Cohen DM, Bankston LA, Bobkov AA, Cadwell GW, Jennings L, et al. Structural basis for vinculin activation at sites of cell adhesion. *Nature* 2004;**430**:583–6.
121. Zhang YJ, Chen K, Tu YZ, Velyvis A, Yang YW, Qin J, et al. Assembly of the PINCH-ILK-CH-ILKBP complex precedes and is essential for localization of each component to cell-matrix adhesion sites. *J Cell Sci* 2002;**115**:4777–86.
122. Delcommenne M, Tan C, Gray V, Rue L, Woodgett J, Dedhar S. Phosphoinositide-3-OH kinase-dependent regulation of glycogen synthase kinase 3 and protein kinase B/AKT by the integrin-linked kinase. *Proc Natl Acad Sci USA* 1998;**95**:11211–6.
123. Desai LP, Wu Y, Tepper RS, Gunst SJ. Mechanical stimuli and IL-13 interact at integrin adhesion complexes to regulate expression of smooth muscle myosin heavy chain in airway smooth muscle tissue. *Am J Physiol Lung Cell Mol Physiol* 2011;**301**: L275–84.
124. Gosens R, Stelmack GL, Bos ST, Dueck G, Mutawe MM, Schaafsma D, et al. Caveolin-1 is required for contractile phenotype expression by airway smooth muscle cells. *J Cell Mol Med* 2011;**15**:2430–42.
125. Jansen SR, Van Ziel AM, Baarsma HA, Gosens R. β-Catenin regulates airway smooth muscle contraction. *Am J Physiol Lung Cell Mol Physiol* 2010;**299**:L204–14.
126. Gosens R, Mutawe M, Martin S, Basu S, Bos ST, Tran T, et al. Caveolae and caveolins in the respiratory system. *Curr Mol Med* 2008;**8**:741–53.
127. Nunes RO, Schmidt M, Dueck G, Baarsma H, Halayko AJ, Kerstjens HA, et al. GSK-3/beta-catenin signaling axis in airway smooth muscle: role in mitogenic signaling. *Am J Physiol Lung Cell Mol Physiol* 2008;**294**:L1110–8.
128. Gosens R, Meurs H, Schmidt M. The GSK-3/beta-catenin-signalling axis in smooth muscle and its relationship with remodelling. *Naunyn Schmiedebergs Arch Pharmacol* 2008;**378**: 185–91.

accompanied by an increase in collagen content (17,21) that accumulates in "gaps" separating two adjacent lamellar units, whereas the relative elastin content decreases (2). With age, aortic elastin modifies its structure (22,23). There is a progressive accumulation of collegenase-resistant, insoluble protein, sensitive to trypsin (22,24). Electron microscopy reveals that this protein has a fibrillar structure associated with elastin which appears to be "encrusted" (22).

With aging, progressive calcification areas were encountered (15), medial elastic laminae appeared stiff and "encrusted" by the calcified deposits, prevalently in the intermediate third of the tunica media; a progressive increase in GAGs was also found (24,25), in particular sulfated ones (26). They were present in most "gaps" among lamellar units, more abundant in the intimal inner layer of the tunica media, often coincident with calcified areas (27).

Aging and Changes of Relationship Between SMC and Endothelium

With aging, progressive modifications of the shape and junctions of vascular endothelial cells have been reported in mammals (18). Similar endothelium alterations are reported with hypertension and hypercholesterolemia (28). Under these three conditions, a decrease in basal and stimulated release of nitric oxide (NO) was observed. Moreover, an increase in endothelin-1 release was found with aging, while the sensitivity to the peptide was markedly decreased under the same conditions (29).

These modifications in the endothelium may have major clinical implications for the pathogenesis of cardiovascular diseases. We have previously reported morphological evidence of an altered permeability of endothelial barrier. In the aortic tunica intima of normocholesterolemic aged rabbits diffuse IT often showed large ground substance storages, more alcianophilic than in the adjacent tunica media (13,17). Focal subendothelial "lakes" of plasma-like material, mostly overlying large diffuse IT, associated with floating foam cells have been also reported in fat-fed monkeys (30) as well as in aged hyperlipemic rabbits (13). They are similar to the gelatinous lesions (Figure 105.1C) described in child aortas (31), that were reported as pre-atherosclerotic lesions, and considered strong evidence in support of the time-honored insudative theory of atherogenesis, first proposed by Rokitansky (32). In fact, changes in form or turnover of the endothelium are associated with an increase in shear forces, most likely linked to age-related increased rigidity of the arterial wall (1,33). On the other hand, the age-related accumulation of collagen and GAGs may induce an increased density of the extracellular matrix thereby blocking the diffusion of solutes (lipoproteins, growth factors, etc.), and favoring their accumulation. The greater influx of plasma lipoproteins and growth and chemotactic factors seems in fact to be related with the initial stages of atherogenesis (34,35). As a matter of fact, albumin, fibrinogen and LDL are described in intimal insudations in human arteries and in aortic and cerebral vascular districts of hypercholesterolemic-hypertensive rabbits (36).

MORPHOLOGICAL AND FUNCTIONAL MODIFICATIONS OF AGING SMCS

Unbalanced Homeostatic Control of SMC Population Growth: Cell Proliferation

Aging may induce an alteration in the mechanisms of control of vascular SMC proliferation, which has also been implicated in the age-dependent susceptibility to atherosclerosis (37,38). The cellular proliferation in the plaque is regulated by synthesis and release of various growth factors (for review see 39). Several reports suggest that SMCs from aged rats have a higher proliferative rate than SMCs from young rats (40). This is associated with an increased platelet-derived growth factor-like and a reduced heparin-like activity (40). Moreover, *in vivo* aged rat aortas incorporate more 3H-thymidine than young animals after disendothelization (41). The high replicative activity of SMCs from old rats is not shared by fibroblasts cultured from the same animals (42), suggesting that cells from different tissues of old animals do not necessarily show a stereotyped increase of replicative potential *in vitro*. The modification in SMCs' proliferative activity with aging is accompanied *in vitro* by a modification in their phenotype (42). SMC cultures from young rats show the characteristic "peaks and troughs" aspect (43), whereas SMCs from old rats have a polygonal shape (44). Moreover, the percentage of α-smooth muscle (α-SM) actin and smooth muscle myosin positive cells, and the amount of α-SM actin by immunoblots and of α-SM actin mRNA were significantly lower in SMCs from old rats as compared with young rats in the presence of fetal calf serum (42,44).

Age-related changes in microenvironmental stimuli (cytokines, extracellular matrix components) and/or in intrinsic properties of target arterial cells influence SMC proliferation. In line with this view, heparin induced a decrease of cell growth percentage which was higher in SMCs cultured from the old rat than the young rat tunica media and associated with a higher increase in α-SM actin and α-SM actin mRNA expression; conversely, transforming growth factor α-1 (TGF α-1) exerted an opposite action (45). McCaffrey and Falcone (38) have demonstrated that SMCs derived from old animals can have a regular basal production of TGF α-1, which exerts an anti-proliferative activity, but fail to respond to the autocrine growth inhibitory effects of this agent, leading to enhanced proliferation.

Unbalanced Homeostatic Control of SMC Population Growth: Cell Apoptosis

Apoptosis contributes to the modulation of intimal cell population size and counteracts exaggerated intimal hyperplasia (46–47). Apoptotic cells are rarely observed within the arterial wall of either young or aged normolipemic animals using traditional methods as TUNEL, electron microscopy, and PCR. This makes verification of age-related differences in apoptotic susceptibility *in vivo* impossible. In addition, Urano et al. (48) reported that rat aortic intimal SMCs from aged rats cultured 15 days after balloon injury undergo 7-ketocholesterol-induced apoptosis *in vitro* more than those from young rats. In contrast, intimal senescent SMCs induced by a second angioplastic injury appear more resistant to apoptosis compared to those obtained after a single injury (49,50).

SMCs from the arteries of aged mice show decreased α-thrombin-induced proliferation but generate higher levels of reactive oxygen species (ROS) and have constitutionally increased mitogen-activated protein kinase activity in comparison with SMCs from young mice (51). These changes result in a preferential accumulation of oxidative damage in the arterial wall of old animals facilitating the greater progression of atherosclerosis in aged animals. Moreover, accumulation of oxidative mitochondrial DNA damage may promote SMC apoptosis. Indirect evidence can be drawn from the consideration that apoptosis is more marked in early fatty streaks of aged rabbits than in those of young animals without differences in plasma cholesterol levels (52). Apoptosis in underlying medial SMCs remains low, with no differences compared to respective normolipemic controls, suggesting that this phenomenon is limited to intimal cells. Nevertheless, it remains difficult to clarify whether the modulation of apoptosis with aging is intrinsic to the whole arterial population or, alternatively, is mediated by a subpopulation that contributes to the progression of intimal thickening in aged animals. It remains to be clarified whether, with aging, a subpopulation of resident or migrating stem cells, which is capable of proliferating in response to microenvironmental changes, prevails in the arterial wall whereas remaining cells undergo senescence.

Differentiation Properties of Aged SMC (Activity of the Synthetic Phenotype, Changes of ECM and Cellular Signaling)

In adult organisms vascular SMC exhibit an extraordinary capacity to undergo profound and reversible changes in phenotype in response to changes in local environmental factors that normally regulate phenotypes (53) (see Chapter 95). SMC heterogeneity has been documented by several laboratories using different criteria (54,55). In addition to the paradigmatic notion of "contractile" and "synthetic" SMCs phenotypes (Figure 105.1D and E) isolated from tunica media and repairing tunica intima, respectively, more recent *in vivo* and *in vitro* studies, using powerful molecular tools, have demonstrated that phenotypic modulation is often related to the entire spectrum of mesenchymal lineage, including, thin tapered SMCs burying themselves in multiple layers of basement-like material (Figure 105.1G,H, and I), and osteoblastic (Figure 105.1F), chondrocytic, and adipocytic cells. Deregulated TGF-β superfamily signaling most likely drives some of these mesenchymal differentiations (56). Whether and how these phenotypes contribute to calcification and altered matrix production in aging is still to be clarified. It is worth noting that patients affected by Hutchinson–Gilford progeria syndrome develop severe premature atherosclerosis characterized by vascular SMCs calcification and attrition (57).

Age-related phenotypic changes with aging also include the increase of tetraploidy, from 8 to 64% of cells, in young compared to old rats (10). Tetraploidy associates with a reduction of matrix protein transcripts as well as inflammatory-associated molecules, such as macrophage inflammatory protein-2 (MIP-2), complement component C4 and Gal/GalNAc-specific lectin (MGL) (7). In addition, both monocyte chemotactic protein-1 (MCP-1) and its receptor CCR2 mRNA and proteins are increased in old versus young rat aortas *in vivo*.

The different SMC reactivity from old animal observations suggests another possibility that can be explored in order to understand SMC adaptation to aging *in vivo*. When two different SMC populations, derived from newborn and old rat aortic tunica media, are seeded into the intima of denuded rat carotid artery, old rat media-derived SMCs continue to produce cellular retinol binding protein-1 but little α-SM actin and smooth muscle myosin heavy chains, while the newborn rat-derived SMCs continue to express α-SM actin and smooth muscle myosin heavy chains but no cellular retinol binding protein-1. This reinforces the notion that arterial SMC phenotypic heterogeneity is controlled genetically and not by local microenvironmental factors and is maintained within an *in vivo* environment. Importantly, VSMC heterogeneity and age-related differences in cytoskeletal protein expression may contribute to the remodeling of the aortic arterial wall with aging (58).

Transactivation of NF-κB in old SMCs on tumor necrosis factor-alpha (TNF-α) stimulation is intense and only weak in SMCs from newborn animals (20–30). These data indicate that the ability to respond to proinflammatory stimuli differs among SMCs at different stages of development. This results in differential capability to express NF-κB-dependent genes such as iNOS and ICAM-1, which could have implications for host defense and the pathogenesis of vascular diseases with aging (20). Aortic SMCs from old rats produce significantly more angiotensinogen (21). The age-related increase of local angiotensin system activity may contribute to vascular tone regulation. In addition, signaling pathways regulating migration of vascular SMCs from older animals are able to bypass the requirement for CamKII activation and, therefore, the need for bFGF release from the underlying medial SMCs (22).

In VSMCs, age-related changes of the response mediated by beta-adrenoreceptors have been intensively investigated. Myoctic beta-adrenoreceptor-mediated relaxation decreases in most arteries with increasing age (23). In contrast, the response to alpha-adrenoreceptor agonists gives conflicting results or appears unchanged with aging. Finally, aging induces changes in the phenotype of rat coronary arterioles, with a decrease of endothelial NOS and increase of iNOS transcript levels, thus contributing to the development of oxidative stress, which impairs nitric oxide-mediated dilations (24).

MODULATION OF SIGNALING PATHWAYS IN AGED SMC

Replicative Senescence

Replicative senescence was originally defined by the finite replicative life span of human somatic cells in culture. Senescent VSMCs that enter irreversible growth arrest display a characteristic morphology: vacuolated, flattened, and enlarged shape. These phenotypic changes associated with senescence have been suggested to be involved in human aging. The growth potential of cultured cells correlates well with the mean maximum life span of the species from which the cells are derived.

Cultured VSMC from old rat aortas display accelerated growth rates compared to VSMC from young rats (59). Additionally, compared to early passage VSMC from young rat aortas, old VSMC from old rat aortas have a greater percentage of their population in the S phase, and a lower percentage in the G0/G1 phase (60). These differences are mediated by deregulation of the cell cycle, in part, via ERK1/2 signaling that occurs during aging (61). Early passage aortic VSMC of old rats exhibit an exaggerated chemotactic PDGF-BB response, whereas cells from young aortas require several additional passages in culture to generate an equivalent response (61). In response to a chemoattractant gradient of PDGF-BB and MCP-1, VSMC isolated from old aortas also exhibit increased invasion relative to young VSMC (62,63). This age difference is abolished or substantially reduced by Losartan, an AT1 antagonist, vCCI, an inhibitor of MCP-1/CCR2 signaling, GM 6001, an MMP inhibitor, and Ci 1, α-calpain inhibitor, or by silencing MFG-E8 (64,65). Thus, the increased age-associated VSMC invasion/migration is modulated by concurrent increases in elements of Ang II biosignaling networks.

Senescent cells express a biomarker of senescence, the senescence-associated β-galactosidase (SAβ-gal) (66) and a set of genes – including negative regulators of the cell cycle such as p53 and p16 – that differs from those normally expressed. SAβ-gal has been described as a marker of senescent cells *in vitro* and *in vivo*. β-galactosidase is a metabolic enzyme highly expressed in pre-senescent and senescent cells (67). SAβ-gal activity corresponds to β-galactosidase activity measured in pH conditions where only high levels of the enzyme are detectable, and proportionally correlate with lysosomalcontent (68). In experimental models such as the old rat arterial wall, SAβ-gal activity is detected in VSMC enriched with p16 and Nox4 (69). In human atherosclerotic plaques, endothelial cells and VSMCs exhibit the morphological features of cellular senescence (70,71). Vascular cells that are positive for SAβ-gal activity have been found in atherosclerotic plaques from the coronary arteries of patients with ischemic heart disease (72). In advanced plaques, however, SAβ-gal-positive VSMCs are only detected in the intima and not in the media (73), possibly the result of extensive replication in these lesions. SAβ-gal-positive VSMCs cells from human atheromas show increased expression of p53 and p16, both markers of cellular senescence (73). These cells also exhibit various functional abnormalities, including decreased expression of endothelial NOS and increased expression of proinflammatory molecules.

Oxidative Stress and ROS

Oxidative stress is one of the most physiologically relevant triggers of cell senescence in pathological conditions. A correlation between aging and the accumulation of oxidatively damaged proteins, lipids, and nucleic acids has been reported (74). This raises the possibility that the accumulation of oxidized proteins during aging reflects a loss of apoptotic capacity (i.e., oxidatively modified proteins persist mainly in cells that have escaped apoptosis). Oxidative modification of proteins causes the introduction of a carbonyl group into the protein, leading to loss of catalytic or structural function of the affected proteins. Therefore, increased levels of oxidatively modified proteins during aging will have deleterious effects on cellular and organ function (74). Numerous studies underscore the importance of deregulated oxidant and antioxidant balance in advancing age (75) and in the development and progression of atherosclerosis in both animal models and in humans (76).

ROS, particularly superoxide anions, hydrogen peroxide (H_2O_2), and hydroxyl radicals, can produce a large variety of DNA damage, including DNA strand breaks and DNA base modifications. ROS can accelerate telomere loss during replication in some cell types (77), but also induce premature senescence independently of telomere shortening (78). *In vitro*, oxidant stress induced by chronic H_2O_2 treatment (79), hyperoxic culture conditions (80) or alterations of the cell's anti-oxidant properties can all accelerate senescence. Treatment of cultured fibroblasts with H_2O_2 can induce telomere single strand breaks that may promote telomere shortening (81) and consequently induce premature cell cycle arrest by triggering pathways converging towards activation of the G1-associated cell cycle inhibitors (p21Cip1, p16ink4). Increased telomere loss per division can also occur in individual cells due to a telomere-specific deficiency in base excision repair. This mechanism leads to preferential accumulation of ROS-induced single-stranded DNA breaks (82), preventing replication of distal segments of chromosomes when cells divide. Alternatively, repeated stress dramatically increases the proportion of cells undergoing growth arrest (83,84), suggesting that oxidative stress may exert selection pressure with replication of a subset of VSMCs *in vivo*. Oxidative stress can also induce premature senescence independently of telomere shortening. Pulsed treatments with low doses of H_2O_2 in fibroblasts can cause irreversible cell cycle arrest accompanied by an increase in SAβG staining without concomitant changes in telomere length (85).

Accumulation of oxidative damage to genomic DNA may contribute to "stress-induced premature senescence" (SIPS), but also to replicative senescence since senescent cells *in vitro* have higher levels of 8-oxoG DNA base modifications (86). These results are consistent with the observation that senescent cells present more DNA damage foci, even in non-telomeric sequences (87). Therefore, the distinction between replicative and oxidative stress-induced senescence is not clearly delineated, and both pathways lead to SAβG overexpression, even though distinct cell cycle inhibitors may be involved.

Oncogene Activation

Cells undergo SIPS in response to activated oncogenes (e.g. Ha-Ras) and suboptimal culture conditions (88). *In vitro*, SIPS can be elicited by overexpressing Ras and Raf oncogenes (89,90), radiation (91,92), or chemical agents producing any form of DNA damage and oxidant stress (93,94).

Replicative senescence and SIPS converge on the tumor suppressor genes p53 and RB, the latter being regulated by cyclin-dependent kinase inhibitors (cdkis), including p16 and p21. pRB, p53, p21, or p16 expression can induce senescence and are often increased in both replicative senescence and SIPS (95). Telomere loss or damage activates p53 via DNA damage-sensing mechanisms (96), with subsequent transcription of p21, whereas stress-induced activation of p16 accelerates replicative senescence independently of telomere length (97). In addition, p16 expression effectively renders telomere-based senescence irreversible (95), in part, by promoting repressive heterochromatin at loci containing targets of E2F transcription factors (98). Although the division between replicative senescence and SIPS is useful, the pathways have multiple areas of overlap. Indeed, both telomere-based DNA damage and stress-induced activation of p16 may occur simultaneously, inducing a growth arrest with cell cycle regulator expression, reflecting activation of both pathways (95).

Telomere Attrition and Telomerase Activity

In most primary cells, the telomeres of chromosomes shorten at each cell division because of incomplete chromosomal replication. Replicative senescence may be induced at critical telomere lengths or structures, such as telomeric fusion or dicentrics or loss of telomere-bound factors (99,100). After repeated divisions, telomeres may reach a critical length or structure whereby irreversible growth arrest or senescence is triggered (101). In addition, there is substantial evidence of a cause and effect relationship between telomerase expression and manifestations of senescence. Ectopic expression of the catalytic subunit of telomerase (hTERT) can prevent replicative senescence in several cell types such as fibroblasts or epithelial cells, despite the fact that telomeres were always protected (102–105). hTERT may also influence the interaction of telomeres with the nuclear matrix, increase chromosome stability, decrease telomere fusion, reduce spontaneous chromosome breaks and enhance DNA repair. These effects are independent of the effects of telomerase on telomere length (106). Telomere uncapping can also cause cell senescence independent of telomere length and telomerase activity. For example, overexpression of a negative mutant of the telomere-capping protein TRF2 causes senescence in fibroblasts or fibrosarcoma cells, even though the cells retain their long telomeres (107–109). These experiments support the idea that as telomeres shorten they lose their protein-binding properties, possibly causing irreversible damage to the T loop structure (110).

Comparative analysis of the transcriptome profiles of early and late passage human arterial VSMC found a total of 327 differentially expressed probe sets. These include IL-1β, IL-8, ICAM-1, and MCP-1. Furthermore, senescent VSMC also secrete IL-1, IL-6/8, MCP-1, PAI-1, and MMP-2, similar to a phenomenon found in senescent fibroblasts, referred to as the senescence-associated secretory phenotype (SASP). Thus, senescent VSMC become "non-conventional" inflammation response (AAASP) cells. Like the SASP, the AAASP also likely allows damaged cells to communicate with the surrounding tissue, providing a complementary signaling role in arterial aging.

AGE-RELATED ACCUMULATION OF ADVANCED GLYCOSYLATION END PRODUCTS IN THE VESSEL WALL

The advanced glycosylation end-products (AGEs) are a heterogeneous group of heterocyclic structured substances with variable spectral properties and cross-linking (for review see 8). They are the result of complex changes occurring in the non-enzymatic glycosylation products, also defined as "early glycosylation products", corresponding to the Schiff's base and the "Amadori product" (111). The latter gives origin to AGEs after further re-arrangements due to oxidation, dehydration, and polymerization reactions (for a review see 112). Today, four AGE components have been characterized, named FFI, AFGP, pyrraline, and pentosidine, all having a few common physico-chemical properties, such as yellow-brown pigmentation, a characteristic fluorescent spectrum, and the ability to establish irreversible links with different proteins, thus producing "cross-linking". Therefore, the amount of AGEs linked to slow-turnover proteins, e.g. collagen and lenses crystals, keeps increasing progressively with time (8). In the vessel wall, because of the high collagen content, AGEs accumulate as a function of age and diabetes.

Possible Biological Effects of AGEs on Vessel Wall

The physiopathological consequences of AGE accumulation on the vessel wall and in serum are not well defined yet. However, accumulation of AGEs seems to substantially contribute to aging of SMCs through increased generation of ROS (previous section). As a matter of fact, recent studies have shown that binding of AGEs to receptor for AGEs (RAGE) generates ROS in several vascular cells and triggers secretion of inflammatory cytokines (113). In addition, the hypothesis that AGEs may play a role in the pathogenesis of atherosclerosis derives from the following circumstantial observations: (i) AGEs accumulate in the arterial wall in aged people and much more in diabetics; (ii) AGEs induce in the vascular wall some biological modifications, many of which are potentially atherogenic. In particular, the cross-linking collagen leads to a decrease in solubility and susceptibility to enzymatic digestion paralleled by an increase in stiffness of the collagen-rich tissues (114).

To what extent AGEs are increased in human vessel wall because of age and their effects on vessel wall physiology is still unknown. It may be hypothesized, however, that similar to what is observed in the rat aortas (115), the reduced arterial elasticity in the elderly people may be mainly due to AGEs accumulation. Moreover, the receptor-mediated uptake of AGE-modified proteins induces in monocytes the release of various cytokines, such as TNF, interleukin-1 (IL-1), platelet-derived growth factor (PDGF) and insulin-like growth factor-1 (IGF-1) (for a review see 8). Finally, *in vivo* and *in vitro* studies have demonstrated that AGE-modified proteins interfere with NO-dependent vasodilation, suggesting that AGEs are major modulators of vessel tone (116). Dysfunctions of endothelium, recruitment of circulating monocytes within the vessel wall, and the release of some cytokines and growth factors are believed to be major elements in atherogenesis (117).

To our present knowledge, however, there are still doubts as to the relevance of circulating or parietal AGEs in the age-related increase of clinical manifestations of atherosclerosis. Moreover, we do not know whether there is a threshold value below which AGEs do not produce effects of any pathogenic relevance or whether low-concentration AGEs are atherogenous because of synergism with risk factors other than diabetes mellitus. The latter hypothesis is somewhat supported by a recent paper of Bucala et al. (118) reporting the *in vitro* formation of phospholipid-like AGEs which appeared to develop in parallel with the oxidation of unsaturated fatty acids. In addition, the authors observed that during glucose incubation of LDL, AGEs moieties were produced that linked both the lipid and apoprotein component, similar to oxidized LDL (118). Aminoguanidine, an inhibitor of advanced glycosylation, would inhibit glycosylation of both apoprotein and lipid components and oxidative modifications (118).

CONCLUSIONS

The data reported above documented that aging-related changes of SMCs are accompanied by a series of structural and physiological alterations of the arterial wall, some of which are relevant for the increased susceptibility and progression of experimental atherosclerosis. Although regarded as a non-modifiable risk factor because related to genetic modifications, circumstantial evidence that SMC aging phenotype can be determined by genotoxic factors, such as ROS or advanced glycation end-products, raises a great interest in studying the molecular mechanisms involved in this biological process in the hope of identifying targets that could be used for the treatment or prevention of life-threatening cardiovascular and cerebrovascular diseases.

REFERENCES

1. Dobrin PB. Mechanical properties of arteries. *Phys Rev* 1978;**58**:397–421.
2. Spina M, Garbisa S, Hinnie J, Serafini-Fracassini A. Age-related changes in composition and mechanical properties of tunica media of the upper thoracic human aorta. *Arteriosclerosis* 1983;**3**:64–76.
3. Movat ZH, More MH, Haust MD. The diffuse intimal thickening of human aorta with aging. *Am J Pathol* 1958;**34**:1023–35.
4. Scebat L, Renais J, Hadjisky P. Histometabolic and structural changes during arterial wall ageing. Possible role of immune process. In: Cavallero C, editor. *The arterial wall in atherogenesis.* Padua: Piccin Medical Book;1975. p. 43–60.
5. Geer JC, Haust MD. *Smooth muscle cells in atherosclerosis. Monographs on Atherosclerosis*, vol. 2. Basle: Karger;1972.
6. Tracy RE, Strong JP, Toca VT, Lopez CR. Variable patterns of non-atheromatous aortic intimal thickening. *Lab Invest* 1979;**41**:553–9.
7. Kritchevsky D. Diet, lipid, metabolism, and aging. *Fed Proc* 1979;**38**:2001–6.
8. Stary HC. Macrophages, macrophage foam cells, and eccentric intimal thickening in the coronary arteries of young children. *Atherosclerosis* 1987;**64**:91–108.
9. Friedman MH. A biologically plausible model of thickening of arterial intima under shear. *Arteriosclerosis* 1989;**9**:511–22.
10. Glagov S, Zarins CK. Is intimal hyperplasia an adaptive response or a pathologic process? Observations on the nature of nonatherosclerotic intimal thickening. *J Vasc Surg* 1989;**10**:571–3.
11. Bucala R, Cerani A. Advanced glycosylation: chemistry, biology, and implications for diabetes and aging. *Adv Pharmacol* 1992;**23**:1–34.
12. Spagnoli LG, Orlandi A, Mauriello A, Santeusanio G, De Angelis C, Lucreziotti R, et al. Aging and atherosclerosis in the rabbit 1. Distribution, prevalence and morphology of atherosclerotic lesions. *Atherosclerosis* 1991;**89**:11–24.
13. Spagnoli LG, Orlandi A, Mauriello A, et al. Age-dependent increase of rabbit aortic wall sensitivity to atherosclerosis: a morphometric approach. *Pathol Res Pract* 1992;**4-5**:637–42.
14. Dietschy JM. The effect of aging on the processes that regulates plasma LDL cholesterol levels in animal and man. In: Bates SR, Gangloff EC, editors. *Atherosclerosis and aging.* New York: Springer-Verlag;1987. p. 104–22.
15. Elliot RJ, McGrath LT. Calcification of the human thoracic aorta during aging. *Calcif Tissue Int* 1994;**54**:268–73.
16. Wolinsky H. Long-term effects of hypertension on the rat aortic wall and their relation to concurrent aging changes. *Circ Res* 1972;**30**:301–9.
17. Orlandi A, Mauriello M, Marino B, et al. Age-related modifications of aorta and coronaries in the rabbit: a morphological and morphometrical assessment. *Arch Gerontol Ger* 1993;**17**:37–53.
18. Nakamura H, Izumiyama N, Nakamura K, et al. Age-associated ultrastructural changes in the aortic intima of rats with diet-induced hypercholesterolemia. *Atherosclerosis* 1989;**79**:101–11.
19. Clarkson TB, Lofland HB, Bullock BC, et al. Atherosclerosis in some species of new world monkeys. *Ann NY Acad Sci* 1969;**162**:103–9.
20. Cliff WJ. The aortic tunica media in aging rats. *Exp Mol Pathol* 1970;**13**:172–89.
21. Mauriello A, Oberholzer M, Orlandi A, et al. Age-related modification of average volume and anisotropy of vascular smooth muscle cells. *Path Res Pract* 1992;**188**:630–6.
22. Nejjar I, Pieraggi MT, Thiers JC, et al. Age-related changes in the elastic tissue of the human thoracic aorta. *Atherosclerosis* 1990;**80**:199–208.
23. John R, Thomas J. Chemical composition of elastins isolated from aortas and pulmonary tissue of humans of different ages. *Biochem J* 1972;**127**:261–6.
24. Spina M, Garbin G. Age related chemical changes in human elastins from non-atherosclerotic areas of thoracic aorta. *Atherosclerosis* 1976;**24**:267–83.
25. Nakamura T, Tokita K, Tateno S, et al. Human aortic acid mucopolysaccharides and glycoprotein. Changes during ageing and the atherosclerosis. *J Atheroscler Res* 1968;**8**:891–902.
26. Wight TR, Ross R. Proteoglycans in primate arteries. Ultrastructural localization and distribution in the intima. *J Cell Biol* 1975;**667**:660–75.
27. Kumar V, Berenson GS, Ruiz M, et al. Acid mucopolysaccharides of human aorta. Part 1: variation with maturation. *J Atheroscler Res* 1967;**7**:573–83.
28. Chobanian AV. The arterial smooth muscle cell in systemic hypertension. *Am J Cardiol* 1987;**60**:94I–8I.
29. Luscher TF, Tanner FC, Age Dohi Y. hypertension and hypercholesterolemia alter endothelium-dependent vascular regulation. *Pharmacol Toxicol* 1992;**70**:S32–9.
30. Faggioto A, Ross R, Harker L. Studies of hypercholesterolemia in the nonhuman primates. I. Changes that led to fatty streak formation. *Arteriosclerosis* 1984;**4**:323–40.
31. Haust MD. The morphogenesis and fate of potential and early atherosclerotic lesions in man. *HumanPathol* 1971;**2**:1–13.
32. Rokitansky C. In: Braunmuller W, Seidel L, editors. *Handbuch der Patologischen Anatomie*, vol. 2; 1844.
33. Hayashi K, Takamizawa K, Nakamura T, et al. Effects of elastase on the stiffness and elastic properties of arterial walls in cholesterol-fed rabbits. *Atherosclerosis* 1987;**66**:259–67.
34. Smith EB, Staples EM. Intimal and medial plasma protein concentrations and endothelial function. *Atherosclerosis* 1982;**41**:295–305.
35. Minick CR, Stemerman MB, Insull Jr. W. Role of endothelium and hypercholesterolemia in intimal thickening and lipid accumulation. *Am J Pathol* 1979;**95**:131–40.
36. Kurozumi T, Imamura T, Tanaka K, et al. Permeation and deposition of fibrinogen and low-density lipoprotein in the aorta and cerebral artery of rabbits – immunoelectron study. *Br J Exp Path* 1984;**65**:355–64.
37. Porreca E, Ciccarelli R, Di Febbo C, et al. Protein kinase C pathway and proliferative responses of aged and young rat vascular smooth muscle cells. *Atherosclerosis* 1993;**104**:137–45.
38. McCaffrey TA, Falcone DJ. Evidence for an age-related dysfunction in the antiproliferative response to transforming growth factor-beta in vascular smooth muscle cells. *Mol Biol Cell* 1993;**4**:315–22.

39. Bobik A, Campbell JH. Vascular derived growth factors: cell biology, pathophysiology and pharmacology. *Pharmacol Res* 1993;**45**:1–42.
40. McCaffrey T, Nicholson AC, Szabo PE, et al. Aging and arteriosclerosis. The increased proliferation or arterial smooth muscle cells isolated from old rats is associated with increased platelet-derived growth factor-like activity. *J Exp Med* 1988;**167**:163–74.
41. Stemerman MB, Weinstein R, Rowe JW, et al. Vascular smooth muscle cell growth kinetics in vivo in aged rats. *Proc Natl Acad Sci USA* 1982;**79**:3863–6.
42. Bochaton-Piallat ML, Gabbiani F, Ropraz P, et al. Age influences the replicative activity and the differentiation features of cultured rat aortic smooth muscle cells populations and clones. *Arterioscler Thromb* 1993;**13**:1449–55.
43. Chamley-Campbell JG, Campbell GR, Ross R. Smooth muscle cells in culture. *Physiol Rev* 1979;**59**:1–61.
44. Orlandi A, Ehrlich HP, Ropraz P, et al. Rat aortic smooth muscle cells isolated from different layers and at different times after endothelial denudation show distinct biological features in vitro. *Arterioscler Thromb* 1994;**14**:982–9.
45. Orlandi A, Ropraz P, Gabbiani G. Proliferative activity and α-smooth muscle actin expression in cultured rat aortic smooth muscle cells are differently modulated by transforming growth factor α-1 and heparin. *Exp Cell Res* 1994;**214**:528–36.
46. Azuma H, Niimi Y, Terada T, Hamasaki H. Accelerated endothelial regeneration and intimal hyperplasia following a repeated denudationof rabbit carotid arteries: morphological and immunohistochemical studies. *Clin Exp Pharmacol Physiol* 1995;**22**: 748–54.
47. Haunstetter A, Izumo S. Apoptosis: basic mechanisms and implications for cardiovascular disease. *Circ Res* 1998;**82**: 1111–29.
48. Urano Y, Shirai K, Watanabe H, et al. Vascular smooth muscle cell outgrowth, proliferation, and apoptosis in young and old rats. *Atherosclerosis* 1999;**146**:101–15.
49. Fenton M, Barker S, Kurz DJ, Erusalimsky JD. Cellular senescence after single and repeated balloon catheter denudations of rabbit carotid arteries. *Arterioscler Thromb Vasc Biol* 2001;**21**:220–6.
50. Pollman MJ, Hall JL. Gibbon GH. Determinants of vascular smooth muscle cell apoptosis after balloon angioplasty injury. *Circ Res* 1996;**84**:113–21.
51. Moon SK, Thompson LJ, Madamanchi N, et al. Aging, oxidative responses, and proliferative capacity in cultured mouse aortic smooth muscle cells. *Am J Physiol Heart Circ Physiol* 2001;**280**: H2779–88.
52. Faggiotto A, Ross R, Harker L. Studies of hypercholesterolemia in the nonhuman primate. I. Changes that lead to fatty streak formation. *Arteriosclerosis* 1984;**4**:323–40.
53. Owens GK, Kumar MS, Wamhoff BR. Molecular regulation of vascular smooth muscle cell differentiation in development and disease. *Physiol Rev* 2004;**84**:767–801.
54. Walker LN, Bowen-Pope DF, et al. Production of platelet-derived growth factor-like molecules by cultured arterial smooth muscle cells accompanies proliferation after arterial injury. *Proc Natl Acad Sci USA* 1986;**83**:7311–5.
55. Orlandi A, Ehrlich HP, Ropraz P, et al. Rat aortic smooth muscle cells isolated from different layers and at different times after endothelial denudation show distinct biological features in vitro. *Arterioscler Thromb* 1994;**14**:982–9.
56. Iyemere VP, Proudfoot D, Weissberg PL, Shanahan CM. Vascular smooth muscle cell phenotypic plasticity and the regulation of vascular calcification. *J Intern Med* 2006;**260**: 192–210.
57. Ragnauth CD, Warren DT, Liu Y, McNair R, Tajsic T, Figg N, et al. Prelamin A acts to accelerate smooth muscle cell senescence and is a novel biomarker of human vascular aging. *Circulation* 2010;**121**:2200–10.
58. Wolinsky H. Long-term effects of hypertension on the rat aortic wall and their relation to concurrent aging changes. Morphological and chemical studies. *Circ Res* 1972;**30**:301–9.
59. Li Z, Cheng H, Lederer WJ, et al. Enhanced proliferation and migration and altered cytoskeletal proteins in early passage smooth muscle cells from young and old rat aortic explants. *Exp Mol Pathol* 1997;**64**:1–11.
60. Hariri RJ, Hajjar DP, Coletti D, et al. Aging and arteriosclerosis. Cell cycle kinetics of young and old arterial smooth muscle cells. *Am J Pathol* 1988;**131**:132–6.
61. Pauly RR, Passaniti A, Crow M, et al. Experimental models that mimic the differentiation and dedifferentiation of vascular cells. *Circulation* 1992;**86**(Suppl.):III68–73.
62. Wang M, Zhang J, Jiang LQ, et al. Proinflammatory profile within the grossly normal aged human aortic wall. *Hypertension* 2007;**50**:219–27.
63. Wang M, Zhang J, de Cabo R, et al. Calorie restriction reduces MMP-2 activity and retards age-associated aortic restructuring in rats. *Circulation* 2006;**114**(Suppl. II) II-335.
64. Fu Z, Wang M, Gucek M, et al. Milk fat globule protein epidermal growth factor-8: a pivotal relay element within the angiotensin II and monocyte chemoattractant protein-1 signaling cascade mediating vascular smooth muscle cells invasion. *Circ Res* 2009;**104**:1337–46.
65. Jiang L, Wang M, Zhang J, et al. Increased aortic calpain-1 activity mediates age-associated angiotensin II signaling of vascular smooth muscle cells. *PLoS ONE* 2008;**3**:e2231.
66. Campisi J. The biology of replicative senescence. *Eur J Cancer* 1997;**33**:703–9.
67. Dimri G, Lee X, Basile G, Acosta M, Scott G, Roskelley C, et al. A biomarker that identifies senescent human cells in culture and in aging skin in vivo. *Proc Natl Acad Sci USA* 1995;**92**: 9363–7.
68. Kurz DJ, Decary S, Hong Y, Erusalimsky JD. Senescence-associated β-galactosidase reflects an increase in lysosomal mass during replicative ageing of human endothelial cells. *J Cell Sci* 2000;**113**: 3613–22.
69. McCrann DJ, Yang D, Chen H, et al. Upregulation of Nox4 in the aging vasculature and its association with smooth muscle cell polyploidy. *Cell Cycle* 2009;**8**:902–8.
70. Burrig KF. The endothelium of advanced arteriosclerotic plaques in humans. *Arterioscler Thromb* 1991;**11**:1678–89.
71. Ross R, Wright TN, Strandness E, Thiele B. Human atherosclerosis: I. cell constitution and characteristics of advanced lesions of the superficial femoral artery. *Am J Pathol* 1984;**114**:79–93.
72. Minamino T, Komuro I. Endothelial cell senescence in human atherosclerosis: role of telomere in endothelial dysfunction. *Circulation* 2002;**105**:1541–4.

73. Minamino T, Yoshida T, Tatero K, Miyauchi H, Zou Y, Toko H, et al. Ras induces vascular smooth muscle cell senescence and inflammation in human atherosclerosis. *Circulation* 2003;**108**:2264–9.
74. Levine RL. Carbonyl modified proteins in cellular regulation, aging, and disease. *Free Rad Biol Med* 2002;**32**:790–6.
75. Moon SK, Thompson LJ, Madamanchi N, Ballinger S, Papaconstantinou J, Horaist C, et al. Aging, oxidative responses, and proliferative capacity in cultured mouse aortic smooth muscle cells. *Am J Physiol Heart Circ Physiol* 2001;**280**:H2779–88.
76. Wassmann S, Wassmann K, Nickenig G. Modulation of oxidant and antioxidant enzyme expression and function in vascular cells. *Hypertension* 2004;**44**:381–6.
77. von Zglinicki T, Saretzki G, Docke W, Lotze C. Mild hyperoxia shortens telomeres and inhibits proliferation of fibroblasts: a model for senescence? *Exp Cell Res* 1995;**220**:186–93.
78. Chen QM, Prowse KR, Tu VC, Purdom S, Linskens MH. Uncoupling the senescent phenotype from telomere shortening in hydrogen peroxidetreated fibroblasts. *Exp Cell Res* 2001;**265**:294–303.
79. von Zglinicki T, Saretzki G, Docke W, Lotze C. Mild hyperoxia shortens telomeres and inhibits proliferation of fibroblasts: a model for senescence? *Exp Cell Res* 1995;**220**:86–93.
80. von Zglinicki T, Pilger R, Sitte N. Accumulation of single-strand breaks is the major cause of telomere shortening in human fibroblasts. *Free Radic Biol Med* 2000;**28**:64–74.
81. Petersen S, Saretzki G, von Zglinicki T. Preferential accumulation of single-stranded regions in telomeres of human fibroblasts. *Exp Cell Res* 1998;**239**:152–60.
82. Toussaint O, Houbion A, Remacle J. Aging as a multi-step process characterized by a lowering of entropy production leading the cell to a sequence of defined stages. II. Testing some predictions on aging human fibroblasts in culture. *Mech Ageing Dev* 1992;**65**:65–83.
83. Dumont P, Burton M, Chen QM, Gonos ES, Frippiat C, Mazarati JB, et al. Induction of replicative senescence biomarkers by sublethal oxidative stresses in normal human fibroblast. *Free Radic Biol Med* 2000;**28**:361–73.
84. Chen QM, Prowse KR, Tu VC, Purdom S, Linskens MH. Uncoupling the senescent phenotype from telomere shortening in hydrogen peroxide-treated fibroblasts. *Exp Cell Res* 2001;**265**:294–303.
85. Chen Q, Fischer A, Reagan JD, Yan LJ, Ames BN. Oxidative DNA damage and senescence of human diploid fibroblast cells. *Proc Natl Acad Sci USA* 1995;**92**:4337–41.
86. d'Adda di Fagagna F, Reaper PM, Clay-Farrace L, Fiegler H, Carr P, von Zglinicki T, et al. A DNA damage checkpoint response in telomere-initiated senescence. *Nature* 2003; **426**:194–8.
87. Harbour JW, Dean DC. The Rb/E2F pathway: expanding roles and emerging paradigms. *Genes Dev* 2000;**14**:2393–409.
88. Serrano M, Lin AW, McCurrach ME, Beach D, Lowe SW. Oncogenic ras provokes premature cell senescence associated with accumulation of p53 and p16INK4a. *Cell* 1997;**88**:593–602.
89. Zhu JY, Woods D, McMahon M, Bishop JM. Senescence of human fibroblasts induced by oncogenic Raf. *Genes Dev* 1998;**12**:2997–3007.
90. Zhu JY, Woods D, McMahon M, Bishop JM. Senescence of human fibroblasts induced by oncogenic Raf. *Genes Dev* 1999;**12**:2997–3007.
91. Chainiaux F, Magalhaes JP, Eliaers F, Remacle J, Toussaint O. UVB-induced premature senescence of human diploid skin fibroblasts. *Int J Biochem Cell Biol* 2002;**34**:331–9.
92. Herskind C, Rodemann HP. Spontaneous and radiation-induced differentiation of fibroblasts. *Exp Gerontol* 2000;**35**:747–55.
93. Ogryzko VV, Hirai TH, Russanova VR, Barbie DA, Howard BH. Human fibroblast commitment to a senescence-like state in response to histone deacetylase inhibitors is cell cycle dependent. *Mol Cell Biol* 1996;**16**:5210–8.
94. Campisi J. Senescent cells, tumor suppression, and organismal aging: good citizens, bad neighbors. *Cell* 2005;**120**:513–22.
95. Beausejour CM, Krtolica A, Galimi F, Narita M, Lowe SW, Yaswen P, et al. Reversal of human cellular senescence: roles of the p53 and p16 pathways. *EMBO J* 2003;**22**:4212–22.
96. Narita M, Nunez S, Heard E, Lin AW, Hearn SA, Spector DL, et al. Rb-mediated heterochromatin formation and silencing of E2F target genes during cellular senescence. *Cell* 2003;**113**:703–16.
97. Harley CB, Futcher AB, Greider CW. Telomeres shorten during ageing of human fibroblasts. *Nature* 1990;**345**:458–60.
98. Blackburn E. Switching and signaling at the telomere. *Cell* 2001;**106**:661–73.
99. Allsopp RC, Chang E, Kashefi-Aazam M, Rogaev EI, Piatyszek MA, Shay JW, et al. Telomere shortening is associated with cell division in vitro and in vivo. *Exp Cell Res* 1995;**220**:194–200.
100. Bodnar AG, Ouellette M, Frolkis M, Holt SE, Chiu CP, Morin GB, et al. Extension of life-span by introduction of telomerase into normal human cells. *Science* 1998;**279**:349–52.
101. Ouellette MM, McDaniel LD, Wright WE, Shay JW, Schultz RA. The establishment of telomerase-immortalized cell lines representing human chromosome instability syndromes. *Hum Mol Genet* 2000;**9**:403–11.
102. Wood LD, Halvorsen TL, Dhar S, Baur JA, Pandita RK, Wright WE, et al. Characterization of ataxia telangiectasia fibroblasts with extended life-span through telomerase expression. *Oncogene* 2001;**20**:278–88.
103. Nakamura H, Fukami H, Hayashi Y, Kiyono T, Nakatsugawa S, Hamaguchi M, et al. Establishment of immortal normal and ataxia telangiectasia fibroblast cell lines by introduction of the hTERT gene. *J Radiat Res (Tokyo)* 2002;**43**:167–74.
104. Sharma GG, Gupta A, Wang H, Scherthan H, Dhar S, Gandhi V, et al. hTERT associates with human telomeres and enhances genomic stability and DNA repair. *Oncogene* 2003;**22**:131–46.
105. van Steensel B, Smogorzewska A, de Lange T. TRF2 protects human telomeres from end-to-end fusions. *Cell* 1998;**92**:401–13.
106. Takai H, Smogorzewska A, de Lange T. DNA damage foci at dysfunctional telomeres. *Curr Biol* 2003;**13**:1549–56.
107. Bakkenist CJ, Drissi R, Wu J, Kastan MB, Dome JS. Disappearance of the telomere dysfunction-induced stress response in fully senescent cells. *Cancer Res* 2004;**64**:3748–52.
108. Griffith JD, Comeau L, Rosenfield S, Stansel RM, Bianchi A, Moss H, et al. Mammalian telomeres end in a large duplex loop. *Cell* 1999;**97**:503–14.
109. McKee JA, Banik SS, Boyer MJ, Hamad NM, Lawson JH, Niklason LE, et al. Human arteries engineered in vitro. *EMBO Rep* 2003;**4**:633–8.
110. Minamino T, Kourembanas S. Mechanisms of telomerase induction during vascular smooth muscle cell proliferation. *Circ Res* 2001;**89**:237–43.

111. Well-Knecht KJ, Zyzak DV, Litchfield JE, et al. Mechanism of autoxidative glycosylation: identification of glyoxal and arabinose as intermediates in the autoxidative modification of proteins by glucose. *Biochemistry* 1995;**34**:3702–9.
112. Vlassara H, Bucala R, Striker L. Pathogenic effects of advanced glycosylation: biochemical, biologic, and clinical implications for diabetes and aging. *Lab Invest* 1994;**70**:138–51.
113. Nam MH, Lee HS, Seomun Y, Lee Y, Lee KW. Monocyte-endothelium-smooth muscle cell interaction in co-culture: proliferation and cytokine productions in response to advanced glycation end products. *Biochim Biophys Acta* 2011;**1810**:907–12.
114. Schneider SL, Kohn RK. Effects of age and diabetes mellitus on the solubility of collagen from human skin, tracheal cartilage and dura mater. *Exp Gerontol* 1982;**17**:185–94.
115. Makita Z, Vlassara H, Cerani A, et al. Immunochemical detection of advanced glycosylation end products in vivo. *J Biol Chem* 1992;**267**:5133–8.
116. Bucala R, Tracey K, Cerani A. Advanced glycosylation products quench nitric oxide and mediate defective endothelium dependent vasodilatation in experimental diabetes. *J Clin Invest* 1991;**87**:432–8.
117. Ross R. The pathogenesis of atherosclerosis: a perspective for the 1990S. *Nature* 1993;**362**:801–9.
118. Bucala R, Makita Z, Vega G, Grundy S, Koschinsky T, Cerami A, et al. Modification of low density lipoprotein by advanced glycation end products contributes to dyslipidemia of diabetes and renal insufficiency. *Proc Natl Acad Sci USA* 1994;**91**:9441–5.

Chapter 106

Vascular Calcification

Linda Demer and Yin Tintut
David Geffen School of Medicine at UCLA, Los Angeles, CA

CLINICAL SIGNIFICANCE

Cardiovascular calcification is prevalent, affecting nearly all patients with cardiovascular disease (1). In asymptomatic adults, the prevalence of coronary calcification corresponds roughly with age (2,3). Coronary calcification is now used as a quantitative marker for atherosclerotic plaque burden, even in early, subclinical stages (4). First recognized as extraskeletal ossification over a century ago (5,6), vascular calcium deposits were, until recently, dismissed as passive, inevitable, unregulated, and degenerative consequences of aging. While the prevalence, significance, and regulatory mechanisms of vascular calcification is increasingly recognized, research and clinical awareness remain at an early stage.

Calcific vasculopathy increases the risk of cardiovascular events even after adjustment for confounding factors (2,3,7). The primary effect of vascular calcification is likely to be impaired vascular compliance and recoil in the aorta and muscular arteries (8,9). Loss of this central hemodynamic function promotes systolic hypertension, coronary insufficiency, and intensifies cardiac energy demand. In peripheral arteries, calcification promotes ischemia, and predicts amputation (10). In microvessels, calcific uremic arteriolopathy blocks autoregulation, leading to infarction of downstream tissues (11). In cardiac valve leaflets, calcification impairs flexibility, leading to life-threatening stenosis (12). Overall, calcium deposition has a profound negative impact on cardiovascular function.

Calcium deposits may arise in the arterial neointima, media, microvessels, or valve leaflets. Neointimal calcification occurs in a patchy distribution, co-localizing with atherosclerotic lesions, whereas medial calcium deposits are distributed more diffusely, often in close association with the elastic laminae. Calcific aortic valve disease shares risk factors and some histological features with atherosclerosis. Mechanisms under investigation include oxidant stress (13), lipids (14,15), and Wnt/β-catenin/LRP5 pathway (16,17).

Histopathologically, the mineralized lesions usually have amorphous features, but about 15% contain fully formed bone (6), marrow sinusoids, or even cartilaginous tissue (18–20). Their resemblance to skeletal bone extends to the nanoscale (21). The role of calcium deposits in atherosclerotic plaque vulnerability is complex. In general, mineralization strengthens tissue; it also concentrates stress at its edges due to compliance mismatch. Finite element analysis suggests that rigid material within a compliant material, such as mineral in an artery, reduces stress in certain adjacent areas and increases it in others. The net effect on stability depends on the relative size and orientation of a mineral deposit with respect to the lumen, the direction of stress, and adjacency of lipid deposits (22).

Calcific vasculopathy is closely tied to metabolic diseases, correlating especially with atherosclerosis burden (23). By far, the most advanced calcific vasculopathy occurs in patients with chronic kidney disease (24), followed by those with type I diabetes (25), and both groups often have superimposed atherosclerosis. A paradoxical association of vascular calcification with osteoporosis has been consistently reported, and, most often, found to be independent of age (26,27). Some evidence suggests that bone loss causes vascular calcification (28,29). Other evidence suggests that inflammation causes both calcific vasculopathy and osteoporosis. Atherogenic lipids, which accumulate in bone tissue (30,31) as well as artery wall, impair differentiation of skeletal osteoblasts but promote osteoblastic differentiation of vascular smooth muscle cells (SMC) (32). Atherogenic lipids also promote bone resorption by enhancing osteoclast differentiation (33–35) and blunting anabolic effects of parathyroid hormone (36).

CLINICAL INTERACTIONS BETWEEN VASCULAR AND BONE THERAPIES

Bisphosphonates, used in osteoporosis to inhibit bone resorption, have the theoretical potential to also prevent any resorption of calcific vasculopathy. However, evidence suggests they are preventive (37), possibly through lowering lipoprotein levels (38). HMG-CoA reductase

Muscle. DOI: http://dx.doi.org/10.1016/B978-0-12-381510-1.00106-X

inhibitors (statins) are reported to inhibit (39,40) as well as promote (41) calcification and induce BMP-2 expression in SMC (42) as they do in skeletal osteoblasts (43). In mice, statins halt progression but promote little regression of calcific aortic stenosis (44). Clinical studies also show limited benefit (16). Statins are known to promote mineralization in osteoblasts, and it has been suggested that, once SMC undergo osteoblastic differentiation, their response to statins may reverse (43). High-dose dietary vitamin D has been used as an experimental model for calcific vasculopathy for decades (39,45).

In Vitro Models

Culture models of calcific vasculopathy and valvulopathy are widely used and include SMC, aortic myofibroblasts, valvular interstitial cells, and pericytes. Calcifying vascular cells, a purified subpopulation of bovine aortic SMC, produce hydroxyapatite mineral spontaneously (46), usually within raised nodules or ridges (Figure 106.1). Primary vascular SMC usually produce calcium mineral from a monolayer in a more diffuse manner but, as with primary osteoblasts, only in the presence of supplemental phosphate. Primary aortic myofibroblasts (17) and valvular interstitial and SMC (19,47) also produce mineral in nodules *in vitro*. Microvascular pericytes were the first vascular cells shown to mineralize in culture (48), and they share multilineage potential with SMC. Most of these cells undergo osteogenic differentiation while some undergo chondrogenic (49).

Regulatory factors governing vascular calcification are diverse and often enigmatic, since factors that bind mineral may have dual roles as activators and inhibitors in a context-dependent manner. Their interactions are complex, multicompartmental, and involve negative and positive feedback control (Figure 106.2).

Lipoproteins are also nanoparticles, and in oxidized form, they trigger oxidant stress, inflammation, atherogenesis, and vascular calcification. In vascular SMC, oxidant stress (50,51) induces the master regulatory, osteogenic transcription factor, Runx2. Oxidant stress due to hyperlipidemia induces pro-osteogenic signaling in the

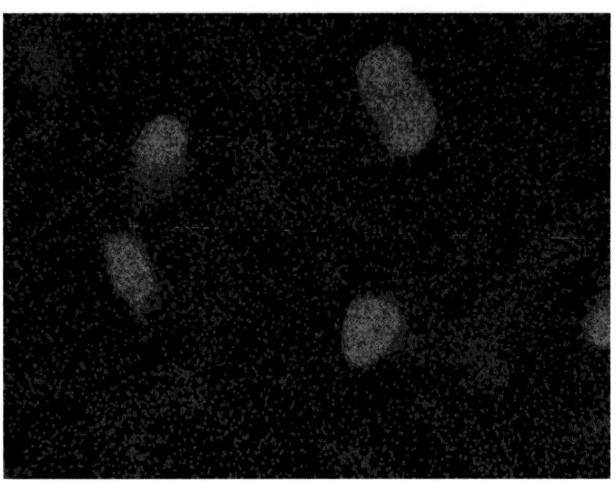

FIGURE 106.1 Nodules produced *in vitro* by calcifying vascular cells, a purified subpopulation of bovine aortic SMC.

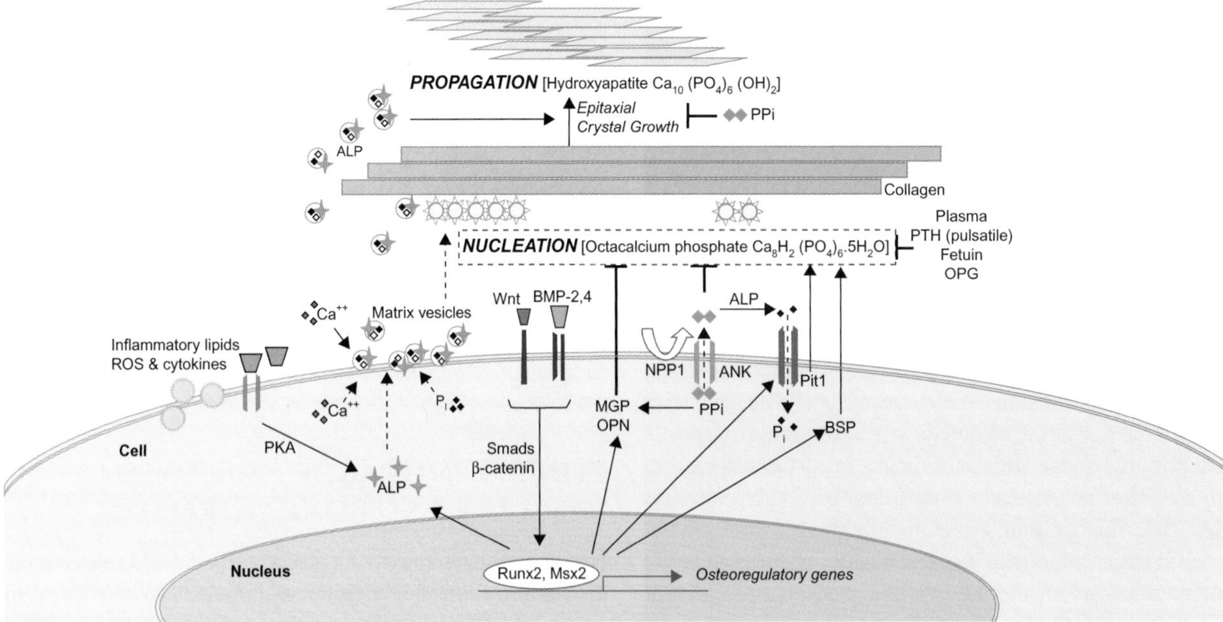

FIGURE 106.2 Schematic diagram of selected regulatory factors and their possible roles in vascular biomineralization. *(Modified from Demer LL, Tintut Y. Vascular calcification: pathobiology of a multifaceted disease. Circulation 2008;**117**:2938–48.)*

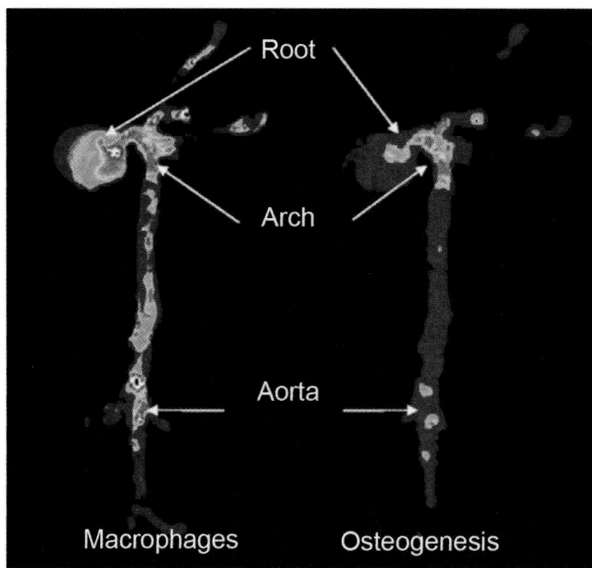

FIGURE 106.3 *In vivo* fluorescence reflectance imaging of the hyperlipidemic mouse aorta showing correspondence between macrophages and a spectrally distinct agent to detect osteogenesis. *(From Aikawa et al., 2007 (56), with permission. © American Heart Association 2007.)*

aortic valve, which can be blocked by reducing the lipid levels (52). A homeobox gene, Msx2, responds to oxidized lipoproteins and governs Wnt signaling (17) and osterix expression (53), leading to osteogenic differentiation in SMC. Mice overexpressing Msx2 develop aortic and coronary calcification through paracrine signaling (17). Calcium deposits colocalize with inflammatory cells *in vitro* (54,55) and *in vivo* (Figure 106.3) (56). Tumor necrosis factor-alpha (TNF-α) induces VSMC calcification via the Msx2/Wnt/β-catenin signaling pathway (57). TNF-α also signals through the protein kinase A pathway (54). *In vivo*, VSMC-specific TNF-α overexpression enhances Msx2-Wnt-induced calcification in hyperlipidemic mice, and its inhibition blocks calcification in these mice (58).

Endothelial cells release bone morphogenetic protein-2 (BMP-2) in response to oxidant stress, mechanical stress, and inflammatory cytokines, such as TNF-α (59). BMP-2 and BMP-4 activate Runx2 and induce ectopic mineralization via Smad signaling (60) and are antagonized by noggin and chordin, as well as matrix gamma-carboxyglutamic acid protein (MGP) (61). In contrast, another member of the transforming growth factor-β superfamily, BMP-7, inhibits vascular calcification (62). Serum levels of MGP associate with conventional cardiovascular risk factors, though not with coronary calcification (63). Expression is increased in areas of calcification (64,65), presumably due to an insufficient compensatory response. The MGP null mouse develops complete aortic chondro-ossification (66). MGP function depends on vitamin K-dependent gamma-carboxylation of glutamate residues (67), a process inhibited by warfarin, treatment with which is linked to femoral artery calcification (3). Another GLA-containing protein, Gas6, and its receptor, Axl, also inhibits VSMC calcification (68,69).

Extracellular matrix components, such as osteopontin and elastin, modulate crystal initiation and growth. Osteopontin is believed to limit hydroxyapatite crystal growth by direct binding (70,71). Elastin damage, such as by matrix metalloproteinases (MMPs), promotes vascular elastocalcinosis, in which crystals deposit along disrupted fibrils (72). MMP inhibitors attenuate aortic calcification *in vivo* (73). Elastin derangements in genetic disorders also cause elastocalcinosis, such as fibrillin deficiency (Marfan syndrome) (74), as well as in mutations of an elastin gene, ABCC6, which leads to the human disorder pseudoxanthoma elasticum (75).

Inorganic phosphate metabolism drives calcific vasculopathy of chronic kidney disease, the main cause of medial calcification, possibly through activation of a sodium-phosphate cotransporter, Pit-1, which drives Runx2 expression (76,77). An inhibitor of Pit-1, phosphonoformic acid, inhibits vascular calcification, but possibly through an independent, pyrophosphate-like, inhibitory effect on crystals (78). Inorganic phosphate is produced extracellularly by the action of alkaline phosphatase on pyrophosphate (PPi), which potently inhibits calcium phosphate mineralization. It is produced intracellularly also in VSMC, in part, by nucleotide pyrophosphatase/phosphodiesterase (NPP1) from nucleotide triphosphates, such as ATP. Disorders of this enzyme account for the fatal congenital condition, generalized arterial calcification of infancy (GACI) (79). Intracellular PPi may be exported via the transmembrane protein, Ank, deficiency of which results in vascular and joint calcification with spontaneous chondrogenic metaplasia in mice (80).

Mineral resorption is governed by three interacting molecules: receptor activator of NF-κB (RANK), its ligand (RANKL), and the ligand's soluble decoy receptor, osteoprotegerin (OPG). Serum levels of OPG correlate positively with coronary calcification (81) even in CKD patients (82–84). Yet, in mice, OPG deficiency accelerates atherosclerotic calcification (85), and RANKL inhibition by OPG or denosumab attenuates vascular calcification (86,87). It is likely that OPG associates with calcific vasculopathy as a mitigating factor, rather than a causal one.

Fetuin A is an abundant serum protein that, like osteopontin, binds and complexes calcium phosphate nanocrystals to limit growth. It accumulates at sites of vascular calcium deposition (88) and promotes scavenging of calcioprotein particles (89). *In vitro*, fetuin A taken up by VSMCs reduces the mineralization potential of secreted matrix vesicles (88,90). Clinically, low fetuin A levels are associated with more severe calcific vasculopathy and mortality in CKD patients (91).

Hormones have pleiotropic effects on calcific vasculopathy. For example, the adipose-derived factor, leptin, promotes vascular calcification *in vitro* (92) and *in vivo* (93). Adiponectin-deficient mice have increased vascular calcification (94). Parathyroid hormone inhibits vascular calcification in diabetic, hyperlipidemic mice (15) and in rats with subtotal nephrectomy (95). Moreover, constitutive activation of PTH receptor-1 (PTH1R) reduces aortic calcification via the Wnt-β-catenin pathway (96). Levels of fibroblast growth factor-23 (FGF23), secreted by bone to inhibit renal phosphate resorption, are elevated in dialysis patients and correlate significantly with vascular calcification (97,98).

Animal Models

Aortic calcification occurs in mice deficient in MGP (66), NPP1 (79), OPG (99), and fibrillin. OPG deficiency in hyperlipidemic mice increases the atherosclerotic burden despite no change in cholesterol levels (85), and OPG treatment reduces vascular calcification in a hyperlipidemic model (87). In contrast, patients with cardiovascular disease tend to have high plasma OPG levels, possibly representing an insufficient compensatory response (81–84,100,101). Osteopontin deficiency enhances the vascular calcification of apoE null mice (102). Mice deficient in the receptor for low-density lipoprotein (LDL), which develop mild hyperlipidemia and diabetes, also display atherosclerotic calcification, after about 20 weeks on a high cholesterol or atherogenic diet (103). The corresponding human disorder, homozygous familial hypercholesterolemia, is characterized by severe, premature calcific vasculopathy and valvulopathy (104). More severe atherosclerotic calcification occurs in LDLR null ($Ldlr^{-/-}$) mice that are genetically modified to synthesize only apolipoprotein B100 (105). Similarly, mice deficient in apolipoprotein E have more severe hyperlipidemia, and their atherosclerotic calcification develops calcified cartilage and a chondrogenic gene profile in their brachiocephalic arteries even on a chow diet by 10–18 months of age (85). As further evidence of the role of lipids, regression of osteogenic signaling and calcium deposition were reversed in mice engineered to genetically switch from hyperlipidemic to normolipemia (Reversa mouse) (52). Several rodent models of vascular calcification have abnormal calcium-phosphate metabolism. Rodents fed high dose adenine develop medial calcific vasculopathy, as do rats fed 1,25-dihydroxyvitamin D (106), an effect enhanced by warfarin (45,107). Mice deficient in FGF23 or its coreceptor, Klotho, also develop vascular calcification (108).

In summary, mineralization and osteogenic differentiation of SMC drives calcific vasculopathy through metabolic, mechanical, and genetic regulatory mechanisms that are shared with and interactive with bone, renal, and endocrine systems. This complex interplay is under active investigation using *in vitro* and *in vivo* models. A systems approach is essential to understanding the mechanisms underlying mineral deposition in the vasculature and avoiding conflicting treatment regimens.

REFERENCES

1. O'Rourke RA, Brundage BH, Froelicher VF, Greenland P, Grundy SM, Hachamovitch R, et al. American College of Cardiology/AHA Expert Consensus document on electron-beam computed tomography for the diagnosis and prognosis of coronary artery disease. *Circulation* 2000;**102**:126–40.
2. Budoff MJ, Shaw LJ, Liu ST, Weinstein SR, Mosler TP, Tseng PH, et al. Long-term prognosis associated with coronary calcification: observations from a registry of 25,253 patients. *J Am Coll Cardiol* 2007;**49**:1860–70.
3. Rennenberg RJ, Kessels AG, Schurgers LJ, van Engelshoven JM, de Leeuw PW, Kroon AA. Vascular calcifications as a marker of increased cardiovascular risk: a meta-analysis. *Vasc Health Risk Manag* 2009;**5**:185–97.
4. Lee CD, Jacobs Jr. DR, Schreiner PJ, Iribarren C, Hankinson A. Abdominal obesity and coronary artery calcification in young adults: the Coronary Artery Risk Development in Young Adults (CARDIA) Study. *Am J Clin Nutr* 2007;**86**:48–54.
5. Bunting CH. The formation of true bone with cellular (red) marrow in a sclerotic aorta. *J Exp Med* 1906;**8**:365–76.
6. Virchow R. *Cellular pathology: As based upon physiological and pathological histology*. New York: Dover;1863.
7. Vliegenthart R, Oudkerk M, Hofman A, Oei HH, van Dijck W, van Rooij FJ, et al. Coronary calcification improves cardiovascular risk prediction in the elderly. *Circulation* 2005;**112**:572–7.
8. Blacher J, Demuth K, Guerin AP, Safar ME, Moatti N, London GM. Influence of biochemical alterations on arterial stiffness in patients with end-stage renal disease. *Arterioscler Thromb Vasc Biol* 1998;**18**:535–41.
9. Demer LL. Effect of calcification on in vivo mechanical response of rabbit arteries to balloon dilation. *Circulation* 1991;**83**:2083–93.
10. Guzman RJ, Brinkley DM, Schumacher PM, Donahue RM, Beavers H, Qin X. Tibial artery calcification as a marker of amputation risk in patients with peripheral arterial disease. *J Am Coll Cardiol* 2008;**51**:1967–74.
11. Milas M, Bush RL, Lin P, Brown K, Mackay G, Lumsden A, et al. Calciphylaxis and nonhealing wounds: the role of the vascular surgeon in a multidisciplinary treatment. *J Vasc Surg* 2003;**37**:501–7.
12. Horstkotte D, Loogen F. The natural history of aortic valve stenosis. *Eur Heart J* 1988;**9**(Suppl. E):57–64.
13. Miller JD, Chu Y, Brooks RM, Richenbacher WE, Pena-Silva R, Heistad DD. Dysregulation of antioxidant mechanisms contributes to increased oxidative stress in calcific aortic valvular stenosis in humans. *J Am Coll Cardiol* 2008;**52**:843–50.
14. Olsson M, Thyberg J, Nilsson J. Presence of oxidized LDL in nonrheumatic stenotic aortic valves. *Arterioscler Thromb Vasc Biol* 1999;**19**:1218–22.

15. Shao JS, Cheng SL, Charlton-Kachigian N, Loewy AP, Towler DA. Teriparatide (human parathyroid hormone (1-34)) inhibits osteogenic vascular calcification in diabetic Ldlr-deficient mice. *J Biol Chem* 2003;**278**:50195–202.
16. Rajamannan NM, Subramaniam M, Caira F, Stock SR, Spelsberg TC. Atorvastatin inhibits hypercholesterolemia-induced calcification in the aortic valves via the Lrp5 receptor pathway. *Circulation* 2005;**112**:1229–34.
17. Shao JS, Cheng SL, Pingsterhaus JM, Charlton-Kachigian N, Loewy AP, Towler DA. Msx2 promotes cardiovascular calcification by activating paracrine Wnt signals. *J Clin Invest* 2005;**115**:1210–20.
18. Hunt JL, Fairman R, Mitchell ME, Carpenter JP, Golden M, Khalapyan T, et al. Bone formation in carotid plaques: a clinicopathological study. *Stroke* 2002;**33**:1214–9.
19. Mohler 3rd ER, Gannon F, Reynolds C, Zimmerman R, Keane MG, Kaplan FS. Bone formation and inflammation in cardiac valves. *Circulation* 2001;**103**:1522–8.
20. Qiao JH, Mertens RB, Fishbein MC, Geller SA. Cartilaginous metaplasia in calcified diabetic peripheral vascular disease. *Hum Pathol* 2003;**34**:402–7.
21. Duer MJ, Friscic T, Murray RC, Reid DG, Wise ER. The mineral phase of calcified cartilage: its molecular structure and interface with the organic matrix. *Biophys J* 2009;**96**:3372–8.
22. Hoshino T, Chow LA, Hsu JJ, Perlowski AA, Abedin M, Tobis J, et al. Mechanical stress analysis of a rigid inclusion in distensible material. *Am J Physiol Heart Circ Physiol* 2009;**297**:H802–10.
23. Simons DB, Schwartz RS, Edwards WD, Sheedy PF, Breen JF, Rumberger JA. Noninvasive definition of anatomic coronary artery disease by ultrafast computed tomographic scanning: a quantitative pathologic comparison study. *J Am Coll Cardiol* 1992;**20**:1118–26.
24. Moe SM, Chen NX. Pathophysiology of vascular calcification in chronic kidney disease. *Circ Res* 2004;**95**:560–7.
25. Shao JS, Cheng SL, Sadhu J, Towler DA. Inflammation and the osteogenic regulation of vascular calcification: a review and perspective. *Hypertension* 2010;**55**:579–92.
26. Persy V, D'Haese P. Vascular calcification and bone disease: the calcification paradox. *Trends Mol Med* 2009;**15**:405–16.
27. Szulc P, Kiel DP, Delmas PD. Calcifications in the abdominal aorta predict fractures in men: MINOS study. *J Bone Miner Res* 2008;**23**:95–102.
28. Barreto DV, Barreto F de C, Carvalho AB, Cuppari L, Draibe SA, Dalboni MA, et al. Association of changes in bone remodeling and coronary calcification in hemodialysis patients: a prospective study. *Am J Kidney Dis* 2008;**52**:1139–50.
29. Price PA, Faus SA, Williamson MK. Bisphosphonates alendronate and ibandronate inhibit artery calcification at doses comparable to those that inhibit bone resorption. *Arterioscler Thromb Vasc Biol* 2001;**21**:817–24.
30. Niemeier A, Niedzielska D, Secer R, Schilling A, Merkel M, Enrich C, et al. Uptake of postprandial lipoproteins into bone in vivo: impact on osteoblast function. *Bone* 2008;**43**:230–7.
31. Tintut Y, Morony S, Demer LL. Hyperlipidemia promotes osteoclastic potential of bone marrow cells ex vivo. *Arterioscler Thromb Vasc Biol* 2004;**24**:e6–e10.
32. Parhami F, Morrow AD, Balucan J, Leitinger N, Watson AD, Tintut Y, et al. Lipid oxidation products have opposite effects on calcifying vascular cell and bone cell differentiation. *Arterioscler Thromb Vasc Biol* 1997;**17**:680–7.
33. Graham LS, Parhami F, Tintut Y, Kitchen CM, Demer LL, Effros RB. Oxidized lipids enhance RANKL production by T lymphocytes: implications for lipid-induced bone loss. *Clin Immunol* 2009;**133**:265–75.
34. Tintut Y, Parhami F, Tsingotjidou A, Tetradis S, Territo M, Demer LL. 8-Isoprostaglandin E2 enhances receptor-activated NFkappa B ligand (RANKL)-dependent osteoclastic potential of marrow hematopoietic precursors via the cAMP pathway. *J Biol Chem* 2002;**277**:14221–6.
35. Tseng W, Lu J, Bishop GA, Watson AD, Sage AP, Demer L, et al. Regulation of interleukin-6 expression in osteoblasts by oxidized phospholipids. *J Lipid Res* 2010;**51**:1010–6.
36. Huang MS, Lu J, Ivanov Y, Sage A, Tseng W, Demer LL, et al. Hyperlipidemia impairs osteoanabolic effects of PTH. *J Bone Miner Res* 2008;**23**:1672–9.
37. Lomashvili KA, Monier-Faugere MC, Wang X, Malluche HH, O'Neill WC. Effect of bisphosphonates on vascular calcification and bone metabolism in experimental renal failure. *Kidney Int* 2009;**75**:617–25.
38. Adami S, Braga V, Guidi G, Gatti D, Gerardi D, Fracassi E. Chronic intravenous aminobisphosphonate therapy increases high-density lipoprotein cholesterol and decreases low-density lipoprotein cholesterol. *J Bone Miner Res* 2000;**15**:599–604.
39. Kizu A, Shioi A, Jono S, Koyama H, Okuno Y, Nishizawa Y. Statins inhibit in vitro calcification of human vascular smooth muscle cells induced by inflammatory mediators. *J Cell Biochem* 2004;**93**:1011–9.
40. Son BK, Kozaki K, Iijima K, Eto M, Kojima T, Ota H, et al. Statins protect human aortic smooth muscle cells from inorganic phosphate-induced calcification by restoring Gas6-Axl survival pathway. *Circ Res* 2006;**98**:1024–31.
41. Trion A, Schutte-Bart C, Bax WH, Jukema JW, van der Laarse A. Modulation of calcification of vascular smooth muscle cells in culture by calcium antagonists, statins, and their combination. *Mol Cell Biochem* 2008;**308**:25–33.
42. Emmanuele L, Ortmann J, Doerflinger T, Traupe T, Barton M. Lovastatin stimulates human vascular smooth muscle cell expression of bone morphogenetic protein-2, a potent inhibitor of low-density lipoprotein-stimulated cell growth. *Biochem Biophys Res Commun* 2003;**302**:67–72.
43. Wu B, Elmariah S, Kaplan FS, Cheng G, Mohler 3rd ER. Paradoxical effects of statins on aortic valve myofibroblasts and osteoblasts: implications for end-stage valvular heart disease. *Arterioscler Thromb Vasc Biol* 2005;**25**:592–7.
44. Miller JD, Weiss RM, Serrano KM, Brooks 2nd RM, Berry CJ, Zimmerman K, et al. Lowering plasma cholesterol levels halts progression of aortic valve disease in mice. *Circulation* 2009;**119**:2693–701.
45. Price PA, June HH, Buckley JR, Williamson MK. Osteoprotegerin inhibits artery calcification induced by warfarin and by vitamin D. *Arterioscler Thromb Vasc Biol* 2001;**21**:1610–6.
46. Bostrom K, Watson KE, Horn S, Wortham C, Herman IM, Demer LL. Bone morphogenetic protein expression in human atherosclerotic lesions. *J Clin Invest* 1993;**91**:1800–9.
47. Rajamannan NM, Subramaniam M, Rickard D, Stock SR, Donovan J, Springett M, et al. Human aortic valve calcification is associated with an osteoblast phenotype. *Circulation* 2003;**107**:2181–4.

48. Canfield AE, Sutton AB, Hoyland JA, Schor AM. Association of thrombospondin-1 with osteogenic differentiation of retinal pericytes in vitro. *J Cell Sci* 1996;**109**(Pt 2):343–53.
49. Neven E, Persy V, Dauwe S, De Schutter T, De Broe ME, D'Haese PC. Chondrocyte rather than osteoblast conversion of vascular cells underlies medial calcification in uremic rats. *Arterioscler Thromb Vasc Biol* 2010;**30**:1741–50.
50. Byon CH, Javed A, Dai Q, Kappes JC, Clemens TL, Darley-Usmar VM, et al. Oxidative stress induces vascular calcification through modulation of the osteogenic transcription factor Runx2 by AKT signaling. *J Biol Chem* 2008;**283**:15319–27.
51. Mody N, Parhami F, Sarafian TA, Demer LL. Oxidative stress modulates osteoblastic differentiation of vascular and bone cells. *Free Radic Biol Med* 2001;**31**:509–19.
52. Miller JD, Weiss RM, Serrano KM, Castaneda LE, Brooks RM, Zimmerman K, et al. Evidence for active regulation of pro-osteogenic signaling in advanced aortic valve disease. *Arterioscler Thromb Vasc Biol* 2010;**30**:2482–6.
53. Taylor J, Butcher M, Zeadin M, Politano A, Shaughnessy SG. Oxidized low-density lipoprotein promotes osteoblast differentiation in primary cultures of vascular smooth muscle cells by upregulating osterix expression in an Msx2-dependent manner. *J Cell Biochem* 2010; ePub ahead of print November 22, 2010, PMID: 21104819.
54. Tintut Y, Patel J, Parhami F, Demer LL. Tumor necrosis factor-alpha promotes in vitro calcification of vascular cells via the cAMP pathway. *Circulation* 2000;**102**:2636–42.
55. Tintut Y, Patel J, Territo M, Saini T, Parhami F, Demer LL. Monocyte/macrophage regulation of vascular calcification in vitro. *Circulation* 2002;**105**:650–5.
56. Aikawa E, Nahrendorf M, Figueiredo JL, Swirski FK, Shtatland T, Kohler RH, et al. Osteogenesis associates with inflammation in early-stage atherosclerosis evaluated by molecular imaging in vivo. *Circulation* 2007;**116**:2841–50.
57. Lee HL, Woo KM, Ryoo HM, Baek JH. Tumor necrosis factor-alpha increases alkaline phosphatase expression in vascular smooth muscle cells via MSX2 induction. *Biochem Biophys Res Commun* 2010;**391**:1087–92.
58. Al-Aly Z, Shao JS, Lai CF, Huang E, Cai J, Behrmann A, et al. Aortic Msx2-Wnt calcification cascade is regulated by TNF-alpha-dependent signals in diabetic Ldlr −/− mice. *Arterioscler Thromb Vasc Biol* 2007;**27**:2589–96.
59. Csiszar A, Smith KE, Koller A, Kaley G, Edwards JG, Ungvari Z. Regulation of bone morphogenetic protein-2 expression in endothelial cells: role of nuclear factor-kappaB activation by tumor necrosis factor-alpha, H_2O_2, and high intravascular pressure. *Circulation* 2005;**111**:2364–72.
60. Li X, Yang HY, Giachelli CM. BMP-2 promotes phosphate uptake, phenotypic modulation, and calcification of human vascular smooth muscle cells. *Atherosclerosis* 2008;**199**:271–7.
61. Zebboudj AF, Imura M, Bostrom K. Matrix GLA protein, a regulatory protein for bone morphogenetic protein-2. *J Biol Chem* 2002;**277**:4388–94.
62. Mathew S, Davies M, Lund R, Saab G, Hruska KA. Function and effect of bone morphogenetic protein-7 in kidney bone and the bone-vascular links in chronic kidney disease. *Eur J Clin Invest* 2006;**36**(Suppl. 2):43–50.
63. O'Donnell CJ, Shea MK, Price PA, Gagnon DR, Wilson PW, Larson MG, et al. Matrix Gla protein is associated with risk factors for atherosclerosis but not with coronary artery calcification. *Arterioscler Thromb Vasc Biol* 2006;**26**:2769–74.
64. Canfield AE, Doherty MJ, Kelly V, Newman B, Farrington C, Grant ME, et al. Matrix Gla protein is differentially expressed during the deposition of a calcified matrix by vascular pericytes. *FEBS Lett* 2000;**487**:267–71.
65. Tyson KL, Reynolds JL, McNair R, Zhang Q, Weissberg PL, Shanahan CM. Osteo/chondrocytic transcription factors and their target genes exhibit distinct patterns of expression in human arterial calcification. *Arterioscler Thromb Vasc Biol* 2003;**23**:489–94.
66. Luo G, Ducy P, McKee MD, Pinero GJ, Loyer E, Behringer RR, et al. Spontaneous calcification of arteries and cartilage in mice lacking matrix GLA protein. *Nature* 1997;**386**:78–81.
67. Schurgers LJ, Spronk HM, Skepper JN, Hackeng TM, Shanahan CM, Vermeer C, et al. Post-translational modifications regulate matrix Gla protein function: importance for inhibition of vascular smooth muscle cell calcification. *J Thromb Haemost* 2007;**5**:2503–11.
68. Collett GD, Sage AP, Kirton JP, Alexander MY, Gilmore AP, Canfield AE. Axl/phosphatidylinositol 3-kinase signaling inhibits mineral deposition by vascular smooth muscle cells. *Circ Res* 2007;**100**:502–9.
69. Son BK, Kozaki K, Iijima K, Eto M, Nakano T, Akishita M, et al. Gas6/Axl-PI3K/Akt pathway plays a central role in the effect of statins on inorganic phosphate-induced calcification of vascular smooth muscle cells. *Eur J Pharmacol* 2007;**556**:1–8.
70. Holt C, Sorensen ES, Clegg RA. Role of calcium phosphate nanoclusters in the control of calcification. *FEBS J* 2009;**276**:2308–23.
71. Wada T, McKee MD, Steitz S, Giachelli CM. Calcification of vascular smooth muscle cell cultures: inhibition by osteopontin. *Circ Res* 1999;**84**:166–78.
72. Basalyga DM, Simionescu DT, Xiong W, Baxter BT, Starcher BC, Vyavahare NR. Elastin degradation and calcification in an abdominal aorta injury model: role of matrix metalloproteinases. *Circulation* 2004;**110**:3480–7.
73. Qin X, Corriere MA, Matrisian LM, Guzman RJ. Matrix metalloproteinase inhibition attenuates aortic calcification. *Arterioscler Thromb Vasc Biol* 2006;**26**:1510–6.
74. Van Herck JL, De Meyer GR, Martinet W, Van Hove CE, Foubert K, Theunis MH, et al. Impaired fibrillin-1 function promotes features of plaque instability in apolipoprotein E-deficient mice. *Circulation* 2009;**120**:2478–87.
75. Le Saux O, Urban Z, Tschuch C, Csiszar K, Bacchelli B, Quaglino D, et al. Mutations in a gene encoding an ABC transporter cause pseudoxanthoma elasticum. *Nat Genet* 2000;**25**:223–7.
76. Jono S, McKee MD, Murry CE, Shioi A, Nishizawa Y, Mori K, et al. Phosphate regulation of vascular smooth muscle cell calcification. *Circ Res* 2000;**87**:E10–7.
77. Li X, Yang HY, Giachelli CM. Role of the sodium-dependent phosphate cotransporter, Pit-1, in vascular smooth muscle cell calcification. *Circ Res* 2006;**98**:905–12.
78. Villa-Bellosta R, Sorribas V. Phosphonoformic acid prevents vascular smooth muscle cell calcification by inhibiting calcium-phosphate deposition. *Arterioscler Thromb Vasc Biol* 2009;**29**:761–6.

79. Rutsch F, Boyer P, Nitschke Y, Ruf N, Lorenz-Depierieux B, Wittkampf T, et al. Hypophosphatemia, hyperphosphaturia, and bisphosphonate treatment are associated with survival beyond infancy in generalized arterial calcification of infancy. *Circ Cardiovasc Genet* 2008;**1**:133–40.
80. Johnson K, Goding J, Van Etten D, Sali A, Hu SI, Farley D, et al. Linked deficiencies in extracellular PP(i) and osteopontin mediate pathologic calcification associated with defective PC-1 and ANK expression. *J Bone Miner Res* 2003;**18**:994–1004.
81. Jono S, Ikari Y, Shioi A, Mori K, Miki T, Hara K, et al. Serum osteoprotegerin levels are associated with the presence and severity of coronary artery disease. *Circulation* 2002;**106**:1192–4.
82. Morena M, Terrier N, Jaussent I, Leray-Moragues H, Chalabi L, Rivory JP, et al. Plasma osteoprotegerin is associated with mortality in hemodialysis patients. *J Am Soc Nephrol* 2006;**17**:262–70.
83. Nitta K, Akiba T, Uchida K, Otsubo S, Takei T, Yumura W, et al. Serum osteoprotegerin levels and the extent of vascular calcification in haemodialysis patients. *Nephrol Dial Transplant* 2004;**19**:1886–9.
84. Rasmussen LM, Tarnow L, Hansen TK, Parving HH, Flyvbjerg A. Plasma osteoprotegerin levels are associated with glycaemic status, systolic blood pressure, kidney function and cardiovascular morbidity in type 1 diabetic patients. *Eur J Endocrinol* 2006;**154**:75–81.
85. Bennett BJ, Scatena M, Kirk EA, Rattazzi M, Varon RM, Averill M, et al. Osteoprotegerin inactivation accelerates advanced atherosclerotic lesion progression and calcification in older ApoE$^{-/-}$ mice. *Arterioscler Thromb Vasc Biol* 2006;**26**:2117–24.
86. Helas S, Goettsch C, Schoppet M, Zeitz U, Hempel U, Morawietz H, et al. Inhibition of receptor activator of NF-kappaB ligand by denosumab attenuates vascular calcium deposition in mice. *Am J Pathol* 2009;**175**:473–8.
87. Morony S, Tintut Y, Zhang Z, Cattley RC, Van G, Dwyer D, et al. Osteoprotegerin inhibits vascular calcification without affecting atherosclerosis in ldlr(−/−) mice. *Circulation* 2008;**117**:411–20.
88. Reynolds JL, Skepper JN, McNair R, Kasama T, Gupta K, Weissberg PL, et al. Multifunctional roles for serum protein fetuin-a in inhibition of human vascular smooth muscle cell calcification. *J Am Soc Nephrol* 2005;**16**:2920–30.
89. Heiss A, Eckert T, Aretz A, Richtering W, van Dorp W, Schafer C, et al. Hierarchical role of fetuin-A and acidic serum proteins in the formation and stabilization of calcium phosphate particles. *J Biol Chem* 2008;**283**:14815–25.
90. Chen NX, O'Neill KD, Chen X, Duan D, Wang E, Sturek MS, et al. Fetuin-A uptake in bovine vascular smooth muscle cells is calcium dependent and mediated by annexins. *Am J Physiol Renal Physiol* 2007;**292**:F599–606.
91. Ketteler M, Bongartz P, Westenfeld R, Wildberger JE, Mahnken AH, Bohm R, et al. Association of low fetuin-A (AHSG) concentrations in serum with cardiovascular mortality in patients on dialysis: a cross-sectional study. *Lancet* 2003;**361**:827–33.
92. Parhami F, Tintut Y, Ballard A, Fogelman AM, Demer LL. Leptin enhances the calcification of vascular cells: artery wall as a target of leptin. *Circ Res* 2001;**88**:954–60.
93. Zeadin M, Butcher M, Werstuck G, Khan M, Yee CK, Shaughnessy SG. Effect of leptin on vascular calcification in apolipoprotein E-deficient mice. *Arterioscler Thromb Vasc Biol* 2009;**29**:2069–75.
94. Luo XH, Zhao LL, Yuan LQ, Wang M, Xie H, Liao EY. Development of arterial calcification in adiponectin-deficient mice: adiponectin regulates arterial calcification. *J Bone Miner Res* 2009;**24**:1461–8.
95. Sebastian EM, Suva LJ, Friedman PA. Differential effects of intermittent PTH(1-34) and PTH(7-34) on bone microarchitecture and aortic calcification in experimental renal failure. *Bone* 2008;**43**:1022–30.
96. Cheng SL, Shao JS, Halstead LR, Distelhorst K, Sierra O, Towler DA. Activation of vascular smooth muscle parathyroid hormone receptor inhibits Wnt/beta-catenin signaling and aortic fibrosis in diabetic arteriosclerosis. *Circ Res* 2010;**107**:271–82.
97. El-Abbadi MM, Pai AS, Leaf EM, Yang HY, Bartley BA, Quan KK, et al. Phosphate feeding induces arterial medial calcification in uremic mice: role of serum phosphorus, fibroblast growth factor-23, and osteopontin. *Kidney Int* 2009;**75**:1297–307.
98. Nasrallah MM, El-Shehaby AR, Salem MM, Osman NA, El Sheikh E, Sharaf El Din UA. Fibroblast growth factor-23 (FGF-23) is independently correlated to aortic calcification in haemodialysis patients. *Nephrol Dial Transplant* 2010;**25**:2679–85.
99. Bucay N, Sarosi I, Dunstan CR, Morony S, Tarpley J, Capparelli C, et al. Osteoprotegerin-deficient mice develop early onset osteoporosis and arterial calcification. *Genes Dev* 1998;**12**:1260–8.
100. Browner WS, Lui LY, Cummings SR. Associations of serum osteoprotegerin levels with diabetes, stroke, bone density, fractures, and mortality in elderly women. *J Clin Endocrinol Metab* 2001;**86**:631–7.
101. Kiechl S, Schett G, Wenning G, Redlich K, Oberhollenzer M, Mayr A, et al. Osteoprotegerin is a risk factor for progressive atherosclerosis and cardiovascular disease. *Circulation* 2004;**109**:2175–80.
102. Matsui Y, Rittling SR, Okamoto H, Inobe M, Jia N, Shimizu T, et al. Osteopontin deficiency attenuates atherosclerosis in female apolipoprotein E-deficient mice. *Arterioscler Thromb Vasc Biol* 2003;**23**:1029–34.
103. Towler DA, Bidder M, Latifi T, Coleman T, Semenkovich CF. Diet-induced diabetes activates an osteogenic gene regulatory program in the aortas of low density lipoprotein receptor-deficient mice. *J Biol Chem* 1998;**273**:30427–34.
104. Awan Z, Alrasadi K, Francis GA, Hegele RA, McPherson R, Frohlich J, et al. Vascular calcifications in homozygote familial hypercholesterolemia. *Arterioscler Thromb Vasc Biol* 2008;**28**:777–85.
105. Heinonen SE, Leppanen P, Kholova I, Lumivuori H, Hakkinen SK, Bosch F, et al. Increased atherosclerotic lesion calcification in a novel mouse model combining insulin resistance, hyperglycemia, and hypercholesterolemia. *Circ Res* 2007;**101**:1058–67.
106. Mizobuchi M, Finch JL, Martin DR, Slatopolsky E. Differential effects of vitamin D receptor activators on vascular calcification in uremic rats. *Kidney Int* 2007;**72**:709–15.
107. Price PA, Faus SA, Williamson MK. Warfarin-induced artery calcification is accelerated by growth and vitamin D. *Arterioscler Thromb Vasc Biol* 2000;**20**:317–27.
108. Shimada T, Kakitani M, Yamazaki Y, Hasegawa H, Takeuchi Y, Fujita T, et al. Targeted ablation of Fgf23 demonstrates an essential physiological role of FGF23 in phosphate and vitamin D metabolism. *J Clin Invest* 2004;**113**:561–8.

Chapter 107

Smooth Muscle Progenitor Cells: A Novel Target for the Treatment of Vascular Disease?

Andreas Schober[1], Zhou Zhe[1] and Christian Weber[2]

[1]*Institute for Molecular Cardiovascular Research, RWTH Aachen University, Aachen, Germany,* [2]*Institut für Prophylaxe und Epidemiologie der Kreislaufkrankheiten, Munich, Germany*

INTRODUCTION

Circulating vascular progenitor cells have attracted much attention in vascular biology, because of their therapeutic potential in cardiovascular diseases. Besides the frequently studied endothelial progenitor subset (EPCs), precursors of smooth muscle cells (SPCs) have been described to play a role in vascular repair and atherosclerosis. EPCs and SPCs appear to have divergent impact on atherosclerosis, allograft vasculopathy, and neointima formation after vascular injury (1). Whereas circulating EPCs promote angiogenesis and are associated with an athero-protective effect, SPCs seem to contribute to lesion formation. Nevertheless, manipulation of the mobilization and local recruitment of SPCs promises to be a valuable strategy for the treatment of different types of atherosclerotic vascular diseases.

Classically, accumulation of medial smooth muscle cells (SMCs) in the tunica intima plays a crucial role in the pathogenesis of atherosclerosis and restenosis following angioplasty or stenting. In the past ten years, this concept has been broadened by evidence that indicates various ancestral cell candidates for neointimal SMCs, e.g., from the bone marrow (BM), the circulation, from medial and adventitial resident stem/progenitor cells (2). In this chapter we will critically review the evidence for SPCs, the mechanisms of their recruitment, and potential therapeutic strategies targeting SPCs.

THE SPC CONTROVERSY

Although EPCs are generally considered to play a significant role in neovascularization, there is still a controversy on whether SPCs are involved in vascular diseases and where they might originate. Part of this debate might be due to the complex biology of SMCs, which show a unique plasticity between a contractile and a synthetic phenotype and are derived even during normal development from multiple sources (3). The first point can make it difficult to accurately define a SPC under pathological conditions. Is the expression of markers for highly differentiated SMCs, such as SMMHC, required to identify a SMC lineage? According to this criterion, it may be difficult to detect SPCs and even SMCs, since in most vascular lesions dedifferentiated SMCs prevail, which may temporarily lose the expression of SMC markers (4,5).

Bone Marrow-Derived SPCs in the Circulation

In mouse models of post-angioplasty restenosis, graft vasculopathy and hyperlipidemia-induced atherosclerosis using bone marrow (BM)-chimeric GFP or LacZ-expressing mice, Sata et al. observed that BM-derived hematopoietic cells give rise to a substantial proportion of SMCs (up to 82% in the neointima) in diseased arteries (6). To circumvent potentially confounding effects of irradiation, parabiotic mice have been subjected to vascular injury. In line with the results from irradiated mice, circulating SPCs contributed to neointima formation in this model. A certain population of SPCs, characterized by the expression of Sca-1 and the absence of hematopoietic lineage markers (lin-) is expanded in the circulation after vascular injury in $ApoE^{-/-}$ mice and after aortic transplantation (7,8). Following injection of peripheral $Sca\text{-}1^{+}/Lin^{-}$ cells into the circulation of mice with injured carotid arteries, these cells home to the neointima and differentiate into SMMHC-expressing SMCs (7). This finding was confirmed by injection of $Sca\text{-}1^{+}/Lin^{-}$ cells, either c-kit^{+} or c-kit^{-}, which express LacZ under the control of the promoter for the SMC-specific SM22a (9). Although the first report from

Muscle. DOI: http://dx.doi.org/10.1016/B978-0-12-381510-1.00107-1

Nagai's group indicated that hematopoietic stem cells give rise to vascular SMCs, they found in a more detailed approach that other BM cell types contain SPCs. Most BM-derived α-SMA$^+$ cells were detected in the neointima after wire-induced vascular injury after transplantation of total bone marrow (6,10). Whereas the transplantation of highly purified hematopoietic stem cells did not lead to the neointimal accumulation of BM-derived SMCs, following transplantation of c-kit$^+$/Sca$^-$1$^+$/Lin$^-$ cells, α^-SMA$^+$ cells from the BM were found in the neointima, although to a lesser extent than with total BM cells. In contrast, CD11b$^+$/Ly$^-$6C$^+$ bone marrow cells, which are also recruited to the neointima, appear to express primarily α-SMA, but not SMMHC (11). Furthermore, CX$_3$CR1 expression appears to be characteristic for circulating SPCs, since CX$_3$CR1$^+$ cells are preferentially recruited to injured arteries and give rise to neointimal smooth muscle cells (12). Neointimal, BM-derived SPC accumulation has also been demonstrated after local incubation with lysophosphatidic acid (LPA) by 2-photon microscopy of BM cells that express LacZ under the SM22 promoter in perfused arteries. The fraction of SPC-derived neointimal SMCs, however, differs significantly between the types of vascular injury (13). Whereas reports on SPCs in neointima formation after mechanical injury are quite consistent, SPCs are rather infrequent in diet-induced atherosclerosis. Using genetic tracking in a mouse model with SMMHC promoter selective LacZ expression, Yu et al. showed that bone marrow-derived-SMC-like cells are present in advanced atherosclerotic plaques at low frequency. However, these cells secrete proinflammatory cytokines and mitogens, thereby promoting atherosclerosis (14). This study clearly shows that the determination only of the number of SPCs in the lesion is not sufficient to assess their functional contribution to plaque growth (2).

Of note, SMC can be differentiated from CD34$^+$ human circulating progenitor cells and bone marrow cells *in vitro,* termed smooth muscle outgrowth cells (SOCs), by the addition of PDGF-BB (15). In patients with coronary in-stent restenosis, circulating CD34$^+$ cells were increased early after stent implantation (16,17). In addition, the number of SMCs differentiated *in vitro* from peripheral blood mononuclear cells (PBMCs) was selectively increased in patients with in-stent restenosis, indicating that injury-induced mobilization of SPCs is critical in neointima formation (16). Furthermore, CD34$^+$ cells, which express the PDGF-BB receptor CD140, but not CD34$^+$KDR$^+$ EPCs, are increased in patients with cardiac allograft vasculopathy and correlate with the degree of angiographically determined transplant arteriosclerosis (18). In addition, a subfraction of PBMCs, which express CD14 and CD105 (the TGF-β coreceptor endoglin), can be differentiated into SMCs *in vitro* by gradual stimulation with PDGF-BB and TGF-β. Interestingly, freshly isolated PBMCs, but not THP-1 monocytes, already express α-SMA and SM22 mRNA and these cells display a pro-inflammatory phenotype, including increased production of INF-γ and MMP-9, following *in vitro* differentiation into SMCs (19). Although CD14$^+$CD105$^+$ cells are increased in patients with coronary artery disease, indicating a pro-atherogenic role, it is unclear whether these cells are actually recruited to atherosclerotic lesions. Myeloid specific-antigens, such as CD14 and CD68, but not CD11b or CD45, were also described on SOCs and in recipient derived SMCs of newly formed arteries in cardiac allografts (6).

Despite these numerous studies demonstrating the role of circulating SPCs, the origin of SPCs and the extent to which they contribute to vascular lesion formation is highly controversial, since several studies reported negative results (20). However, this might be partially due to a simplified concept of vascular repair by SPCs, which expects SPCs to be present under all circumstances in a high number and in different vascular disease models. Tanaka et al. have shown that the recruitment of SPCs crucially depends on the type of vascular injury and the degree of apoptosis of the medial SMCs (21). This study indicates that the recruitment of circulating SPCs is required, if the vascular repair through resident SMCs is precluded due to extensive apoptosis of medial SMCs. This might also explain the controversial findings in various models of transplant arteriosclerosis. This concerns the type of transplantation, e.g. aorta to aorta, aorta to carotid, carotid to carotid, cardiac transplantation, or vein grafting, and the mouse strains used, e.g. BALB/c into C57BL/6 mice with B6 bone marrow, C57BL/6 grafts into BALB/c mice with transplanted BALB/c bone marrow, or BALB/c grafts into B6 mice with SM22-LacZ expressing bone marrow. Although all of these models lead to lesion formation, the exact mechanism of neointimal SMC accumulation may vary due to different degrees of medial SMC apoptosis. Furthermore, each method to identify SPCs has its own limitation and the interpretation of the findings must take this into account. Currently, reporter gene expression under a SMC-specific promoter appears to be the most advanced technology, because the difficulties of interpreting overlays from different types of stainings, which may occur, for example, in the combination of in situ hybridization for the Y chromosome and the immunostainings for SMC markers, are avoided. Promoters of SMC markers, such as SMMHC or SM22, which are expressed during advanced stages of SMC differentiation, have been used primarily to drive the reporter gene expression (22). However, this may underestimate the real contribution of SPCs due to an early stage of differentiation of neointimal SMCs where these markers are not expressed. A further source of variability relates to often-used bone marrow transplantation studies. Various irradiation protocols exist and the susceptibility of different mouse strains to irradiation is distinct (23). Although most studies grossly determine the chimerism rate in peripheral blood cells, it is unclear how fast specific progenitor cells from the BM recover following transplantation. In some mouse strains, the usual interval of 3–4 weeks between irradiation and the start of the experiment may not be enough to allow full recovery of SPCs (or only of a subpopulation of SPCs) in the BM. This is especially problematic if negative findings are generalized. In summary, considering the numerous reports that convincingly demonstrated the contribution of circulating SPCs in vascular disease models, studies reporting negative results might rather provide clues for specific mechanisms of SPC-mediated repair that are absent in these models than to disprove the whole concept.

Alternative Sources of SPCs

Heterogeneous SMCs subpopulations have been found in the media of arterial vessels (5,24,25). Frid et al. (26) described a non-muscle medial cell population with unique growth characteristics *in vitro*. These cells might probably be related to the progenitor cells, termed "side population", isolated from the media of murine aortas characterized by the expression of the stem cell antigen (Sca)-1 in the absence of c-kit and hematopoietic lineage markers (lin-) (27). Of note, these media-derived SP cells did not differentiate into lymphoid of myeloid cells *in vitro*, but develop an endothelial or SMC phenotype when stimulated with VEGF or TGF-β/PDGF-BB, respectively (27). In addition, mesenchymal stem cells have been retrieved from the media of adult human and animal aortas, which express smooth muscle cell markers upon stimulation with serum (28). Although these reports raise the possibility that arterial vessels harbor the potential of repair by endogenous SPCs, most studies rely on *in vitro* findings. Thus, the role of media-derived SPCs in the normal vessel homeostasis and the contribution to neointimal lesion formation remains to be determined (25). Resident vascular progenitors, which differentiate into endothelial cells and SMCs *in vitro*, have been detected in human coronary vessels. Injection of these human VPCs into dogs with myocardial ischemia resulted in the incorporation into newly formed large coronary arteries, primarily as SMCs (29).

Several studies have highlighted the role of the adventitia in vascular remodeling after mechanical injury, which induces an inflammatory reaction in the perivascular area (5,25). The contribution of α-SMA negative adventitial cells to SMC-like cells in the neointima has been described at least after severe endoluminal injury. Hu et al. (30) found in the adventitia of the aortic root, in contrast to other tissues, an enrichment of cells that express murine stem cell markers, such as Sca-1, c-kit, or Flk-1. Isolated $Sca^{-}1^{+}$ adventitial cells from the aortic root differentiate into SMCs *in vitro* after stimulation with PDGF-BB. Even more intriguing, the perivascularly transplanted $Sca^{-}1^{+}$ cells contributed significantly to the SMCs in neointimal lesions of vein grafts indicating that these cells migrate through the vessel wall and differentiate to SMCs upon atherogenic stimuli. This would explain previous findings that recipient, but not BM-derived cells were found in the neointima of transplant arteriosclerosis. Moreover, Sonic hedgehog (Shh) signaling appears to play a major role in the function of $Sca^{-}1^{+}$ cells of the aortic root, since adventitial $Sca^{-}1^{+}$ cells were dramatically reduced in $Shh^{-/-}$ mice (31). In humans, $CD44^{+}$ multipotent progenitors have been identified in the vessel wall, which can differentiate into SMCs and contribute to vessel formation in Matrigel (32).

However, clear evidence for a role of endogenous adventitial or vessel wall resident SPCs in atherosclerotic vascular diseases is still lacking.

SPCs IN VASCULAR DISEASES

SPCs in Atherosclerosis

SMC accumulation in atherosclerotic lesions is characteristic for advanced atherosclerotic plaques and is supposed to enhance plaque stability. During early lesion development, however, SMCs are known to play a role in the progression of atherosclerosis, partly due to proinflammatory effects. The chronic apoptosis of smooth muscle cells due to IL-1β-induced inflammation, however, accelerates atherosclerosis suggesting that lesional SMCs may limit atherogenesis (18).

Sata et al. (6) reported that a significant amount of cells immunopositive for α-SMA in murine atherosclerotic plaques originate from BM-derived progenitors (between 40 and 60%, respectively) as determined in $ApoE^{-/-}$ mice expressing either eGFP or β-galactosidase in BM cells. In addition, Nagai's group also studied the expression of SMC differentiation markers in BM-derived lesional cells of hyperlipidemic $ApoE^{-/-}$ mice by transplantation of BM cells, which express a reporter gene under the control of the SMMHC or the α-SMA promoter. In contrast to their previous study, only a minor fraction of plaque cells expressed EGFP driven by the human α-SMA promoter. This suggests that the two methods used to detect SPCs, double immunostaining and the α-SMA-driven expression of the EGFP transgene, do not match quantitatively. Either the immunostainings were not quite specific or the expression of the α-SMA EGFP transgene was lower than the actual endogenous α-SMA protein expression, probably due to differences between the human and mouse α-SMA promoter activity. Moreover,

ApoE$^{+/+}$ BM cells were used for transplantation into ApoE$^{-/-}$ mice in these studies, which is known to result in a reduced size and deviant composition of the plaques due to reduced serum cholesterol levels compared to mice which are also ApoE$^{-/-}$ in BM cells (33). In addition, in both studies plaque analysis was performed after 8 weeks of a high fat diet. After this short time of hyperlipidemia the plaques are usually small and contain only a limited number of SMCs. In contrast, Bentzon et al. studied ApoE$^{-/-}$ mice after transplantation of ApoE$^{-/-}$ BM cells that ubiquitously express eGFP after 12 and 24 weeks of a high fat diet (34). They were not able to detect α-SMA/eGFP double-positive cells in atherosclerotic plaques. Furthermore, when they studied collar-induced plaque formation after syngenic carotid artery grafting in ApoE$^{-/-}$ mice with eGFP-expressing BM cells, only resident α-SMA-positive cells were detected in the plaques (34). The difficulties of reporting negative findings are illustrated by the study of Yu et al. (8), where 0.7% of plaque cells were BM-derived SMCs expressing β-galactosidase through SMMHC-specific Cre-recombinase activation. This elegant study performed BMT of SMMHC-Cre/ROSA26R/ApoE$^{-/-}$ cells into ApoE$^{-/-}$ mice and studied the atherosclerotic lesions after 22 weeks of a high fat diet. Thereby, the authors confirmed that, although infrequently, SPCs are recruited to atherosclerotic plaques and, moreover, express markers of highly differentiated SMCs, which contrasts with the findings of Iwata et al., probably due to their use of a model of very early atherosclerosis (22). Even more interesting, Yu et al. found a proatherogenic role of SPCs, since apoptosis of lesional SPCs induced by chronic diphtheria toxin treatment of ApoE$^{-/-}$ mice with SM22a-hDTR/ApoE$^{-/-}$ BM significantly reduced atherosclerosis (14). This suggests that even a small number of SPCs might have a great impact on lesion formation, for example, due to secretion of proinflammatory cytokines and promotion of SMC proliferation and collagen synthesis (22).

In attempt to investigate the role of circulating SPCs in the healing of ruptured atherosclerotic plaques (2,5), Bentzon et al. analyzed atherosclerotic plaques of ApoE$^{-/-}$ mice that were transplanted with eGFP^{+}/ApoE$^{-/-}$ BM cells at the age of 18 months. Subsequently, the arteries were collected within 24 hours after the spontaneous death of the mice. Intraplaque hemorrhage, which was considered as a sign of recent plaque disruption, was observed in some plaques. In these hemorrhagic plaques no bone marrow-derived α-SMA positive cells were detected. Taking into account the debate about the difficulties of studying plaque rupture in mouse models of atherosclerosis (35,36), the cause for the intraplaque hemorrhage, especially after irradiation of advanced plaques, remains to be determined. Furthermore, the delay between the death of the mice and the harvesting of the arteries in this study might favor post mortem accumulation of red blood cells in the plaques. To further corroborate these findings, plaque rupture was initiated by inserting a needle from the luminal side. Again, no α-SMA positive bone marrow cells were detected 4 weeks after the needle-induced plaque rupture (37). Of note, histological sections were taken at 100 μm intervals, which does not rule out that SPCs were missed. Thus, it remains questionable if these findings can be generalized and allow the conclusion that SPCs do not contribute to the healing of ruptured plaques. In addition, the data from Yu et al. regarding the proatherogenic role of SPCs would be compatible with the view that endogenous SPCs actually promote plaque rupture rather than being involved in the healing process (22).

In humans with sex-mismatched BM transplantation because of hematologic neoplasia, Caplice et al. found by combined *in situ* hybridization and immunostaining that up to 10% of the SMCs in atherosclerotic plaques in coronary arteries were actually BM-derived (38). Interestingly, human SPCs derived from the circulation of patients with coronary artery disease and differentiated *in vitro* by PDGF-BB into SMMHC^{+} SMCs, were significantly reduced in patients with acute coronary syndrome compared with stable coronary artery disease (39). Of note, chronic treatment with culture expanded human SPCs derived from CD34^{+}-enriched human umbilical cord blood significantly reduced atherosclerotic lesion formation in ApoE$^{-/-}$/RAG$^{-/-}$ mice, but did not affect the progression of already established lesions (39). The cellular composition of the plaques following SPC injections was in both groups characterized by diminished macrophage content. The number of recruited human SPCs, however, was scarce at day 4 and no longer detectable at 2 weeks after SPC treatment, indicating that these SPCs only temporarily enter the plaques (2,5,40). Interestingly, treatment with EPCs had no effect on lesion development and formation.

SPCs in Transplant Arteriosclerosis

After transplantation of vascularized organs, such as the heart or kidney, chronic rejection characterized by accelerated arteriosclerosis in the graft is a major limitation of the long-term survival of patients. This graft vasculopathy is mediated by T-cell-dependent injury to the medial SMCs and subsequent progressive intimal thickening due to the accumulation of mostly SMCs (41).

The first evidence for the contribution of SPCs to neointimal lesions came from small animal studies following vascular or cardiac transplantation as a model for graft arteriopathy, which allows the proper tracking of the origin of lesional cells by using transgenic mice as hosts that express a reporter gene, such as β-galactosidase, or by sex-mismatched transplantation (42,43). Murine aortic transplantation into β-galactosidase expressing recipients showed that intimal SMCs can be derived from host cells. Hillebrands and co-workers also found by immunostaining and single-cell PCR that neointimal SMCs in murine transplant arteriosclerosis are host-derived (44). Similarly, heterotopic cardiac transplantation in mice (129/SvJ hearts to C57BL/6x129/S recipients) showed that the majority of neointimal SMCs originate from the recipient (up to 88%) and expressed the full range of SMC differentiation markers, such as SMMHC, calponin, h-caldesmon, and α-SMA. Interestingly, the same group could not confirm this finding when C3H/HeN hearts were transplanted into C57BL/6 recipients, because no recipient-derived neointimal cells were found which express SMMHC (14). Furthermore, BM transplantation of β-galactosidase- or eGFP-expressing cells into aortic or cardiac allograft recipients demonstrated that host-derived intimal SMCs, which express α-SMA, but not SMMHC, can originate from the BM (6,11). This is in accordance with a previous study by Hu et al. using aortic allografts (BALB/c aortas into C57BL/6 mice), which showed that 5–10% of the neointima cells were α-SMA$^+$ BM-derived cells. However, none of the BM-derived neointimal cells exhibited SM22 promoter activity (45). The BM origin of neointimal SMCs has also been reported in a model of aortic allotransplantation in rats following sex-mismatched BM transplantation. Of note, the allogenic immune response appears to be critical for both the destruction of the medial SMCs and the intimal accumulation of host-derived SMCs. Transplantation of carotid arteries from BALB/c mice into eGFP$^+$/ApoE$^{-/-}$ (C57BL/6) mice was performed as an additional model of allograft vasculopathy. In this model, allografts were repopulated by recipient cells primarily from the region flanking the grafted artery (20). Apart from potential differences due to the vessels used for transplantation, the latter study in particular raises the question of whether, at least for studying the role of SPCs in transplant arteriosclerosis, the transplantation of whole organs, such as the heart, is the superior model, because it more closely resembles the clinical situation, where ingrowth of vascular cells from the recipient into the coronary tree may hardly occur.

In humans, graft vasculopathy in transplanted kidneys, for instance, is characterized by a significant accumulation of host-derived SMCs in the vessel wall. Furthermore, Quaini et al. (46) showed a high frequency of recipient-derived cells in the myocardium, coronary arterioles, including SMCs, and capillaries of eight hearts that were transplanted from a female donor to male recipient. Similarly, various studies demonstrated that SMCs in pathologic coronary arteries from transplanted hearts are to a significant extent host-derived (2,40).

SPCs in Mechanical Vascular Injury

Wire- or balloon-induced mechanical vascular injury induces apoptosis of medial SMCs and the adhesion of platelets and leukocytes to the denuded arterial wall (2,47). The vascular repair is characterized by the intimal accumulation of mainly phenotypically distinct SMCs. An exacerbated vascular repair leads to critical narrowing of the injured vessel, clinically encountered as in-stent restenosis.

Because large parts of the medial layer become acellular after injury, it has been supposed that medial SMCs can hardly account for the generation of neointimal SMCs. The first report showing that BM-derived cells are a source for neointimal SMCs (44%) following mechanical injury already indicated the central role of the severity of the vascular injury (48). Sata et al. confirmed this finding after femoral wire injury in mice with β-galactosidase expressing BM cells. Double positivity for β-galactosidase and α-SMA revealed the recruitment of SPCs to the injured artery. Tanaka et al. investigated the contribution of BM cells in a variety of vascular injury models and found that the origin of intimal cells is diverse and that the contribution of BM-derived cells to neointimal hyperplasia was most prominent after wire injury (21). Neointimal SPCs, however, were also detected after cuff-induced injury and ligation of the carotid artery (21). The number of recruited SPCs was closely related to the degree of apoptosis in the injured vessel wall (21). A diverse pattern of neointimal SPCs was revealed in parabiotic mice after femoral wire injury, including CD45$^+$ and CD45$^-$ subpopulations (49). In a carotid wire injury model, CX3CR1$^+$ SPCs, expressing α-SMA, calponin, or SMMHC, formed 5–7% of the neointimal SMCs (12). Iwata et al (11), however, observed that BM-derived SMC-like cells in the neointima remain in a poorly differentiated state expressing α-SMA but not SMMHC. Furthermore, SPC recruitment into neointimal lesions appears to occur primarily in the early phase following injury and to decline substantially in chronic lesions (11). Interestingly, α-SMA expressing neointimal BM-derived cells, in contrast to medial SMCs, were found to express surface markers of inflammatory monocytes (11). It was deduced from this finding that monocytes/macrophages are a major source for the BM derived α-SMA positive cells. It remains, however, unclear if these cells are really comparable to "monocytes/macrophages", because macrophages were previously reported to be absent in lesions after wire-induced injury of the femoral artery in non-hyperlipidemic mice (11). Moreover, the mutually exclusive expression of macrophage markers and α-SMA has been used in several studies to discriminate lesional macrophages from BM-derived SPCs, which makes a considerable expression of α-SMA in monocytes/macrophages highly unlikely (2,47).

Taken together, the evidence for the contribution of SPCs to neointima formation following mechanical vascular injury is quite consistent, although the terminal differentiation into SMCs is under debate. Interestingly, the presence of SPCs in the neointima seems to vanish over time, indicating the requirement for progenitor cell-mediated repair in the early phase after the injury. Furthermore, different phenotypes of SPCs might be able to contribute to vascular healing.

MOLECULAR MECHANISMS OF INTIMAL SPC ACCUMULATION

The CXC chemokine stromal cell-derived factor-1α (SDF-1α, CXCL12) and its receptor CXCR4 have been shown to play a crucial role in the mobilization and homing of BM-derived progenitors after vascular injury (18,50). CXCL12 is constitutively expressed in various tissues and was originally found in the supernatant of BM stromal cells (51). CXCL12 binds to the G protein-coupled seven transmembrane receptor (GPCR) CXCR4 and to CXCR7 (RDC1/Cmkor1). Under normal conditions, the high CXCL12 expression in the BM retains hematopoietic progenitor cells and disruption of the CXCL12 gradient between the peripheral blood and the BM, e.g. by increased circulating CXCL12 levels or inhibition of CXCR4, induces mobilization of stem cells (52). It has been reported that increased CXCL12 expression particularly in SMCs and transient rise of CXCL12 in plasma levels occur after different types of vascular injury (53). The wire-induced carotid injury resulted in prominent CXCL12 expression in the media within 24 hours which remains increased throughout the vessel wall during neointima formation. This injury-induced CXCL12 expression is inhibited by blocking caspase-dependent apoptosis of medial SMCs (50). In addition, vascular injury activates platelets which subsequently release CXCL12 or immobilize CXCL12 on their surface after adhesion to the denuded vessel wall. Lack of the Angiotensin II type 1 receptor (Agtr1) on platelets reduces the release of CXCL12, which appears responsible for the diminished recruitment of vascular progenitor cells to the injured artery in mice with $Agtr1^{-/-}$ BM (54). The increase in circulating CXCL12 induces the mobilization of $Sca\text{-}1^{+}/Lin^{-}$ SPCs, preferentially $c\text{-}kit^{-}/Sca\text{-}1^{+}/Lin^{-}$ SPCs expressing the PDGF receptor β, which lack the long-term repopulating potential of hematopoietic stem cells. The local/system blockade or genetic deficiency of CXCL12 or CXCR4, e.g. by local gene transfer of a CXCL12 antagonist peptide or BM reconstitution with fetal hematopoietic stem cells from $CXCR4^{-/-}$ mice, alleviated the neointima formation induced by vascular injury due to a reduced recruitment of circulating SPCs (50,55). Injury-induced apoptosis of medial SMCs triggers, by releasing apoptotic bodies, the expression of CXCL12 which might signal the demand for BM-derived SPCs in vascular repair to overcome the cellular deficit (50). Compared to carotid ligation and periarterial cuff placement, wire-induced arterial injury causes more extensive apoptosis of medial cells and induces the highest neointimal CXCL12 levels. The molecular mechanism of CXCL12 expression through apoptotic bodies, however, remains to be determined. Lysophosphatidic acid (LPA) is generated during shedding of membrane microvesicles and induces neointima formation after short-term intravascular incubation even without any mechanical injury (56). Interestingly, treatment of murine carotid arteries with LPA induced CXCL12 expression and the CXCL12-dependent mobilization of SPCs through activating the LPA receptors LPA1 and LPA3 in the vessel wall. Furthermore, the neointimal recruitment of SPCs by LPA was detected in mice with SM22-LacZ expressing BM cells by 2-photon microscopy of *ex vivo* perfused carotid arteries. Accordingly, pharmacological inhibition of LPA1 and LPA3 reduced the neointima formation after carotid wire-injury mainly by reducing the SMC content, suggesting that LPA plays a critical role after vascular injury (13). In addition to a diminished CXCL12 expression, treatment with an LPA1/LPA3 reduced HIF-1α in the neointima (13). HIF-1α is known to transcriptionally upregulate CXCL12 and to mediate the injury-induced neointimal CXCL12 expression (57). Silencing of the increased HIF-1α expression reduces neointimal hyperplasia and blocks the mobilization of SPCs after vascular injury (57). In summary, these results suggest that the formation of apoptotic bodies from medial SMCs following mechanical injury leads to the formation of LPA, which in turn triggers the HIF-1α-dependent CXCL12 expression via LPA1 and LPA3 (Figure 107.1).

The PI3K/Akt antagonist PTEN (phosphatase and tensin homolog) is critically for the suppression of PI3K-dependent HIF-1α activation in normal SMCs. Deletion of PTEN in SMCs leads to medial hyperplasia by SMC proliferation and progenitor cell recruitment through HIF-1α mediated upregulation of CXCL12 (58). Following wire-induced femoral injury, PTEN-deficiency in SMCs leads to exacerbated neointima formation mediated by CXCL12, primarily due to the recruitment of Mac3-positive bone marrow cells (59). It remains unclear, however, whether PTEN is actually downregulated in SMCs following vascular injury and thus really contributes to the injury-induced upregulation of HIF-1α and CXCL12 in the artery.

Several other molecules have been identified that affect the CXCL12-mediated neointima formation and SPC recruitment. Syndecan-4, which mediates CXCL12 signalling, expressed in the vascular wall and on BM cells is involved in SPC mobilization and promotes neointima

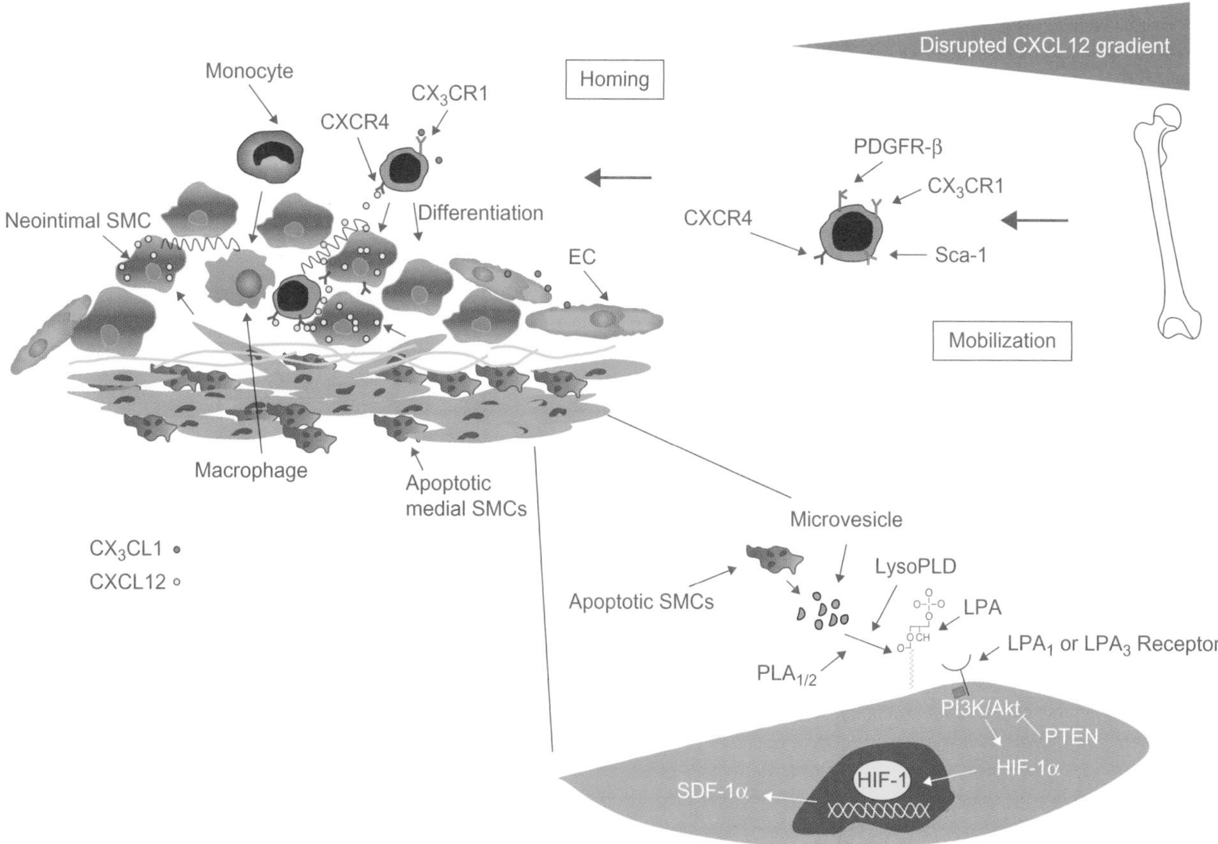

FIGURE 107.1 The CXCL12/CXCR4 axis controls vascular repair by smooth muscle progenitor cells (SPCs). The formation of apoptotic bodies from medial SMCs following mechanical injury leads to the formation of LPA, presumably through PI3K/Akt, which in turn triggers the HIF-1α-dependent CXCL12 expression via LPA1 and LPA3. CX3CR1/ CX3CL1 may also be functionally involved in the accumulation of BM-derived SPCs in neointimal lesions by inducing the differentiation of SPCs into SMCs.

formation (60). Furthermore, the adenosine receptor (A2b) suppresses the expression of CXCR4 in BM-derived cells (61). Hence, neointima formation in mice with A2b adenosine receptor deficiency was significantly increased (61). The deficiency of eNOS increased the expression of CXCL12 in ligated carotid arteries and induced a prolonged mobilization of Sca-1^+/Lin-/c-kit-cells into the circulation (62). This implicates a central role of eNOS in the regulation of CXCL12 expression in a vascular injury model without endothelial denudation.

In addition to the CXCL12/CXCR4 axis, Kumar et al. have shown that the chemokine CX_3CR1 is functionally involved in the accumulation of bone marrow-derived SPCs in neointimal lesions (6). This may be attributed to the effect of CX_3CL1 on the differentiation of SPCs.

THERAPEUTIC OPTIONS OF TARGETING SPCs

Neointimal SMC accumulation crucially contributes to the lesion formation in atherosclerosis, restenosis, and transplant arteriosclerosis. In restenotic neointima formation and allograft vasculopathy, neointimal SMCs appear to primarily be a part of the response to the acute injury (mechanical after stent implantation or immunological in transplanted organs) to the vessel wall, especially the media, and the subsequent loss of medial SMCs. If this vascular repair is exacerbated, stenosis of the vessels forms and may limit the blood and oxygen supply. Therefore, therapeutic strategies predominantly focus on limiting the SMC accumulation in the intima to avoid the critical reduction of the blood flow. In atherosclerosis, however, the role of SMCs seems more complex. Atherosclerotic lesions develop within decades and progress from early, macrophage-rich plaques into complex lesions with a lipid core and a SMC containing fibrous cap. In addition, there is no acute loss of or injury to the medial SMCs, but instead there is endothelial dysfunction, for instance through modified LDL particles and subsequent monocyte infiltration (63). Different functional roles of SMCs in terms of atherosclerosis outcome have been discussed. Whereas SMCs in early lesions might contribute to lesion formation, e.g. through a pro-inflammatory phenotype, the SMC content in the fibrous cap of advanced lesions has been suggested to stabilize the plaques and prevent the catastrophic event of plaque rupture and acute, thrombotic obstruction of the artery.

Currently, the therapeutic options to modify the lesional SMC content are limited. Statins are well established in the prevention of atherosclerosis through lowering lipid levels and effects on vascular cells. One of those pleiotropic effects of statins has been related to vascular progenitor cells: statins increase the circulation of endothelial progenitor cells and the number of SOCs from peripheral mononuclear cells (64,65). In hypoxia-induced pulmonary hypertension, pravastatin reduces the recruitment of bone marrow-derived SPCs and prevents the hypoxia-induced up-regulation of CXCL12 (66). Therefore, the therapeutic benefits of statins might be partially related to its effects on SPCs.

The current mainstay of the prevention of in-stent restenosis (ISR) is the use of drug-eluting stents. Sirolimus has been extensively studied as an antiproliferative compound coated in DES and prevents very effectively the ISR in the clinical setting. Of note, sirolimus reduces the outgrowth of SM- and endothelial-like cells from mononuclear cells from the peripheral blood (2). Furthermore, local application of sirolimus to an injured artery results in diminished neointima formation with a decreased number of SPCs. Accordingly, sirolimus-eluting stents appear to prevent the mobilization of $CD34^+$ cells after stent implantation, which typically occurs in patients with ISR. In addition, the outgrowth of α-SMA^+ cells from circulating mononuclear cells typically increased in patients with ISR, was not observed after sirolimus-eluting stent implantation. Hence, part of the beneficial effect of sirolimus in the prevention of ISR may be actually due to the suppression of SPCs. Sirolimus, however, has been shown to delay re-endothelization and to promote the formation of lipid rich lesions, which both are discussed to increase the risk for late stent thrombosis (67). This may be explained by the unspecific antiproliferative effect of sirolimus, which affects SMCs and endothelial cells. Therefore, drugs for the coating of stents that selectively prevent the intimal accumulation of SMCs without targeting the endothelium would be desirable. In this regard, inhibition of neointimal SPC recruitment is a reasonable therapeutic strategy. Interestingly, blocking CXCR4 through systemic application of the CXCR4 antagonist AMD3465 has been shown to effectively reduce neointima formation and impair SPC mobilization after carotid injury in $ApoE^{-/-}$ mice. The re-endothelization, however, was not affected by AMD3465 (50). The interference with the CXCL12/CXCR4 axis might therefore be a promising therapeutic alternative in the prevention of ISR, e.g. through stent coating of drugs that inhibit CXCR4. Moreover, $CD34^+CD140^+$ peripheral cells, which express α-SMA, correlate with the degree of cardiac allograft vasculopathy and circulating CXCL12 levels in patients after heart transplantation (18). This indicates that the CXCL12/CXCR4 axis mediates the recruitment of SPCs in human transplant arteriosclerosis, similar to what has been observed in mice. Chronic inhibition of CXCR4 by systemic administration of a CXCR4 antagonist, however, might not be applicable for transplant atherosclerosis, since neutrophilia, which exacerbates naïve atherosclerosis, has been found after treatment with AMD3465 in $ApoE^{-/-}$ mice (68). The full contribution of CXCL12 in atherogenesis is, however, still incompletely understood. In genome-wide association studies two SNPs associated with coronary artery disease have been identified that result in increased plasma CXCL12 levels indicating a proatherogenic function (69).

Besides a strategy that aims to interfere with the recruitment of SPCs, cellular therapies to stabilize atherosclerotic plaques or promote ischemic neovascularization by SPCs have been investigated (5,50). More studies, however, are required due to the potentially pro-atherogenic function of endogenous SPCs to address these issues. Especially the identification of the molecular mechanisms involved in SPC recruitment and differentiation might aid in this respect.

REFERENCES

1. Hristov M, Weber C. Ambivalence of progenitor cells in vascular repair and plaque stability. *Curr Opin Lipidol* 2008;**19**:491–7.
2. van Oostrom O, Fledderus JO, de Kleijn D, Pasterkamp G, Verhaar MC. Smooth muscle progenitor cells: friend or foe in vascular disease? *Curr Stem Cell Res Ther* 2009;**4**:131–40.
3. Owens GK, Kumar MS, Wamhoff BR. Molecular regulation of vascular smooth muscle cell differentiation in development and disease. *Physiol Rev* 2004;**84**:767–801.
4. Kane NM, Xiao Q, Baker AH, Luo Z, Xu Q, Emanueli C. Pluripotent stem cell differentiation into vascular cells: a novel technology with promises for vascular re(generation). *Pharmacol Ther* 2011;**129**:29–49.
5. Orlandi A, Bennett M. Progenitor cell-derived smooth muscle cells in vascular disease. *Biochem Pharmacol* 2010;**79**:1706–13.
6. Sata M, Saiura A, Kunisato A, Tojo A, Okada S, Tokuhisa T, et al. Hematopoietic stem cells differentiate into vascular cells that participate in the pathogenesis of atherosclerosis. *Nat Med* 2002;**8**: 403–9.
7. Schober A, Knarren S, Lietz M, Lin EA, Weber C. Crucial role of stromal cell-derived factor-1alpha in neointima formation after vascular injury in apolipoprotein E-deficient mice. *Circulation* 2003;**108**:2491–7.
8. Zernecke A, Weber C. Chemokines in the vascular inflammatory response of atherosclerosis. *Cardiovasc Res* 2010;**86**:192–201.
9. Zernecke A, Schober A, Bot I, von Hundelshausen P, Liehn EA, Mopps B, et al. SDF-1alpha/CXCR4 axis is instrumental in

neointimal hyperplasia and recruitment of smooth muscle progenitor cells. *Circ Res* 2005;**96**:784–91.

10. Sahara M, Sata M, Matsuzaki Y, Tanaka K, Morita T, Hirata Y, et al. Comparison of various bone marrow fractions in the ability to participate in vascular remodeling after mechanical injury. *Stem Cells* 2005;**23**:874–8.
11. Iwata H, Manabe I, Fujiu K, Yamamoto T, Takeda N, Eguchi K, et al. Bone marrow-derived cells contribute to vascular inflammation but do not differentiate into smooth muscle cell lineages. *Circulation* 2010;**122**:2048–57.
12. Kumar AH, Metharom P, Schmeckpeper J, Weiss S, Martin K, Caplice NM. Bone marrow-derived CX3CR1 progenitors contribute to neointimal smooth muscle cells via fractalkine CX3CR1 interaction. *FASEB J* 2010;**24**:81–92.
13. Subramanian P, Karshovska E, Reinhard P, Megens RTA, Zhou Z, Akhtar S, et al. Lysophosphatidic acid receptors LPA1 and LPA3 promote CXCL12-mediated smooth muscle progenitor cell recruitment in neointima formation. *Circ Res* 2010;**107**:96–105.
14. Yu H, Stoneman V, Clarke M, Figg N, Xin HB, Kotlikoff M, et al. Bone marrow-derived smooth muscle-like cells are infrequent in advanced primary atherosclerotic plaques but promote atherosclerosis. *Arterioscler Thromb Vasc Biol* 2011;**31**:1291–9.
15. Kashiwakura Y, Katoh Y, Tamayose K, Konishi H, Takaya N, Yuhara S, et al. Isolation of bone marrow stromal cell-derived smooth muscle cells by a human SM22alpha promoter: in vitro differentiation of putative smooth muscle progenitor cells of bone marrow. *Circulation* 2003;**107**:2078–81.
16. Inoue T, Sata M, Hikichi Y, Sohma R, Fukuda D, Uchida T, et al. Mobilization of CD34-positive bone marrow-derived cells after coronary stent implantation: impact on restenosis. *Circulation* 2007;**115**:553–61.
17. Schober A, Hoffmann R, Opree N, Knarren S, Iofina E, Hutschenreuter G, et al. Peripheral CD34+ cells and the risk of in-stent restenosis in patients with coronary heart disease. *Am J Cardiol* 2005;**96**:1116–22.
18. Schober A, Weber C. Bone marrow-derived smooth muscle cells are breaking bad in atherogenesis. *Arterioscler Thromb Vasc Biol* 2011;**31**:1258–9.
19. Sugiyama S, Kugiyama K, Nakamura S, Kataoka K, Aikawa M, Shimizu K, et al. Characterization of smooth muscle-like cells in circulating human peripheral blood. *Atherosclerosis* 2006;**187**:351–62.
20. Hagensen MK, Shim J, Falk E, Bentzon JF. Flanking recipient vasculature, not circulating progenitor cells, contributes to endothelium and smooth muscle in murine allograft vasculopathy. *Arterioscler Thromb Vasc Biol* 2011;**31**:808–13.
21. Tanaka K, Sata M, Hirata Y, Nagai R. Diverse contribution of bone marrow cells to neointimal hyperplasia after mechanical vascular injuries. *Circ Res* 2003;**93**:783–90.
22. Yu H, Stoneman V, Clarke M, Figg N, Xin HB, Kotlikoff M, et al. Bone marrow-derived smooth muscle-like cells are infrequent in advanced primary atherosclerotic plaques but promote atherosclerosis. *Arterioscler Thromb Vasc Biol* 2011;**31**:1291–9.
23. Cui YZ, Hisha H, Yang GX, Fan TX, Jin T, Li Q, et al. Optimal protocol for total body irradiation for allogeneic bone marrow transplantation in mice. *Bone Marrow Transplant* 2002;**30**:843–9.
24. Psaltis PJ, Harbuzariu A, Delacroix S, Holroyd EW, Simari RD. Resident vascular progenitor cells – diverse origins, phenotype, and function. *J Cardiovasc Transl Res* 2011;**4**:161–76.
25. Torsney E, Xu Q. Resident vascular progenitor cells. *J Mol Cell Cardiol* 2011;**50**:304–11.
26. Frid MG, Aldashev AA, Dempsey EC, Stenmark KR. Smooth muscle cells isolated from discrete compartments of the mature vascular media exhibit unique phenotypes and distinct growth capabilities. *Circ Res* 1997;**81**:940–52.
27. Sainz J, Al Haj Zen A, Caligiuri G, Demerens C, Urbain D, Lemitre M, et al. Isolation of "side population" progenitor cells from healthy arteries of adult mice. *Arterioscler Thromb Vasc Biol* 2006;**26**:281–6.
28. Pasquinelli G, Pacilli A, Alviano F, Foroni L, Ricci F, Valente S, et al. Multidistrict human mesenchymal vascular cells: pluripotency and stemness characteristics. *Cytotherapy* 2010;**12**:275–87.
29. Bearzi C, Leri A, Lo Monaco F, Rota M, Gonzalez A, Hosoda T, et al. Identification of a coronary vascular progenitor cell in the human heart. *Proc Natl Acad Sci USA* 2009;**106**:15885–90.
30. Hu Y, Zhang Z, Torsney E, Afzal AR, Davison F, Metzler B, et al. Abundant progenitor cells in the adventitia contribute to atherosclerosis of vein grafts in ApoE-deficient mice. *J Clin Invest* 2004;**113**:1258–65.
31. Passman JN, Dong XR, Wu SP, Maguire CT, Hogan KA, Bautch VL, et al. A sonic hedgehog signaling domain in the arterial adventitia supports resident sca1$^+$ smooth muscle progenitor cells. *Proc Natl Acad Sci USA* 2008;**105**:9349–54.
32. Klein D, Weisshardt P, Kleff V, Jastrow H, Jakob HG, Ergun S. Vascular wall-resident CD44$^+$ multipotent stem cells give rise to pericytes and smooth muscle cells and contribute to new vessel maturation. *PLoS One* 2011;**6**:e20540.
33. Linton MF, Atkinson JB, Fazio S. Prevention of atherosclerosis in apolipoprotein e-deficient mice by bone marrow transplantation. *Science* 1995;**267**:1034–7.
34. Bentzon JF, Weile C, Sondergaard CS, Hindkjaer J, Kassem M, Falk E. Smooth muscle cells in atherosclerosis originate from the local vessel wall and not circulating progenitor cells in apoe knockout mice. *Arterioscle Thromb Vasc Biol* 2006;**26**:2696–702.
35. Falk E, Schwartz SM, Galis ZS, Rosenfeld ME. Putative murine models of plaque rupture. *Arterioscler Thromb Vasc Biol* 2007;**27**:969–72.
36. Jackson CL, Bennett MR, Biessen EA, Johnson JL, Krams R. Assessment of unstable atherosclerosis in mice. *Arterioscler Thromb Vasc Biol* 2007;**27**:714–20.
37. Bentzon JF, Sondergaard CS, Kassem M, Falk E. Smooth muscle cells healing atherosclerotic plaque disruptions are of local, not blood, origin in apolipoprotein E knockout mice. *Circulation* 2007;**116**:2053–61.
38. Caplice NM, Bunch TJ, Stalboerger PG, Wang S, Simper D, Miller DV, et al. Smooth muscle cells in human coronary atherosclerosis can originate from cells administered at marrow transplantation. *Proc Natl Acad Sci USA* 2003;**100**:4754–9.
39. Zoll J, Fontaine V, Gourdy P, Barateau V, Vilar J, Leroyer A, et al. Role of human smooth muscle cell progenitors in atherosclerotic plaque development and composition. *Cardiovasc Res* 2008;**77**:471–80.
40. Campagnolo P, Wong MM, Xu Q. Progenitor cells in arteriosclerosis: good or bad guys? *Antioxid Redox Signal* 2011;**15**:1013–27.
41. Rahmani M, Cruz RP, Granville DJ, McManus BM. Allograft vasculopathy versus atherosclerosis. *Circ Res* 2006;**99**:801–15.
42. Religa P, Bojakowski K, Bojakowska M, Gaciong Z, Thyberg J, Hedin U. Allogenic immune response promotes the accumulation

of host-derived smooth muscle cells in transplant arteriosclerosis. *Cardiovasc Res* 2005;**65**:535–45.

43. Saiura A, Sata M, Hirata Y, Nagai R, Makuuchi M. Circulating smooth muscle progenitor cells contribute to atherosclerosis. *Nat Med* 2001;**7**:382–3.
44. Hillebrands JL, Klatter FA, van den Hurk BM, Popa ER, Nieuwenhuis P, Rozing J. Origin of neointimal endothelium and alpha-actin-positive smooth muscle cells in transplant arteriosclerosis. *J Clin Invest* 2001;**107**:1411–22.
45. Hu Y, Davison F, Ludewig B, Erdel M, Mayr M, Url M, et al. Smooth muscle cells in transplant atherosclerotic lesions are originated from recipients, but not bone marrow progenitor cells. *Circulation* 2002;**106**:1834–9.
46. Quaini F, Urbanek K, Beltrami AP, Finato N, Beltrami CA, Nadal-Ginard B, et al. Chimerism of the transplanted heart. *N Engl J Med* 2002;**346**:5–15.
47. Daniel JM, Sedding DG. Circulating smooth muscle progenitor cells in arterial remodeling. *J Mol Cell Cardiol* 2011;**50**:273–9.
48. Han CI, Campbell GR, Campbell JH. Circulating bone marrow cells can contribute to neointimal formation. *J Vasc Res* 2001;**38**:113–9.
49. Tanaka K, Sata M, Natori T, Kim-Kaneyama JR, Nose K, Shibanuma M, et al. Circulating progenitor cells contribute to neointimal formation in nonirradiated chimeric mice. *FASEB J* 2008;**22**:428–36.
50. Schober A. Chemokines in vascular dysfunction and remodeling. *Arterioscler Thromb Vasc Biol* 2008;**28**:1950–9.
51. Bleul CC, Fuhlbrigge RC, Casasnovas JM, Aiuti A, Springer TA. A highly efficacious lymphocyte chemoattractant, stromal cell-derived factor 1 (SDF-1). *J Exp Med* 1996;**184**:1101–9.
52. Petit I, Szyper-Kravitz M, Nagler A, Lahav M, Peled A, Habler L, et al. G-csf induces stem cell mobilization by decreasing bone marrow sdf-1 and up-regulating cxcr4. *Nat Immunol* 2002;**3**:687–94.
53. Shiba Y, Takahashi M, Yoshioka T, Yajima N, Morimoto H, Izawa A, et al. M-csf accelerates neointimal formation in the early phase after vascular injury in mice: the critical role of the SDF-1-CXCR4 system. *Arterioscler Thromb Vasc Biol* 2007;**27**:283–9.
54. Yokoi H, Yamada H, Tsubakimoto Y, Takata H, Kawahito H, Kishida S, et al. Bone marrow at1 augments neointima formation by promoting mobilization of smooth muscle progenitors via platelet-derived SDF-1. *Arterioscler Thromb Vasc Biol* 2009;**30**:60–7.
55. Karshovska E, Zagorac D, Zernecke A, Weber C, Schober A. A small molecule CXCR4 antagonist inhibits neointima formation and smooth muscle progenitor cell mobilization after arterial injury. *J Thromb Haemost* 2008;**6**:1812–5.
56. Yoshida K, Nishida W, Hayashi K, Ohkawa Y, Ogawa A, Aoki J, et al. Vascular remodeling induced by naturally occurring unsaturated lysophosphatidic acid in vivo. *Circulation* 2003;**108**: 1746–52.
57. Karshovska E, Zernecke A, Sevilmis G, Millet A, Hristov M, Cohen CD, et al. Expression of hif-1alpha in injured arteries controls SDF-1alpha mediated neointima formation in apolipoprotein E-deficient mice. *Arterioscler Thromb Vasc Biol* 2007;**27**:2540–7.
58. Nemenoff RA, Simpson PA, Furgeson SB, Kaplan-Albuquerque N, Crossno J, Garl PJ, et al. Targeted deletion of pten in smooth muscle cells results in vascular remodeling and recruitment of progenitor cells through induction of stromal cell-derived factor-1alpha. *Circ Res* 2008;**102**:1036–45.
59. Nemenoff RA, Horita H, Ostriker AC, Furgeson SB, Simpson PA, VanPutten V, et al. SDF-1alpha induction in mature smooth muscle cells by inactivation of pten is a critical mediator of exacerbated injury-induced neointima formation. *Arterioscler Thromb Vasc Biol* 2011;**31**:1300–8.
60. Ikesue M, Matsui Y, Ohta D, Danzaki K, Ito K, Kanayama M, et al. Syndecan-4 deficiency limits neointimal formation after vascular injury by regulating vascular smooth muscle cell proliferation and vascular progenitor cell mobilization. *Arterioscler Thromb Vasc Biol* 2011;**31**:1066–74.
61. Yang D, Koupenova M, McCrann DJ, Kopeikina KJ, Kagan HM, Schreiber BM, et al. The A2b adenosine receptor protects against vascular injury. *Proc Natl Acad Sci USA* 2008;**105**:792–6.
62. Zhang LN, Wilson DW, da Cunha V, Sullivan ME, Vergona R, Rutledge JC, et al. Endothelial no synthase deficiency promotes smooth muscle progenitor cells in association with upregulation of stromal cell-derived factor-1alpha in a mouse model of carotid artery ligation. *Arterioscler Thromb Vasc Biol* 2006;**26**:765–72.
63. Weber C, Zernecke A, Libby P. The multifaceted contributions of leukocyte subsets to atherosclerosis: lessons from mouse models. *Nat Rev Immunol* 2008;**8**:802–15.
64. Dimmeler S, Aicher A, Vasa M, Mildner-Rihm C, Adler K, Tiemann M, et al. Hmg-coa reductase inhibitors (statins) increase endothelial progenitor cells via the PI3-kinase/Akt pathway. *J Clin Invest* 2001;**108**:391–7.
65. Kusuyama T, Omura T, Nishiya D, Enomoto S, Matsumoto R, Murata T, et al. The effects of hmg-coa reductase inhibitor on vascular progenitor cells. *J Pharmacol Sci* 2006;**101**:344–9.
66. Satoh K, Fukumoto Y, Nakano M, Sugimura K, Nawata J, Demachi J, et al. Statin ameliorates hypoxia-induced pulmonary hypertension associated with down-regulated stromal cell-derived factor-1. *Cardiovasc Res* 2009;**81**:226–34.
67. Pendyala LK, Yin X, Li J, Chen JP, Chronos N, Hou D. The first-generation drug-eluting stents and coronary endothelial dysfunction. *JACC Cardiovasc Interv* 2009;**2**:1169–77.
68. Zernecke A, Bot I, Djalali-Talab Y, Shagdarsuren E, Bidzhekov K, Meiler S, et al. Protective role of CXC receptor 4/CXC ligand 12 unveils the importance of neutrophils in atherosclerosis. *Circ Res* 2008;**102**:209–17.
69. Mehta NN, Li M, William D, Khera AV, Derohannessian S, Qu L, et al. The novel atherosclerosis locus at 10q11 regulates plasma cxcl12 levels. *Eur Heart J* 2011;**32**:963–71.

Chapter 108

Smooth Muscle: Novel Targets and Therapeutic Approaches

Mark W. Majesky
Departments of Pediatrics and Pathology, Center for Cardiovascular Biology, Institute for Stem Cell and Regenerative Medicine, Seattle Children's Research Institute, University of Washington, Seattle, WA

INTRODUCTION

Smooth muscle cells (SMCs) are an abundant type of specialized contractile cell distributed throughout the body. In addition to the well-studied contractile properties of slow phasic or tonic smooth muscle, these cells are also capable of robust cell proliferation, growth factor secretion, abundant extracellular matrix production, and cell migration in both embryonic and adult tissues. These non-contractile properties of smooth muscle tissues offer novel targets for therapeutic application. Recent advances in our understanding of how smooth muscle cells (SMCs) develop, differentiate, interact within a mechanically active environment, communicate with their neighbors, repair tissue injury, and respond to pathogens provide specific opportunities for intervention in congenital defects and chronic disease processes. This chapter will highlight examples of recent advances in our understanding of smooth muscle development, differentiation, and signaling that offer new targets for therapeutic intervention.

NOVEL APPROACHES TO THERAPEUTIC TARGETING OF SMOOTH MUSCLE TISSUES

Smooth Muscle Lineage Diversity

High-resolution fate mapping studies of developing vertebrate embryos reveal that vascular smooth muscle is actually a mosaic tissue composed of subtypes of smooth muscle cells (SMCs) arising from at least eight independent origins (1,2). This fact implies the existence of SMC lineage-specific pathways that may provide unique targets for the development of novel therapeutics with intrinsic vascular bed-specific profiles of activity. For example, coronary smooth muscle arises from progenitors in the proepicardium (3,4). No other blood vessels in the vascular system are composed of proepicardial-derived SMCs. Likewise, SMCs in the walls of the ascending aorta, pulmonary trunk, common carotid arteries and ductus arteriosus originate from progenitors in the cranial neural crest (5–7) (Figure 108.1). A number of studies now show that SMCs from different embryonic origins respond in lineage-specific ways to a common systemic stimulus. Thus, cranial neural crest-derived SMCs in the thoracic aorta proliferate in response to activation of transforming growth factor-beta (TGF-β) signaling whereas somite-derived SMCs in the abdominal aorta are growth inhibited by TGF-β under identical conditions *in vitro* (8). Smooth muscle lineage-dependent responses have now been reported for signaling by angiotensin II (9) and sphingosine-1-phosphate (10). Similarly, arterial SMCs of neural crest origin have selective requirements for myocardin-related transcription factor-B (MRTF-B) for transcriptional activation of SMC-specific contractile and cytoskeletal proteins when compared to arterial SMCs of non-neural crest origin *in vivo* (11,12). The proximal segments of major lymphatic vessels are coated with a specialized form of smooth muscle that is essential for returning lymphatic fluid to the great veins that drain into the heart (13). Defects in formation or function of lymphatic smooth muscle can lead to lymphedema, a condition characterized by excessive fluid retention and localized tissue swelling (14). Lymphatic return is driven by extrinsic pumps, typically the compression and expansion of surrounding tissues (e.g., skeletal muscle), and intrinsic pumps, the lymphatic SMCs that surround conduit lymphatic vessels. Intrinsic pump activity is activated by stretch on the wall due to lymphatic vessel filling and is characterized by rapid phasic contractions. Although the developmental origins of lymphatic smooth muscle are not well studied, the unique physiology of their contractile activity argues for the function of tissue-specific gene products, similar to the lymphatic endothelial cell-specific molecules described previously (15).

Muscle. DOI: http://dx.doi.org/10.1016/B978-0-12-381510-1.00108-3

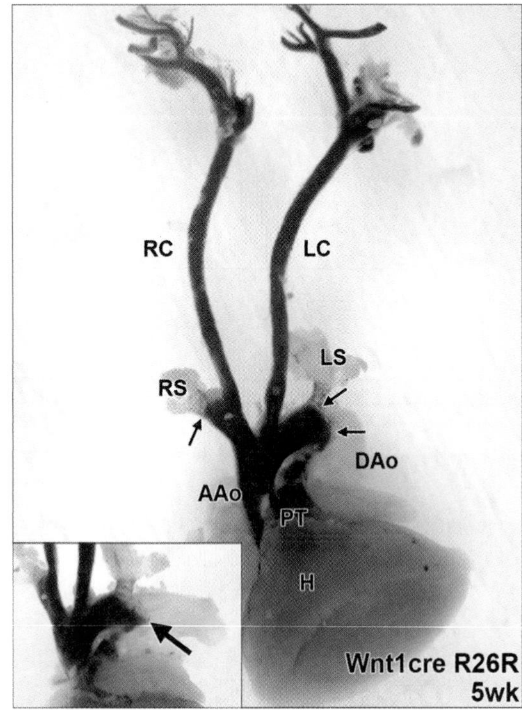

FIGURE 108.1 Smooth muscle lineage diversity. Progenitors arising from the cranial neural crest form the smooth muscle layers surrounding the great arteries. Wnt1-cre is selectively expressed in cranial neural crest cells. When intercrossed with an R26R reporter strain of mice, Wnt1-cre activity permanently marks these progenitors and their progeny with constitutive β-galactosidase (β-gal) activity. The sharply demarcated border (arrows) between neural crest-derived SMCs (blue) and non-neural crest-derived SMCs (white) can be detected by a β-gal histochemical stain. Inset: a higher power image of SMC lineage boundaries in the aortic arch region at 5 weeks after birth. Note that the transition from neural crest-derived SMCs (blue) to somite-derived SMCs (white) in the transverse aorta (arrow) is abrupt with little or no mixing of the two types of SMC. AAo, ascending thoracic aorta; Dao, descending thoracic aorta; PT, pulmonary trunk; LS, left subclavian artery; LC, left common carotid artery; RC, right common carotid artery; RS, right subclavian artery; H, heart.

Superimposed on the mosaic pattern of lineage diversity described above is a form of anterior–posterior positional identity provided by the *Hox* code (16). Most, if not all, cells acquire this positional identity during morphogenesis. The importance of positional identity in guiding progenitor cells to appropriate cell fates is highlighted by the dramatic transformations seen in homeotic mutants of *Drosophila* (17). Smooth muscle is an interesting case in this regard since smooth muscle tissues extend throughout the body and have generally been "targeted" therapeutically with very broad approaches that affect smooth muscle function systemically. Recent studies have provided evidence of *Hox* gene-dependent positional identity in vascular smooth muscle (18), airway smooth muscle (19), and enteric smooth muscle (20). The natural diversity of vascular smooth muscle offers the exciting possibility of vascular bed-specific targeting and of novel therapeutics based on intrinsic properties of different subtypes of vascular SMCs themselves. Such a strategy is currently being discussed as a therapeutic approach for treatment of aortic aneurysms (21). Similar strategies based on a more detailed understanding of the natural diversity of other (non-vascular) smooth muscle types will also improve the specificity of therapeutic targeting of those smooth muscle tissues as well.

Resident Smooth Muscle Progenitor Cells in the Vessel Wall

Like most tissues, blood vessels activate intrinsic pathways for tissue repair when damaged or diseased. This capacity for repair is substantial and involves all three layers of the vessel wall. For example, when injured by balloon catheter overdilation, replication rates in all layers of rat carotid or porcine coronary artery can increase over one hundred-fold (22,23). Repair of arterial smooth muscle damage is accomplished by acquisition of a proliferative and migratory phenotype of vascular SMCs accompanied by downregulation of expression of SMC differentiation marker genes in a process known as phenotypic switching (24–26). In addition, a very rapid activation of adventitial cells occurs shortly after distension injury that results in robust increases in cell proliferation, myofibroblast formation, and extracellular matrix production, in part, via TGF-β-dependent pathways (27).

Among the multiple cell types found in normal arterial adventitia is a recently discovered population of resident SMC progenitor cells that forms clusters near the border of the adventitia with the smooth muscle-containing medial layer. In 2004, Hu et. al. (28) reported that adult *ApoE*$^{-/-}$ mice maintained stem cell antigen-1 (Sca1, also called *Ly6A/E*)-positive cells in the aortic root adventitia that differentiated to a SMC-like cell type when removed from the adventitia and stimulated with PDGF-BB *in vitro* (28). In 2006, Zengin et al. reported that a "vasculogenic zone" could be identified in human internal thoracic artery that contained CD34^{+} progenitor cells capable of forming vascular structures in arterial ring explant cultures *in vitro* and promoting microvessel formation in a transplantable tumor model *in vivo* (29). In 2007, Pasquinelli et al. reported finding two distinct progenitor cell populations between the media and the adventitia, one CD34^{+} and the other c-kit^{+}, in human aortas and femoral arteries (30). Together, these progenitor cells could form capillary-like vascular structures when tested in the presence of vascular endothelial growth factor (VEGF) *in vitro*.

In 2008, Passman et al. reported a localized zone of sonic hedgehog (Shh) signaling that was almost entirely

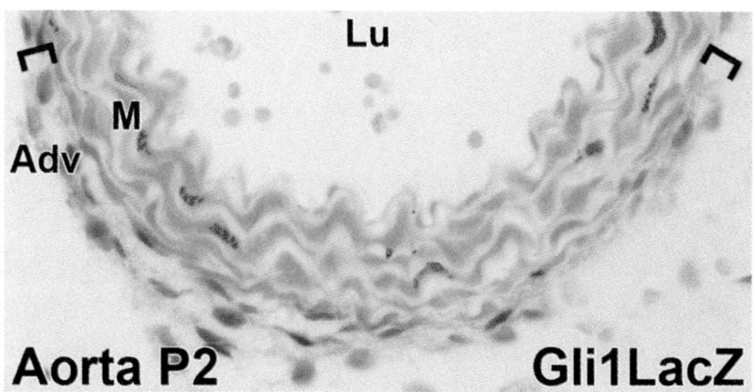

FIGURE 108.2 Smooth muscle progenitors in the adventitial niche. A cross-section of the descending thoracic aorta from a *Gli1*$^{lacZ/+}$ transgenic mouse at postnatal day 2. The tissue was stained in whole mount for β-galactosidase activity, fixed, embedded in paraffin, sectioned and counterstained with nuclear fast red. Gli1-positive cells (blue), an indicator of sonic hedgehog (Shh) signaling, are confined to the adventitial layer (brackets). Previous work showed that P2 aortic adventitia is also positive for two other reporters of Shh signaling activity, Patched1-lacZ (*Ptc1*$^{lacZ/+}$) and *Ptc2*$^{lacZ/+}$ in the same pattern as shown above for *Gli1*$^{lacZ/+}$ (31). Moreover, a population of stem cell antigen 1 (Sca1)-positive SMC progenitor cells has been shown to reside within this Shh signaling niche *in vivo* (28,31). Lu, lumen; M, media; Adv, adventitia.

restricted to the adventitial layer of blood vessels in late fetal and perinatal mice (31) (Figure 108.2). Shh protein itself was localized to the adventitia and concentrated close to the border between the media and the adventitia. Clustered within this zone of Shh signaling in the adventitia was a population of Sca1$^+$ smooth muscle progenitor cells (AdvSca1 cells). Analysis of *Shh*$^{-/-}$ mice and exposure of isolated AdvSca1 cells to Shh or the Hh signaling antagonist cyclopamine provided evidence that Hh signaling stimulates proliferation and promotes survival of these progenitor cells (31). When removed from the stem/progenitor "niche" environment in the adventitia and placed into a serum-containing culture medium *in vitro*, about 50% of isolated AdvSca1 cells differentiated into SMCs, about 25% proliferated and maintained *Sca1* expression (i.e., self-renewal), and the remaining 25% lost expression of *Sca1* but did not express detectable levels of either SMC or endothelial cell markers (31). These observations suggest that AdvSca1 are a heterogeneous population of progenitor cells with different potentials for self-renewal versus differentiation. Finally, Campagnolo et al. isolated a population of CD34$^+$/CD31$^-$ cells from the adventitia of human saphenous veins obtained during coronary artery bypass surgery (32). These CD34$^+$ progenitor cells possessed multilineage differentiation potential and formed osteoblasts, adipocytes, pericytes, and SMCs under selective differentiation-promoting conditions in culture. Taken together, these findings suggest that the adventitia of adult blood vessel walls maintains several types of progenitor cells that are capable of acting in concert to maintain or repair existing blood vessels and promote the formation of new ones (33–35). These natural resident progenitor cells are potential novel targets for mobilization to repair SMC defects that accompany degenerative diseases of the artery wall, including aneurysms, medial dissections, fibrosis, and progressive medial calcification (36–38). Since the adventitia forms the outer layer of blood vessels, it follows that the adventitia also forms a border with the tissue in which it resides. Moreover, because blood vessels are found in nearly all tissues, adventitial progenitor cells may respond to injury or disease in virtually all tissues and acquire tissue-specific potentials for differentiation (39). If so, then adventitial progenitor cells may represent novel targets for therapeutics that spare the mature contractile SMCs and the surrounding tissue cells by specifically targeting the progenitor cells or their niche environment (40).

Differentiation of SMC progenitor cells is preceded by a sequence of specification steps that are mediated by specific epigenetic modifications to SMC chromatin (41). For example, an epigenetic histone modification that correlates with SMC identity in progenitor cells is H3K4 dimethylation (H3K4Me2) (42). Chromatin immunoprecipitation (ChIP) assays showed that transcription factor complexes containing serum response factor (SRF) and myocardin that are capable of activating the expression of SMC differentiation marker genes physically associate with H3K4Me2. By contrast, transcription-silencing complexes consisting of SRF and Elk1 do not associate with H3K4Me2 in ChIP assays (42). Thus histone methyltransferases responsible for the dimethyl modification of H3K4 would be key targets of one or more pathways that confer SMC specification on multipotential progenitor cells in embryonic or adult tissues. Recent evidence suggests that a DNA binding homeodomain protein called Pituitary homeobox protein-2 (Pitx2) physically associates with SRF and recruits histone acetyltransferase activity to SMC target genes. Pitx2 also binds WD repeat-containing protein 5 (WDR5), a component of the Mixed Lineage Leukemia methyltransferase family, and directs histone methylation of SMC marker gene loci (43). As the molecular mechanisms and signaling pathways for SMC specification become more completely understood, it will be possible to more specifically promote or interfere with SMC differentiation by targeting subtypes of SMC progenitors *in vivo*.

Chemorepulsive Signaling Pathways for Cell Migration

Migration of SMCs and their progenitors is an important step in smooth muscle development, repair of tissue injury, and the progression of various diseases in smooth muscle tissues. For many years, cell-matrix adhesion receptors and matrix degrading enzymes have been the focus of studies whose goal was to identify mechanisms of cell migration within vascular, as well as non-vascular, smooth muscle tissues *in vivo*. Little attention was paid to the large family of genes encoding chemorepulsive ligands and their receptors in smooth muscle. The dependence of SMCs on molecules of this gene family for the assembly of smooth muscle tissues in development and for SMC migration *in vitro* and *in vivo* has been demonstrated for a few of the family members. For example, ephrin B2-deficient-SMCs are defective in spreading, focal adhesion formation, and polarized cell migration *in vitro* (44). Ephrin-B2 is selectively expressed in arterial, and not in venous, smooth muscle within the vascular system (45). Moreover, ephrin-B2 expression by mural cells *in vivo* is required for vascular development and angiogenesis (44). Ephrin-B2-deficient SMCs and pericytes are defective in interactions with microvascular endothelial cells resulting in a poorly organized and leaky vascular network and perinatal lethality in mice (44). Members of the Slit/Robo gene families are also expressed in smooth muscle tissues (46,47). Isolated airway SMCs express Slit2, Slit3, Robo1, Robo2, and Robo4 (48). Addition of exogenous soluble Slit2N to activate Robo receptors *in vitro* inhibited airway SMC proliferation and reduced PDGF-stimulated lamellipodia formation, actin rearrangement, and cell migration in part by inhibition of PDGF-induced activation of WASP and Arp2/3 proteins required for actin-based cytoskeletal reorganization (48). Similarly, addition of soluble ephrin A1 to cultures of rat vascular SMCs strongly inhibited cell spreading, an effect that was correlated with repression of Rac1 and p21-activated kinase (PAK1) activity (49). Liu et al. reported that intact blood vessels expressed Slit2 and Robo receptors, and observed that recombinant Slit2 blocked PDGF-stimulated SMC migration *in vitro* via inhibition of Rac1 activation (47). These findings suggest that chemorepulsive guidance mechanisms that direct development of the nervous system play functionally conserved roles in the assembly of smooth muscle tissues in the airway and vascular system (46).

Mechanochemical Signaling via the Primary Cilium

The primary cilium was discovered almost a century ago (50) but was regarded for many years as a non-motile evolutionary remnant of motile cilia. We now know that primary cilia are specialized microtubule-based cell organelles that are adapted for mechanochemical signaling in vertebrates (reviewed in 51,52,53,54). Odorant receptors and visual pigments in the rod outer segment are examples of sensory molecules that are trafficked into primary cilium (52). Significant advances in our understanding of functions of the primary cilium have been motivated by two important findings. One is that the multiple defects seen in polycystic kidney disease were shown to arise from defects in the structure or function of primary cilia (reviewed in 55). The other is the discovery based on genome-wide mutagenesis screens in mice that the vertebrate hedgehog (Hh) family of morphogens requires primary cilia for signaling (56,57; reviewed in 58). Subsequent reports showed that the primary cilium also mediates signaling through the PDGF α-receptor, a ligand-activated tyrosine kinase (but not the PDGF β-receptor) (59), and the G-protein-coupled receptors (GPCRs) serotonin HTr6 receptor, and somatostatin Sstr3 receptor (60).

The primary cilium contains a microtubule-based core structure called an axoneme composed of nine peripheral doublets of microtubules (54) (Figure 108.3). Cilia extend from the basal body, a structure derived from the mother centriole that serves as the MTOC (microtubule organizing center) in the cell. Microtubule-based motor systems transport proteins to the ciliary tip (anterograde transport, kinesin-2 motor, and intraflagellar transport (IFT) complex B proteins) and away from the cilia tip (retrograde transport, dynein motor, and IFT complex A proteins) (reviewed in 61). The vertebrate Hh signaling protein smoothened (Smo) is thought to be functional when it is transported to the tip region of the primary cilia to engage signal transduction machinery that is located there (62). Smo has the molecular structure of a GPCR (63) and recent studies have shown Smo signaling is mediated by heterotrimeric G proteins (64,65). Moreover, Smo activity is regulated by G-protein-coupled receptor kinase-2 (66–68) and β-arrestin-2, in part by facilitating the transport of Smo into the primary cilium via interaction with Kif3A, a kinesin motor protein of the anterograde ciliary transport system (69).

Both vascular and airway SMCs have been reported to contain primary cilia *in vivo* (70–72). Lu et al. showed that vascular SMCs in the artery wall contained primary cilia and that the cilia were aligned with their long axis projecting into the extracellular matrix (ECM) at a 58-degree angle in relation to the cross-sectional plane of the artery. These cilia contained $\alpha_2\beta_1$ integrins and when stimulated with collagen (a cognate ligand for $\alpha_2\beta_1$ integrins), or when deflection of the primary cilia was induced mechanically, a transient rise in intracellular Ca^{2+} was observed (71). These data argue that primary cilia in vascular SMCs may be directly linked to the ECM and thus may serve as important mechanosensors of artery wall deformation and thus may be important signaling elements in artery wall homeostasis, growth and remodeling in response to changes in radial and longitudinal wall stress (Figure 108.3). In airway smooth muscle, a similar interaction with the ECM was evident with localization of

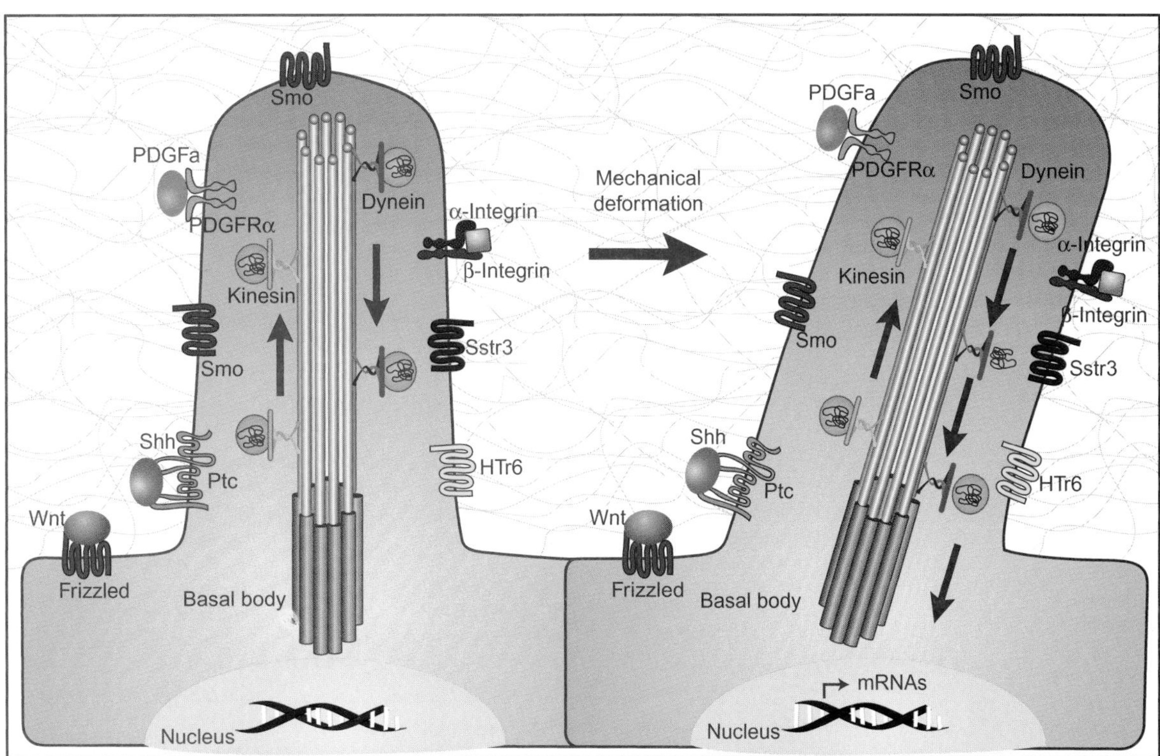

FIGURE 108.3 Primary cilia. Primary cilia are microtubule-based projections of the cell surface that have important mechanochemical sensing and signaling functions (left side). Primary cilia have been reported in arterial and in airway smooth muscle tissues where they are seen projecting into the extracellular matrix (ECM). Primary cilia are known to contain ECM-binding integrins, and are also known to respond to mechanical deformation by increases in intracellular Ca^{2+} concentrations, changes in gene expression, and modifications of cell phenotype (right side). In addition, primary cilia also contain receptors for Shh (Ptc), PDGF-AA (PDGFRα), serotonin (HTr6), somatostatin (Sstr3), and a constitutively active form of smoothened (Smo) that is required for Shh signaling.

$\alpha_2\beta_1$ and $\alpha_5\beta_1$ integrins to primary cilia *in vivo* (72). Cell migration assays *in vitro* showed a repositioning of primary cilia in the direction of migration takes place as SMCs begin to move, and cells with cilia migrated more efficiently than cells without primary cilia. Previous observations had also observed a polarity of the SMC cytoskeleton during cell migration following scratch injury *in vitro* (73). Using antibodies to γ-tubulin, Langille and co-workers showed that the mother centriole and basal body reorient to the leading edge of the migrating SMCs (73). Since primary cilia are extensions of the microtubule-based cytoskeleton that are positioned by the basal body (54,61), it may explain why primary cilia are found to be oriented in the direction of cell migration *in vitro*. These findings extend the role of primary cilia to a second type of smooth muscle *in vivo*, and further support a mechanosensory role for primary cilia in smooth muscle tissue homeostasis and wound repair (72).

SUMMARY AND CONCLUSIONS

Considerable intrinsic diversity is found among smooth muscle subtypes as a result of differences in their embryonic origins and lineage histories. This epigenetic diversity is evident in adult tissues and prepatterns responses obtained to a common stimulus, e.g., activation of TGF-β signaling pathways (1,8,21). These intrinsic differences in SMC subtypes present attractive therapeutic targets as they offer advantages of inherent specificity over current broadly acting systemic agents. Novel approaches to smooth muscle degenerative diseases, particularly for vascular smooth muscle, are suggested by the recent characterization of resident SMC progenitor cells in the adventitia of mouse and human artery wall. These SMC progenitor cells are dependent on Shh signaling for proliferation and survival in the adventitia. Directed expansion of this progenitor pool may provide additional tools to repair large artery walls whose integrity or function is compromised by medial dissection, progressive calcification or aneurysmal dilation. Genetic analysis of polycystic kidney disease in humans and patterning of the neural axis in mice led to the common finding that primary cilia are specialized vertebrate mechanochemical signaling organelles present in a wide variety of cell types, including smooth muscle. The functions of primary cilia in smooth muscle tissues are just beginning to be defined but the possibilities for their roles as biosensors of mechanical forces suggest a potentially rewarding area for future studies. Finally, advances in our understanding of molecular genetic mechanisms for stage-specific SMC specification in embryonic and adult progenitor cells will provide the information necessary to target direct somatic cell reprogramming approaches and cell-based therapies to smooth muscle tissues in the near future.

ACKNOWLEDGMENTS

I thank present and former members of my laboratory for their input and many helpful discussions. I also thank Xiu Rong Dong, Jenna Regan, and Virginia Hoglund for help preparing and editing the figures. The author's work was supported by NIH grants HL-93594 and HL-19242, and the Seattle Children's Research Institute, University of Washington.

REFERENCES

1. Majesky MW. Developmental basis of vascular smooth muscle diversity. *Arterioscler Thromb Vasc Biol* 2007;**27**:1248–58.
2. Wasteson P, Johansson BR, Jukkola T, Breuer S, Akyurek LM, Partanen J, et al. Developmental origin of smooth muscle cells in the descending aorta in mice. *Development* 2008;**135**:1823–32.
3. Mikawa T, Fishman D. Retroviral analysis of cardiac morphogenesis: discontinuous formation of coronary vessels. *Proc Natl Acad Sci USA* 1992;**89**:9504–8.
4. Majesky MW. Development of coronary vessels. *Curr Top Dev Biol* 2004;**62**:225–59.
5. Le Lievre C, Le Douarin N. Mesenchymal derivatives of the neural crest: analysis of chimeric quail and chick embryos. *J Embryol Exp Morphol* 1975;**34**:125–54.
6. Kirby M, Gale T, Stewart D. Neural crest cells contribute to normal aorticopulmonary septation. *Science* 1983;**220**:1059–61.
7. Li J, Liu KC, Jin F, Lu MM, Epstein JA. Transgenic rescue of congenital heart disease and spina bifida in Splotch mice. *Development* 1999;**126**:2495–503.
8. Topouzis S, Majesky MW. Smooth muscle lineage diversity in the chick embryo: two types of aortic smooth muscle cell differ in growth and receptor-mediated transcriptional responses to transforming growth factor-β. *Dev Biol* 1996;**178**:430–45.
9. Owens III AP, Subramanian V, Moorleghen JJ, Guo Z, McNamara CA, Cassis LA, et al. Angiotensin II induces a region-specific hyperplasia of the ascending aorta through regulation of inhibitor of differentiation 3. *Circ Res* 2010;**106**:611–9.
10. Grabski AD, Shimizu T, Deou J, Mahoney Jr. WM, Reidy MA, Daum G. Sphingosine-1-phosphate receptor-2 regulates expression of smooth muscle alpha-actin after arterial injury. *Arterioscler Thromb Vasc Biol* 2009;**29**:1644–50.
11. Oh J, Richardson JA, Olson EN. Requirement of myocardin-related transcription factor-B for remodeling of branchial arch arteries and smooth muscle differentiation. *Proc Natl Acad Sci USA* 2005;**102**:15122–7.
12. Li J, Zhi X, Chen M, Cheng L, Zhou D, Lu MM, et al. Myocardin-related transcription factor B is required in cardiac neural crest for smooth muscle differentiation and cardiovascular development. *Proc Natl Acad Sci USA* 2005;**102**:8916–21.
13. Zawieja DC. Contractile physiology of lymphatics. *Lymphatic. Res. Biol* 2009;**7**:87–96.
14. Petrova TV, Karpanen T, Norrmen C, Mellor R, Tamakoshi T, Finegold D, et al. Defective valves and abnormal mural cell recruitment underlie lymphatic vascular failure in lymphedema distichiasis. *Nat Med.* 2004;**10**:974–81.
15. Tammela T, Alitalo K. Lymphangiogenesis: molecular mechanisms and future promise. *Cell* 2010;**140**:460–76.
16. McGinnis W, Krumlauf R. Homeobox genes and axial patterning. *Cell* 1992;**68**:283–302.
17. Gehring WJ. Homeo boxes in the study of development. *Science* 1987;**236**:1245–62.
18. Pruett ND, Visconti RP, Jacobs DF, Scholz D, McQuinn T, Sundberg JP, et al. Evidence for Hox-specified positional identities in adult vasculature. BMC. *Dev Biol* 2008;**8**:93.
19. Maeda Y, Dave V, Whitsett JA. Transcriptional control of lung morphogenesis. *Physiol Rev* 2007;**87**:219–44.
20. Kapur RP, Gershon MD, Milla PJ, Pachnis V. The influence of Hos genes and three intercellular signaling pathways on enteric neuromuscular development. *Neurogastroenterol Motil* 2004;**16** (Suppl. 1):8–13.
21. Lindsay ME, Dietz HC. Lessons on the pathogenesis of aneurysm from heritable conditions. *Nature* 2011;**473**:308–16.
22. Clowes AW, Reidy MA, Clowes MM. Kinetics of cellular proliferation after arterial injury. I. Smooth muscle growth in the absence of endothelium. *Lab Invest* 1983;**49**:327–33.
23. Scott NA, Cipolla CE, Ross CE, Dunn B, Martin FH, Simonet L, et al. Identification of a potential role for the adventitia in vascular lesion formation after overstretch balloon injury of porcine coronary arteries. *Circulation* 1996;**93**:2178–87.
24. Chamley-Campbell J, Campbell GR, Ross R. The smooth muscle cell in culture. *Physiol Rev* 1979;**59**:1–61.
25. Owens G, Kumar M, Wamhoff B. Molecular regulation of vascular smooth muscle cell differentiation in development and disease. *Physiol Rev* 2004;**84**:767–801.
26. Miano J, Long S, Fujiwara K. Serum response factor: master regulator of the actin cytoskeleton and contractile apparatus. *Am J Physiol Cell Physiol* 2007;**292**:C70–81.
27. Smith JD, Bryant SR, Couper LL, Vary CP, Gotwals PJ, Koteliansky VE, et al. Soluble transforming growth factor-β type II receptor inhibits negative remodeling, fibroblast transdifferentiation, and intimal lesion formation but not endothelial growth. *Circ Res* 1999;**84**:1212–22.
28. Hu Y, Zhang Z, Torsney AR, Afzal F, Davison B, Metzler B, et al. Abundant progenitor cells in the adventitia contribute of atherosclerosis of vein grafts in ApoE-deficient mice. *J Clin Invest* 2004;**113**:1258–62.
29. Zengin E, Chalajour F, Gehling UM, Ito WD, Treede H, Lauke H, et al. Vascular wall resident progenitor cells: a source for postnatal vasculogenesis. *Development* 2006;**133**:1543–51.
30. Pasquinelli G, Tazzari PL, Vaselli C, Foroni L, Buzzi M, Storci G, et al. Thoracic aortas from multiorgan donors are suitable for obtaining resident angiogenic mesenchymal stromal cells. *Stem Cells* 2007;**25**:1627–34.
31. Passman JN, Dong XR, Wu SP, Maguire CT, Hogan KA, Bautch VL, et al. A sonic hedgehog signaling domain in the arterial

adventitia supports resident Sca1+ smooth muscle progenitor cells. *Proc Natl Acad Sci USA* 2008;**105**:9349–54.

32. Campagnolo P, Cesselli D, Al Haj Zen A, Beltrami AP, Krankel N, Katare R, et al. Human adult vena saphena contain perivascular progenitor cells endowed with clonogenic and proangiogenic potential. *Circulation* 2010;**121**:1735–45.
33. Tilki D, Hohn H, Ergun B, Rafii S, Ergun S. Emerging biology of vascular wall progenitor cells in health and disease. *Trends Mol Med* 2009;**15**:501–9.
34. Torsney E, Xu Q. Resident vascular progenitor cells. *J Mol Cell Cardiol* 2011;**50**:304–11.
35. Majesky MW, Dong XR, Hoglund VJ, Mahoney Jr WM, Daum G. The adventitia: a dynamic interface containing resident progenitor cells. *Arterioscler Thromb Vasc Biol* 2011;**31**:1530–9.
36. Shao JS, Cai J, Towler DA. Molecular mechanisms of vascular calcification: lessons learned from the aorta. *Arterioscler. Thromb. Vasc. Biol.* 2006;**26**:1423–30.
37. Olive M, Harten I, Mitchell R, Beers JK, Djabali K, Cao MR, et al. Cardiovascular pathology in Hutchinson–Gilford progeria: correlation with vascular aging. *Arterioscler Thromb Vasc Biol* 2010;**30**:2301–9.
38. Lindsey ME, Dietz HC. Lessons on the pathogenesis of aneurysm from heritable conditions. *Nature* 2011;**473**:308–16.
39. Tian H, Callahan CA, DuPree KJ, Darbonne WC, Ahn CP, Scales SJ, et al. Hedgehog signaling is restricted to the stromal compartment during pancreatic carcinogenesis. *Proc Natl Acad Sci USA* 2009;**106**:4254–9.
40. Scadden DT. The stem-cell niche as an entity of action. *Nature* 2006;**441**:1075–9.
41. Majesky MW, Dong XR, Regan JN, Hoglund VJ. Vascular smooth muscle progenitor cells: building and repairing blood vessels. *Circ Res* 2011;**108**:365–77.
42. McDonald O, Wamhoff B, Hoofnagle M, Owens GK. Control of SRF binding to CArG box chromatin regulates smooth muscle gene expression in vivo. *J Clin Invest* 2006;**116**:36–48.
43. Gan Q, Thiebaud P, Theze N, Jin L, Xu G, Grant P, et al. WD repeat-containing Protein 5, a ubiquitously expressed histone methyltransferase adaptor protein, regulates smooth muscle cell selective gene activation through interaction with pituitary homeobox 2. *J Biol Chem* 2011;**286**:21853–64.
44. Foo SS, Turner CJ, Adams S, Compagni A, Aubyn D, Kogata N, et al. Ephrin-B2 controls cell motility and adhesion during blood-vessel-wall assembly. *Cell* 2006;**124**:161–73.
45. Gale NW, Baluk P, Pan L, Kwan M, Holash J, DeChiara TM, et al. Ephrin-B2 selectively marks arterial vessels and neovascularization sites in the adult, with expression in both endothelial and smooth-muscle cells. *Dev Biol* 2001;**230**:151–60.
46. Adams R. Nerve cell signposts in the blood vessel roadmap. *Circ Res* 2006;**98**:440–2.
47. Liu D, Hou J, Hu X, Wang X, Xiao Y, Mou Y, et al. Neuronal chemorepellant Slit2 inhibits vascular smooth muscle cell migration by suppressing small GTPase Rac1 activation. *Circ Res* 2006;**98**:480–9.
48. Ning Y, Sun Q, Dong Y, Xu W, Zhang W, Huang H, et al. Slit2-N inhibits PDGF-induced migration in rat airway smooth muscle cells: WASP and Arp2/3 involved. *Toxicology* 2011;**283**:32–40.
49. Deroanne C, Vouret-Craviari V, Wang B, Pouyssegur J. EphrinA1 inactivates integrin-mediated vascular smooth muscle cell spreading via the Rac/PAK pathway. *J Cell Sci* 2003;**116**:1367–76.
50. Zimmerman KW. Contributions to knowledge of some glands and epithelium. *Arch Mikr Anat* 1898;**52**:552–706.
51. Pazour GJ, Whitman GB. The vertebrate primary cilium is a sensory organelle. *Curr Opin Cell Biol* 2003;**15**:105–10.
52. Singla V, Reiter JF. The primary cilium as the cell's antenna: signaling at a sensory organelle. *Science* 2006;**313**:629–33.
53. Eggenschwiler JT, Anderson KV. Cilia and developmental signaling. *Annu Rev Cell Dev Biol* 2007;**23**:345–73.
54. Berbari NF, O'Conner AK, Haycraft CJ, Yoder BK. The primary cilium as a complex signaling center. *Curr Biol* 2009;**19**:R526–35.
55. Waters AM, Beales PL. Ciliopathies: an expanding disease spectrum. *Pediatric Nephrol* 2011;**26**:1039–56.
56. Huangfu D, Anderson KV. Cilia and hedgehog responsiveness in the mouse. *Proc Natl Acad Sci USA* 2005;**106**:4254–9.
57. Corbit KC, Aanstad P, Singla V, Norman AR, Stainier DYR, Reiter JF. Vertebrate smoothened functions at the primary cilium. *Nature* 2005;**437**:1018–21.
58. Ingham PW, Nakano Y, Seger C. Mechanisms and functions of Hedgehog signaling across the metazoa. *Nat Rev Genet* 2011;**12**:393–406.
59. Schneider L, Clement CA, Teilmann SC, Pazour GJ, Hoffmann EK, Satir P, et al. PDGFRαα signaling is regulated through the primary cilium in fibroblasts. *Curr Biol* 2005;**15**:1861–6.
60. Berbari NF, Johnson AD, Lewis JS, Askwith CC, Mykytym K. Identification of ciliary localization sequences within the third intracellular loop of G protein-coupled receptors. *Mol Biol Cell* 2008;**19**:1540–7.
61. Gerdes JM, Davis EE, Katsanis N. The vertebrate primary cilium in development, homeostasis and disease. *Cell* 2009;**137**: 32–45.
62. Rohatgi R, Milenkovic L, Scott MP. Patched1 regulates hedgehog signaling at the primary cilium. *Science* 2007;**317**:372–6.
63. Alcedo J, Ayzenzon M, Von Ohlen T, Noll N, Hooper JE. The Drosophila smoothened gene encodes a seven-pass membrane protein, a putative receptor for the hedgehog signal. *Cell* 1996;**86**:221–32.
64. Ogden SF, Kei DL, Schilling NS, Ahmed YF, Hwa J, Robbins DJ. G protein Galpha(i) functions immediately downstream of Smoothened in Hedgehog signaling. *Nature* 2008;**456**:967–70.
65. Barzi M, Kostrz D, Menendez A, Pons S. Sonic hedgehog-induced proliferation requires specific Gα inhibitory proteins. *J Biol Chem* 2011;**286**:8067–74.
66. Chen W, Ren XR, Nelson CD, Barak LS, Chen JK, Beachy PA, et al. Activity-dependent internalization of smoothened mediated by beta-arrestin 2 and GRK2. *Science* 2004;**306**:2257–60.
67. Meloni AR, Fralish GB, Kelly P, Salahpour A, Chen JK, Wechsler-Reya RJ, et al. Smoothened signal transduction is promoted by G protein-coupled receptor kinase 2. *Mol Cell Biol* 2006;**26**:7550–60.
68. Philipp M, Caron MG. Hedgehog signaling: is Smo a G protein coupled receptor? Curr. *Biol* 2009;**19**:R125–7.
69. Kovacs JJ, Whalen EJ, Liu R, Xiao K, Kim J, Chen M, et al. Beta-arrestin-mediated localization of smoothened to the primary cilium. *Science* 2008;**320**:1777–81.
70. Poole CA, Jensen CG, Snyder JA, Gray CG, Hermanutz VL, Wheatley DN. Confocal analysis of primary cilia structure and colocalization with the Golgi apparatus in chondrocytes and aortic smooth muscle cells. *Cell Biol Int* 1997;**21**:483–94.

71. Lu CJ, Du H, Wu J, Jansen DA, Jordon KL, Xu N, et al. Non-random distribution and sensory functions of primary cilia in vascular smooth muscle cells. *Kidney Blood Press Res* 2008;**31**:171–84.
72. Wu J, Du H, Wang X, Mei C, Sieck GC, Qian Q. Characterization of primary cilia in human airway smooth muscle cells. *Chest* 2009;**136**:561–70.
73. Sabatini PJ, Zhang M, Silverman-Gavrila R, Bendeck MP, Langille BL. Homotypic and endothelial cell adhesions via N-cadherin determine polarity and regulate migration of vascular smooth muscle cells. *Circ. Res.* 2008;**103**:405–12.

Glossary

AAV adeno-associated vector

AC adenylyl cyclase

actin isoforms (isoactins) actin is an acidic 43 kDa cytoskeletal protein involved in a plethora of functions in most of the cells, which is impressively conserved across species. Higher vertebrates display six actin isoforms: the two striated muscle actins, α-SKA and α-CAA; the two smooth muscle actins, α-SMA and γ-SMA; and the two cytoplasmic actins, β-CYA and γ-CYA. Isoactins exhibit highly conserved primary sequences, with only few differences, mainly located at their N-terminus.

activation (of channels) the process by which an ion channel transitions from a closed non-conducting state to the open state that allows the flow of ionic current through the channel pore.

activin type II receptors receptors that mediate the initial binding of myostatin to target cells; contain intracellular serine/threonine kinase domains that phosphorylate the type I receptors.

adeno-associated virus non-enveloped dependovirus that is less immunogenic than adenovirus; packaging capacity is limited.

adenovirus a non-enveloped virus in the family Adenoviridae; can target striated muscle, but is highly immunogenic.

AGEs advanced glycation end-products.

aggresomes clusters of intracellular misfolding proteins sequestered with other intracellular proteins at perinuclear sites.

α-myosin heavy chain the major, or larger, subunit of an ATP-dependent motor protein involved in muscle contraction and actin-dependent motility.

amyloidosis refers to a specific pathologic state wherein soluble protein precursors aggregate within the extracellular space to produce insoluble amyloid fibrils.

amyotrophic lateral sclerosis (ALS) pathogenesis also known as Lou Gehrig's disease; the most common adult motor neuron disease, it causes the deterioration of the upper and lower motor neurons. The hallmark of this disease is the dysfunction and eventual death of motor neurons, leading to muscle atrophy, paralysis of lower limb and respiratory muscles, and death.

anaplerosis replenishment of moiety cycles.

angioplasty a procedure that opens clogged arteries by compressing plaque against the artery wall. A catheter with a small balloon at its tip is moved to where the artery is clogged. The balloon is inflated and deflated a few times. This compresses the plaque, opens the artery, and increases blood flow. Then the balloon-tipped catheter is removed.

angiotensin-1 receptor autoantibody (AT1-AA) agonistic autoantibodies to the angiotensin-1 receptor. These antibodies are commonly observed in preeclamptic women, and have been shown to contribute to the associated hypertension in experimental models.

ANT adenine nucleotide translocator.

anti-fibrotics classes of compounds that reduce fibrosis in muscular dystrophy. Many act through the TGFβ pathway.

antigen presenting cells cells that express major histocompatibility complex (MHC) and other proteins necessary to activate naïve T cells. These cells are found in lymphoid and epithelial tissues and present peptides in the context of MHC to naïve T and B cells to mount an immune response.

aponeurosis a sheet-like tendinous expansion, mainly serving to connect a muscle with the parts it moves.

apoptosis the process of programmed (orchestrated) cell death.

arterioles terminal vessels of the arterial tree that have a single layer of smooth muscle in their walls and are embedded in the tissue that they perfuse. First-order arterioles branch from feed arteries, followed by 3–5 divergent branchings. The smallest arterioles are termed terminal arterioles from which capillaries arise.

arteriosclerosis a group of diseases characterized by thickening or hardening of the arteries and loss of blood flow to the heart due to plaque; can lead to angina (chest pain) or myocardial infarction (heart attack).

ARVC arrhythmogenic RV cardiomyopathy.

ARVD arrhythmogenic RV dysplasia.

atherosclerosis a disease process that leads to the buildup of fat and cholesterol, called plaque, inside blood vessels.

atrophy the loss of muscle mass, either through inactivity, aging, or disease.

autophagy an evolutionarily conserved process of cellular cannibalization involving an intricate cascade of molecular events leading to intracellular cargo sequestration, delivery to lysosomes, and subsequent degradation.

autosomal dominant inheritance inheritance pattern in which one abnormal copy of a pair of genes in the human genome results in the development of a disease. When transmitted to offspring, the abnormal gene is passed with 50% likelihood.

autosome a non-sex chromosome.

β-AR beta-adrenergic receptor

β-subunit one of the smaller regulatory subunits of an ion channel that can bind to the pore-foring α-subunit to modify its expression level or gating.

Becker muscular dystrophy (BMD) a recessive X-linked inherited disorder characterized by slowly progressive muscle weakness. Becker muscular dystrophy is related to

Duchenne muscular dystrophy (DMD) (q.v.) in that both result from mutations in the dystrophin gene, but mutations that lead to BMD result in a truncated or reduced expression of dystrophin. Thus, dystrophin expression is still partially maintained in BMD making BMD less severe than DMD.

bFGF basic fibroblast growth factor.

biglycanan extracellular matrix protein that requires utrophin for its action in treating muscular dystrophy.

Ca^{2+} clearance the lowering of cytosolic $[Ca^{2+}]_i$ by extrusion across the cell membrane and/or uptake into intracellular stores, such as the sarcoplasmic reticulum.

Ca^{2+} indicators dye molecules that change their fluorescence or absorbance properties in response to binding Ca^{2+}.

Ca^{2+}-induced Ca^{2+} release (CICR) the process whereby Ca^{2+} entry into the cardiomyocyte, through opening of L-type Ca^{2+} channels, activates the RyR2 and causes further release of Ca^{2+} from the SR.

$[Ca^{2+}]_m$ mitochondrial $[Ca^{2+}]$.

Ca^{2+} sparks and Ca^{2+} puffs the Ca^{2+} signals that depend on Ca^{2+} release from clusters of ryanodine receptors (RYRs) or inositol tris-phosphate receptors (Ins(1,4,5)P_3Rs) that are located on the endoplasmic/sarcoplasmic reticulum (ER/SR).

Ca^{2+} transient rise and fall of myoplasmic free Ca^{2+} concentration in response to muscle fiber depolarization.

calcific valvulopathy mineral deposition in the vasculature and cardiac valve leaflets.

calcium-sensitive ion channel a transmembrane ion channel that has binding sites for Ca^{2+}, which can modulate channel gating to increase or decrease the open-state probability of the channel.

calcium sensitization refers to biochemical processes that increase the contractile responsiveness of a cell to intracellular calcium.

calstabins small molecules that stabilize the ryanodine receptor leak.

CamKII Ca^{2+}/calmodulin-dependent protein kinases II.

cAMP cyclic adenosine monophosphate.

capillaries vessels that branch from terminal arterioles which consist of an endothelial cell tube. No smooth muscle cells are present, but the vessels may be invested with pericytes.

carbohydrates a group of organic compounds including glucose, lactate and glycogen.

cardiomyopathy heart muscle disorder that results in dysfunction of the heart. Cardiomyopathies are subdivided into those with enlarged chambers and poor pumping (dilated cardiomyopathy), thickened walls (hypertrophic cardiomyopathy), enlarged atria due to abnormal heart relaxation (restrictive cardiomyopathy), abnormal heart rhythm (arrhythmogenic cardiomyopathy), and abnormal strips of muscle (trabeculations) in the left ventricle (noncompaction cardiomyopathy).

carotid artery a major artery on the right and left side of the neck supplying blood to the brain.

cartilaginous metaplasia transformation of non-cartilage tissue to cartilage.

CCR2 monocyte chemotactic protein-1 receptor.

cell cycle the growth cycle of a eukaryotic cell, consisting of four phases termed G1, S, G2, and M.

cell migration the movement of cells over time.

cell proliferation the growth and division of cells.

centronuclear myopathy (CNM) a group of congenital myopathies characterized by muscle weakness and abnormal centralization of nuclei in muscle fibers.

channelopathy any disease caused by a defect of ion channel function. Channelopathies may be acquired (e.g., myasthenia gravis) or inherited (e.g., myotonia congenita).

chemorepulsive signaling the pathway of cell migration is shaped by two opposing types of chemical signals, e.g., chemoattraction and chemorepulsion. Chemorepulsive signaling is mediated by a large family of cell surface guidance proteins consisting of the ephrins, netrins, plexins, robos, semaphorins, and neuropilins. First described in the developing nervous system, chemorepulsive guidance pathways have also been shown to be critical for assembly and repair of smooth muscle tissues.

chromatin a nucleo-protein complex comprised of DNA, RNA, histone proteins, and non-histone proteins (e.g., RNA polymerase II and transcription factors).

CLCN1 chloride channel 1.

CMR cardiac magnetic resonance (imaging).

CMV cytomegalovirus.

complement group of small inactive precursor proteins in serum that are synthesized in liver. Immune complexes (classical pathway), specific antigens (alternate pathway) and lectins (mannose-binding lectins) activate the complement cascade that ultimately results in the formation of membrane attack complex (MAC) and release of anaphylotoxins (C5a and C3a) that enhance vascular permeability and facilitate chemotaxis and inflammation to the site of injury.

concentric contraction an isotonic muscle contraction during which the muscle shortens.

congenital muscular dystrophy (CMD) term used to describe autosomal recessive muscular dystrophies that are clinically present at birth.

congestive heart failure the clinical syndrome that may develop when the myocardium for any number of reasons is no longer able to maintain adequate blood flow without also allowing the intracardiac pressure to rise. The most common cause of congestive heart failure in the United States, and the focus of most cell therapy trials, is coronary artery disease leading to myocardial infarction and subsequent left ventricular systolic dysfunction. Congestive heart failure symptoms vary from patient to patient and depend also on which chambers of the heart are involved. However, for patients with heart failure symptoms arising from left ventricular systolic dysfunction, dyspnea on exertion is typical.

connexin member of protein family that compose gap junction channels. They are named with a suffix number according to their predicted molecular mass (e.g., connexin40).

cooperativity of cross-bridge cycling the ability of detached dephosphorylated cross-bridges to reattach due to a population of attached phosphorylated or rigor cross-bridges which facilitates reattachment of the former. Cooperativity is thought to contribute to the maintenance of high levels of tension at low phosphorylation levels termed the latch state.

COP9 signalosome (CSN) the CSN is a protein complex that was initially identified in Arabidopsis. The COP9 stands for constitutive photomorphogenesis 9. The COP9 mutant of Arabidopsis when growing in dark displays the morphology of the wild-type counterpart grown in light. The CSN holocomplex consists of eight unique protein subunits (CSN1 through CSN8). The biochemical function of the CSN is cullin deneddylation.

copy number variant large region of the genome that is found either deleted or duplicated in the population; copy number variants can encompass multiple genes or involve regions that contain no genes, leading to decreased or increased gene dosage. They may also disrupt the structure of genes at the boundaries of the affected region.

coronary artery an artery of the heart that supplies oxygenated blood.

corpus cavernosum either of two masses of erectile tissue in the penis of mammals. The engorgement of the corpora cavernosa with blood is a key process in the development of an erection.

creatine kinase (CK) an ATP-dependent enzyme that catalyzes the conversion of creatine to phosphocreatine. Regulatory elements from the muscle–creatine kinase gene have been utilized to generate muscle-specific expression cassettes for muscle gene therapy.

CsA cyclosporin A

CUGBP1 CUG binding protein 1.

cyclic strain the cyclic stress–strain curve defines the relationship between stress and strain under cyclic loading conditions.

CyP-D cyclophilin D.

cytokine signaling proteins that activate or repress immune cells.

Δp protonmotive force.

$\Delta\psi_m$ mitochondrial inner membrane electrical potential.

deneddylation a biochemical process that removes NEDD8 (neural precursor cell expressed, developmentally down-regulated 8), a ubiquitin-like protein, from its modified proteins.

depolarization a change in transmembrane potential (voltage) that makes the inside of the cell more positive.

dermomyotome dorsal epithelial part of the mature somite that gives rise to the muscles of the trunk and the limbs, as well as other mesodermal derivatives.

desmin-related myopathy a heterogeneous family of myopathies with the predominant pathological feature being the presence of desmin-positive aberrant protein aggregates in muscle cells.

differentiation process whereby cells acquire their mature morphological and biochemical characteristics.

diffuse vasculopathy describes the pattern of vascular diseases found in patients with ACTA2 mutations; these patients can be afflicted with both aneurysmal disease (e.g., TAAD, intracranial aneurysms) and occlusive disease (e.g., early onset coronary artery disease and stroke).

dihydropyridine receptor (DHPR) (in skeletal muscle) voltage-dependent Ca^{2+} channel (Cav1.1) that works primarily as the voltage sensor for SR Ca^{2+} release.

DM dystrophia myotonica (myotonic dystrophy).

DMPK dystrophia myotonica protein kinase.

DNA replication a natural process, occurring in all living organisms, beginning with one double-stranded DNA molecule which serves as a template to generate two identical copies of the DNA molecule.

domain region of a protein with a distinct tertiary structure and characteristic function or activity.

dominance a mode of inheritance in which only one allele of a gene is required to manifest a phenotype.

dosage screen a systematic search of the human genome for deletions, duplications, translocations, and inversions at the DNA sequence level. It is assumed that the majority of these sequence variations lead to loss or gain of genetic material relative to the wild-type to cause a mutant phenotype. Some translocations and inversions can be balanced (with no loss of DNA) and lead to a mutant phenotype from position effects (from placing a coding sequence adjacent to the regulatory elements of a different gene).

DRP DNAse-resistant particles.

Drp1 dynamin-related protein 1.

drug-eluting stent (DES) a peripheral or coronary stent (a scaffold) placed into narrowed, diseased peripheral or coronary artery that slowly releases a drug to block cell proliferation. The stent is left behind in the artery to keep it open.

Duchenne muscular dystrophy Duchenne muscular dystrophy (DMD) is a recessive X-linked form of muscular dystrophy, which results in progressive muscle weakness and degeneration. Mutations that cause DMD are within the dystrophin gene and lead to a complete loss of expression of dystrophin, and thus complete functional loss of the protein.

duty cycle the duty cycle is a measure of the fraction of the total cross-bridge cycle time that cross-bridges spend attached to actin and generating force or motion.

dysferlin the protein product of the limb girdle muscular dystrophy type 2B gene. Dysferlin is a membrane-associated protein important for vesicle trafficking including vesicles needed for resealing membrane disruption in muscle.

dystocia (labor) an abnormal or difficult childbirth often associated with poor, uncoordinated contractions of the uterus smooth muscle.

dystroglycan the dystroglycan is the core component of the dystrophin–glycoprotein complex. Dystroglycan consists of α- and β-dystroglycan and provides a transmembrane linkage between the basal lamina and F-actin of the sub-sarcolemmal cytoskeleton. α-dystroglycan binds to laminin, agrin, and perlecan of the basement membrane, while β-dystroglycan is a transmembrane protein and binds α-dystroglycan outside the cell to dystrophin inside the cell.

dystrophin the 427 kDa protein product of the Duchenne muscular dystrophy (DMD) gene. Dystrophin is a rod-shaped membrane-associated protein that binds F-actin in the subsarcolemmal cytoskeleton and dystroglycan at the sarcolemma.

ECCE excitation-coupled calcium entry.

eccentric contraction an isotonic contraction during which the muscle lengthens as it resists being stretched by an external force

ECM extracellular matrix; structural and bioactive proteins.

economy a term used when comparing the energy usage for contraction, calculated as the force/cross-sectional area divided by the rate of high energy phosphate usage.

Eisenmenger's syndrome a form of cyanotic congenital heart disease that is considered as a form of WHO Group 1 PH. Eisenmenger's syndrome results from an intracardiac shunt. Eisenmenger's physiology occurs late in the natural history of the shunt by which time right-to-left shunting occurs as a result of obstructive pulmonary vascular remodeling. Thus, Eisenmenger's syndrome patients are cyanotic. Eisenmenger's syndrome most commonly occurs with untreated ventricular septal defects (in response to pressure and volume overload) but can occur with atrial septal defects (where volume overload usually predominates).

elastin-contractile unit the basic unit of contraction in the aorta; comprised of smooth muscle cell contractile filaments linked via integrin receptor-containing focal adhesions at the cell surface to similarly aligned microfibrils in the extracellular matrix. The herringbone pattern formed by these aligned contractile units allows the vessel to contract coordinately to oppose blood flow.

electromechanical mapping an interventional cardiology technique which allows three-dimensional mapping of the left ventricle to determine areas of viable myocardium and areas of scar. This is often used as an aid to localizing optimal sites of cell injection in cell therapy trials using an intramyocardial approach for cell delivery.

EMT epithelial-to-mesenchymal transition.

endMT endothelial-to-mesenchymal transition.

endochondral ossification type of bone formation that occurs by replacement of a cartilage scaffold with bone tissue involving vascular invasion; source of long bones.

endothelin-1 (ET-1) small protein produced by the endothelium. One of the most potent vasoconstrictors ever discovered. ET-1 production is a final common pathway shared by multiple pathogenic factors produced during preeclampsia.

endothelium the endothelium is the thin layer, comprised of endothelial cells, that lines the interior surface of vessels forming an interface between circulating blood and the vascular wall. The endothelium lines the entire circulatory system from the heart to capillaries. The endothelium modulates tone, growth, hemostasis, and inflammation throughout the circulatory system and forms a thromboresistant layer between blood and subendothelial tissue.

endothelium-dependent dilation dilation that requires the release of endothelial mediators which act on the smooth muscle to elicit dilation (e.g., nitric oxide and prostaglandins).

energy usage the suprabasal high-energy phosphate utilization calculated from direct measurements of ATP, phosphocreatine, and adenosine monophosphate concentrations as (ΔATP + ΔPCr − ΔAMP).

eNOS endothelial nitric oxide synthases.

epigenetic heritable changes in cell phenotype produced by mechanisms that are not directly due to changes in the DNA sequence of a cell. Most epigenetic regulation of cell phenotype occurs at the level of chromatin, and more specifically by an array of covalent modifications on core histone proteins that are essential components of stable nucleosomes.

epigenetic code the combination of histone modifications that defines the transcriptional status of chromatin.

epigenetic therapy a therapy aimed at modulating the epigenetic profile of cells through the use of drugs capable of inhibiting epigenetic enzymes.

epigenetics mechanisms that control gene expression in a potentially heritable way without a modification in the DNA sequence.

ER endoplasmic reticulum.

erectile dysfunction the inability to achieve or maintain an erection sufficient for satisfactory sexual performance.

euchromatin a loosely-packed form of chromatin that is associated with active gene expression.

excitation–contraction coupling (EC coupling) the signaling process whereby depolarization of the sarcolemma leads to muscle contraction.

extracellular matrix the extracellular material (largely composed of proteins and proteoglycans) of tissue that provides both structural support and a functional connectivity between the intra- and extracellular environments.

fat a group of organic compounds including fatty acids of different chain lengths and triglycerides.

fibrosis pathological build-up of connective tissue.

Fis1 fission 1.

FKBP12.6 (also known as calstabin2) a small (12.6 kDa) cytosolic binding partner of RyR2, is a member of the immunophilin family of prolyl isomerases.

flow cytometry a method used to identify and quantitate types of immune cells based on their cell surface markers. To carry out this technique, cell suspensions are labeled (usually with fluorescently-tagged antibodies that recognize cell surface markers) and cells are passed through a tube, excited by a laser beam and detected by a fluorimeter.

focal adhesion an assembly of specialized proteins at the plasma membrane that mediates attachment of the cell to its substrate by linking the cytoskeleton to the extracellular matrix. Also called "adhesion plaque" and, in smooth muscle, sometimes called "dense plaque".

follistatin a circulating protein that is a naturally-occurring inhibitor of myostatin.

functional electrical stimulation technique that uses electrical currents to directly activate muscle-nerves innervating extremities affected by paralysis.

GAG glycosaminoglycans.

GAP GTPase activating protein. A protein that increases the GTPase activity (GTP $\rightarrow$ GDP + Pi) of small GTP-binding proteins, thus converting them to the inactive state.

gap junction a specialized intercellular connection or channel composed of transmembrane proteins called connexins which connect the cytoplasm of two adjacent cells and permit the passage of action potentials, ions, and small molecules between them.

gating (of channels) the process by which a channel transitions between conformational states that affect the flow of ionic current. The term "gating" is derived from the notion that a hypothetical gate in the channel opens and shuts to regulate conduction through the pore.

gene transcription the process of creating a complementary RNA copy of a sequence of DNA. It is the first step leading to gene expression.

genome and exome sequencing the use of chemical DNA sequencing methods to deduce the nucleotide sequence of the complete diploid human genome or only that part of the genome that codes for protein-encoding genes (exome) through specific capture of these sequences using template-based hybridization.

genome the entirety of an organism's hereditary information.

genome-wide association study (GWAS) a systematic search of the human genome for common sequence variation in a gene that is statistically associated with variation in a measured phenotype or a categorical disease. The genetic basis for detecting the association is linkage disequilibrium (LD) whereby a disease or trait or some other functional allele occurs on a specific genetic background (haplotype) characterized by the pattern of neighboring sequence variants. Over time, with ensuing genetic recombination between the functional allele and neighboring sequence variants, this association declines as recombination brings in new marker alleles. In this method, a million or more polymorphisms are tested for association with a phenotype and only those markers that survive the multiple test correction (the "Bonferroni" correction owing to the chance association when numerous tests are conducted) are deemed associated and termed genome-wide significant. A conventional threshold is $P < 5 \times 10^{-8}$.

Glagov phenomenon ability of a vessel wall to outwardly remodel to preserve blood flow.

Glut1 the most widely distributed facilitated glucose transport protein. Catalyzes much of the basal glucose uptake in skeletal muscle.

Glut4 the "insulin-responsive" glucose transporter. Retained in cells in the basal state but redistributes to the cell surface in response to insulin. Expressed at highest levels in insulin target tissues such as skeletal muscle, adipose tissue and heart.

GPCR G-protein-coupled receptor.

GRK G-protein-coupled receptor kinase.

Gs stimulatory heterotrimeric G protein.

GSV Glut4 storage vesicles. The intracellular compartment in which Glut4 is stored in the basal state.

hematopoietic stem cell (HSC) precursor of mature blood cells that give rise to all red and white blood cells and platelets.

heme oxygenase-1 (HO-1) protein that catalyzes the rate-limiting step in the conversion of the oxidant molecule heme into the antioxidant molecule bilirubin. Heme oxygenase has been shown to have significant antihypertensive properties in experimental models, and remains a subject of intense research.

hemichannel six connexins assemble to form a hemichannel, which is integrated into the cell membrane. It is a symmetric ring structure with a central pore that docks together with a partner from the adjacent neighboring cell creating an intercellular channel.

hemodynamic deals with simultaneously acquired and processed blood flow and blood pressure.

heterochromatin a tightly-packed form of chromatin that is associated with repressed gene expression.

HF heart failure.

homeostasis maintenance by the highly coordinated, regulated actions of the body systems of relatively stable chemical and physical conditions in the internal fluid environment that bathes the body's cells

homolog, ortholog, paralog genes related by common ancestry are called homologs; orthologs are homologous genes in different species while paralogs are homologous genes in the same species, all arising from common ancestry.

hTERT catalytic subunit of telomerase.

hyperglycemia a condition wherein there is an excess amount of glucose circulating in blood plasma. *Hyper* = excess; *glyc* = sweet; *emia* = blood.

hyperpolarization a change in a cell's membrane potential making it more negative. The negative membrane potential dampens cell excitation.

hypertrophy the increase in muscle mass, normally driven by the increase in muscle fiber girth. It can arise normally through exercise training, or be a compensatory change in the musculature to counter muscle weakness.

I-1 protein phosphatase inhibitor-1.

ICAM-1 inter-cellular adhesion molecule 1.

ICD implantable cardiac defibrillators.

ion channel a transmembrane protein with an aqueous pore.

IMM inner mitochondrial membrane.

IMS mitochondrial intermembrane space.

inactivation (of channels) the process by which an ion channel enters a non-conducting inactive state. The inactive state is distinct from the closed one, because while both are non-conducting, channels cannot be opened from the inactive state by activation (i.e. depolarization of a voltage-gated channel). Channels must first recover from inactivation in response to membrane hyperpolarization before they can be opened. Inactivation causes the refractory period and sets the maximal firing rate of excitable cells.

Indo-1 a fluorescent indicator, sensitive to calcium, used to measure changes in calcium concentration in muscle cells, e.g., during myometrial contractions.

infarct expansion an increase in the length of the infarcted myocardial segment in the absence of additional myocardial necrosis.

inflammasome a multiprotein platform in cells whose activation results in secretion of the proinflammatory cytokine IL-1beta.

iNOS inducible nitric oxide synthase.

in-stent restenosis recurrent blockage or narrowing of a previously implanted stent.

insulin resistance a condition wherein the hormone insulin is unable to lower systemic circulating blood glucose levels.

An alternative definition is the reduced ability of the hormone insulin in glucose uptake in a particular cell or tissue for energy utilization.

integrin $\alpha 7$ an alternative link between the cytoskeleton, membrane and matrix in muscle.

integrin a transmembrane protein that possesses an extracellular domain, which binds to the extracellular matrix, and an intracellular signaling domain, which is linked to the cytoskeleton.

integrins family of heterodimeric proteins possessing an extracellular domain that binds extracellular matrix proteins and a short cytoplasmic tail that associates with focal adhesion molecules including various kinases and cytoskeletal proteins.

intercellular Ca^{2+} waves the Ca^{2+} signal that spreads through the smooth muscle tissue that depends on Ca^{2+} entry via voltage gated Ca^{2+} channels responsible for the upstroke of the action potential propagating across gap junctions.

intracellular Ca^{2+} oscillations the Ca^{2+} signal that spreads through the cytoplasm as a regenerative wave that makes up Ca^{2+} oscillations and depends on successive rounds of Ca^{2+} release and diffusion from clusters of Ins(1,4,5)P_3Rs or RYRs that are located on the ER/SR.

intraflagellar transport complex (IFT) a multiprotein complex that associates with the microtubule motor proteins kinesin and dynein to transport signaling proteins into and out of the primary cilium.

intramembrane charge movement (in skeletal muscle) electrical manifestation of the voltage-dependent movements of positively charged amino acid residues embedded in the dihydropyridine receptor, an integral membrane protein concentrated in the transverse tubular system.

iPAH idiopathic pulmonary arterial hypertension.

IRS insulin receptor substrate. The major substrate of the tyrosine protein kinase insulin receptor. Phosphorylated IRS serves as a docking site for signaling molecules.

ischemic heart disease a group of clinical syndromes characterized by myocardial ischemia, an imbalance between blood supply and demand.

ischemic preconditioning the protective effect of multiple cycles of brief intermittent ischemia and reperfusion prior to an episode of sustained ischemia.

isometric contraction a muscle contraction in which the development of tension occurs at a constant muscle length.

isotonic contraction a muscle contraction with negligible change in the force of contraction but shortening of the distance between the origin and insertion.

IT intimal thickening.

lamellipodia actin-rich protrusions at the mobile edge of a migrating cell.

laminin 111 an extracellular protein that is being tested for treatment in muscular dystrophy.

laminin laminins are major proteins in the basal lamina, a protein network surrounding muscle fibers. Laminins are heterotrimeric proteins that contain an α-chain, a β-chain, and a γ-chain.

LARGE glycosyltransferase-like protein that is putative glycotransferase which functions in the post-translational modification of α-dystroglycan.

latch state a tonic force maintenance state in SM with very low energy consumption and shortening velocity and with markedly reduced RLC_{20} phosphorylation levels.

lateral plate mesoderm a type of mesoderm that is found at the periphery of the embryo. It will split into two layers, the somatic layer and the splanchnic layer. The somatic layer forms the future body wall. The splanchnic layer forms the circulatory system and the future gut wall.

lentivirus an enveloped virus in the family *Retroviridae* which can be utilized to permanently modify the host genome of targeted cells.

lesion a blockage in a blood vessel that is interrupting blood flow to the heart or brain often due to plaque; also called stenosis.

limb-girdle muscular dystrophy an autosomal recessive class of muscular dystrophy that is similar but distinct from Duchenne muscular dystrophy and Becker's muscular dystrophy.

lineage diversity an important element of cell identity is its embryonic origin and subsequent developmental history (e.g., its lineage) which becomes recorded in epigenetic modifications that pattern the genome and control nuclear gene expression. How cells respond to a common stimulus can differ dramatically based on differences in their intrinsic lineage history.

linkage disequilibrium the allelic association between two loci whereby a specific allele at one locus occurs preferentially with a specific allele at the second locus. The association can be maintained for long periods of time owing to the rarity of recombination between the two loci. This degree of association depends on the allele frequencies at the two loci, genetic distance (and, thus, recombination rate) between the loci and the time period across which recombination occurs. LD is transient and disappears asymptotically over time.

linkage study a study of the co-segregation of genetic markers across the genome with a trait or phenotype within families or pedigrees containing multiple members who share a mutant phenotype, usually a Mendelian disease. By identifying all markers that co-segregate with the putative mutant allele one identifies (maps) a genomic location that must contain the disease gene.

L-type Ca^{2+} channel (also known as the DHPR) the main voltage-gated Ca^{2+} channel in the cardiomyocyte. A central molecular component of the Ca^{2+}-induced Ca^{2+} release process.

lumen the cavity or hollow space inside a blood vessel.

LVAD left ventricular assist device.

lymphoid cells bone marrow-derived cells of the adaptive immune response. Also known as lymphocytes. B and T cells are examples of lymphocytes. These cells respond to peptide or lipid antigen presented in the context of major histocompatability complex (that present peptide to T and B cells) or in the context of CD1d molecules (that present glycolipid to NKT cells).

macrosatellite a large tandem repeat sequence in the human genome.

MAO monoamine oxidase.

matricellular proteins a family of extracellular matrix proteins that do not serve a primary structural role but serve as dynamic integrators of microenvironmental signals, modulating cell–cell and cell–matrix interactions.

MBNL muscleblind-like.

MCP-1 monocyte chemotactic protein-1.

Mdx mouse the mouse model for Duchenne muscular dystrophy (C57BL/10ScSn-Dmdmdx/J). The mouse has a point mutation in exon 23 that introduces a stop codon. The mRNA for dystrophin is made but there is no detectable protein. The mouse undergoes a predictable pattern of disease, beginning with the first bout of necrosis at age 3 weeks, leading to low levels of necrosis, inflammation and regeneration throughout most of the mouse's lifespan. These mice have a slightly reduced lifespan than wild-type mice.

mechanosensor cellular element, analogous to a receptor, which initiates signal transduction processes in response to a mechanical stimulus.

mechanotransduction the ability of cells to sense and translate mechanical force into biochemical signals, thereby affecting downstream signaling pathways and gene regulation.

membrane adhesion junctions localized regions of the cell membrane where extracellular matrix proteins bind to transmembrane integrins, which in turn connect to cytoskeletal filaments within the cell.

mesenchymal stem cells (MSCs) cells from the immature embryonic connective tissue. A number of cell types come from mesenchymal stem cells, including chondrocytes, which produce cartilage.

metabolic cycles cycles of energy transfer requiring fixed moieties.

Mfn mitofusin

MG53 a small protein recruited to sites of muscle membrane damage.

MGL Gal/GalNAc specific lectin.

microcirculation network of branching vessels composed of arterioles, capillaries and venules.

microdomain any of several small regions of a cell membrane that has a distinct structure and a distinct function, for example proteins grouped in caveolae or a subsarcolemmal region bordering between the plasmalemma and sarcoplasmic reticulum.

microRNA (miRNAs) a class of $\sim$22 nucleotide non-coding RNAs that are evolutionarily conserved from plants to mammals and negatively regulate gene targets by inhibiting protein translation or enhancing mRNA degradation.

microRNA biogenesis miRNAs are transcribed by RNA polymerase II as pre-miRNAs, which are processed in the nucleus by Drosha into hairpins, known as pre-miRNAs. Dicer, the RNase essential for miRNA biogenesis, processes pre-miRNAs into miRNAs.

migration directional movement of cells from one region to another, often in response to a chemical gradient.

MIP-2 macrophage inflammatory protein-2.

mitochondria membrane-bound organelles that provide the energy a cell needs to move, divide, contract. They are the power centers of the cell.

molecular chaperones facilitate the folding and translocation of nascent polypeptides in the cell.

motor unit a motoneuron and all of the muscle fibers that it innervates.

muscle fascicle a bundle of muscle fibers surrounded by perimysium.

muscle action potential brief and sudden change in membrane potential initiated at the neuromuscular junction and propagated along and into a skeletal muscle fiber.

myeloid cells bone marrow-derived cells of the innate immune response. Macrophages, neutrophils, eosinophils and basophils are examples of myeloid cells.

myocardial hibernation a state of persistent regional contractile ventricular dysfunction in patients with chronic ischemic heart disease that is reversible with revascularization.

myocardial infarction (heart attack) occurs when one of more regions of the heart muscle experience a severe or prolonged decrease in oxygen supply caused by a blocked blood flow to the heart muscle.

myocardial stunning post-ischemic dysfunction that persists after reperfusion despite the absence of irreversible cardiomyocyte injury and despite restoration of normal coronary flow.

myocardin a cardiac myocyte- and smooth muscle cell-restricted transcriptional coactivator that binds directly to SRF activating a subset of SRF-regulated genes encoding cytoskeletal and muscle contractile proteins.

myoepithelial cells myoepithelial cells are modified epithelial cells found in sweat, mammary, salivary, lacrimal, and tracheobronchial glands. These cells present some architectural characteristics of SMCs, including caveolae, microfilaments, dense bodies and α-SMA, and display contractile properties which allow fluid ejection such as sweat or milk.

myofibrillar disorders forms of muscular dystrophies characterized by intracellular aggregation of misfolded protein localized at Z-disc structures.

myofibroblast the myofibroblast is a mesenchymal cell sharing features of the fibroblast and of the SMC. Under the influence of mechanical tension, ED-A fibronectin and TGF-β, fibroblasts develop stress fibers and cell-matrix connections; moreover, they express SM-specific protein (e.g., α-SMA). The presence of myofibroblasts has been described in numerous physiological and pathological conditions such as wound healing, fibrosis and stromal response to neoplasia.

myogenesis formation of skeletal muscle.

myogenic (muscle) describes a muscle capable of contracting without an outside stimulus such as hormonal or nerve innervations. A "myogenic" contraction refers to a myocyte contraction that originates from a property of the myocyte itself.

myogenic response temporal response of smooth muscle cells in arterioles and other arteries to changes in luminal pressure in which a step increase in pressure leads to initial passive dilation of the vessels, followed by activation of smooth muscle contraction which returns vessel diameter back to, or below the initial diameter.

myogenic tone the steady-state contractile activity of smooth muscle cells in arterioles and arteries due to pressure in the lumen of the vessels.

myoid cells myoid cells are myofibroblastic cells surrounding several structures including crypts in the gastrointestinal system, seminiferous tubules in the testis, or oocytes (mature follicles). These cells, which are known as pericryptal, peritubular or thecal cells respectively, display several SM-specific differentiation markers and confer contractile features to these various systems.

myometrium the muscular layer (smooth muscle) of the uterus.

MyomiRs refers to a family of intronic miRNAs consisting of miR-208, miR-208b, and miR-499, which are embedded in the introns of three muscle-specific myosin genes (Myh6, Myh7, and Myh7b).

myosin heavy chain isoforms myosin II, the major myosin type in muscle cells, contains two heavy chains, each about 2000 amino acids in length, which constitute the head and tail domains. Each of these heavy chains contains an N-terminal head domain and the C-terminal tail. The two tails take on a coiled-coil morphology, holding the two heavy chains. The intermediate neck domain is the region creating the angle between the head and tail. In smooth muscle, there is a single gene (MYH11) that codes for the heavy chains myosin II, but there are splice variants of this gene that result in four distinct isoforms.

myosin light chains myosin II contains 4 light chains, resulting in 2 per head, weighing 20 (MLC_{20}) and 17 (MLC_{17}) kDa. These bind the heavy chains in the "neck" region between the head and tail. The MLC_{20} is known as the "regulatory light chain" and actively participates in regulating smooth muscle contraction. The MLC_{17} is known as the "essential light chain" and may contribute to the structural stability of the myosin head.

myostatin a member of the TGF-β family that is a naturally occurring inhibitor of muscle growth. Anti-myostatin molecules may be useful for sarcopenia and muscle disease.

myostatin latency inactive state in which the mature myostatin peptide is bound to the propeptide; myostatin appears to be activated from this latent state *in vivo* by proteolytic cleavage of the propeptide by members of the BMP-1/TLD family of metalloproteases.

myostatin propeptide the N-terminal fragment of the myostatin precursor protein following proteolytic processing; remains bound to the mature C-terminal domain and inhibits its activity.

myotonia involuntary after-contraction of skeletal muscle that follows voluntary muscular effort or may be elicited by direct percussion of muscle. Myotonia is caused by prolonged bursts of action potentials in the muscle fiber that persist for seconds to minutes after cessation of motor neuron activity.

myotome central compartment of the somite where skeletal muscle first forms in the embryo.

NAb neutralizing antibodies.

NCX sodium/calcium (Na^{+}/Ca^{2+}) exchanger.

neddylation a process similar to ubiquitination that covalently attaches NEDD8 to the side chain of a lysine residue in a target protein.

neointima the scar tissue made up of cells and cell secretions that often forms as a result of vessel injury following angioplasty or stent placement as part of the natural healing process.

neural crest multipotent progenitor cells arising from the border of the neural plate. These cells undergo epithelial to mesenchymal transition, delaminate and migrate to specific locations throughout the embryo where they differentiate into smooth muscle cells, cardiomyoctes, melanocytes, craniofacial structures as well as peripheral and enteric neurons and glia.

neural crest cells multipotent neurectodermal progenitor cells that derive from the dorsal neural tube and give rise to derivatives such as the peripheral nervous system, including dorsal root ganglia, or the connective tissue of the head.

neuromuscular synapse reinnervation denervation of motor neurons in skeletal muscle causes axon degeneration and muscle atrophy. Subsequently, the motor axons regenerate through the nerve stump to the skeletal muscle and form new neuromuscular junctions.

neuronal nitric oxidase synthase (nNOS) an enzyme that catalyzes the production of nitric oxide (NO) from L-arginine.

nitric oxide (NO) a cellular messenger molecule that regulates many physiological and pathological processes and is synthesized from synthases (NOS) enyzymes from L-arginine, oxygen, and NADPH.

nuclear hormone receptor a class of proteins found within cells that have the ability to directly bind DNA and regulate the expression of adjacent genes, hence are classified as transcription factors.

nucleosome the base unit of chromatin structure, formed by a segment of 145–147 base pairs of DNA wrapped around a histone octamer containing two molecules of each core histone (H2A, H2B, H3, and H4).

OMM outer mitochondrial membrane.

Opa1 optic atrophy 1.

osteoblast cell that produces bone matrix (osteoid), which is permissive for mineralization.

osteoclast bone-resorbing cell derived from monocytes.

osteogenesis bone formation, which may be skeletal or extraskeletal.

osteoprotegerin soluble decoy receptor for "receptor activator of nuclear-factor kappa-B ligand" (RANKL); prevents RANKL from stimulating osteoclast.

outside-in signaling transduction of force or information from the substrate through focal adhesions to the interior of the cell.

paramyotonia myotonic stiffness that paradoxically worsens with repeated muscular activity and is often aggravated by muscle cooling. In contrast, myotonia diminishes with repeated voluntary contractions (warm-up phenomenon).

paraxial mesoderm thick bands of mesodermal cells that lie on either side of the neural tube which separate into blocks of cells called somites. Somites organize the segmental pattern of vertebrate embryos and give rise to skeletal muscle, smooth muscle, vertebrae, ribs, and dermis of the dorsal skin.

parturition the act or process of giving birth (labor).

PCR polymerase chain reaction.

PDGF platelet-derived growth factor.

PDH pyruvate dehydrogenase complex.

PDK pyruvate dehydrogenase kinase.

pericyte cells of mesodermal origin that function in the maintenance of microvascular structure and angiogenesis. These cells demonstrate significant plasticity and may assume characteristics resembling endothelial cells, smooth muscle cells or fibroblasts.

periodic paralysis disorder of skeletal muscle characterized by episodic attacks of muscle weakness that may be generalized or focal. Attacks typically last for hours and are caused by a transient loss of fiber excitability. Periodic paralysis may be acquired (e.g., from severe electrolyte imbalance) or inherited (e.g., hyperkalemic periodic paralysis).

pharmacomechanical coupling a physiological highly important mechanism of activation of contraction in SM that operates through multiple cellular signaling mechanisms that can change the level of force without a necessary change in membrane potential. The major mechanisms of pharmacomechanical coupling are Ca^{2+}release by InsP3 and modulation of the sensitivity to Ca^{2+} of MLC_{20} phosphorylation.

phasic smooth muscle smooth muscle characterized by spontaneous rapid, cyclical mechanical activity, such as portal vein.

phenotypic adaptation the ability of a cell, such as a vascular smooth muscle cell, to modify its normal program of gene expression and function in response to local signaling inputs

phenotypic modulation ability of a vascular smooth muscle cell to change from a contractile cell to one that is more synthetic, migratory, and proliferative in nature.

phosphagen energy storage compounds; in muscle, the major one is creatine phosphate.

phosphodiesterase-5 inhibitors phosphodiesterase-5 catalyzes the breakdown of cGMP. The highly successful oral treatments for erectile dysfunction, Viagra (sildenafil), Cialis (tadalafil) and Levitra (vardenafil), are inhibitors of this enzyme, and result in increased levels of cGMP following sexual stimulation.

PLGA poly (lactic-co-glycolic) acid (PLGA).

PLN phospholamban.

PMCA plasmalemma Ca^{2+} ATPase.

positional cloning a molecular genetic set of technologies for physically cloning the genomic segment containing a disease gene of interest, for example after linkage mapping. The search for a gene and its mutation within the segment leading to a disease has now been replaced with reading the DNA sequence in the genomic segment from reference sequence databases and subjecting the segment, or parts thereof, to nucleotide sequencing.

post-infarction cardiac remodeling the geometric changes of the ventricle that occur after a large myocardial infarction, involve both infarcted and non-infarcted myocardium and result in dilation and increased sphericity of the chamber, thinning of the infarct, and hypertrophy of non-infarcted segments.

precursor cells in fetal or adult tissues, these are partly differentiated cells that divide and give rise to differentiated cells, e.g. smooth muscle cells. Also known as progenitor cells.

preeclampsia pregnancy-specific hypertensive order characterized by proteinuria and maternal endothelial dysfunction. The underlying mechanisms leading to the disease are not certain, but are believed to derive through placental hypoperfusion and hypoxia/ischemia.

priapism a persistent, often painful, penile erection that continues hours beyond, or is unrelated to, sexual stimulation that can eventually lead to erectile dysfunction.

primary cilium a microtubule-based cell organelle that is specialized for mechanical and chemical signal transduction. There is usually a single primary cilium per cell.

proepicardium a transient source of cardiovascular progenitor cells located near the septum transversum in the embryo. The proepicardium contributes to formation of the coronary vasculature giving rise to coronary endothelial cells, smooth muscle cells and cardiac fibroblasts.

progenitor cell an incompletely differentiated cell type capable of giving rise to one or more differentiated cell types. This term designates a cell more differentiated and therefore more committed to a particular lineage than a stem cell.

proliferation growth of a cell population characterized by completion of the cell cycle to create daughter cells.

protein-induced diseases acquired or inheritable disorders with predominant pathogenic features of misfolding proteins and protein aggregates.

proteostasis normal processing of intracellular proteins, including biosynthesis, folding, transport to the appropriate site(s) of action within the cell, and elimination when they are damaged.

PTP permeability transition pore

pulse pressure the rhythmic contraction and expansion of an artery due to the surge of blood from the beat of the heart. The pulse is most often measured by feeling the arteries of the wrist. There is also a pulse, although far weaker, in veins.

RAGE receptor for AGEs.

RCA right coronary artery.

reactive oxygen species chemically reactive molecules containing oxygen.

refractory angina chest pain caused by obstruction of the coronary arteries that persists despite maximal therapy with medications and mechanical interventions to restore blood flow to the heart, including angioplasty and coronary artery bypass grafting.

remodeling alterations in ventricular architecture and function in the setting of changes in workload demand. Elements of this response can include cellular hypertrophy, changes in ventricular geometry, cell death, and fibrosis.

renin-angiotensin-aldosterone system a hormone system that regulates sodium and water homeostasis as well as blood pressure regulation.

respiration the reaction of protons with molecular oxygen to form water.

restenosis the re-narrowing of an artery in the same location of a previous treatment; clinical restenosis is the manifestation of an ischemic event, usually in the form of recurrent angina.

resting membrane potential the transmembrane potential gradient that exists in a cell in the absence of excitatory stimuli. The resting membrane potential is dominated in most cells by K^+ conductance across the plasma membrane.

rhabdomyosarcoma (RMS) the most common soft tissue sarcomas in children and young adults. The defining characteristic of RMS is expression of myogenic differentiation markers.

ROS reactive oxygen species.

RVF right ventricular failure.

RVH right ventricular hypertrophy.

ryanodine receptor (RyR) (in skeletal muscle) Ca^{2+} release channel located in the junctional SR which is regulated by the TT depolarization via the TT voltage sensor.

ryanodine receptor type 2 (RyR2) the SR Ca^{2+} release channel in the heart. A large homotetrameric protein that forms a macromolecular complex with multiple regulatory proteins.

RYR1 skeletal sarcoplasmic reticulum calcium release channel.

sarcoglycan the sarcoglycans are a family of transmembrane proteins (α, β, γ, δ) with a single transmembrane domain and N-linked glycosylation. The sarcoglycans interact along with sarcospan to form a subcomplex within the dystrophin–glycoprotein complex. This subcomplex helps to stabilize other components of the dystrophin–glycoprotein complex.

sarcolemma membrane of muscle cells.

sarcomere contractile apparatus of the heart.

sarcopenia age-related loss of muscle mass, strength, and functional decline.

sarcoplasmic reticulum (SR) a specialized form of the endoplasmic reticulum found in muscle cells, that stores a high concentration of Ca^{2+}.

sarcospan the 25 kDa transmembrane protein located in the dystrophin–glycoprotein complex of skeletal muscle. It contains four transmembrane spanning helices with both N- and C-terminal domains located intracellularly.

SASP senescence associated secretory phenotype.

satellite cells a stem cell-like population residing close to muscle fibers and a source for replenishing nuclear content of the muscle.

SAβ-gal senescence-associated β-galactosidase.

scAAV self complementary AAV.

scaffold a protein, generally without enzyme function, that assembles components of a signaling pathway into a functional signaling module by binding to several signaling proteins simultaneously.

SCF complex the abbreviation for Skp1, Cullin1, F-box-containing complex, a class of cullin-RING ubiquitin E3 ligases in which Skp1 is a bridging protein essential to recognition and binding of the F-box. The F-box protein is substrate-specific and functions to recruit the substrate for ubiquitination. Cullin1 serves as a scaffold linking Skp with Fbx1 that contains the RING finger, to which the E2 ubiquitin conjugating enzyme binds.

SDF-1 stromal cell-derived factor 1.

second heart field located anterior and dorsal to the cardiogenic mesoderm and serves as the origin of cardiovascular progenitor cells giving rise to structures of the outflow tract and right ventricle.

seed sequences these are nucleotides 2–8 at the 5′ end of the miRNA, which are essential for target recognition and binding.

SERCA sarcoplasmic/endoplasmic reticulum ATPase.

serum response factor (SRF) a DNA-binding transcription factor that binds a CArG box.

SIPS stress-induced premature senescence.

skeletal muscle-specific miRNAs these are miRNAs that are expressed in skeletal muscle and consist of the miR-1/206 family (miR-1-1, miR-1-2, and miR-206), and the miR-133 family (miR-133a-1, miR-133a-2, and miR-133b).

SMC smooth muscle cells.

smooth muscle cell mechanotransduction the signaling networks induced in smooth muscle cells upon stimulation with mechanical stress. The function of these pathways as sensors of environmentally increased pressures or genetically defective contractile function may play a key role in the pathogenesis of vascular disease.

SOCE store-operated calcium entry.

soluble activin type IIB receptor a fusion protein consisting of an Fc domain and the extracellular ligand-binding domain of the activin type IIB receptor; functions as a potent inhibitor of myostatin activity and can induce dramatic muscle growth when administered systemically to mice.

soluble fms-like tyrosine kinase-1 (sFlt-1) soluble form of the VEGF receptor Flt-1. Arises by alternative splicing of the transcript deleting the transmembrane anchoring domain. A potent VEGF antagonist, sFlt-1 sequesters VEGF and leaves it unavailable for receptor activation. sFlt-1 is believed to be a major pathogenic factor in preeclampsia.

somites transitory structures formed during development by the segmentation of paraxial mesoderm; they give rise to a number of tissues such as bone, cartilage, and all the muscles of the trunk and limbs.

spinal cord isolation surgical procedure where the lumbar region of the spinal cord is functionally isolated via complete spinal cord transections at two levels and bilateral dorsal rhizotomy between the two transection sites. Thus, this model eliminates supraspinal, infraspinal, and peripheral afferent input to motoneurons located in the isolated cord segments while leaving the motoneuron–skeletal muscle fiber connections intact, but electrically silent.

spontaneously hypertensive rat (SHR) an animal model of essential (or primary) hypertension that develops high blood pressure spontaneously. The SHR strain was obtained by breeding Wistar–Kyoto rats selected with high blood pressure.

SR sarcoplasmic reticulum.

stem cell a cell type that exists in multiple locations of the body and is capable of both self-renewal and the generation of a variety of terminally differentiated cell types. They are clonally expandable and exist along a continuum of potency, with stem cells capable of giving rise to all embryonic lineages termed pluripotent stem cells, and those yielding progressively more limited subsets of embryonic lineages termed multipotent or oligopotent stem cells. The terms progenitor cell and oligopotent stem cell are often used interchangeably.

stem/progenitor cell niche classic studies of hematopoietic stem cells showed that the survival and function of these stem cells is largely governed by neighboring "niche" cells via the soluble signals and ECM proteins that niche cells produce. The adventitial layer of blood vessels exhibits properties resembling a stem/progenitor cell niche for resident smooth muscle progenitor cells.

stenosis inward remodeling often coupled with hypertrophic growth of the vessel wall with a resultant narrowing in lumen diameter.

stent a tiny mesh cylindrical device that is placed permanently inside an artery during angioplasty. It expands within the blood vessel and props open a previously clogged artery.

STR simple tandem repeat.

stretch-activated ion channels ion channels that undergo conformational changes upon exposure to mechanical strain thereby allowing ion flux through the channel.

surface couplings excitation–contraction coupling sites where the sarcoplasmic reticulum (SR) tubules at the periphery of the cell establish close couplings with the surface membrane. Periodic bridging structures span the 12–20 nm junctional gap separating the two membranes. InsP3 receptors localize to the junctional SR that stores Ca.

syncitium coupled cells that act in synchrony due to intercellular communication.

synthetic surfactant small molecule that serves as a molecular band aid or resealant. An example is Poloxamer 188.

TBC1D4 also known as AS160, a putative Rab GAP and substrate of Akt. Signaling intermediate in the pathway by which insulin regulates Glut4 translocation.

TBC1D41 putative Rab GAP and signaling intermediate in the pathway by which AMPK or contraction regulated glucose transport into muscle.

Telomere a region of repetitive DNA at the end of a chromosome.

tensegrity a word fusion of "tension" and "integrity". The term denotes the underlying principle of structures that are held together by the balanced forces of compression and tension acting on rigid and elastic elements.

TGF transforming growth factor.

Th2 cytokines Th2 cytokines may play an important role in the pathophysiology of allergic diseases, including asthma. The cytokines IL-4, IL-5, IL-9, and IL-13 are derived primarily from T helper type 2 (Th2) cells and more specific to allergic inflammation as opposed to those secreted by Th1 cells, which secrete IL-2 and interferon-γ, although the clear distinction between Th1 and Th2 cells is not always distinct in humans.

tidal volume the lung volume representing the normal volume of air displaced between normal inspiration and expiration when extra effort is not applied.

tonic smooth muscle smooth muscle characterized by slow and sustained contraction. The reproductive, digestive, respiratory, and urinary tracts, skin, eye, and vasculature all contain this tonic muscle type. This type of smooth muscle can maintain force for prolonged time with only little energy utilization.

TRAF6 the abbreviation for tumor necrosis factor (TNF) receptor-associated factor 6, a RING domain ubiquitin E3 ligase that is known to catalyze K63-linked polyubiquitination.

transcription factor a protein that binds to specific DNA sequences, thereby controlling the rate of gene transcription.

transcriptional co-activator a gene regulatory protein that responds to specific intracellular and extracellular signals by binding directly to a transcription factor and activating transcription of sets of genes.

transdifferentiation the transformation of a previously committed stem, progenitor, or differentiated cell into a cell type outside its established potential.

transduction successful expression of a gene product in a cell following gene delivery.

translocation hypothesis a model which posits that the major control of glucose transport involves the redistribution of a pool of glucose carrier proteins form the interior of the cell to the cell surface.

TRPC canonical transient receptor potential channels.

TUNEL terminal deoxy nucleotidyl transferased UTP nick end labeling.

unitary conductance a measure of an ion channel's ability to conduct current as a function of the transmembrane voltage.

URE unstable repeat expansion.

USP14 the abbreviation for ubiquitin carboxyl-terminal hydrolase 14, the mammalian ortholog of yeast Ubp6 (ubiquitin-specific processing protease 6), a deubiquitination enzyme that is associated with the 19S proteasome.

utrophin a homolog of dystrophin that is normally concentrated at the neuromuscular and myotendinous junctions in skeletal muscle fibers. Upregulated expression of utrophin can partially compensate for loss of dystrophin in striated muscle.

variant, polymorphism and haplotype a "variant" is an alternative name for an allele and refers to a nucleotide that is different from that in the reference sequence. Polymorphism refers to a locus that harbors two or more alleles and where the least frequent allele has frequency of

1% or greater. A haplotype, or haploid genotype, refers to the allelic status of multiple loci at the level of individual chromosomes or DNA segments.

vascular hyperplasia a proliferative pathology of the smooth muscle cells, currently most often associated with *ACTA2* mutations.

vascular media the middle layer of the vessels wall composed primarily of smooth muscle cells and elastic tissue. It accounts for the bulk of the vessel wall.

vascular remodeling ability of the vessel wall to adapt under pathological conditions to maintain blood flow. Remodeling can be hypertrophic (e.g. increase of cross-sectional area), eutrophic (no change in cross-sectional area), or hypotrophic (e.g. decrease of cross-sectional area). These forms of remodeling can be inward (i.e., reduction in lumen diameter), or outward (i.e., increase in lumen diameter). In hypertension, changes in small artery structure are mainly of two kinds: (1) inward eutrophic remodeling, and (2) hypertrophic remodeling.

vascular resistance the term used to define the resistance to flow that must be overcome to drive blood through the circulatory system. The resistance offered by the peripheral circulation is referred to as the systemic vascular resistance (SVR) and is determined primarily by vasoconstriction and vasodilation of resistance arteries.

vasoconstriction refers to narrowing of blood vessels due to contraction of vascular smooth muscle cells in arteries, arterioles and large veins to reduce flow of blood and increase vascular resistance in order to regulate perfusion and maintain mean arterial pressure.

vasodilation widening of blood vessels due to relaxation of vascular smooth muscle cells in arteries, arterioles, and large veins to allow for increased flow of blood.

VDAC voltage-dependent anion channel.

ventilation perfusion matching in respiratory physiology, the ventilation/perfusion ratio (or V/Q ratio) is a measurement used to assess the efficiency and adequacy of the matching of two variables, and is defined as the ratio of the amount of air reaching the alveoli to the amount of blood reaching the alveoli.

venules vessels that drain capillaries. Comprised of post-capillary venules that are formed by the joining of two or more capillaries, and collecting venules formed from the joining of post-capillary venules. Post-capillary and collecting venules are invested with pericytes. Collecting venules drain into muscular venules, which have 1–2 layers of smooth muscle in their walls.

Vg viral genomes.

voltage sensor domains of an integral membrane protein that sense and respond to changes in transmembrane potential in voltage-gated ion channels, transporters, enzymes, and receptors.

voltage-sensitive ion channel a transmembrane ion channel whose activity (open-state probability) is sensitive to changes in membrane potential.

voltage-clamp electrophysiological technique that allows the control of membrane potential in any desired command waveform.

VSMC vascular smooth muscle cells.

WHO World Health Organization.

X-linked inheritance this inheritance pattern occurs when an abnormal gene located on the X-chromosome causes disease in males due to their single X-chromosome. Males can pass the abnormal gene to females only. Females, due to having two X chromosomes, become "carriers" and can also pass the abnormal gene to offspring, either males or females.

ZNF9 zinc finger 9.

Index

Note: Page numbers followed by *f* indicate a figure; page numbers followed by *t* indicate a table.

D

E

G

H

I

J

K

L

M

N

O

P

R

T

U

V

W

X

Z